Peterson's Principles of Oral and Maxillofacial Surgery - Third Edition
VOLUME TWO

Editors

Michael Miloro, DMD, MD, FACS
G. E. Ghali, DDS, MD, FACS
Peter E. Larsen, DDS
Peter D. Waite, MPH, DDS, MD, FACS

2012
PEOPLE'S MEDICAL PUBLISHING HOUSE—USA
SHELTON, CONNECTICUT

People's Medical Publishing House-USA

2 Enterprise Drive, Suite 509
Shelton, CT 06484
Tel: 203-402-0646
Fax: 203-402-0854
E-mail: info@pmph-usa.com

PMPH-USA

11 12 13 14/9 8 7 6 5 4 3 2 1

ISBN-13: 978-1-60795-111-7
ISBN-10: 1-60795-111-8

Printed in China by People's Medical Publishing House
Copyeditor/Typesetter: Spearhead Global, Inc.
Cover designer: Mary McKeon

Library of Congress Cataloging-in-Publication Data
Peterson's principles of oral and maxillofacial surgery.—3rd ed. / editors, Michael Miloro ... [et al.].
   p. ; cm.
  Principles of oral and maxillofacial surgery
  Includes bibliographical references and index.
  ISBN 978-1-60795-111-7
  I. Miloro, Michael. II. Peterson, Larry J., 1942 III. Title: Principles of oral and maxillofacial surgery.
  [DNLM: 1. Oral Surgical Procedures. 2. Face—surgery. 3. Facial Bones—surgery. 4. Stomatognathic System—surgery. WU 600]
  LC classification not assigned
  617.5′2059—dc23   2011032524

Notice: The authors and publisher have made every effort to ensure that the patient care recommended herein, including choice of drugs and drug dosages, is in accord with the accepted standard and practice at the time of publication. However, since research and regulation constantly change clinical standards, the reader is urged to check the product information sheet included in the package of each drug, which includes recommended doses, warnings, and contraindications. This is particularly important with new or infrequently used drugs. Any treatment regimen, particularly one involving medication, involves inherent risk that must be weighed on a case-by-case basis against the benefits anticipated. The reader is cautioned that the purpose of this book is to inform and enlighten; the information contained herein is not intended as, and should not be employed as, a substitute for individual diagnosis and treatment.

Sales and Distribution

Canada
McGraw-Hill Ryerson Education
Customer Care
300 Water St
Whitby, Ontario L1N 9B6
Canada
Tel: 1-800-565-5758
Fax: 1-800-463-5885
www.mcgrawhill.ca

Foreign Rights
John Scott & Company
International Publisher's Agency
P.O. Box 878
Kimberton, PA 19442
USA
Tel: 610-827-1640
Fax: 610-827-1671

Japan
United Publishers Services Limited
1-32-5 Higashi-Shinagawa
Shinagawa-ku, Tokyo 140-0002
Japan
Tel: 03-5479-7251
Fax: 03-5479-7307
Email: hayashi@ups.co.jp

United Kingdom, Europe, Middle East, Africa
McGraw Hill Education
Shoppenhangers Road
Maidenhead
Berkshire, SL6 2QL
England
Tel: 44-0-1628-502500
Fax: 44-0-1628-635895
www.mcgraw-hill.co.uk

Singapore, Thailand, Philippines, Indonesia
Vietnam, Pacific Rim, Korea
McGraw-Hill Education
60 Tuas Basin Link
Singapore 638775
Tel: 65-6863-1580
Fax: 65-6862-3354
www.mcgraw-hill.com.sg

Australia, New Zealand, Papua New Guinea, Fiji, Tonga,
Solomon Islands, Cook Islands
Woodslane Pty Limited
Unit 7/5 Vuko Place
Warriewood NSW 2102
Australia
Tel: 61-2-9970-5111
Fax: 61-2-9970-5002
www.woodslane.com.au

Brazil
SuperPedido Tecmedd
Beatriz Alves, Foreign Trade
Department
R. Sansao Alves dos Santos, 102 | 7th floor
Brooklin Novo
Sao Paolo 04571-090
Brazil
Tel: 55-16-3512-5539
www.superpedidotecmedd.com.br

India, Bangladesh, Pakistan, Sri Lanka, Malaysia
CBS Publishers
4819/X1 Prahlad Street 24
Ansari Road, Darya Ganj,
New Delhi-110002
India
Tel: 91-11-23266861/67
Fax: 91-11-23266818
Email:cbspubs@vsnl.com

People's Republic of China
People's Medical Publishing House
International Trade Department
No. 19, Pan Jia Yuan Nan Li
Chaoyang District
Beijing 100021
P.R. China
Tel: 8610-67653342
Fax: 8610-67691034
www.pmph.com/en/

Contents

Preface   ix
Editors   xiii
Contributors   xv

VOLUME ONE

SECTION 1

Medicine, Surgery, and Anesthesia   1

Section Editor: Peter E. Larsen, DDS

CHAPTER 1
Wound Healing   3
Vivek Shetty and Charles N. Bertolami

CHAPTER 2
Medical Management and Preoperative Patient
Assessment   17
Steven M. Roser and Gary F. Bouloux

CHAPTER 3
Pharmacology of Outpatient Anesthesia
Medications   43
Steven I. Ganzberg

CHAPTER 4
Outpatient Anesthesia   63
Kevin J. Butterfield, Jeffrey D. Bennett, and Jeffrey B. Dembo

SECTION 2

Dentoalveolar and Implant Surgery   95

Section Editor: Peter D. Waite, MPH, DDS, MD, FACD

CHAPTER 5
Impacted Teeth   97
Gregory M. Ness

CHAPTER 6
Preprosthetic and Reconstructive Surgery   123
Daniel B. Spagnoli and John C. Nale

CHAPTER 7
Pediatric Dentoalveolar Surgery   159
Carl Bouchard, Maria J. Troulis, and Leonard B. Kaban

CHAPTER 8
Utilization of Three-dimensional Imaging
Technology to Enhance Maxillofacial
Surgical Applications   179
Scott D. Ganz

CHAPTER 9
Implant Prosthodontics   201
Thomas J. Salinas

CHAPTER 10
The Science of Osseointegration   229
Craig M. Misch and Carl E. Misch

CHAPTER 11
Comprehensive Implant Site Preparation   269
Ole T. Jensen

CHAPTER 12
Soft Tissue Management in Implant Therapy   283
Anthony G. Sclar

CHAPTER 13
Craniofacial Implant Surgery   303
Douglas P. Sinn, Edmond Bedrossian, and Allison Vest

SECTION 3

Maxillofacial Trauma   323

Section Editor: Peter E. Larsen, DDS

CHAPTER 14
Initial Management of the Trauma Patient   325
Michael P. Powers and John R. Gusz

CHAPTER 15
Soft Tissue Injuries   357
Alan S. Herford and G.E. Ghali

CHAPTER 16
Rigid versus Nonrigid Fixation   373
Edward Ellis III

CHAPTER 17
Management of Alveolar and Dental Fractures   387
Richard D. Leathers and Reginald E. Gowans

CHAPTER 18
Contemporary Management of Mandibular Fractures   407
R. Bryan Bell

CHAPTER 19
Fractures of the Mandibular Condyle   441
Leon A. Assael

CHAPTER 20
Management of Maxillary Fractures 455
Larry L. Cunningham, Jr.

CHAPTER 21
Management of Zygomatic Complex Fractures 465
Jonathan S. Bailey

CHAPTER 22
Orbital and Ocular Trauma 483
Deepak G. Krishnan and Mark W. Ochs

CHAPTER 23
Management of Frontal Sinus and
Naso-orbitoethmoid Complex Fractures 519
Stephen P. R. MacLeod and Larry L. Cunningham, Jr.

CHAPTER 24
Nasal Fractures 539
Tirbod Fattahi

CHAPTER 25
Gunshot Injuries 545
Jon D. Holmes

CHAPTER 26
Pediatric Facial Trauma 565
Bruce B. Horswell and Daniel Meara

CHAPTER 27
Management of Panfacial Fractures 593
Patrick J. Louis

SECTION 4
Maxillofacial Pathology/Infections 609
Section Editor: G.E. Ghali, DDS, MD, FACS

CHAPTER 28
Differential Diagnosis of Oral Disease 611
John R. Kalmar and Carl M. Allen

CHAPTER 29
Odontogenic Cysts and Tumors 625
Eric R. Carlson

CHAPTER 30
Benign Nonodontogenic Lesions of the Jaws 653
M. Anthony Pogrel

CHAPTER 31
Oral Cancer: Etiology, Diagnosis, Classification
and Staging 677
Christopher M. Harris and G. E. Ghali

CHAPTER 32
Oral Cancer Treatment 693
Jon D. Holmes and Eric J. Dierks

CHAPTER 33
Lip Cancer 727
David M. Montes and G. E. Ghali

CHAPTER 34
Head and Neck Skin Cancer 743
Michael F. Zide and Yan Trokel

CHAPTER 35
Salivary Gland Disease 773
Antonia Kolokythas and Robert Ord

CHAPTER 36
Mucosal and Related Dermatologic Diseases 795
John M. Wright, Harvey P. Kessler, and Yi-Shing Lisa Cheng

CHAPTER 37
Pediatric Maxillofacial Pathology 821
Antonia Kolokythas

CHAPTER 38
Principles of Management of Maxillofacial Infections 841
Thomas R. Flynn

CHAPTER 39
Osteomyelitis, Osteoradionecrosis, and BRONJ 861
George M. Kushner and Brian Alpert

VOLUME TWO

SECTION 5
Maxillofacial Reconstruction 875
Section Editor: G.E. Ghali, DDS, MD, FACS

CHAPTER 40
Local and Regional Flaps 877
Alan S. Herford and G. E. Ghali

CHAPTER 41
Vascularized and Nonvascularized Hard and
Soft Tissue Reconstruction 893
D. David Kim and Rui Fernandes

CHAPTER 42
Microneurosurgery 919
Michael Miloro

CHAPTER 43
Cleft Lip and Palate 945
Bernard J. Costello and Ramon L. Ruiz

CHAPTER 44
Reconstruction of the Alveolar Cleft 965
Kelly Kennedy and Peter E. Larsen

CHAPTER 45
Nonsyndromic Craniosynostosis   979
G. E. Ghali and Andrew R. Banker

CHAPTER 46
Craniofacial Dysostosis Syndromes: Evaluation &
Treatment of the Skeletal Deformities   995
Paul S. Tiwana, Ramon L. Ruiz, and Jeffrey C. Posnick

SECTION 6
Temporomandibular
Joint Disease   1031
Section Editor: Michael Miloro, DMD, MD, FACS

CHAPTER 47
Anatomy and Pathophysiology of the
Temporomandibular Joint   1033
Mark C. Fletcher, Joseph F. Piecuch, and Stuart E. Lieblich

CHAPTER 48
Nonsurgical Management of Temporomandibular
Disorders   1049
Vasiliki Karlis and Robert Glickman

CHAPTER 49
Arthroscopy and Arthrocentesis of the
Temporomandibular Joint   1069
Joseph McCain and Luciano Stroia

CHAPTER 50
Internal Derangement of the
Temporomandibular Joint   1123
Luis G. Vega, Florencio Monje Gil, and Rajesh Gutta

CHAPTER 51
Hypomobility and Hypermobility Disorders of the
Temporomandibular Joint   1155
Meredith August, Maria J. Troulis, and Leonard B. Kaban

CHAPTER 52
End-Stage Temporomandibular Joint Disease   1173
Louis G. Mercuri

SECTION 7
Orthognathic Surgery   1187
Section Editor: Michael Miloro, DMD, MD, FACS

CHAPTER 53
Craniofacial Growth and Development   1189
Peter M. Spalding

CHAPTER 54
Orthognathic Database Acquisition   1239
Marc B. Ackerman and David M. Sarver

CHAPTER 55
Orthodontics for Orthognathic Surgery   1263
*Larry M. Wolford, Eber L. L. Stevao, C. Moody Alexander,
Joao Roberto Goncalves, and Daniel B. Rodrigues*

CHAPTER 56
Model Surgery and Virtual Planning
for Orthognathics   1295
Martin B. Steed, Vincent J. Perciaccante, and Robert A. Bays

CHAPTER 57
Mandibular Orthognathic Surgery   1317
Dale S. Bloomquist and Jessica J. Lee

CHAPTER 58
Principles of Maxillary Orthognathic Surgery   1365
Vincent J. Perciaccante and Robert A. Bays

CHAPTER 59
Facial Asymmetry   1393
Peter D. Waite and Scott D. Urban

CHAPTER 60
Soft Tissue Changes Associated
with Orthognathic Surgery   1411
Stephen Schendel, Richard Jacobson, and Dror Aizenbud

CHAPTER 61
Complications of Orthognathic Surgery   1427
Joseph E. Van Sickels

CHAPTER 62
Cleft Orthognathic Surgery   1455
Kevin S. Smith

CHAPTER 63
Distraction Osteogenesis of the
Maxillofacial Skeleton   1467
Michael Miloro

CHAPTER 64
Surgical and Nonsurgical Management
of Obstructive Sleep Apnea   1493
B. D. Tiner and Peter D. Waite

SECTION 8
Facial Aesthetic Surgery   1513
Section Editor: Peter D. Waite, MPH, DDS, MD, FACD

CHAPTER 65
Blepharoplasty   1515
Tirbod Fattahi

Chapter 66
Basic Principles of Rhinoplasty   1531
James Koehler and Peter D. Waite

Chapter 67
Rhytidectomy   1555
G. E. Ghali and Andrew R. Banker

Chapter 68
Forehead and Brow Procedures   1571
Angelo Cuzalina

Chapter 69
Otoplastic Surgery for the Protruding Ear   1597
Todd G. Owsley

Chapter 70
Adjunctive Facial Aesthetic Procedures   1609
Joseph Niamtu

Index

Preface

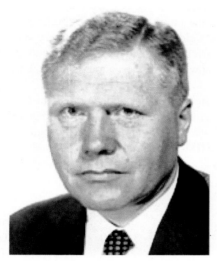

Dr. Gustav O. Kruger

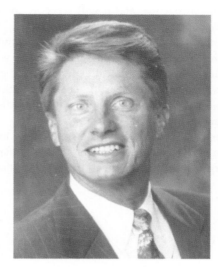

Dr. Larry J. Peterson

Dr. Larry J. "Pete" Peterson was a teacher, and nothing would please him more than knowing that the legacy of this textbook and its teachings still continues posthumously today. Dr. Peterson began to assemble the editors and authors for the *Principles of Oral and Maxillofacial Surgery* textbook in the late 1980s, and the 1st edition was published in 1992.

Pete considered this a tribute to one of his mentors, Dr. Gustav O. Kruger, Chairman at Georgetown University School of Dentistry where Pete completed his oral and maxillofacial surgery residency training program. Dr. Kruger died in 2010 at the age of 93.

Like Dr. Peterson, whose car license plate read "OSUTCHR" (for "Ohio State University Teacher"), Dr. Kruger believed his role as an educator was most important to him. "Father really felt education was the key to a better world and instilled that in all of us," he said.

Dr. Kruger had edited his own *Textbook of Oral and Maxillofacial Surgery* in 1959, and this masterpiece underwent several editions, and enjoyed its final 6th edition in 1984. This textbook provided the basis for undergraduate and postgraduate education in the specialty of oral and maxillofacial surgery for dental students and residents throughout the country for three decades, until Dr. Peterson resurrected the idea of continuing to produce a comprehensive and complete reference in oral and maxillofacial surgery that was clinically applicable and easily readable for students and residents studying the principles of the specialty of oral and maxillofacial surgery.

This 3rd edition of the *Principles* textbook proudly continues the student and resident teachings that began by Dr. Kruger more than a half century ago.

The 3rd Edition of *Peterson's Principles of Oral and Maxillofacial Surgery,* reflects the efforts of many people, including leading oral and maxillofacial surgeons throughout the country and abroad. Although it was not an easy task to enlist the authors who have contributed to this textbook, the breadth of experience and talent of the contributing authors make this 3rd edition very special.

Oral and maxillofacial surgery encompasses an ever-expanding range of diverse topics that makes it unique among the medical and dental specialties. Dr. Kruger's *Textbook of Oral and Maxillofacial Surgery* was the first reference textbook to cover the full scope of the specialty and was available for students, residents, and surgeons to use as a reference for clinical practice.

The 3rd Edition of *Peterson's Principles of Oral and Maxillofacial Surgery* continues this tradition and provides an organized and systematic approach to the entire specialty for residents and clinicians who practice full-scope oral and maxillofacial surgery. The 3rd edition of this textbook is unique in many respects, with the inclusion of contributions from more than 100 oral and maxillofacial surgeons and other dental and medical specialists. The clear purpose of this textbook is to provide a concise, authoritative, easy-to-read, currently referenced, contemporary survey of the entire specialty of oral and maxillofacial surgery that contains the information that a competent surgeon should possess and understand. Although some of the information may be outside of the scope of an individual practitioner, the material contained in this textbook is clearly within the scope of the specialty.

This textbook should be considered a reference for the oral and maxillofacial surgeon not only during residency but also into clinical practice, and it will serve as an excellent resource for examination preparation purposes.

As with the 1st and 2nd editions of this textbook, the authors, primarily oral and maxillofacial surgeons, were chosen because of their broad clinical experience and expertise in each specific area of the specialty. The contributions from these national and international authors clearly reflect their knowledge and expertise.

Whenever appropriate, each chapter attempts to review etiology, diagnosis, patient assessment, treatment plan development, surgical and nonsurgical treatment options, and recognition and management of complications. The information contained in this textbook is based upon a thorough evaluation of the current literature, as well as clinical expertise, and, as much as possible, is free from commercial and personal bias.

If additional information is required, suggested references have been provided so that other resources may be consulted. Considering the rapid technological advances and developments in the fields of medicine and surgery, a constant survey of the current published literature is required to maintain a working knowledge of the standards of diagnosis and treatment.

Future editions of this textbook will also reflect these changes in clinical practice. *Peterson's Principles of Oral and Maxillofacial Surgery* has established itself as *the* authoritative textbook for the specialty of oral and maxillofacial surgery.

Michael Miloro
G.E. Ghali
Peter E. Larsen
Peter D. Waite

Dedications

To my wife, Beth, and daughter, Macy, for your love, support, and understanding, and to my parents for their inspiration and encouragement. To the students and residents of oral and maxillofacial surgery for providing the impetus for this textbook, and to Pete for your mentorship.

Michael Miloro

To my wife, Hope, and my children, Gregor, Gracie, Gabrielle, and Garrisyn. To my parents, who inspired me to enter dentistry. And finally, to my residents and fellows who make it fun every day.

G. E. Ghali

To my wife, Patty, and my sons, Michael, Matthew, and Mark, for reminding me that my most important role is that of father and husband. To my father, who inspired me to enter medicine and to my mother, who convinced me that I could accomplish whatever I put my mind to. Lastly, to my colleagues and friends, who have supported me throughout my career.

Peter Larsen

I dedicate this textbook to my father, Daniel Waite, Professor and chair of OMS. His love and commitment to the specialty continue to inspire me. I thank my loving wife, Sallie, and children, for giving me the time to follow my surgical and teaching ambitions. Thanks to the residents who challenge me every day.

Peter D. Waite

Editors

Michael Miloro, DMD, MD, FACS
Professor and Head
Program Director
Department of Oral and Maxillofacial Surgery
University of Illinois at Chicago
Chicago, Illinois

G.E. Ghali, DDS, MD, FACS
Gamble Professor and Chairman
Department of Oral and Maxillofacial Surgery
Head and Neck Surgery
Louisiana State University Health Sciences Center
Shreveport, Louisiana

Peter E. Larsen, DDS
Larry J. Peterson Endowed Professor and
Chair, Division of Oral and Maxillofacial Surgery,
Anesthesiology, and Oral and Maxillofacial Pathology
The Ohio State University College of Dentistry
Columbus, Ohio

Peter D. Waite, MPH, DDS, MD
Professor and Chairman, Department of Oral and
Maxillofacial Surgery
Endowed Charles McCallum Chair
University of Alabama at Birmingham
School of Dentistry and School of Medicine
Birmingham, Alabama

Contributors

Marc B. Ackerman, DMD, MBA
Director of Orthodontics, Children's Hospital Boston
Lecturer, Department of Developmental Biology
Harvard School of Dental Medicine
Boston, Massachusetts

C. Moody Alexander, DDS, MS
Texas A&M University Health Science Center
Baylor College of Dentistry
Dallas, Texas

Carl M. Allen, DMD, MSD
Professor and Director, Division of Oral and Maxillofacial
Surgery, Pathology, and Dental Anesthesiology
College of Dentistry, The Ohio State University,
Columbus, Ohio

Brian Alpert, DDS
Chair and Professor, Oral and Maxillofacial Surgery
University of Louisville School of Dentistry
Chief, Oral and Maxillofacial Surgery and Dentistry
University of Louisville Hospital
Louisville, Kentucky

Dror Aizenbud, DMD, MSC
Orthodontic and Craniofacial Center, School of
Graduate Dentistry
Rambam Health Care Campus
Bruce and Ruth Rappaport Faculty of Medicine
Technion - Israel Institute of Technology
Haifa, Israel

Leon A. Assael, DMD
Professor of OMFS and Surgery
Department Chair
Medical Director, Hospital Dentistry
Oregon Health and Science University
Portland, Oregon

Meredith August, DMD, MD
Associate Professor, Harvard School of Dental Medicine
Visiting Oral and Maxillofacial Surgeon, Oral and
Maxillofacial Surgery,
Massachusetts General Hospital
Boston Massachusetts

Jonathan S. Bailey, DMD, MD, FACS
Clinical Associate Professor, OMS Program Director,
Division of Oral and Maxillofacial Surgery
Division of Head and Neck Cancer,
Carle Foundation Hospital
Carle Clinic, Division of Oral and Maxillofacial
Surgery, Head and Neck Cancer
Urbana, Illinois

Andrew R. Banker, DDS, MD
Assistant Professor
Department of Oral and Maxillofacial Surgery
Louisiana State University Health Sciences Center
Shreveport, Louisiana

Robert A. Bays, DDS
Professor and Chairman (Retired) Division of Oral and
Maxillofacial Surgery,
Department of Surgery, School of Medicine
Emory University
Atlanta, Georgia

Edmond Bedrossian, DDS, FACS, FACOMS
Assistant Professor, Dugoni School of Dentistry
Director, Implant Training
Department Oral Maxillofacial Residency Training Program
Private Practice, San Francisco, California

R. Bryan Bell, MD, DDS, FACS
Clinical Associate Professor
Oregon Health and Science University
Attending Head and Neck Surgeon and Director of
Resident Education
Oral and Maxillofacial Surgery Service
Legacy Emanuel Medical Center
Portland, Oregon

Jeffrey D. Bennett, DMD
Professor and Chair
Department of Oral Surgery and Hospital Dentistry
Indiana University School of Dentistry
Indianapolis, Indiana

Charles N. Bertolami, DDS, D. Med. Sc.
Professor and Dean
College of Dentistry
New York University
New York, New York

Dale Bloomquist, DDS, MS
Acting Chairman, Department of Oral and
Maxillofacial Surgery
University of Washington
Private Practice - Orthognathic Surgery
Seattle, Washington

Carl Bouchard, DMD, MSc, FRCD (C)
Clinical Professor, Department of Oral and
Maxillofacial Surgery
Laval University
Centre Hospitalier Affilié Universitaire de Québec
Quebec, Canada

Gary F. Bouloux, MD, DDS, MDSc, FRACDS (OMS)
Division of Oral and Maxillofacial Surgery
Emory University School of Medicine
Atlanta, Georgia

Kevin J. Butterfield, DDS, MD, FRCD (C)
Argyle Associates Oral and Maxillofacial Surgery
Division Chief, Dentistry/Oral and Maxillofacial Surgery
The Ottawa Hospital
Ottawa, Canada

Eric R. Carlson, DMD, MD, FACS
Professor and Chairman, Department of Oral and
Maxillofacial Surgery
Director of Oral and Maxillofacial Surgery Residency
Program
University of Tennessee Graduate School of Medicine
University of Tennessee Cancer Institute
Knoxville, Tennessee

Yi-Shing Lisa Cheng, DDS, MS, PhD
Associate Professor, Department of Diagnostic Sciences
Texas A&M Health Science Center
Baylor College of Dentistry
Dallas, Texas

Bernard J. Costello, DMD, MD, FACS
Chief, Division of Craniofacial and Cleft Surgery
Professor and Program Director
Department of Oral and Maxillofacial Surgery
University of Pittsburgh School of Dental Medicine
Pittsburgh, Pennsylvania

Larry L. Cunningham, Jr., DDS, MD, FACS
Associate Professor, Residency Director, and
Chief, Division of Oral and Maxillofacial Surgery
University of Kentucky College of Dentistry
Lexington, Kentucky

Angelo Cuzalina, MD, DDS
Private Practice - Tulsa Surgical Arts
President, American Academy of Cosmetic Surgery 2011
Chairman, AACS Cosmetic Surgery Fellowship Program
Adjunct Clinical Assistant Professor of Surgery, Oklahoma
State University
Tulsa, Oklahoma

Jeffrey B. Dembo, DDS
Professor, Oral and Maxillofacial Surgery
University of Kentucky College of Dentistry
Professor, Anesthesiology
University of Kentucky College of Medicine
Division of Oral and Maxillofacial Surgery
Lexington, Kentucky

Eric J. Dierks, MD, DMD, FACS
The Head and Neck Surgical Associates
Portland, Oregon
Director of Fellowship in Head and Neck Oncologic Surgery
Legacy Emanuel and Portland Providence Hospital
Affiliate Professor of Oral and Maxillofacial Surgery
Oregon Health and Science University
Affiliate Professor of Oral and Maxillofacial Surgery
University of Washington

Edward Ellis III, DDS, MS
Professor and Chair, Department of Oral and
Maxillofacial Surgery
University of Texas Health Science Center
San Antonio, Texas

Tirbod Fattahi, DMD, MD, FACS
Associate Professor and Chief, Division of Oral and
Maxillofacial Surgery
University of Florida Health Science Center
Jacksonville, Florida

Rui Fernandes, DMD, MD, FACS
Assistant Professor, Chief, Section of Head and
Neck Surgery
Department of Surgery
Divisions of Oral and Maxillofacial Surgery and
Surgical Oncology
Director of Microvascular Fellowship Program
University of Florida College of Medicine
Jacksonville, Florida

Mark C. Fletcher, DMD, MD
Division of Oral and Maxillofacial Surgery
University of Connecticut School of Dental Medicine
Avon Oral and Maxillofacial Surgery
Avon, Connecticut

Thomas R. Flynn, DMD
Former Associate Professor, Department of Oral and
Maxillofacial Surgery
Harvard School of Dental Medicine
Boston, Massachusetts

Scott D. Ganz, DMD
Clinical Assistant Professor, Department of Restorative
Dentistry
University of Medicine and Dentistry of New Jersey
Newark, NJ
Prosthodontics, Maxillofacial Prosthetics &
Implant Dentistry
Fort Lee, New Jersey

Steven I. Ganzberg, DMD, MS
Clinical Professor of Anesthesiology
School of Dentistry
University of California at Los Angeles
Los Angeles, California

Florencio Monje Gil, MD
Head, Department of Oral and Maxillofacial Surgery
Hospital Infanta Cristina
Complejo Hospitalario Universitario de Badajoz
Badajoz, Spain

Robert S. Glickman, DMD
Professor and Chair, Department of Oral and
Maxillofacial Surgery
New York University College of Dentistry
New York, New York

Joao Goncalves, DDS, PhD
Departamento de Clinica Infantil Faculdade de Odontologia
de Araraquara-UNESP,
Araraquara-SP, Brazil

Reginald E. Gowans, DDS
Division of Oral and Maxillofacial Surgery, Harbor-UCLA
Medical Center
Torrance, California

John R. Gusz, MD, FACS
Private Practice - Portage Surgical Associates
Trauma Services Director
Robinson Memorial Hospital
Ravenna, OH

Rajesh Gutta, BDS, MS
Assistant Professor, Division of Oral and Maxillofacial
Surgery, Department of Surgery, University of Cincinnati
Cincinnati, Ohio

Christopher M. Harris, DMD, MD
Residency Program Director
Oral and Maxillofacial Surgery
Naval Medical Center Portsmouth
Portsmouth, VA

Alan S. Herford, DDS, MD, FACS
Associate Professor, Department of Oral and
Maxillofacial Surgery
School of Dentistry, Loma Linda University
Loma Linda, California

Jon D. Holmes, DMD, MD, FACS
Assistant Clinical Professor, Department of Oral and
Maxillofacial Surgery
University of Alabama at Birmingham
Private Practice - Oral and Facial Surgery of Alabama
Birmingham, Alabama

Bruce B. Horswell, MD, DDS, MS, FACS
Director, FACES, Department of Surgery
Charleston Area Medical Center
CAMC Women and Children's Hospital
Charleston, West Virginia

Richard Jacobson, DMD, MS
Clinical Instructor of Orthodontics, School of Dentistry
Department of Orthodontics
University of California, Los Angeles

Ole T. Jensen, DDS, MS
Private Practice, Implant Dentistry Associates of Colorado
Greenwood Village, Colorado

Leonard Kaban, DMD, MD, FACS
Walter C Guralnick Professor and Chairman
Department of Oral and Maxillofacial Surgery
Harvard School of Dental Medicine
Chief, Department of Oral and Maxillofacial Surgery
Massachusetts General Hospital
Boston, Massachusetts

John R. Kalmar, DMD, PhD
Clinical Professor, Division of Oral and Maxillofacial
Surgery, Pathology, and Dental Anesthesiology
College of Dentistry, The Ohio State University
Columbus, Ohio

Vasiliki Karlis, DMD, MD, FACS
Associate Professor, Director of Advanced Education
Program
Department of Oral and Maxillofacial Surgery
New York University College of Dentistry
New York, New York

Kelly Kennedy, DDS, MS
Assistant Professor, Division of Oral and
Maxillofacial Surgery
The Ohio State University College of Dentistry
Columbus, Ohio

Harvey P. Kessler, DDS, MS
Professor and Director of Pathology, Department of
Diagnostic Sciences
Texas A&M Health Science Center
Baylor College of Dentistry
Dallas, Texas

D. David Kim, DMD, MD, FACS
Associate Professor, Department of Oral and
Maxillofacial Surgery
Louisiana State University Health Sciences Center
Shreveport, Louisiana

James Koehler, DDS, MD
Private Practice - Tulsa Surgical Arts
Adjunct Clinical Assistant Professor of Surgery,
Oklahoma State University
Tulsa, Oklahoma

Antonia Kolokythas, DDS, MSc
Assistant Professor, Director of Research
Department of Oral and Maxillofacial Surgery
College of Dentistry, Department of Oral and
Maxillofacial Surgery
University of Illinois at Chicago
Chicago, Illinois

Deepak G. Krishnan, DDS
Assistant Professor of Surgery, Residency Program
Director, Division of Oral Maxillofacial Surgery,
University of Cincinnati Medical Center
Cincinnati, Ohio

George M. Kushner, DMD, MD
Professor of Oral and Maxillofacial Surgery
University of Louisville School of Dentistry
Louisville, Kentucky

Richard D. Leathers, DDS
Division of Oral and Maxillofacial Surgery, Harbor-UCLA
Medical Center
Torrance, California

Jessica J. Lee, DDS
University of Washington
Department of Oral and Maxillofacial Surgery
Seattle, Washington

Stuart E. Lieblich, DMD
Associate Professor, University of Connecticut
Farmington, Conneticut
Visiting Assistant Professor, Tufts University
Boston, Massachusetts
Private Practice - Avon Oral and Maxillofacial Surgery
Avon, Connecticut

Patrick J. Louis, DDS, MD
Professor and Program Director, Oral and
Maxillofacial Surgery
University of Alabama at Birmingham
Birmingham, Alabama

Stephen P. MacLeod, BDS, MBCHB, FDSRCS
(ED&ENG), FRCS (ED)
Director of Dentistry and Oral and Maxillofacial Surgery
Associate Professor
Denver Health
Denver, CO

Joseph P. McCain, DMD
Adjunct Professor of Oral and Maxillofacial Surgery
Nova Southeastern University, School of Dental Medicine
Fort Lauderdale, Florida
Chief of Oral and Maxillofacial Surgery, Private Practice
Baptist Hospital
Miami, Florida

Daniel J. Meara, MS, MD, DMD
Program Director
Oral and Maxillofacial Surgery
Christiana Care Health System
Wilmington, Delaware

Louis G. Mercuri, DDS, MS
Clinical Consultant, TMJ Concepts
Ventura, California

Carl E. Misch, DDS, MD
Private Practice, Prosthodontics, Beverly Hills, Michigan
Clinical Professor, Department of Periodontology and
Oral Implantology
Temple University Kornberg School of Dentistry
Philadelphia, Pennsylvania

Craig M. Misch, DDS, MDS
Clinical Associate Professor, Department of Implant Dentistry
New York University College of Dentistry
New York, New York
Private Practice - Oral and Maxillofacial Surgery and
Prosthodontics
Sarasota, Florida

David M. Montes, DDS
Chairman, Department of Maxillofacial/Head and
Neck Surgery
Sanford Health System
Fargo, North Dakota

John C. Nale, DMD, MD
University Oral and Maxillofacial Surgery
Charlotte, North Carolina

Gregory M. Ness, DDS
Professor, Department of Oral and Maxillofacial Surgery
School of Dentistry
Virginia Commonwealth University
Richmond, Virginia

Joseph Niamtu III, DMD
Cosmetic Facial Surgery
Richmond, Virginia

Mark W. Ochs, DMD, MD
Professor and Chair, Oral and Maxillofacial Surgery
University of Pittsburgh School of Dental Medicine
Pittsburgh, Pennsylvania

Robert A. Ord, DDS, MD, FRCS, FACS
Professor and Chairman, Department of Oral and
Maxillofacial Surgery
University of Maryland
Professor, Oncology Program
Greenebaum Cancer Center, University of Maryland
Medical Center
Baltimore, Maryland

Todd Owsley, DDS, MD
Greensboro, North Carolina

Vincent J. Percciacante, DDS
Clinical Assistant Professor, Division of Oral and
Maxillofacial Surgery
Department of Surgery, Emory University School of
Medicine
Atlanta, Georgia

Joseph F. Piecuch, DMD, MD
Clinical Professor, Division of Oral and
Maxillofacial Surgery
Department of Craniofacial Sciences
University of Connecticut Health Center
Farmington, Connecticut

M. Anthony Pogrel, DDS, MD, FRCS, FACS
William Ware Endowed Professor and Chairman
Associate Dean for Hospital Affairs
Department of Oral and Maxillofacial Surgery
University of California - San Francisco
San Francisco, California

Jeffrey C. Posnick, DMD, MD, FACS, FRCS(C)
Clinical Professor of Surgery and Pediatrics
Georgetown University, Washington, DC
Adjunct Professor of Orthodontics
Baltimore College of Dental Surgery
University of Maryland
Adjunct Professor of Oral and Maxillofacial Surgery
Howard University College of Dentistry
Washington, DC

Michael P. Powers, DDS, MS
Private Practice, Oral and Maxillofacial Surgery
Kent, Ohio
Department of Oral and Maxillofacial Surgery
Robinson Memorial Hospital
Ravenna, Ohio

Daniel B. Rodrigues, DDS
Texas A&M University Health Science Center
Baylor College of Dentistry
Dallas, Texas

Steven Roser, DDS, MD, FACS
DeLos Hill Professor and Chief
Division of Oral and Maxillofacial Surgery
Emory University School of Medicine
Atlanta, Georgia

Ramon L. Ruiz, DMD, MD
Medical Director, Pediatric Craniomaxillofacial Surgery
Vice Chair, Department of Children's Surgery
The Arnold Palmer Hospital for Children
Associate Professor of Surgery,
University of Central Florida College of Medicine
Orlando, Florida

Thomas J. Salinas, DDS
Associate Professor of Dentistry
Mayo Clinic College of Medicine
Department of Dental Specialties
Rochester, Minnesota

David M. Sarver, DMD, MS
Clinical Professor, Department of Orthodontics
University of North Carolina
Chapel Hill, North Carolina

Stephen A. Schendel. MD, DDS, FACS
Stanford University Medical Center, Professor Emeritus
of Surgery
Menlo Park, California

Anthony G. Sclar, DMD
Director, Clinical Research and Postgraduate Dental
Implant Surgery
Department of Oral and Maxillofacial Surgery
Nova Southeastern University College of Dental Medicine
Fort Lauderdale, Florida
Chairman, Department of Education
Sclar Center for Empowered Dental Implant Learning
Miami, Florida

Vivek Shetty, DDS, Dr. Med. Dent.
Professor, Section of Oral and Maxillofacial Surgery
School of Dentistry, University of California Los Angeles
Los Angeles, California

Douglas P. Sinn, DDS
Clinical Professor University of Texas
Southwestern Medical Center
Private Practice Division of Oral and Maxillofacial Surgery
Mansfield, Texas

Kevin S. Smith, DDS
Professor and Residency Program Director
Division of Oral and Maxillofacial Surgery
University of Oklahoma
The Oral Facial Surgery Center
Oklahoma City, Oklahoma

Peter M. Spalding, DDS, MS, MS
Department of Growth and Development
University of Nebraska Medical Center College of Dentistry
Lincoln, Nebraska

Daniel B. Spagnoli, DDS, PhD
University Oral and Maxillofacial Surgery
Charlotte, North Carolina

Martin B. Steed, DDS
Assistant Professor and Residency Program Director,
Department of Surgery,
Division of Oral and Maxillofacial Surgery
Emory University School of Medicine
Atlanta, Georgia

Eber L. Stevao, DDS, PhD
Department of Oral and Maxillofacial Surgery
Texas A&M University Health Science Center
Baylor College of Dentistry
Dallas, Texas

Luciano Stroia, DDS
Endoscopic Oral and Maxillofacial Foundation
Fellowship 2010
Private Practice - Oral and Maxillofacial Surgery
San Antonio, Texas

B.D. Tiner, DDS, MD
Clinical Professor Department of Oral and
Maxillofacial Surgery
University of Texas Health Science Center
San Antonio, Texas

Paul S. Tiwana, DDS, MD, MS, FACS
Associate Professor and Graduate Program Director
Division of Oral and Maxillofacial Surgery
University of Texas Southwestern Medical Center
Dallas, Texas

Yan Trokel, MD, DDS
Clinical Instructor
Department of Oral and Maxillofacial Surgery
Mount Sinai Medical School
Medical Director
The Yan Center for Corrective & Cosmetic Surgery
New York, New York

Maria Troulis, DDS, MSc
Associate Professor
Harvard School of Dental Medicine
Director of Residency Program, Oral and
Maxillofacial Surgery
Massachusetts General Hospital
Boston, Massachusetts

Scott Urban, MDM, MD
Private Practice - Utah Facial Surgical Arts
Jordan, Utah

Joseph E. Van Sickels, DDS
Professor of Oral and Maxillofacial Surgery
Assistant Dean and Chair of Hospital Dentistry
University of Kentucky
Lexington, Kentucky

Luis Vega, DDS
Assistant Professor, Assistant Program Director
OMS Residency
Division of Oral and Maxillofacial Surgery?
University of Florida Health Science Center
Jacksonville, Florida

Allison K. Vest, MS, CCA
Medical Art Prosthetics, L.L.C.
Dallas, Texas

Larry M. Wolford, DMD
Department of Oral and Maxillofacial Surgery
Texas A&M University Health Science Center
Baylor College of Dentistry
Dallas, Texas

John M. Wright, DDS, MS
Regents Professor and Chair, Department of
Diagnostic Sciences
Texas A&M Health Science Center
Baylor College of Dentistry
Dallas, Texas

Michael F. Zide, DMD
Clinical Assistant Professor, OMFS (Retired)
University of Texas Southwestern Medical Center
Dallas, Texas

Maxillofacial Reconstruction

Local and Regional Flaps

Alan S. Herford, DDS, MD, and G. E. Ghali, DDS, MD

FLAP PRINCIPLES

Over the past 50 years, the development and application of several different flaps has led to reliable reconstruction of facial defects. Most defects can be reconstructed immediately, leading to better restoration of form and function with early rehabilitation.[1] Reconstructing facial defects can be both challenging and rewarding. Missing tissue most often results from either trauma or oncologic surgery. Commonly, a wide range of options is available for repairing a given defect, including healing by secondary intention, primary closure, placement of a skin graft, or mobilization of local or regional tissue. Compared with skin grafts, local flaps often produce superior functional and aesthetic results.[2–6] A great advantage of local tissue transfer is that the tissue closely resembles the missing skin in color and texture. These flaps can be rotated, advanced, or transposed into a tissue defect. Regional tissue can also be recruited to repair facial defects.

When deciding which option to use, there should be a progression from simple to complex treatments. Consideration should be given to primary closure or the use of skin grafts first, followed by local, then regional, and finally, distant pedicled or microsurgical free tissue transfer. Flaps require additional incisions and tissue movement, which increase the risks of postoperative bleeding, hematoma, pain, and infection. Confirmation of tumor-free margins should be done before flap reconstruction if a malignant lesion has been excised.[7]

Some defects are amenable to closure with a single flap, but others require a combination of flaps for optimal results.[8] An advantage of using multiple flaps is that they can be harvested from separate aesthetic units. This decreases the size of the secondary defect and may allow placement of scars between aesthetic units, thus improving scar camouflage, leading to better cosmesis. Often, separated repair of individual facial subunits with separate flaps provides a better cosmetic result than if a single flap is used to reconstruct the entire defect.

Flaps differ from grafts in that they maintain their blood supply as they are moved. Abundant dermal and subdermal plexus allow for predictable elevation of random cutaneous flaps. A cutaneous flap may also have its arterial supply based on a dominant artery in the subcutaneous layer. Muscular perforating arteries are important contributors to the cutaneous vascular bed. The most important variable for flap viability is not the length-to-width ratio but, rather, the perfusion pressure and vascularity at the pedicle base.[9] Because local flaps provide their own blood supply, they are particularly useful in patients with compromised recipient sites such as those that have been irradiated.

As local flaps heal, regaining of blood flow and cutaneous sensibility increases. The rate of blood flow and two-point discrimination on the surface of local flaps is statistically no different when compared with the corresponding area of the unoperated side.[10] The recovery of sensory nerve function in facial flaps is dependent on the intimacy of contact between the flap and the recipient bed and on the viability of the type of restoration.

Relaxed skin tension lines (RSTLs) result from vectors within the skin that reflect the intrinsic tension of the skin at rest. They are due to the microarchitecture of the skin and represent the directional pull on wounds. The RSTLs are generally parallel to the facial rhytids. Lines of minimal tension (rhytids) result from repeated bending of the skin from muscular contraction. A permanent crease results from the adhesions between the dermis and the deeper tissues. These natural skin creases run perpendicular to the direction of muscle pull and can guide incision orientation for optimal scar camouflage and cosmesis.

The face is composed of aesthetic subunits.[11,12] The areas where these subunits meet are referred to as *anatomic borders*. The aesthetic subunit principle is based on the fact that our eyes see objects as a series of block images that are spatially organized. Scars that are located at the junction of two adjacent anatomic subunits are inconspicuous because one expects to see a delineation between these areas.

FLAP NOMENCLATURE

Many methods are described for classifying cutaneous flaps: by the arrangement of their blood supply, their configuration, location, tissue content, and method of transferring the flap.

Blood Supply

Cutaneous flaps consist of skin and subcutaneous tissue and can be characterized by their predominant arterial supply. These include random pattern, axial pattern, and pedicle flaps (Figure 40-1). *Random flaps* are supplied by the dermal and subdermal plexus alone and are the most common type of flap used for reconstructing facial defects. *Axial pattern flaps* are supplied by more dominant superficial vessels oriented longitudinally along the flap axis. *Pedicle flaps* are supplied by large named arteries that supply the skin paddle through muscular perforating vessels. *Free tissue transfer* refers to flaps that are harvested from a remote region and have the vascular connection reestablished at the recipient site.

Location

Another means of classification is by the region from which the tissue is mobilized. This includes local, regional, and distant flaps. *Local flaps* imply use of tissue adjacent to the defect, whereas *regional flaps* refer to those flaps recruited

from different areas of the same part of the body. *Distant flaps* are harvested from different parts of the body.

Configuration

Flaps are often referred to by their geometric configuration. Examples of these flaps include *bilobed, rhombic,* and *Z-plasty.*

Tissue Content

The layers of tissue contained within the flap can also be used to classify a flap. *Cutaneous flap* refers to those flaps that contain the skin only. When other layers are incorporated into the flap they are classified accordingly. Examples include *myocutaneous* and *fasciocutanous flaps.*

Method of Transfer

The most common method of classifying flaps is based on the method of transfer. *Advancement flaps* are mobilized along a linear axis toward the defect (Figure 40-2). *Rotation flaps* pivot around a point at the base of the flap (Figure 40-3). Although most flaps are moved by a combination of rotation and advancement into the defect, the major mechanism of tissue transfer is used to classify a given flap. *Transposition flap* refers to one that is mobilized toward an adjacent defect over an incomplete bridge of skin. Examples of transposition flaps include rhombic flaps and bilobed flaps (Figure 40-4). *Interposition flaps* differ from transposition flaps in that the incomplete bridge of adjacent skin is also elevated and mobilized. An example of an interposition flap is a Z-plasty. *Interpolated flaps* are those flaps that are mobilized either over or beneath a complete bridge of intact skin

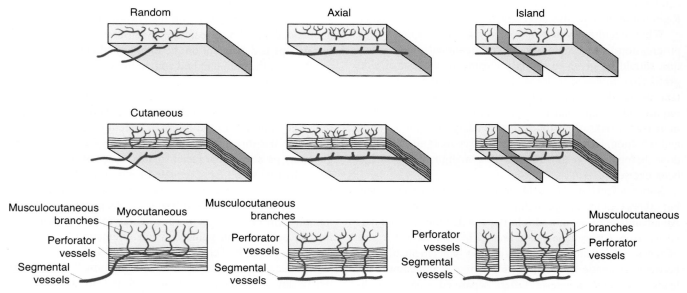

FIGURE 40-1. Diagrammatic representation of cutaneous blood supply in skin and myocutaneous flaps. (Adapted from Ariyan S. Pectoralis major, sternomastoid, and other musculocutaneous flaps for head and neck reconstruction. Clin Plast Surg 1980;7:89–109.)

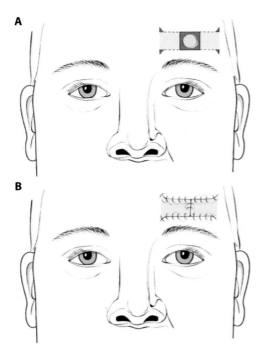

FIGURE 40-2.   **A,** Double advancement flaps with Burow's triangles. **B,** Closure of the defect.

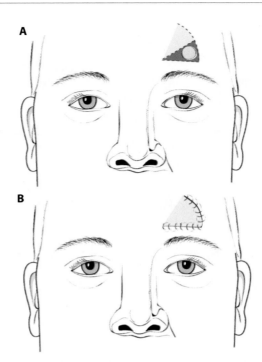

FIGURE 40-3.   **A,** Rotation flap for closure of a forehead defect. **B,** Closure of the defect.

via a pedicle. These flaps often require a secondary surgery for pedicle division. Microvascular free tissue transfer from a different part of the body relies on reanastomosis of the vascular pedicle.

DESIGNING THE FLAP

Many options are available for reconstructing facial defects. Often, the optimal method is not readily apparent. A stepwise approach can be helpful in selecting and designing a flap. The characteristics of the defect and adjacent tissue must be analyzed. These include color, elasticity, and texture of the missing tissue. The defect size, depth, and location are evaluated as well as the availability and characteristics of adjacent or regional tissue. It is important to determine the mobility of adjacent structures and to identify those anatomic landmarks that must not be distorted. The orientation of the RSTLs and aesthetic units should by analyzed closely.

Potential flap designs should be drawn on the skin surface, being careful to avoid those designs that obliterate or distort anatomic landmarks. The final location of the resultant scar should be anticipated by previsualizing suture lines and choosing flaps that place the lines in normal creases.

The secondary defect created as the tissue is transferred into the primary defect must be able to be closed easily. When designing a flap, it is important to avoid secondary deformities that distort important facial landmarks or affect function. Avoid obliterating critical anatomic lines that are essential for normal function and appearance.

Proper surgical technique involves gentle handling of the tissue by grasping the skin margins with skin hooks or fine-toothed tissue forceps. Avoid traumatizing the vascular supply by twisting or kinking the base of the flap. Deep pexing sutures minimize tension on the flap and eliminate dead space. Excessive tension on the flap may decrease blood flow and cause flap necrosis. Meticulous hemostasis should be achieved before final suturing so that a hematoma does not develop beneath the flap. It is important to adequately mobilize and extend the flap, which should be of adequate size to remain in place without tension to minimize the chance of dehiscence, scarring, or ectropion.

TYPES OF FLAPS

Local Flaps

Advancement Flaps

Advancement flaps have a linear configuration and are advanced into the defect along a single vector. These flaps can be single or double. Advancement flaps are often chosen when the surrounding skin exhibits good tissue laxity and the resulting incision lines can be hidden in natural creases. Advancement flaps limit wound tension to a single vector with minimal perpendicular tension. They are often helpful in reconstructing defects involving the forehead, helical rim, lips, and cheek. In these areas, advancement flaps capitalize on the natural forehead furrows without causing vertical distortion of the hairline superiorly or the eyebrow inferiorly (Figure 40-5).

Advancement flaps are created by parallel incisions approximately the width of the defect. Standing cutaneous

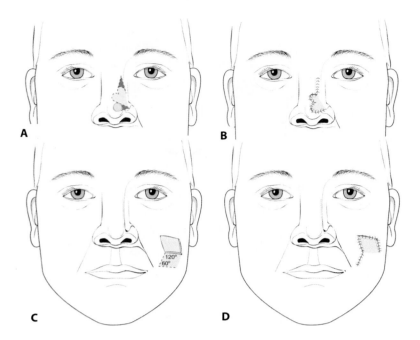

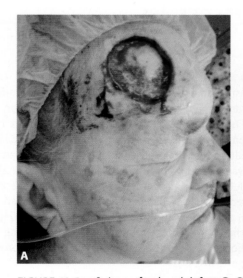

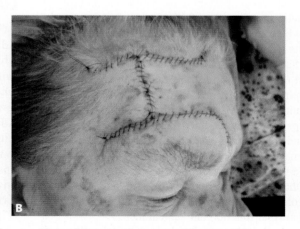

FIGURE 40-4. **A,** Bilobed flap for closure of a nasal tip defect. **B,** Closure of the defect. **C,** Rhombic flap for closure of a check defect. Note the 120- and 60-degree angles. **D,** Closure of the defect.

deformities ("dog-ears") are usually created and are managed with excision. A Z-plasty incision or Burow's triangle may be performed at the base of the flap, reducing the standing cutaneous deformities.

A variation of the advancement flap is the V-Y flap. A triangular island of tissue adjacent to the defect is isolated and attached only to the subcutaneous tissue. It relies on a subcutaneous pedicle for blood supply. As it is advanced into the defect, the secondary defect is closed primarily in a simple V-Y manner. These flaps are especially amenable for cheek defects along the alar facial groove and are generally avoided where there are superficial nerves because of the depth of the incisions.

Local flaps are also useful for staged recostruction of ear defects. Advancement of local tissue can be used to rebuild the missing tissue including the helical rim (Figure 40-6).

Intraoral uses of advancement flaps include covering oroantral fistulae and alveolar clefts. A disadvantage of buccal advancement flaps is the decrease in vestibular sulcus depth (Figure 40-7).

Rotation Flaps

Rotation flaps have a curvilinear configuration. Defects reconstructed with rotation flaps should be somewhat triangular or modified by removing normal tissue to create a triangular defect. These flaps have a large base and are usually

FIGURE 40-5. **A,** Large forehead defect. **B,** Closure utilizing bilateral advancement flaps combined with Burow's triangles.

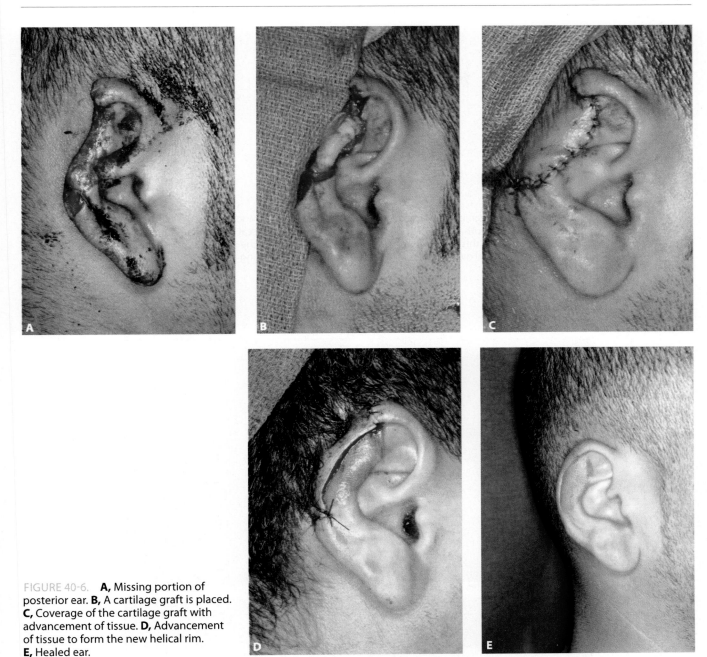

FIGURE 40-6. **A,** Missing portion of posterior ear. **B,** A cartilage graft is placed. **C,** Coverage of the cartilage graft with advancement of tissue. **D,** Advancement of tissue to form the new helical rim. **E,** Healed ear.

random in their vascularity but may be axial. One or more rotation flaps are often used to reconstruct scalp defects. Because of the relative inelasticity of the scalp tissue, these flaps must be large relative to the size of the defect. Scoring of the galea is helpful in gaining additional rotation and advancement (Figure 40-8).

The axial frontonasal flap is a modified simple rotation flap with a back cut.[13–16] It is useful for closing nasal defects (Figure 40-9). The flap is based on a vascular pedicle at the level of the medial canthus. This pedicle consists of a branch of the angular artery and the supraorbital artery.

Rotated palatal flaps are helpful for closing large oroantral fistulae.[8,17] Fistulae less than 5 mm in diameter usually close spontaneously.[18,19] Local flaps or grafts can be used to close larger fistulae. Two-layer closures are less prone to developing recurrence of oroantral fistulae. Approximately 75% of the palatal soft tissue can be rotated to cover adjacent defects.

Transposition Flaps

These flaps are rotated and advanced over adjacent skin to close a defect. Examples of transposition flaps include rhombic flaps and bilobed flaps. These flaps are advantageous in areas where it is desired to transfer the tension away from closure of the primary defect and into the repair of the secondary defect. Transposition flaps have a straight linear

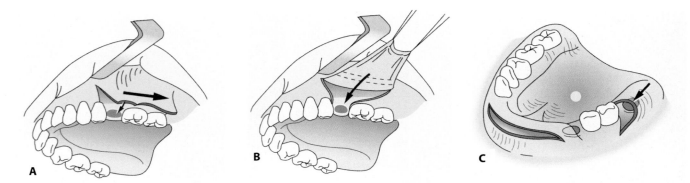

FIGURE 40-7. Buccal advancement flaps can be used to cover an oroantral fistula. **A,** A Moczair buccal sliding trapezoidal flap is slid *(arrow)* to use the papilla of the adjacent tooth to rotate into the defect. **B,** Rehrman's buccal advancement flap uses a flap that has vertical extensions. To adequately mobilize this flap to cover the defect without tension, the periosteum must be incised *(broken line)* along its base and the flap advanced *(arrow)* over the defect. **C,** If the fistula is present along an edentulous region, a transverse flap or bipedicle flap can be used.

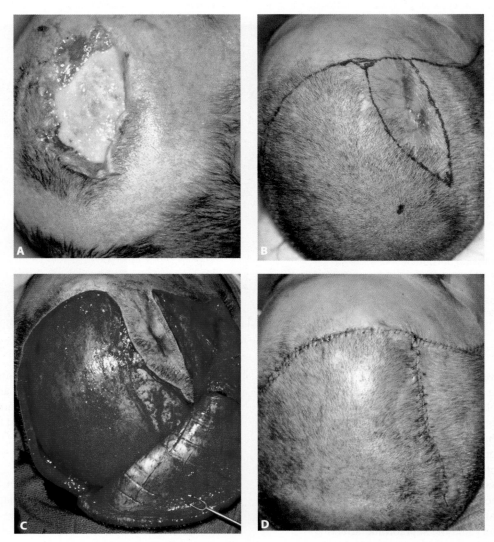

FIGURE 40-8. **A,** A large scalp defect secondary to trauma. **B,** Outline of scalp flaps. **C,** Elevation of flaps with scoring of the galea. **D,** Closure of the defect.

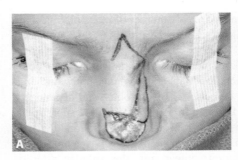
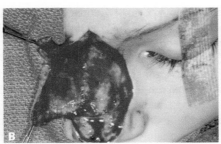
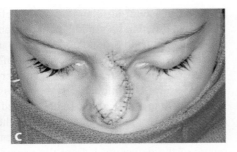

FIGURE 40-9. **A,** Axial frontonasal flap for repair of a nasal defect. **B,** Elevation of the flap with thorough undermining. **C,** Closure of the defect

axis and are usually designed so that one border of the flap is also a border of the defect. An advantage of this type of flap is that it can be developed at variable distances. Areas where these flaps are often used include the nasal tip and ala, the inferior eyelid, and the lips.

The rhombic flap is a precise geometric flap that is useful for many defects of the face.[20,21] The traditional rhombic ("Limberg") flap is designed with 60- and 120-degree angles and equal-length sides. The angle of the leading edge of the rhombic flap is approximately 120 degrees but may vary. The

flap is begun by extending an incision along the short axis of the defect that is equal to the length of one side of the rhombic defect. Another incision is then made at 60 degrees to the first and of equal length (Figure 40-10). Disadvantages of the rhombic flap are the significant tension at the closure point as well as the amount of discarded tissue to transform a circular defect into a rhombus.

The bilobed flap is a transposition flap with two circular skin paddles (see Figure 40-4).[22,23] Esser is credited with the design of the bilobed flap in 1918. It is useful for skin

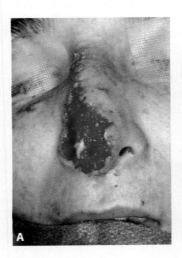
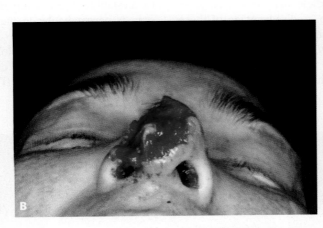
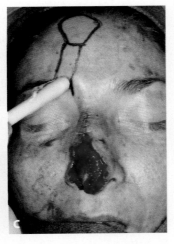
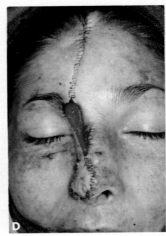
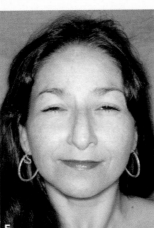

FIGURE 40-10. **A,** Nasal defect with missing skin and exposure of lower lateral cartilages. **B,** Inferior view of missing tissue. **C,** Use of Doppler to isolate the supratrochlear vessels to incorporate into the flap. **D,** The flap is secured in place with the blood supply intact. **E,** After the flap has been taken down and the incisions have healed.

repairing of lateral nose and nasal tip defects up to 1.5 cm. The bilobed flap has a random pattern blood supply. The flap is primarily rotated around a pivot point and the paddles are transposed over an incomplete bridge of skin. The second lobe allows the transfer of tension further from the primary defect closure. The bilobed design rotates around an arc that is usually 90 to 100 degrees. In the bilobed flap, the first lobe closes the defect and the second closes the first lobe defect. The flap is designed with a pivot point approximately a radius of the defect away from the wound margin. The first lobe is usually the same size as the defect, and the second lobe is slightly smaller with a triangular apex to allow for primary closure. The axis of the second flap is roughly 90 to 100 degreees from the primary defect and undermined widely to distribute the tension.

An advantage of the bilobed flap is that one can construct a flap at some distance from the defect with an axis that is independent of the linear axis of the defect. A disadvantage of this flap is that it leaves a circular scar that does not blend with the existing skin creases. During healing, the flap may become elevated ("pin cushioning") because of the narrow pedicle that is prone to congestion, scar tissue that impedes lymphatic drainage, and curvilinear scars that tend to bunch the flap up as they shorten.

Interpolation Flaps

Interpolation flaps contain a pedicle that must pass over or under intact intervening tissue. A disadvantage of these types of flaps is that for those passing over bridging skin, the pedicle must be detached during a second surgical procedure. Occasionally, it is possible to perform a single-stage procedure by deepithelializing the pedicle and passing it under the intervening skin. Advantages of interpolation flaps include their excellent vascularity and their skin color and texture match.

The forehead flap (median and paramedian) is a commonly used interpolation flap and remains the workhorse flap for large nasal defects.[24-27] It is a robust and dependable flap. The forehead flap is primarily based on the supratrochlear vessel, is relatively narrow, and uses a skin paddle from the forehead region. The flap is supplied by a rich anastomosis between the supratrochlear and the angular arteries. Because of the marked vascularity, it is possible to incorporate cartilage or tissue grafts for nasal reconstruction. The forehead flap has abundant tissue available, allowing resurfacing of the entire nasal unit with a single flap, and provides a good texture and color match to the native nose.

The technique for elevating the forehead flap is straightforward. The flap can be designed directly in the midline or in a paramidline location. A template of the defect is used to outline the flap. Elevation of the flap proceeds in either a subgaleal or a subcutaneous plane. The pedicle is always elevated in such a way as to incorporate the frontalis muscle. The width of the pedicle is usually 1.0 to 1.5 cm, which allows for easy rotation of the pedicle. Before inset, the skin paddle is selectively thinned to match the native skin thickness. The pedicle is divided approximately 3 weeks later, with the base of the pedicle inset into the glabellar area to reestablish brow symmetry. The incision, and resulting scar, is perpendicular to the RSTLs but tends to heal well (Figure 40-11).

The nasolabial flap (melolabial) is useful for reconstructing defects involving the oral cavity and those involving the lower third of the nose (Figure 40-12).[28-31] It can be used

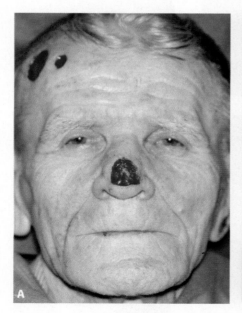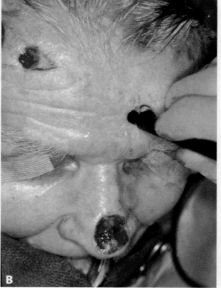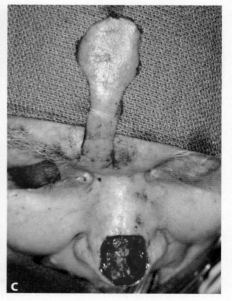

FIGURE 40-11.   **A,** Nasal defect after excision of a squamous cell carcinoma lesion. **B,** Use of Doppler ultrasonography to locate the supratrochlear artery. **C,** The forehead flap has been elevated. *(Continued)*

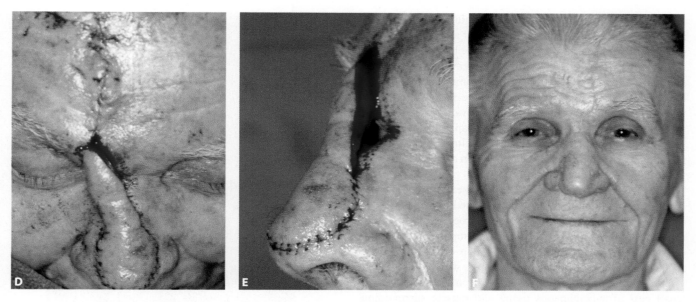

FIGURE 40-11.   *(Continued)* **D,** The flap is turned 180 degrees and sutured into place. **E,** The pedicle is divided 2 to 3 weeks later. **F,** Postoperative result.

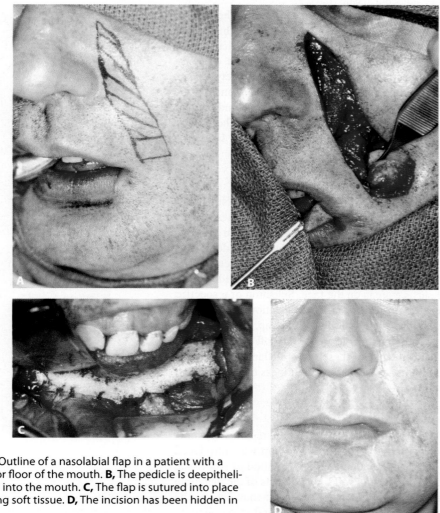

FIGURE 40-12.   **A,** Outline of a nasolabial flap in a patient with a defect in the anterior floor of the mouth. **B,** The pedicle is deepithelialized and tunneled into the mouth. **C,** The flap is sutured into place to restore the missing soft tissue. **D,** The incision has been hidden in the nasolabial fold.

as an interpolation flap with either a single or a staged technique. The flap is supplied by the angular artery, intraorbital artery, and infratrochlear artery and can be based either superiorly or inferiorly. The area of recruitment for nasal reconstruction is in closer proximity to the primary defect than is the forehead flap. A disadvantage of the nasolabial flap is that there is a limited amount of tissue available, and asymmetry can occur along the nasolabial flap folds. When the pedicle is divided, the defect can be closed primarily by placing the scar in the nasal facial junction and the nasolabial flap fold.

The lip-switch flap (Abbé) can be taken from either lip, but it is most commonly switched from the lower to the upper lip.[32-34] This flap can be used to reconstruct as much as one third of the upper lip. The lower lip can supply a flap of one quarter of its length, and the Abbé flap offers immediate replacement of total lip anatomy (Figure 40-13). The labial artery supplies the flap and should be maintained with a small cuff of subcutaneous tissue and muscle surrounding the vascular pedicle. The pedicle is divided after approximately 2 to 3 weeks.

Tongue flaps are excellent flaps for intraoral reconstruction. They use adjacent tissue, have an excellent blood supply, and are associated with minimal morbidity. The tongue has excellent axial and collateral circulation, with the lingual artery providing the main blood supply. Up to one half of the tongue can be rotated for tissue coverage without compromising speech, mastication, or deglutition.[35] A variety of flap designs have been described including anterior- and posterior-based tongue flaps (Figure 40-14). Some indications include repair of oral defects and fistula closure. These flaps are helpful for providing closure of large oroantral fistulae.

Regional Flaps

For large facial defects, local flaps may not provide sufficient tissue to adequately restore the missing tissue. In these cases, consideration should be given to using a regional flap.[36,37] *Regional flaps* are defined as those located near a defect but not in the immediate proximity. They are frequently harvested from the neck, chest, or axilla and can provide coverage of large surface areas on the face. Selection of a specific regional flap depends on the size and location of the defect and also on the intrinsic properties of the flap. Advantages of regional flaps include the large amount of soft tissue and skin available. Disadvantages of these types of flaps include poor color and texture match, excessive bulkiness of the flap, and donor site morbidity.

Pectoralis Major Myocutaneous Flap

The pectoralis major myocutaneous flap remains a workhorse of reconstructive surgery[38-40] The flap was introduced by Ariyan[41] and has provided a reliable method of soft tissue reconstruction of bone and soft tissue defects of the mandible and maxilla. The pectoralis major myocutaneous flap can be rotated around a pivot point 180 degrees and is supplied by

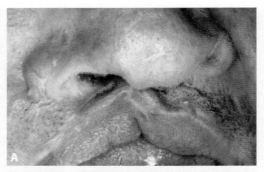
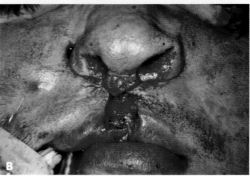
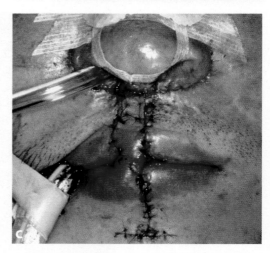
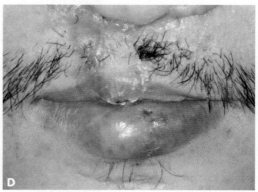

FIGURE 40-13. **A,** Patient with a traumatic lip deformity with avulsion of a portion of his upper lip. **B,** Reapproximation of the orbicularis oris muscles and perialar advancement flaps to reestablish upper lip length. **C,** An Abbé flap is used to restore the missing philtrum. **D,** Postoperative result.

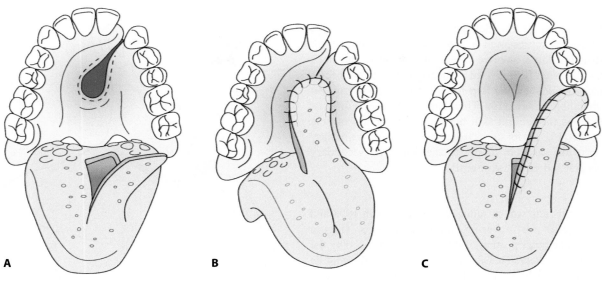

A   **B**   **C**

FIGURE 40-14.   **A** and **B,** Use of an anteriorly based tongue flap to cover the soft tissue deficit resulting from an alveolar cleft. **C,** This type of flap is also useful for closing large oroantral fistulas.

two separate blood supplies (Figure 40-15). The thoracoacromial artery arises from the second portion of the axillary artery and forms four branches as it penetrates the fascia. The pectoral branch is the major artery that supplies the pectoralis major myocutaneous flap. The position of the vascular pedicle can be approximated by drawing a line from the shoulder point to the xiphoid. The pectoral branch descends at a right angle from the middle of the clavicle until it meets this line. Branches of the internal mammary artery supply the medial portion of the muscle and skin over the sternum. The flap provides good coverage for the carotid artery when combined with a neck dissection.

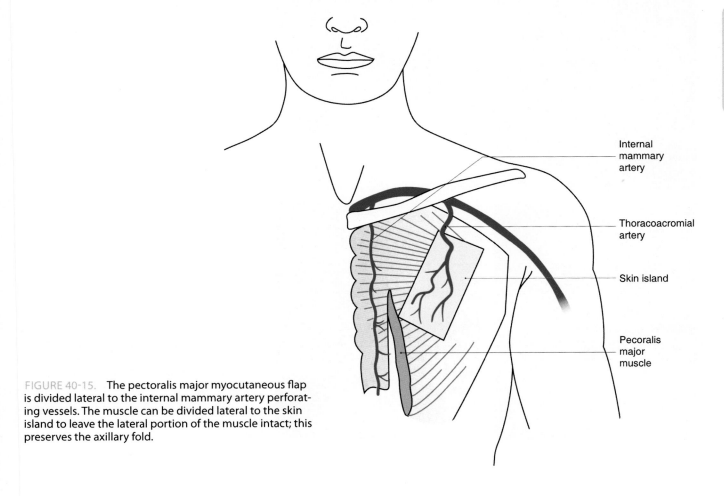

Internal mammary artery

Thoracoacromial artery

Skin island

Pecoralis major muscle

FIGURE 40-15.   The pectoralis major myocutaneous flap is divided lateral to the internal mammary artery perforating vessels. The muscle can be divided lateral to the skin island to leave the lateral portion of the muscle intact; this preserves the axillary fold.

Deltopectoral Flap

The introduction of the deltopectoral flap by Bakamjian and colleagues represented a significant improvement for reconstructing large ablative resections for head and neck cancer.[42–44] Currently, it is used as an alternative to the pectoralis major myocutaneous flap for soft tissue reconstruction of the mandible and maxilla. This flap is composed of fascia, subcutaneous tissue, and skin but does not contain muscle (Figure 40-16). Perforators from the internal mammary artery provide vascular supply to the flap. The secondary defect is covered with a skin graft.

Temporalis Flap

The temporalis flap was introduced by Golovine in 1898 and remains useful for covering intraoral defects (Figure 40-17).[45–48] The outer portion of the muscle is invested by the deep temporal fascia. This fascia is supplied by the middle temporal vessel, which originates just below the zygomatic arch. The temporalis muscle is supplied by both the anterior and the posterior deep temporal arteries, which arise from the second portion of the internal maxillary artery. This dual

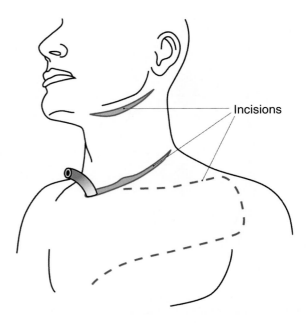

FIGURE 40-16. Incisions for a deltopectoral flap.

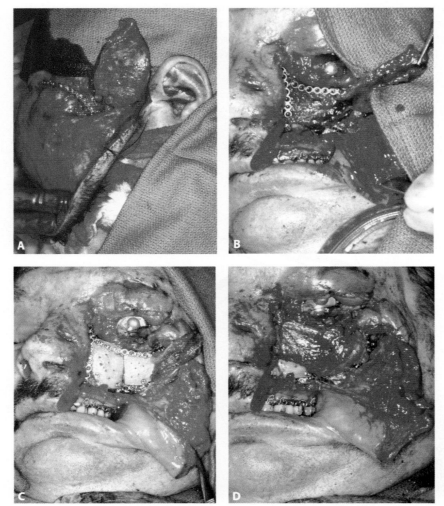

FIGURE 40-17. **A,** Temporalis muscle flap for repair of a midface defect caused by a shotgun wound. **B,** The temporalis muscle is divided, and the posterior portion is sutured into place. **C,** Cranial bone is used to restore the missing tissue. **D,** The anterior portion of the temporalis flap is sutured into place to "sandwich" the bone grafts.

blood supply allows for splitting of the muscle into anterior and posterior flaps.

When elevating the muscle, it is important to remain on the deep temporal fascia beneath the superficial temporal fascia to avoid damage to the frontal branch of the facial nerve. Elevation of the inferior portion of the flap is performed in a subperiosteal plane to avoid damage to the deep temporal arteries, which lie on the undersurface of the muscle. An osteotomy of the zygomatic arch is often helpful to facilitate placement of the muscle into the mouth. The arch can be put back into place and secured with plates and screws. A disadvantage of the temporalis flap is the minimal cosmetic deformity of hollowing in the temporal region; this can be corrected with autogenous or alloplastic materials and can be minimized by using either an anterior or a posterior flap.

Sternocleidomastoid Flap

First described by Jinau in 1909[49] for facial reanimation, the sternocleidomastoid flap was repopularized by Owens.[50-55] The muscle is invested by the deep cervical fascia and is supplied by three arteries. The dominant vessel is the occipital artery, which enters the muscle below the mastoid tip and supplies the superior portion of the muscle. The superior thyroid artery supplies the middle portion, and the thyrocervical trunk supplies the inferior third of the muscle.

The muscle is elevated over the deep cervical fascia superior to the carotid sheath. It is recommended to maintain two of the three vessels when elevating the flap to enhance the viability of the flap. The spinal accessory nerve enters the deep portion of the muscle approximately at the carotid bifurcation and should be preserved to prevent denervation atrophy of the muscle (Figure 40-18). Advantages of the sternocleidomastoid flap include its close proximity to the defect and minimal donor site defect (Figures 40-19 and 40-20).

Trapezius Myocutaneous Flap

The trapezius myocutaneous flap is supplied by three arteries, allowing several flaps to be used. The main vessel supplying

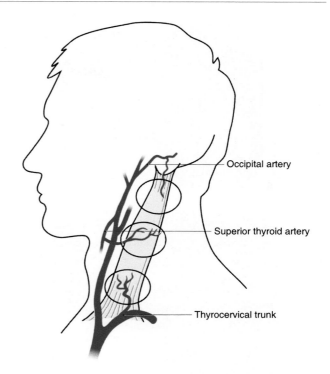

FIGURE 40-18.   Blood to the sternocleidomastoid muscle is supplied through three arteries.

the trapezius muscle is the transverse cervical artery, which is a branch of the thyrocervical trunk. The upper portion of the muscle is supplied by the occipital artery. The trapezius myocutaneous flap is a ready source of skin of uniform thickness without excessive muscle bulk.[56] The main disadvantage is the limited rotation and the short pedicle.

Latissimus Dorsi Myocutaneous Flap

Quillen and colleagues[57] first described the use of the latissimus dorsi myocutaneous flap for head and neck reconstruction in 1978.[57] The flap is not commonly used for head and

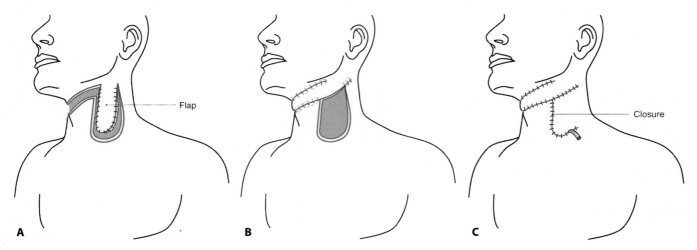

FIGURE 40-19.   **A,** A superiorly based flap with a skin pedicle. **B,** Transposition of the flap. **C,** Closure of the donor defect.

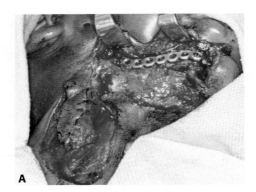

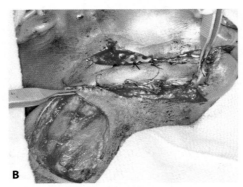

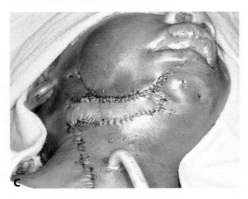

FIGURE 40-20. **A,** The sternocleidomastoid flap is elevated with a superior base. **B,** The flap is rotated in place to provide soft tissue coverage over the reconstruction plate. **C,** The flap is sutured into place and the donor site closed primarily.

neck reconstruction unless other flaps are unavailable or there are very large defects requiring coverage. The muscle is supplied by the thoracodorsal artery, which is the dominant vessel, and also by four to six perforators from the posterior intercostals and lumbar vessels. The main advantage of the latissimus dorsi flap is the large amount of skin provided. The main disadvantages are the need to reposition the patient during the operation and morbidity from the donor site.

COMPLICATIONS

Postoperative complications can be minimized with careful preoperative planning of flap design and by early recognition of problems.[59] A medical history can be used to identify patients with risk factors involving small vessels. These risk factors include smoking, diabetes, hypertension, previous radiation, and preexisting scars.[60,61] Complications may be reversible or irreversible. Early recognition and treatment can minimize complications and prevent them from becoming irreversible. Two main unwanted outcomes are flap failure and unacceptable cosmetic results.

Flap survival depends on early recognition of flap compromise. *Ischemia* is defined as an inadequacy of perfusion in providing tissue needs. Signs of arterial ischemia include a pale and cool flap that does not blanch with pressure and typically does not bleed with a pinprick. Flaps are somewhat ischemic initially because the original tissue perfusion has been compromised by flap elevation. Most tissue can survive on 10% of its average blood flow.[59] Whether the flap will undergo necrosis depends on patient-related and surgery-related factors that influence the risk of necrosis in facial flaps. Smoking is associated with an increased risk of flap failure. The deleterious effects of smoking on flap survival include hypoxemia and vasoconstriction. Patients should be advised to quit smoking during the perioperative period.

Common causes of bleeding in facial reconstruction with local flaps include inadequate hemostasis and drug-induced coagulopathy. Hematoma formation should be identified and decompressed within 24 hours.[62] Decompression can be accomplished with aspiration using a 22-gauge needle or by taking out one or two sutures and applying gentle compression on the flap. Hematoma formation may diminish tissue perfusion and can lead to ischemia or necrosis by inducing vasospasm, stretching the subdermal plexus, or separating the flap from its recipient bed. Patients should be questioned carefully about the use of medications that affect coagulation such as acetylsalicylic acid, nonsteroidal anti-inflammatory drugs, and vitamin E. If possible, these medications should be avoided for 2 weeks before and 1 week after surgery.

Congestion is the most common vascular problem associated with facial flaps. Signs of a congested flap include warmth, edema, and a purple color that blanches with pressure then immediately refills. A pinprick will cause release of dark venous blood. Venous congestion can lead to arterial compromise and flap necrosis. Management of congested flaps may include temporarily releasing sutures to allow decompression at the flap edges or possible impingement involving the flap pedicle. Tight bandages around the flap pedicle should be removed. Medicinal leeches *(Hirudo medicinalis)* may be useful in decompressing congested flaps.[63,64] Saliva from the leech contains an anticoagulant and a vasodilator that facilitate continued oozing from the site even up to 6 hours after they detach.

Hyperbaric oxygen (HBO) has been shown to be beneficial in improving the vascularity of marginal tissues.[65] Prophylactic HBO therapy in cutaneous flap surgery in the irradiated tissue bed may be particularly helpful to combat the hypoxia and hypocellularity. HBO is beneficial in treating both venous congestion and arterial ischemia by creating a local arterial vasoconstriction through the rise in arterial oxygen content, which reduces the amount of inflow. The tissue oxygen levels continue to rise owing to the improved diffusion even though there is vasoconstriction and a reduction in vascular perfusion. The flap can maintain viability while continued neovascularization occurs. Other options include the use of heparin and dipyridamole to help increase the survival of an ischemic flap.[66]

Infection can complicate flap healing.[67] The postoperative infection rate for clean wounds in facial surgery is as low as 2.8%, with higher rates in facial reconstruction with local flaps.[68] Tissue oxygenation is an important factor in prevention of wound infection and is closely related to blood supply. Infections involving local flaps may result in flap failure or poor cosmetic outcome secondary to wound dehiscence and scarring.

CONCLUSION

A variety of facial flaps are available to the reconstructive surgeon for repairing facial defects. The goal of flap surgery is to restore form, function, and aesthetics. There are many advantages to using local and regional flaps, which can lead to optimal aesthetic results.

References

1. Schliephake H, Furrert K, Schneller T. Prospective study of the quality of life of cancer patients after intraoral tumor surgery. J Oral Maxillofac Surg 1996;54:664–669.
2. Kruger E. Reconstruction of bone and soft tissue in extensive facial defects. J Oral Maxillofac Surg 1982;40:714–720.
3. Summers BK, Siegle RJ. Facial cutaneous reconstructive surgery: general aesthetic principles. J Am Acad Dermatol 1993;29:669–681.
4. Baker SR. Resurfacing flaps in reconstructive rhinoplasty. Aesthetic Plast Surg 2002; 26:17–23.
5. Baker SR. Local cutaneous flaps. Otolaryngol Clin North Am 1994;27:139–159.
6. Baker SR. Regional flaps in facial reconstruction. Otolaryngol Clin North Am 1990;23:925–946.
7. Escobar V, Zide MF. Delayed repair of skin cancer defects. J Oral Maxillofac Surg 1999;57:271–279.
8. Ducic Y, Herford AS. The use of palatal island flaps as an adjunct to microvascular free tissue transfer for reconstruction of complex oromandibular defects. Laryngoscope 2001;111: 1666–1669.
9. Milton S. Pedicled skin-flaps: the fallacy of the length:width ratio. Br J Surg 1970;57:502–508.
10. Schliephake H, Schmelzeisen R, Neukam FW. Long-term results of blood flow and cutaneous sensibility of flaps used for the reconstruction of facial soft tissues. J Oral Maxillofac Surg 1994;52:1247–1252.
11. Gonzalez-Ulloa M. Restoration of the face covering by means of selected skin in regional aesthetic units. Br J Plast Surg 1956;9:212–221.
12. Burget GC, Menick FJ. The subunit principle in nasal reconstruction. Plast Reconstr Surg 1985;76:239–247.
13. Rieger RA. A local flap for repair of the nasal tip. Plast Reconstr Surg 1967;40:147–149.
14. Marchac D, Toth B. The axial frontonasal flap revisited. Plast Reconstr Surg 1985;76:686–694.
15. Haneke E. Surgical treatment of defects on the tip of the nose. Dermatol Surg 1998;24:711–717.
16. Herford AS, Zide MF. Reconstruction of superficial skin cancer defects of the nose. J Oral Maxillofac Surg 2001;59:760–767.
17. Millard DR. The island flap in cleft palate surgery. Surg Gynecol Obstet 1963;116:197–198.
18. Liposky RB. Immediate repair of the oroantral communication: a preventative dental procedure. J Am Dent Assoc 1981; 103:727–729.
19. Yih WY, Merrill RG, Howerton DW. Secondary closure of oroantral and oronasal fistulas: a modification of existing techniques. J Oral Maxillofac Surg 1988;46:357–364.
20. Limberg AA, editor. Planimetrie und Stereometrie der Hautplastik. Jena, Germany: Fischer Verlag; 1967.
21. Borges AF. Choosing the correct Limberg flap. Plast Reconstr Surg 1978;62:542–545.
22. Zitelli JA. The bilobed flap for nasal reconstruction. Arch Dermatol 1989;125:957–959.
23. Iida N, Ohsumi N, Tonegawa M, et al. Simple method of designing a bilobed flap. Plast Reconstr Surg 1999;104:495–499.
24. Shumrick KA, Smith TL. The anatomic basis for the design of forehead flaps in nasal reconstruction. Arch Otolaryngol Head Neck Surg 1992;118:373–379.
25. The paramedian forehead flap. In Burget GC, Medick FJ, editors. Aesthetic Reconstruction of the nose. St. Louis: Mosby; 1994; pp. 57–92.
26. Burget GC. Aesthetic restoration of the nose. Clin Plast Surg 1985;12:463–480.
27. McCarthy JG, Lorenc ZP, Cutting C, et al. The median forehead flap revisited: the blood supply. Plast Reconstr Surg 1985; 76:866–869.
28. Ducic Y, Burye M. Nasolabial flap reconstruction of oral cavity defects: a report of 18 cases. J Oral Maxillofac Surg 2000;59:1104–1108.
29. Kakinuma H, Iwasawa U, Honjoh M, Koura T. A composite nasolabial flap for an entire ala reconstruction. Dermatol Surg 2002;28: 237–240.
30. Maurer P, Eckert AW, Schubert J. Functional rehabilitation following resection of the floor of the mouth: the nasolabial flap revisited. J Craniomaxillofac Surg 2002;30:369–372.
31. Lazaridis N, Zouloumis L, Venetis G, et al. The inferiorly and superiorly based nasolabial flap for reconstruction of moderate-sized oronasal defects. J Oral Maxillofac Surg 1998;56: 1255–1259.
32. Zide MF, Fuselier C. The partial-thickness cross-lip flap for correction of postoncologic surgical defects. J Oral Maxillofac Surg 2001;59:760–767.
33. Yih WY, Howerton DW. A regional approach to reconstruction of the upper lip. J Oral Maxillofac Surg 1997;55:383–389.
34. Schulte DL, Sherris DA, Kasperbauer JL. The anatomical basis of the Abbé flap. Laryngoscope 2001;111:382–386.
35. Massengill R, Pickrell K, Mladick R. Lingual flaps: effect on speech articulation and physiology. Ann Otol Rhinol Laryngol 1970;179:853–857.
36. Motamedi MH, Behnia H. Experience with regional flaps in the comprehensive treatment of maxillofacial soft-tissue injuries in war victims. J Craniomaxillofac Surg 1999;27:256–265.

37. Blackwell KE, Buchbinder D, Biller HF, Urken ML. Reconstruction of massive defects in the head and neck: the role of simultaneous distant and regional flaps. Head Neck 1997;19: 620–628.

38. Ariyan S. The pectoralis major myocutaneous flap. A versatile flap for reconstruction in the head and neck. Plast Reconstr Surg 1979;63:73–81.

39. Ariyan S. Further experiences with the pectoralis major myocutaneous flap for the immediate repair of defects from excisions of head and neck cancers. Plast Reconstr Surg 1979;65: 605–612.

40. Marx RE, Smith BR. An improved technique for development of the pectoralis major myocutaneous flap. J Oral Maxillofac Surg 1990;48:1168–1180.

41. Ariyan S. Pectoralis major, sternomastoid, and other musculocutaneous flaps for head and neck reconstruction. Clin Plast Surg 1980;7:89–109.

42. Bakamjian VY. Total reconstruction of pharynx with medially based deltopectoral skin flap. N Y State J Med 1968;68:2771–2778.

43. Sasaki K, Nozaki M, Honda T, et al. Deltopectoral skin flap as a free skin flap revisited: further refinement in flap design, fabrication and clinical usage. Plast Reconstr Surg 2001;107: 1134–1141.

44. Lazaridis N, Tilaverdis I, Dalambiras S, et al. The fasciocutaneous cervicopectoral rotation flap for lower cheek reconstruction: report of three cases. J Oral Maxillofac Surg 1997;55: 1166–1171.

45. Golovine SS. Procede de cloture plastique de l'orbite après l'exenteration. Arch Ophthal 1898;18:679.

46. Alonso del Hoyo J, Fernandez Sanroman J, GilDiez JL, et al. The temporalis muscle flap: an evaluation and review of 38 cases. J Oral Maxillofac Surg 1994;52:143–147.

47. Burggasser G, Happak W, Gruber H, Freilinger G. The temporalis: blood supply and innervation. Plast Reconstr Surg 2002;109:1862–1869.

48. Abubaker AO, Abouzgia MB. The temporalis muscle flap in reconstruction of intraoral defects: an appraisal of the technique. Oral Surg Oral Med Oral Pathol Oral Radiol Endod 2002;94:24–30.

49. Jinau A. Die Chirurgishe behanolung der facialislachmung. Dtsch ZF Chin 1909;102:377–381.

50. Owens NA. A compound neck pedicle designed for the repair of massive facial defects. Plast Reconstr Surg 1955;15:369–389.

51. Zhao YF, Zhang WF, Ahao JH. Reconstruction of intraoral defects after cancer surgery using cervical pedicle flaps. J Oral Maxillofac Surg 2001;59:1142–1146.

52. Ariyan S. Further experience with the sternocleidomastoid myocutaneous flap. Plast Reconstr Surg 2003;111:381–382.

53. Kerawala CJ, McAloney N, Stassen LF. Prospective randomized trial of the benefits of a sternocleidomastoid flap after superficial parotidectomy. Br J Oral Maxillofac Surg 2002;40: 468–472.

54. Kierner AC, Zelenka I, Gstoettner W. The sternocleidomastoid flap—its indications and limitations. Laryngoscope 2001; 111:2201–2204.

55. Marx RE, McDonald DK. The sternocleidomastoid muscle as a muscular or myocutaneous flap for oral and facial reconstruction. J Oral Maxillofac Surg 1985;43:155–162.

56. Papadopoulos O, Tsakoniatis N, Georgiou P, Christopoulos A. Head and neck soft-tissue reconstruction using the vertical trapezius musculocutaneous flap. Ann Plast Surg 1999;42:457–458.

57. Quillen CG, Shearing JG, Georgiade NG. Use of the latissimus dorsi myocutaneous island flap for reconstruction in the head and neck area. Plast Reconstr Surg 1978;62:113–117.

58. Posnick JC, McCraw JB, Magee W Jr. Use of a latissimus dorsi myocutaneous flap for closure of an orocutaneous fistula of the cheek. J Oral Maxillofac Surg 1988;46:224–228.

59. Vural E, Key JM. Complications, salvage, and enhancement of local flaps in facial reconstruction. Otolaryngol Clin North Am 2001;34:39–51.

60. Goldminz D, Bennett RG. Cigarette smoking and flap and full-thickness graft necrosis. Arch Dermatol 1991;127:1012–1015.

61. Kinsella JB, Rassekh CH, Wassmuth ZD, et al. Smoking increases facial skin flap complications. Ann Otol Rhinol Laryngol 1999;108:139–142.

62. Mulliken JB, Healey NA. Pathogenesis of skin flap necrosis from an underlying hematoma. Plast Reconstr Surg 1979; 63:540–545.

63. Utley DS, Koch RJ, Goode RL. The failing flap in facial plastic and reconstructive surgery: role of the medicinal leech. Laryngoscope 1998;108:1129–1135.

64. Dabb RW, Malone JM, Leverett LC. The use of medicinal leeches in the salvage of flaps with venous congestion. Ann Plast Surg 1992;29:250–256.

65. Zamboni WA, Roth AC, Russell RC, et al. The effect of hyperbaric oxygen on reperfusion of ischemic axial skin flaps: a laser Doppler analysis. Ann Plast Surg 1992;28:339–341.

66. Kerrigan CL, Daniel RK. Pharmacologic treatment of the failing skin. Plast Reconstr Surg 1982;70:541–548.

67. Bumpous JM, Johnson JT. The infected wound and its management. Otolaryngol Clin North Am 1995;28:987–1001.

68. Sylaidis P, Wood S, Murray DS. Postoperative infection following clean facial surgery. Ann Plast Surg 1997;39:342–346.

Vascularized and Nonvascularized Hard and Soft Tissue Reconstruction

D. David Kim, DMD, MD, FACS, and Rui Fernandes, DMD, MD, FACS

INTRODUCTION

Reconstruction of the oral cavity involves restoration of complex functional, anatomic, and aesthetic characteristics that can make this a daunting task. The reconstructive surgeon has many techniques at his or her disposal for realizing these goals; often, this requires complex decision making as to which techniques will yield the best outcome. These decisions should be made by evaluating the patient and the defect on a case-by-case basis. Clearly, the myriad of techniques available to the reconstructive surgeon each have their own merits and demerits and the most ideal technique for one patient may not be adequate for the next.

This chapter outlines many of the major options in soft tissue and bony reconstruction. Many smaller defects of the oral cavity may be amenable to simpler techniques for reconstruction such as primary closure, skin grafting, secondary intention, or random pattern local flaps. These techniques are described in numerous articles throughout our literature and are not covered in this chapter. Instead, the authors focus on the use of regional or distant soft tissue and bone for reconstruction of more complex defects in the head and neck. The authors have attempted to detail the procedures, advantages, and disadvantages in a concise and objective manner.

Flaps can be classified based on their proximity to the recipient site. This results in the clinically useful terms: local, regional, and distant flaps. Most regional and distant flaps are based on a vascular pedicle that provides the nutrient inflow and outflow of blood to the transferred tissue. Understanding the variations of the different classifications of muscle-containing flaps is extremely important for the reconstructive surgeon; the studies of the blood supply to muscles reported by Mathes and Nahai[1] are primary to this understanding (Table 41-1). Of course, this classification system involves only muscles, but the understanding of the blood supply to the skin has been elucidated Taylor and Palmer's

TABLE 41-1. **The Classification of Muscle Flaps**

Type 1	One vascular pedicle	Gastrocnemius, rectus femoris, tensor fascia lata
Type 2	One dominant vascular pedicle plus minor pedicles (most common pattern)	Abductor digiti minimi, abductor hallucis, biceps femoris, flexor digitorum brevis, gracilis, peroneus longus, peroneus brevis, platysma, semitendinosis, soleus, sternocleidomastoid, temporalis, trapezius, vastus lateralis
Type 3	Two dominant pedicles	Gluteus maximus, rectus abdominis, serratus anterior, semimembranosus
Type 4	Segmental vascular pedicles	Extensor digitorum longus, extensor hallucis longus, flexor digitorum longus, flexor hallucis longus, sartorius, tibialis anterior
Type 5	One dominant vascular pedicle and secondary segmental vascular pedicles	Pectoralis major, latissimus dorsi

Adapted from Mathes SJ, Nahai F. Classification of the vascular anatomy of muscles: experimental and clinical correlation. Plast Reconstr Surg 1981;67:177–187.

anatomic study[2] of the human body's angiosomes. The angiosome theory proposes that the human body is composed of approximately 40 blocks of composite tissue, each with its own cutaneous territory supplied by a discrete source vessel. Simply stated, all arteries to the skin travel either directly to their destination (direct perforators) or first travel through other tissues, usually muscle (indirect perforators). These studies allow the reconstructive surgeon to classify flaps according to the type of vascular supply and predictably determine the vascular territory of the flap's pedicle.

Reconstruction of the craniomaxillofacial complex has been a cornerstone of the specialty of oral and maxillofacial surgery, and the reconstructive options for bony defects continue to expand. Currently, the surgeon has a vast array of autologous and autogenous options. This chapter covers the available autogenous options.

The use of nonvascularized bone has always been within the everyday realm of maxillofacial surgeons. Recently, the use of microvascular free tissue transfer has become an established and routine reconstructive option in head and neck surgery. Furthermore, it has been embraced by oral and maxillofacial units worldwide wherein free flap reconstruction of such defects is now considered the gold standard of care.[3] The use of nonvascularized bone grafts continues to be the workhorse for the majority of defects encountered by maxillofacial surgeons. As such, this chapter also reviews the commonly used nonvascularized grafts and highlights the advantages as well as disadvantages of their use. Equally, the chapter highlights commonly used microvascular bone flaps and their associated advantages and disadvantages.

TECHNIQUES FOR SOFT TISSUE RECONSTRUCTION OF THE ORAL CAVITY

Regional Soft Tissue Flaps

Regional flaps have historically been the mainstay technique for head and neck soft tissue reconstruction. These techniques take advantage of the flap's proximity to the ablative or injured site and generally rely on an "arc of rotation" as the limiting factor for utilization of these flaps. Their popularity is undeniable owing to proximity, ease of harvest, general reliability, and elimination of the need for specialized instruments and skills for microvascular anastomosis. The main drawbacks of these flaps are the relative limited area of application due to the arc of rotation as well as a limited volume of soft tissue available for reconstruction. Some flaps such as the pectoralis major, temporalis, and latissimus flaps require removal of a relatively large volume of tissue with only a small portion of it used for the actual reconstruction. The combination of these drawbacks has led to an increase in utilization of free tissue reconstruction techniques for head and neck defects.

Submental Island Flap

The submental island flap was introduced by Martin and coworkers in 1993[4] and has rapidly increased in popularity in

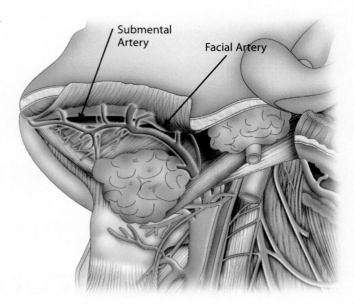

FIGURE 41-1. The course of the submental artery. (From Clement CD. Anatomy Regional Atlas of the Human Body. 3rd ed. Baltimore: Urban & Schwarzenberg; 1987; Fig. 581.)

head and neck reconstruction owing to its ease of harvest, accessibility, quality of available tissue, and overall versatility. It can be raised as a cutaneous, musculocutaneous, fasciocutaneous, or osteocutaneous flap and can be utilized as a rotational flap for oral or facial defects as distant as the upper third of the face.[5] The flap may also be harvested as a free flap for more distant recipient sites. The submental flap is an axial patterned flap based on the submental branch of the facial artery and vein (Figure 41-1). This is a consistent branch of the facial artery and arises behind the submandibular gland and crosses anteriorly along the mylohyoid muscle. Here, the artery may pass superficially across the anterior belly of the digastric muscle but passes deep to this muscle 70% of the time.[6] The artery ends at the symphysis of the mandible where it sends terminal branches to the lower lip and sublingual gland. The artery gives off one tow four cutaneous perforators throughout its course,[7] which travels through the platysma muscle to the subdermal plexus where it anastomoses with the contralateral artery. This pattern of perfusion allows for reliable skin paddle design that can extend from one mandibular angle to the other. Many times, the dimensions of the flap may be limited by the remainder of the neck skin's mobility to achieve primary closure of the donor site defect. However, split- or full-thickness skin grafting may be utilized in cases in which primary closure cannot be obtained. The potential skin paddle for this flap has been described as large as 18 × 7 cm and the vascular pedicle length can be as long as 8 cm.[8]

Several descriptions of increasing the flap's vascular pedicle have been offered. The facial artery may be ligated distal to the take-off of the submental artery, providing a modest increase in pedicle length. The facial artery may also be ligated proximal to the take-off of the submental artery, relying on reversed flow from the distal facial artery, resulting in a reverse-flow flap. Finally, one or both of the submental artery or vein may be divided and anastomosed to a suitable recipient vessel nearer to the defect.[9]

The submental skin is very pliable and thin. The quality of this donor site is analogous to the skin of the radial forearm flap. Therefore, this flap is well suited for moderate-sized defects of the tongue, floor of mouth, and buccal mucosa. In facial reconstruction, the hair-bearing nature of the submental skin in males and some females must be considered before its use.

Owing to this donor site's location, its use for reconstruction of oncologic defects of the oral cavity may be limited. If a neck dissection is included in the treatment of an oral cavity malignancy, the vascular pedicle must be dissected through the primary lymphatic drainage basin of many of these, tumors which may compromise the oncologic safety of the resection. Some authors have advocated close dissection of the pedicle of this flap in these circumstances to avoid leaving a significant amount of fibroadipose tissue surrounding the vessels.[7] This flap has even been advocated in cases in which cervical node involvement is known or suspected.[10] Others have recommended a more prudent approach to donor site selection owing to the vast array of available reconstructive options; the risk of using this flap in this circumstance is difficult to justify.[11]

Flap Harvesting

With the patient in the supine position and the neck extended, the skin paddle is designed along the inferior border of the mandible at a distance of approximately 1 cm inferior to this landmark. This provides a relatively hidden scar and decreases the chance of pulling the lower lip down upon closure of the defect (Figure 41-2). The neck skin can be pinched to determine the maximum dimension of the flap that will facilitate

primary closure; otherwise, skin grafting will be required.[10] Dissection of the flap may begin on the ipsilateral or contralateral side of the vascular pedicle to be utilized and also either the inferior or the superior border of the flap. The dissection is in the subplatysmal plane on the contralateral side of the skin paddle, and because this dissection proceeds toward the pedicle, it is carried over the contralateral anterior belly of the digastric muscle and the mylohyoid muscle in the midline of the neck. The ipsilateral anterior belly of the digastric muscle is detached at the inferior border of the mandible and at the common tendon and included in the flap. The ipsilateral portion of the mylohyoid muscle may be preserved by meticulous dissection of the submental vessels, or a portion of this muscle may be removed along with the pedicle, which may facilitate passage of the flap to an intraoral site (Figure 41-3). The facial artery is usually easily identified behind the submandibular gland as it passes behind the posterior belly of the digastric muscle. It can then be traced distally either through or posterior to the submandibular gland where numerous glandular branches will be encountered and ligated. The submental artery is then dissected off its deep attachments and the distal facial artery can be ligated.

Applications

The flap has many indications for head and neck reconstruction including coverage for any intraoral defect including maxillectomies. The nature of the submental skin makes it particularly useful for tongue, floor of mouth, and buccal mucosa defects. Facial skin can be reconstructed ranging from lips and cheeks as well as the temporal region.[7]

Temporalis Flap

The temporalis muscle flap has extensive applications for head and neck reconstructions. The flap is well described for use in facial reanimation as well as skull base and midfacial

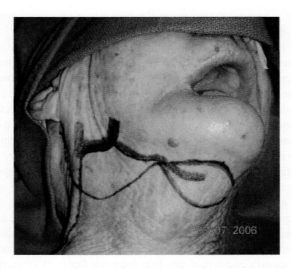

FIGURE 41-2.   Submental flap elevated in the subplatysmal plane until the ipsilateral anterior belly of the digastric. This muscle is incorporated into the flap by detaching from the mandible and at the common digastric tendon.

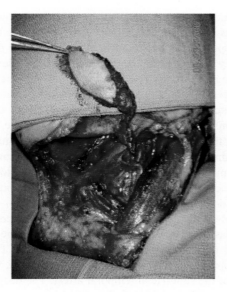

FIGURE 41-3.   Elevated submental flap with ipsilateral anterior belly of digastric tendon.

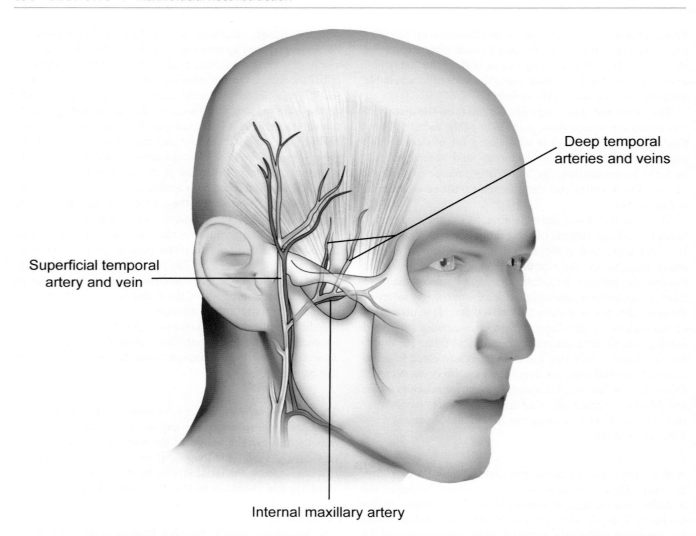

Deep temporal
arteries and veins

Superficial temporal
artery and vein

Internal maxillary artery

FIGURE 41-4.   Blood supply to the temporalis muscle. Anterior and posterior deep temporal arteries and the middle temporal artery (branch off the superficial temporal).

reconstruction. First introduced in 1898 by Golovine,[12] it is known as one of the oldest muscular flaps in use today. The flap's popularity is bolstered by its relative ease of harvest, proximity to maxillofacial applications, and flexibility in harvesting all or only a portion of the muscle. The main disadvantages include a relative lack of soft tissue available for reconstruction, minimal application due to arc of rotation limitations, as well as a contour deformity of the donor site and over the zygoma. Of course, these last two concerns have been addressed by alloplastic implants or autogenous tissue to minimize the donor site defect and by osteotomy of the zygomatic arch to pass the temporalis muscle and prevent a contour deformity.

Based on the deep temporal arteries, the temporalis muscle is classified by Mathes and Nahai[1] as a type 2 muscle with one dominant pedicle plus minor pedicles. The second blood supply is from the middle temporal artery, which is a branch of the superficial temporal artery. The deep temporal arteries arise from the internal maxillary artery and enter the muscle from its deep surface and provide a segmental blood supply because there are usually separate anterior and posterior deep temporal arteries (Figure 41-4).

The muscle originates from the superior temporal line and coalesces to a dense tendon at its insertion to the coronoid process. In terms of the layers of the scalp, the temporalis muscle lies directly on the temporal bone and is covered by the deep temporal fascia, which also inserts into the superior temporal line and is analogous to the pericranium covering the remainder of the skull (Figure 41-5). Caudally, the fascia splits into superficial and deep layers approximately 2 cm above the zygomatic arch; a layer of fat exists between the two layers. The deep and superficial layers continue caudally to fuse with the periosteum of the zygomatic arch. The zygomatic and temporal branches of the facial nerve cross the zygomatic arch in the layer of the temporoparietal fascia, which is superficial to the superficial layer of the deep temporal fascia. By incising the superficial layer of the deep temporal fascia at the root of the zygoma and extending it anterosuperiorly at a 45-degree angle, the entire zygomatic arch can be exposed while adequately protecting the facial nerve.

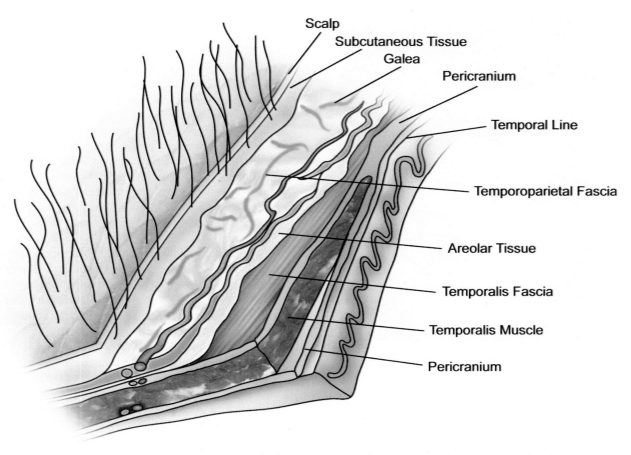

FIGURE 41-5. Layers of scalp at the superior temporal line. Note the confluence of the deep temporal fascia with the pericranium.

FLAP HARVESTING

Many techniques for exposing and harvesting a temporalis muscle flap exist for specific indications. Some of the more common uses include a small strip of temporalis muscle harvested for interpositional reconstruction of the temporomandibular joint (TMJ) after ankylosis release or diskectomy and temporalis muscle for facial reanimation surgery. This narrative deals with harvesting the entire temporalis muscle for intraoral reconstruction. With the patient in a supine position, the head should be placed on a Mayfield headrest to allow for easy access to the scalp. The authors do not recommend shaving the patient's head for this procedure, but long hair may be trimmed so it does not interfere with the dissection. A coronal or hemicoronal incision within the hair-bearing scalp can be planned based on the particular needs of the reconstruction or ablative defect location. Likewise, the planned incision can be combined with a preauricular, endaural, or retroaural incision and injected with 1% lidocaine with 1:100,000 epinephrine for hemostasis. The incision is carried through all the layers of the scalp except for the pericranium and deep temporal fascia. Raney clips may be used for hemostasis of the incised scalp. The scalp is bluntly elevated anteriorly above this layer until a point 2 cm above the lateral orbital rim is reached and posteriorly until the most posterior portions of

the superior temporal line is identified. The root of the zygomatic arch is palpated and the deep temporal fascia is cut at a 45-degree angle upward from the root of the arch, anteriorly to the point approximately 2 cm above the lateral orbital rim. This exposes the temporal fat pad between the superficial and the deep layers of the deep temporal fascia and allows for exposure of the entire zygomatic arch in a subperiosteal plane from the root of the arch to the lateral orbital rim while adequately protecting the frontal branch of cranial nerve VII.

At this point, the entire temporalis muscle and deep temporal fascia is visualized and separated from its origin at the superior temporal line. The whole muscle may be raised and used if necessary. Alternatively, if a smaller defect is present, the muscle may be split into an anterior third and a posterior two thirds and utilizing the thinner and longer posterior portion of the muscle while leaving the anterior portion attached to the temporal fossa, thus decreasing the cosmetic deformity of the donor site depression (Figure 41-6). The dissection elevates the muscle off the temporal bone along with its fascia down to the infratemporal fossa. Although the superior portion of the deep temporal fascia is elevated with the flap, its blood supply is derived mainly from the middle temporal artery, which is usually sacrificed during this dissection. Therefore, this fascia may not be reliable for oral cavity

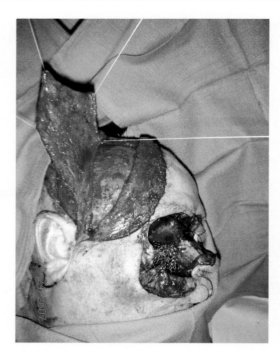

FIGURE 41-6.   Temporalis muscle flap elevated.

relining as described by Wong and colleagues.[13] The muscle itself without a fascial covering is adequate for most oral reconstructions.

Several techniques for introducing the flap into the oral cavity have been offered. These include zygomatic arch osteomy, coronoidectomy,[14] and passage over or under the zygomatic arch. These are all viable techniques depending on the clinical indication and can be performed fairly easily without compromise of the vascular pedicle to the muscle flap. For many defects, the simplest method of transfer is to create a tunnel through the infratemporal fossa between the coronoid process and the remaining lateral wall of the maxilla by blunt dissection. A silk suture can be placed on the free edge of the temporalis muscle and grasped by a long clamp introduced through the tunnel from the oral cavity. Gentle passage through the tunnel can allow the muscle to unfold and adequately line the defect.

APPLICATIONS

The temporalis muscle is well suited for relining defects of the maxilla, ipsilateral hard and soft palate, pharynx, retromolar trigone, and buccal mucosa. It has also been used for tongue and floor of mouth reconstructions.

Pectoralis Major Myocutaneous Flap

The pectoralis major myocutaneous flap (PMMF) has earned the title of the "workhorse flap" for head and neck reconstruction since its introduction in 1979 by Ariyan.[15] The popularity of this soft tissue flap has decreased significantly with the generalized acceptance of microvascular fasciocutaneous, musculocutaneous, and perforator flaps. However, the flap remains popular for reconstruction in patients who may

have one or more contraindications to microvascular surgery, in facilities that lack microvascular capabilities, or as a rescue flap for failed microvascular reconstructions. The main reasons for this flap's popularity include its relative ease of harvest, proximity to the head and neck, hearty and consistent vascular supply, low donor site morbidity, and good versatility for head and neck defects.

The pectoralis major is a fan-shaped muscle that originates at the sternum, clavicle, and external oblique aponeurosis and inserts via a thick tendon to the greater tubercle of the humerus. The muscle medially rotates and adducts the arm with some flexion (upper fibers) and extension (lower fibers) of the arm. The loss of this muscle is tolerated well with most of the muscle's function compensated by the latissimus dorsi.

According to Mathes and Nahai,[1] the pectoralis major is a type 5 muscle with one dominant pedicle, the pectoral branch of the thoracoacromial artery, and a secondary segmental blood supply through the internal mammary artery's parasternal perforators. Both the lateral thoracic and the superior thoracic arteries provide some vascularity to the pectoralis major but both are usually sacrificed to obtain a greater arc of rotation. Notably, the lateral thoracic has been shown to provide a substantial vascular supply to the pectoralis major muscle and has a caliber as large as or larger than the pectoral branch of the thoracoacromial artery. Some authors have advocated the preservation of this artery to improve the flap's blood supply.[16] Cadaver injection studies suggest that the thoracoacromial artery supplies the lateral and proximal portions of the muscle and the inferior and medial sections of the muscle are dependent on the lateral thoracic artery.[17,18] Though these studies provide less than conclusive data for the preservation of the lateral thoracic artery, they do offer compelling evidence for further study regarding the optimum blood supply to this flap.

The use of the PMMF for head and neck reconstruction usually involves the harvest of a skin paddle along with the muscle. The skin of the anterior chest wall is adequately supplied by the thoracoacromial axis superiorly and laterally by the fourth intercostal space. However, inferior and medially, the skin is supplied by direct musculocutaneous perforators from the internal mammary vessels. The use of an inferiorly and medially placed skin paddle relies on a network of "choke" vessels that link the adjacent angiosomes (Figure 41-7). This skin paddle can be compromised when based on the thoracoacromial artery if these "choke" vessels are insufficient or become occluded. This may be the anatomic reason for skin paddle necrosis with intact blood supply to the underlying muscle.[19] An even more tenuous situation occurs when the skin paddle is extended onto the abdominal skin by including a portion of the underlying rectus fascia. This orientation introduces an area of "random" skin in an angiosome "once removed" from the angiosome of the main arterial pedicle. The use of a laterally placed skin paddle along the free edge of the pectoralis major muscle in the area of the inframammary fold may allow for more predictable

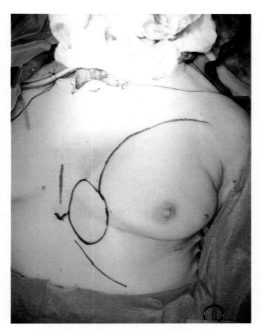

FIGURE 41-7.   Patient markings for pectoralis major myocutaneous flap with a medially based skin paddle.

cutaneous blood supply. According to Reid and Taylor's ink injection studies,[18] this region derives its blood supply through direct fasciocutaneous perforators from the thoracoacromial axis (Figure 41-8). This benefit would come with a slightly decreased arc of rotation.

FLAP HARVESTING

The patient's chest should be prepared for surgery to include the upper abdomen, past midline of the chest, as well as the ipsilateral shoulder and axilla. The ipsilateral arm may be placed on an arm board and extended to facilitate dividing the humeral attachment. Design of the skin paddle should take into consideration the shape and extent of the defect as well as the anatomic position to maximize the vascularity of

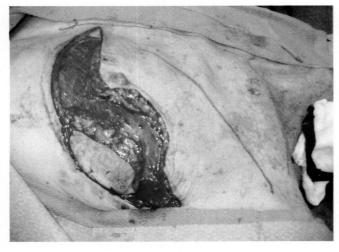

FIGURE 41-8.   Laterally based skin paddle.

the skin paddle. The most common location of the skin paddle for head and neck reconstruction is a parasternal skin paddle, which utilizes the "choke" vessel system between the thoracoacromial artery and the internal mammary perforators (see Figure 41-7). Alternatively, a laterally positioned skin paddle takes advantage of the direct fasciocutaneous perforators from the thoracoacromial axis (see Figure 41-8). Next, the arc of rotation for the desired skin paddle should be estimated using a lap sponge or suture held at the junction of the middle and lateral third of the clavicle and estimating the length of pedicle necessary by extending it to the farthest point of the defect. This length of lap sponge can then be transposed to the chest by rotating around the point held at the clavicle. The point estimated on the chest represents the distalmost point of the necessary soft tissue reconstruction. Finally, access to the anterior chest wall can be designed in a curvilinear fashion from the ipsilateral axilla (see Figure 41-7) across the anterior chest wall to the medially placed skin paddle. This incision design allows for direct exposure of pectoralis major muscle with minimal undermining, and less tunneling is necessary to pass the flap over the clavicle. In female patients or those adverse to a scar across the chest, an inframammary skin incision can be utilized (see Figure 41-8), but this limits access and visualization of the upper portions of the muscle and requires significant undermining to pass the flap to the head and neck.

The skin is incised from the shoulder to the superior margin of the proposed skin paddle and extended down the lateral portion of the skin paddle. All layers are incised until the pectoralis major muscle is exposed. The skin is then undermined laterally to visualize the lateral and inferior borders of the pectoralis major muscle. This allows the surgeon to evaluate the position of the skin paddle's orientation over the muscle and can be adjusted as necessary to minimize the amount of "random" skin that is harvested. The circumference of the skin paddle is then incised down to the muscle and the skin should be sutured down to the muscle to prevent shearing of the perforators during harvest. The skin and fascia of the access incision are then undermined cephalad to communicate with the neck incision and a wide tunnel (four fingers wide) over the clavicle should be created for adequate passage of the flap pedicle without compression.

Separation of the pectoralis major from the anterior chest wall is then started at the lateral border of the muscle where a plane between the pectoralis major and minor muscles can be identified. This is continued inferiorly to detach the pectoralis major from the ribs. Care must be taken to identify and ligate the intercostal perforators, and monopolar cautery should be avoided. This dissection is carried cephalad by detaching the sternal origins of the muscle. The second and third intercostal perforators can be preserved by moving the dissection of the muscle at this point more lateral to avoid these arteries, which supply the deltopectoral flap. As this dissection progresses superiorly, the pectoral branch of the thoracoacromial artery will come into view on the undersurface of the pectoralis major along the medial aspect of the pectoralis minor muscle. One or two branches of the pectoral nerve will also be seen in this area and should be divided to provide a greater arc of rotation.

Once the pedicle is in view, the humeral attachment can be divided with meticulous hemostasis to prevent post-operative hematoma formation. During this dissection, the lateral thoracic artery can be identified. The decision to preserve the lateral thoracic for additional blood supply to the flap should be made at this point. This dissection can be carried up to the clavicle while preserving the thoracoacromial artery. Once complete, the flap can be turned over the clavicle and passed through the tunnel to reach the head and neck site. The donor site should be evaluated for hemostasis and primary closure obtained over suction drains with wide undermining if necessary.

Applications

The usefulness of the pectoralis major myocutaneous flap is limited by its arc of rotation, character and quantity of skin available for reconstruction, and bulk of tissue in the neck. However, the flap is well suited for reconstruction of floor of mouth and lateral mandibular defects when a delayed bone reconstruction is considered. Essentially, any defect of the lower third of the face can be reached with this flap. However, it is not ideal for partial glossectomy defects owing to the relative immobility of the flap.

Latissimus Dorsi Myocutaneous Pedicled Flap

The latissimus dorsi myocutaneous flap (LDMF) is a very versatile flap for head and neck reconstruction. Owing to its flat, broad nature and large amounts of soft tissue available, this flap can cover huge defects of the head and neck. Indeed, the LDMF was the first musculocutaneous flap to be reported in the literature in 1896,[20] but it was not reported for use in the head and neck until 1978.[21]

The latissimus dorsi muscle arises from the thoracic spine (T6–12), the lower four ribs, the iliac crest, and the thoracolumbar fascia. The muscle converges around the teres major and inserts into the intertubular groove of the humerus. Like the pectoralis major, the latissimus dorsi is classified as a type 5 muscle by Mathis and Nahai[1] with its one dominant pedicle being the thoracodorsal artery and its segmental secondary pedicles consisting of the paraspinal perforators. The thoracodorsal artery is a branch of the subscapular artery, which is itself a branch of the third part of the axillary artery. The thoracodorsal artery also gives off branches to the teres major, serratus anterior, and subscapularis muscles as well as the angular branch to the inferior tip of the scapula. The vascular territories of the skin can be divided into three angiosomes. Zone I is the superior third of the muscle, which is supplied by perforators from the thoracodorsal artery. Zone II is the middle third of the muscle, which is mainly supplied by the paraspinal perforators. Zone III is the caudal third, which is fed by the lumbar arteries.[2] Placement of a skin paddle over this distal zone may be at risk of necrosis owing to this "once removed" relationship of that angiosome. It is the anterior free margin of zone II where an abundance of perforators exist and the skin paddle can be most ideally placed.

Flap Harvesting

The most cumbersome aspect of utilizing this flap is patient positioning. The flap can be approached in a supine position with the ipsilateral arm extended across the chest and rolls placed under the ipsilateral shoulder and hip to expose the back. However, a lateral decubitus position allows for easier access to this flap, although it requires multiple preparing and draping of the head and neck to avoid contamination. Once properly positioned, the surface landmarks should be identified and marked. These include the midpoint of the axilla, the midpoint between the anterior and the posterior superior iliac spines, the scapular tip, and the spinous processes of the vertebrae. A line connecting the midpoint of the axilla and the midpoint of the iliac crest approximates the anterior free border of the latissimus dorsi muscle. The thoracodorsal artery runs 3 to 4 cm posterior to the edge of the muscle and divides into a horizontal and vertical branch just below the scapular tip. A skin paddle can be designed over the anterior edge of the muscle overlying zone II as described previously (Figure 41-9). This design provides adequate perfusion of the overlying skin as well as good length of pedicle for rotation into the head and neck.

Incision of the anterior margin of the skin paddle and extension along the line estimating the anterior edge of the muscle up to the axilla allows for identification of the muscle's leading edge. At this point, an attempt to identify the pedicle can be made by elevating the muscle off the posterior chest wall. A branch off the thoracodorsal pedicle will be encountered supplying the serratus anterior muscle and can be traced proximally to identify the main thoracodorsal pedicle. Once the thoracodorsal artery is identified, the branch to the serratus is ligated. Alternatively, the remainder of the skin paddle can be incised down to the underlying muscle and can be sutured down to the underlying fascia to prevent shearing of the cutaneous perforators. The surrounding skin is then undermined to expose the origins of the muscle and can be

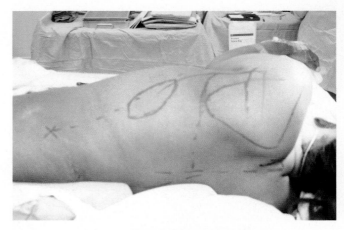

FIGURE 41-9. Patient markings for latissimus myocutaneous flap with the patient in the lateral decubitus position.

detached from its origins using electrocautery. Working from inferior to superior, the muscle is raised off the posterior chest wall with identification of the vascular pedicle on the undersurface of the muscle near the tip of the scapula. Once identified, the pedicle can be followed proximally ligating and dividing the muscular branches as well as the angular branch to the tip of the scapula. The humeral attachment of the latissimus dorsi muscle must be detached carefully to avoid damage to the underlying pedicle. Finally, the circumflex scapular vessels will be identified at the most proximal portion of the pedicle dissection and can be ligated to provide even more mobilization.

Once the flap is elevated, a tunnel must be prepared to pass the flap to the head and neck region. This is accomplished by identifying the lateral edges of the pectoralis major and minor muscles and creating a plane between them. This dissection continues until the level of the clavicle where a separate incision is necessary. The attachments of the pectoralis major to the clavicle must be incised while attempting to preserve the thoracoacromial vascular pedicle to the pectoralis major muscle. A generous passage into the neck should be achieved and can be estimated by the ease of passage of three or four fingers through the tunnel. The flap can then be passed through the tunnel with care not to twist the pedicle.

Applications

Like the pectoralis major myocutaneous flap, the utility of the latissimus dorsi flap is limited by its arc of rotation. However, the area that the latissimus can reach in the head and neck is quite broad, extending as far superiorly as the apex of the skull. Owing to the large surface area of available muscle and skin, this flap is well suited for use in defects where a large surface area of soft tissue is necessary for reconstruction.

Microvascular Soft Tissue Flaps

The continued penetration of microvascular reconstructive techniques into head and neck surgery has been astounding. Once thought to be radical, last-resort procedures that were fraught with failure and complications, these procedures have come to the forefront of head and neck reconstruction and have unsurpassed reliability and versatility. These reconstructive techniques have allowed for customized reconstruction options for tumor and trauma patients in whom previously a "one-size-fits-all" approach was the norm. The use of microvascular reconstruction often allows for more comprehensive ablative surgery without the limitations placed on the ablative surgeon that local or regional flaps have incurred in the past. Furthermore, in anatomic regions like the maxilla, midface, and skull base where reconstructive options were particularly limited and resulted in poor cosmetic and functional outcomes, free tissue transfer has proved to be invaluable in providing meaningful surgical outcome improvements. Finally, several studies have shown that microvascular reconstruction does not incur higher cost for treatment compared with conventional reconstructive techniques.[22,23]

Though the benefits of microvascular surgery are numerous, the limitations of these techniques are also clearly delineated. The need for specialized training and instrumentation are certainly obstacles that are becoming decreasingly prevalent, with more training facilities exposing residents and fellows to microvascular reconstruction. Also, patient factors such as hypercoagulability states or vessel depletion after ablative surgery must be taken into consideration. Finally, the increased operative time required for these procedures may make medically compromised patients poor candidates for this type of reconstruction.

It is difficult to classify many microvascular flaps into soft tissue or bone flaps because many have variations in harvesting that can easily incorporate composite tissue. However, this section attempts to describe some of the more common flaps used in soft tissue reconstruction of the head and neck.

Radial Artery Fasciocutaneous Flap

In many institutions, the radial artery fasciocutaneous flap (RAFF) or radial forearm free flap has supplanted the pectoralis major myocutaneous flap as the "workhorse" soft tissue flap for head and neck reconstruction. Popularized by Soutar and associates in 1983,[24] the RAFF has become one of the most commonly used and reliable soft tissue free flaps for head and neck reconstruction. This versatile flap offers thin, pliable skin that can be as large as nearly the entire forearm from the flexor crease of the wrist to the antecubital fossa except for a small strip over the ulnar aspect of the forearm. The flap may also be harvested with partial-thickness radial bone, palmaris longus tendon, brachioradialis muscle, and lateral antebrachial cutaneous nerve. The characteristics of the skin of the forearm allows for this flap to be nearly ideal for reconstruction of areas in the head and neck that require thin, mobile tissue such as the tongue, floor of mouth, and soft palate. The skin paddle should be centered over the radial vessels, but the design of the flap can be tailored to the particular reconstructive situation. Bilobed, double paddle, folded, tubed, and fascia-only flaps have been described.

The radial and ulnar arteries are the terminal branches of the brachial artery and supply the hand and fingers through an arterial array known as the *superficial and deep palmar arches*. The radial artery ends in the deep palmar arch and the ulnar artery ends in the superficial palmar arch. In most individuals, the superficial palmar arch alone can supply adequate blood to the hand and fingers either directly by sending branches to all five digits or by communicating branches to the deep palmar arch to supply the thumb and forefinger. However, in an estimated 12% of individuals,[25] the superficial palmar arch is incomplete *and* no communication between the deep and the superficial palmar arches exists. It is in these patients that harvesting the radial artery along with a RAFF can have catastrophic consequences to the distal upper extremity. If the ulnar distribution is undisturbed, the third, fourth, and fifth digits should still remain viable but the thumb and forefinger are at risk for ischemia should the previously described circumstances be present.

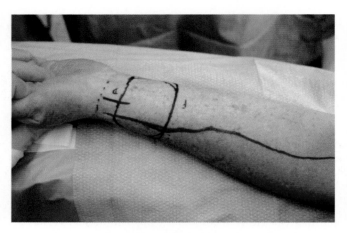

FIGURE 41-10. Skin markings for radial artery fasciocutaneous flap

To avoid this complication, the performance of an accurate Allen's test is essential and in cases in which this test is equivocal, radial and ulnar artery duplex studies may be performed to objectively observe the pattern of flow and the reversal of flow with total occlusion of the radial artery.

FLAP HARVESTING

The arm should be prepared circumferentially up to the axilla and draped accordingly for access to the entire arm. The distal portion of the radial artery should be palpated and marked as well as the distal location of the cephalic vein in the "snuffbox" region. Flap design should be carefully considered to approximately center the flap over the radial vessels as much as possible, with particular care in selecting the orientation of the pedicle relative to the skin paddle (Figure 41-10). Once marked, the arm is exsanguinated with an elastic wrap and the tourniquet inflated to 250 mmHg. The tourniquet time should be recorded, as should the overall ischemia time to the flap.

The initial incision is along the palmar crease of the forearm, and initial identification of the distal radial artery and venae commitantes as well as the cephalic vein is performed. These should then be isolated and ligated. The superficial branches of the radial nerve will also be encountered here and can be preserved or transected, leaving an area of anesthesia over the dorsum of the thumb and forefinger. Once the distal vasculature is secured, the remainder of the skin paddle incisions can be made. The flap is then raised off the deep forearm muscles and tendons from medial to lateral in a subfascial plane. This dissection will traverse the flexor tendons of the forearm, which must maintain a thin layer of paratenon to facilitate skin graft healing. This dissection continues until the lateral intermuscular septum is approached. Similarly, on the radial side, the flap is elevated from lateral to medial in the same subfascial plane. Here the superficial branches of the radial nerve can again be preserved by breaking the subfascial plane of dissection or sacrificed. Once complete, the flap can then be elevated from distal to proximal by carefully elevating the radial artery and veins along

the intermuscular septum. Vascular clips are necessary to control the numerous branches to the surrounding muscles and radial bone.

The remainder of the vascular pedicle is dissected by first making a curvilinear incision from the antecubital fossa to the proximal portion of the skin paddle. This incision is taken to subcutaneous tissue only and the skin is undermined in this subcutaneous plane medially and laterally. Care must be taken not to injure the proximal cephalic vein during this dissection. The cephalic vein is identified as it exits the skin paddle and circumferentially dissected. A vessel loop is passed around the vein and the entire length of vein is dissected up to the desired length. Finally, the proximal radial pedicle is accessed by separating the brachioradialis and the flexor carpi radialis muscles and retracting the brachioradialis laterally. The remainder of the pedicle can then be elevated up to the brachial artery if necessary (Figure 41-11).

The flap is then allowed to reperfuse for 15 to 20 minutes by releasing the tourniquet. Hemostasis can also be achieved at this time. The flap is then harvested and passed to the ablative field. A suction drain should be placed in the deep tissues in the proximal forearm and the curvilinear incision can be closed primarily. A full- or split-thickness skin graft is normally required to close the skin paddle site. The skin graft is covered with a nonadherent dressing, the arm is then padded generously with cast padding, and a volar splint is fabricated to immobilize the arm during skin graft healing.

APPLICATIONS

The quality of the skin of the forearm lends itself for use in a wide variety of head and neck reconstruction applications. Most commonly used for reconstruction of tongue, floor of mouth, and buccal mucosa defects, this flap also has the versatility for use in facial skin or scalp reconstructions. The generous pedicle length allows for placement in areas quite remote from recipient vessels, and the relatively low morbidity of the procedure make the radial artery fasciocutaneous flap a workhorse in microvascular soft tissue reconstruction.

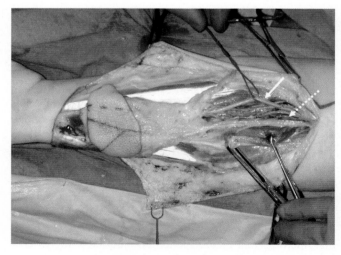

FIGURE 41-11. Radial artery fasciocutaneous flap elevated up to antecubital fossa.

Anterolateral Thigh Flap

The anterolateral thigh flap (ALTF) is based on the cutaneous perforators of the descending branch of the lateral circumflex femoral artery, a branch of the profunda femoris. The pedicle travels in the intermuscular septum between the rectus femoris and the vastus lateralis muscles along with the motor nerve to the vastus lateralis. The cutaneous perforators may travel through the intermuscular septum between these muscles (septocutaneous perforators) or through a portion of the vastus lateralis (musculocutaneous perforators). This latter variation appears to be the more common configuration. The skin of the lateral thigh may also be supplied by the transverse branch of the lateral circumflex femoral artery or directly from the deep femoral artery. Though the flap has enjoyed a recent explosion in popularity, it is these variations in vascular anatomy that have detracted from the flap's overall acceptance in head and neck reconstruction.

The pedicle to this flap can support a large area of relatively thin and flexible skin, depending on the patient's overall body habitus. Up to 800 cm^2 has been reported,[26] encompassing an area from the greater trochanter of the femur to a line 3 cm above the patella. No preoperative evaluation is required before flap harvesting[27]; however; the use of a handheld Doppler can identify the dominant perforator to the thigh skin. The most likely position of this perforator can be estimated by drawing a line from the anterior superior iliac spine (ASIS) to the superolateral corner of the patella. At the midpoint of this line, a 3-cm-radius circle is drawn and the most likely position of the skin perforator will be in the inferolateral quadrant of this circle. The skin paddle should be centered on this point (Figure 41-12).

The main disadvantage to this flap is the inconsistent size and location of the cutaneous perforators. These perforators have been reported to be completely missing.[27] Celik and coworkers[28] argue that many of these reports result in a lack of recognitions of small perforators or due to the surgeon's inability to dissect the musculocutaneous perforators through the vastus lateralis muscle.[25] The reconstructive surgeon should be prepared to convert to an anteromedial thigh flap or a tensor fascia lata flap if this situation arises.[28]

Flap Harvesting

The surface landmarks for the ALTF are drawn as described previously. A Doppler probe is used to confirm the location of this perforator. The flap's skin paddle is designed to be centered on this perforator. The initial incision is made on the medial aspect of the skin paddle down through the deep fascia to the rectus femoris muscle. The flap is elevated laterally off the muscle until a cutaneous perforator is identified. Once the perforator is identified, the remainder of the skin paddle can be incised. The perforator is followed through the intermuscular septum between the rectus femoris and the vastus lateralis (septocutaneous perforators) or through the vastus lateralis muscle (musculocutaneous perforators) until the source artery is identified (Figure 41-13). The descending branch of the lateral circumflex femoral artery can be dissected proximally for the desired pedicle length or up to 16 cm.[29] Running along with the source vessels is the nerve to the vastus lateralis muscle. This nerve must be preserved to maintain motor innervation to this muscle.

Once the flap is harvested, any muscular dissection should be reapproximated and a suction drain placed in the deep tissues. The area of the skin paddle can generally be closed primarily with a modest amount of undermining of the surrounding skin if the skin paddle's dimensions do not exceed 6 to 9 cm.

Applications

For many reconstructive surgeons, this flap has supplanted the radial forearm flap as the primary soft tissue flap for head and neck reconstruction. Indeed, the low morbidity and the ability to primarily close the donor site are key advantages to utilizing this flap. However, the inconsistent nature of the perforators remains as the primary deterrent for the widespread adoption of this flap. Furthermore, the nature of the thigh skin varies with the patient's overall body habitus

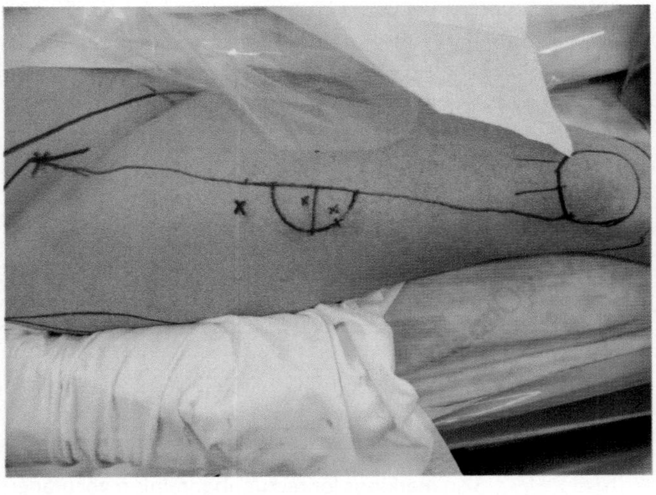

FIGURE 41-12. Skin markings for anterolateral thigh flap.

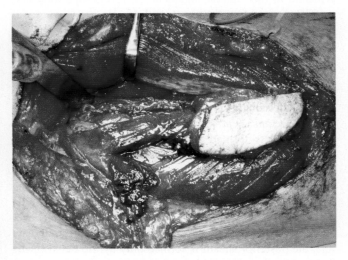

FIGURE 41-13. Dissection through vastus lateralis muscle for musculocutaneous perforators.

and is generally thicker and less pliable than the radial fore-arm skin. In patients who have had axillary node dissection, radial artery harvested for coronary bypass grafting, or previous trauma to the forearm, the ALTF can be an excellent alternative source of soft tissue for head and neck reconstruction.

Rectus Abdominis Myocutaneous Flap

The rectus abdominis myocutaneous flap (RAMF) is based on the deep inferior epigastric artery and vein (DIEA and DIEV) and has been a reliable flap for many areas of reconstruction. These vessels are of good caliber and a fairly long vascular pedicle can be obtained. The flap can transfer a large volume of skin, fat, muscle, and fascia, which is dependent on the patient's body habitus. This volume will decrease over time because the denervated muscle will atrophy significantly. The RAMF is well suited to cover defects that require a large volume of tissue such as total maxillectomy, total glossectomy, skull base, or scalp defects. Pedicled and free flaps based on the inferior or superior epigastric arteries have been well described for breast reconstruction. A variety of different skin paddle orientations are available for this flap depending on the needs of the reconstruction.

A perforator flap based on the DIEA and DIEV allows for harvesting the skin, subcutaneous tissue and fascia without the rectus muscle.[31] In this flap (DIEP), the cutaneous perforators are dissected through the rectus muscle to the vascular source, allowing for a much thinner flap.

The rectus muscle receives its blood supply from both the deep superior epigastric artery and vein (DSEA and DSEV) and the DIEA and DIEV. The DIEA and DIEV have approximately twice the diameter of the DSEA and DSEV and the paraumbilical musculocutaneous perforators are directly associated with the DIEA and DIEV, whereas they must anastomose to the DSEA and DSEV through a series of small vessels where flow can be reversed.[32]

The DIEA branches from the external iliac artery just cephalad to the inguinal ligament. It travels superiorly and medially to penetrate the transversalis fascia 3 to 4 cm caudal to the arcuate line on the undersurface of the rectus muscle. It courses superiorly through the muscle, giving off branches to the skin near the umbilicus.

The anatomy of the anterior abdominal wall is important when harvesting this flap because preservation of fascial sheaths is crucial to preventing postoperative hernia formation. The rectus sheath extends from the pubis to the xiphoid process and is formed by the fibrous aponeurosis of the abdominal muscles. The arcuate line is estimated by a line connecting the ASISs and indicates the change in composition of the posterior rectus sheath. Above the arcuate line, the posterior sheath is composed of the transversalis fascia and a portion of the internal oblique aponeurosis. This double layer of fascia is adequate to prevent hernias. Below the arcuate line, the posterior sheath is formed only by the transversalis fascia. If not reinforced, this area is prone to bulging or hernia formation. In this region, the anterior rectus sheath must

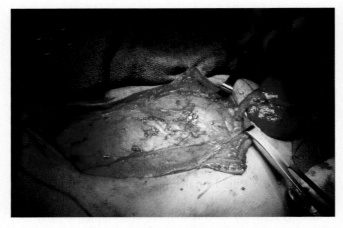

FIGURE 41-14. Elevated rectus abdominis myocutaneous flap. Note the bulging of the abdominal contents below the arcuate line.

be preserved and used to reinforce the transversalis fascia (Figure 41-14).

FLAP HARVESTING

Surface landmarks for the RAMF include the midline of the abdomen and the estimated width of the rectus abdominis muscle as well as both ASISs with a line connecting them to estimate the arcuate line. The ipsilateral femoral vessels should be palpated and marked as well as the costal margin (Figure 41-15). A concentration of cutaneous perforators exists around the umbilicus and the skin paddle design should be centered in this area. Flap elevation begins by creating the superior and inferior skin paddle incisions down through the anterior rectus sheath to expose the rectus muscle. The rectus sheath is divided horizontally until the medial and lateral edges of the muscle are identified. The lateral edge of the muscle indicates the linea semilunaris and the medial edge of the muscle indicates the linea alba. Once these fascial divisions are identified, the lateral skin paddle incision can be created down to Scarpa's fascia and then undermined from lateral to medial to the linea

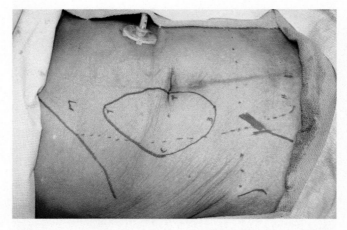

FIGURE 41-15. Skin markings for rectus abdominis myocutaneous flap.

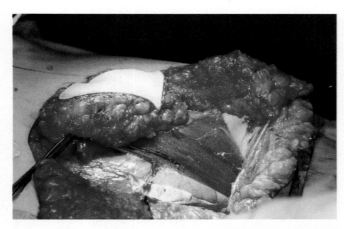

FIGURE 41-16. Caudal portion of rectus abdominis muscle exposed.

semilunaris. The same can be performed medially. The rectus sheath is then incised along the linea semilunaris and the linea alba.

To access the DIEA and DIEV, a vertical incision is made from the inferior portion of the skin paddle down toward the femoral vessels down to the anterior rectus sheath. The rectus sheath is incised at the midpoint of the long axis of the muscle and undermined laterally and medially to expose the caudal portion of the muscle (Figure 41-16). This split anterior rectus sheath will serve as the hernia-preventing layer inferior to the arcuate line to preserve the integrity of the abdominal wall. Once the incision is completed and the caudal rectus muscle is exposed, the flap may be elevated from superior to inferior off the posterior rectus sheath. The mixed motor/sensory nerve supply from the intercostals nerves will be encountered laterally as the flap is elevated and can be ligated and divided. These nerves have been reported to be useful in segmentally reinnervating the rectus muscle. On the undersurface of the muscle, the DIEA and DIEV will come into view. The pedicle should be protected while the inferior portion of the rectus muscle is transected at any point inferior to the vascular pedicle. The pedicle is followed inferiorly until the desired length is achieved or the external iliac vessels are reached. The DIEVs usually join to become a single vein just before its take-off from the external iliac vein, which may be beneficial depending on the size of the recipient vein. The pedicle is then divided and the flap passed to the ablative field.

Closure of the donor site begins with reapproximation of the inferior portion of the cut anterior rectus sheath. Again, this layer will serve to restore the integrity of the abdominal wall inferior to the arcuate line. The superior portion of the anterior sheath that was harvested with the flap may also be reapproximated by large, slowly absorbable suture. Care should be exercised to prevent visceral injury with suture needles or other sharp instruments. Finally, a layered primary closure of the skin can be achieved with wide undermining with suction drains placed in the dead space.

APPLICATIONS

Owing to the large volume of skin and muscle available for reconstruction, the RAMF is ideally suited for applications in which a large bulk of tissue is necessary. Total maxillectomy and total glossectomy defects are the most common indications, though it may also be useful in scalp or facial skin reconstructions. The potential for reinnervation of the muscle by anastomosis of the segmental nerves to a recipient nerve in the ablative field makes this flap feasible for facial reanimation surgery.

Latissimus Myocutaneous Free Flap

The latissimus myocutaneous free flap shares the anatomic and flap harvesting details with the latissimus rotational flap. Obviously, a tunnel through the axilla is not necessary for use as a free flap and the thoracodorsal vessels are divided. The flap is useful in head and neck reconstruction when a large surface area of soft tissue is necessary and the ability to anastomose the pedicle to local recipient vessels eliminates the bulk of the pedicle traversing the axilla and neck (Figure 41-17).

Lateral Arm Free Flap

Introduced in 1982 by and colleagues,[32] the lateral arm free flap derives its blood supply from several septocutaneous perforators through the lateral intermuscular septum from the posterior radial collateral artery and vein (PRCA and PRCV, respectively). The PRCA is itself a branch of the profunda brachii artery, which is a branch off of the brachial artery. The flap has the potential for dual outflow with the PRCV venae commitantes serving as the deep venous system and the cephalic vein as the superficial system. The flap may be harvested with skin, soft tissue, nerve (posterior cutaneous nerve of the arm [PCNA]), muscle (triceps), and bone (partial thickness humerus). Large amounts of skin and soft tissue have been reported , the largest being 18 × 11 cm,[33] but most are limited to one third of the upper arm

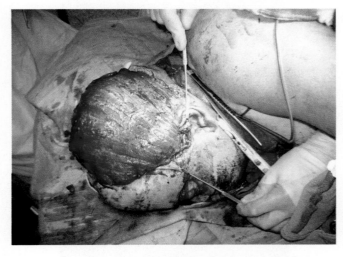

FIGURE 41-17. Latissimus muscle flap for near-total scalp reconstruction.

circumference in order to facilitate primary closure of the donor site defect.

The lateral arm flap's primary advantage is a potentially thin, pliable soft tissue paddle without the concern of ischemic injury to the upper extremity as with the radial forearm flap. Also, the donor site defect can often be closed primarily without the need for an additional skin graft donor site. The primary disadvantages to this flap are the relatively short vascular pedicle and the proximity of the profunda brachii artery to the radial nerve with potential for injury during dissection.

FLAP HARVESTING

The arm should be circumferentially prepared and draped exposing the upper forearm to the axilla. The surface landmarks include the lateral epicondyle of the humerus and the V-shaped insertion of the deltoid muscle. A line is drawn between the point of the V, and the lateral epicondyle represents an area 1 cm anterior to the lateral intermuscular septum (Figure 41-18). The skin paddle is designed in a fusiform shape with its long axis 1 cm posterior to this line.

The initial incision is made at the anterior margin of the skin paddle down to the brachioradialis and brachialis muscles. The posterior cutaneous nerve of the forearm (PCNF) may be encountered in the distal portion of this incision and may be preserved or sacrificed, creating an area of anesthesia in the upper forearm. The dissection continues in a subfascial plane posteriorly toward the intermuscular septum where septocutaneous perforators will be identified. The posterior skin paddle incision can then be made down to the triceps muscle and dissected in the subfascial plane anteriorly toward the intermuscular septum and identification of the septocutaneous perforators. Following these perforators proximally will lead to the source artery and vein (PRCA and PRCV). The same vessels are then identified from the ante-

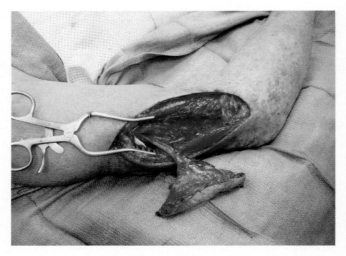

FIGURE 41-19.   Elevated lateral arm flap with generous pedicle length.

rior dissection by separating the brachioradialis from the intermuscular septum. The radial nerve will be encountered in this dissection and must be preserved.

The flap is elevated from distal to proximal by first ligating the continuation of the PCRA distally to become the recurrent interosseous artery and separating the septum from the humerus. The PCNA and the PCNF run along with the pedicle. The pedicle is followed proximally through the intermuscular septum toward the spiral groove of the humerus. Part of the deltoid attachment to the humerus may be divided to allow access to the proximal pedicle (Figure 41-19). The pedicle is severed when the desired pedicle length is achieved.

A suction drain may be placed in the deep tissues. The brachialis and triceps muscles can be lightly reapproximated and primary closure can be achieved in most cases.

APPLICATIONS

The applications for the lateral arm flap mirror those of the radial forearm and ALTF. The skin quality of the upper arm is generally thin and pliable and a generous vascular pedicle is available for harvest. The main advantage of this flap over the radial forearm is that the distal circulation of the arm and hand is not dependent upon the PRCA and, like the ALTF, may serve as an effective alternative in patients in whom a radial forearm flap is contraindicated.

TECHNIQUES FOR HARD TISSUE RECONSTRUCTION OF THE ORAL CAVITY

Nonvascularized Bone Grafts

The most commonly used nonvascularized bone grafts in the head and neck are the anterior iliac crest, posterior iliac crest, tibial bone, and cranial bone. When the quantity of needed bone is small, intraoral sites can also be a source for harvesting. Sites in the oral cavity such as the ramus of the mandible, the anterior symphysis region, and the maxillary

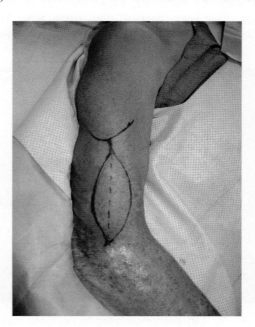

FIGURE 41-18.   Skin markings for lateral arm flap.

tuberosity region are commonly used for these purposes. Owing to chapter length constraints, the intraoral donor sites are not covered and the readers are encouraged to review other chapters within this text covering dental implants to obtain details of intraoral bone harvesting. This chapter focuses more on larger bone grafts for use in maxillofacial reconstruction.

Iliac Crest (Anterior and Posterior)

The iliac crest system has for a number of years been the most popular site for the harvesting of nonvascularized bone grafts for use in the maxillofacial region. Reconstruction of defects measuring less than 5 cm in size can be accomplished with a single anterior iliac crest, whereas greater defects warrant either bilateral harvest or harvesting of the posterior iliac crest. An established guideline is that the anterior iliac crest allows for the harvest of approximately 50 cc of uncompressed bone, and the posterior iliac crest allows for 100 cc of bone.

The overview of the anatomy is divided into the anterior iliac regional anatomy and the posterior iliac anatomy.

ANTERIOR CREST

The anterior ilium is located between the ASIS and the tubercle of the ilium. The inguinal ligament attaches to the ASIS laterally and to the pubic symphysis medially. Inferior to the attachment of the inguinal ligament is the sartorius muscle attachment; the muscle then travels in a diagonal fashion to insert along the medial aspect of the tibial head. Lateral to the sartorius is the origin of the tensor fascia latae muscle. This muscle attaches along the inferior aspect of the lateral crest for a few centimeters in a lateral direction. Directly lateral to the tensor fascia latae is the iliotibial tract. Behind the iliotibial tract is the gluteus medius muscle. The medial surface of the ilium is covered by the iliacus muscle.

The main blood vessel in this region is the deep circumflex iliac artery, which courses superficial to the iliacus muscle medially. Several sensory nerves traverse this area but only two are of significance; the lateral cutaneous branch of the iliohypogastric nerve (L1, L2), and the lateral cutaneous branch of the subcostal nerve (T12, L1).

POSTERIOR CREST

The muscles attached to the posterior aspect of the iliac crest are fewer than those attached to the anterior. The main muscles are the gluteus medius and maximus. The gluteus maximus has the more medial attachment. The sensory nerves in this region are the superior and middle cluneal nerves. The superior cluneal nerve (L1–3) pierces the lumbodorsal fascia superior to the posterior iliac crest and innervates the skin over the posterior buttocks. The middle cluneal nerves (S1–3) emerge from the sacral foramina and course laterally to innervate the medial buttocks. The sciatic nerve is the only motor nerve in this region and it runs deep to the gluteus maximus. It emerges between the piriformis muscle and the superior gemellus muscle on its inferior course to the lower limb.

The blood vessels in the region are the superior and inferior gluteal arteries. The terminal branches of the superior gluteal artery may be encountered because they may be found between the gluteus maximus and medius.

GRAFT HARVESTING

Anterior crest   The patient is placed in a supine position with a bump under the hip to be harvested. This maneuver elevates the iliac crest and facilitates the palpation as well as the harvest of the bone. Once the patient is prepared and draped, the skin marking is made. Care should be taken to place the incision in a location where it will not interfere with wearing pants or skirts. This is accomplished by rolling the skin in a cephalad/cranial manner before making the mark. The incision should be a couple of centimeters lateral to the ASIS and should follow the curvature of the ilium. The skin and subcutaneous fascia and Scarpa's fascia are incised and the periosteum overlying the crest is incised and reflected. The medial aspect of the iliac is addressed by reflecting the iliacus. The exposure is maintained by placing a Taylor retractor. The amount of bone needed is then marked with an oscillating saw, taking care to make the medial cut in an oblique fashion away from the ASIS. This oblique cut away from the ASIS prevents the undermining of the ASIS and fracture. Several approaches to the harvest as it relates to the crest have been reported. Irrespective of the approach used, if the cortical bone is to be harvested, the amount needed is outlined and harvested. The cancellous bone is harvested with the aid of large curettes until the desired quantity is obtained.

Posterior crest   Harvesting of the posterior iliac crest necessitates that the patient be placed in a prone position. Once in prone position and the airway secured, the hip ipsilateral to the donor site should be elevated using a bump made of folded linen or an intravenous bag. The patient is then prepared and draped. The hip is palpated and marked. An exact palpation is difficult in obese patients. In these cases, the palpation should begin at the inferior rib cage bilaterally and move caudally until the lateral projection of the iliac bone is felt. The midline is marked and the curvature of the posterior iliac is also marked. A linear incision is made closer to the medial aspect, and the dissection is continued through the subcutaneous fat until the fascia overlying the muscle is encountered. At this point, the periosteum is reflected and the bone is exposed. A self-retaining retractor is placed and the bone is harvested in a similar manner to that for the anterior iliac crest.

The closure of the site for either anterior or posterior harvesting is straightforward. The bleeding is often diminished when the cancellous bone is completely harvested at the site, causing the marrow bleed to stop. Use of hemostatic agents such as microfibrillar collagen is often done in order to maintain hemostasis. Some surgeons advocate the use of resorbable mesh to re-create the contour of the crest in cases in which this was harvested. A drain is placed and the closure is continued by reapproximating the fascia and dermis followed by skin. The posterior closure is done in a similar fashion (Figure 41-20).

SECTION 5

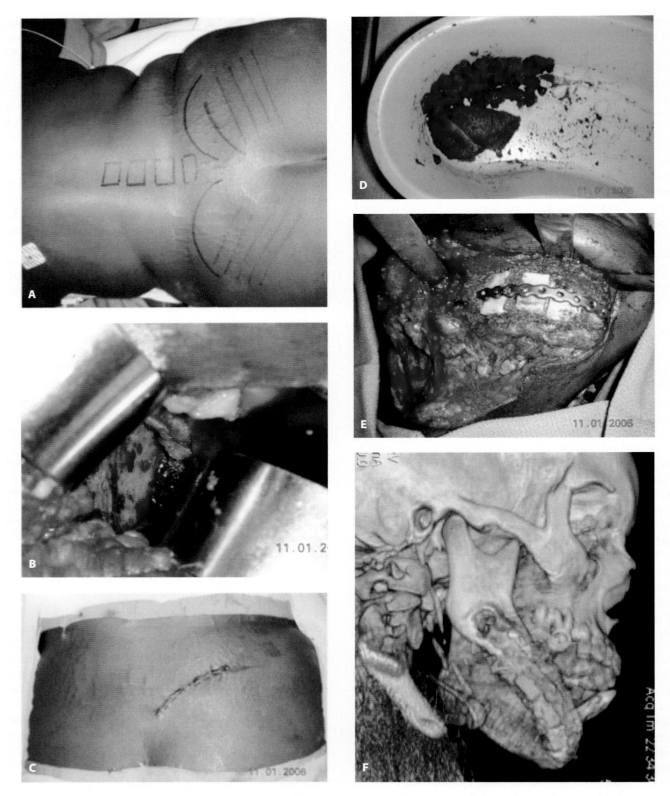

FIGURE 41-20. **A,** Patient positioned in a prone fashion with markings made depicting the posterior iliac crest. **B,** Exposure of the posterior iliac crest bone with placement of a deep retractor. **C,** Closure of the donor site. **D,** Harvested bone consisting of both cortical and cancellous bone. **E,** Insetting of the harvested bone to re-create the mandibular contour. **F,** Postoperative computed tomography (CT) scan depicts the newly reconstructed mandible.

The anterior iliac crest has specific advantages and disadvantages that are not shared by the posterior iliac crest. Its main advantages are the ease of harvest and ability to have a two-team approach. The main drawback for the anterior iliac is the limited quantity of available bone. The possibility for gait disturbances exists if too much reflection of the tensor fascia lata is performed. This scenario results in pain on ambulation and possible delays in rehabilitation.

The posterior iliac crest has a distinct advantage of greater quantity of available bone to be harvested. The amount of bone on each side is around 100 cc, thus allowing for reconstruction of large defects. The main disadvantage of the posterior harvest is the need for repositioning of the patient. This fact increases the operative time while making it impossible to have a two-team approach. Another potentially serious problem associated with the posterior iliac crest is the possible displacement of the endotracheal tube when the patient is moved. This can lead to a disastrous outcome.

Tibial Bone Graft

The tibial bone graft was initially described for use in maxillofacial reconstruction by Catone and associates.[34] Since that description, it has become very popular and is routinely performed in the office setting under intravenous sedations.

The tibia is the main bone of the lower leg. It provides support for weight bearing, and it is medial to the fibula. The superior aspect of the bone has the tuberosity, which serves as the point of insertion for the quadriceps femoris; it is medial to the sartorius, gracilis, and semitendinosus muscles. Lateral to the tuberosity is the origin of the tibialis anterior muscle. The patellar ligament inserts superiorly. Anteriorly and laterally, the proximal tibia exists an oval protuberance called Gerdy's tubercle. This is the main target for the bone graft.

The main blood supply to the region is the inferior medial genicular artery and the inferior lateral genicular artery. Both of the genicular arteries are branches of the popliteal artery. The saphenous nerve is the only sensory nerve in the region.

Graft Harvesting

The patient's knees should be elevated with a bump so as to cause a moderate degree of flexion. The area is then prepared and draped. Local anesthesia is infiltrated along the palpated Gerdy's tubercle in an oblique line of approximately 3 cm. The skin is incised down to the subcutaneous fascia; the periosteum is then incised and reflected. A bone window is marked with a surgical drill and a fine bur. The cortical bone is removed, thus gaining access to the marrow space. Using a curette, the bone is harvested. Usually the amount of bone that can be harvested is around 20 to 40 cc. Once the harvest is completed, a hemostatic agent may be placed in the area, if so desired, followed by approximation and closure of the periosteum. The remaining closure is as usual.

Minimal complications exist with the harvesting of the tibial bone. A fairly common sequelae is the formation of ecchymosis along the lower leg extending to the ankle. Given that this is almost an expected sequelae, the patient should be informed of it before the surgery.

Cranial Bone Graft

Cranial bone grafts have long been used in maxillofacial reconstruction. Their use has been largely associated with the reconstruction of craniofacial defects. More recently, they have been used for mandibular and maxillary alveolar ridge augmentation in cases of severe atrophy. One of the major advantages of the cranial bone is its ability to withstand intraoral exposure and resist resorption.

The cranial vault is made up of several bones, each with a contralateral match. The bones that make up the skull are the frontal, parietal, temporal, sphenoid, and occipital. The sagittal sinus is directly inferior to the midline of the skull along the vertex. This area is to be avoided during cranial bone harvesting. The parietal bone has the greatest thickness and also the best location for ease of harvest.

Graft Harvesting

The cranial bone graft may be harvested in one of three ways: particulate, split thickness, or full thickness. The most commonly harvest method is the split thickness and, therefore, the one covered in this chapter.

The parietal bone is the most commonly harvested cranial bone. The approach is made either via a hemicoronal, a coronal, or a horizontal incision over the area to be harvested. Once the incision is made, it is extended to the pericranium. The scalp is retracted and the area to be harvested is marked with a thin bur, usually multiple strips are marked out. Following this, a round bur is used to feather the bone outside of the markings in order to create a bevel and facilitate the saw cut. Using a thin reciprocating saw, the strips are harvested, taking care not to break them.

The closure of the donor site is begun by first establishing hemostasis. The bone bleed can be controlled with the aid of bone wax and the soft tissue bleeds may be cauterized, taking care not to damage the hair follicles. A suction drain is placed and the incision is closed in a layered fashion. The scalp may be closed with staples or sutures (Figure 41-21).

The most commonly encountered complication is the formation of a hematoma. A hematoma is more often seen in cases in which a drain is not placed. The more feared complication of a cranial bone graft is an inadvertent cranial penetration with or without dural tear. This complication is rare if care is taken to harvest small strips and bevel the bone so as to have a less acute angle of harvest. A rare but dreaded complication is a subdural bleed. Given this, the patient should be monitored for altered mental status for several hours after cranial bone harvest.

Vascularized Flaps

Osteocutaneous Radial Forearm Flap

The radial forearm flap has enjoyed tremendous popularity since its initial description. The vast majority of radial forearm flaps (RFFFs) used in head and neck reconstruction are soft tissue–only flaps. The use of these flaps as bone-containing flaps was first described by Soutar and coworkers.[35] The use of the RFFF as an osteocutaneous flap is

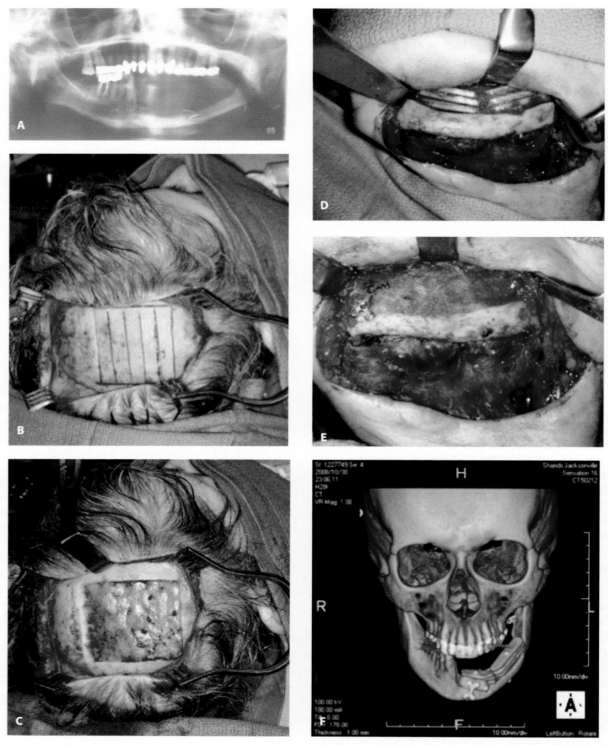

FIGURE 41-21.   **A,** Panoramic radiograph of a mandible after a left marginal mandibulectomy was performed secondary to a squamous cell carcinoma. **B,** Harvesting of the cranial bone with markings of the planned strips. **C,** Use of bone wax to improve hemostasis after split calvaria bone harvest. **D,** Insetting of the harvested cranial bone in a stacked fashion. **E,** The cranial bone stack is secured to the native mandible using titanium plates and screws. **F,** Postoperative CT depicts the reconstructed left hemimandible using the harvested cranial bone. (**B–F,** Courtesy of Dr. Luis Vega.)

surpassed by other bone flaps such as the fibula and the deep circumflex femoral artery (DCIA) flap. The reason for the poor performance of the osteocutaneous RFFF in head and neck reconstruction has been twofold: (1) its poor bone quantity and (2) its potential for significant donor site morbidity.

The anatomy of the RFFF has been covered earlier in this chapter. The surgical anatomy of the bone-containing RFFF is related to the bone perforators from the radial artery. The nutrition to the bone is by the periosteal and direct bone perforating the flexor pollicis longus muscle.

FLAP HARVESTING

The harvest begins under tourniquet control distally and proceeds in a proximal fashion. An incision is made at the most distal point of the flap and is carried to the subcutaneous fascia, directly overlying the muscles and the tendons. The tendons of the flexor carpi radialis, the brachioradialis, and the palmaris longus are identified. A subfascial plane is dissected while maintaining the paratenon over the tendons. The radial artery and the accompanying venae commitantes are identified and isolated using an angled clamp. Two 2-0 silk sutures are passed under the vessels. The vessels are then ligated and divided. Dissection continues on the radial side and the cephalic vein is identified, ligated, and divided. The cephalic vein is commonly harvested by the author in order to increase the venous drainage to the flap. Continued subfascial dissection is carried out toward the radial pedicle while taking care to identify and preserve the sensory branches of the radial nerve. At this point, attention is turned to the ulnar aspect. The skin paddle on the ulnar side is incised to the fascia and a subfascial elevation of the flap is similarly carried out toward the radial vascular pedicle.

At this point, the proximal portion of the flap is incised and a subcutaneous flap is elevated toward the antecubital fossa. The cephalic vein is further dissected until the desired length is exposed. An Allis clamp is used to retract the flexor carpi radialis muscle and dissection of the vascular bundle is carried out between the flexor carpi radialis and the brachioradialis. Dissection in this region is performed in a very meticulous fashion, taking care to preserve the perforators to the muscle and the radius. A cuff of the muscle is then incised so as to maintain the perforators to the bone. Using a periosteal elevator, the bone is exposed from both sides. A measurement of the desired bone length is marked. Using the oscillating saw, the bone is cut from the opposite side of the pedicle and in a curved fashion so as to avoid a sharp angle and, therefore, stress risers. Once the bone cut is performed, the desired length of pedicle is dissected, the tourniquet is deflated, and the flap is allowed to reperfuse. The residual radius bone can be plated using the dynamic compression plate over the harvested bone site. Prophylactic plating diminishes the incidence of radius bone fracture. The arm is closed by reapproximating the proximal flap and closing it over a suction drain. The proximal donor site defect is repaired with a full-thickness skin graft. A volar splint is placed with the wrist in a 45-degree extension. The splint is left in place for at least 2 weeks.

This flap has rapidly lost popularity and has been superseded by superior bone flaps owing to its limited bone stock and significant incidence of postoperative radius fracture. Early reports showed an incidence of fracture as high as 28% to 43%,[36–39] whereas larger series reported incidences of 23%[40] and 31%.[41] Refinements in osteotomy technique and prophylactic internal fixation have reduced this functionally disabling complication to 15%.[42] Serious frequent sequelae of pathologic radius fracture include wrist deformity and reduced wrist and grip strength from impaired flexor pollicis longus function. Postoperative radius fracture can be minimized by strictly adhering to bony dimensions not exceeding 30% of its cross-sectional area and 40% of its circumference.[43] Additional radius protection can be offered by external support with an above elbow cast or by splint to ensure 6 to 8 weeks of immobilization. However, fracture rates remain as high as 19%.[44] Prophylactic internal fixation with dynamic compression plate (DCP) is the most effective method of increasing both the torsional and the bending strength of the osteotomized radius, supported by several large clinical series.[45–48]

Osteocutaneous Fibula Flap

Hidalgo in 1989[49] performed the first case of mandibular reconstruction with the fibula using multiple defined osteotomies to reproduce the shape of almost an entire mandible. Since then, the fibula free flap has enjoyed much popularity in mandibular reconstruction and has continued to undergo technical developments.

The fibula is a long, thin, non–weight-bearing bone of the lower extremity. It has a tubular shape with a thick circumference of cortical bone providing it with significant inherent strength. Approximately 22 to 25 cm of bone may be harvested, while preserving 6 to 7 cm of bone proximally and distally to maintain integrity and functional stability of both the knee and the ankle joints, respectively. Proximally, the common peroneal nerve is encountered as it wraps around the neck of the fibula.

The fibula can be harvested as a free osseous or free osteoseptocutaneous flap. The inclusion of an overlying skin paddle is possible because septocutaneous or musculocutaneous perforators from the peroneal artery and vein provide a viable blood supply to this area of skin.

The peroneal artery and vein compose the dominant blood supply and vascular pedicle to the fibula osteocutaneous flap. Classically, the popliteal artery divides into the anterior and posterior tibial arteries below the knee, with the latter vessel subsequently giving rise to the peroneal artery. The peroneal artery and its paired venae commitantes descend in the lower leg between the flexor hallucis longus and the tibialis posterior muscles as they course toward the foot.

The peroneal artery via a nutrient medullary artery provides a rich endosteal vascular supply to the fibula along with multiple periosteal feeding vessels. The vascular supply to the skin over the fibula arises from numerous fasciocutaneous perforators running in the posterior crural septum.

Their position and course may be highly variable. The amount of skin that can be harvested is usually limited by the ability to primarily close the defect, although skin grafting the donor site defect is also frequently performed successfully.

The sensory supply to the skin over the lateral calf is derived from the lateral sural cutaneous nerve, a branch of the common peroneal nerve, arising within or above the popliteal fossa. When harvested as part of the osteocutaneous fibula flap, it can provide variable sensation to the accompanying skin paddle.

The goal of preoperative arteriography with respect to the free fibula flap is to identify patients in whom the harvest of this flap would result in either a nonviable flap or a compromised extremity.

Noninvasive clinical assessment begins with a thorough patient history and general physical examination. Claudication with walking should alert the clinician of underlying arteriocclusive disease. A more detailed examination of the perfusion status of the lower leg and foot is performed looking for signs of limb deformity, previous surgery, or trauma. Stigmata of peripheral arterial and/or venous vascular disease include skin pallor or cyanosis, ulceration, cool skin temperature, sparse hair growth, and thickened nail beds. Palpation of popliteal, posterior tibial, and dorsalis pedis pulses is mandatory. Questionable or absent pulses should be investigated further with Doppler flow assessment.

Conventional angiography, computed tomography (CT) angiography, or magnetic resonance angiography (MRA), although more invasive, provides superior anatomic detail and functional assessment of limb perfusion adequacy and quality of the donor vessels (Figure 41-22).

FLAP HARVESTING

The fibula free flap can be harvested as an osseous or osteocutaneous flap. The latter is described first because the former does not require preservation of cutaneous perforator vessels.

The patient is positioned supine on the operating table with the hip and knee slightly flexed and internally rotated and maintained in that position. The entire lower extremity is prepared and draped in the standard fashion with circumferential exposure up to the groin. The sole of the foot is supported with a sandbag or a 1-L saline bag. Pertinent landmarks such as the head of the fibula, lateral malleolus, and peroneal nerve are outlined on the skin. A vertical mark joining the proximal and distal fibula represents the intermuscular septum. The necessary skin island is outlined over the junction of the middle and lower thirds of the fibula to capture the largest possible caliber septocutaneous perforators. A Doppler will frequently and reliably aid in identifying these perforators, ensuring the skin island is centered over them. A sterile tourniquet is applied, the lower extremity is exsanguinated, and the tourniquet inflated to 350 mmHg.

The incision begins at the anterior margin of the skin island and extends proximally and distally to within 6 cm of the fibula head and lateral malleolus, respectively, to a level below the superficial fascia. Subfascial dissection in the lateral compartment proceeds toward the intermuscular septum where attention focuses on identifying and ensuring incorporation of the relevant perforators. Exposure and anterior retraction of the peroneus longus and brevis muscles allows their dissection off the fibula directed toward the anterior crural septum. Incision through the anterior crural septum

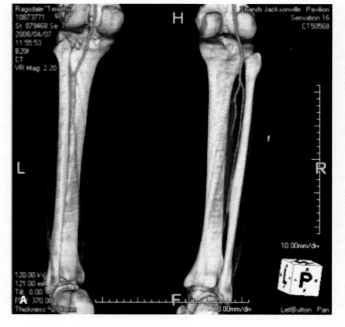
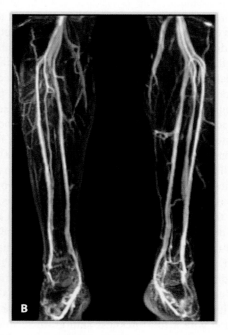

FIGURE 41-22. **A,** CT angiogram used to evaluate the lower extremity vasculature. **B,** Magnetic resonance angiography (MRA) used to evaluate the lower extremity vasculature.

provides entry into the anterior compartment, exposing the anterior tibial vessels and deep peroneal nerve beneath, which are preserved and gently retracted anteriorly. The interosseous membrane is exposed and incised to reveal the tibialis posterior muscle and its typical chevron-appearing fibers. Further dissection through this muscle will reveal the peroneal vessels lying beneath running close to the medial aspect of the fibula. Attention now focuses on proximal and distal exposure of the fibula with subperiosteal dissection 6 cm below the fibula head and 8 cm proximal to the lateral malleolus. With the aid of curved periosteal elevators protecting the peroneal vessels immediately deep to the fibula, appropriate osteotomies can be made with the oscillating saw removing a 1-cm segment of fibula. The pedicle can now be ligated and divided distally, and the fibula is now able to be rotated laterally enabling easier and safer dissection of the pedicle in a distal to proximal fashion. Upon reaching the tibioperoneal trunk, the peroneal artery and venae commitantes are isolated. The posterior incision of the skin island can now be performed down to the soleus muscle where it is optional to include a small cuff of soleus and flexor hallucis longus in cases in which musculocutaneous perforators are encountered. With the composite flap now isolated on its pedicle, the tourniquet is deflated and hemostasis of the donor bed is achieved (Figure 41-23).

In instances in which a bone-only flap is required, one need only make a linear skin incision without inclusion of a skin island. When dissection is directed toward the intermuscular septum, the remainder of the flap harvest technique proceeds as described previously (Figure 41-24).

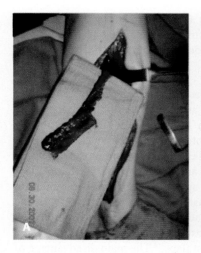
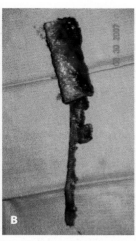

FIGURE 41-24.   **A,** Harvesting of a bone-only fibula flap, flap in situ with dissected vascular pedicle. **B,** Harvested bone-only fibula flap. Note the length of the vascular pedicle.

Donor site closure is performed with loose approximation of muscles, with the flexor hallucis longus sutured to the tibialis posterior to optimize postoperative great toe flexion. A suction drain is placed and secured. A split-thickness skin graft harvested from the thigh is sutured to the skin paddle donor defect, followed by application of a bolster and posterior splint. While the patient is nonambulatory, leg elevation is advised to minimize dependent edema. The cast and bolster are removed after 7 days, at which time ambulation may commence.

Following division of the pedicle, the flap is transferred to the prepared recipient site. Preparation of the fibula at this stage is dependent upon the site of the mandibular defect. For reconstruction of straight segments, fibula preparation is minimal, often with no osteotomies required. For defects in which osteotomies are required to reproduce mandibular contour, one or more osteotomies may be necessary. The osteotomized fibula is then fixed to a preadapted reconstruction plate using fixation screws and subsequently fixed in situ to the native mandibular defect.

Acquired vascular insufficiency of the lower extremities is frequently associated with atherosclerosis particularly in elderly patients. Preoperative imaging with CT angiography, MRA, or routine angiography can avoid limb-threatening ischemia. Compartment syndrome from wound closure under excessive tension can produce disastrous ischemic complications.

Almost all patients develop limited flexion capability of the hallux consistent with inclusion of the flexor hallucis longus muscle with the flap.

The common peroneal nerve is the nerve at risk during fibula flap harvest. It has both sensory and motor functions, with sensory disturbance reported in up to 24% of cases in either the superficial or the deep peroneal nerve distribution.[50] Motor disturbances lead to weakness in dorsiflexion in about 7% of cases resulting from damage to peroneal nerve branches and associated equinovarus deformity.[51] Common

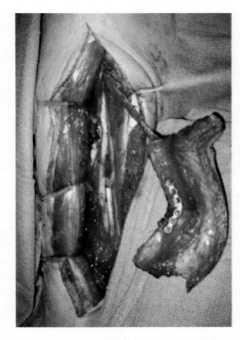

FIGURE 41-23.   Harvesting of an osteocutaneous fibula flap. The proximal cuts were already done and plated, re-creating the mandible to be reconstructed. Note the skin paddle and the dissected vascular pedicle.

peroneal nerve damage is avoided by limiting proximal dissection to greater than 6 cm from the fibula head and avoidance of overzealous traction during proximal dissection.

Scapula Free Flap

The scapula free flap was first transferred by Gilbert in 1979.[52] This was after the anatomic description by Saijo.[53]

The scapula free flap has proved to be an extremely valuable reconstructive option in head and neck surgery. Its ability to carry multiple skin flaps, latissimus dorsi muscle, serratus anterior muscle, and scapula bone, all based on a single pedicle, makes this system of flaps uniquely suited for the complex three-dimensional sculpting necessary in the head and neck. A distinct advantage in the elderly population is the unimpeded early postoperative ambulation not shared by the fibula and iliac crest flaps.[54] The main disadvantage of this flap is the need to reposition the patient in order to harvest the flap, preventing a two-team approach.

The scapula is a triangular bone. A number of muscles attach and originate from the scapula. The triceps brachii muscle, teres minor, and teres major originate along the lateral aspect of the scapula from a superior to inferior direction. The medial aspect of the bone is the location of the insertion of the rhomboid major, rhomboid minor, and levator scapula in an inferosuperior direction. The infraspinatus occupies the regions inferior to the spine of the scapula and the supraspinatus is in the superior portion. The deltoid muscle originates along the inferior aspect of the spine of the scapula and the superior region is the location for the insertion of the trapezius muscle.

The blood supply to the region begins with the subscapular artery, a branch of the axillary artery. The circumflex scapular artery originates from the subscapular artery and divides into the superficial skin branches: a transverse and a descending branch and a deep periosteal branch. The deep periosteal branch travels along the lateral border of the scapula, giving perforators to the periosteum and bone.

Flap Harvesting

The harvesting of the scapula flap is done by placing the patient in a lateral decubitus position with the arm fully prepped.

In cases in which a scapular skin paddle is to be included in the harvest, the area is marked, taking advantage of the transverse cutaneous branch from the circumflex scapular artery, or a dual skin flap may be designed, taking advantage of the descending cutaneous branch in addition to the transverse.

The incision is begun medially and progresses laterally toward the lateral border of the scapula. The skin flap is raised in a suprafascial plane, taking care to identify and not injure the transverse branch. Once the lateral border of the scapula is approached, the dissection is directed in the triangular space to identify the deep branch of the circumflex scapular artery. The bone feeders are identified and preserved. The teres minor and major muscles are disinserted from the bone, taking care not to injure the periosteal feeders.

The latissimus muscle is reflected from the inferior border of the scapula and the subscapularis muscle is freed. The area of bone to be harvested is marked out and the infraspinatus is reflected to expose the bone. A malleable retractor is placed under the scapula to protect the thoracic cavity and the bone cut is then made. Care should be taken superiorly to make sure that this cut does not encroach on the joint nor compromise the vascular pedicle to the bone or skin paddle. With the bone cut completed, the subscapularis muscle is then divided. The pedicle is then dissected toward the circumflex scapular artery and vein and the flap is mobilized and harvested (Figure 41-25).

The closure of the scapula demands special attention in order to prevent winging of the scapula. Several bone holes are placed along the lateral aspect of the scapula, and the teres muscles are then approximated to the scapula. The skin is mobilized and suction drains are placed followed by closure in a layered fashion.

Shoulder weakness results from division of the rotator cuff muscles teres major and minor, from the lateral border of the scapula during flap harvest. Restricted arm elevation, extension, and adduction are the most common impaired shoulder movements.[55] The most significant and feared complication associated with the scapula flap harvest is compromise of the joint space during the osteotomy. Another potential complication is the winging of the scapula, which can result from poor attention to closure with lack of approximation of the teres muscles to the bone using drilled holes or from injury to the long thoracic nerve. Intense postoperative physical therapy has also been shown to maximize shoulder mobility with return to premorbid function by 6 months after surgery.[56,57]

Iliac Crest Free Flap

The iliac crest free flap arguably provides the greatest quantity of bone stock for head and neck reconstruction. Its site distant from the ablative head and neck team permits synchronous harvest, and its inherent shape is well suited for reconstruction of the facial bones.[58] This flap is often avoided owing to an apparent technically demanding flap harvest, relatively short vascular pedicle, and small-caliber vessels. Others, however, have shown excellent outcomes with this flap.[59]

Taylor and colleagues[60] and Sanders and Mayou[61] in 1979 separately identified and reported the DCIA and DCIV as the most reliable and favorable pedicle for free transfer of the ilium. Taylor and associates[62] further elucidated the endosteal and periosteal blood supply of the ilium through dye injection studies. Experimental work by Ramasastry and coworkers in 1984[63] identified the ascending branch of the DCIA as the primary blood supply to the internal oblique muscle allowing for composite flap transfer.

The iliac crest possesses a natural curvature that makes it ideal for reconstruction of mandibular defects. The height of bone that can be harvested from this site allows for the restoration of the height of a native dentate mandible.

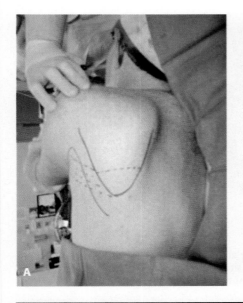
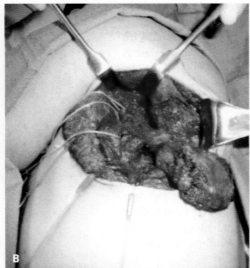
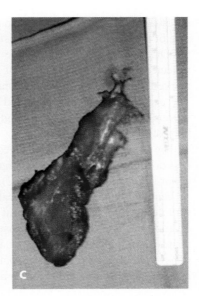
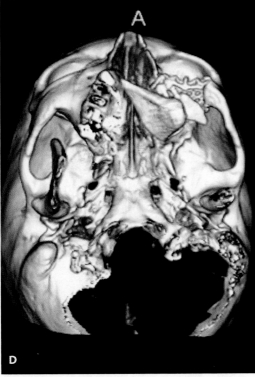
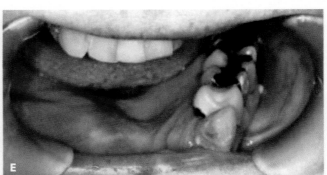

FIGURE 41-25.   **A,** patient positioned for flap harvest, note the skin markings. *B,* Harvested angle of scapula flap with dissected vascular pedicle. **C,** Harvested flap. Note the length of the vascular pedicle. **D,** Postoperative CT scan shows the position of the scapula used to reconstruct the maxillectomy defect. **E,** Intraoperative healing. After the scapula flap, the muscle mucosalizes to resemble normal oral mucosa.

The anatomy of this region has been described previously in this chapter. Additional to the bony and muscular anatomy, the vascular pedicle to the flap is the deep circumflex iliac artery and vein. The lateral femoral cutaneous nerve crosses over the artery medially as it approaches its take-off from the external iliac vessels.

FLAP HARVEST
The patient is placed in a supine position with a bump under the hip to be harvested. The incision for the harvest of the DCIA flap is begun just lateral and above the palpable femoral pulse. The incision in then continued in a curved fashion, following the contour of the iliac bone in a posterosuperior direction.

After the incision of the skin and subcutaneous fat, the external oblique muscle is incised allowing for the visualization of the internal oblique muscle. This muscle is readily identified owing to the direction of the muscle fibers, which run in an opposite direction from the external oblique muscle. The internal oblique is incised 2 cm cephalad and along the crest. Once the oblique muscles are transected, the iliacus is visualized. The DCIA may be palpated at this time. Incision of the iliacus is done a safe distant inferior to the path of the DCIA. The muscles along the lateral/gluteal aspect are reflected. The planned amount of bone to be harvested is marked. The bone cuts are made while protecting the pedicle. The pedicle dissection is extended toward the external iliac vessels. Once adequate vessel length is dissected, the flap is harvested (Figure 41-26).

The bone harvest can be achieved in two forms, full thickness or split thickness. The advantage of the latter is decreased donor site deformity (Figure 41-27).

Ventral hernias result from weakening of the abdominal wall through harvest of the internal oblique muscle and denervation of the rectus muscle whose motor nerves run in the neurovascular plane between the internal oblique and the transversus abdominis.[64] Mesh repair to reinforce the abdominal wall can eliminate this phenomenon.

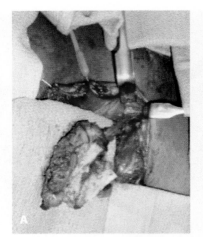
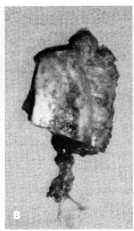

FIGURE 41-26. **A,** Harvesting of a deep circumflex femoral artery (DCIA) flap in situ with vascular pedicle still connected. **B,** Harvested DCIA; note the short pedicle length.

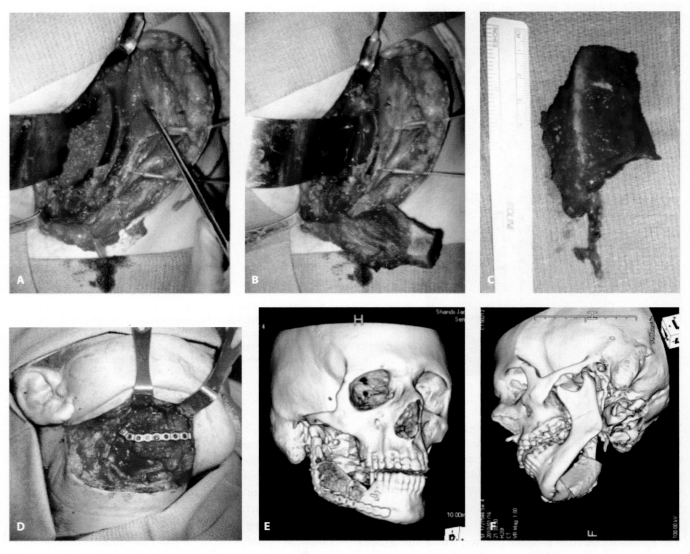

FIGURE 41-27. **A,** Markings for a harvesting of a split DCIA flap. **B,** Donor site defect after harvesting of a split DCIA flap. Note the preservation of the contour of the iliac crest. **C,** Harvested flap. **D,** Inset of the split DCIA flap. **E,** CT scan of the flap in place. **F,** CT scan depicting the lingual view of the reconstructed mandible. Note the amount of bone in terms of not only height but also width.

Immediate postoperative and short-term effects on ambulation are common following iliac crest free flaps, with antalgic gait and weakness of the operated hip being usual sequelae. Reports in the literature have demonstrated through controlled orthopedic objective testing that ambulation resolves by 6 months postoperatively.[65,66]

References

1. Mathes SJ, Nahai F. Classification of the vascular anatomy of muscles: experimental and clinical correlation. Plast Reconstr Surg 1981;67:177–187.

2. Taylor G, Palmer J. The vascular territories (angiosomes) of the body: experimental study and clinical applications. Br J Plast Surg 1987;40:113–141.

3. Brown, JS, Magennis P, Rogers SN, et al. Trends in head and neck microvascular reconstructive surgery in Liverpool (1992–2001). Br J Oral Maxillofac Surg 2006;44:364–370.

4. Martin D, Pascal J, Baudet J, et al. The submental island flap: a new donor site. Anatomy and clinical applications as a free or pedicled flap. Plast Reconstr Surg 1993;92:867–873.

5. Abouchadi A, Capon-Degardin N, Patenotre P, et al. The submental flap in facial reconstruction: advantages and limitations. J Oral Maxillofac Surg 2007;65:863–869.

6. Tan O, Atik B, Parmaksizoglu D. Soft tissue augmentation of the middle and lower face using the deepithelialized submental flap. Plast Reconstr Surg 2007;119:873–879.

7. Multinu A, Ferrari S, Bianchi B, et al. The submental island flap in head and neck reconstruction. Int J Oral Maxillofac Surg 2007;36:716–720.

8. Merten S, Jiang R, Caminer D. The submental artery island flap for head and neck reconstruction. Aust N Z J Surg 2002; 72:121–124.

9. Steme G, Januszkiewicz J, Hall P, Bardsley A. The submental island flap. Br J Plast Surg 1996;49:85–89.

10. Sebastian P, Thomas S, Varghese B, et al. The submental island flap for reconstruction of intraoral defects in oral cancer patients. Oral Oncol 2008;44:1014–1018.

11. Parmar PS, Goldstein DP. The submental island flap in head and neck reconstruction. Curr Opin Otolaryngol Head Neck Surg 2009;17:263–266.

12. Golovine SS. Procede de cloture plastique de l'orbite après l'exenteration. J Fr Ophtalmol 1898;18:679.

13. Wong TY, Chung CH, Huang JS, Chen HA. The inverted temporalis muscle flap for intraoral reconstruction: its rationale and the results of its application. J Oral Maxillofac Surg 2004; 62:667–675.

14. Koranda FC, McMahon MF, Jernstrom VR. The temporalis muscle flap for intraoral reconstruction. Arch Otolaryngol Head Neck Surg 1987;113:740–743.

15. Ariyan S. The pectoralis major myocutaneous flap: A versatile flap for reconstruction in the head and neck. Plast Reconstr Surg 1979;63:73–81.

16. Moloy P, Gonzales F. Vascular anatomy of the pectoralis major myocutaneous flap. Arch Otolaryngol Head Neck Surg 1986;112:66–69.

17. Freeman JL, Walker EP, Wilson J, et al. The vascular anatomy of the pectoralis major myocutaneous flap. Br J Plast Surg 1981;34:3–10.

18. Reid CD, Taylor GI. The vascular territory of the acromiothoracic axis. Br J Plast Surg 1984;37:194–212.

19. Rikimaru H, Kiyokawa K, Inoue Y, et al. Three-dimensional anatomical vascular distribution in the pectoralis major myocutaneous flap. Plast Reconstr Surg 2005;115:1342–1352.

20. Tansini I. Spora il mio muovo processo di amputazione della mammaella per cancre. Riforma Med (Palermo, Napoli) 1896;12:3.

21. Quillen C, Shearin J, Georgiade N. Use of the latissimus dorsi myocutaneous island flap for reconstruction in the head and neck area. Plast Reconstr Surg 1978;62:113–117.

22. Brown MR, McCullough TM, Funk GF, et al. Resource utilization and patient morbidity in head and neck reconstruction. Laryngoscope 1997;107:1028–1031.

23. Huang RD, Silver SM, Hussain A, et al. Pectoralis major myocutaneous flap: analysis of complications in a VA population. Head Neck 1992;14:102–106.

24. Soutar DS, Scheker CR, Tanner NSB, et al. The radial forearm flap: a versatile method for intraoral reconstruction. Br J Plast Surg 1983;36:1–8.

25. Urken ML. Free flaps: fascial and fasciocutaneous flaps. Radial forearm. In Atlas of Regional and Free Flaps for Head and Neck Reconstruction. New York: Raven; 1995; pp. 149–168.

26. Song YG, Chen GZ, Song YL. The free thigh flap: a new free flap concept based on the septocutaneous artery. Br J Plast Surg 1984;37:149–159.

27. Kimata Y, Uchiyama K, Ebihara S, et al. Anatomic variations and technical problems of the anterolateral thigh flap: a report of 74 cases. Plast Reconstr Surg 1998;102:1517–1523.

28. Celik N, Wei FC, Lin CH, et al. Technique and strategy in anterolateral thigh perforator flap surgery, based on an analysis of 15 complete and partial failures in 439 cases. Plast Reconstr Surg 2002;109:2211–2216.

29. Wei FC, Jain V, Celik N, et al. Have we found an ideal soft-tissue flap? An experience with 672 anterolateral thigh flaps. Plast Reconstr Surg 2002;109:2219–2226.

30. Koshima I, Moriguchi T, Fukuda H, et al. Free thinned paraumbilical perforator-based flaps. J Reconstr Microsurg 1991;7: 313–316.

31. Boyd JB, Taylor GI, Corlett R. The vascular territories of the superior epigastric and the deep inferior epigastric systems. Plast Reconstr Surg 1984;73:1–14.

32. Song R, Song Y, Yu Y, Song Y. The upper arm free flap. Clin Plast Surg 1982;9:27–35.

33. Rivet D, Buffet M, Martin D, et al. The lateral arm flap: an anatomic study. J Reconstr Microsurg 1987;3:121–132.

34. Catone GA, Reimer BL, McNeir D, Ray R. Tibial autogenous cancellous bone as an alternative donor site in maxillofacial surgery: a preliminary report. J Oral Maxillofac Surg 1992;50:1258–1263.

35. Soutar DS, Scheker LR, Tanner NS, McGregor IA. The radial forearm flap: a versatile method for intra-oral reconstruction. Br J Plast Surg 1983;36:1–8.

36. Soutar DS, McGregor IA. The radial forearm flap in intraoral reconstruction: the experience of 60 consecutive cases. Plast Reconstr Surg 1986;78:1–8.

37. McGregor IA. Fasciocutaneous flaps in intraoral reconstruction. Clin Plast Surg 1985;12:453–461.

38. Timmons MJ, Missotten FE, Poole MD, et al. Complications of radial forearm flap donor sites. Br J Plast Surg 1986;39: 176–178.

39. Boorman JG, Brown JA, Sykes PJ. Morbidity in the forearm flap donor arm. Br J Plast Surg 1987;40:207–212.

40. Bardsley AF, Soutar DS, Elliot D, et al. Reducing morbidity in the radial forearm flap donor site. Plast Reconstr Surg 1990;86:287–294.

41. Vaughan ED. The radial forearm free flap in orofacial reconstruction. Personal experience in 120 consecutive cases. J Craniomaxillofac Surg 1990;18:2–7.

42. Thoma A, Khadaroo R, Grigenas O, et al. Oromandibular reconstruction with the radial-forearm osteocutaneous flap: experience with 60 consecutive cases. Plast Reconstr Surg1999;104: 368–380.

43. Collyer J, Goodger NM. The composite radial forearm free flap: an anatomical guide to harvesting the radius. Br J Oral Maxillofac Surg 2005;43:205–209.

44. Clark S, Greenwood M, Banks RJ, et al. Fracture of the radial donor site after composite free flap harvest: a ten-year review. Surgeon 2004;2:281–286.

45. Avery CM, Danford M, Johnson PA. Prophylactic internal fixation of the radial osteocutaneous donor site. Br J Oral Maxillofac Surg 2007;45:576–578.

46. Werle AH, Tsue TT, Toby EB, et al. Osteocutaneous radial forearm free flap: its use without significant donor site morbidity. Otolaryngol Head Neck Surg 2000;123:711–717.

47. Villaret DB, Futran NA. The indications and outcomes in the use of osteocutaneous radial forearm free flap. Head Neck 2003;25:475–481.

48. Kim JH, Rosenthal EL, Ellis T, et al. Radial forearm osteocutaneous free flap in maxillofacial and oromandibular reconstructions. Laryngoscope 2005;155:1697–1701.

49. Hidalgo DA. Fibula free flap: A new method of mandible reconstruction. Plast Reconstr Surg 1989;84:71–79.

50. Anthony JP, Rawnsley JD, Benhaim P, et al. Donor leg morbidity and function after fibula free flap mandible reconstruction. Plast Reconstr Surg 1995;96:146–152.

51. Goodacre TE, Walker CJ, Jawad AS, et al. Donor site morbidity following osteocutaneous free fibula transfer. Br J Plast Surg 1990;43:410–412.

52. Gilbert A. Free vascularized bone grafts. Int Surg 1979;66:27.

53. Saijo M. The vascular territories of the dorsal trunk: a reappraisal for potential donor sites. Br J Plast Surg 1978;31:200.

54. Hallock GG. Permutations of combined free flaps using the subscapular system. J Reconstr Microsurg 1997;13:47–54.

55. Swartz WM, Banis JC, Newton ED, et al. The osteocutaneous scapular flap for mandibular and maxillary reconstruction. Plast Reconstr Surg 1986;77:530.

56. Clark JR, Vesely M, Gilbert R. Scapular angle osteomyogenous flap in postmaxillectomy reconstruction: defect, reconstruction, shoulder function, and harvest technique. Head Neck 2008;30:10–20.

57. Nkenke E, Vairaktaris E, Stelzle F, et al. Osteocutaneous free flap including medial and lateral scapular crests: technical aspects, viability and donor site morbidity. J Reconstr Microsurg 2009;25:545–554.

58. Brown JS. Deep circumflex iliac artery free flap with internal oblique muscle as a new method of immediate reconstruction of maxillectomy defect. Head Neck 1996;18:412–421.

59. Urken ML, Vickery C, Weinberg H, et al. The internal oblique–iliac crest osseomyocutaneous free flap in oromandibular reconstruction: report of 20 cases. Arch Otolaryngol Head Neck Surg 1989;115:339.

60. Taylor GI, Townsend P, Corlett R. Superiority of the deep circumflex iliac vessels as the supply for free groin flaps: experimental work. Plast Reconstr Surg 1979;64:595–604.

61. Sanders R, Mayou B. A new vascularized bone graft transferred by microvascular anastomosis as a free flap. Br J Surg 1979;66:787.

62. Taylor GI, Townsend P, Corlett R. Superiority of the deep circumflex iliac vessels as the supply for free groin flaps: clinical work. Plast Reconstr Surg 1979;64:745.

63. Ramasastry SS, Tucker JB, Swartz WM, et al. The internal oblique muscle flap: an anatomic and clinical study. Plast Reconstr Surg 1984;73:721.

64. Urken ML, Weinberg H, Vickery C, et al. The internal oblique–iliac crest free flap in composite defects of the oral cavity involving bone, skin and mucosa. Laryngoscope 1991; 101:257.

65. Boyd JB, Rosen I, Rotstein L, et al. The iliac crest and the radial forearm flap in vascularized oromandibular reconstruction. Am J Surg 1990;159:301–308.

66. Rogers SN, Lakshmiah SR, Narayan B, et al. A comparison of the long-term morbidity following deep circumflex iliac and fibula free flaps for reconstruction following head and neck cancer. Plast Reconstr Surg 2003;112:1517–1525.

42

Microneurosurgery

Michael Miloro, DMD, MD, FACS

Injuries to the terminal branches of the trigeminal nerve may occur commonly after routine oral and maxillofacial surgical procedures, and the overwhelming majority of these injuries undergo spontaneous neurosensory recovery without intervention. Third molar surgery accounts for most of the injuries that occur to both the inferior alveolar nerve (IAN) and the lingual nerve (LN). The reported incidence of iatrogenic nerve injury varies in the literature, but both temporary and permanent rates of paresthesia must be considered. Potential for nerve injury involves mandibular and maxillary orthognathic surgery, maxillofacial trauma, dental implant placement, endodontic therapy, facial fractures, and treatment of benign and malignant head and neck pathologic lesions. The anatomy of the trigeminal nerve system is unique because it carries, in some branches, both general sensory information and special (e.g., taste) sensation. Injury to a nerve may result in neuroma formation, which can manifest with a wide spectrum of objective clinical signs and subjective patient symptoms. Nerve injuries are classified by two different classification schemes (Seddon and Sunderland, described later), which are based on the degree of axonal injury at the histologic light microscopic level but, more important, upon the likelihood that an injured nerve will recover spontaneously after injury. A basic understanding of nerve terminology (see Appendix) and normal neural wound healing anatomy and physiology is essential to most appropriately managed clinical situations.

The initial clinical evaluation of patients with nerve injuries should proceed in an structured and orderly fashion, with the performance of several levels of objective testing to most accurately determine the degree of individual nerve injury. A standardized clinical neurosensory test (CNT) may be used for most patients; however, some advanced testing is also available for special circumstances (e.g., gustatory testing). It should be remembered that there are many nonsurgical, including pharmacologic, treatments available for the patient who sustains a nerve injury, and for the majority of patients with dysesthesia or painful neuropathies, drug therapy is considered the mainstay of treatment and may involve other medical professionals, including a neurologist.

Once the decision is made that the patient is a surgical candidate to potentially improve sensation with microneurosurgery, an orderly sequence of surgical steps must be followed meticulously. Specific surgical techniques depend on which nerve is involved as well as the estimated extent of the injury. In general, microneurosurgical repair of a trigeminal nerve injury involves neurolysis (surgical manipulation of the nerve) and preparation of the nerve stumps to perform neurorrhaphy (nerve repair). The deleterious effects of tension on a nerve repair site have been well documented, so the inability to perform a primary, tension-free, repair warrants consideration for an autogenous nerve graft or another option for nerve gap management, such as entubulation (gap or conduit repair). Following microneurosurgery, postoperative sensory reeducation may play an important role in the neural regenerative process. The overall success rates of microneurosurgical repair of the trigeminal nerve vary considerably based upon individual surgeon reports and a lack of consensus regarding "success criteria." However, an important factor that affects the success of microneurosurgery is the length of time from injury to repair, because this affects the degree of trigeminal ganglion cell death, wallerian degeneration of the distal axon, and cortical somatosensory reorganization of the information from the target site (lower lip and chin or tongue). The American Association of Oral and Maxillofacial Surgeons Clinical Interest Group on Maxillofacial Neurologic Disorders has promulgated treatment time recommendations for the patient who sustains a trigeminal nerve injury, and these are based upon allowing sufficient time for spontaneous neurosensory recovery, while considering the impact of delayed treatment on final functional neurosensory outcome.[1]

The field of microneurosurgery is in its infancy considering the current rapid advances in technology and growth factor research, and as more surgeons become adept at the diagnosis and treatment of patients who sustain trigeminal nerve injuries, more clinical, laboratory, and radiologic information will become available to guide the therapeutic decision-making process. Also, postgraduate training programs in oral and maxillofacial surgery will become more capable of training surgical residents in the principles and practice of microneurosurgery, and this will hopefully foster access to this aspect of specialty care throughout the country and abroad.

DEMOGRAPHICS

Trigeminal nerve injuries result from a variety of routine oral and maxillofacial surgical procedures, such as third molar odontectomy, management of facial trauma, orthognathic surgery, endosseous dental implant placement, salivary duct and gland surgery, treatment of benign and malignant lesions of the head and neck, preprosthetic surgery, and endodontic and periradicular surgery. Complications of third molar removal are responsible for the majority of injuries to the terminal branches of the third division of the trigeminal nerve.[2] These can occur during any phase of third molar surgery, including local anesthetic injection, incision and flap design, the use of a high-speed drill for bone removal or tooth sectioning, elevation of the tooth with trauma to the lingual soft tissues, socket curettage with exposed neurovascular tissue, removal of remnants of an assumed "dental follicle" that may contain neural or vascular tissue, the use of medicaments in the extraction site to aid healing or prevent alveolar osteitis (e.g., tetracycline-containing compounds[3,4]), and the placement of sutures. The efficacy of LN retraction during lower third molar surgery has shown that, although the incidence of temporary LN paresthesia is increased owing to a slight stretching or manipulation (6.4% with retraction vs. 0.6% without retraction), the difference in long-term dysfunction is not significant (0.6% with retraction vs. 0.2% without retraction).[5] Other studies have indicated a temporary paresthesia rate of approximately 10% to 15% with LN retraction and protection, with a permanent paresthesia rate of less than 1%.

The incidence of trigeminal nerve injury may be estimated based on a review of the available literature. Overall, the incidence of IAN injury from third molar surgery is 0.41% to 7.5% and from sagittal split osteotomy is 0.025% to 84.6%, whereas the LN is affected 0.06% to 11.5% of the time after third molar removal. However, the more important clinical distinction is to differentiate temporary from permanent paresthesia rates. For sagittal split osteotomies, temporary IAN paresthesia may be as high as 80% to 100%, but permanent rates, which are age-dependent, are typically less than 1% to 5%. For third molar surgery, both IAN and LN temporary paresthesias range from 2% to 6%, whereas permanent rates are approximately one fourth of the temporary

rates, or 0.5% to 2% overall. Many risk factors for nerve injury during third molar surgery have been reported in addition to the vulnerable position of the IAN and LN and include advanced patient age, female gender, depth of impaction, mesiodistal angulation of the tooth (distoangular), lingual angulation of the tooth, lack of integrity of the lingual cortex, the need for tooth sectioning, removal of bone distal to the third molar, longstanding pericoronitis that may result in scarring of the soft tissue and LN compression postoperatively, and surgeon experience. It has been postulated that a right-handed surgeon standing on the right side of the patient during third molar removal would experience more injuries to the LN on the right side (associated with the mandibular right third molar) because visualization of the LN is partially obstructed, and more IAN injuries on the left side (associated with the mandibular left third molar) owing to visual obstruction of the buccal aspect of the left posterior mandible. Certainly, the risk of an IAN injury may be influenced by so-called Rood and Shehab[6] radiographic predictors of potential tooth proximity to the inferior alveolar canal, although these were described earlier by Howe and Poynton in 1960.[7] These seven radiographic predictors on panoramic radiograph may indicate the potential for increased risk of injury to the IAN, and they are listed in Table 42-1. Of the seven radiographic predictors, Rood and Shehab[6] noted that three of these were more significant: root darkening, root deflection, and interruption of the white line of the canal. It has been suggested that the lack of any radiographic finding would correlate with a minimal risk of IAN injury (<1%), whereas a finding of one or more predcitors would increase the risk of IAN injury up to 10%. With the current increased use of cone beam computed tomography (CT) scanning, the assessment of the proximity of the third molar to the IAN has improved significantly. In cases with a high index of suspicion of nerve injury (e.g., deep impaction, advanced age), intentional coronectomy with close observation should be considered.[8] As opposed to the relatively consistent course of the IAN, the LN position is variable; and it is injured less often than the IAN after third molar surgery.[9-13] The position of the LN has been documented clinically,[13] in cadaveric dissections,[15,16] and radiologically.[17] On average, in the third molar region, the LN lies 2.5 mm medial to the lingual plate of the mandible and 2.5 mm inferior to the lingual crest. The LN may be in direct contact with the lingual plate in 25% of

TABLE 42-1. **Rood's Radiographic Predictors of Potential Tooth Proximity to the Inferior Alveolar Canal**

1. Darkening of the root
2. Deflection of the root
3. Narrowing of the root
4. Dark and bifid root apex
5. Interruption of the white line of the canal
6. Diversion of the canal
7. Narrowing of the canal

Adapted from Rood JP, Shehab AAN. The radiological prediction of inferior alveolar nerve injury during third molar surgery. Br J Oral Maxillofac Surg 1990;28:20.

cases (Kisselbach and Chamberlain reported 62%[14]) and may lie above the lingual crest in 10% to 15% of cases (Kisselbach and Chamberlain reported 17.6%[14]) based on an undisturbed radiographic assessment of the nerve.

Mandibular blocks may result in IAN and LN injuries; however, the incidence is unknown owing to a significant number of unreported cases. An estimated 1 in 100,000 to 1 in 500,000 blocks result in paresthesia. Perhaps the largest study of its kind, Harn and Durham's study of 9587 mandibular blocks[18] showed a 3.62% incidence of temporary paresthesia and a 1.8% incidence of long-term paresthesia lasting longer than 1 year. Several theories have been proposed to explain the mechanism of injury. Direct neural trauma is unlikely owing to abundant interfascicular neural components resulting in separation of the fascicles by a needle or suture without direct neural disruption.[19] The resultant edema may be responsible for the transient paresthesia that resolves spontaneously. Local anesthetic toxicity may be responsible for prolonged paresthesia after a mandibular block, especially if the solution is deposited within the confines of the epineurium. Several reports indicate that prilocaine and articaine may be associated with an increased risk of long-term paresthesia, especially with mandibular block anesthesia, compared with other local anesthetic solutions owing to a concentration gradient effect, but further investigation is warranted.[20–22] The third potential mechanism of injury involves the formation of an epineurial hematoma. The epineurium and perineurium contain a vast plexus of vessels that nurture the neural elements, and a needle may cause disruption of one or more vessels. The localized bleeding most certainly tamponades itself owing to the surrounding epineurium, and the pressure may impinge on select groups of fascicles contained within the nerve. The resultant clinical signs and symptoms of localized paresthesia, not involving the entire distribution of the IAN/mental nerve, nicely match the expected histologic situation, making this theory plausible. Also, lymphatic drainage of the localized hematoma over the few days to weeks after surgery coincides with the clinical resolution of symptoms in most cases. The final theory is that of the needle-barb mechanism of injury.[23] During a mandibular block injection, the needle may be advanced to the medial ramus where a small barb may form at the needle tip. On withdrawal, if the needle has passed through or in the vicinity of the LN or IAN, fascicular disruption may occur with potentially longstanding clinical consequences. Recent trends in our clinical understanding of injection-related nerve injuries include the following:

1. Injection nerve injuries are difficult to predict and prevent.
2. The classic electric shock sensation upon injection is reported uncommonly by patients who sustain these injuries.
3. Injection injuries are more likely to result in dysesthesia than are other causes of nerve injuries.
4. There may be a nonanatomic distribution of nerve involvement (including the second and third divisions of the trigeminal nerve) due to progressive demyelination along the nerve.
5. Persistent symptoms after injection injuries occur more commonly in female patients.
6. The LN, which is stretched more upon mouth opening than is the IAN, is more commonly affected.
7. The majority of cases resolve within 8 weeks, and if paresthesia persists for longer than 8 weeks, then only one third of those injuries resolve spontaneously.

Microneurosurgery is a poor option for patients with injection-related nerve injuries not only because most of these patients have a component of dysesthesia but also because surgical access is extremely difficult; therefore, most cases are managed with pharmacologic therapy. One of the clinical dilemmas is to differentiate a mandibular block injury to the IAN from a third molar injury to the IAN. On rare occasions, the third molar site of the IAN has been explored after third molar removal and resultant lower lip and chin paresthesia and the IAN is found to be normal at the third molar site, with the assumption at that point that the injury occurred as a result of injection rather than extraction.[24] However, again, it is difficult to estimate the incidence of mandibular block injuries to the IAN and LN or to precisely define the etiology.

It is well known that orthognathic surgery may result in nerve injury. The IAN is affected more often than is the LN, and rarely, the facial nerve may be affected (0.67% with sagittal split osteotomy in one study[25]). Certainly, a great deal is known about the risks of IAN injury associated with sagittal split osteotomy as well as screw overpenetration injury or manipulation injury to the LN.[26,27] Unfortunately, the reported incidence of immediate and long-term neurosensory deficit varies considerably (from < 5% to > 90%) owing to poorly controlled factors inherent in the study designs or case reports, such as individual surgeon experience, technical variability in the surgery, lack of standardization of neurosensory testing, lack of control sites for normal cutaneous facial sensibility (in bilateral cases), and variation in the time periods when neurosensory testing is performed. Several studies have examined the specific parameters for neurosensory recovery after bilateral sagittal split osteotomy by using objective and subjective assessment criteria.[28] One study found a 39% incidence of neurosensory dysfunction after sagittal ramus surgery,[29] and others have shown less than 15% dysfunction at 6 months.[30] Although the incidence of nerve dysfunction varies, there are well-known risk factors for nerve injury,[31] including patient age[32]; increased length of the surgical procedure; proximal or distal segment fractures ("bad splits"); concomitant third molar removal; concomitant genioplasty procedures; compression during fixation (e.g., lag screw technique); inadvertent use of chisels in the osteotomy site; nerve entrapment in the proximal segment; nerve manipulation in the area of the osteotomy as well as the region of the lingula during the medial dissection (based on intraoperative recordings of IAN somatosensory evoked potentials)[33]; the location of the inferior alveolar canal close to the inferior border; low mandibular body corpus height

SECTION 5

and retrognathism in class II deformities (the IAN tends to be closer to buccal cortex and more vulnerable to injury)[34]; and frank nerve transection during surgery, especially with a large mandibular advancement. Unfortunately, long-term neurosensory dysfunction after orthognathic surgery is not generally amenable to microneurosurgical correction. However, most patients tolerate the paresthesia well after correction of a significant dentofacial deformity. Three caveats to remember regarding orthognathic surgery-related nerve injuries: (1) that the older the patient the more severe the potential paresthesia; (2) that patients tolerate "mild" paresthesia after "major" surgery well (with appropriate informed consent); and (3) that the magnitude of neurosensory dysfunction decreases as the time from injury increases.

Craniomaxillofacial trauma may result in injury to any of the terminal branches of the trigeminal nerve. Orbitozygomatic and zygomaticomaxillary complex fractures may involve the infraorbital canal and the second division of the trigeminal nerve. The small fibers of the infraorbital nerve as it exits the infraorbital foramen are less than ideal for surgical manipulation and repair. Mandible fractures that violate the IAN canal result in temporary or permanent paresthesia, depending upon the degree of fracture displacement. Treatment of mandible fractures with inadvertent placement of screws that traverse the inferior alveolar canal may cause iatrogenic transien or permanent paresthesia. In general, reduction and stabilization of the fracture segments aid in realigning the natural bony conduit (i.e., the IAN canal or the infraorbital canal) that will help to guide spontaneous neurosensory recovery, even in cases of partial or complete transection injuries.

Also, the presence and/or biopsy and treatment of head and neck pathologic lesions may result in nerve injury. The use of Carnoy's solution (ferric chloride 0.1 g/mL, absolute alcohol 6 mL, chloroform 3 mL, glacial acetic acid 1 mL) after treatment of pathology has been shown to have a critical exposure time in an animal model of 5 minutes, after which time there may be long-term irreversible neural injury.[35,36] After a resection procedure, consideration should be given to immediate or delayed neural reconstruction using autogenous or allogeneic nerve grafts or conduits.

Although preprosthetic surgery is performed less frequently today than in the past, procedures such as torus mandibularis reduction and maxillary or mandibular vestibuloplasty place the terminal branches of the mental nerve and infraorbital nerve at risk for injury. As mentioned, surgical repair of the small terminal nerve fibers of the infraorbital and mental nerves is difficult and often results in scarring of the nerve and adjacent soft tissues and a poor chance of neurosensory recovery. The maxilla and mandible are excellent sources of autogenous bone grafts; however, they are not performed without potential morbidity. The majority of patients who undergo genial bone graft harvest complain of desensitization of the mandibular anterior teeth, when present. Depending on the specific technique employed for posterior mandibular ramus bone graft harvesting, the IAN may be at risk of iatrogenic injury; the anatomic position of the IAN laterally within the ascending ramus contributes to its vulnerability. Mandibular endodontic therapy and periapical surgery may result in an injury to the IAN, depending on the proximity of the root apex to the canal. Some endodontic filling materials may be neurotoxic (paraformaldehyde-containing pastes [Sargenti paste, N2, AH26], or eugenol-containing cements [ZOE, PCS]); to prevent irreversible paresthesia that in many cases results in dysesthesia, consideration should be given to prompt exploration (12–24 hr) and débridement of medicaments that have permeated through the root apex and are in direct contact with the nerve. Distraction osteogenesis of the mandible has been shown to induce transient changes in neuronal conduction without significant long-term nerve dysfunction.[37,38] Because age is a factor in spontaneous neurosensory recovery after injury, a younger patient would certainly tolerate a "stretch-type" of injury to the nerve better than an adult. Some data indicate that with a true corticotomy (vs. osteotomy) and distraction rates of 1 mm/day, permanent neural changes are unlikely, but that distraction rates greater than this may be deleterious to nerve function. However, more studies are necessary.[39]

Finally, implant-related injuries to the IAN are common (30–40%) and difficult to manage appropriately; however, with current technqiues of advanced imaging and computer treatment planning with surgical implant guides, the incidence of iatrogenic nerve injury may be declining. Unfortunately, there is a lack of data regarding appropriate patient assessment and management, with a lack of consensus on treatment protocols. In the posterior mandible, the likely cause of nerve damage may be that the initial pilot (depth) drill penetrates the superior cortex of the canal and violates the IAN vein (or artery, which is less likely). This results in some bleeding that, on placement of the implant, will tamponade itself. However, the resultant increased pressure in the closed environment of the inferior alveolar canal creates a "compartment syndrome," with harmful effects on neurosensory function. This type of compression injury commonly results in long-term unpleasant altered sensation (dysesthesia) rather than simple decreased sensation (hypoesthesia). The recognition postoperatively that the patient has paresthesia and that the implant is within the confines of the canal warrants the clinician to consider removal of the implant, with or without immediate replacement with a shorter implant. If, however, the injury was due to a compartment syndrome effect, implant removal without replacement may be the more prudent option. For patients with persistent paresthesia, referral to a microneurosurgeon or neurologist may be warranted for consideration for pharmacotherapy. The procedure of IAN repositioning (lateralization and transpositioning) is an option that theoretically would induce a "controlled" injury to the nerve and protect it during implant preparation. With lateral decortication of the mandible and nerve exposure, a compartment syndrome would not be possible. Despite the potential advantages of nerve repositioning, there is a high incidence of long-term paresthesia ranging from 0% to 77%, with a mean of approximately 30% to 40%.[39] With appropriate surgeon experience, proper patient selection, the presence of a strong indication for the procedure (e.g., lack of interocclusal clearance in the posterior mandible), and an adequate and informed consent discussion, this procedure remains an option for posterior mandibular implant reconstruction.

TRIGEMINAL NERVE ANATOMY AND PHYSIOLOGY

A review of trigeminal nerve anatomy and physiology is necessary in order to understand clinical patient presentation and diagnosis and management. The trigeminal nerve (Figure 42-1) is composed of a mesoneurium that suspends the nerve within the surrounding tissues and is continuous with the outer epineurium that defines and surrounds the nerve trunk. This epineurium contains a vast plexus of blood vessels called the *vasa nervorum* as well as lymphatic channels. The epineurium is divided into both outer and inner components; the inner layer is composed of a loose connective tissue sheath with longitudinal collagen bundles that protect against compressive and stretching forces imposed on the nerve. Individual fascicles are defined by the perineurium, which is a continuation of the pia-arachnoid layer of the central nervous system. This perineurium functions to provide structural support and act as a diffusion barrier, similar to the blood-brain barrier that prevents the transport of certain molecules. The individual nerve fibers and Schwann cells are surrounded by the endoneurium, which is composed of collagen, fibroblasts, and capillaries. In the peripheral nervous system, there are three types of neural fascicular patterns: monofascicular (one large fascicle), oligofascicular (2–10 fascicles), and polyfascicular (>10 fascicles) (Figure 42-2). The IAN and LN are, for the most part, polyfascicular in nature. Polyfascicular nerves have abundant interfascicular connective tissue; the importance of this fact is twofold: first, needle penetrations rarely cause direct neural trauma to the fascicles themselves because the needle would pass preferentially through the interfascicular spaces, and second,

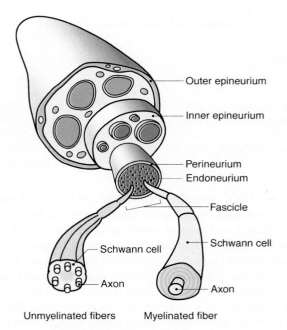

FIGURE 42-1. Trigeminal nerve anatomy.

nerve repair with realignment of the fascicles (coaptation) is challenging to perform on polyfascicular nerves.

The trigeminal nerve is composed of a functional unit with differing fiber types that transmit a variety of information (Table 42-2). The A-alpha fibers are the largest myelinated fibers with the fastest conduction velocity; they mediate position and fine touch through muscle spindle afferents and skeletal muscle efferents. The A-beta fibers mediate proprioception sense. The smallest myelinated fibers are the A-delta fibers that carry pain ("first" or "fast" pain) and temperature information. The smaller-diameter and slower-conducting unmyelinated C fibers mediate "second" or "slow" pain and temperature sensations. The Schwann cells surround both myelinated (one Schwann cell per nerve fiber) and unmyelinated (one Schwann cell per several nerve fibers) nerves, and they play a major role in nerve survival and regeneration after injury. Although the myelin sheath may not survive a nerve injury, the Schwann cells do, and

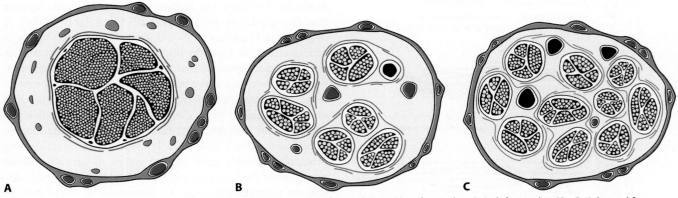

FIGURE 42-2. Three types of neural fascicular patterns. **A,** Monofascicular. **B,** Oligofascicular. **C,** Polyfascicular. (**A–C,** Adapted from Lundborg G. The nerve trunk. In Lundborg G, editor. Nerve Injury and Repair. New York: Churchill Livingstone; 1998; p. 198.)

TABLE 42-2. **Trigeminal Nerve Fibers**

Fiber	Size (μ)	Conduction Velocity (m/sec)	Function
A alpha (myelin)	12–20	70–120	Position, fine touch
A beta (myelin)	6.0–12	35–170	Proprioception
A delta (thin myelin)	1.0–6.0	2.5–3.5	Superficial (first) pain, temperature
C (unmyelinated)	0.5–1.0	0.7-1.5	Deep (second) pain, temperature

they provide a supportive role in the production of neurotrophic and neurotropic factors (such as nerve growth factor) that enhance and support neural recovery. In a myelinated axon, the nodes of Ranvier are the 0.3- to 2.0-μm unmyelinated segments between the myelin sheaths that are responsible for the diffusion of certain ions that cause nerve depolarization and repolarization as well as the rapid saltatory conduction of a nerve impulse along the nerve fiber.

Following nerve injury, many neural changes occur, but the basic process of nerve healing involves both degeneration and regeneration (Figure 42-3).[41,42] The nerve cell body responds with an increased metabolic phase with a heightened production of RNA (protein synthesis) and breakdown of Nissl's substance for export from the cell body. At the site

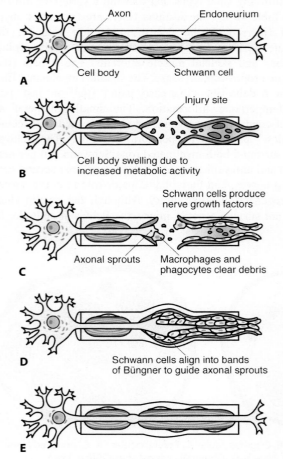

A Axon   Endoneurium
Cell body   Schwann cell

B Injury site
Cell body swelling due to increased metabolic activity

C Schwann cells produce nerve growth factors
Axonal sprouts   Macrophages and phagocytes clear debris

D Schwann cells align into bands of Büngner to guide axonal sprouts

E

FIGURE 42-3. **A–E,** Neural wound healing mechanisms.

of injury, there is edema and accumulation of particulate cellular debris. In addition, there is a proliferation of phagocytes and macrophages that begin to clean the area of this debris. Within days, axonal sprouts begin to bud and extend from the proximal nerve stump in the area of injury. Each axon may have as many as 50 collateral sprouts from the proximal nerve stump with random orientation toward the distal nerve stump. There is proliferation and a high level of activity of Schwann cells as well. These Schwann cells begin to form new myelin "conduits" in anticipation of the arrival of the new axonal sprouts. In addition, nerve growth factors are produced that influence the direction of sprouting and guide the new axons into the newly formed myelin sheath conduits, known as the *bands of Büngner.* In the event that all of these interrelated processes occur appropriately, spontaneous neural regeneration will occur. If one or more of the reparative processes fail to occur at the appropriate time and location, there may formation of a neuroma and lack of spontaneous neurosensory recovery. This failure may be due to a variety of reasons including advanced local tissue scarring, insufficient neurotrophic and neurotropic factor production, or malaligned nerve stumps separated beyond the critical size defect to allow sponatenous reconnection. A neuroma is simply a disorganized mass of collagen fibers and randomly oriented small nerve fascicles (sprouts that could not find the distal target). Neuromas are classified by gross morphology into the following types (Figure 42-4): amputation (stump) neuroma, neuroma-in-continuity (central or fusiform neuroma), and lateral neuromas that are either lateral exophytic neuromas or lateral adhesive neuromas. From a surgical perspective, the neuroma must be excised completely both proximally and distally to allow the neurorrhaphy a chance for success rather than suturing a neuromatous proximal segment to a neuromatous distal stump with no chance of improvement in functional neurosensory recovery.

NERVE INJURY CLASSIFICATION

Two classification schemes are used to describe the anatomic and histologic changes that occur after nerve injury. Seddon described a three-stage classification system in 1943,[43] and Sunderland revised and further subclassified nerve injuries into five grades in 1951 (Figure 42-5 and Table 42-3).[44] A neurapraxia (Seddon) or first-degree (Sunderland) injury is characterized as a conduction block from transient anoxia due to acute epineurial/endoneurial vascular interruption resulting from mild nerve manipulation (traction or compression), with rapid and complete recovery of sensation and no axonal degeneration. Damage is confined to within the endoneurium. Sunderland[44] further subdivides first-degree injuries into types I, II, and III. Type I results from mild nerve manipulation with rapid (hours) return of sensation when neural blood flow is restored. Type II is due to moderate traction or compression with the formation of transudate or exudate fluid and intrafascicular edema, with return of sensation after resolution of edema (days). Type III injuries result

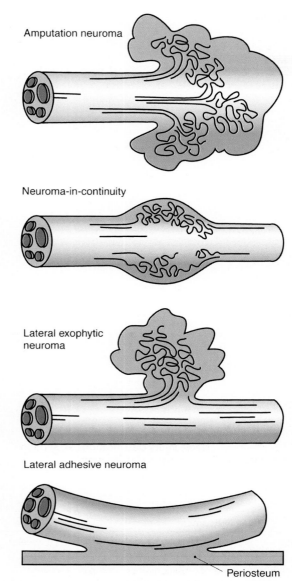

Amputation neuroma

Neuroma-in-continuity

Lateral exophytic
neuroma

Lateral adhesive neuroma

Periosteum

FIGURE 42-4. Neuroma types: amputation neuroma, neuroma-in-continuity, lateral exophytic neuroma, lateral adhesive neuroma.

from more severe nerve manipulation that may cause segmental demyelination, with recovery within days to weeks. An axonotmesis (Seddon) corresponds to second-, third-, and fourth-degree (Sunderland) injuries, with the difference being the degree of axonal damage. Second-degree injuries are due again to traction or compression that results in ischemia, intrafascicular edema, or demyelination. This damage extends through and includes the endoneurium with no significant axonal disorganization. Recovery is slow and may take weeks to months, and it may not be complete. Third-degree injuries continue the spectrum of more advanced neural injury due to more significant neural trauma with variable degrees of intrafascicular architectural disruption and damage extending to the perineurium. Recovery is variable; it may take months and be incomplete. Fourth-degree

injuries result in damage to the fascicle that extends through the perineurium to the epineurium, but the epineurium remains intact as a near-complete transection injury. There is axonal, endoneurial, and perineurial damage with disorganization of the fascicles. Spontaneous recovery is unlikely, but minimal improvement may occur in 6 to 12 months. Finally, neurotmesis (Seddon) and fifth-degree (Sunderland) injuries result from complete transection of the nerve (traverses the entire width of the fascicle) with epineurial discontinuity and likely subsequent neuroma formation during attempted spontaneous regeneration of the nerve, making spontaneous neurosensory recovery unlikely. For completeness, in 1988, Dellon and Mackinnon[45] described a sixth-degree injury, which recognizes that many nerve injuries exhibit features of different degrees of injury according to Sunderland (Table 42-4). The Seddon and Sunderland classification schemes attempt to correlate histologic changes of nerve injury with expected clinical outcomes (see Table 42-3).

CLINICAL NEUROSENSORY TESTING

The patient who sustains an injury to the trigeminal nerve may present with a variety of signs and symptoms. These may be divided into nonpainful anesthesia, hypoesthesia, hyperesthesia or painful anesthesia (anesthesia dolorosa), hypoesthesia, or hyperesthesia (allodynia, pain from a nonpainful stimulus, or hyperpathia, increased pain due to a painful or nonpainful stimulus). The history usually indicates the etiologic event, and the chief complaint may include the following: "numbness," "itchy," "crawling," "stretched," "drooling," "painful," "tingling," "tickling," "pulling," "burning," "stinging," "pins and needles," "hot sensation," "cold sensation," inability to feel food on lip, inability to taste, inability to shave, inability to smile, and loss of consortium. The history of present illness should be explored in depth with a comprehensive description of the onset and progression of symptoms, change in symptoms, treatment received and response to that treatment, any aggravating and alleviating factors, and current symptoms.

The McGill Pain Questionnaire (MPQ) may be used to assess pain and altered sensation, and it is a useful tool for monitoring progression of neurosensory recovery. The MPQ uses three classes to assess the level of dysfunction and interference with activity: sensory class (temporal, spatial, thermal, punctate, incisive, constrictive, traction pressure), affective class (tension, fear, autonomic properties, punishment), and evaluative class (patient perception). Perhaps the simplest and most reliable measure of subjective patient assessment is the use of a visual analogue scale. Typically, this is a 10-cm five-degree scale, with a degree marked every 2.5 cm (Figure 42-6). This is a useful tool for monitoring subjective improvement. It must be remembered that subjective and objective nerve test results are rarely at the same level. For example, in one study of nerve testing after sagittal split osteotomy, the subjective neurosensory deficit was 26.0%, whereas objective testing revealed an 89.5% deficit.[46]

SECTION 5

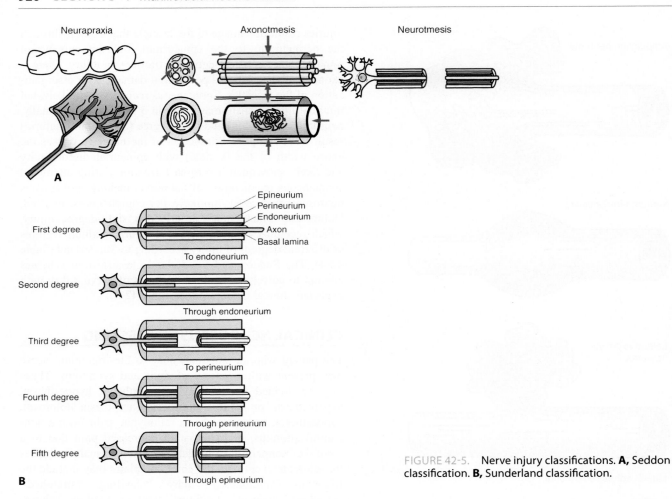

FIGURE 42-5. Nerve injury classifications. **A,** Seddon classification. **B,** Sunderland classification.

TABLE 42-3. **Nerve Injury Classifications: Seddon versus Sunderland**

Seddon	Sunderland	Histology	Outcomes
Neurapraxia	First degree	No axonal damage, no demyelination, no neuroma	Loss of sensation, rapid recovery (days to weeks), no microneurosurgery
Axonotmesis	Second, third, and fourth degrees	More axonal damage, demyelination, possible neuroma	Loss of sensation, slow incomplete recovery (weeks to months), possible microneurosurgery
Neurotmesis	Fifth degree	Severe axonal damage, epineurial discontinuity, neuroma formation	Loss of sensation, spontaneous recovery unlikely, microneurosurgery

TABLE 42-4. **Sunderland Grade and Recovery Patterns**

Degree of Injury	Recovery Pattern	Rate of Recovery	Treatment
First degree	Complete	Fast (days–wk)	None
Second degree	Complete	Slow (wk)	None
Third degree	Variable	Slow (wk–mo)	Possible nerve exploration
Fourth degree	None	Unlikely recovery	Microneurosurgery
Fifth degree	None	No recovery	Microneurosurgery
Sixth degree*	Varies†	Varies†	Varies†

*Sixth-degree injury data from Dellon AL, Mackinnon SE. Basic scientific and clinical applications of peripheral nerve regeneration. Surg Annu 1988;20:59.
†Depending on specific injury pattern.

Treatment planning decisions must be based on a thorough assessment of both the subjective and the objective testing results. Also, a radiographic assessment may reveal the presence of radiographic predictors of root proximity to the inferior alveolar canal, retained root fragments, evidence of distal bone removal, or the presence of foreign bodies in the extraction sites, which should be ruled out in the initial assessment of the patient's nerve injury.

The CNT begins with inspection of the oral cavity, which may show signs of self-induced trauma to the tongue or lower lip and chin, a lingually positioned third molar incision scar, or atrophic changes of the tongue fungiform papillae.[47] Palpation in the area of the suspected nerve injury (e.g., lingual aspect of the third molar extraction site) may induce Tinel's sign, which is a provocative test of regenerating nerve

Right	1	2	3	4	5
	Complete absence of sensation	Almost no sensation	Reduced sensation	Almost normal sensation	Fully normal sensation

Left	1	2	3	4	5
	Complete absence of sensation	Almost no sensation	Reduced sensation	Almost normal sensation	Fully normal sensation

FIGURE 42-6. Visual analogue scale.

sprouts that is performed by light palpation over the area of suspected injury. This maneuver elicits a distal referred "tingling" sensation at the target site of the nerve (tongue or lower lip). This Tinel's sign is thought to indicate small-diameter nerve fiber recovery; however, it is poorly correlated with functional recovery and is often confused with neuroma formation. To perform the CNT appropriately, the patient should be seated comfortably in a quiet room, and the specific testing procedures should be explained clearly to the patient, with confirmation that there is an understanding of what the patient is being asked to do and what possible responses are acceptable. The specific tests are performed with the patient's eyes closed, and the contralateral uninjured side serves as the control, when appropriate, to establish a baseline for assessment of the injured side.

The CNT is performed at three levels: levels A, B, and C (Table 42-5).[48] The CNT involves a dropout algorithm that attempts to correlate the results of the CNT with the level of nerve injury (Figure 42-7). This level of nerve injury may be correlated with the Sunderland classification and expected outcomes. If the results of level A testing are normal, the CNT is terminated and the patient is considered normal; this would correspond to a Sunderland first-degree injury. An abnormal result at level A indicates the need to proceed to level B testing. If the results of level B testing are normal, the patient is considered mildly impaired (Sunderland second-degree injury). If level B results are abnormal, level C testing is performed. If level C results are normal, the patient is considered to have a moderate impairment of the nerve (Sunderland third-degree injury). If level C results are abnormal, the patient is considered severely impaired (Sunderland fourth-degree injury). If the patient's test results are abnormal at levels A, B, and C and there is no response

to any noxious stimulus at level C, the patient is considered completely impaired (Sunderland fifth-degree injury). Level A testing includes brushstroke directional and static two-point discrimination. These two tests assess function of the larger myelinated A-alpha and A-beta fibers. These fibers are the most sensitive to compression and traction injuries; therefore, the CNT is terminated if level A is normal, indicating that these fibers are uninvolved in the injury. Brushstroke directional discrimination is performed with a fine sable or camel hair brush. The brush is stroked gently across the area of involvement at a constant rate and pressure, and the patient is asked to indicate the direction of movement (i.e., to the left or to the right) and the correct number of patient responses out of 10 strokes is recorded. Two-point discrimination is performed in a static fashion (vs. a moving two-point discrimination test) and with blunt tips to avoid A-delta and C fiber stimulation. This test can be performed with any device capable of allowing the distance between two points to be measured consistently (e.g., a Boley gauge). The closest distance (in millimeters) at which the patient can consistently discern the two points is recorded at the control site for reference and then the affected area is tested. At level B testing, contact detection is performed with Semmes-Weinstein monofilaments or von Frey hairs, which also assess the A-beta fiber integrity and function. These devices are acrylic resin or plastic transparent/translucent rods with nylon filaments of varying diameters. The stiffness of each filament determines the force necessary to deflect or bend the filament. The narrowest diameter filament that requires the least amount of force to deflect that is detected consistently by the patient is recorded. At level C testing, pinprick nociception and thermal discrimination assess the smaller A-delta and C fibers, which are most resistant to injury. Pinprick nociception may be performed simply with a dental explorer tip or a 30-gauge needle; however, a pressure-sensitive device is more appropriate in order to quantify the test result rather than achieving an all-or-none response, which would vary depending upon depth of penetration of the needle. Thermal discrimination is usually performed with suprathreshold temperature devices such as an ice cube or ethyl chloride spray or hot water placed on a cotton swab, but other options are available, such as

TABLE 42-5. **Clinical Neurosensory Testing**

Subjective assessment: visual analogue scale
Objective assessment
Level A: static two-point discrimination, brush-stroke directional discrimination
Level B: contact detection
Level C: pinprick nociception, thermal discrimination

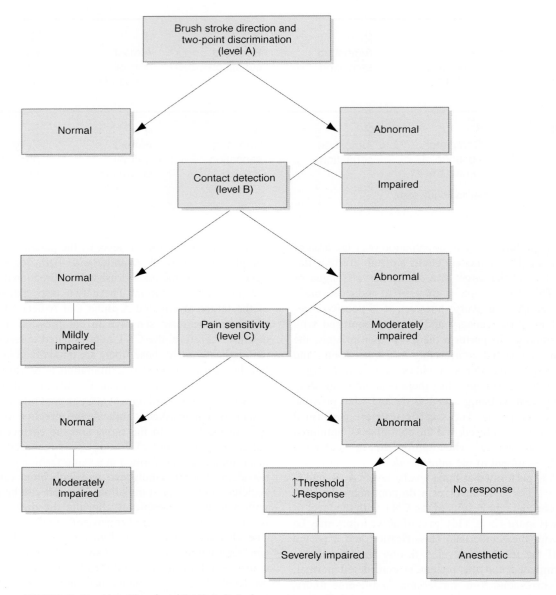

FIGURE 42-7. Algorithm for objective clinical neurosensory test.

Minnesota thermal disks made of copper, stainless steel, glass, and polyvinyl chloride.

Although these five tests employed in the CNT are considered "objective" tests, they are, in reality, "subjective" because they require a "subjective" patient response. Few purely objective tests of nerve function are available, and these include trigeminal somatosensory evoked potentials and magnetic source imaging.[49] Unfortunately, these tests are not readily available and are not considered a part of the routine assessment of a nerve-injured patient. Also, there are little data on the trigeminal nerve and the patterns of responses to these objective tests based on specific types of nerve injuries.

Finally, taste may be assessed by a variety of methods, but, it is performed as either whole -mouth or localized taste

testing. Solutions such as 1 M sodium chloride (salt), 1 M sucrose (sweet), 0.4 M acetic acid (sour), and 0.1 M quinine (bitter) are used. There are many difficulties and limitations with gustatory assessment in the patient with an LN injury. The perception of taste alteration (cranial nerve VII) is extremely variable and has little correlation with the degree of LN (cranial nerve V) injury. For example, a patient with a fourth- or fifth-degree LN injury may not report any taste alteration subjectively but may test abnormally upon formal taste testing. The complex sense of taste is mediated not only by the chorda tympani branch of the facial nerve but also through feedback mechanisms in the nasopharynx, oropharynx, and hypopharynx as well as the nucleus tractus solitarius in the brainstem.[50] Taste buds are located throughout the oral cavity, not solely on the anterior two thirds of the tongue surface, but the palate, buccal mucosa, and floor of mouth. Also, after microneurosurgical LN repair, the objective and subjective neurosensory recovery of tongue sensation and taste perception also are inconsistent.[51]

Diagnostic nerve blocks can be a useful component of the patient evaluation when dysesthesia or unpleasant sensations predominate the clinical scenario. The goals of the diagnostic nerve block is to localize the source of nerve injury, determine whether delivery of peripheral anethesia resolves the painful symptoms, and estimate the prognosis for recovery after either pharmacologic or surgical therapy. If surgical management includes consideration for a nerve transection procedure for pain relief, the nerve block may use a long-acting local anesthetic solution to allow the patient several hours to determine whether permanent anesthesia is tolerable. The preferred local anesthetic solution for a routine nerve block, however, is of a low concentration (e.g., 0.25% lidocaine) to selectively block the smaller A-delta and C fibers while not affecting the larger myelinated fibers. If the low concentration fails to relieve the pain, a higher concentration is used in the same location. Diagnostic blocks begin in the most central location and proceed with progressively more peripheral injections along the course of the nerve with constant reassessment of the area of involvement both objectively and subjectively. If the patient presents with symptoms consistent with sympathetically mediated pain or causalgia, a stellate ganglion block may be performed as well, but these symptoms usually indicate a problem not amenable to peripheral microneurosurgery. Other painful syndromes that generally are not relieved with diagnostic nerve blocks include anesthesia dolorosa and deafferentation pain, and similar to other neuropathies with predominating symptoms of dysesthesia, these syndromes are used managed with pharmacotherapy.

NONSURGICAL TREATMENT

Pharmacologic management of peripheral nerve injuries is reserved for patients who present with unpleasant abnormal sensations or dysesthesia. In the majority of these cases, pharmacologic treatment should be managed with a consultation from an experienced individual such as a neurologist or facial pain specialist. Many systemic (Table 42-6) and topical (Table 42-7) medications are available.[51] Whereas the systemic drugs may have significant side effects, topical

TABLE 42-6. **Systemic Pharmacologic Agents**

Local anesthetics
Corticosteroids
Nonsteroidal anti-inflammatory agents
Antidepressants
Narcotic analgesics
Anticonvulsants
Muscle relaxants
Benzodiazepines
Antisympathetic agents

TABLE 42-7. **Topical Medications**

Category	Example
Topical anesthetics	5% viscous lidocaine gel; 20% benzocaine gel; 2.5% lidocaine with 2.5% prilocaine
Neuropeptides	Capsaicin cream (0.025% or 0.075%)
Nonsteroidal anti-inflammatory drugs	Ketoprofen 10–20% PLO base; diclofenac 10–20% PLO base
Sympathomimetics	Clonidine 0.01% PLO base or patch
N-methyl-D-aspartate blocking agents	Ketamine 0.5% PLO base
Anticonvulsants	Carbamazepine 2% PLO base
Tricyclic antidepressants	Amitriptyline 2% PLO base
Antispasmodics	Baclofen 2% PLO base

PLO = pleuronic lecithin organogel.

agents offer the advantages of little systemic absorption, possibly only minor irritation (which can be relieved with a period of abstinence), and over-the-counter availability in many cases. There are also many combinations of topical agents that can be used, such as a eutectic mixture of local anesthetics (EMLA) that contains 2.5% lidocaine and 2.5% prilocaine. Many of the topical agents are prepared in a pleuronic lecithin organogel base. For most oral and maxillofacial surgeons, long-term pharmacologic management with drug dosage adjustments based upon clinical response is not part of their routine practice, so the prompt referral to a microneurosurgeon or neurologist may offer the best chance for long-term successful patient management. Pharmacotherapy for dysesthesia includes the use of membrane-stabilizing agents, such as antidepressants and anticonvulsants, and many neurologists and surgeons consider gabapentin (neurontin) as a first-line agent. There are also dorsal horn inhibitors or γ-aminobutyirc acid (GABA) agonists, including muscle relaxants and benzodiazepines. Consideration may be given to a trial of a topical agent such as capsaicin cream 0.025% or 0.075% three times a day and/or a systemic medication with few side effects, such as baclofen (Lioresal) 10 mg orally three times a day, pregabalin (Lyrica) 50 mg orally three times a day, or gabapentin (Neurontin) 100 mg orally three times a day. The most common side effect of these medications is sedation or drowsiness that may require frequent daily dose adjustments. Again, surgeons unfamiliar with the drugs, as well as the spectrum of pharmacologic options, should consider obtaining a neurology consultation.

It may be appropriate to manage perioperative paresthesia after third molar removal or implant placement with a short course of systemic corticosteroid therapy in an attempt to decrease perineural edema caused by the local response to the nerve injury. Although there is little evidence to suggest that systemic steroids actually provide any effect, the use of steroids when a nerve injury occurs indicates that the surgeon has recognized the problem and has taken some initiative to potentially improve outcome based upon a knowledge of neural anatomy and injury physiology, which is advantageous when considering medicolegal involvement issues.

TABLE 42-8. **Microneurosurgeon Referral Indications**

Observed nerve transection
Complete postoperative anesthesia
Persistent paresthesia (lack of improvement in symptoms) at 4 wk
Presence or development of dysesthesia

Perhaps the most important initial consideration in patient management should be prompt referral, when indicated, to a specialist for pharmacologic or surgical management. The indications for referral include but are not limited to those listed in Table 42-8.

In the past, before considering surgical management, a variety of neuroablative techniques had been used to ameliorate painful neuropathies. Some of these included radiofrequency thermal neurolysis, cryoneurolysis, and alcohol and glycerol injections at the site of injury as well as at the gasserian (trigeminal) ganglion. Based on the published complications of these types of procedures as well as the recurrence rates of the symptoms of dysesthesia, caution should be employed when considering these options.[53,54] The use of a low-level ("soft") laser (gallium-aluminum-arsenide, wavelength of approximately 820 nm) holds promise in the area of neural healing. Several studies have shown improvement in objective and subjective neurosensory function with the use of laser therapy in some of the more difficult clinical scenarios, such as longstanding nerve injuries, orthognathic-related IAN paresthesia, and prolonged dysesthesia unresponsive to pharmacologic or surgical therapy.[55-57] However, the current limited availability of the low-level laser and the lack of approval by the U.S. Food and Drug Administration (FDA) preclude its routine use for patients with nerve injuries, although clinical trials continue.

TRIGEMINAL NEURALGIA

Whereas it is not the intention of this chapter to cover the various facial pain syndromes, it is appropriate to discuss briefly the subject of trigeminal neuralgia (TN), which is typically not amenable to microneurosuregry but should be ruled out in the assessment of patients who present with complaints related to the trigeminal nerve system. The reported incidence of TN is 4/100,000 as a spontaneous occurrence. Female patients older than 50 years are more commonly affected by TN symptoms, and the right side of the face is involved more often than the left. The typical symptoms are lancinating or stabbing ("electric shock"–like) paroxysms of facial pain involving the second and third divisions of the trigeminal nerve (V2 and V3). Although various theories have been proposed, including arterial compression of the trigeminal nerve in the pons region (Janetta), the etiology of TN is unknown in most cases and, therefore, has been designated idiopathic trigeminal neuralgia (ITN). The diagnosis of TN is made based upon the Sweet diagnostic criteria, 1969, that includes paroxysmal pain, pain provoked by light touch (with trigger zones), pain confined to the trigeminal distribution, unilateral pain, and a normal clinical neurosensory test. The International Classification of Headache Disorders (ICHD) has established criteria to differentiate two forms of TN, classic TN and symptomatic TN. *Classic TN* is the most common form with paroxysmal attacks lasting from 1 second to 2 minutes affecting the trigeminal nerve. The pain has at least one of the following features: intense, sharp, superficial or stabbing, or precipitated by a trigger point or area. The attacks in classic TN are stereotyped in each individual patient occurring at the same time and location each day. There is no clinical neurologic deficit on examination. Finally, the symptoms of classic TN cannot be attributed to another disorder. The second form, *symptomatic TN,* has all of the features of classic TN with the additional finding of a causative lesion, other than vascular compression, identified by special studies (magnetic resonance imaging [MRI], lumbar puncture, evoked potentials, hematologic studies) or exploration of the posterior cranial fossa. Another form of TN is known as *atypical TN* because it may meet most, but not all, of the Sweet diagnostic criteria of classic TN. TN is managed with pharmacologic therapy, and usually multidrug regimens are used. A variety of medications have been used, including antiepileptic drugs, gabapentin, baclofen, clonezepam, lamotrigine, oxcarbazepine, toprimate, and carbamezepine. For acute exacerbations of TN symptoms, several treatment options include peripheral local anesthetic nerve block, intravenous lidocaine (100 mg over 20 min), intravenous antiepilepric drugs (dilantin, fosphenytoin, or valproic acid), and analgesics (opioid and nonopioid) that may have little clinical effect. Surgical options for TN are limited to a few specialized procedures, with minimal morbidity, that may provide some form of symptomatic relief in 80% to 85% of patients. These include percutaneous stereotactic radiofrequency thermal lesioning of the trigeminal ganglion, posterior fossa exploration and microvascular decompression of the trigeminal root, and gamma knife radiation to the trigeminal nerve root entry zone, which has shown promising results.

TREATMENT ALGORITHMS

The decision to proceed with microneurosurgery must be made after a careful patient assessment over a defined period of time. The dilemma for clinicians is that sufficient time must be given to allow for spontaneous neurosensory recovery but that prompt surgical intervention may afford the best chance for recovery. Time is a critical issue in the management of nerve injuries for three main reasons. First, at the site of injury, distal nerve degeneration (wallerian degeneration—named for Augustus Waller, 1892) occurs owing to an interruption of anterograde and retrograde axonal transport across the site of injury. This results in a progressive loss of neural tissue due to lack of stimulation that may compromise future repair attempts by causing a greater length of neuromatous nerve segment requiring resection at the time of nerve repair. Second, at the nerve cell bodies, there is ganglion cell death that occurs early after injury.[58] This may result in a large percentage (>50%) of cell body death in a short period of time after the injury (weeks to months), so that any "peripheral" attempt at microneurosurgical repair would have, at best, a 50% functional neurosensory recovery. Third, as the time from the nerve injury increases, there is a higher likelihood that central intracranial somatosensory cortical changes may occur, and these would make peripheral repair ineffective.[59] The central nervous system remains "plastic" in that longstanding peripheral painful neuropathies become "expected" in the area of the brain devoted to that region and, despite peripheral nerve transection as an attempt at painful symptom resolution,

the brain will continue to interpret the information not as "anesthesia," but as "dysesthesia" (similar to "phantomlimb" pain syndromes).

Microneurosurgery is indicated for persistent paresthesia that fails to improve over successive examinations, including both subjective and objective interval assessments. Microneurosurgery is not indicated if there is continued improvement at each interval assessment. The currently accepted recommendations are to consider microneurosurgery, when indicated, for the LN within 1 to 3 months after the injury and for the IAN within 3 to 6 months after the injury (Figure 42-8). The rationale for the difference in time is that the IAN lies within a bony canal or "physiologic conduit" that can

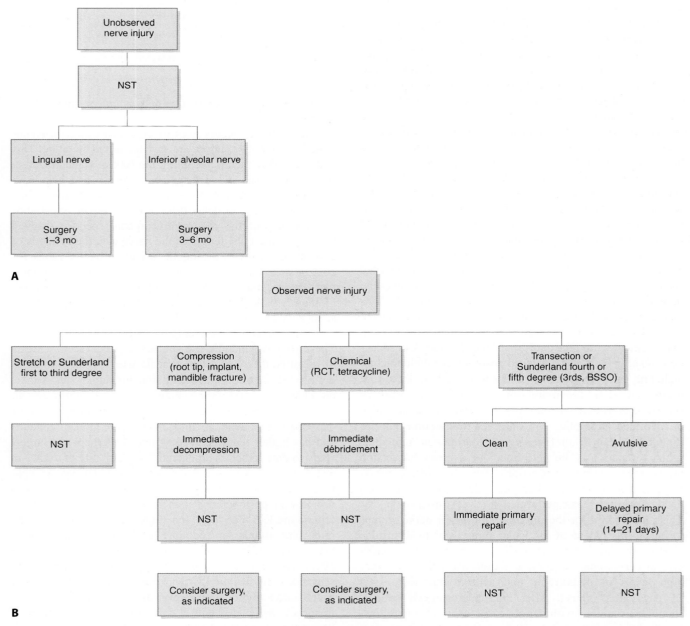

FIGURE 42-8.   Nerve treatment algorithms. **A,** Unobserved nerve injury. **B,** Observed nerve injury. BSSO = bilateral sagittal split osteotomy; NST = neurosensory testing; RCT = root canal therapy.

guide spontaneous regeneration, so more time is allotted for that process to occur, whereas an LN injured within soft tissue does not have a "conduit" to guide spontaneous regeneration. In general, the oral and maxillofacial surgeon should schedule weekly follow-up examinations with the patient over a period of approximately 4 weeks. If there is persistent paresthesia or a worsening of symptoms, referral should be made to a microneurosurgical specialist for prompt definitive evaluation and management.

The indications for microneurosurgery include the complete (100%) postoperative anesthesia, or less than 50% residual sensation in an injury classified as a Sunderland grade III, IV, or V. Some surgeons consider another indication to be the level of sensation, which is unacceptable to the patient, even if the objective tests show greater than 50% residual sensation of a Sunderland I or II injury. In these cases, the patient must be informed of the reasonable expectation for recovery after microneurosurgery, which, according to the literature, may be at or below their current level of sensibility. Also, whereas as a general rule unpleasant sensations are managed pharmacologically and decreased sensations are managed surgically, some cases of early dysesthesia or hyperpathic pain may indicate the early formation of a neuroma at the site of nerve injury, and consideration should be given toward early microneurosurgical intervention.

For an unobserved nerve injury, the plan should be to continue neurosensory testing for 1 month and then to refer for surgery in the 1- to 3-month (LN) or 3- to 6-month (IAN) time periods. For an observed nerve injury, treatment should focus on the specific etiology. For a suspected traction injury (Sunderland first-, second-, and third-degree injuries), the patient should be tested for 1 month for signs of expected spontaneous recovery. In the case of nerve compression, immediate decompression should be considered. This includes removal of a root displaced into the IAN canal, removal or replacement when there is evidence of implant impingement within the confines of the IAN canal, or reduction and alignment of a displaced posterior mandible fracture including the IAN canal. Neurosensory testing should be performed after decompression, and microneurosurgery should be considered as indicated. Chemical injuries should be débrided promptly. For observed transection injuries (Sunderland fourth- or fifth-degree injuries), an immediate primary repair may be performed for a clean transection injury (e.g., scalpel transection). For an avulsive injury (e.g., LN entangled in a bur), consideration is given to a delayed primary repair performed at 3 weeks after the injury. This allows time for the proximal and distal nerve stumps to define the extent of fascicular injury and to determine whether the immediate surrounding environment is conducive to nerve repair surgery, at a time when there are very high levels of neurotropic and neurotrophic factors (at 21 days after injury). After microneurosurgery, patients should be examined with repeat neurosensory testing following the first signs or symptoms of return of sensation. Sensory reeducation exercises should be considered early in

TABLE 42-9. **Classification of Sensory Recovery (Medical Research Council System)**

Grade (Stage)	Recovery of Sensibility
S0	No recovery
S1	Recovery of deep cutaneous pain
S1+	Recovery of some superficial pain
S2	Return of some superficial pain and tactile sensation
S2+	S2 with overresponse
S3*	Return of some superficial pain and tactile sensation without overresponse; two-point discrimination > 15 mm
S3+	S3 with good stimulus localization; two-point discrimination = 7–15 mm
S4	Complete recovery, S3+; two-point discrimination = 2–6 mm

*S3 score indicates significant clinical recovery (from Wyrick JD, Stern PJ. Secondary nerve reconstruction. Hand Clin 1992;8:587).
Adapted from Mackinnon SE. Surgical management of the peripheral nerve gap. Clin Plast Surg 1989;16:587.

the postoperative period to potentially augment neurosensory recovery.

The reported success rates of microneurosurgical reconstruction after nerve injury are variable in the literature. This is due to many factors including the lack of standardization in the diagnosis and management process and also with wide variations of the following[60]: patient age, etiology of the nerve injury, time of delay from injury to repair, experience and training of the microneurosurgeon, specific surgical techniques used, the length of the nerve gap, the methods of clinical neurosensory testing, the use of normative values for control sites, the length of the follow-up period, and important, the criteria used by the surgeon to define "success" (Table 42-9). A global review of the literature might indicate a success rate of 30% to 50% after microneurosurgery, including direct and indirect (gap or graft) repair techniques. These studies generally use subjective patient assessments to quantify the results into a scale used by the patient to define the sensation after microneurosurgery as worse, no change, some improvement, or good improvement. In general, direct repair (neurorrhaphy) is preferred over gap repair (e.g., using an autogenous nerve graft or conduit) and has higher reported success rates.[61] Perhaps the largest study to date indicates an overall "success" rate of 76.2% in 521 patients.[62] The success criteria were defined as light touch detected more than 80% of the time and a 30% decrease in postoperative pain level. Although the success criteria are less than ideal, the study results suggested some important trends in outcome after microneurosurgery: hypoesthetic (decreased sensation) injuries improved more after microneurosurgery than did hyperesthetic (unpleasant sensation) injuries; the LN recovered more than did the IAN overall after microneurosurgery; and there was a decrease in success associated with a delay from injury to repair of longer than 6 months. Another report of 51 microneurosurgical reconstructions (direct and gap repairs) found that

10 patients subjectively reported good improvement, 18 patients some improvement, 22 patients no improvement, and 1 patient reported feeling worse after surgery.[63] This indicates that 55% of patients (28/51) showed some improvement, or "success." In another study of 53 surgical patients, with a mean follow-up of 13 months, light touch improved from 0% to 51% and pinprick nociception improved from 34% to 77%. Patients in this study also experienced improved taste and an increased number of fungiform papillae, and there was a decrease in incidence of accidental tongue biting. Interestingly, there was no correlation of success with delay from time of injury to repair. No patient became completely normal, and there was no reduction in dysesthesia; however, most patients considered the surgery worthwhile. In order to most appropriately interpret the literature and allow proper assessment and management of patients who sustain nerve injuries based upon a critial review of evidence-based medicine, there is certainly a need for standardization in all aspects of evaluation and management of the nerve-injured patient.

SURGICAL TREATMENT

Microneurosurgical reconstruction surgery involves an orderly sequence of surgical procedures including nerve identification and exposure (either via access through soft tissues for the LN [Figure 42-9] or via an osteotomy for the IAN [Figure 42-10]), dissection of the nerve from the surrounding tissues, assessment of the degree of injury, manipulation of the nerve (neurolysis), which may include neuroma resection, débridement of the nerve stumps as required, and repair with a direct anastomosis or the use of a nerve graft or

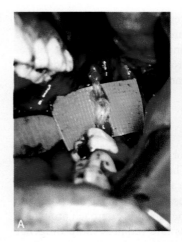
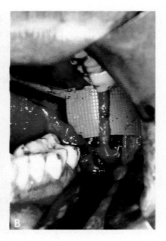

FIGURE 42-9.   Lingual nerve (LN) direct repair. **A,** Left LN neuroma after exposure. **B,** Direct repair of left LN after neuroma resection.

conduit. Many of the techniques of trigeminal nerve repair closely mimic those of hand surgery (although access is more limited) and use similar microneurosurgical instrumentation. In general, surgical loupe magnification (×3.5 magnification) is adequate for most microneurosurgeons. An operating microscope (×12 magnification) provides a higher magnification, but it is cumbersome and difficult to use effectively with a transoral exposure in the posterior oral cavity, although it may be more useful with a transfacial approach to the IAN. Most experienced microneurosurgeons have had some form of advanced training in the technical aspects of this specific type of surgery, including the use of microinstruments and an operating microscope for both vascular and

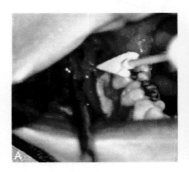
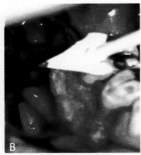
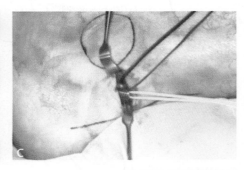
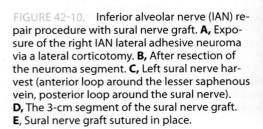
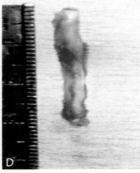
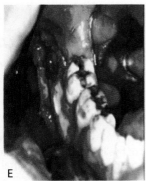

FIGURE 42-10.   Inferior alveolar nerve (IAN) repair procedure with sural nerve graft. **A,** Exposure of the right IAN lateral adhesive neuroma via a lateral corticotomy. **B,** After resection of the neuroma segment. **C,** Left sural nerve harvest (anterior loop around the lesser saphenous vein, posterior loop around the sural nerve). **D,** The 3-cm segment of the sural nerve graft. **E,** Sural nerve graft sutured in place.

neural tissue handling and repair, although, as mentioned previously, these techniques are becoming more widespread with dissemination of the principles and practice of micro-neurosurgery, as well as microvascular surgery, in oral and maxillofacial surgery residency training programs in the United States and abroad.

Exposure

Surgical access to the LN or IAN may be accomplished transfacially or transorally. The transfacial approach to the IAN in the posterior mandible affords wide surgical exposure and access; however, it necessitates a facial incision with subsequent scar formation. The intraoral approach provides a more difficult surgical access and requires more diligence during the procedure involving the posterior regions of the oral cavity, but it avoids a facial scar. The decision regarding surgical access depends on an individual patient's anatomy; the site of nerve injury; planned surgical procedures; patient preference; and surgeon's preference, skill, and experience.

External Neurolysis

Microdissection of the nerve once exposed involves liberation of the nerve from the surrounding tissues to facilitate inspection. For the LN, this procedure may commonly involve the release of the nerve from a lateral adhesive neuroma in the area of the lingual plate in the third molar region or from within the healing third molar extraction site itself, whereas for the IAN, a lateral corticotomy is generally required in order to perform an external neurolysis and mobilization of the IAN from within the inferior alveolar canal. Several techniques have been described for lateral decortication in the area of the third molar for IAN exposure, ranging from a simple nerve transpositioning procedure to a modified buccal corticotomy or a unilateral sagittal split ramus osteotomy (Figure 42-11).[64] The specific location of the injury as well as the surgeon's preference frequently dictate the specific approach used. The LN is usually exposed via a modified incision used for third molar surgery with a gingival sulcular lingual extension (Figure 42-12). As another

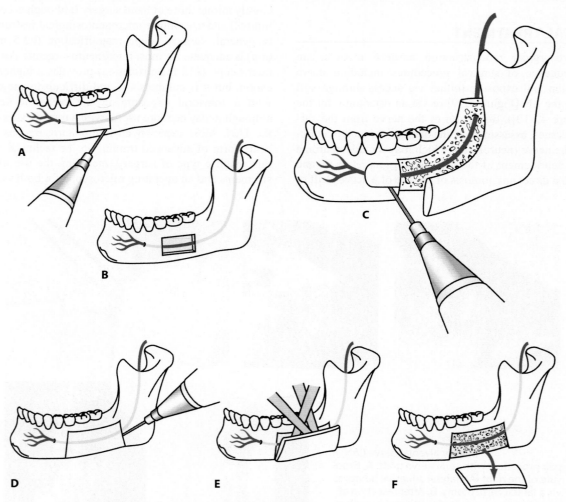

FIGURE 42-11. Exposure techniques for the IAN. **A,** Lateral decortication of the mandible. **B,** With exposure of the inferior alveolar neurovascular bundle. **C,** Sagittal ramus osteotomy with anterior extension via lateral decortication to the mental foramen. **D,** Lateral mandibular decortication. **E,** Bone removal with chisels. **F,** Wide exposure of the neurovascular bundle.

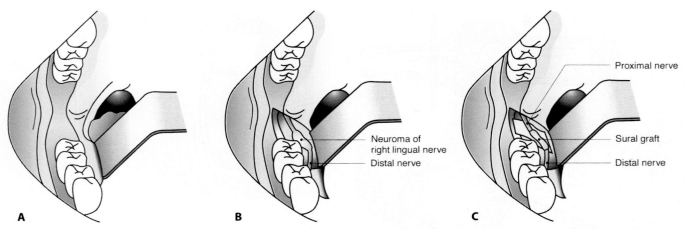

FIGURE 42-12.   LN exposure. **A,** Incision design via a distobuccal extension and lingual gingival sulcus approach. **B,** Right LN exposure with neuroma. **C,** Right LN repair with an interpositional nerve graft.

example, external neurolysis of the infraorbital nerve (V2) may be performed via reduction and fixation of the displaced zygomaticomaxillary complex fracture impinging on the neurovascular bundle at its exit through the infraorbital foramen. It has been suggested that external neurolysis may provide definitive treatment for a nerve injury if the nerve compression is less than 25% of the normal diameter, if the paresthesia is of short duration (<6 mo), and if there is no evidence of neuroma formation.[65] Typically, external neurolysis is followed by techniques of "internal" neurolysis that will address the specific fascicular injury by internal nerve manipulation.

Internal Neurolysis

The term *internal neurolysis* refers to surgical manipulation within the confines of the epineurium that is done in order to prepare the nerve for subsequent repair. Sophisticated maneuvers that involve attempts to dissect the individual fascicles of the nerve (especially in a polyfascicular nerve) may compromise repair by unnecessary removal of tissue

and/or induction of cicatrix formation owing to excessive manipulation in the interfascicular spaces. Several methods of internal neurolysis have been described, including epifascicular epineurotomy, epifascicular epineurectomy, and interfascicular epineurectomy (Figure 42-13). The first two techniques prepare the epineurium for repair, and the third technique involving interfascicular dissection may cause further fascicular disruption and tissue scarring. Extensive internal neurolysis procedures should be used with caution, with the goal of doing no further harm to the uninvolved segments of the proximal and distal nerve stumps.

Nerve Stump Preparation

Perhaps the most critical portion of the microneurosurgical procedure involves thorough inspection of the proximal and distal nerve stumps via magnification. It should be noted that there may already be an existing discontinuity from a transection injury to the nerve and identification of the proximal and distal stumps may be difficult owing to scar tissue formation. When a neuroma of any type is present,

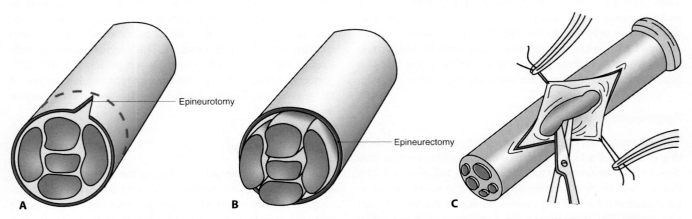

FIGURE 42-13.   Internal neurolysis. **A,** Epifascicular epineurotomy. **B,** Epifascicular epineurectomy. **C,** Interfascicular epineurectomy. (**A** and **B,** Adapted from LaBanc JP. Reconstructive microneurosurgery of the trigeminal nerve. In Peterson **L J,** Indresano AT, Marciani RD, Roser SM, editors. Principles of Oral and Maxillofacial Surgery. Vol 2. Philadelphia: JB Lippincott; 1992; p. 1067.)

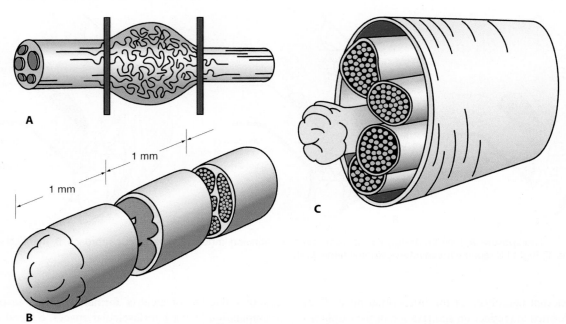

FIGURE 42-14.   Nerve stump preparation. **A,** Neuroma; resection at the "clinical margin" of the neuroma fails to complete nerve preparation. **B,** Neuroma resection in 1-mm increments. **C,** Mushrooming fascicle.

meticulous attention to detail is required in order to remove all neuromatous tissue (Figure 42-14). It must be recognized that with any neuroma, the clinical appearance of neuronal edema or atrophy may be less apparent than the actual, more severe internal fascicular disruption (see Figure 42-14A). The failure by the microneurosurgeon to resect enough nerve tissue to encounter normal nerve fascicular tissue will inevitably result in a failure of neurosensory recovery. Once the nerve is divided, when necessary, into proximal and distal stumps, care must be taken to sequentially resect small (1-mm) portions of the nerve trunk in both directions (see Figure 42-14B) until healthy glistening white "mushrooming" fascicles are seen to herniate through the edges of the epineurium (see Figure 42-14C). The microneurosurgeon should be confident that the repair will be performed in order to anastomose healthy nerve tissues, rather than neuromatous tissue, and this requires an aggressive approach at this point and may result in a greater need for consideration of indirect (graft) repair over direct neurorrhaphy. The informed consent process for all microneurosurgical procedures should include a discussion of options for gap repair in the event that this becomes necessary during the surgical procedure.

Approximation

The trigeminal nerve is similar to other peripheral nerves in that it does not tolerate tension well; therefore, tension-free closure after microneurosurgical repair is mandatory.[66] The deleterious effects of tension on a repair site result from vascular compromise and subsequent fibrosis at the nerve repair site, essentially resulting in the formation of a surgically induced neuroma. Approximation is the act of bringing the nerve stumps into direct contact and assessing the degree of

tension that may be present. At the time of approximation, a decision must be made regarding whether to use an interpositional graft or conduit. In general, mobilization with primary epineurial repair is usually possible when the LN gap is less than 10 mm and when the IAN gap is less than 5 mm. The difference in acceptable gap length is due to the relative immobility of the IAN within the confines of the inferior alveolar canal, whereas there is usually more mobility of the LN stumps with dissection into the pterygomandibular space in a posterior direction and the floor of the mouth in an anterior direction.

Coaptation

Coaptation is the process of aligning the proximal and distal nerve stumps into the correct premorbid cross-sectional fascicular orientation. This is a very difficult maneuver to accomplish with a polyfascicular nerve that has undergone any degree of proximal or distal nerve structural alteration in diameter or fascicular pattern. This surgical step of coaptation of the LN or IAN is usually not performed with diligence in because of the complex polyfascicular pattern of the nerve as well as the limited visualization in the posterior oral cavity.

Neurorrhaphy

Neurorrhaphy is the act of bringing the nerve ends together and maintaining this position with sutures. A *direct neurorrhaphy* is performed with the proximal and distal nerve stumps, and an *indirect neurorrhaphy* is performed when using an interpositional graft between the nerve stumps, such as a nerve graft or conduit. The polyfascicular trigeminal

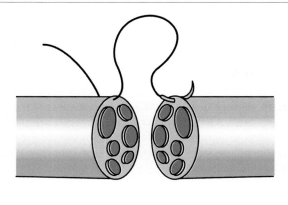

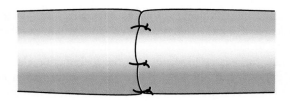

FIGURE 42-15.   Direct epineurial neurorrhaphy.

nerve is repaired using epineurial sutures, not perineurial sutures (Figure 42-15), because any attempt to suture the individual fascicles would be technically difficult as well as prone to induce excessive scar tissue in the area of nerve repair. Generally, 8-0 to 10-0 monofilament nonresorbable nylon suture is preferred, because a resorbable suture material would tend to invoke an inflammatory response and disturb the area of anticipated neural healing. At least two sutures should be used per anastomosis site to prevent rotation of the nerve stumps, but no more than three or four sutures should be used per anastomosis. The first suture is usually placed on the medial side of the anastomosis because it is the more difficult site of repair to access. The epineurium is pierced with the needle approximately 0.5 to 1.0 mm from the edge of the nerve stump. The second suture is placed 180 degrees from the first suture row on the lateral aspect of the repair site, and then an assessment is made regarding the necessity for the placement of one or two additional sutures.

Nerve Grafts

When neurorrhaphy is not possible without tension and a nerve gap exists, an interpositional graft must be considered for indirect neurorrhaphy.[67] The options for autogenous nerve grafting include, but are not limited to, the sural nerve, the greater auricular nerve, and possibly the medial antebrachial cutaneous nerve.[68] The sural nerve is preferred for grafting because it most appropriately matches the nerve diameter and the fascicular number and pattern of the trigeminal nerve (Table 42-10).[69] The area of the nerve superior to the lateral malleolus exhibits less branching than at or below the lateral malleolus. The sural nerve, or medial sural cutaneous nerve, is a branch of the sacral plexus (S1, S2) and supplies sensory

TABLE 42-10. **Size of Donor Nerve Grafts Relative to Injured Nerve**

Injured Nerve	Donor Nerve		
	Sural (2.1 mm)	Greater Auricular (1.5 mm)	Greater Auricular Cable (3.0 mm)
Inferior alveolar (2.4 mm)	88%	63%	125%
Lingual (3.2 mm)	66%	47%	94%

Adapted from Brammar JP, Epker BN. Anatomic-histologic survey of the sural nerve: implications for inferior alveolar nerve grafting. J Oral Maxillofac Surg 1988;46:111.

information to the posterior lower extremity and the dorsolateral foot. Sural grafts up to 20 cm in length are possible, and patients tolerate the donor site deficit well.[70] The greater auricular nerve is a poor choice for trigeminal repair. As a branch of the cervical plexus (C1, C2), the greater auricular nerve supplies sensation to the pre- and postauricular regions, the lower third of the ear, and the skin overlying the posteroinferior border at the angle of the mandible. Patients are generally not amenable to sacrificing sensation of one facial region to regain sensation in another neighboring location. In addition, the small diameter of the greater auricular nerve makes it useful only when used as a cable graft (Figure 42-16). The sole advantage of a greater auricular graft over a sural graft is in situations when it can be harvested via the same incision for another procedure, such as the repair of an extraoral mandibular fracture or management of pathology. The basic premise with graft repair is that the nerve graft will supply the Schwann cell conduit sheaths and the growth factors necessary to support and encourage axonal sprouting through the graft toward the target site. In addition, there are currently available FDA-approved human allogeneic nerve grafts from cadaveric donors that may be used for repair of IAN and LN discontinuties; early studies show promising results. This allograft is avialble in various lengths and diameters that can be used for the trigeminal system. Although the allograft is decellularized, it mainatins certain neurotrophic and neurotropic factors such as basement membrane laminin.

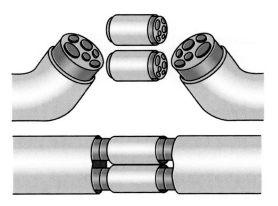

FIGURE 42-16.   Greater auricular nerve cable graft.

SECTION 5

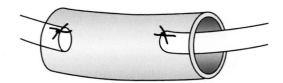

FIGURE 42-17. Entubulation (conduit) nerve repair.

Entubulation Techniques

In an attempt to avoid donor site morbidity, a variety of entubulation techniques have been proposed to create conduits to support nerve regeneration (Figure 42-17). These conduits include both autogenous and alloplastic materials (Table 42-11). The autogenous options include vein,[71–73] collagen,[74,75] and muscle grafts.[76] Alloplastic materials include polyglycolic acid,[77] polymeric silicone,[78] and expanded polytetrafluoroethylene.[79–82] It appears that the use of these alloplastic materials has a high success in the animal model, but poor human clinical outcomes. Perhaps this is due to the fact that these materials have no inherent strength to prevent compression during the postoperative period, although newer bioabsorbable synthetic materials for nerve conduits are under investigation.

POSTSURGICAL MANAGEMENT

In the majority of cases, patients experience a variable period of complete anesthesia after nerve repair. In general, the nerve regeneration process progresses at approximately 1 mm/day (~3 cm/mo) from the cell body to the target site. For example, with a direct IAN repair, the approximate distance from the trigeminal ganglion to the lower lip and chin is nearly 10 cm; therefore, complete nerve regeneration of an IAN repair would take about 100 days, or 12 weeks, after microneurosurgical repair. With graft or conduit indirect repair, the time frame is lengthened owing to slowed regeneration through the graft site, and recovery is variable. As mentioned, the use of sensory reeducation exercises ("biofeedback") in the postoperative period may improve or

TABLE 42-11. **Materials for Entubulation (Conduit) Repair**

Autogenous Materials
Collagen
Muscle
Fascia
Vein
Alloplastic Materials
Polyglycolic acid
Polyester
PTFE
ePTFE
Silicone, polymeric silicone
Allogeneic Materials
Cadaveric nerve allograft

ePTFE = expanded polytetrafluoroethylene; PTFE = polytetrafluoroethylene.

accelerate neurosensory recovery. For the LN or IAN, this may simply involve self-performance of a two-point discrimination or brushstroke directional discrimination test while looking in a mirror, using the uninvolved side of the tongue or lower lip and chin as the control site in order to quantify normalcy. It should be remembered that a poor outcome after attempted microneurosurgery may preclude future surgical options; therefore, the best chance for microneurosurgical success occurs at the first (and most likely, last) surgical intervention.

MEDICOLEGAL ISSUES

Oral and maxillofacial surgeons recognize the potential medicolegal issues related to nerve injuries that occur secondary to third molar removal, and these adverse outcomes account for a large proportion of the malpractice claims in this country and abroad.[83] Based on the information contained in this chapter and recent trends in liability defense, all oral and maxillofacial surgeons should have a minimum understanding of the diagnosis and management of nerve injuries according to the so-called legal parameters of care, with which the legal profession is familiar.[84] These are summarized as follows:

- Spontaneous sensory recovery occurs in most, but not all patients. It is difficult to predict early, it may not be "complete," and it may not be to the patient's satisfaction. Nerves in soft tissue (LN) have a lower rate of spontaneous regeneration than do those in bony canals (IAN).
- All nerve injuries should be documented and evaluated with a history, examination, and neurosensory testing (objective and subjective). The injury should be classified (Seddon or Sunderland). In cases of observed or known nerve injury, prompt referral for microsurgery provides the best opportunity for sensory recovery.
- Repeat examinations at frequent intervals may be necessary. Patients should be followed up for at least 1 month. Complete recovery in 1 month indicates neurapraxia, and no further treatment is indicated. Neurosensory dysfunction that lasts longer than 1 month indicates a higher-grade injury with uncertain spontaneous neurosensory recovery. Microneurosurgical consultation should be considered.
- Nerve injuries that show improvement (objective and/or subjective) may be followed up expectantly. Once improvement stops for a period of time, it usually does not begin again.
- Most nerve injuries resolve within 3 to 9 months, but *only* if improvement begins before 3 months. Patients who are anesthetic at 3 months usually do not achieve significant neurosensory recovery. Prompt microsurgery is usually indicated.
- Patients with partial sensory loss and/or painful sensations *that they find unacceptable* should be considered for microsurgery if objective and subjective findings have not improved or returned to normal by 4 months. Microsurgical delay decreases the chance of success because

progressive distal nerve degeneration and/or the development of a central pain syndrome occur.

- Some painful neuropathies may be managed nonsurgically under the supervision of a microneurosurgeon or other experienced individual (e.g., neurologist).

- Angry uninformed patients with nerve injuries are less likely to improve with any treatment, surgical or nonsurgical. A discussion regarding options and the risk of nerve injury should be provided so that the patient can give informed consent. Local anesthetic injections carry a risk of nerve injury.

- Early surgical intervention (i.e., at 3–4 mo) is *more likely* to produce neurosensory improvement than is late intervention. Surgery delayed beyond 12 months is seriously compromised by distal nerve degeneration and the development of chronic pain syndromes.

- Surgery is *more likely* to improve responses to objective sensory testing and/or to reduce functional impairment than it is to reduce pain or subjective feelings of numbness.

References

1. American Association of Oral and Maxillofacial Surgeons. Parameters and pathways: clinical practice guidelines for oral and maxillofacial surgery (AAOMS ParPath 01), Version 3.0. J Oral Maxillofac Surg 2001;59(Suppl).
2. Pogrel MA, Thamby S. The etiology of altered sensation in the inferior alveolar, lingual, and mental nerve as a result of dental treatment. J Calif Dent J 1999;27:531,534–538.
3. Zuniga JR, Leist JC. Topical tetracycline-induced neuritis: a case report. J Oral Maxillofac Surg 1995;53:196.
4. Leist JC, Zuniga JR. Experimental topical tetracycline-induced neuritis in the rat. J Oral Maxillofac Surg 1995;53:427.
5. Pichler JW, Beirne OR. Lingual flap retraction and prevention of lingual nerve damage associated with third molar surgery: a systematic review of the literature. Oral Surg Oral Med Oral Pathol Oral Radiol Endod 2001;91:395.
6. Rood JP, Shehab AAN. The radiological prediction of inferior alveolar nerve injury during third molar surgery. Br J Oral Maxillofac Surg 1990;28:20.
7. Howe G, Poynton HG: Prevention of damage to the inferior alveolar nerve during the evaluation of mandibular third molars. Br Dent J 1960;109:355.
8. Pogrel MA, Lee JS, Muff DF. Coronectomy in lower third molar removal. J Oral Maxillofac Surg 2003;61(Suppl 1):25.
9. Alling CC. Dysesthesia of the lingual and inferior alveolar nerves following third molar surgery. J Oral Maxillofac Surg 1986;44:454.
10. Gulicher D, Gerlach KL. Sensory impairment of the lingual and inferior alveolar nerves following removal of impacted third molars. Int J Oral Maxillofac Surg 2001;30:306.
11. Carmichael FA, McGowan DA. Incidence of nerve damage following third molar removal: a West Scotland Oral Surgery Research Group study. Br J Oral Maxillofac Surg 1992;30:78.
12. Valmaseda-Castellon E, Berini-Aytes L, Gay-Escoda C. Lingual nerve damage after third lower molar surgical extraction. Oral Surg Oral Med Oral Pathol Oral Radiol Endod 2000;90:567.
13. Valmaseda-Castellon E, Berini-Aytes L, Gay-Escoda C. Inferior alveolar nerve damage after lower third molar surgical extraction: a prospective study of 1117 surgical extractions. Oral Surg Oral Med Oral Pathol Oral Radiol Endod 2001;92:377.
14. Kisselbach JE, Chamberlain JG. Clinical and anatomic observations on the relationship of the lingual nerve to the mandibular third molar region. J Oral Maxillofac Surg 1984;42:565.
15. Pogrel MA, Renaut A, Schmidt B, Ammar A. The relationship of the lingual nerve to the mandibular third molar region: an anatomic study. J Oral Maxillofac Surg 1995;53:1178.
16. Holzle FW, Wolff KD. Anatomic position of the lingual nerve in the mandibular third molar region with special consideration of an atrophied mandibular crest: an anatomical study. Int J Oral Maxillofac Surg 2001;30:333.
17. Miloro M, Halkias LE, Slone HW, Chakeres DW. Assessment of the lingual nerve in the third molar region using magnetic resonance imaging. J Oral Maxillofac Surg 1997;55:134.
18. Harn SD, Durham TM. Incidence of lingual nerve trauma and postinjection complications in conventional mandibular block anesthesia. J Am Dent Assoc 1990;121:519.
19. Pogrel MA, Bryan J, Regezi J. Nerve damage associated with inferior alveolar nerve blocks. J Am Dent Assoc 1995;126:1150.
20. Pogrel MA, Thamby S. Permanent nerve involvement resulting from inferior alveolar nerve blocks. J Am Dent Assoc 2000;131:901.
21. Pogrel MA, Schmidt BL, Sambajon V, et al. Lingual nerve damage due to inferior alveolar nerve blocks: a possible explanation. J Am Dent Assoc 2003;134:195.
22. Van Eeden SP, Patel MF. Letter: prolonged paraesthesia following inferior alveolar nerve block using articaine. Br J Oral Maxillofac Surg 2002;40:519.
23. Stacy GC, Hajjar G. Barbed needle and inexplicable paresthesias and trismus after dental regional anesthesia. Oral Surg Oral Med Oral Pathol 1994;77:585.
24. Pogrel MA, Schmidt BL. Trigeminal nerve chemical neurotrauma from injectable materials. Oral Maxillofac Surg Clin North Am 2001;13:247.
25. Behrman S. Complications of sagittal osteotomy of the mandibular ramus. J Oral Surg 1972;35:554.
26. Hegdvedt AK, Zuniga JR. Lingual nerve injury as a complication of sagittal ramus osteotomy. J Oral Maxillofac Surg 1990;48:647.
27. Schow SR, Triplett RG, Solomon JM. Lingual nerve injury associated with overpenetration of bicortical screws used for rigid fixation of a bilateral sagittal split osteotomy. J Oral Maxillofac Surg 1996;54:1451.
28. August M, Marchena J, Donady J, Kaban L. Neurosensory deficit and functional impairment after sagittal ramus osteotomy: a long-term follow-up study. J Oral Maxillofac Surg 1998;56:1231.
29. Westermark A, Bystedt H, von Konow L. Inferior alveolar nerve function after mandibular osteotomies. Br J Oral Maxillofac Surg 1998;36:425.
30. Karas ND, Boyd SB, Sinn DP. Recovery of neurosensory function following orthognathic surgery. J Oral Maxillofac Surg 1990;48:124.
31. Teerijoki-Oksa T, Jaaskelainen SK, Forssell K, et al. Risk factors of nerve injury during mandibular sagittal split osteotomy. Int J Oral Maxillofac Surg 2001;31:33.
32. Nishioka GJ, Zysset MK, van Sickels JE. Neurosensory disturbance with rigid fixation of the bilateral sagittal split osteotomy. J Oral Maxillofac Surg 1987;45:20.

33. Jones DL, Wolford LM. Intraoperative recording of trigeminal evoked potentials during orthognathic surgery. Int J Adult Orthodon Orthognath Surg 1990;5:167.

34. Hallikainen D, Iizuka T, Lindqvist C. Cross-sectional tomography in evaluation of patients undergoing sagittal split osteotomy. J Oral Maxillofac Surg 1992;50:1269.

35. Frerich B, Cornelius C-P, Wietholter H. Critical time of exposure of the rabbit inferior alveolar nerve to Carnoy's solution. J Oral Maxillofac Surg 1994;52:599.

36. Loescher AR, Robinson PP. The effect of surgical medicaments on peripheral nerve function. Br J Oral Maxillofac Surg 1998;36:327.

37. Block MS, Daire J, Stover J, Matthews M. Changes in the inferior alveolar nerve following mandibular lengthening in the dog using distraction osteogenesis. J Oral Maxillofac Surg 1993;51:652.

38. Hu J, Zou S, Tang Z, et al. Response of Schwann cells in the inferior alveolar nerve to distraction osteogenesis: an ultrastructural and immunohistochemical study. Int J Oral Maxillofac Surg 2003;32:318.

39. Hu J, Tang Z, Wang D, Buckley MJ. Changes in the inferior alveolar nerve after mandibular lengthening with different rates of distraction. J Oral Maxillofac Surg 2001;59:1041.

40. Louis P. Inferior alveolar nerve transposition for endosseous implant placement: a preliminary report. Oral Maxillofac Surg Clin North Am 2001;13:265.

41. Zuniga JR. Normal response to nerve injury: histology and psychophysics of degeneration and regeneration. Oral Maxillofac Surg Clin North Am 1992;4:323.

42. Muller HW, Stoll G. Nerve injury and regeneration: basic insights and therapeutic interventions. Curr Opin Neurol 1998;11:557.

43. Seddon JJ. Three types of nerve injury. Brain 1943;66:237.

44. Sunderland S. A classification of peripheral nerve injuries produced by loss of function. Brain 1951;74:491.

45. Dellon AL, Mackinnon SE. Basic scientific and clinical applications of peripheral nerve regeneration. Surg Annu 1988;20:59.

46. Coglan KM, Irvine GH. Neurological damage after sagittal split osteotomy. Int J Oral Maxillofac Surg 1986;15:369.

47. Zuniga JR, Cheng N, Miller I, Phillips C. Regeneration of taste receptors and recovery of taste after lingual nerve repair. J Oral Maxillofac Surg 1994;52(Suppl 2):128.

48. Zuniga JR, Meyer RA, Gregg JM, et al. The accuracy of clinical neurosensory testing for nerve injury diagnosis. J Oral Maxillofac Surg 1998;56:2.

49. McDonald AR, Roberts TPL, Rowley HA, Pogrel MA. Noninvasive somatosensory monitoring of the injured inferior alveolar nerve using magnetic source imaging. J Oral Maxillofac Surg 1996;54:1968.

50. Scrivani SJ, Moses M, Donoff RB, Kaban LB. Taste perception after lingual nerve repair. J Oral Maxillofac Surg 2000;58:3.

51. Hillerup S, Hjorting-Hansen E, Reumert T. Repair of the lingual nerve after iatrogenic injury: a follow-up study of return of sensation and taste. J Oral Maxillofac Surg 1994;52:1028.

52. Padilla M, Clark GT, Merrill RL. Topical medications for orofacial neuropathic pain: a review. J Am Dent Assoc 2000;131:184.

53. Gregg JM, Small EW. Surgical management of trigeminal pain with radiofrequency lesions of peripheral nerves. J Oral Maxillofac Surg 1986;44:122.

54. Fardy MJ, Patton DW. Complications associated with peripheral alcohol injections in the management of trigeminal neuralgia. Br J Oral Maxillofac Surg 1994;32:387.

55. Khullar S, Emami B, Westermark A, Haanes H. Effect of low-level laser treatment on neurosensory deficits subsequent to sagittal ramus osteotomy. Oral Surg Oral Med Oral Pathol Oral Radiol Endod 1996;82:132.

56. Khullar S, Brodin E, Barkvoll B, Haanes H. Preliminary study of low-level laser treatment of long-standing sensory aberrations of the inferior alveolar nerve. J Oral Maxillofac Surg 1996;54:2.

57. Miloro M, Repasky M. Low-level laser effect on neurosensory recovery after sagittal ramus osteotomy. Oral Surg Oral Med Oral Pathol Oral Radiol Endod 2000;89:12.

58. Zuniga JR. Trigeminal ganglion cell response to mental nerve section and repair in the rat. J Oral Maxillofac Surg 1999;57:427.

59. Pons TP. Massive cortical reorganization after sensory deafferentation in adult macaques. Science 1991;252:1159.

60. Dodson TB, Kaban LB. Recommendations for management of trigeminal nerve defects based on a critical appraisal of the literature. J Oral Maxillofac Surg 1997;55:1380.

61. Smith KG, Roninson PP. An experimental study of three methods of lingual nerve defect repair. J Oral Maxillofac Surg 1995;53:1052.

62. LaBanc JP, Gregg JM. Trigeminal nerve injuries: basic problems, historical perspectives, early successes, and remaining challenges. Oral Maxillofac Surg Clin North Am 1992;4:277.

63. Pogrel MA. The results of microneurosurgery of the inferior alveolar and lingual nerve. J Oral Maxillofac Surg 2002;60:485.

64. Miloro M. Surgical access for inferior alveolar nerve repair. J Oral Maxillofac Surg 1995;53:1224.

65. Joshi A, Rood JP. External neurolysis of the lingual nerve. Int J Oral Maxillofac Surg 2002;31:40.

66. Millesi H, Terzis JK. Nomenclature in peripheral nerve surgery. Clin Plast Surg 1984;11:3.

67. Eppley BL, Snyders RV. Microanatomic analysis of the trigeminal nerve and potential nerve graft donor sites. J Oral Maxillofac Surg 1991;49:612.

68. McCormick SU, Buchbinder D. Microanatomic analysis of the medial antebrachial cutaneous nerve as a potential donor nerve in maxillofacial grafting. J Oral Maxillofac Surg 1994;52:1022.

69. Brammar JP, Epker BN. Anatomic-histologic survey of the sural nerve: implications for inferior alveolar nerve grafting. J Oral Maxillofac Surg 1988;46:111.

70. Miloro M. Subjective outcomes following sural nerve harvest. J Oral Maxillofac Surg 2002;60 Suppl 1:75.

71. Miloro M. Inferior alveolar nerve regeneration through an autogenous vein graft. J Oral Maxillofac Surg 1996;54:65.

72. Pogrel MA, Maghen A. The use of autogenous vein grafts for inferior alveolar and lingual nerve reconstruction. J Oral Maxillofac Surg 2001;59:985.

73. Miloro M. Discussion: the use of autogenous vein grafts for inferior alveolar and lingual nerve reconstruction. J Oral Maxillofac Surg 2001;59:988.

74. Kitahara AK, Suzuki Y, Qi P. Facial nerve repair using a collagen conduit in cats. Scand J Plast Reconstr Surg Hand Surg 1999;33:187.

75. Eppley BL, Delfino JJ. Collagen tube repair of the mandibular nerve: a preliminary investigation in the rat. J Oral Maxillofac Surg 1996;46:41.

76. DeFranzo AJ, Morykwas MJ, LaRosse JR. Autologous denatured muscle as a nerve graft. J Reconstr Microsurg 1994;10:145.

77. Mackinnon SE, Dellon AL. Clinical nerve reconstruction with a bioabsorbable polyglycolic acid tube. Plast Reconstr Surg 1990;85:419.

78. Eppley BL, Snyders RV, Winkelmann T. Efficacy of nerve growth factor in regeneration of the mandibular nerve: a preliminary report. J Oral Maxillofac Surg 1991;49:61.

79. Miloro M, Macy J. Expanded polytetrafluoroethylene entubulation of the rabbit inferior alveolar nerve. Oral Surg Oral Med Oral Pathol 2000;89:292–298.

80. Miloro M, Halkias L, Mallery S, et al. Low level laser effect on neural regeneration in Gore-Tex tubes. Oral Surg Oral Med Oral Pathol Oral Radiol Endod 2002;93:27–34.

81. Pitta MC, Wolford LM, Mehra P, Hopkin J. Use of Gore-Tex tubing as a conduit for inferior alveolar and lingual nerve repair: experience with 6 cases. J Oral Maxillofac Surg 2001;59:493.

82. Pogrel MA, McDonald AR, Kaban LB. Gore-Tex tubing as a conduit for repair of lingual and inferior alveolar nerve continuity defects: a preliminary report. J Oral Maxillofac Surg 1998;56:319.

83. Lydiatt DD. Litigation and the lingual nerve. J Oral Maxillofac Surg 2003;61:197.

84. Deegan AE. The numbing truth. Monitor 1998;9:1.

Appendix
Nerve Terminology Review[*]

allodynia: Pain due to a stimulus that does not normally provoke pain.

analgesia: Absence of pain in the presence of stimulation that would normally be painful.

anesthesia: Absence of any sensation in the presence of stimulation that would normally be painful or nonpainful.

anesthesia dolorosa: Pain in an area or a region that is anesthetic.

atypical neuralgia: A pain syndrome that is not typical of classic nontraumatic trigeminal neuralgia.

axonotmesis (Seddon) or second- through fourth-degree injuries (Sunderland): Nerve injury characterized by axonal injury with subsequent degeneration and regeneration. *Third-degree injury:* Characterized by axonal damage and a breach of the endoneurial sheath, resulting in intrafascicular disorganization. The perineurium and epineurium remain intact. The mechanism is typically traction or compression. *Fourth-degree injury:* Characterized by disruption of the axon, endoneurium, and perineurium, resulting in severe fascicular disorganization. The epineurium remains intact. Possible mechanisms include traction, compression, injection injury, and chemical injury.

causalgia: Burning pain, allodynia, and hyperpathia after a partial injury of a nerve.

central pain: Pain associated with a primary central nervous system lesion (spinal cord or brain trauma, vascular lesions, tumors).

chemoreceptor: A peripheral nerve receptor that is responsive to chemicals, including catecholamines.

deafferentation pain: Pain occurring in a region of partial or complete traumatic nerve injury in which there is interruption of afferent impulses by destruction of the afferent pathway or other mechanism.

dysesthesia: An abnormal sensation, either spontaneous or evoked, that is unpleasant. All dysesthesias are a type of paresthesia but not all paresthesias are dysesthesias.

endoneurium: A connective tissue sheath surrounding individual nerve fibers and their Schwann cells.

epineurium: A loose connective tissue sheath that encases the entire nerve trunk.

fascicle: A bundle of nerve fibers encased by the perineurium.

hyperalgesia: An increased response to a stimulus that is normally painful.

hyperesthesia: An increased sensitivity to stimulation, excluding the special senses (i.e., seeing, hearing, taste, touch, and smell).

hyperpathia: A painful syndrome characterized by increased reaction to a stimulus, especially a repetitive stimulus. The threshold is increased as well.

hypoalgesia: Diminished pain in response to a normally painful stimulus.

hypoesthesia: Decreased sensitivity to stimulation, excluding the special senses (i.e., seeing, hearing, taste, touch, and smell).

mechanoreceptor: A peripheral nerve receptor preferentially activated by physical deformation from pressure and associated with large sensory axons.

mesoneurium: A connective tissue sheath, analogous to the mesentery of the intestine, that suspends the nerve trunk within soft tissue.

---

*Adapted from LaBanc JP, Gregg JM. Glossary. Trigeminal nerve injury: diagnosis and management. Oral Maxillofac Surg Clin North Am 1992;4:563.

monofascicular pattern: Characteristic cross-section of a nerve containing one large fascicle.

neuralgia: Pain in the distribution of a nerve or nerves.

neurapraxia (Seddon) or first-degree injury (Sunderland): Nerve injury characterized by a conduction block, with rapid and virtually complete return of sensation or function and no axonal degeneration.

neuritis: A special case of neuropathy now reserved for inflammatory processes affecting nerves.

neurolysis: The surgical separation of adhesions from an injured peripheral nerve.

neuroma: An anatomically disorganized mass of collagen and nerve fascicles, and a functionally abnormal region of a peripheral nerve resulting from a failed regeneration after injury.

neuropathy: A disturbance of function or a pathologic change in a nerve.

neurotization: Axonal invasion of the distal nerve trunk.

neurotmesis (Seddon) or fifth-degree injury (Sunderland): Nerve injury characterized by severe disruption of the connective tissue components of the nerve trunk, with compromised sensory and functional recovery. *Fifth-degree injury:* Characterized by complete disruption of the nerve trunk with considerable tissue loss. Possible mechanisms include laceration, avulsion, and chemical injury.

nociceptor: A receptor preferentially sensitive to a noxious stimulus or to a stimulus that would become noxious if prolonged.

oligofascicular pattern: Characteristic cross-section of a nerve containing 2 to 10 rather large fascicles.

paresthesia: An abnormal sensation, either spontaneous or evoked, that is not unpleasant. A global term used to encompass all types of nerve injuries.

perineurium: A thick connective tissue sheath surrounding fascicles.

polyfascicular pattern: Characteristic cross-section of a nerve containing greater than 10 fascicles of different sizes, with a prevalence of small fascicles.

protopathia: The inability to distinguish between two different modes of sensation, such as a painful and a nonpainful pinprick.

sympathetically mediated pain: A general term that refers to a family of related disorders including causalgia, reflex sympathetic dystrophy, minor causalgia, Sudeck's atrophy, and postherpetic neuralgia, which may be sympathetically maintained.

synesthesia: A sensation felt in one part of the body when another part is stimulated.

wallerian degeneration: The distal degeneration of the axon and its myelin sheath following injury.

Cleft Lip and Palate

Bernard J. Costello, DMD, MD, and Ramon L. Ruiz, DMD, MD

The comprehensive treatment of cleft lip and palate deformities requires thoughtful consideration of the anatomic complexities of the deformity and the delicate balance between intervention and growth. Comprehensive and coordinated care from infancy through adolescence is essential in order to achieve an ideal outcome, and surgeons with formal training and experience in all of the phases of care must be actively involved in the planning and treatment.[1-3] Specific goals of surgical care for children born with cleft lip and palate include the following:

- Normalized esthetic appearance of the lip and nose
- Intact primary and secondary palate
- Normal speech, language, and hearing
- Nasal airway patency
- Class I occlusion with normal masticatory function
- Good dental and periodontal health
- Normal psychosocial development

Successful management of the child born with a cleft lip and palate requires coordinated care provided by a number of different specialties including oral/maxillofacial surgery, otolaryngology, genetics/dysmorphology, speech/language pathology, orthodontics, prosthodontics, and others.[4] In most cases care of patients with congenital clefts has become a subspecialty area of clinical practice within these different professions. In addition to surgery for cleft repair, treatment plans routinely involve multiple treatment interventions to achieve the above-stated goals. Because care is provided over the entire course of the child's development, long-term follow-up is critical under the care of these different health care providers. The formation of interdisciplinary cleft palate teams has served two key objectives of successful cleft care: (1) coordinated care provided by all of the necessary disciplines, and (2) continuity of care with close interval follow-up of the patient throughout periods of active growth and ongoing stages of reconstruction. The best outcomes are achieved when the team's care is centered on the patient, family, and community rather than a particular surgeon, specialty, or hospital. The idea of having an objective team that does not revolve around the desires of one particular individual or discipline is sometimes impeded by competitive interactions between surgical specialties. Historic battles over surgical domains between surgical specialties and economic factors contribute to these conflicts and negatively affect the work of the team. Healthy team dynamic and optimal patient care are achieved when all members are active participants, when team protocols and referral patterns are equitable and based on the surgeons' formal training and experience instead of specialty identity, and when the needs of the child are placed above the needs of the team.

This chapter presents an overview of the concepts for reconstruction of the cleft lip and palate deformity. The surgical reconstruction of clefts requires that the surgeon undertaking this important work maintain a cognitive understanding of the complex malformation itself, the varied operative techniques employed, facial growth considerations, and the psychosocial health of the patient and family. The objectives of this chapter will be to present the overall staged reconstructive approach for repair of cleft lip and palate from infancy through the time of skeletal maturity, as well as a focused discussion of the specific surgical procedures involved in primary cleft lip and palate repair. Secondary revision procedures, bone graft reconstruction of the cleft maxilla, and orthognathic surgery for cleft-related dysmorphology are discussed in Chapter 42, "Reconstruction of the Alveolar Cleft," Chapter 43, "Reconstruction of Cleft Lip and Palate: Secondary Procedures," and Chapter 60, "Orthognathic Surgery in the Patient with Cleft Palate."

HISTORY OF CLEFT LIP AND PALATE REPAIR

The history of cleft lip and palate care has always been closely linked to dentistry and oral and maxillofacial surgery. The birth and roots of what is now the American Cleft Palate-Craniofacial Association are strongly rooted in dentistry.

The first documented cleft lip repair was performed in ' c 390 on a patient who later became the Governor General of several regions in China, although nothing is known about the actual surgeon.[5,6] Jehan Yperman is believed to have been the first to describe unilateral and bilateral cleft lip repair.[6,7] The first diagrammatic representation of cleft lip repair and cleft palate obturator use is credited to Ambrose Pare in the fourteenth century.[6,8] Much later the first documented successful cleft palate repair was performed by a dentist, Le Monnier, in 1766 in Paris.[6,9] The concepts of cleft lip and palate repair have evolved from straight line repairs to a variety of techniques using various cutbacks, triangles, and Z-plasties.[6-14] During the 1950s, Asensio, an oral and maxillofacial surgeon from Guatemala, developed a novel technique for cleft lip repair, which involved the rotation of the philtral segment inferiorly and advancement of the lateral segment medially using a quadrangular flap. Although he used this approach in Guatemala throughout the 1950s, he did not report it until much later.[15,16] Ralph Millard of Miami described his classic rotational-advancement technique in the mid-1950s, and his concepts changed cleft repair forever.[17,18] Millard is credited with perhaps the most important technical development related to cleft lip repair, and today the majority of surgeons use his original technique or some close modification of it.

In the mid-nineteenth century, Hullihen, recognized as the father of American oral and maxillofacial surgery, published a treatise on comprehensive care of cleft lip and palate deformities.[19] Another pioneer, Truman Brophy, was the professor of oral surgery and dean of the Chicago College of Dentistry and contributed greatly to the care of many patients with clefts. Brophy published a text detailing his experiences with the management of various malformations of the mouth and their surgical repairs including the details of cleft repair.[20] One of his pupils was Chalmers Lyons who started a residency program in oral surgery at the University of Michigan in 1917.[20] Lyons developed the largest cleft practice in America and contributed extensively to the literature.[20]

Many of the concepts related to interdisciplinary care with a cleft palate team care were introduced by Robert Ivy, an oral and maxillofacial surgeon who later became dually qualified in plastic surgery.[20] Robert Ivy trained both in dentistry and medicine at the University of Pennsylvania. After his training in dentistry, Ivy further developed his interests in maxillofacial surgery as an assistant to his uncle, Matthew Cryer, who was a professor in oral surgery at the University of Pennsylvania. Robert Ivy became interested in clefts during his training as the first dental intern at Philadelphia General Hospital at the University of Pennsylvania. His interests in maxillofacial injury led him to serve in France in World War I as an assistant to Vilray Blair. After the war Ivy and Blair's collaboration resulted in two landmark publications by Ivy, *Essentials of Oral Surgery* and *Fractures of the Jaws*. Through work with his state representatives in Harrisburg, Pennsylvania, he was able to start the very first cleft palate clinics in Lancaster, Pittsburgh, Philadelphia, Erie, and Scranton that provided interdisciplinary care to children for cleft lip and palate deformities. When Reed Dingman put forth a resolution of the American Society of Maxillofacial Surgeons condemning oral and maxillofacial surgeons practicing in the hospital setting, Ivy resigned his membership and sent a letter of protest to the organization that he helped build in support of his dental colleagues.[20]

In the 1950s the concept of primary or early bone grafting of the cleft maxillary defect was introduced by Schmid.[21] Although the concept was initially met with enthusiasm from a number of surgeons, primary bone grafting was eventually abandoned due to unfavorable outcomes. During the decades that followed, the negative skeletal, dental, and growth-related consequences of primary bone grafting became better understood.[22,23] During the early 1970s oral and maxillofacial surgeons Boyne and Sands were the first to publish their favorable outcomes using autogenous particulate bone grafts for reconstruction of the cleft maxilla/alveolus later in childhood during the mixed dentition rather than earlier in life.[24] Although their work and results represented a landmark discovery in the field of cleft reconstruction, cleft palate teams were slow to integrate his approach into their treatment protocols because of the negative associations that lingered following the days of primary bone grafting. Today their principles of secondary bone grafting represent the standard approach for almost all of the world's cleft centers.[24,25]

Orthognathic reconstruction of the patient with cleft deformities has been discussed by many authors.[26-36] Early techniques limited some surgeons' options to procedures centered on mandibular setback.[37] During the 1970s the use of total maxillary osteotomy was pioneered by Bell.[38] His novel ideas provided oral and maxillofacial surgeons with an understanding of the biologic basis for maxillary osteotomy, described the vascular supply that allowed the procedures to be performed safely, and as a result incorporated the Le Fort I osteotomy into modern-day practice.[38] Since that time a number of technical refinements have been described for use of the Le Fort I osteotomy specifically in the cleft patient. Much of this work has been done by two of Bell's former pupils, Fonseca and Turvey, who went on to make substantial contributions to the skeletal reconstruction of patients with clefts.[39] Another dual qualified oral and maxillofacial surgeon, Posnick, has published the most complete descriptions of surgical technique modifications for patients undergoing midfacial advancement in the absence of prior bone graft reconstruction and his extensive experiences with the long-term stability of midfacial advancement after correction of various types of cleft deformities with orthognathic techniques.[26–30] Distraction osteogenesis has gained recent popularity for correction of midfacial hypoplasia but has yet to show significant advantages over traditional techniques for the majority of patients.[32,33,40–42]

Comprehensive and coordinated care has become more prevalent across the world, involving many different types of specialty care for children with clefts. Posnick has provided the most comprehensive, succinct, and evidenced-based discussions on the topic of cleft lip and palate reconstruction from infancy through adolescence.[26] These efforts as well as craniofacial training programs associated with oral and maxillofacial surgery have helped to solidify the role of oral and maxillofacial surgery in the comprehensive care of patients with clefts.

EMBRYOLOGY

To understand the goals of lip and palate repair from an anatomic standpoint the cleft surgeon must have an appreciation for the failure of embryogenesis that results in clefting. There are critical points in the development of the fetus when the fusion of various prominences creates continuity and form to the lip, nose, and palate. Anomalies occur when the normal developmental process is disturbed between these components. Each of these prominences is made up of ectomesenchyme derived from neural crest tissue of the mesencephalon and rhombencephalon. Mesoderm is also present within these prominences as mesenchymal tissue. The prescribed destiny of each of these cells and tissues is controlled by various genes to alter the migration, development, and apoptosis and form the normal facial tissues of the fetus. At the molecular level there are many interdependent factors such as signal transduction, mechanical stress, and growth factor production that affect the development of these tissues. Currently only portions of this complex interplay of growth, development, and apoptosis are clear.

At approximately 6 weeks of human embryologic development the median nasal prominence fuses with the lateral nasal prominences and maxillary prominences to form the base of the nose, nostrils, and upper lip. The confluence of these anterior components becomes the primary palate. When this mechanism fails, clefts of the lips and/or maxilla occur. At approximately 8 weeks the palatal shelves elevate and fuse with the septum to form the intact secondary palate. When one palatal shelf fails to fuse with the other components, then a unilateral cleft of the secondary palate occurs. If both of the palatal shelves fail to fuse with each other and the midline septum, then a bilateral cleft of the palate occurs.

Fusion occurs when programmed cell death (apoptosis) occurs at the edges of the palatal shelves. The ectodermal component disintegrates and the mesenchyme fuses to form the intact palate. Soon after this the anterior primary palate fuses with the secondary palate and ossification occurs. At any point, if failure of fusion occurs with any of the above components, a cleft will occur of the primary and/or secondary palates. Clefts may be complete or incomplete based on the degree of this failure of fusion.

GENETICS AND ETIOLOGY

Clefts of the upper lip and palate are the most common major congenital craniofacial abnormality and are present in approximately 1 in 700 live births.[43] Although inheritance may play a role, cleft lip and palate is not considered a single-gene disease. Instead clefts are thought to be of a multifactorial etiology with a number of potential contributing factors. These factors may include chemical exposures, radiation, maternal hypoxia, teratogenic drugs, nutritional deficiencies, physical obstruction, or genetic influences. One prevailing theory relates the process of clefting as a threshold in which multiple factors come together to raise the individual above a threshold at which time the mechanism of fusion fails.[44,45] Recently multiple genes have been implicated in the etiology of clefting.[46–48] Some of these genes include the *MSX*, *LHX*, *goosecoid*, and *DLX* genes. Additional disturbances in growth factors or their receptors that may be involved in the failure of fusion include fibroblast growth factor, transforming growth factor-, platelet-derived growth factor, and epidermal growth factor.

Clefts of the lip occur more commonly in males than in females.[49] In addition left-sided cleft lips are more common than right-sided cleft lips, and unilateral cleft lips are more common than the bilateral cleft of the lip.[50] Bilateral clefts of the lip are most often associated with clefting of both the primary and secondary palates. Cleft palate alone is seen in approximately 1 in 2,000 live births and this incidence is similar in all racial groups.[51] Significant differences in the prevalence of clefts exist when specific ethnic/racial populations are examined. For example, African Americans have a birth prevalence that is less common than the total population, but Asians tend to have a higher prevalence.

In the majority of cases unilateral cleft lip and palate is an isolated nonsyndromic birth defect that is not associated with any other major anomalies.[43,52,53] By comparison a much greater proportion of patients with an isolated cleft palate will have an associated syndrome or sequence.[43,53] Some of the more common syndromes seen in this group include Stickler's, Van der Woude's, or DiGeorge syndromes. It is important to identify the diagnosis early, as functional issues may arise early in life and go unnoticed. For example, patients with an isolated cleft palate should be evaluated early by an experienced pediatric ophthalmologist to evaluate the possibility of Stickler's syndrome. Patients with Stickler's syndrome may have ocular abnormalities that lead to retinal detachment. In an otherwise healthy-appearing child these findings may be difficult to diagnose and so early visual loss

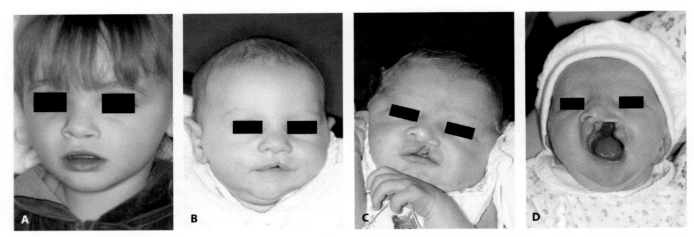

FIGURE 43-1.   Cleft lips come in a variety of configurations, such that each repair must be customized to establish the most normal morphology. **A,** Microform left unilateral cleft lip only, not requiring primary repair. **B,** Minor left incomplete unilateral cleft lip only. **C,** Left incomplete unilateral cleft lip and palate with a Simonart's band. **D,** Wide left complete unilateral cleft lip and palate.

may go unnoticed. In many cases long-term genetics follow-up is necessary to make a definitive diagnosis and to provide genetic counseling.

The chances of a recurrence of clefting within a family are dependent on many factors, including family history, severity, gender, degree of relationship to the affected individual, and the expression of a syndrome. Predicting the inheritance patterns of families who have a history of cleft lip and/or palate can be complicated. A skilled geneticist/dysmorphologist is best equipped to make these determinations based on pedigree analysis and genetic testing. Since most clefts are sporadic the chances of a family having another child with a cleft after having a child with a unilateral cleft lip and palate in which there was no family history of clefting is approximately 2 to 4%. The chances are higher if additional family history is present or if the cleft is bilateral.[54,55] The nature of any genetic influence will have an effect on the presence of a cleft. Such is the case in patients with autosomal dominant syndromes such as Stickler syndrome where 50% of the children may express the syndrome if one of the parents carries the altered gene.

CLASSIFICATION

The typical classification system used clinically to describe standard clefts of the lip and palate is based on careful anatomic description. Clefts can be unilateral or bilateral; microform, incomplete, or complete; and may involve the lip, nose, primary palate, and/or secondary palates (Figure 43-1). The presentation of clefts is extremely variable, and the individual repairs are custom-tailored to achieve the best symmetry and balance. More severe facial clefting is most commonly described using Tessier's orbitocentric system of numbering (Figure 43-2).[56] Other systems exist that are based on embryologic fusion planes, but these are cumbersome to use in routine clinical practice.[57]

PRENATAL COUNSELING

Recent advances in ultrasound imaging have revolutionized prenatal care and maternal-fetal medicine. Currently ultrasound images of clefts of the lip can be visualized as early as 16 weeks.[58–60] Diagnostic images of the palate are more difficult to acquire, making the correct prenatal diagnosis of a cleft palate less predictable. Palatal structures may be visualized using sagittal and coronal views, but this currently requires the very latest technology and a skilled ultrasonographer with experience performing this type of study.

When the diagnosis of cleft lip is made during pregnancy the family can then be referred to an experienced surgeon for a prenatal discussion. A prenatal consultation provides an excellent opportunity to explain the diagnosis, review the different stages of cleft lip and palate reconstruction that may be necessary, and prepare the parents for practical considerations such as feeding of a child with a cleft palate. This gives the family the opportunity to ask questions, calm fears, and learn about feeding techniques that will be important during the first week of life for their baby. Parents are empowered with this new knowledge, and the preparations made during a prenatal consultation allow them to anticipate the delivery of their baby with a greater comfort level regarding the necessary care of the child during the early postnatal period. The family is then referred to a cleft and craniofacial team in order to undergo a more thorough interdisciplinary approach.

Critical to this process is consultation with a geneticist/dysmorphologist to further discuss the issues associated with the birth and the possibility of other associated deformities. Additional testing may be warranted to evaluate the possibility of associated deformities, syndromes, or sequences that could affect the birthing process. Exceptionally skilled ultrasonographers can visualize airway development and other abnormalities that may require early intervention with fetal

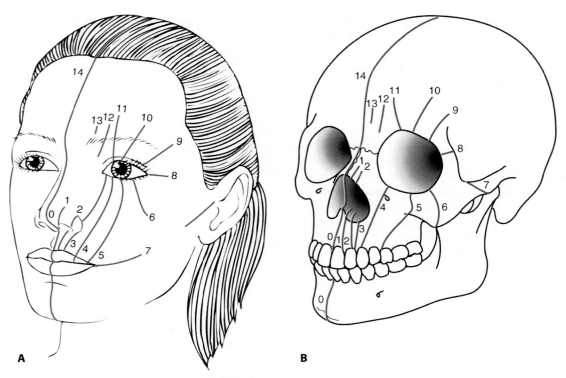

FIGURE 43-2. **A** and **B,** Complex facial clefts can be classified based on Tessier's original orbitocentric system of numbering. Clefts may involve all tissue planes including skin, mucosa, bone, teeth, muscle, brain, peripheral nerve, and other specialized tissues.

surgery, exit procedures, extracorporeal membrane oxygenation, or surgical airway management (tracheotomy) at the time of delivery.

In some medical centers fetal diagnosis and treatment teams are in place to deal with issues associated with various deformities diagnosed in the prenatal period. These teams foster a cohesive environment where information is exchanged through consultation. Much like in the environment of a cleft and craniofacial team, families can get the best information available to consider their child's treatment decisions using an interdisciplinary care model that is patient (mother and fetus), family, and community oriented.

FEEDING CONCERNS

Children born with isolated cleft lip can feed quite well and even have the opportunity to breastfeed in most instances. However, infants with cleft palate can have difficulty feeding due to the inability to form an adequate seal between the tongue and palate for creation of sufficient negative pressure to suck fluid from a bottle. Nasal regurgitation and inefficient handling of secretions and foodstuffs may also be observed during early development. Specialized nipples and bottles are necessary to improve feeding immediately after birth. The most useful devices combine oversized nipples with reservoir spaces and large openings, a squeezable bottle to push fluid into the nipple assembly, and a one-way valve that allows the

bolus of fluid to pass from the bottle to the nipple only in order to minimize the amount of work the child must perform to feed. These include a variety of nipples with reservoirs that collect a variable volume of liquid that can be expressed more easily when sucking is inefficient or not possible. Bottles that can be squeezed to allow for manual flow of liquid to the infant are helpful for improving feeding. No single bottle and nipple combination tends to work better than another, but trials with a variety of types using different techniques are helpful in optimizing feeding early in life. Close attention to weight gain is necessary for these children. Generally, in 24 hours each infant should have approximately 2 to 3 ounces of milk for each pound of weight. Feeding sessions should last no longer than 35 minutes as longer sessions are fatiguing and burn more calories than the baby can consume. Infants should be weighed at least weekly using the same scale, preferably at their pediatrician's office.

The subject of breast-feeding an infant with a cleft palate is controversial, with some practitioners encouraging the practice and others strongly opposed to it. There are clear advantages to breast-feeding a newborn, including passive immunologic contribution of the mother to the child in the form of secretory immunoglobulin A and an experience that enhances bonding between the mother and child during such a critical period.[61,62] At the same time the infant's inability to create negative oral pressure will often make successful nursing difficult, if not impossible. It is relatively common to encounter an exclusively breast-fed infant with severe dehydration and failure to thrive secondary to these difficulties. This is especially a concern in infants that have a wide cleft of the secondary palate, where breast-feeding may not be possible. The authors' approach with regard to breast-feeding in the presence of a cleft palate is to use a combined protocol that includes intermittent feeding with the use of a specialized bottle (as described above) and attempts at nursing. Breast milk may be pumped for use with the specialized nipple and bottle that will provide the nutritional and immunologic benefits desired. This also allows the parents to keep a more quantitative record of how many ounces have been ingested over the course of the day since this is normally difficult with breast-feeding alone. At the same time the mother and baby are not deprived of an opportunity to incorporate breast-feeding into the daily regimen. This approach obviously requires rigorous documentation of the child's weight, consultation with a lactation consultant and infant feeding specialist, and frequent follow-up evaluations through the surgeon and/or pediatrician.

TREATMENT PLANNING AND TIMING: OVERVIEW

The timing of cleft lip and palate repair is controversial. Despite a number of meaningful advancements in the care of patients with cleft lip and palate, a lack of consensus exists regarding the timing and specific techniques used during each stage of cleft reconstruction. Surgeons must continue to carefully balance the functional needs, esthetic concerns, and the issue of ongoing growth when deciding how and when to intervene. In no other type of surgical problem is the issue of early surgery's effect on growth more apparent than in the treatment of cleft lip and palate deformities. The decision to surgically manipulate the tissues of the growing child should not be made lightly and should take into account the possible growth restriction that can occur with early surgery. Nevertheless many patients with congenital deformities will benefit from surgical intervention based on functional or psychosocial reasons. Understanding the growth and development of the craniofacial skeleton is critical to the treatment planning process.[33] In many cases waiting for a greater degree of growth to occur is advantageous unless compelling functional or esthetic issues are present that can not or should not wait.

Due to many different treatment philosophies the timing of treatment interventions is considerably variable amongst cleft centers. Therefore, it is difficult to produce a timing regimen that everyone agrees on. Each stage of surgical reconstruction and the suggested timing based on the patient's age are presented in Table 43-1. Special considerations may alter the sequencing or timing of the various procedures based on individual functional or esthetic needs.

Cleft lip repair is generally undertaken at some point after 10 weeks of age. One advantage of waiting until the child is 10 to 12 weeks of age is that it allows a complete medical evaluation of the patient so that any associated congenital

TABLE 43-1. **Staged Reconstruction of Cleft Lip and Palate Deformities**

Procedure	Timing
Cleft lip repair	After 10 weeks
Cleft palate repair	9–18 months
Pharyngeal flap or pharyngoplasty	3–5 years or later based on speech development
Maxillary/alveolar reconstruction with bone grafting	6–9 years based on dental development
Cleft orthognathic surgery	14–16 years in girls, 16–18 years in boys
Cleft rhinoplasty	After age 5 years but preferably at skeletal maturity; after orthognathic surgery when possible
Cleft lip revision	Anytime once initial remodeling and scar maturation is complete but best performed after age 5 years

defects affecting other organ systems (eg, cardiac or renal anomalies) may be uncovered. The surgical procedure itself may be easier when the child is slightly larger and the anatomic landmarks more prominent and well defined. Historically the anesthetic risk-related data suggested that the safest time period for surgery in this population of infants could be outlined simply by using the "rule of 10's." This referred to the idea of delaying lip repair until the child was at least 10 weeks old, 10 pounds in weight, and with a minimum hemoglobin value of 10 dL/mg.[63,64] Today more sophisticated pediatric techniques, advances in intraoperative monitoring, and improved anesthetic agents have all resulted in the ability to provide safe general anesthesia much earlier in life.[65] Despite the ability to provide safe anesthesia earlier in life, there is no measurable benefit to performing lip repair prior to 3 months of age.[64,66,67] Some surgeons have advocated that lip repair be carried out in the first days of infancy based on the idea of capitalizing on early "fetal-like" healing. Unfortunately these hoped-for benefits have not been observed, and problems with excessive scarring and less favorable outcomes have been encountered instead.[68–70] Children may have more scarring at this early age, and their tissues are smaller and more difficult to manipulate. Consequently the esthetic outcomes may be worse if surgery is performed at an earlier age, and since there are no clear benefits to earlier repair the recommendations for repair stand at approximately 3 months of age.

Cleft palate repair is usually performed at approximately 9 to 18 months of age. In deciding the timing of repair the surgeon must consider the delicate balance between facial growth restriction after early surgery and speech development that requires an intact palate. Most children will require an intact palate to produce certain speech sounds by 18 months of age. If developmental delay is present and speech will not likely develop until later, then the repair can be delayed further. There is little evidence to suggest any benefit to palate repair prior to 9 months of age.[71–73] Repairs prior to this time are associated with a much higher incidence of maxillary hypoplasia later in life and show no improvements in speech. For these reasons most surgeons will perform primary palate repair at approximately 9 to 12 months of age.

As the child continues to develop, approximately 20% of children will have inadequate closure of the velopharyngeal mechanism (velopharyngeal insufficiency or VPI), and this may produce hypernasal speech.[74] These children are usually diagnosed at 3 to 5 years of age when a detailed speech examination can be obtained by a skilled speech pathologist familiar with clefts. When VPI is shown to be consistent and due to a definable anatomic defect, surgery is often helpful in correcting this problem. A pharyngeal flap or sphincter pharyngoplasty may be used to treat VPI, with the goal of improving closure between the oral and nasal cavities and reducing nasal air escape during the production of certain sounds. The details of assessment, diagnosis, and treatment of VPI associated with cleft palate are discussed in Chapter 43, "Reconstruction of Cleft Lip and Palate: Secondary Procedures." Approximately 75% of patients with any type of cleft will present with clefting of the maxilla and alveolus.[24–26] Bone graft reconstruction of this site is performed during the mixed dentition prior to the eruption of the permanent canine and/or the permanent lateral incisor. The timing of this procedure is based on dental development and not chronologic age. Based on work by Boyne and Sands, most surgeons reconstruct this area during the mixed dentition prior to eruption of the permanent canine. Earlier reconstruction of this area has been associated with a high degree of maxillary growth restriction requiring orthognathic correction later in life in a much higher percentage of patients.[22,24] The gold standard for reconstruction in this area is autogenous bone from the anterior iliac crest. Cranial bone, rib, tibia, symphysis of the mandible, zygoma, and allogeneic bone have all been studied, but none have been shown to be appreciably better than the iliac crest.[26,75,76]

Orthognathic reconstruction of maxillary and mandibular discrepancies is performed at 14 to 18 years of age based on individual growth characteristics.[26–36,38] This is done in conjunction with orthodontics prior to and after surgery. However, in some cases of severe maxillary hypoplasia, early Le Fort I osteotomy may be performed to optimize facial esthetics and occlusion with the supposition that revision osteotomies will likely be necessary. These early osteotomies may complicate later treatment. Early orthognathic correction is reserved for the most severe dysmorphology, and in most cases the authors prefer standard orthognathic techniques.[31–33] Attempts at using distraction osteogenesis have been associated with a higher complication rate than with standard orthognathic techniques.[32,42,77] Orthognathic correction of the deformities associated with cleft lip and palate defects is discussed in Chapter 60, "Orthognathic Surgery in the Patient with Cleft Palate."

As with the timing of other interventions, lip and nasal revision is best reserved until after the majority of growth is complete. Most of the lip and nasal growth is complete after age 5 years. Lip revision can be considered prior to school age at about 5 years of age. However, this may be performed earlier if the deformity is severe. Nasal revision is performed after age 5 years as most of the nasal growth is also complete by this time. If orthognathic reconstruction is likely, then rhinoplasty is usually best performed after orthognathic surgery as maxillary advancement improves many characteristics of nasal support. However, when nasal deformity is particularly severe, rhinoplasty can be considered earlier even if orthognathic surgery is expected. Multiple early revisions of the lip or nose should be avoided so that excess scarring does not potentially impair ongoing growth. Secondary revisions of cleft lip and palate deformities are discussed in Chapter 43, "Reconstruction of Cleft Lip and Palate: Secondary Procedures."

CLEFT LIP AND PALATE REPAIR

Presurgical Taping and Presurgical Orthopedics

Facial taping with elastic devices is used for application of selective external pressure and may allow for improvement of lip and nasal position prior to the lip repair procedure. In the authors' opinions these techniques often have greater impact in cases of wide bilateral cleft lip and palate where manipulation of the premaxillary segment may make primary repair technically easier. Although one of the basic surgical tenets of wound repair is to close wounds under minimal tension, attempts at improving the arrangement of the segments using taping methods have not shown a measurable improvement.[78–80]

Some surgeons prefer presurgical orthopedic (PSO) appliances rather than lip taping to achieve the same goals.[81,82] PSO appliances are composed of a custom-made acrylic base plate that provides improved anchorage in the molding of lip, nasal, and alveolar structures during the presurgical phase of treatment (Figure 43-3). Although the use of appliances probably makes for an easier surgical repair, there

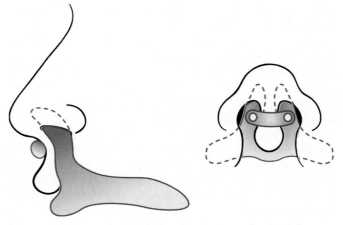

FIGURE 43-3. Frontal and lateral views of the Grayson nasoalveolar molding appliance showing the nasal projections that help to theoretically mold the nasal cartilages and maxillary segments into a more appropriate configuration prior to repair.

has been a lack of clinical evidence to demonstrate that there is any measurable improvement in esthetics of the nose or lip, dental arch relationship, tooth survival, or occlusion. Studies have looked at the dental arch relationship outcomes in patients who have infant presurgical orthopedic devices, and no improvement in dental arch relationship was seen.[83,84] Additionally no long-term improvement in speech outcome has be demonstrated in patients who had PSOs.[85] Furthermore concerns regarding potential negative consequences with these types of appliances have been raised.[86] PSOs also add significant cost and time to treatment early in the child's life. Many appliances require a general anesthetic for the initial impression used to fabricate the device. Frequent appointments are necessary for monitoring of the anatomic changes and periodic appliance adjustment.

The Latham appliance was popular for expanding and aligning the maxillary segments of the patient with a cleft palate.[87] It is a pin-retained device that is inserted into the palate with acrylic extensions onto the alveolar ridges. A screw mechanism is then used to manipulate the segments as desired. The Latham appliance has been shown to be associated with significant growth restriction of the midface when used in infancy to approximate the segments prior to definitive repair.[86] Children who have had Latham appliances have been shown to have significant midfacial growth restriction in adolescence 100% of the time whereas children who have not had the Latham appliance have midface hypoplasia 25 to 35% of the time.[42,80,86]

The nasoalveolar molding appliance has become popular with some surgeons in attempts to manipulate the segments without pin retention prior to lip and nose repair (see Figure 43-3). The appliance popularized by Grayson is adjustable by removing or adding acrylic and manipulating protrusive elements that attempt to mold the nasal cartilages. This device attempts to align the alveolar segments, lip structures, and nasal cartilages to optimize repair. Unfortunately the hoped-for advantages of this appliance have not been realized. Additionally no long-term data are available regarding growth in the craniofacial skeleton after using this protocol. The limited short-term data that are available cannot be extrapolated to determine the ultimate outcome on growth, function, or esthetics. Some surgeons use gingivoperiosteoplasty in conjunction with the PSO, using limited flaps to close the alveolus cleft during the primary repair of the lip or palate. Many surgeons who use this appliance in conjunction with their primary lip repairs will perform a gingivoperiosteoplasty in attempts to have bone form at the alveolus. This is more easily performed with the segments aligned in close proximity as the flaps are small.[82] Experiences with similar techniques in the 1960s involving primary bone grafting were poor with respect to growth.[22,23] Additionally there has been no convincing long-term objective data showing improvement in either lip or nose esthetics.

In their current state of technical refinement there is no evidence that any of the PSOs offer an improved outcome with respect to esthetics, function, or growth in patients with cleft lip and palate. Coupled with the fact that appliances are time-consuming and have a high cost of fabrication and utilization, it is difficult to advocate their uniform use. As with other interventions considered for patients with clefts, costly and unproven interventions should be avoided, although they may prove to be helpful in some select cases.[88] Hopefully, long-term data will be forthcoming and positive to help determine which patients may benefit from PSO appliance treatment.

Lip Adhesion

Some surgeons attempt to surgically approximate the segments of the cleft lip prior to definitive lip repair in an attempt to achieve a better relationship of both the lip structures and the dental arches.[89–91] This is achieved by advancing small flaps of tissue across the cleft site. While some surgeons advocate the use of this technique in wide bilateral clefts, it is rarely performed in unilateral cases. When used, the lip adhesion is usually completed at 3 months of age. In most cases this will convert a wide complete cleft into a wide incomplete cleft as the scar will eventually be excised from the cleft site recreating a similar wide deformity. The definitive lip repair is then completed 3 to 9 months later by excising the scar and reapproximating the remaining lip structures. Furthermore at the second procedure there is usually less supple tissue to work with when performing the definitive repair due to scarring. As with most endeavors in cleft surgery, repeated early interventions tend to complicate later refinements due to excessive scarring. In general adequate mobilization of the flaps in one stage will make tension-free skin closure possible in almost every case without the need for taping, presurgical orthopedic appliances, and/or lip adhesion.

Unilateral Cleft Lip Repair

Clefts of the lip and nose that are unilateral present with a high degree of variability, and thus each repair design is unique (see Figure 43-1).[26,92] The repair technique preferred by the authors for cleft lip and nasal deformities is shown in Figures 43-4 and 43-5 and is usually performed after 10 weeks of age.[17,18,26,63] The basic premise of the repair is to create a three-layered closure of skin, muscle, and mucosa that approximates normal tissue and excises hypoplastic tissue at the cleft margins. Critical in the process is the reconstruction of the orbicularis oris musculature into a continuous sphincter. The Millard rotation-advancement technique has the advantage of allowing for each of the incision lines to fall within the natural contours of the lip and nose. This is an advantage because it is difficult to achieve "mirror image" symmetry in the unilateral cleft lip and nose with the normal side immediately adjacent to the surgical site. A Z-plasty technique such as the Randall-Tennison repair may not achieve this level of symmetry because the

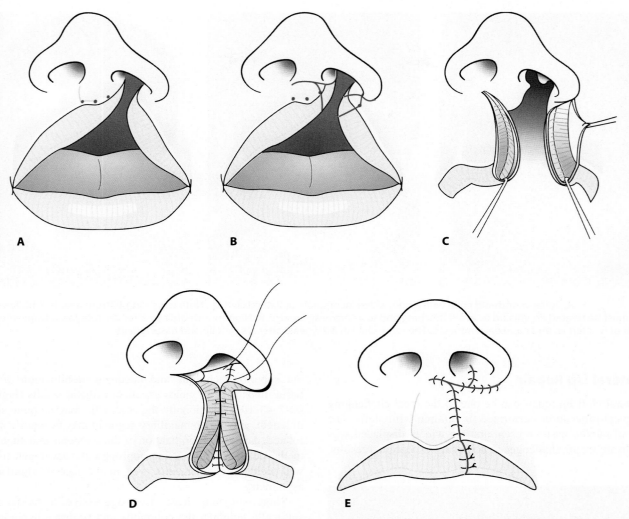

FIGURE 43-4.   **A,** A complete unilateral cleft of the lip is shown highlighting the hypoplastic tissue in the cleft site that is not used in the reconstruction. Note the nasal deformities that are typical in the unilateral cleft, including displaced lower lateral nasal cartilages, deviated anterior septum, and nasal floor clefting. **B,** The typical markings for the authors' preferred repair are shown highlighting the need to excise the hypoplastic tissue and approximate good vermilion and white roll tissue for the repair. **C,** Once the hypoplastic tissue has been excised, the three layers of tissue are dissected (skin, muscle, and mucosa). It is important to completely free the orbicularis oris from its abnormal insertions on the anterior nasal spine area and lateral alar base. Nasal flaps are also incorporated into the dissection to repair the nasal floor (not shown). **D,** The orbicularis oris muscle is approximated with multiple interrupted sutures, and the vermilion border/white roll complex is reconstructed. The nasal floor and mucosal flaps are approximated. **E,** The lateral flap is advanced and the medial segment is rotated downward to create a healing scarline that will resemble the natural philtral column on the opposite side. The incision lines are hidden in natural contours and folds of the nose and lip.

Z-shaped scar is directly adjacent to the linear nonclefted philtrum (Figure 43-6). Achieving symmetry is more difficult when the rotation portion of the cleft is short in comparison to the advancement segment.

Primary nasal reconstruction may be considered at the time of lip repair to reposition the displaced lower lateral cartilages and alar tissues. Several techniques are advocated, and considerable variation exists with respect to the exact nasal reconstruction performed by each surgeon.[93,94] The primary nasal repair may be achieved by releasing the alar base, augmenting the area with allogeneic subdermal grafts, or even a formal open rhinoplasty. Since lip repair is done at such an early point in growth and development, the authors prefer minimal surgical dissection due to the effects of scarring on the subsequent growth of these tissues. McComb described a technique that has become popular, consisting of dissecting the lower lateral cartilages free from the alar base and the surrounding attachments through an alar crease incision.[93,95–97] This allows the nose to be bolstered and/or stented from within the nostril to improve symmetry.

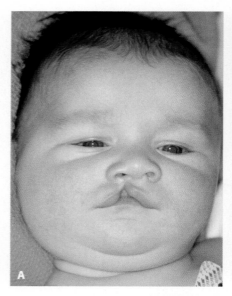
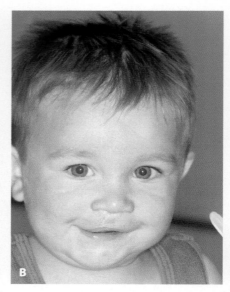
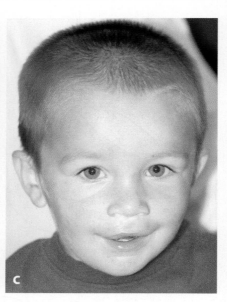

FIGURE 43-5.   **A,** Three-month-old child with a right-sided incomplete unilateral cleft lip. Note the short philtrum near the midline that must be rotated downward to avoid notching and to improve symmetry. **B,** Nine-month-old boy after the rotation-advancement repair of his cleft lip and nasal deformities. **C,** The same child in B 2½ years after his cleft lip and nasal repairs.

Bilateral Lip Repair

Bilateral cleft lip repair can be one of the most challenging technical procedures performed in children with clefts. The lack of quality tissue present and the widely displaced segments are major challenges to achieving exceptional results,

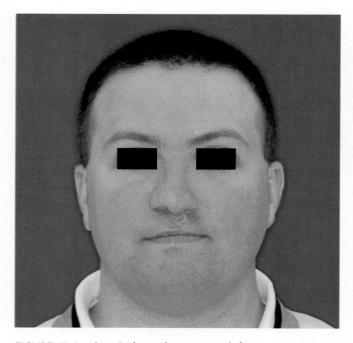

FIGURE 43-6.   A typical scar that may result from a Z-type lengthening repair. Although the length and symmetry of the lip is good, an unnatural contour can occur due to the Z shape of the closure.

but superior technique and adequate mobilization of the tissue flaps usually yields excellent esthetic results (Figures 43-7–43-10). Additionally the columella may be quite short in length, and the premaxillary segment may be significantly rotated. Adequate mobilization of the segments and attention to the details of only using appropriately developed tissue will yield excellent results even in the face of significant asymmetry.

Some surgeons have used aggressive techniques to surgically lengthen the columella and preserve hypoplastic tissue using banked fork flaps.[98,99] Early and aggressive tissue flaps in the nostril and columella areas do not look natural after significant growth has occurred and result in abnormal tissue contours. While surgical attempts at lengthening the columella may look good initially, they frequently look abnormally long and excessively angular later in life (Figure 43-11). Revision of these iatrogenic deformities is difficult and some of the contour irregularities will not be able to be revised adequately. Usually if the hypoplastic tissue is excised and incisions within the medial nasal base and columella are avoided, the long-termes thetic results are excellent.

The authors prefer a primary nasal reconstruction that can be performed in a similar fashion to the unilateral technique described by McComb.[100] This allows for release and repositioning of the lower lateral cartilages and alar base on both sides without aggressive degloving of the entire nasal complex. Other open rhinoplasty techniques have been suggested using either direct incision on the nasal tip or through prolabial unwinding techniques.[100–103] As with most early maneuvers aggressive rhinoplasty at this time may incur early scarring that affects the growth potential of the surrounding

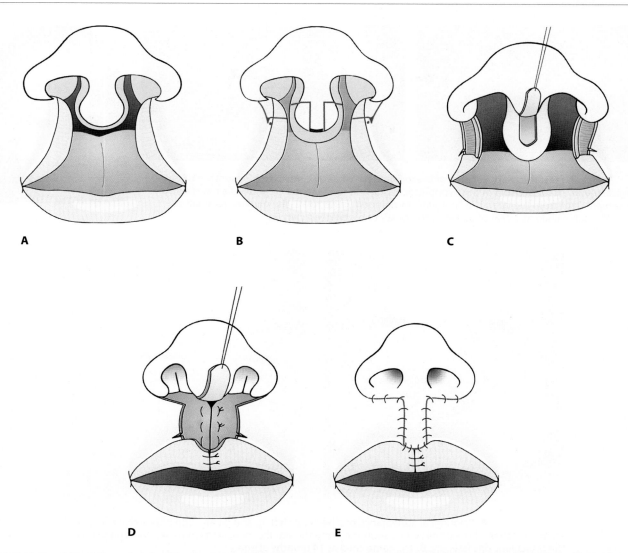

FIGURE 43-7.   **A,** The bilateral cleft of the lip and maxilla shown here is complete and highlights the hypoplastic tissue along the cleft edges. The importance of the nasal deformity is evident in the shorter columella and disrupted nasal complexes. **B,** Markings of the authors' preferred repair are shown with an emphasis on excision of hypoplastic tissue and approximating more normal tissue with the advancement flaps. **C,** A new philtrum is created by excising the lateral hypoplastic tissue and elevating the philtrum superiorly. Additionally the lateral advancement flaps are dissected into three distinct layers (skin, muscle, and mucosa). Nasal floor reconstruction is also performed. **D,** The orbicularis oris musculature is approximated in the midline with multiple interrupted and/or mattress sutures. This is a critical step in the total reconstruction of the functional lip. There is no musculature present in the premaxillary segment, and this must be brought to the midline from each lateral advancement flap. The nasal floor flaps are sutured at this time as well. The new vermillion border is reconstructed in the midline with good white-roll tissue advanced from the lateral flaps. **E,** The final approximation of the skin and mucosal tissues is performed leaving the healing incision lines in natural contours of the lip and nose.

tissues, making revision more difficult and long-term esthetics less than ideal.

Cleft Palate Repair

The term *primary palate* is used to describe the anatomic structures anterior to the incisive foramen (eg, the alveolar ridge, maxilla, piriform rim). The term *secondary palate* refers to those structures posterior to the incisive foramen.

Therefore, when surgeons refer to the initial or "primary" cleft palate repair, they are actually describing the closure of the secondary palate structures that include the hard palate, soft palate, and uvula. The structures of the embryologic primary palate are reconstructed later in childhood during the cleft maxillary/ alveolar bone graft procedure.

There are two main goals of cleft palate repair during infancy: (1) the water-tight closure of the entire oronasal communication involving the hard and soft palate; and (2) the

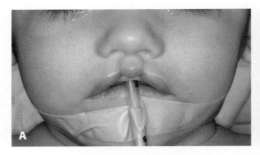
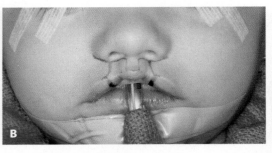
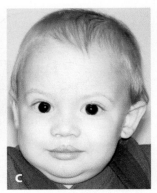

FIGURE 43-8.   **A,** Presurgical appearance of the incomplete bilateral cleft lip of a 3-month-old boy. **B,** Surgical markings for excision of the hypoplastic tissue and the planned creation of a new philtrum. Advancement flaps from the lateral lip segments bring good white-roll to the midline via small cutbacks. **C,** The same child at 1 year of age after the repair of his bilateral cleft lip.

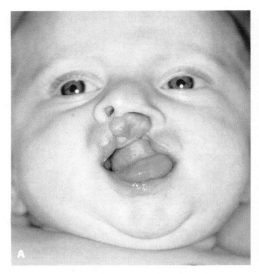
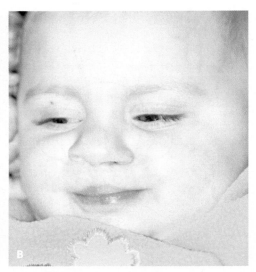

FIGURE 43-9.   **A,** Presurgical appearance of a bilateral cleft lip and palate with impressive asymmetry and rotation of the premaxillary segment. Note the significant nasal asymmetry and bunching of the orbicularis oris laterally. **B,** The same child at 14 months of age.

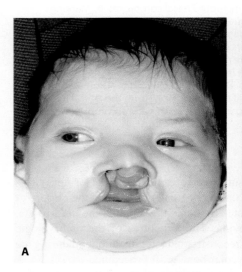
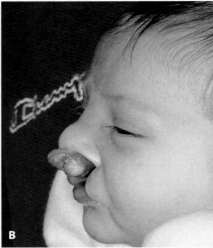
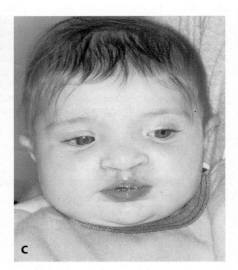

FIGURE 43-10.   **A,** Presurgical frontal view of a wide bilateral cleft lip and palate with significant asymmetry and lack of columella length. **B,** Presurgical left lateral view of a wide bilateral cleft lip and palate with a protrusive premaxillary segment. Note the short columella length. **C,** The same child at 10 months of age after repair of her bilateral cleft lip and palate. No presurgical taping or orthopedic appliances were used.

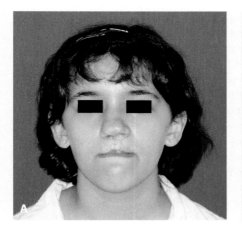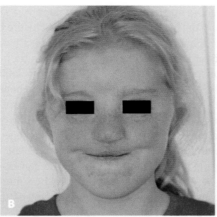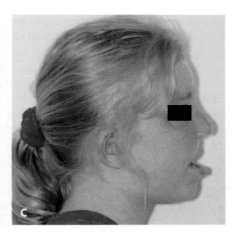

FIGURE 43-11. **A,** Frontal view of a teenage girl who had undergone columella lengthening and banked fork flaps during her initial repair and multiple attempts at secondary rhinoplasty by another surgeon prior to orthognathic surgery. **B,** Frontal view of a patient who underwent columella lengthening and banked fork flaps during her initial repair. **C,** Lateral view of the patient from B with a columella that is curved upwards and abnormally angular.

anatomic repair of the musculature within the soft palate that is critical for normal creation of speech. The soft palate, or velum, is part of the complex coupling and decoupling of the oral and nasal cavities involved in the production of speech. When a cleft of the soft palate is present there are abnormal muscle insertions located at the posterior edge of the hard palate. Surgery must not simply be aimed at closing the palatal defect but rather at the release of abnormal muscle insertions. Muscle continuity with correct orientation should be established so that the velum may serve as a dynamic structure.

The exact timing of repair of a palate cleft is controversial. Generally the velum must be closed prior to the development of speech sounds that require an intact palate. On average this level of speech production is observed by about 18 months of age in the normally developing child. If the repair is completed after this time, compensatory speech articulations may result. Repair completed prior to this time allows for the intact velum to close effectively, appropriately separating the nasopharynx from the orophayrynx during certain speech sounds.[104–107]

In patients with cleft palate, concerns for normal speech development are frequently balanced with the known biologic consequences of surgery during infancy; namely, the problem of surgery during the growth phase resulting in maxillary growth restriction.[33,72,73,108] When repair of the palate is performed between 9 and 18 months of age, the incidence of associated growth restriction affecting the maxillary development is approximately 25%.[31,33,109–111] If repair is carried out earlier than 9 months of age, then severe growth restriction requiring future orthognathic surgery is seen with greater frequency.[22,26,31,33,109,112–114] At the same time proceeding with palatoplasty prior to 9 months of age is not associated with any increased benefit in terms of speech development so the result is an increase in growth-related problems with an absence of any functional benefit.[115,116] Using only the chronologic age it seems that carrying out the

operation during the 9 to 18 months timeline best balances the need to address functional concerns such as speech development with the potential negative impact on growth. To date no case-controlled rigorous clinical trial has examined what is likely the most critical factor in dictating the exact timing of cleft repair—the individual child's true language age. In cases where significant developmental delay is present surgery should be delayed since speech formation is not yet an issue and there is a likely benefit in terms of growth of the maxilla. Delaying palatal closure is relevant in situations where the cleft palate is associated with other complex medical conditions, neurodevelopmental delay, complex craniofacial anomalies, and/or the presence of a tracheotomy.

Another approach used to balance speech issues with growth-related concerns is to stage the closure of the secondary palate with two operations. Generally this involves the repair of the soft palate early in life as an initial step, followed by closure of the hard palate later in infancy. The idea is that timely repair of the soft palate, which is critical for speech, is accomplished while hard palate repair with mucoperiosteal stripping is delayed until growth is further along.[117,118] Although this technique is not advocated by the majority of surgeons, some surgeons may feel that repairing the hard palate portion later may offer the advantages of less growth restriction, easier repair of larger clefts, and less chance for fistula formation. No convincing data exist to favor this approach over a single-stage repair, but the practice is continued by some centers where anecdotal evidence suggests that there may be some benefit. In contrast most North American speech and language pathologists prefer closure of the palate as a single operation.[117]

Cleft palate reconstruction requires the mobilization of multilayered flaps to reconstruct the defect due to the failure of fusion of the palatal shelves. Generally when the initial palate closure is performed, this refers to closure of the tissues posterior to the incisive foramen. This is done in a layered fashion by first closing the nasal mucosa and then the oral mucosa. Since the main function of the palate is to close the space between the nasopharynx and oropharynx during certain speech sounds, the surgeon must also reconstruct the musculature of the velopharyngeal mechanism. The musculature of the levator palatini is abnormally inserted on the posterior aspect of the hard palate and therefore must be disinserted and reconstructed in the midline.[26,119] Therefore, the soft palate is closed in three layers by approximating the nasal mucosa, levator musculature, and the oral mucosa. The hard palate portion is closed in two layers using nasal mucosa flaps and then oral mucosa flaps. Both the hard and soft palate repairs must be done in a tension-free manner to avoid wound breakdown and fistula formation. Adequate mobilization of the flaps during the dissection is essential to achieve tension-free closure. At times some surgeons may elect to incorporate vomer flaps into the repair if there is difficulty in mobilizing the lateral flaps to the midline.

Many techniques have been described for repair of the palate.[120–127] The Bardach two-flap palatoplasty uses two large full-thickness flaps that are mobilized with layered dissection and brought to the midline for closure (Figure 43-12).[26,120] This technique preserves the palatal neurovascular bundle as well as a lateral pedicle for adequate blood supply. The von Langenbeck technique is similar to the Bardach palatoplasty but preserves an anterior pedicle for increased blood supply

to the flaps.[26,121] This technique is also successful in achieving a layered closure but may be more difficult when suturing the nasal mucosa near the anteriorly based pedicle attachments. The authors do not favor push-back techniques as they may incur more palatal scarring, restrict growth, and do not show a measurable benefit in speech.

Another common technique is the Furlow double-opposing Z plasty, which attempts to lengthen the palate by taking advantage of a Z-plasty technique on both the nasal mucosa and the oral mucosa (Figure 43-13).[26,124–127] This technique can be effective at closing the palate but has been reported by some to have a higher rate of fistula formation at the junction of the soft and hard palates where theoretical lengthening of the soft palate may compromise the closure.[26,128–133] No benefit has been convincingly demonstrated with any particular repair technique when one looks at dental arch form, speech outcome, feeding, or any other functional variable. At this point in our understanding surgeons often consider their own experiences and training when repairing clefts, since definitive data suggesting that one repair is preferable over another are lacking.

In very wide clefts some surgeons will advocate the consideration of a pharyngeal flap at the primary palatoplasty procedure to assist in closure since revision palatoplasty is sometimes unsuccessful in eradicating fistulas. Those who use this technique usually perform it in extremely wide clefts

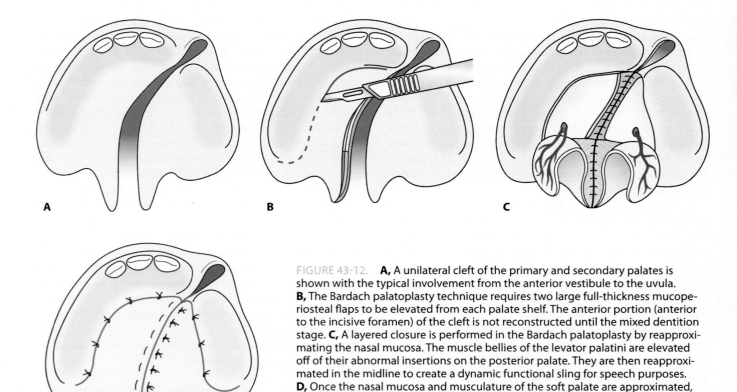

FIGURE 43-12. **A,** A unilateral cleft of the primary and secondary palates is shown with the typical involvement from the anterior vestibule to the uvula. **B,** The Bardach palatoplasty technique requires two large full-thickness mucoperiosteal flaps to be elevated from each palate shelf. The anterior portion (anterior to the incisive foramen) of the cleft is not reconstructed until the mixed dentition stage. **C,** A layered closure is performed in the Bardach palatoplasty by reapproximating the nasal mucosa. The muscle bellies of the levator palatini are elevated off of their abnormal insertions on the posterior palate. They are then reapproximated in the midline to create a dynamic functional sling for speech purposes. **D,** Once the nasal mucosa and musculature of the soft palate are approximated, the oral mucosa is closed in the midline. The lateral releasing incisions are quite easily closed primarily due to the length gained from the depth of the palate. In rare cases, in very wide clefts a portion of the lateral incisions may remain open and granulate by secondary intention.

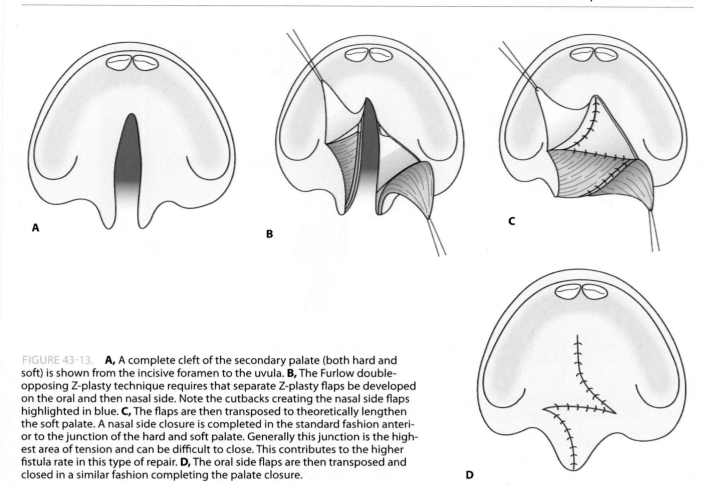

FIGURE 43-13. **A,** A complete cleft of the secondary palate (both hard and soft) is shown from the incisive foramen to the uvula. **B,** The Furlow double-opposing Z-plasty technique requires that separate Z-plasty flaps be developed on the oral and then nasal side. Note the cutbacks creating the nasal side flaps highlighted in blue. **C,** The flaps are then transposed to theoretically lengthen the soft palate. A nasal side closure is completed in the standard fashion anterior or to the junction of the hard and soft palate. Generally this junction is the highest area of tension and can be difficult to close. This contributes to the higher fistula rate in this type of repair. **D,** The oral side flaps are then transposed and closed in a similar fashion completing the palate closure.

and do so very selectively. This allows the central portion of the closure to be filled with posterior pharyngeal wall tissue making the closure of the nasal and palatal mucosa easier. Patients with Pierre Robin syndrome or Treacher Collins syndrome may have exceptionally wide clefts that are difficult to close with no tension, and this technique may be considered. The drawbacks of using a pharyngeal flap during the repair of the palate include a significantly increased risk for complications such as bleeding, snoring, obstructive sleep apnea, or hyponasality. The details of pharyngeal flap surgery and revision palatoplasty techniques are discussed in Chapter 43, "Reconstruction of Cleft Lip and Palate: Secondary Procedures."

COMPLEX FACIAL CLEFTING

Clefting of the facial structures other than the typical nasolabial region is rare and often presents difficult challenges to the reconstructive cleft surgeon. Therefore it is important to consider referring patients with complex facial clefting to surgeons with experience in this particular area. Comprehensive interdisciplinary care is mandatory to achieve the best results including involvement of neurosurgery, ophthalmology, orthodontics, speech pathology, and other members

of the craniofacial team. Some interventions such as eye lubrication may be necessary within hours after birth, and accurate prenatal diagnosis of severe facial clefting is helpful in planning for early care.

The etiology of the various facial clefts may be related to failure of embryologic fusion, physical obstruction in fetal life, association with an encephalocele or tumor, amniotic bands, or other anatomic disruptions during fetal life.[55] The vast majority of complex facial clefts are sporadic events and not related to a single gene disease. Many complex facial clefts involve the orbit, and the classification system most often used is orbitocentric in design (see Figure 43-2). Paul Tessier described a numbering system for facial clefting phenomena to make description and surgical planning more easily discussed.[56] Other systems exist but have a more cumbersome nomenclature.[57]

Primary repair of severe facial clefts is often more difficult than even the most difficult standard bilateral clefts.[134–136] While mobilization of the lip and nose structures is rather straightforward, the closure of clefts in the orbital region can be challenging due to the lack of eyelid and adjacent tissue for advancement and/or rotation. Revision surgery is the norm in this group and should include a skilled ophthalmologic surgeon early in the process for the best results.

SECTION 5

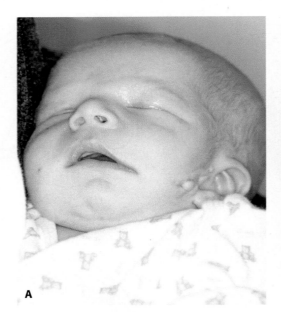 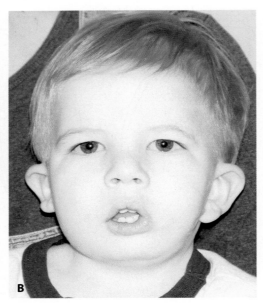

FIGURE 43-14. **A,** A 2-month-old boy with a Tessier no. 7 left facial cleft associated with craniofacial microsomia (Kaban type IIb), congenital ear anomalies, a lateral tongue cleft, and a left-sided epibulbar dermoid. **B,** The same child at 8 months after the primary repair.

The staged reconstruction of these types of severe facial clefts is similar to the more common cleft lip and palate protocols. However, several functional issues are present in patients with complex facial clefting that require more immediate attention. For example, patients with large Tessier no. 7 clefts may have problems with retaining foodstuffs in their oral cavities due to the discontinuity of the orbicularis oris (Figure 43-14). This may prompt early repair and reestablishment of the orbicularis oris musculature for functional concerns.

For those patients with orbital clefts a skilled pediatric ophthalmologist should evaluate the child early to avoid severe corneal abrasion and desiccation. Immediate lubrication of the globes is necessary to prevent severe irreversible corneal damage until eyelid structures can be mobilized to cover the globe adequately. Early after birth tarsorrhaphy stitches can be used to gain adequate closure of the lids for corneal protection. Ignoring the need for eye protection may result in severe corneal scarring that may cause blindness and prompt consideration for corneal transplantation. Corneal transplants in infants are often not successful but are possible in patients with severe orbitofacial clefts. Another concern is the support of the globes at the orbit floor that may be involved in some facial clefts. The timing of orbital reconstruction is dependent on the functional needs of the cleft area in each patient. These are just some of the concerns present in complex facial clefting, and a customized treatment plan must be formulated for each patient.

OUTCOME ASSESSMENT

Decision-making in cleft care should be based on evidenced-based research and a critical look at outcomes. Unfortunately there is little evidenced-based research available to guide clinicians through the many treatment protocols for cleft care.[113] Although the clinical experience of the surgeon certainly has value, this must be integrated with a constant review of evidence-based research. Typically enthusiasm by a surgeon or a particular group of surgeons regarding a specific intervention because of personal experiences may help popularize that intervention but with little outcome data to support its use. Too frequently the long-term results are not forthcoming, and the treatment regimen may still persist. Unfortunately some of the treatment regimens used today are based on the poor outcomes and mishaps of previous surgeons rather than regimens chosen as a consequence of published evidence of the actual success of a particular treatment.

Additionally the pressures of a costly health care system have made treatment decision questions even harder to investigate.[88] A need to understand the outcome differences between treatment philosophies will be critical to help determine which protocols will be most beneficial to the patient without extending valuable health care resources on unproven or ineffective methods. For this reason among many others, the need to discard unproven and unnecessary interventions has never been greater. Outcomes studies based on functional results such as appearance, facial growth, occlusion, patient satisfaction, and psychosocial development are all critical in this process. Surgeons involved in the care of patients with clefts must critically review the literature on a regular basis and not be tempted by poorly evaluated techniques popularized by clinical reports.

CONCLUSIONS

The comprehensive care of patients with clefts requires an interdisciplinary approach that demands precise surgical execution of the various procedures necessary to correct cleft deformities, as well as frequent long-term follow-up. Clinicians experienced in the comprehensive interdisciplinary care of patients with clefts are best equipped to deal with these concerns. The treatment of patients with cleft and craniofacial deformities should be free of bias and should demand team care that is patient, family, and community oriented. Only in this fashion can the overall treatment be optimally successful. This type of care maximizes the patient's ability to grow into adulthood and succeed in life without focusing on their deformity.

References

1. Adams GR. The effects of physical attractiveness on the socialization process. In: Lucker GW, Ribbens KA, McNamara JA, editors. Psychological aspects of facial form. Craniofacial growth series monograph no. 11. Ann Arbor: University of Michigan Press; 1981. p. 25–47.

2. Kapp K. Self concept of the cleft lip and or palate child. Cleft Palate J 1979;16:171.

3. Kapp-Simon KA. Psychological interventions for the adolescent with cleft lip and palate. Cleft Palate Craniofac J 1995; 32:104–8.

4. American Cleft Palate-Craniofacial Association. Parameters for the evaluation and treatment of patients with cleft lip/palate or other craniofacial anomalies. Cleft Palate Craniofac J 1993;30 Suppl 1:4.

5. Boo-Chai K. An ancient Chinese text on a cleft lip. Plast Reconstr Surg 1966;38:89.

6. Rogers BO. Harelip repair in colonial America: a review of 18th century and earlier surgical techniques. Plast Reconstr Surg 1964;34:142.

7. Bushe G. An essay on the operation for cleft palate. New York (NY): William Jackson; 1835.

8. Pare A. Dix Livres de la Chirurgie. Paris: Iean le Royer; 1564. p. 211.

9. LeMesurier AB. Method of cutting and suturing lip in complete unilateral cleft lip. Plast Reconstr Surg 1949;4:1.

10. Veau V. Operative treatment of complete double harelip. Ann Surg (Paris) 1922;76:143.

11. Tennison CW. The repair of unilateral cleft lip by the stencil method. Plast Reconstr Surg 1952;9:115.

12. Skoog T. A design for the repair of unilateral cleft lip. Am J Surg 1958;95:223.

13. Brauer RO. Repair of unilateral cleft lip. Triangular flap repairs. Clin Plast Surg 1985;12:595.

14. Randall P. Long-term results with the triangular flap technique for unilateral cleft lip repair. In: Bardach J, Morris H, editors. Multidisciplinary management of cleft lip and palate. Philadelphia (PA): W.B. Saunders; 1990. p. 173.

15. Asensio OE. Labioleporino y paladar heindido. Acta Odontol Venez 1971;3:229–42.

16. Asensio OE. A variation of the rotation-advancement operation for repair of wide unilateral cleft lips. Plast Reconstr Surg 1974;53:167–73.

17. Millard DR. Cleft craft. Vol 1. Boston (MA): Little Brown; 1976. p. 165–73.

18. Millard DR. A primary camouflage of the unilateral harelip. In: Transactions of the international congress of plastic surgeons. Baltimore (MD): Williams & Wilkins; 1957. p. 160–6.

19. Hullihen SP. A treatise on hare-lip and its treatment. Baltimore (MD): Woods and Crane; 1844.

20. The building of a specialty: oral and maxillofacial surgery in the United States 1918–1998. J Oral Maxillofac Surg. 1998;7 Suppl 56.

21. Schmid E. Die Annaherung der Kieferstumpfe bei Lippen-Kiefer-Gaumenspalten: Ihre schadlichen Folgen und Vermeidung. Fortschr Kiefer Gesichtschir 1955;1:37.

22. Pruzansky S. Presurgical orthopaedics and bone grafting for infants with cleft lip and palate: a dissent. Cleft Palate J 1964; 1:164.

23. Robertson NR, Jolleys A. Effects of early bone grafting in complete clefts of the lip and palate. Plast Reconstr Surg 1968;42: 414–21.

24. Boyne PJ, Sands NR. Secondary bone grafting of residual alveolar and palatal clefts. J Oral Surg 1972;30:87–92.

25. Millard DR. Cleft craft: the evolution of its surgery. Alveolar and palatal deformities. Vol 3. Boston (MA): Little Brown; 1980.

26. Posnick JC. The staging of cleft lip and palate reconstruction: infancy through adolescence. In: Posnick JC, editor. Craniofacial and maxillofacial surgery in children and young adults. Philadelphia (PA): W.B. Saunders; 2000. p. 785–826.

27. Posnick JC, Tompson B. Cleft-orthognathic surgery. Complications and long-term results. Plast Reconstr Surg 1995;96:255.

28. Posnick JC. Cleft-orthognathic surgery: the unilateral cleft lip and palate deformity. In: Posnick JC, editor. Craniofacial and maxillofacial surgery in children and young adults. Philadelphia (PA): W.B. Saunders; 2000. p. 860–907.

29. Posnick JC. Cleft-orthognathic surgery: the bilateral cleft lip and palate deformity. In: Posnick JC, editor. Craniofacial and maxillofacial surgery in children and young adults. Philadelphia (PA): W.B. Saunders; 2000. p. 908–50.

30. Posnick JC. Cleft-orthognathic surgery: the isolated palate deformity. In:Posnick JC, editor. Craniofacial and maxillofacial surgery in children and young adults. Philadelphia (PA): W.B. Saunders; 2000. p. 951–78.

31. Ruiz RL, Costello BJ, Turvey T. Orthognathic surgery in the cleft patient. In: Ogle O, editor. Oral and maxillofacial surgery clinics of North America: secondary cleft surgery. Philadelphia (PA): W.B. Saunders; 2002. p. 491–507.

32. Costello BJ, Ruiz RL. The role of distraction osteogenesis in orthognathic surgery of the cleft patient. Selected Readings Oral Maxillofac Surg 2002;10(3):1–27.

33. Costello BJ, Shand J, Ruiz RL. Craniofacial and orthognathic surgery in the growing patient. Selected Readings Oral Maxillofac Surg 2003;11(5):1–20.

34. Braun TW, Sotereanos GC. Orthognathic and secondary cleft reconstruction of adolescent patients with cleft palate. J Oral Surg 1980;38:425–34.

35. Kiehn CL, DesPrez JD, Brown F. Maxillary osteotomy for late correction of occlusion and appearance in cleft lip and palate patients. Plast Reconstr Surg 1968;42:203–7.

36. Westbrook MT, West RA, McNeill RW. Simultaneous maxillary advancement and closure of bilateral alveolar clefts and oronasal fistulas. J Oral Maxillofac Surg 1983;41:257–60.

37. Georgiade NG. Mandibular osteotomy for the correction of facial disproportion in the cleft lip and palate patient. Symposium on management of cleft lip and palate and associated deformities. Am Plast Reconstr Surg 1974;8:238.

38. Bell WH. Le Fort I osteotomy for correction of maxillary deformities. J Oral Surg 1975; 33:412–26.

39. Fonseca RJ, Turvey TA, Wolford LM. Orthognathic surgery in the cleft patient. In: Fonseca RJ, Baker SJ, Wolford LM, editors. Oral and maxillofacial surgery. Philadelphia (PA): W.B. Saunders; 2000. p. 87–146.

40. Polley JW, Figueroa AA, Charbel FT, et al. Monoblock craniomaxillofacial distraction osteogenesis in a newborn with severe craniofacial synostosis: a preliminary report. J Craniofac Surg 1995;6:421–3.

41. Polley JW, Figueroa AA. Rigid external distraction: its application in cleft maxillary deformities. Plast Reconstr Surg 1998;102:1360–72.

42. Posnick JC, Ruiz RL. Management of secondary orofacial cleft deformities [discussion]. In: Goldwyn RM, Cohen MN, editors. The unfavorable result in plastic surgery: avoidance and treatment. 3rd ed. Philadelphia (PA): Lippincott Williams & Wilkins; 2000.

43. Tolarova MM, Cervenka J. Classification and birth prevalence of orofacial clefts. Am J Med Genet 1998;75: 126–37.

44. Tolarova M. Etiology of clefts of lip and/or palate: 23 years of genetic follow-up in 3660 individual cases. In: Pfeifer G, editor. Craniofacial abnormalities and clefts of the lip, alveolus, and palate. Stuttgart: Thieme; 1991.

45. Gundlach KKH, Abou Tara N, von Kreybig T. Tierexperimentelle Ergebnisse zur Entstehung und Pravention von Geischtsspalten und anderen kraniofazialen Anomalien. Fortschr Kieferorthop 1986;47:356–61.

46. Prescott NJ, Lees MM, Winter RM, Malcolm S. Identification of susceptibility loci for nonsyndromic cleft lip with or without cleft palate in a two stage genome scan of affected sib pairs. Hum Genet 2000;106:345–50.

47. Suzuki K, Hu D, Bustos T, et al. Mutations of PVRL1 encoding a cell-cell adhesion molecule/herpesvirus receptor, in cleft lip/ palate-ectodermal dysplasia. Nat Genet 2000;25:427–30.

48. Van den Boogaard MJ, Dorland M, Beemer FA, van Amstel HKP. MSX1 mutation is associated with orofacial clefting and tooth agenesis in humans. Nat Genet 2000;24:342–3.

49. Oliver-Padilla G, Martinez-Gonzales V. Cleft lip and palate in Puerto Rico: a 33 year study. Cleft Palate J 1986;23:48–57.

50. Lettieri J. Human malformations and related anomalies. In: Stevenson RE, Hall JG, Goodman RM, editors. New York (NY): Oxford University Press; 1993. p. 367–81.

51. Wyszynski DF, Beaty TH, Maestri NE. Genetics of nonsyndromic and syndromic oral clefts revisited. Cleft Palate Craniofac J 1996;33:16406–17.

52. Saal HM. Syndromes and malformations associated with cleft lip with or without cleft palate. Am J Hum Genet 1998;64:A118.

53. Jones MC. Etiology of facial clefts: prospective evaluation of 428 patients. Cleft Palate J 1988;25:16–20.

54. Gorlin R, Cohen MJ, Levin L. Syndromes of the head and neck. 4th ed. New York (NY): Oxford University Press; 2003.

55. Cohen MM. Etiology and pathogenesis of orofacial clefting. Cleft lip and palate: a physiological approach, Oral Maxillofac Clin North Am 2000;12:379–97.

56. Tessier P. Anatomical classification of facial, cranio-facial, and latero-facial clefts. J Maxillofac Surg 1976;4:69–92.

57. Van der Meulen J, Mazzola B, Vermey-Keers, et al. A morphogenetic classification of craniofacial malformations. Plast Reconstr Surg 1983;71:560.

58. Pretorius DH, House M, Nelson TR, Hollenbach KA. Evaluation of normal and abnormal lips in fetuses: comparison between three- and two-dimensional sonography. Am J Roentgenol 1995;165:1233–7.

59. Pretorius DH, Nelson TR. Fetal face visualization using three-dimensional ultrasonography. J Ultrasound Med 1995;14: 349–56.

60. Shaikh D, Mercer NS, Sohan K, et al. Prenatal diagnosis of cleft lip and palate. Br J Plast Surg 2001;54:288–9.

61. Lawrence RA. Breastfeeding: benefits, risks, and alternatives. Curr Opin Obstet Gynecol 2000;12:519–24.

62. Hamosh M, Peterson JA, Henderson TR, et al. Protective function of human milk: the milk fat globule. Semin Perinatol 1999;23:242–9.

63. Thompson JE. An artistic and mathematically accurate method of repairing the defect in cases of harelip. Surg Gynecol Obstet 1912;14:498.

64. Marsh JL. Craniofacial surgery: the experiment on the experiment of nature. Cleft Palate Craniofac J 1996;33:1.

65. Van Boven MJ, Pendeville PE, Veyckemans F, et al. Neonatal cleft lip repair: the anesthesiologist's point of view. Cleft Palate Craniofac J 1993;30:574–7.

66. Eaton AC, Marsh JL, Pigram TK. Does reduced hospital stay affect morbidity and mortality rates following cleft lip and palate repair in infancy? Plast Reconstr Surg 1994;94:916–18.

67. Field TM, Vega-Lahr N. Early interactions between infants with craniofacial anomalies and their mothers. Infant Behav Dev 1984;7:527.

68. Estes JM, Whitby DJ, Lorenz HP, et al. Endoscopic creation and repair of fetal cleft lip. Plast Reconstr Surg 1992;90:743–6.

69. Hallock GG. Endoscopic creation and repair of fetal cleft lip [discussion]. Plast Reconstr Surg 1992;90:747.

70. Hedrick MH, Rice HE, Vander Wall KJ, et al. Delayed in utero repair of surgically created fetal cleft lip and palate. Plast Reconstr Surg 1996;97:906–7.

71. Dorf DS, Curtin JW. Early cleft palate repair and speech outcome. Plast Reconstr Surg 1982;70:74–81.

72. Dorf DS, Curtin JW. Early cleft palate repair and speech outcome: a ten year experience. In: Bardach J, Morris HL. Multidisciplinary management of cleft lip and palate. Philadelphia (PA): W.B. Saunders; 1990. p. 341–8.

73. Copeland M. The effect of very early palatal repair on speech. Br J Plast Surg 1990; 43:676.

74. Costello BJ, Ruiz RL, Turvey T. Surgical management of velopharyngeal insufficiency in the cleft patient. In: Oral and maxillofacial surgery clinics of North America: secondary cleft surgery. Philadelphia (PA): W.B. Saunders; 2002. p. 539–51.

75. Sadove AM, Nelson CL, Eppley BL, et al. An evaluation of calvarial and iliac donor sites in alveolar cleft grafting. Cleft Palate J 1990;27:225–8.

76. Sindet-Pedersen S, Enemark H. Reconstruction of alveolar clefts with mandibular or iliac crest bone graft: a comparative study. J Oral Maxillofac Surg 1990;48:554–8.

77. Lo LJ, Hung KF, Chen YR. Blindness as a complication of LeFort I osteotomy for maxillary disimpaction. Plast Reconstr Surg 2002;109:688–98.

78. Poole R, Farnworth TK. Preoperative lip taping in the cleft lip. Ann Plast Surg 1994; 32:243–9.

79. Shaw WC, Semb G. Current approaches to the orthodontic management of cleft lip and palate. J R Soc Med 1990;83:30–3.

80. Ross RB, MacNamera MC. Effect of presurgical infant orthopedics on facial esthetics in complete bilateral cleft lip and palate. Cleft Palate Craniofac J 1994;31: 68–73.

81. Grayson BH, Cutting CB, Wood R. Preoperative columella lengthening in bilateral cleft lip and palate. Plast Reconstr Surg 1993;92:1422–3.

82. Grayson BH, Santiago PE, Brecht LE, et al. Presurgical nasoalveolar molding in infants with cleft lip and palate. Cleft Palate Craniofac J 1999;36:486–98.

83. Prahl C, Kuijpers-Jagman AM, Van'tHof MA, et al. A randomized prospective clinical trial of the effect of infant orthopedics in unilateral cleft lip and palate: prevention of collapse of the alveolar segments (Dutchcleft). Cleft Palate Craniofac J 2003;40:337–42.

84. Chan KT, Hayes C, Shusterman S, et al. The effects of active infant orthopedics on occlusal relationships in unilateral complete cleft lip and palate. Cleft Palate Craniofac J 2003;40:511–7.

85. Konst EM, Rietveld T, Peters HFM, et al. Language skills of young children with unilateral cleft lip and palate following infant orthopedics: a randomized clinical trial. Cleft Palate Craniofac J 2003;40:356–62.

86. Berkowitz S. The comparison of treatment results in complete cleft lip/palate using conservative approach vs. Millard-Latham PSOT procedure. Semin Orthod 1996;2:169.

87. Georgiade NG, Latham RA. Maxillary arch alignment in the bilateral cleft lip and palate infant, using the pinned coaxial screw appliance. Plast Reconstr Surg 1975; 56:52–60.

88. Strauss RP. Health policy and craniofacial care: issues in resource allocation. Cleft Palate Craniofac J 1994;31:78–80.

89. Randall P, Graham WP. Lip adhesion in the repair of bilateral cleft lip. In: Grabb WC, Rosenstein SW, Bzoch KR, editors. Cleft lip and palate. Boston (MA): Little Brown; 1971.

90. Millard DR. A preliminary adhesion. In: Cleft craft, Vol 1: the unilateral deformity. Boston (MA): Little Brown; 1976.

91. Vander Woude DL, Mulliken JB. Effect of lip adhesion on labial height in two-stage repair of unilateral complete cleft lip. Plast Reconstr Surg 1997;100:567–72.

92. Mulliken JB, Pensler JM, Kozakewich HPW. The anatomy of cupid's bow in normal and cleft lip. Plast Reconstr Surg 1993; 92:395–403.

93. McComb H. Primary correction of unilateral cleft lip nasal deformity: a 10 year review. Plast Reconstr Surg 1985;75: 791–9.

94. Horswell BB, Pospisil OA. Nasal symmetry after primary cleft lip repair: comparison between Delaire cheilorhinoplasty and modified rotation-advancement. J Oral Maxillofac Surg 1995;53:1025–30.

95. Schendel SA. Nasal symmetry after primary cleft lip repair: comparison between Delaire cheilorhinoplasty and modified rotation-advancement [discussion]. J Oral Maxillofac Surg 1995;53:1031.

96. Trier WC. Bilateral complete cleft lip and nasal deformity: an anthropometric analysis of staged to synchronous repair [discussion]. Plast Reconstr Surg 1995;96:24.

97. Takato T, Yonehara Y, Mori Y, et al. Early correction of the nose in unilateral cleft lip patients using an open method: a 10-year review. J Oral Maxillofac Surg 1995;53:28–33.

98. Millard DR. Columella lengthening by a forked flap. Plast Reconstr Surg 1958;22:454.

99. Cronin TD. Lengthening the columella by use of skin from nasal floor and alae. Plast Reconstr Surg 1958;21:417.

100. McComb H. Primary repair of the bilateral cleft lip nose: a 15-year review and a new treatment plan. Plast Reconstr Surg 1990;86:882–9.

101. Mulliken JB. Bilateral complete cleft lip and nasal deformity: an anthropometric analysis of staged to synchronous repair. Plast Reconstr Surg 1995;96:9–23.

102. Trott JA, Mohan NA. A preliminary report on one-stage open tip rhinoplasty at the time of lip repair in bilateral cleft lip and palate. The Alo Setar experience. Br J Plast Surg 1993;46: 215–22.

103. Cutting C, Grayson B. The prolabial unwinding flap method for one-stage repair of bilateral cleft lip, nose and alveolus. Plast Reconstr Surg 1993;91:37–47.

104. Maher W. Distribution of palatal and other arteries in cleft and non-cleft human palates. Cleft Palate J 1977;14:1–12.

105. Ross RB, Johnston MC. Cleft lip and palate. Baltimore (MD). William & Wilkins; 1972.

106. Broomhead I. The nerve supply of the soft palate. Br J Plast Surg 1957;10:81.

107. Riski JE, DeLong E. Articulation development in children with cleft lip/palate. Cleft Palate J 1984;21:57–64.

108. Devlin HB. Audit and the quality of clinical care. Ann R Coll Surg Engl 1990;72 Suppl 1:3–14.

109. Trotman CA, Ross RB. Craniofacial growth in bilateral cleft lip and palate: ages six years to adulthood. Cleft Palate Craniofac J 1993;30:261–73.

110. Bishara SE. Cephalometric evaluation of facial growth in operated and unoperated individuals with isolated clefts of the palate. Cleft Palate J 1973;10:239–46.

111. Bardach J, Kelly KM, Salyer KE. Relationship between the sequence of lip and palate repair and maxillary growth. An experimental study in beagles. Plast Reconstr Surg 1994;93: 269–78.

112. Semb G. A study of facial growth in patients with bilateral cleft lip and palate treated by the Oslo CLP team. Cleft Palate Craniofac J 1991;28:22–48.

113. Shaw WC, Asher-McDade C, Brattstrom V, et al. A six-center international study of treatment outcome in patients with clefts of the lip and palate. Part 5. General discussion and conclusions. Cleft Palate Craniofac J 1992;29:413–8.

114. Canaday JW, Thompson SA, Colburn A. Craniofacial growth after iatrogenic cleft palate repair in a fetal ovine model. Cleft Palate Craniofac J 1997;34:69–72.

115. Peterson-Falzone SJ. Speech outcomes in adolescents with cleft lip and palate. Cleft Palate Craniofac J 1995;32:125–8.

116. Dalston RM. Timing of cleft palate repair: a speech pathologist's viewpoint. In: Lehman JA, editor. Problems of plastic surgery in cleft palate surgery. Philadelphia (PA): J.B. Lippincott; 1992. p. 30–8.

117. Witzel MA, Salyer KE, Ross RB. Delayed hard palate closure: the philosophy revisited. Cleft Palate J 1984;21:263–9.

118. Schweckendiek W. Primary veloplasty: long-term results without maxillary deformity. A twenty-five year report. Cleft Palate J 1991;15:268–74.

119. Kriens O. Fundamental anatomic findings for an intravelar veloplasty. Cleft Palate Journal 1970;7:27–36.

120. Bardach J, Nosal P: Geometry of the two-flap palatoplasty. In: Bardach J, Salyer K, editors. Surgical techniques in cleft lip and palate. 2nd ed. St. Louis (MO): Mosby-Year Book; 1991.

121. Von Langenbeck B. Operation der angeborenen totalen spaltung des harten gaumens nach einer neuen methode. Dtsch Klin 1861;8:231.

122. Wardill WFM. Cleft palate: results of operation for cleft palate. Br J Plast Surg 1928;16:127.

123. Wardill WFM. The technique of operation for cleft palate. Br J Surg 1937;25:117.

124. Furlow LT. Cleft palate repair by double opposing Z-plasty. Plast Reconstr Surg 1986;78:724–38.

125. Furlow LT. Bilateral buccal flaps with double opposing Z-plasty for wider palatal clefts [discussion]. Plast Reconstr Surg 1997;100:1144–5.

126. Randall P, LaRossa D, Solomon M, Cohen M. Experience with the Furlow double-reversing Z-plasty for cleft palate repair. Plast Reconstr Surg 1986;77:569–76.

127. Horswell BB, Castiglione CL, Poole AE, et al. The double-reversing z-plasty in primary palatoplasty: operative experience and early results. J Oral Maxillofac Surg 1993; 51:145–9.

128. Reid DA. Fistulae in the hard palate following cleft palate surgery. Br J Plast Surg 1986; 77:569.

129. Abyholm FE. Palatal fistulae following cleft palate surgery. Scand J Plast Reconstr Surg 1979;13:295–300.

130. Cohen SR, Kalinowski J, La Rossa D, et al. Cleft palate fistulas: a multivariate statistical analysis of prevalence, etiology, and surgical management. Plast Reconstr Surg 1991; 87:1041–7.

131. Emory RE, Clay RP, Bite U, et al. Fistula formation and repair after palatal closure: an institutional perspective. Plast Reconstr Surg 1997;99:1535–8.

132. Rintala AE. Surgical closure of palatal fistulae: follow-up of 84 personally treated cases. Scand J Plast Reconstr Surg Hand Surg 1980;14:235–8.

133. Schultz RC. Management and timing of cleft palate fistula repair. Plast Reconstr Surg 1986;78:739–47.

134. Tessier P. Colobomas: vertical and oblique complete facial clefts. Panminerva Med 1969;11:95–101.

135. Kawamoto HK. The kaleidoscopic world of rare craniofacial clefts: order out of chaos (Tessier Classification). Clin Plast Surg 1976;3:529–72.

136. Posnick JC. Rare craniofacial clefts: evaluation and treatment In: Posnick JC, editor. Craniofacial and maxillofacial surgery in children and young adults. Philadelphia (PA): W.B. Saunders; 2000. p. 487–502.

44

CHAPTER

Reconstruction of the Alveolar Cleft

Kelly Kennedy, DDS, and Peter E. Larsen, DDS

In the management of patients with cleft lip and cleft palate, the decision regarding alveolar cleft grafting is one of the most controversial. Is grafting of the residual alveolar defect indicated? If so, at what age is it most appropriate, what material is most ideal, and should adjunctive procedures such as orthodontic expansion be used before or after grafting? Lastly, what are appropriate measures of success? This chapter reviews what is known, discusses these controversies, and provides a rationale for the approach to the residual alveolar cleft defect.

RATIONALE FOR GRAFTING

Although some authors have advocated nongrafting techniques[1] or prosthodontic approaches, the general consensus is that achieving continuity between the cleft alveolar segments has significant advantages, regardless of how and when this is accomplished. Potential advantages include[2]

1. Grafting achieves stability of the arch and prevents collapse of the alveolar segments. This provides improved orthodontic stability.
2. Grafting preserves the health of the dentition. Grafting provides room for the canine and lateral incisors to erupt into the arch into stable alveolar bone and maintains bony support of teeth adjacent to the cleft.[3,4]
3. Grafting restores continuity not only of the alveolus but also of the maxilla at the piriform rim. This supports the ala and provides improved stability and support for the nose. This may have a direct aesthetic benefit and may also prove to be of long-term benefit when formal rhinoplasty procedures are performed.[3]
4. Palatal and nasolabial fistulae are often present even after palatoplasty. Grafting of the alveolar defect provides an opportunity for the surgeon to address the residual oronasal fistula. This may have potential benefit for both hygiene and speech. Many cleft patients present with chronic upper respiratory and sinus disease, which may be related to reflux into the nasal cavity and sinus. There is some evidence that the residual fistula, whether labial or palatal, can have an effect on speech articulation and nasality. There is evidence that closure of the fistula and grafting the cleft defect can improve nasal emission and nasality.[5]

MEASURING OUTCOMES

Before discussing the controversies associated with reconstruction of the residual alveolar cleft, it is important to accept some consistent measure of successful outcome. Most reports rely on descriptive data. This makes comparison of different approaches difficult. To evaluate bone graft success, Bergland and colleagues[6] described a semiquantitative approach that divided grafts into four types based on alveolar crest height. Although this is effective, it has been suggested that occlusal alveolar bone height does not adequately measure success.[7] Support of the ala and opportunity for successful tooth movement into the site or placement of an endosseous implant also require apical bone formation. A modification of the Bergland scale that measures both occlusal and basal bone height may be a better tool for evaluating graft success. Although the Bergland scale and modifications of it rely on a two-dimensional radiograph to evaluate bone fill within a three-dimensional cleft, studies show good correlation between bone volume as predicted by these two-dimensional radiographs and that shown on three-dimensional computed tomography (CT) scans.[8] Recently, investigators have used three-dimensional imaging almost exclusively to quantify the results of alveolar cleft bone grafting techniques.[9–11] To date, no research has been conducted to show that a critical volume of bone is required at an alveolar cleft site in order for the graft to meet success criteria. Therefore, it appears at this time that three-dimensional imaging certainly has its place in research but two-dimensional imaging continues to be sufficient for routine monitoring of clinical outcomes. An exception to this might include evaluation of the grafted site for the treatment planning of dental implants after skeletal maturity has been achieved.

TIMING OF THE GRAFT

Perhaps the most controversial topic in managing the alveolar cleft is when grafting should be performed. In the traditional literature, terminology is not consistent. Outcome measures for various approaches are also defined inconsistently, which makes comparison difficult. Here, alveolar grafting is grouped according to timing as defined later (Table 44-1).

Primary Grafting

Some define primary alveolar bone grafting as that which is performed simultaneously with lip repair.[12] Others have stated that any grafting that is performed at younger than 2 years of age is considered primary grafting. Still others have defined primary grafting as grafting performed before the palate is repaired.[13,14]

Primary grafting performed at the time of lip repair has failed to result in acceptable outcome. Long-term studies show abnormal maxillary development with maxillary retrognathia, concave profile, and increased frequency of crossbite compared with patients without grafts.[15,16]

Primary grafting performed after the closure of the lip and before the closure of the palate has proved successful in a limited number of centers when a very specific protocol is followed.[13,14] A prosthesis is placed before the lip is closed to mold the alveolar segments into close proximity. The lip is then closed, which further aids in molding the segments. The segments must be in close proximity with good arch form before an onlay rib graft is placed across the labial

TABLE 44-1. **Timing of Alveolar Bone Grafting**

<2 Years of Age: Primary Grafting
After lip repair
Before palate repair

≥2 Years of Age: Secondary Grafting
2–5 yr: Early secondary
6–12 yr: Mixed dentition secondary (after central incisor eruption
   and before the canine erupts)
   6–8 yr: Early mixed dentition
   9–12 yr: Late mixed dentition
>12 yr: Late secondary grafting

surface of the cleft in a subperiosteal tunnel that is developed by limited dissection.

Advocates of this approach have not experienced problems with altered facial growth and malocclusion, most likely the result of the limited dissection used in these cases. They have reported improved occlusion and graft success in these patients compared with patients grafted at other ages.[17] It is still difficult to wholeheartedly endorse this approach. Several additional anesthetics and surgeries are needed at a young age. This technique may not be possible in all patients, such as those with isolated alveolar clefts without palatal clefting or those in whom segments cannot be orthopedically aligned. In one center, because of these limitations, nearly one half of patients could not be treated with primary grafting.[13] Outcomes may also not be as good as with other approaches. In one study, there was an increased incidence of malformation of permanent lateral incisors in the primary graft group and decreased success of the graft, with only 41% of primary grafts (54% if pregrafting orthopedics was included) resulting in adequate bone height when measured with a Bergland scale.[18] This was compared with 73% success of those sites grafted in the mixed-dentition stage (after eruption of the permanent central incisors and before eruption of the maxillary canines).

Early Secondary Grafting

Grafting after the child reaches 2 years of age and before 6 years is considered early secondary grafting. The literature does not support early secondary grafting.

Secondary Grafting during the Mixed Dentition (After Eruption of the Maxillary Central Incisors and before Eruption of the Canines)

Alveolar reconstruction with grafting during the eruption of the permanent dentition may be best for various reasons. Rationale for grafting and for timing of grafting during this time period include

1. There is minimal maxillary growth after age 6 to 7 years, and the effect of grafting at this time will result in minimal to no alteration of facial growth.[19,20]
2. Cooperation with orthodontic and perioperative care is predictable. General anesthesia is not required for routine orthodontic procedures such as expansion.
3. The donor site for graft harvest is of acceptable volume for predictable grafting with autogenous bone.
4. Bone volume may be improved by eruption of the tooth into the newly grafted bone.[21]
5. Grafting during this phase allows placement of the graft before eruption of permanent teeth into the cleft site, which achieves one of the primary goals of grafting—to enhance the health of teeth in and adjacent to the alveolar cleft

The landmark papers by Boyne and Sands[22,23] established that grafting in the mixed dentition achieves many of the goals of

TABLE 44-2. **Factors Contributing to Timing of Grafting during the Mixed Dentition**

Dental age vs. chronologic age
Presence of the lateral incisor
Position of the lateral incisor
Degree of rotation/angulation of the central incisor
Trauma/mobility of premaxillary segment (bilateral clefts)
Social issues
Size of the patient and of the cleft
Occlusion
Need for adjunctive procedures
Dynamic of the team

reconstruction of the cleft alveolus. The ideal patient is between the ages of 8 and 12 years with a maxillary canine root that is one half to two thirds developed. This timing is supported by several well-documented studies.[6,24-28] However, some authors have suggested that earlier grafting should be considered as a means of preserving the lateral incisor as well.[15,29,30] These authors have suggested that grafting be considered as early as 6 years of age. There is some evidence that grafting between the ages of 6 and 8 years, in addition to achieving the expected goal of preserving the canine, can preserve the lateral incisor as well, but this remains controversial. Despite clear indications that grafting in the mixed dentition is preferable to either primary, early secondary, or late secondary grafting, it is not entirely clear whether this grafting should be performed early (age 6–8 yr) or late (age 8–12 yr). Various individual factors should be evaluated when determining the ideal time for grafting during the mixed dentition (Table 44-2).

Dental versus Chronologic Age

Many outcomes of grafting are related to preserving health of the dentition adjacent to and erupting into the cleft site. It makes sense that the timing of the graft be determined on the basis of dental rather than chronologic age. When the maxillary central incisors begin to erupt, regardless of chron-

ologic age, the patient should be evaluated for grafting, taking into consideration the other factors discussed later. In some patients, this may be much earlier than the traditionally recommended age for evaluation.

Presence of the Lateral Incisor

Many proponents of earlier mixed-dentition grafting advocate this timing because of the opportunity to salvage the lateral incisor.[15,27,29] During the evaluation, attention should be directed to the presence of the lateral incisor and to whether this tooth appears to be normally formed. The incidence of congenitally missing permanent lateral incisors within the alveolar cleft is between 35% and 60%.[18,31] If a lateral incisor is present and appears to be well formed, earlier grafting may be beneficial. Even if the tooth is not perfectly formed, it may still be beneficial to attempt to preserve it. The grafted alveolus will often thin to the point that alveolar width is not adequate for definitive reconstruction with an endosseous implant without additional grafting.[32] Retaining the lateral incisor will maintain bone width and perhaps eliminate the need for yet another graft at the time of implant placement.

Position of the Lateral Incisor

If the lateral incisor is mesial to the cleft, it often has adequate space for eruption. However, if the lateral incisor is located in the posterior segment, earlier grafting may be necessary to preserve the lateral incisor.[12] In one review, 36% of patients with cleft lip and alveolus had missing lateral incisors.[31] Of the 64% who had lateral incisors, 90% of the lateral incisors were located distal to the cleft. In the same series of patients, 57% of those with cleft lip and palate had missing lateral incisors, and of the remaining 43%, 86% of the lateral incisors were located distal to the cleft.[31] Therefore, a significant number of patients may benefit from earlier grafting to preserve the lateral incisor (Figure 44-1).

Rotation of the Central Incisor

The maxillary permanent central incisor will often erupt in a rotated and angled position (Figure 44-2). This reflects the

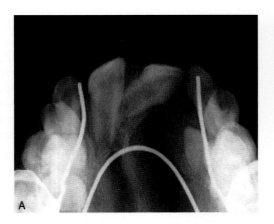
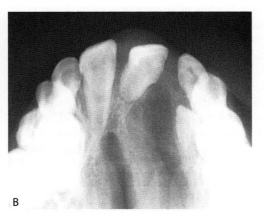

FIGURE 44-1.   **A,** Occlusal radiograph shows lateral incisor distal to the cleft. **B,** Grafting which was performed at age 7 years to facilitate eruption of the lateral incisor.

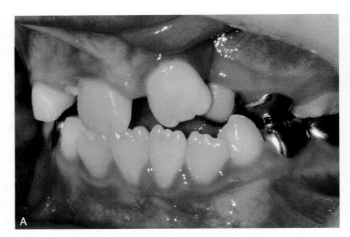 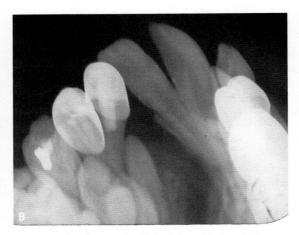

FIGURE 44-2.   **A,** Photograph of a typical unilateral cleft. There is rotation of the central incisor and angulation of the crown toward the cleft. This maintains bone support for the root of the tooth. **B,** Occlusal radiograph shows that the cleft defect is larger than it appears clinically and support for the incisor root is provided by only a thin margin of bone.

morphology of the underlying bone. In extreme cases, the crowding of the two incisors can preclude normal oral hygiene methods, and this can result in decay of the central incisor. The patient or parent may also be concerned with the position of the incisors for aesthetic reasons. If a decision is made to rotate these teeth into alignment, it may be necessary to graft the alveolar defect before this orthodontic tooth movement.[33] Failure to consider the morphology of the bone on the distal surface of the erupted central incisor can result in bone loss and periodontal defects as a result of orthodontic tooth movement. Because the incisor teeth erupt at approximately age 6 years, the surgeon may choose to graft at an earlier age so that orthodontic movement of the incisors can be accomplished.

Social Issues

The window for mixed-dentition grafting is large (age 6–12 yr). This is also during a period of tremendous social development for the patient. If a graft is necessary, the timing of surgery should respect the social and educational development of the child. Slightly earlier grafting, when it may cause less interference with education or other important opportunities for social development, may be preferable to grafting at an exact stage of dental development.

Size of the Patient and of the Cleft

Petite patients with large cleft defects are challenging. Adequate closure of the defect may be difficult, and harvesting an adequate amount of graft material may be challenging as well. This is particularly true for large bilateral cleft defects. In these patients, the lateral incisor is often absent, the oronasal communication is often quite large, and the premaxilla is frequently in less than ideal position. In these large defects, later grafting is often better, to wait for growth of the patient and orthodontic alignment of the cleft segments.

Need for Other Procedures

Patients are often evaluated for velopharyngeal incompetence, minor aesthetic revision of the nose or the lip, and pressure-equalizing tubes for otitis media. It is reasonable to coordinate the timing of surgery for the alveolar cleft with other procedures that may be necessary. If velopharyngeal flap surgery is planned during the mixed-dentition phase, it should take precedence over the alveolar graft. Improved speech is more important to the child's development than achieving continuity of the alveolus. Alveolar grafting would be compromised if performed simultaneously with velopharyngeal flap surgery, and in these patients, it is appropriate to delay the graft until the velopharyngeal flap surgery is accomplished and speech therapy re-instituted. Minor soft tissue, nasal, and lip revision are often desired by the patient and parents. These can be accomplished with alveolar grafting. The grafting process can distort the nose and soft tissue; these soft tissue procedures should be performed first with alveolar grafting undertaken in the same setting and with care not to disrupt the aesthetic procedures already performed.

Dynamic of the Team

Cleft management should always involve a multidisciplinary team, with the wide expertise to develop a proper treatment plan. Difficulties may arise when the priorities of one specialty compete with those of another. If the surgical team is faced with an orthodontic provider who feels strongly that it is appropriate to align the maxillary central incisors as soon as they erupt, it will be necessary for the alveolar defect to be grafted earlier to prevent compromise of osseous support for the central incisors. Some orthodontists and surgeons believe that palatal expansion is necessary before grafting. These teams may find that it is more appropriate to graft patients at a later age, because it may take months to achieve the desired expansion before the graft.

Secondary Grafting after Eruption of the Permanent Canine (Late Secondary Grafting)

Late secondary grafting has received some support; however, data show that when all the goals of alveolar reconstruction are considered, it has a less than acceptable outcome. Patients older than 12 years of age who undergo grafting have been reported to have decreased success when evaluated using the Bergland scale,[6,18,28,30,34,35] loss of osseous support of teeth adjacent to the cleft,[21] and increased morbidity.[30] There is less opportunity to salvage the lateral incisor, and there is a delay in correction of the orthodontic condition. This delayed grafting does allow for increased options with regard to donor site for graft material because harvest of the mandibular symphysis becomes possible. Such grafts are difficult in the mixed-dentition stage, where it is difficult to obtain adequate bone without damaging unerupted teeth.

SOURCE OF BONE GRAFT

The selection of the ideal grafting material is somewhat dependent on the timing of the graft. In primary bone grafting, the rib is the only site for adequate quantity of bone with acceptable morbidity. In the mixed-dentition stage, the rib is not as appropriate as other sites such as the calvaria or iliac crest. These options would also be possible sources for bone for late secondary grafting, as well as grafts from the mandibular symphysis and possibly the tibia.

Because the data suggest that grafting during the mixed dentition is ideal, discussion focuses on comparing various sources of graft material for this group of patients. The advantages and disadvantages of various potential sources of bone are outlined in Table 44-3.

Iliac Crest

Potential advantages of the iliac crest bone graft include low morbidity and high volume of viable osteoblastic cells (cancellous bone); two teams may work simultaneously, and this procedure is well accepted by the patient.

Bone can be harvested from the iliac crest through various approaches. Some have suggested that a lateral approach is appropriate in the growing patient.[36] This procedure disrupts the iliotibial tract and has a higher incidence of gait disturbance and postoperative pain.[37] In theory, it may be appropriate to avoid the anterior crest, which does not complete its growth until after age 20 years.[37] However, the cartilaginous cap overlying the crest is reduced in thickness to about 1 cm by age 9 years. Damage to the crest at this time could lead to disturbance in growth and cosmetic deformity of the crest; however, splitting the crest longitudinally, which allows access to the underlying cancellous marrow, has been used for harvest of bone in this age group with no reported growth alteration and less postoperative gait disturbance than with the lateral subcrestal approach.[38,39]

Calvarial Bone

Calvarial bone has been recommended by some as an alternative to iliac crest grafting.[40,41] Some authors have concerns about the potential for success when the calvarium is used as a graft source.[42,43] This may be related to the technique of harvest. Bone grafts consisting of diploic bone have been shown to be more successful than those grafts harvested using a high-speed rotary device to shave off primarily cortical bone from the surface of the calvarium.[43] However, even when harvesting calvarial bone in such a way as to maximize diploic bone, results may not be as good as with iliac crest bone. In one study in which primarily diploic bone was carefully harvested from the calvarium, the results were still less successful (80% graft success) than with traditional iliac crest bone (93% graft success).[44] It is likely that either source is effective as long as primarily diploic bone is used. This limitation may render calvaria as a less useful source for large clefts and bilateral clefts.

Calvarial grafts may have decreased morbidity compared with iliac crest harvest. There is less postoperative pain and no gait disturbance. Other potential advantages include decreased surgery time. Cranial bone grafts can be harvested more quickly than iliac crest grafts. If a single team is

TABLE 44-3. **Comparison of Graft Sources**

Site	Advantage	Disadvantage	Considerations
Ilium	Large quantity cancellous bone, two teams	Mild transient gait disturbance	All clefts, particularly large and bilateral clefts
Calvaria	Minimal postoperative discomfort, incision hidden, low morbidity	Limited cancellous/diploic bone, increased operative time	Unilateral clefts, lower success
Mandibular symphysis	Same operative field, rapid procurement, minimal pain	Limited bone	Older children with small defects
Rib	Two teams	Poor source cancellous bone, postoperative pain, visible scar, risk of pneumothorax	Not recommend except for primary grafting
Proximal tibia	Abundant cancellous bone, easy procedure, mild postoperative pain, two teams		Not recommend in patients who have not completed growth

Adapted from Ochs MW. Alveolar cleft bone grafting (part 2): secondary bone grafting. J Oral Maxillofac Surg 1996;54:83–88.

performing surgery, this may be significant. However, it is not possible to harvest the cranial graft simultaneously with the alveolar cleft repair. Grafting from the iliac crest if two teams are used can decrease overall operating time compared with calvarial grafting. Lastly, the incision for graft harvest is hidden in the hairline, which may have a cosmetic advantage.

Grafting from the calvarium has potential disadvantages. There is a perceived increased risk by patients and their families, although several studies show that the morbidity of bone harvest from the calvaria is minimal.[37] As mentioned previously, the volume of diploic bone is limited, making this less predictable for large or bilateral clefts.

Allogeneic Bone

In an effort to eliminate the morbidity and time necessary to harvest bone from any autogenous site, some authors have evaluated allogeneic bone as a potential source of graft material. Studies have shown that allogeneic bone can be used successfully to graft secondary alveolar cleft defects and that results can be compared favorably with those achieved with autogenous bone.[45] However, the demands of bone healing in the alveolar defect where there is potential communication between the graft and the nasal and oral cavity may make this less predictable in large cleft defects or bilateral clefts. In general, bone healing with autogenous bone is biologically different than with allogeneic bone. Autogenous bone grafts initiate an angioblastic response early in the healing process, and some of the transplanted cells remain viable, resulting in a more rapid formation of new bone. In contrast, allogeneic bone grafts demonstrate slower revascularization, because no viable cells are transferred with the graft.[45,46] There is also a theoretical risk of disease transmission from allogeneic sources of bone. Mathematically, the risk is quite small but may be of concern to patients and families.

Bone Morphogenic Protein

Bone morphogenic protein (BMP) and its use in maxillofacial reconstruction have recently become topics of interest in oral and maxillofacial surgery. The potential benefits of avoiding a secondary surgical site and obtaining the same results as those with autogenous grafting have prompted surgeons to use the material in a variety of maxillofacial bony defects. The U.S. Food and Drug Administration (FDA) has approved the use of BMP for specific maxillofacial applications in adults but has conducted no research for its use in skeletally immature patients. (INFUSE Bone Graft package insert, Medtronic).

The off-label use of BMP for alveolar cleft grafting in skeletally immature patients with cleft lip and palate has been investigated in several clinical trials.[9,11] In these trials, the investigators compared the results of cleft sites grafted with an autogeneous iliac crest bone graft (AICBG) and sites grafted with BMP on an absorbable collagen sponge (BMP/ACS) in the same sample population. The mature bone volume obtained in both groups was measured by comparing pre- and postoperative CT scans. The cleft sites grafted with BMP on an ACS resulted in bone volume that was comparable with that in group grafted with autogenous bone in both the horizontal and vertical dimensions. In addition, teeth erupted normally through these BMP-grafted sites. As expected, both the length of hospital stay and the amount of postoperative pain were less for those patients grafted with BMP than for those grafted with an AICBG.[9,11] As has been previously seen with the use of BMP in the maxillofacial region, a few patients in each study who received a BMP graft developed severe swelling in the postoperative period that was not consistent with cellulitis and that resolved without intervention.[9,11]

The preparation of the cleft site for BMP/ACS mirrors the technique used to prepare the site for a conventional bone graft. The buccal advancement flaps, palatal flaps, and nasal floor are developed followed by repair of the nasal floor and palatal tissue. The absorbable collagen sponge is cut into small squares and soaked according to manufacturer's guidelines (INFUSE Bone Graft, Medtronic). After the sponge has soaked for the recommended time period, it is placed into the defect and the buccal flaps are advanced and the four-cornered flaps are closed.

The potential advantages of using BMP are all related to eliminating a second surgical site. The patient will likely have a shorter hospital stay due to less postoperative pain. Gait and sensory disturbances can be completely avoided. Complications at a secondary surgical site are eliminated and overall surgical time may be shortened. There are several potential disadvantages of using BMP in the reconstruction of alveolar clefts. Although it resolves spontaneously, severe postoperative swelling that is unique to this material can be both worrisome to the patient as well as place tension across suture lines. In addition, the lack of structural integrity of the absorbable collagen sponge can lead to an unsupported ala.[9] Also, at this point, the refining process to manufacture BMP is extremely expensive, which makes its routine use somewhat unlikely.

The results of using an AICBG or BMP/ACS are similar in the amount of bone obtained as well as the ability to achieve dental eruption through the graft. Unfortunately, the ACS does not have the structural integrity to support the ala and the use of BMP makes this technique quite costly. At this point in time, it seems that even with the advantages that come with avoiding a secondary surgical site, autogenous bone grafts for the reconstruction of alveolar clefts continues to be the gold standard.

Pre-versus Postsurgical Orthodontics

Controversy exists regarding the use of orthopedic expansion of the cleft segments and the relationship between expansion and grafting. This issue has not been entirely settled. Most authors prefer presurgical expansion, citing easier expansion because of less resistance, improved access to the cleft for closure of the nasal floor, better postoperative hygiene, and less chance of reopening the oronasal fistula.[26,27] Presurgical expansion may also allow orthopedic movement of the

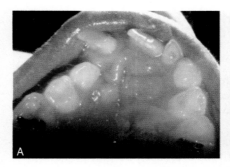
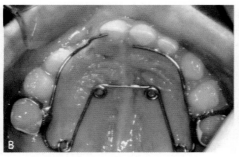
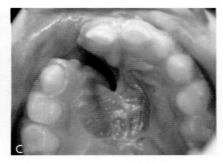

FIGURE 44-3.   **A,** Occlusal photograph of a typical unilateral cleft. There is rotation of the central incisors and collapse of the lesser segment. Expansion of the lesser segment will bring the arch into better form and facilitate grafting without widening the cleft. **B,** Similar cleft that has been expanded. **C,** This cleft is already wide without any expansion. It would not be appropriate to expand this cleft before grafting even if a cross-bite is present.

premaxillary segment in the bilateral cleft patient, which can eliminate traumatic occlusion that can negatively affect graft success. Proponents of expansion after grafting cite advantages of improved bone consolidation when the graft is placed under a dynamic load during healing, a smaller soft tissue defect to close, less difficulty in procuring an adequate volume of bone, and a narrower defect, which will regenerate bone more quickly.[29] Both approaches have been used in conjunction with autogenous grafting in the mixed-dentition stage with success.[12]

In practice, both approaches are valid, and the decision should be based on individual clinical presentation.[34] Small unilateral clefts with collapse of the arch may be easier to graft with some presurgical expansion. In these cases, such expansion may not increase the size of the defect appreciably, and better alignment of the segments can improve hygiene of the teeth adjacent to the cleft and improve access (Figure 44-3). In these cases, the end point of presurgical expansion is improved arch form, not necessarily resolution of cross-bite. Bilateral clefts with collapse of the lateral segments may also benefit from presurgical expansion. Expanding the lateral segments may allow the premaxilla, which is often anteriorly positioned, to be brought back into better relation with the arch, improving arch form, and in some cases, eliminating traumatic occlusion (Figure 44-4). If this is not done before grafting, it may be difficult to obtain ideal arch

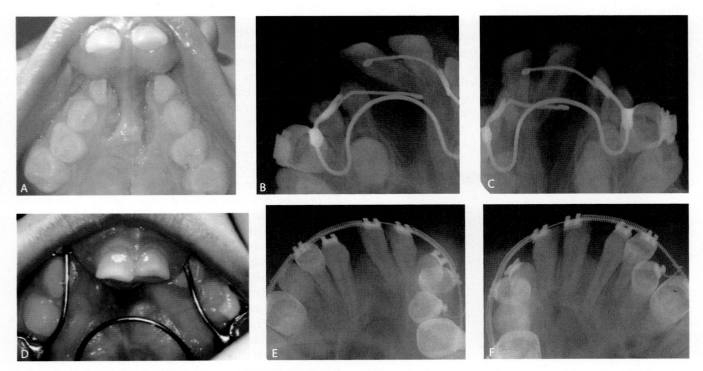

FIGURE 44-4.   **A,** Occlusal photograph of bilateral cleft with collapse of the lateral segments and protrusion of the premaxilla. **B** and **C,** Right and left oblique occlusal radiographs show the cleft defect. **D,** Expansion of the bilateral cleft allows the premaxilla to move posteriorly and improves arch form and alignment of the segments. **E** and **F,** Occlusal radiographs of the same patient after grafting with eruption of the canine.

continuity and positioning of the segments after grafting may be difficult. In patients with reasonable arch form, good alignment of the segments, and dental development corresponding to ideal timing for grafting, it makes little sense to delay grafting in order to expand preoperatively, even in the presence of a buccal cross-bite. These cross-bites may be related only to the anterior-posterior discrepancy, and even if they are truly representative of transverse deficiency, they can be treated easily with expansion after the graft. These clefts can be expanded without opening the oronasal fistula or having a negative effect on the graft.

Not only is there controversy regarding pre-versus post-surgical expansion, there are also two schools of thought regarding orthodontic movement of the erupted teeth adjacent to the cleft. Some authors suggest that aligning the teeth adjacent to the cleft produces better hygiene and an improved result.[26] However, orthodontic movement of teeth adjacent to the cleft is not typically desired.[47] Orthodontic movement of teeth adjacent to the cleft before grafting increases the risk of moving these teeth into the cleft site, compromising osseous support. Studies have directly correlated the success of grafting with the presence of adequate bone on the distal surface of the central incisor preoperatively.[48] These defects cannot subsequently be grafted because the bone graft will not adhere to the tooth surface. The central incisor adjacent to the cleft site is usually rotated and angled with the crown tipped toward the cleft. This rotation and angulation decreases the mesial-distal dimension of the tooth and allows for the best bony support of the tooth (see Figure 44-2). Orthodontic forces of rotation and tipping will have the undesirable effect of increasing the mesial-distal dimension, encroaching on the bony support at the cementoenamel junction of the tooth. Orthodontic root torque to correct the angulation of the tooth will have the undesired effect of pushing the apical portion of the root toward the cleft site. The underlying osseous cleft is frequently much larger than the overlying soft tissue defect may indicate, giving a false sense of security to the orthodontist who may want to move these teeth in the absence of a graft (Figure 44-5).

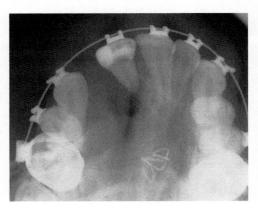

FIGURE 44-5. Occlusal radiograph of a patient who had orthodontic rotation of the maxillary central incisor adjacent to the cleft before grafting the defect. There is loss of bone on the distal surface of the root to the apex. The tooth required removal.

SURGICAL TECHNIQUE FOR GRAFTING THE CLEFT ALVEOLUS

The ideal technique will meet the following criteria:

1. Predictable closure of the nasal floor produces a watertight barrier between the graft and the nasal cavity.
2. There is access to closure of residual palatal and labial fistula.
3. Keratinized attached tissue is maintained around the teeth adjacent to the cleft and in the site where the yet unerupted lateral incisor and canine will erupt.
4. Mobilization of tissue is adequate to close large defects without tension, when such defects are present.
5. The vestibule is not shortened, and scarring is not excessive.

Given these requirements, the technique most often used employs advancing buccal gingival and palatal flaps. This approach has some disadvantages including

1. Difficulty obtaining closure in large bilateral clefts.
2. Defects at the site of the releasing incision created by advancing the flap heal by secondary intention.
3. A four-corner suture line that approximates the flaps directly overlying the graft, which may lead to dehiscence.
4. The possibility that elevating large full-thickness mucoperiosteal flaps leads to growth alteration in young patients. However, when compared with finger flaps and trapezoidal flaps, which can shorten the vestibule and place non-keratinized tissue around the dentition, this approach remains the best.

The procedure can be broken down as follows. The first step requires development of full-thickness mucoperiosteal buccal flaps (Figure 44-6). Consideration may be given to a papilla preserving incision, but this is not required in the mixed dentition. Palatal flaps are then developed, incorporating whatever residual palatal defect may be present to allow for closure of the residual palatal fistula. Some diagrams show this incision being made from a palatal approach. This may be possible in wide clefts but, in practice, is more easily accomplished by starting reflection of the palatal flaps from a sulcular incision placed on the palatal side of the dentition followed by reflection of full-thickness palatal flaps toward the palatal defect. The palatal flaps can then be separated from the nasal tissue along the cleft margin by sharp dissection with scissors from the anterior extending posteriorly as the flaps are elevated (Figure 44-7A). In this manner, the maximum palatal soft tissue is preserved for closure, while assuring adequate nasal mucosa to obtain a watertight nasal closure. Once the buccal and palatal flaps have been developed, access is readily obtained to the nasal mucosa, which is then reflected and sutured, burying the knots to obtain a watertight nasal closure (see Figure 44-7B and C). Most schematic diagrams of cleft closure show this portion of the procedure being performed from the palatal aspect. However, it is generally most readily accomplished in narrow clefts from the anterior through the cleft defect. Once the nasal

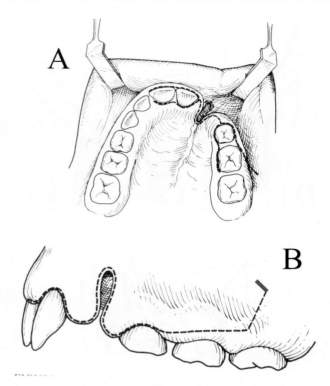

A

B

FIGURE 44-6. **A** and **B,** Sulcular incision used to develop sliding flaps for closure over the graft. (**A** and **B,** Adapted from Hall HD, Posnick JC. Early results of secondary bone grafts in 106 alveolar clefts. J Oral Maxillofac Surg 1983;41:289–294.)

mucosa is closed, the palatal defect is closed by first closing the palatal flaps, converting the cleft palate into a single flap (see Figure 44-7D). The graft material is then placed into the cleft from the anterior, making certain to fill all voids completely to the piriform rim. Graft material can be condensed using an orthodontic band pusher or periosteal elevator (see Figure 44-7E). It is helpful to place a malleable retractor to protect the nasal floor as the bone is packed into place. Finally, the labial flaps can be advanced, and they are sutured to each other and then to the palatal flap, producing the classic four-corner closure over the crest of the ridge (see Figure 44-7F and G). In most cases, the sliding flaps will be advanced one papilla on either side of the cleft, or in some cases, only a single papilla advancement from the posterior segment is necessary. It may be necessary to perform a small backcut or to release or score the periosteum to obtain a tension-free closure. It is best to use a resorbable monofilament suture.

A palatal stent can be used to stabilize the cleft and protect the soft tissue closure. This may compromise hygiene and blood supply to the palatal flaps and, in most cases, is not required for success. In the bilateral cleft, if there is a traumatic occlusion to the anterior maxillary dentition, a mandibular bite plane is helpful to open the bite and prevent mobility of the premaxilla.

It is appropriate to use intraoperative antibiotics. Previous studies show that graft success and incidence of infection

are not improved by the use of postoperative antibiotics.[49] Some surgeons feel more comfortable with a 1-week course of antibiotics, particularly when the soft tissue closure is questionable.

The postoperative diet should be limited to full liquids for approximately 5 days. This can be advanced to a soft mechanical diet. However, it is critical that the patient refrain from incising food with the anterior dentition; rather the patient should cut food into small pieces and masticate primarily on the posterior teeth. In bilateral cases, this is particularly important because any trauma to the premaxilla will cause mobility of the segment, leading to graft failure. Radiographic evidence of graft consolidation should be visible within 8 weeks. The surgeon should confirm successful consolidation of the graft before any orthodontic manipulation of the teeth adjacent to the cleft.

OVERVIEW

This chapter has outlined historic benefits of grafting, discussed many of the controversies, and provided data on the benefits and disadvantages of several approaches.

The following is a stepwise approach to managing the alveolar cleft from one perspective:

1. At age 5 to 6 years, an orthodontic evaluation is performed. The ability of the patient to cooperate with orthodontic treatment is assessed, the arch is evaluated for collapse, and erupted supernumerary teeth in the area of the cleft are identified. Radiographic examination should include a panoramic film as well as an intraoral view that allows detailed evaluation of the cleft site. Periapical films can be used for this, but a lateral oblique occlusal film is best. An occlusal film is placed in the standard position while directing the beam obliquely to the midline along the long axis of the cleft (Figure 44-8).
2. If erupted supernumerary teeth are identified in the area of the cleft, these are extracted now or, at a minimum, 8 weeks before the graft (Figure 44-9A).
3. Orthodontic expansion is performed if there are specific goals that can be met before grafting. These would include decreasing traumatic occlusion to the premaxillary segment in bilateral cleft patients and correcting arch collapse that will compromise grafting. No attempt is made to correct the cross-bite at this stage, and there is no attempt to orthodontically correct rotation of the permanent central incisor (see Figure 44-9A).
4. The alveolar cleft is grafted when the patient is between 6 and 8 years of age. Two teams perform the surgery with graft harvest from the iliac crest simultaneous with the cleft closure.
5. The graft is evaluated with a lateral oblique occlusal radiograph 3 months after surgery (see Figure 44-9B).
6. Final orthodontic expansion is performed if indicated, and permanent incisor teeth are then rotated into proper alignment.

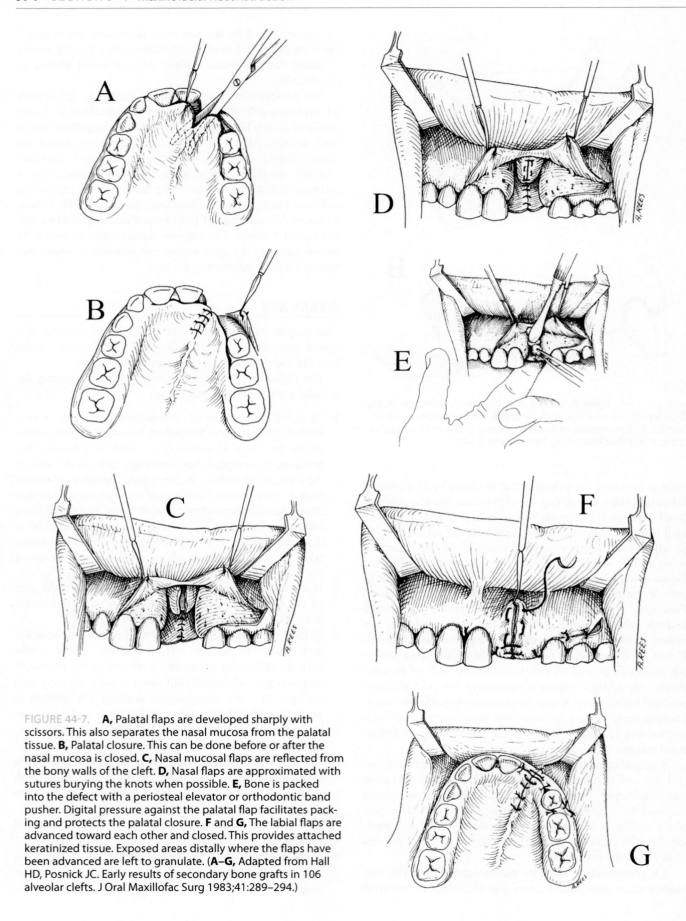

FIGURE 44-7. **A,** Palatal flaps are developed sharply with scissors. This also separates the nasal mucosa from the palatal tissue. **B,** Palatal closure. This can be done before or after the nasal mucosa is closed. **C,** Nasal mucosal flaps are reflected from the bony walls of the cleft. **D,** Nasal flaps are approximated with sutures burying the knots when possible. **E,** Bone is packed into the defect with a periosteal elevator or orthodontic band pusher. Digital pressure against the palatal flap facilitates packing and protects the palatal closure. **F** and **G,** The labial flaps are advanced toward each other and closed. This provides attached keratinized tissue. Exposed areas distally where the flaps have been advanced are left to granulate. (**A–G,** Adapted from Hall HD, Posnick JC. Early results of secondary bone grafts in 106 alveolar clefts. J Oral Maxillofac Surg 1983;41:289–294.)

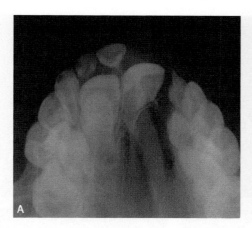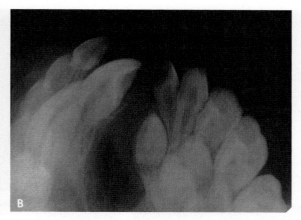

FIGURE 44-8. **A,** Traditional maxillary occlusal radiograph. The cleft is identifiable, but overlap of the bone makes it difficult to determine the size of the defect and relationship of the teeth to the defect. **B,** Oblique occlusal radiograph is exposed by directing the beam obliquely to the midline, along the long axis of the cleft. Note that the morphology of the cleft is better identified, as is the relationship of unerupted teeth to the defect.

7. Conventional orthodontic treatment is performed at a more traditional age, after eruption of the remaining permanent dentition. Patients are periodically monitored for eruption of the canine in the cleft. Some authors have indicated that in 30% to 73% of patients, eruption of the canine into the alveolar graft requires surgical uncovering of the tooth or uncovering and orthodontic assistance.[15,50,51] Others have reported that nearly all of these teeth can be expected to erupt without surgical intervention[27] (see Figure 44-9C). If uncovering is necessary, techniques to preserve attached tissue are used as would be appropriate for impacted canines in noncleft patients.

8. Missing lateral incisors are managed with space development and implant placement as opposed to canine substitution. This is accomplished after definitive orthodontic treatment and orthognathic surgery, if indicated, after maxillary growth is complete. Even when bone height is

adequate and teeth adjacent to the graft have good support, the graft undergoes resorption, resulting in a narrow ridge. This is not unlike the bone resorption found with congenitally absent lateral incisors in noncleft patients. Successful implant restoration is possible, but further grafting is likely needed before adequate labial-palatal width is available for implant placement[33] (Figure 44-10). Attention to soft and hard tissue is critical in these patients to achieve aesthetic results.

CONCLUSION

Restoration of the cleft alveolus and maxilla by grafting is a critical part of the overall management of the patient with cleft palate. A systematic approach can improve predictability. This is best accomplished during the mixed-dentition stage. Adjunctive expansion may be accomplished before or after grafting, depending on the needs of the patient.

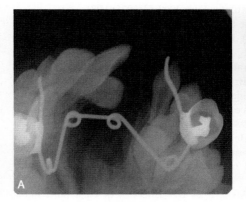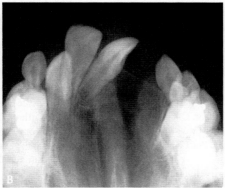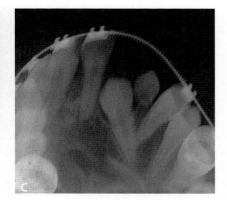

FIGURE 44-9. **A,** The cleft has been expanded. The canine is in position to begin eruption. There is a supernumerary/malformed lateral incisor erupting horizontally into the cleft. **B,** The supernumerary tooth has been removed. The defect was grafted 2 months after extraction and the film shows good bone consolidation. **C,** The maxillary canine can be seen erupting into the graft.

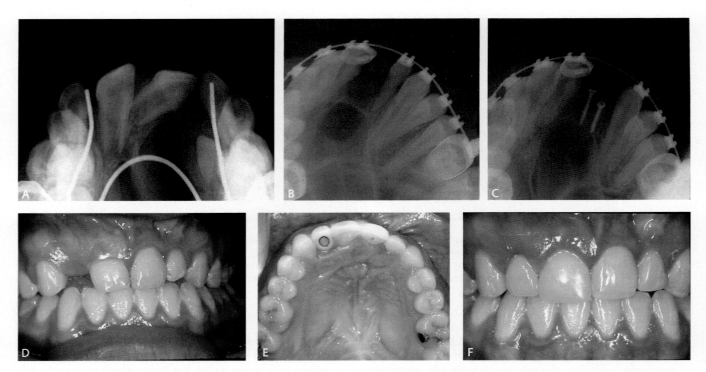

FIGURE 44-10. **A,** Occlusal radiograph shows thin bridge of bone with inadequate height. A malformed lateral incisor was maintained to preserve as much width as possible. **B,** The tooth was removed. **C,** After 2 months of healing, an onlay bone graft was placed. **D,** Clinical view after grafting. **E** and **F,** View after placement of the implant and reconstruction.

References

1. Santiago PE, Grayson BH, Cutting CB, et al. Reduced need for alveolar bone grafting by pre-surgical orthopedics and primary gingivoperiosteoplasty. Cleft Palate Craniofac J 1998;35:77–80.
2. Horswell BB, Henderson JM. Secondary osteoplasty of the alveolar cleft defect. J Oral Maxillofac Surg 2003;61:1082–1090.
3. Kalaaji A, Lilja J, Friede H. Bone grafting at the stage of mixed and permanent dentition in patients with clefts of the lip and primary palate. Plast Reconstr Surg 1994;93:690–696.
4. Teja A, Persson R, Omnell ML. Periodontal status of teeth adjacent to nongrafted unilateral alveolar clefts. Cleft Palate Craniofac J 1992;29:357–362.
5. Bureau S, Penko M, McFadden L. Speech outcome after closure of oronasal fistulas with bone grafts. J Oral Maxillofac Surg 2001;59:1408–1413.
6. Bergland O, Semb G, Abyholm RD. Elimination of the residual alveolar cleft by secondary bone grafting and subsequent orthodontic treatment. Cleft Palate J 1986;23:175–205.
7. Hynes PJ, Earley MJ. Assessment of secondary alveolar bone grafting using a modification of the Bergland grading system. Br J Plast Surg 2003;56:630–636.
8. Dado DV, Rosenstein SW, Adler ME, Kernahan DA. Long term assessment of early alveolar bone grafts using three-dimensional computer assisted tomography: a pilot study. Plast Reconstr Surg 1997;99:1840–1845.
9. Alonso N, Tanikawa D, Freitas R, et al. Evaluation of maxillary alveolar reconstruction using a resorbable collagen sponge with recombinant human bone morphogenetic protein-2 in cleft lip and palate patients. Tissue Eng Part C Methods 2010;16:1183–1189.
10. Fallucco MA, Carstens MH. Primary reconstruction of alveolar clefts using recombinant human bone morphogenic protein-2: clinical and radiographic outcomes. J Craniofac Surg 2009;20:1759–1764.
11. Herford A. Bone morphogenetic protein-induced repair of the premaxillary cleft. J Oral Maxillofac Surg 2007;65;2136–2141.
12. Vig KWL, Turvey TA, Fonseca RJ. Orthodontic and surgical considerations in bone grafting in the cleft maxilla and palate. In Turvey TA, Vig KWL, Fonseca RJ, editors. Facial Clefts and Craniosynostosis: Principles of Management. Philadelphia: WB Saunders; 1996; p. 396.
13. Eppley B. Alveolar cleft bone grafting (part 1): primary bone grafting. J Oral Maxillofac Surg 1996;54:74–82.
14. Rosenstein SW. Early bone grafting of alveolar cleft deformities. J Oral Maxillofac Surg 2003;61:1078–1081.
15. Kwon JK, Waite DE, Stickel FR, Chisholm T. The management of alveolar cleft defects. J Am Dent Assoc 1981;102:848–853.
16. Robertson NRE, Jolleys A. An 11-year follow-up of the effects of early bone grafting in infants born with complete clefts of the lip and palate. Br J Plast Surg 1983;36:438–443.
17. Helms JA, Speidel M, Denis KL. Effect of timing on long-term clinical success of alveolar cleft bone grafts. Am J Orthod Dentofac Orthop 1987;92:232–240.
18. Brattstrom V, McWilliam J. The influence of bone grafting age on dental abnormalities and alveolar bone height in patients with unilateral cleft lip and palate. Eur J Orthod 1989;11:351–358.
19. Daskalogiannakis J, Ross RB. Effect of alveolar bone grafting in the mixed dentition on maxillary growth in complete unilateral cleft lip and palate patients. Cleft Palate Craniofac J 1997;34:455–458.

20. Witsenburg B. The reconstruction of anterior residual bone defects in patients with cleft lip, alveolus and palate: a review. J Maxillofac Surg 1985;13:197–208.

21. Dempf R, Teltzrow T, Kramer FJ, Hausamen JE. Alveolar bone grafting in patients with complete clefts: a comparative study between secondary and tertiary bone grafting. Cleft Palate Craniofac J 2002;39:18–25.

22. Boyne PJ, Sands NR. Combined orthodontics-surgical management of residual palato-alveolar cleft defects. Am J Orthod 1976;70:20–37.

23. Boyne PJ, Sands NR. Secondary bone grafting of residual alveolar and palatal clefts. J Oral Surg 1972;30:87–92.

24. Abyholm RE, Bergland E, Semb G. Secondary bone grafting of alveolar clefts. Scand J Plast Reconstr Surg 1981;15:127–140.

25. Broude D, Waite DE. Secondary closure of alveolar defects. Oral Surg 1974;37:829.

26. Hall HD, Posnick JC. Early results of secondary bone grafts in 106 alveolar clefts. J Oral Maxillofac Surg 1983;41:289–294.

27. Turvey TA, Vig K, Moriarty J. Delayed bone grafting in the cleft maxilla and palate: a multidisciplinary analysis. Am J Orthod 1984;86:244–256.

28. Yi-Lin J, James DR, Mars M. Bilateral alveolar bone grafting: a report of 55 consecutively treated patients. Eur J Orthod 1998;20:299–307.

29. Boyne PJ. Bone grafting in the osseous reconstruction of alveolar and palatal clefts. Oral Maxillofac Clin North Am 1991;3:589–597.

30. Hall HD, Werther JR. Conventional alveolar cleft bone grafting. Oral Maxillofac Clin North Am 1991;3:609–616.

31. Suzuki A, Watanabe M, Nakano M, Takahama Y. Maxillary lateral incisors of subjects with cleft lip and or palate: part 2. Cleft Palate Craniofac J 1992;29:380–384.

32. Kearns G, Perrott DH, Sharma A, et al. Placement of endosseous implants in grafted alveolar clefts. Cleft Palate Craniofac J 1997;34:520–525.

33. Vig KWL. Alveolar bone grafts: the surgical/orthodontic management of the cleft maxilla. Ann Acad Med Singapore 1999;28:721–727.

34. Enemark H, Sindet-Pedersen S, Bundgaard M. Long-term results after secondary bone grafting of alveolar clefts. J Oral Maxillofac Surg 1987;45:913–918.

35. Paulin G, Astrand P, Rosenquist JB, Bartholdson L. Intermediate bone grafting of alveolar clefts. J Craniomaxillofac Surg 1988;16:2–7.

36. Crockford DA, Converse JM. The ilium as a source of bone grafts in children. Plast Reconstr Surg 1972;50:270–274.

37. Larsen PE. Sources of autogenous bone grafts in pediatric patients. Oral Maxillofac Clin North Am 1994;6:137–152.

38. Rudman RA. Prospective evaluation of morbidity associated with iliac crest harvest for alveolar cleft grafting. J Oral Maxillofac Surg 1997;55:219–223.

39. Wolfe SA, Kawamoto HK. Taking the iliac bone graft. J Bone Joint Surg 1978;60:411.

40. Harsha BC, Turvey TA, Powers SK. Use of autogenous cranial bone grafts in maxillofacial surgery. J Oral Maxillofac Surg 1986;44:11–15.

41. Turvey TA. Donor site for alveolar cleft bone grafts (letter). J Oral Maxillofac Surg 1997;45:834.

42. Jackson IT, Helden G, Marx R. Skull bone grafts in maxillofacial and craniofacial surgery. J Oral Maxillofac Surg 1986;44:949–956.

43. Kortebein MJ, Nelson CL, Sadove MA. Retrospective analysis of 135 secondary alveolar cleft grafts using iliac or calvarial bone. J Oral Maxillofac Surg 1991;49:493–498.

44. Sadove MA, Nelson CL, Epply BL, Nguyen B. An evaluation of calvarial and iliac donor sites in alveolar cleft grafting. Cleft Palate Craniofac J 1990;27:225–229.

45. Maxson BB, Baxter SD, Vig KWL, Fonseca RJ. Allogeneic bone for secondary alveolar cleft osteoplasty. J Oral Maxillofac Surg 1990;48:933–941.

46. Marx RE, Miller RI, Ehler WJ, et al. A comparison of particulate allogeneic and particulate autogenous bone grafts into maxillary alveolar clefts in dogs. J Oral Maxillofac Surg 1984;42:3–9.

47. Vig KWL, D'orth RCS, Turvey TA. Orthodonticsurgical interaction in the management of cleft lip and palate. Clin Plast Surg 1985;12:735–748.

48. Aurouze C, Moller KT, Bevis RR, et al. The presurgical status of the alveolar cleft and success of secondary bone grafting. Cleft Palate Craniofac J 2000;37:179–184.

49. Larsen PE, Myers G, Beck MF. Morbidity of alveolar cleft grafting in the early mixed dentition (<8 years). J Oral Maxillofac Surg 1997;55(Suppl 3):127.

50. Eldeeb M, Messer LB, Lehnert MW, et al. Canine eruption into grafted bone in maxillary alveolar cleft defects. Cleft Palate J 1988;19:9–16.

51. Enemark H, Sindet-Pedersen S, Bundgaard M, Simonsen EK. Combined orthodontic-surgical treatment of alveolar clefts. Ann Plast Surg 1988;21:127–133.

52. Ochs MW. Alveolar cleft bone grafting (part 2): secondary bone grafting. J Oral Maxillofac Surg 1996;54:83–88.

SECTION 5

45

Nonsyndromic Craniosynostosis

G. E. Ghali, DDS, MD, and Andrew R. Banker, DDS, MD

In its basic form, craniosynostosis represents premature suture fusion. It occurs in approximately 1 per 1000 live births in the United States. Craniosynostosis may be classified as *nonsyndromic* or *syndromic*. Most forms of craniosynostosis are isolated and not associated with any other conditions and are, therefore, nonsyndromic. Syndromic craniosynostosis is covered in Chapter 46. The pathogenesis of craniosynostosis is complex and probably multifactorial.[1] Moss theorized that craniosynostosis such as seen in Apert's and Crouzon's syndromes results from abnormal tensile forces transmitted to the dura from an anomalous cranial base through key ligamentous attachments.[2] This hypothesis fails to explain craniosynostosis in patients with a normal cranial base configuration. The cause of craniosynostosis may be postulated to be the result of either primary suture abnormalities, sufficient extremes of forces that overcome the underlying expansive forces of the brain, inadequate intrinsic growth forces of the brain, or various genetic and environmental factors.[3] Cranial vault growth achieves approximately 80% of the adult size at birth and definitive size by 2.5 to 3 years of age.[4] The existence of the six major sutural regions allows for head expansion as well as transvaginal head deformation.[5] Recall that posterior fontanelle closure (3–6 mo) generally precedes anterior fontanelle closure (9–12 mo).

FUNCTIONAL CONSIDERATIONS

The major functional problems associated with craniosynostosis are intracranial hypertension, visual impairment, limitation of brain growth, and neuropsychiatric disorders.[6] In general, the functional problems increase as the number of sutures involved increases.[6] These functional abnormalities are gradual in their development, difficult to detect, and often irreversible in nature.

Intracranial Hypertension

Intracranial hypertension is defined as a pressure of greater than 15 mmHg. Studies by Marchac and Renier[7] have demonstrated a 13% incidence of intracranial hypertension with single-suture stenosis and up to a 42% incidence in multisuture-stenosed children. The clinical symptoms of intracranial hypertension include headaches, irritability, and difficulty sleeping. The radiographic signs may include cortical thinning or a lückenschädel (hammered metal) appearance of the inner table of the skull; these clinical and radiographic signs are relatively late developments. If intracranial hypertension goes untreated, it affects brain function; if persistent, this may necessitate early operative intervention during the first few months of life. Intracranial hypertension most likely affects those with the greatest disparity between brain growth and intracranial capacity and may occur in as many as 42% of untreated children with more than one suture affected. Currently, intracranial volume is measured using computed tomography (CT) scans, a noninvasive method appropriate for use in children with craniosynostosis.[8] It might be possible to identify individuals who are at a greater risk for developing intracranial hypertension and would benefit the most from early surgery.

Visual Impairment

Untreated intracranial hypertension in the acute phase may lead to papilledema, and chronically, to some degree of optic atrophy causing a partial to complete blindness.[9] Some forms of craniosynostosis may involve orbital hypertelorism and may lead to compromised visual acuity and restricted binocular vision.

Limitation of Brain Growth

Brain volume in the normal child almost triples during the first year of life. By 2 years of age, the cranial capacity is four times that at birth. If brain growth is to proceed unhindered, open sutures at the level of the cranial vault and base must spread during phases of rapid growth for marginal ossification.

In craniosynostosis, premature suture fusion is combined with continuing brain growth. Depending on the number and location of prematurely fused sutures and the timing of closure, the growth potential of the brain may be limited. Surgical intervention can provide suture release and reshaping to restore a more normal intracranial volume. In general, this does not completely reverse craniosynostosis and diminished volume is often the end result.

Neuropsychiatric Disorders

Neuropsychiatric disorders are believed to be secondary to cerebral compression. Disorders range from mild behavioral disturbances to overt mental retardation. It has been shown that children with craniosynostosis and associated neuropsychiatric disorders often improve after cranial vault reconstruction.[10]

DIAGNOSIS

One should suspect craniosynostosis in any infant with an abnormal head shape. Definitive diagnosis is based on clinical and radiographic evaluations. The clinical evaluation involves the palpation of the skull for any movement, ridging, and presence of the anterior and posterior fontanelles. Quantitative measurements of the superior orbital rims, relative to the most anterior aspect of the cornea, also may help in planning treatment for superior orbital rim advancements.

The radiographic evaluation of craniosynostosis is used to define quantitatively aberrant anatomy, plan surgical procedures, and most important, provide a means to demonstrate to the parents the difference between stenosed and nonstenosed sutures. Conventional skull radiographs, such as plain skull films and lateral cephalograms, are inexpensive and widely available. The preoperative assessment of patients with suspected or known craniosynostosis is based on these conventional radiographs. Most cases of synostosis can be demonstrated on plain skull films. Normal or patent cranial sutures manifest as a line. The absence of a radiolucent line in the normal anatomic position of a suture may suggest craniosynostosis.

Currently, CT scans provide improved hard tissue imaging. The definition of these elements of the bony facial structures on high-resolution CT images with or without three-dimensional reconstruction is unmatched by other imaging techniques (Figure 45-1). The development of CT scanning, particularly three-dimensional reformatting, and the maturation of readily available means of craniofacial surgery have led to a close dependence on CT scanning for

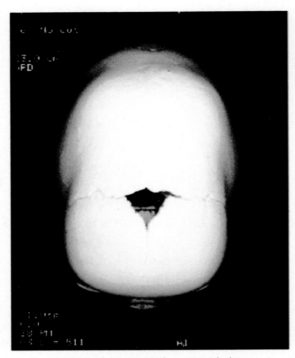

FIGURE 45-1. Computed tomography scan with three-dimensional reconstruction. Patency of metopic and coronal sutures as well as anterior fontanelle; premature fusion of sagittal suture. (Reproduced with permission from Ghali GE, Sinn DP, Tantipasawasin S. Management of nonsyndromic craniosynostosis. Atlas Oral Maxillofac Surg Clin North Am 2002;10:3.)

preoperative surgical planning. CT scanning also has been used to document surgical changes in vivo and to follow developments longitudinally.[11–22]

CLASSIFICATION

The classification of craniosynostosis is based on the shape of the skull, which usually reflects the underlying prematurely fused suture or sutures.[23,24] The major cranial vault sutures that may be involved include the left and right coronal, metopic, sagittal, and lambdoid.

Unilateral Coronal Synostosis

Unilateral coronal synostosis results in flatness on the ipsilateral side of the forehead and supraorbital ridge region. The head is inherently asymmetrical in shape with a flattened or retropositioned forehead on the ipsilateral side, especially when viewed from the top (Figure 45-2). The term for this deformity is *anterior plagiocephaly*. One should rule out infant molding or positional plagiocephaly and congenital torticollis as other possible diagnoses. Premature fusion of the unilateral coronal suture represents 20% of the isolated or nonsyndromic cases of synostosis in the United States. Characteristic morphologic features occur on the ipsilateral side. The frontal bone is flat, and the supraorbital ridge and lateral orbital rim are recessed (Figure 45-3). The orbit is shallow,

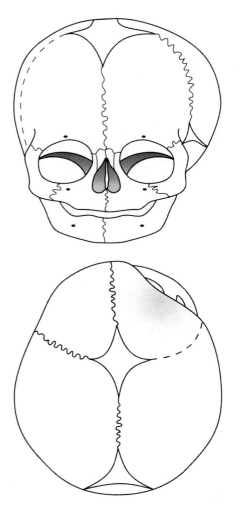

FIGURE 45-2.   Frontal and superior views. Characteristic right anterior plagiocephaly. (Adapted from Ghali GE, Sinn DP, Tantipasawasin S. Management of nonsyndromic craniosynostosis. Atlas Oral Maxillofac Surg Clin North Am 2002;10:4.)

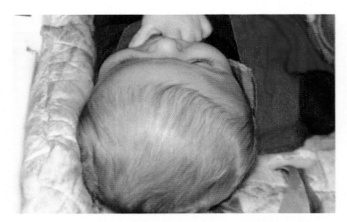

FIGURE 45-3.   Superior view. Recessed frontal bone, supraorbital ridge, and lateral orbital rim on patient's right side. (Reproduced with permission from Ghali GE, Sinn DP, Tantipasawasin S. Management of nonsyndromic craniosynostosis. Atlas Oral Maxillofac Surg Clin North Am 2002;10:5.)

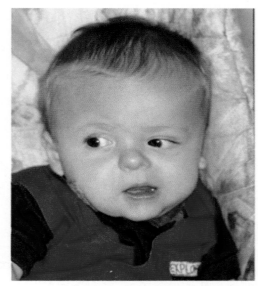

FIGURE 45-4.   Frontal view. Nasal bridge and root deviation to the affected (right) side characteristic in plagiocephaly. (Reproduced with permission from Ghali GE, Sinn DP, Tantipasawasin S. Management of nonsyndromic craniosynostosis. Atlas Oral Maxillofac Surg Clin North Am 2002;10:5.)

and the anterior cranial base is short in the anteroposterior dimension. The root of the nose may be constricted and deviated to the affected side (Figure 45-4). The ipsilateral zygoma and infraorbital rim also may be flat and recessed.

Bilateral Coronal Synostosis

Bilateral coronal synostosis is the most common cranial vault suture synostosis pattern associated with Apert's and Crouzon's syndromes. Bilateral coronal synostosis results in recession of the supraorbital ridges, which causes the overlying eyebrows to sit posterior to the corneas. In addition to the recessed supraorbital bone, the forehead appears to be lower and there is sagittal shortening of the skull (Figure 45-5). The term for this cranial vault deformity is *brachycephaly.* The anterior cranial base is short in the anteroposterior dimension and wide transversely. The overlying cranial vault is high in the superoinferior dimension, with anterior bulging of the upper forehead that results from compensatory growth of the patent metopic suture (Figure 45-6). The orbits are also shallow (exorbitism), with the eyes bulging (exophthalmus) and abnormally separated (orbital hypertelorism). Brachycephaly represents 20% of the isolated craniosynostosis cases in the United States and is the most common syndrome-associated synostosis.

Metopic Synostosis

Metopic synostosis usually occurs in isolation and results in a triangular shape to the skull (Figure 45-7). The term for this cranial vault deformity is *trigonocephaly.* The associated cranial vault deformity consists of relative hypotelorism, an elevated supraorbital ridge medially, and posteroinferior

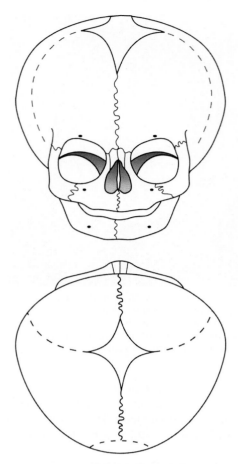

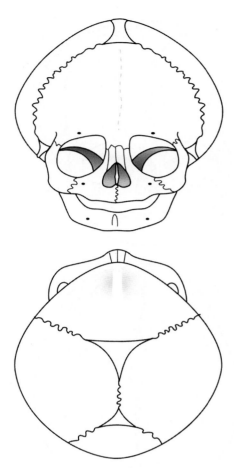

FIGURE 45-5. Frontal and superior views. Characteristic brachycephaly. (Adapted from Ghali GE, Sinn DP, Tantipasawasin S. Management of nonsyndromic craniosynostosis. Atlas Oral Maxillofac Surg Clin North Am 2002;10:4.)

FIGURE 45-7. Frontal and superior views. Characteristic trigonocephaly. (Adapted from Ghali GE, Sinn DP, Tantipasawasin S. Management of nonsyndromic craniosynostosis. Atlas Oral Maxillofac Surg Clin North Am 2002;10:8.)

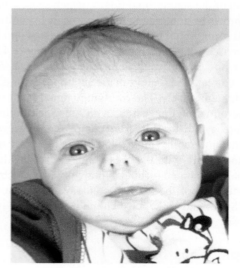

FIGURE 45-6. Frontal view. High cranial vault and transverse widening characteristic of brachycephaly. Note visible ridging in the bicoronal suture region. (Reproduced with permission from Ghali GE, Sinn DP, Tantipasawasin S. Management of nonsyndromic craniosynostosis. Atlas Oral Maxillofac Surg Clin North Am 2002;10:7.)

recession of the lateral orbital rims and lateral aspect of the supraorbital ridges. Palpation often reveals a prominent midline keel in the region of the metopic suture (Figure 45-8). The bitemporal width is decreased, which results in an abnormal anterior cranial vault shape and decreased anterior cranial vault volume. The overlying forehead is sloped posteriorly to approximately the level of the coronal sutures. Trigonocephaly represents 10% of the nonsyndromic craniosynostosis cases in the United States.

Sagittal Synostosis

Sagittal synostosis, the most common form, is rarely associated with increased intracranial pressure. The skull typically has anteroposterior elongation with a compensatory transverse narrowing (Figure 45-9). The term for this cranial vault deformity is *scaphocephaly.* The deformity consists of an elongated anteroposterior dimension and a narrow transverse dimension to the cranial vault (Figure 45-10). Usually, the midface and anterior cranial vault sutures are not affected. Scaphocephaly represents 50% of all single-suture craniosynostosis cases in the United States.

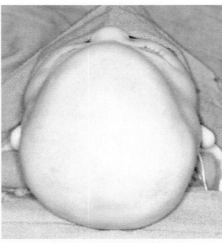

FIGURE 45-8.   Intraoperative view after shaving of the head demonstrates prominent midline ridging associated with trigonocephaly. (Reproduced with permission from Ghali GE, Sinn DP, Tantipasawasin S. Management of nonsyndromic craniosynostosis. Atlas Oral Maxillofac Surg Clin North Am 2002;10:9.)

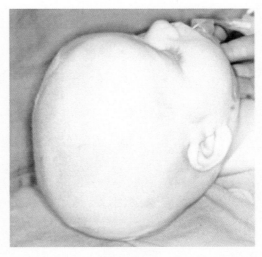

FIGURE 45-10.   Intraoperative view after shaving of the head demonstrates prominent sagittal suture ridging associated with scaphocephaly. (Reproduced with permission from Ghali GE, Sinn DP, Tantipasawasin S. Management of nonsyndromic craniosynostosis. Atlas Oral Maxillofac Surg Clin North Am 2002;10:11.)

Unilateral Lambdoid Synostosis

Unilateral lambdoid synostosis results in flatness of the affected ipsilateral parietooccipital region. The location of

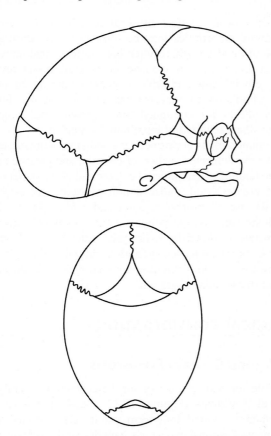

FIGURE 45-9.   Lateral and superior views. Characteristic scaphocephaly. (Adapted from Ghali GE, Sinn DP, Tantipasawasin S. Management of nonsyndromic craniosynostosis. Atlas Oral Maxillofac Surg Clin North Am 2002;10:10.)

the ear canal and external ear is more posterior and inferior on the ipsilateral side than on the contralateral side. This configuration is more noticeable when the patient is examined from the superior view and is relatively inconspicuous from the frontal or profile views. The term for this cranial vault deformity is *posterior plagiocephaly*. One should rule out infant molding and congenital torticollis (Figure 45-11). With positional (or deformational) plagiocephaly, the ipsilateral ear and forehead are positioned anteriorly, and the ear is not inferiorly displaced as it is with true unilateral lambdoid fusion. The use of head-molding helmet therapy has received renewed interest in the past decade as the preferred treatment of children with positional head shape abnormalities.[25,26] The overall incidence of true unilateral lambdoid synostosis is less than 3% of all isolated synostosis cases in the United States.

PRINCIPLES OF MANAGEMENT

Multidisciplinary Team Approach

The multidisciplinary team approach was developed in response to the failures that commonly occurred when various aspects of care were not coordinated and when the relationships among coexisting problems were not known.[4,27] The objectives of this approach are diagnosis, formulation, and execution of treatment plans and longitudinal follow-up for patients with craniofacial deformities; the team should meet at least monthly for regular outpatient evaluations. Transcripts of these evaluations are forwarded with recommendations to primary care providers and appropriate agencies. Children younger than 5 years are usually evaluated annually, whereas children older than 5 years are seen every other year.

SECTION 5

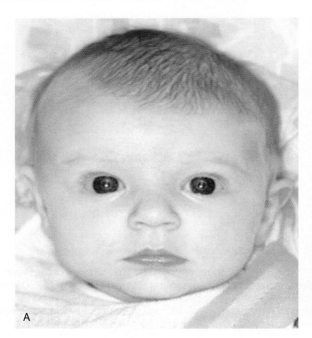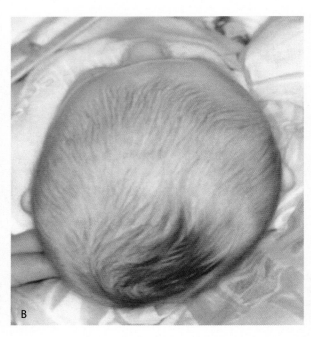

FIGURE 45-11.   Frontal **(A)** and superior **(B)** views of a child with positional plagiocephaly. Radio-graphic and clinical examination demonstrated no evidence of craniosynostosis; note asymmetry of external ear position.

The frequency of evaluation varies with the stability of the deformity and its consequences.

The craniofacial team should consist of a pediatric anesthesiologist, a pediatric ophthalmologist, a surgeon, an audiologist, a maxillofacial prosthodontist, an orthodontist, a psychologist, a geneticist, an otolaryngologist, a pediatrician, social workers, a speech pathologist, and a nurse.[28–32] All these team members have integral roles at various times in the child's development.[33,34]

Current Surgical Approach

The goals of craniosynostosis suture release are twofold. The first goal is to allow the brain to grow and expand without restriction. The second goal is to establish a more normal contour to the forehead, supraorbital ridges, and skull.[35–37] In most cases, an intracranial approach is used for cranial vault and orbital osteotomies, with reshaping and advancement of bony segments for ideal age-appropriate bony morphology. When planning the time and type of surgical intervention, one must consider the functions, future growth and development of the craniofacial skeleton, and the maintenance of normal body image. Simple cranio-synostosis can be managed successfully with frontocranial remodeling.

Although the timing of craniosynostosis repair remains controversial and individualized, we prefer early surgical repair between the ages of 4 and 8 months.[38,39] Early surgical repair allows for rapid frontal lobe growth, which supports the forehead and supraorbital ridge advancement. At this age, the cranium is highly malleable and, therefore, easier to

contour; a positive effect on facial growth may be achieved and future deformities may be lessened. Also, during this period of rapid growth, residual bony defects heal more rapidly. In severe forms of craniosynostosis, additional revision of the cranial vault and orbit is necessary during infancy or early childhood to increase intracranial volume further, which allows for continued brain growth and avoids or reduces the likelihood of intracranial hypertension.

A craniotomy is performed by a pediatric neurosurgeon to remove the deformed section of cranium and provide access for the additional craniofacial osteotomies. The skeletal segments are reshaped, replaced into position, and stabilized with the use of resorbable plates and screws. These plates, which are composed of polylactic and polyglycolic acid, are completely resorbed by hydrolysis within 9 to 14 months while maintaining tensile strength for initial stabilization.[40–43] As a result, growth restrictions are minimized as is the potential for transcranial migration.

SURGICAL CONSIDERATIONS

Unilateral Coronal Synostosis

Multiple surgical approaches for the correction of unilateral coronal synostosis (Figures 45-12 and 45-13) have been described.[44–46] Good long-term results are obtained when treatment of coronal synostosis includes suture release along with cranial vault and orbital osteotomies for reshaping and advancement in infancy. At the Louisiana State University Health Sciences Center in Shreveport, unilateral orbital

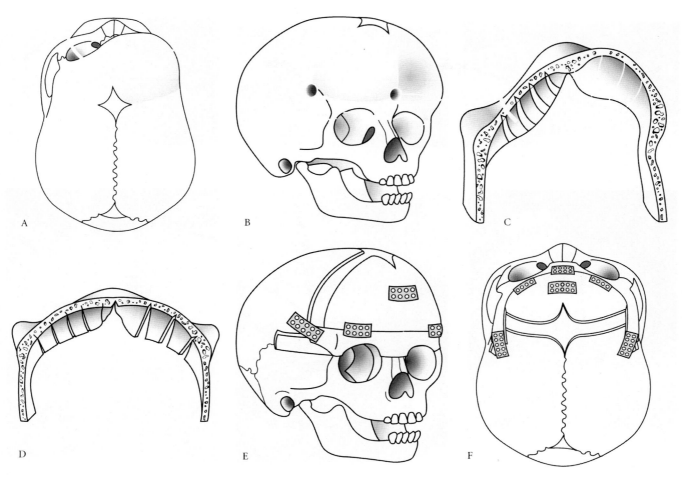

FIGURE 45-12.   A child with unilateral coronal synostosis resulting in left-sided anterior plagiocephaly. **A,** Asymmetrical forehead and orbit viewed from above. Note marked left supraorbital retrusion and right forehead and cranial vault bulging. **B,** Bur holes prepared for bifrontal craniotomy at the level of the supraorbital region, allowing a 1 cm fronto-orbital unit (bandeau), which extends into the temporal fossa via tongue-in-groove (tenon) extensions. Note that the degree of extension into the lateral and inferior orbital rims is variable based on aesthetics. **C,** The removed bandeau is contoured bilaterally via removal of wedges from the left orbital roof and scoring the right orbital roof. **D,** The bandeau is reshaped to achieve symmetry by bending the left side and straightening the right side. **E** and **F,** Stabilization of forehead and bandeau achieved via resorbable plates and screws. (A–F, Adapted from Ghali GE, Sinn DP, Tantipasawasin S. Management of nonsyndromic craniosynostosis. Atlas Oral Maxillofac Surg Clin North Am 2002;10:14–15.)

rim advancement and frontal bone reshaping are ideally performed at 6 to 8 months of age. Other centers have reported good results when treatment is provided between the ages of 2.5 and 3 years. To achieve optimal symmetry, we prefer to use a bilateral surgical approach. Symmetry of the cranial vault and orbit must be achieved during surgery because results generally do not improve over time. Stabilization is achieved by using direct intraosseous wires or resorbable plates and screws.

Bilateral Coronal Synostosis

The treatment of bilateral coronal synostosis (Figures 45-14 and 45-15) requires suture release and simultaneous bilateral orbital rim and frontal bone advancements.[47,48] Surgery is performed when the patient is between 6 and 8 months of age. Other centers have reported good results with children

treated between the ages of 2.5 and 3 years of age. The osteotomies for the bilateral orbital rim advancement are made superior to the nasofrontal and frontozygomatic sutures and extend to the squamous portion of the temporal bone. Stabilization is achieved with direct transosseous wires or resorbable plates and screws. The more normalized shape provides the needed increase in intracranial volume within the anterior cranial vault.

Metopic Synostosis

Surgical treatment of metopic synostosis (Figures 45-16 and 45-17) involves metopic suture release, simultaneous bilateral orbital rim advancements, and lateral widening via frontal bone advancement. These procedures are usually performed at 6 to 8 months of age.[49] Orbital hypotelorism is corrected by splitting the supraorbital ridge unit vertically in

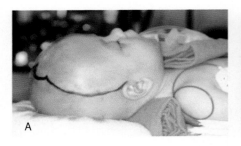

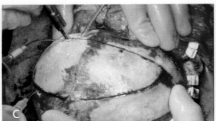

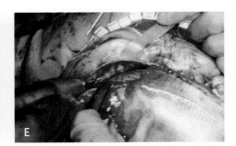

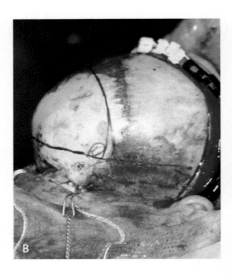

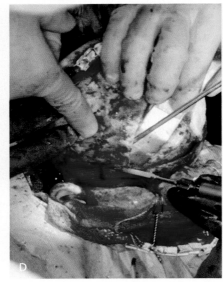

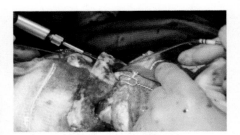

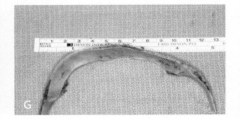

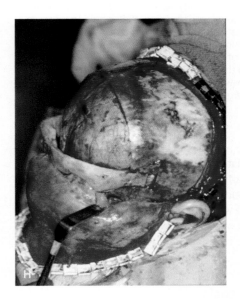

FIGURE 45-13. **A,** A 6-month-old patient with right anterior plagiocephaly placed in the supine position and the head secured in a Mayfield headrest. A coronal incision is used and the anterior scalp flap is elevated subperiosteally along with the temporalis muscle. Extension may be carried pre- or postauricular as needed. **B,** Subperiosteal dissection is achieved bilaterally circumferentially in the periorbital, lateral canthal, lateral orbital, and zygomatic buttresses. Care is taken to maintain the integrity of the medial canthal ligaments. Posterior scalp flap is dissected subperiosteally to between the coronal and the lambdoid sutures. Area of proposed bifrontal craniotomy and bur holes are marked. **C,** Neurosurgeon performs bifrontal craniotomy using a Midas Rex drill. **D,** Frontal and temporal lobes of the brain are gently repositioned to perform upper orbital and temporal osteotomies through the skull base. Reciprocating saw is used to perform bilateral tongue-in-groove extensions from external approach to the level of pterion. **E,** Attention is turned to the anterior skull base osteotomy and the saw is directed internally across the skull base anterior to the olfactory bulbs while retracting the frontal lobe. **F,** In addition to frontal lobe retraction, the orbital contents must be protected via retraction at this time. The level of the osteotomy at the lateral orbital rim is customized as needed from as high as the frontozygomatic suture to as low as the lateral aspect of the orbital floor into the inferior orbital fissure. **G,** Bandeau has been removed and asymmetry noted before reshaping. **H,** Left oblique view after remodeling and recontouring of the bandeau but before frontal bone placement. Resorbable plates and screws are used for fixation. *(Continued)*

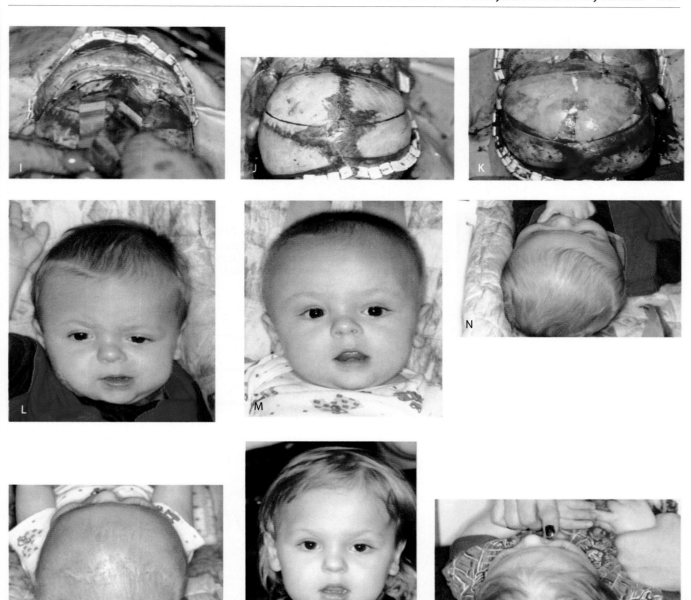

FIGURE 45-13. *(Continued)* **I,** Retraction of bifrontal lobes demonstrates differential degree of advancement on the right side at anterior skull base. **J,** Superior view of anterior cranial vault before reshaping. **K,** Superior view of the anterior cranial vault after osteotomies, reshaping, and resorbable plate and screw fixation of the bone segments. Barrel-staving cuts may be made in the temporal and parietal bones as needed for reshaping purposes. **L,** A 6-month-old boy with right unilateral plagiocephaly. He underwent anterior cranial vault and bilateral superior orbital rim osteotomies with reshaping and advancement by the procedure described. Preoperative frontal view is shown. **M,** Frontal view 6 weeks after reconstruction. **N,** Preoperative superior view. **O,** Superior view 6 weeks after reconstruction. **P,** Frontal view 2 years after reconstruction. **Q,** Superior view 2 years after reconstruction. *(Continued)*

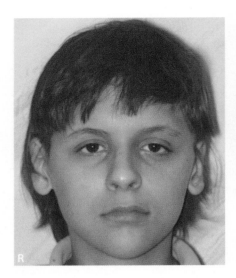

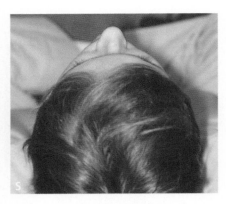

FIGURE 45-13. *(Continued)* **R,** Frontal view 12 years after reconstruction. **S,** Superior view 12 years after reconstruction. (**A–S,** Reproduced with permission from Ghali GE, Sinn DP, Tantipasawasin S. Management of nonsyndromic craniosynostosis. Atlas Oral Maxillofac Surg Clin North Am 2002;10:16–24.)

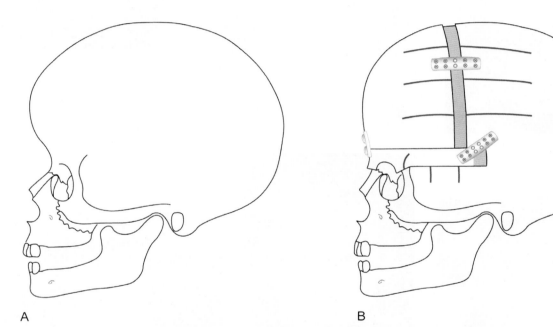

A

B

FIGURE 45-14. Brachycephaly before and after anterior cranial vault and bilateral superior orbital rim osteotomies, reshaping, and advancements. **A,** Site of osteotomies as indicated. Dissection and osteotomies are similar to those previously described for plagiocephaly repair. **B,** After osteotomies, reshaping, and fixation of bandeau and frontal plates. (**A** and **B,** Adapted from Ghali GE, Sinn DP, Tantipasawasin S. Management of nonsyndromic craniosynostosis. Atlas Oral Maxillofac Surg Clin North Am 2002;10:25.)

the midline and placing autogenous cranial bone grafts to increase the intraorbital distance. Stabilization is achieved with direct transosseous wires or resorbable microplate fixation. The microplate fixation is usually placed at the inner surface of the cranial bone. The abnormally shaped bone that has been removed is cut into sections of appropriate shape for the new forehead configuration. The anterior cranial base, anterior cranial vault, and orbit are given a more aesthetic shape, and the volume of the anterior cranial vault is increased, which allows the brain adequate space. Autogenous bone may be taken from the posterior cranium, when required, to enhance frontal reconstruction.

Sagittal Synostosis

Historically, when premature closure of a sagittal suture (Figures 45-18 and 45-19) was recognized in early infancy, most neurosurgeons believed that simple release of the

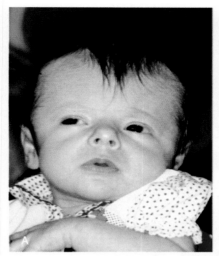

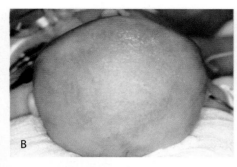

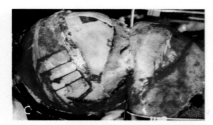

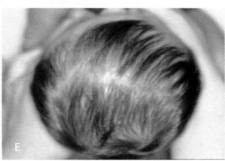

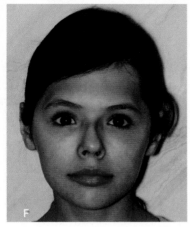

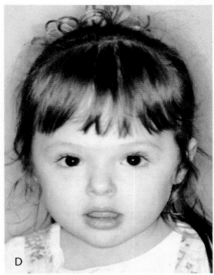

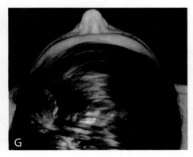

FIGURE 45-15.   A female infant born with bilateral coronal synostosis and apparent normal growth of her midface. She underwent anterior cranial vault and bilateral superior orbital rim osteotomies with reshaping at 6 months of age as previously described. **A,** Frontal view soon after birth. **B,** Superior view preoperatively at 6 months of age. **C,** Intraoperative lateral view of anterior cranial vault and orbits after osteotomies, reshaping, and fixation of segments. **D,** Frontal view at 3 years of age. **E,** Superior view at 1 year of age. **F,** Frontal view at 14 years of age. **G,** Superior view at 14 years of age. (**A–F,** Reproduced with permission from Ghali GE, Sinn DP, Tantipasawasin S. Management of nonsyndromic craniosynostosis. Atlas Oral Maxillofac Surg Clin North Am 2002;10:25–27.)

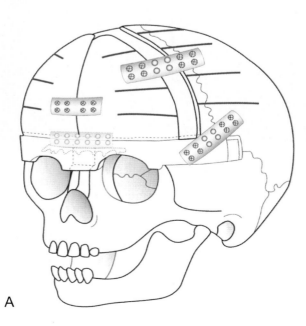

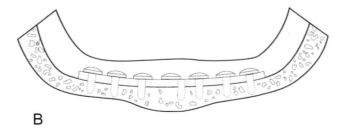

FIGURE 45-16.   Trigonocephaly repair after anterior cranial vault and superior orbital rim osteotomies. For the most part, the surgical approach is similar to that previously described for anterior cranial vault and superior orbital rim osteotomies and reshaping. **A,** As part of the reshaping, the bandeau is often split vertically at the midline and an interpositional autogenous cranial bone graft placed to correct hypotelorism. **B,** Resorbable forms of fixation lend themselves to internal plating of the bandeau as shown. (**A** and **B,** Adapted from Ghali GE, Sinn DP, Tantipasawasin S. Management of nonsyndromic craniosynostosis. Atlas Oral Maxillofac Surg Clin North Am 2002;10:28.)

SECTION 5

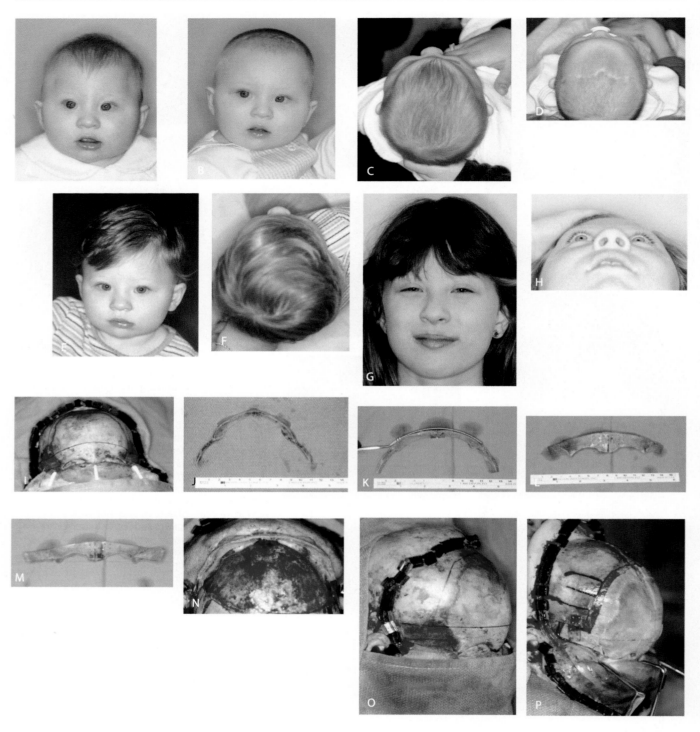

FIGURE 45-17.   A 10-month-old girl with metopic synostosis resulting in trigonocephaly. She underwent anterior cranial vault re-shaping, bilateral superior orbital rim advancements, and bitemporal widening via barrel-staving osteotomies. **A,** Frontal view before surgery. **B,** Frontal view after reconstruction. **C,** Superior view before surgery. **D,** Superior view after reconstruction. **E,** Frontal view at 2 years of age. **F,** Superior view at 2 years of age. **G,** Frontal view at 7 years of age. **H,** Inferior view at 7 years of age. **I,** Intraoperative frontal view outlining proposed osteotomy and bifrontal craniotomy sites. **J,** Superior view of bandeau before reshaping. **K,** Superior view of bandeau after reshaping and resorbable plate and screw stabilization. **L,** Frontal view of bandeau after reshaping and resorb-able plate fixation. **M,** View of same bandeau from cranial aspect. **N,** Superior view after fixation of bandeau. Pivoting point of rotation is about the glabellar region. Observation of the gap between the bandeau and the anterior cranial base assists in assessing ideal placement and bitemporal expansion. **O,** Superior oblique view of anterior cranial vault prior to reshaping. **P,** Superior oblique view of anterior cranial vault after osteotomies, reshaping, and fixation. (**A–P,** Reproduced with permission from Ghali GE, Sinn DP, Tantipasa-wasin S. Management of nonsyndromic craniosynostosis. Atlas Oral Maxillofac Surg Clin North Am 2002;10:28–34.)

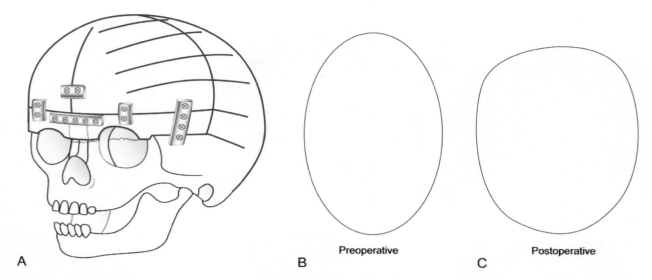

FIGURE 45-18. A child after total cranial vault and upper orbital osteotomies for the treatment of scaphocephaly. **A,** Forehead is symmetrically tilted back. The occiput is symmetrically tilted forward. The anteroposterior dimension is thereby shortened and secured via resorbable plates and screws. Barrel-stave cuts are made laterally to widen the transverse dimension or the squamous portion of the temporal plates as osteotomized, interchanged, and stabilized with resorbable plates and screws. Superior view preoperatively **(B)** and postoperatively **(C).** Total cranial vault reshaping as well as orbital rim alteration is accomplished to increase the biparietal width and decrease the frontal and occipital prominences. **(A–C,** Adapted from Ghali GE, Sinn DP, Tantipasawasin S. Management of nonsyndromic craniosynostosis. Atlas Oral Maxillofac Surg Clin North Am 2002;10:35.)

sagittal suture through a strip craniectomy without simultaneous skull reshaping was adequate treatment. [4,5,40,50] Our results using this technique alone have been less than favorable, and a residual cranial vault deformity usually results. If improvements in cranial vault shape are to be achieved, most cases require a formal total cranial vault reshaping at the age of 4 to 8 months. In our center, a recent trend toward earlier surgery (≤4 mo) involving removal of the stenosed suture along with extensive barrel-staving and postoperative helmet-molding is gaining popularity. Early results using this protocol have shown promising outcomes with less blood loss and shorter operative times. Variations in the degree of the scaphocephalic deformity are common, depending on the extent of sagittal suture stenosis. When the posterior half is fused, the patient is treated in the prone position with the posterior two thirds of the cranial vault reshaped. When the anterior half is fused, the patient is treated in the supine position with the anterior two thirds of the cranial vault reshaped, with or without superior orbital rim reshaping. When the entire suture is fused, a combination of both approaches may be necessary. Unless a significant concomitant supraorbital deformity exists, we prefer to treat full sagittal suture stenosis (anterior and posterior) at one operative setting in the prone position via a total cranial vault reshaping. For older children (>1 yr) or children with a need for upper orbital reconstruction, we prefer the supine position at one operative setting or, rarely, in two stages, with posterior reconstruction preceding anterior and orbital reconstruction

by 4 to 6 months. Other centers have reported good results when routinely staging full sagittal synostosis.

Unilateral Lambdoid Synostosis

Many surgeons consider simple strip craniectomy of the involved suture or partial craniectomy of the region to be adequate treatment. More extensive vault craniectomy and reshaping are generally necessary. If improvements in cranial vault shape are required after 10 to 12 months of age, formal posterior cranial vault reshaping is performed.

SUMMARY

In approximately 1 in 1000 live births in the United States, an infant has some variant of a craniofacial deformity. If cleft lip and palate deformities are included, the incidence is even greater. Surgical management of these patients has been advocated to occur from the first few weeks after birth until well into the teens. Many of these patients require multiple, staged procedures that involve movements of the bone and soft tissue from both the intracranial and the extracranial approaches. The surgical approach to most of these congenital deformities was radically changed by techniques introduced to the United States by Paul Tessier of France in 1967. From his imaginative intracranial and extracranial approaches, numerous advances have been made that have improved the management of these complex pediatric craniofacial deformities.

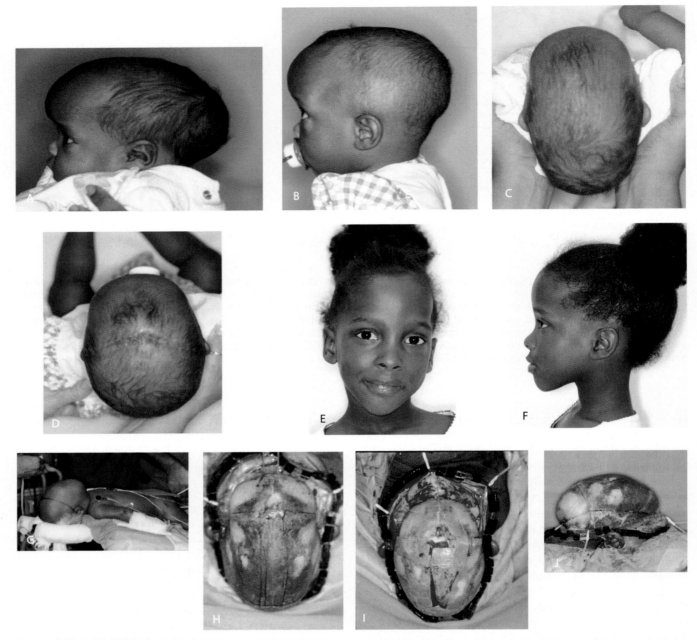

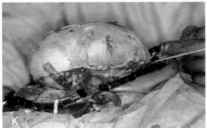

FIGURE 45-19. A 6-month-old girl with anterior and posterior sagittal suture synostosis resulting in scaphocephaly. She underwent total cranial vault reshaping without the need for any orbital osteotomies. A prone position was used throughout the procedure. **A,** Lateral view before surgery. **B,** Lateral view after reconstruction. **C,** Superior view before surgery. **D,** Superior view after reconstruction. **E,** Frontal view 6 years after reconstruction. **F,** Lateral view 6 years after reconstruction. **G,** Prone positioning is necessary and requires careful protection of both the airway and the globes. **H,** Intraoperative superior view of proposed osteotomy sites for total cranial vault reshaping. **I,** Intraoperative superior view of the osteotomies, reshaping, and resorbable plate fixation. **J,** Intraoperative left lateral view before reshaping. **K,** Intraoperative left lateral view after osteotomies, reshaping, and resorbable plate fixation. (**A–K,** Reproduced with permission from Ghali GE, Sinn DP, Tantipasawasin S. Management of nonsyndromic craniosynostosis. Atlas Oral Maxillofac Surg Clin North Am 2002;10:36–40.)

References

1. Cohen MM Jr. Perspectives on craniosynostosis: sutural biology, some well-known syndromes, and some unusual syndromes. J Craniofac Surg 2009;20:646–651.

2. Moss ML. The pathogenesis of premature cranial synostosis in man. Acta Anat (Basel) 1959;37:351.

3. Zeiger JS, Beaty TH, Hetmanski JB, et al. Genetic and environmental risk factors for sagittal craniosynostosis. J Craniofac Surg 2002;13:602–606.

4. Ghali GE, Sinn DP, Tantipasawasin S. Management of nonsyndromic craniosynostosis. Atlas Oral Maxillofac Surg Clin North Am 2002;10:1–41.

5. Graham JM, de Saxe M, Smith DW. Sagittal craniosynostosis: fetal head constraint as one possible cause. J Pediatr 1979;95:747–750.

6. Magge SN, Westerveid M, Pruzinsky T, Persing JA. Long-term neuropsychologic effects of sagittal craniosynostosis on child development. J Craniofac Surg 2002;13:99–104.

7. Marchac D, Renier D. Treatment of craniosynostosis in infancy. Clin Plast Surg 1987;14:61–72.

8. Heller JB, Heller MM, Knoll B, et al. Intracranial volume and cephalic index outcomes for total calvarial reconstruction among nonsyndromic sagittal synostosis patients. Plast Reconstr Surg 2008;121:187–195.

9. Florisson JM, van Veelen ML, Bannink N, et al. Papilledema in isolated single-suture craniosynostosis: prevalence and predictive factors. J Craniofac Surg 2010;21:20–24.

10. Chieffo D, Tamburrini G, Massimi L, et al. Long-term neuropsychological development in single-suture craniosynostosis treated early. J Neurosurg Pediatr 2010;5:232–237.

11. Cutting C, Grayson B, Bookstein F, et al. Computer-aided planning and evaluation of facial and orthognathic surgery. Clin Plast Surg 1986;13:449–462.

12. Gault D, Brunelle F, Renier D, Marchac D. The calculation of intracranial volume using CT scans. Childs Nerv Syst 1988; 4:271–273.

13. Lo LJ. Craniofacial computer-assisted surgical planning and simulation. Clin Plast Surg 1994;21:501–516.

14. Kirmi O, Lo SJ, Johnson D, Anslow P. Craniosynostosis: a radiological and surgical perspective. Semin Ultrasound CT MR 2009;30:492–512.

15. Marsh JL, Vannier MW. Computer-assisted imaging in the diagnosis, management and study of dysmorphic patients. In Vig KWL, Burdi AR, editors. Craniofacial Morphogenesis and Dysmorphogenesis. Ann Arbor: University of Michigan Press; 1988; pp. 109–126.

16. Marsh JL, Vannier MW. The "third" dimension in craniofacial surgery. Plast Reconstr Surg 1983;71:759–767.

17. Marsh JL, Vannier MW. Three-dimensional surface imaging from CT scans for the study of craniofacial dysmorphology. J Craniofac Genet Dev Biol 1989;9:61–75.

18. Marsh JL, Vannier MW, Stevens WG, et al. Computerized imaging for soft tissue and osseous reconstruction in the head and neck. Clin Plast Surg 1985;12:279–291.

19. Marsh JL, Vannier MW, Bresina S, Hemmer KM. Application of computer graphics in craniofacial surgery. Clin Plast Surg 1986;13:441–448.

20. Posnick JC, Bite U, Nakamo P. Comparison of direct and indirect intra-cranial volume measurements. In Proceedings of the 6th International Congress on Cleft Palate and Related Craniofacial Anomalies. 1989;June 15–18, Jerusalem, Israel.

21. Posnick JC. Indirect intracranial volume measurements using CT scans: clinical applications for craniosynostosis. Plast Reconstr Surg 1992;89:34–45.

22. Vannier MW, Marsh JL, Warren JO. Three dimension CT reconstruction images for craniofacial surgical planning and evaluation. Radiology 1984;150:179–84.

23. Longacre JJ, Destafano GA, Holmstrand K. The early versus the late reconstruction of congenital hypoplasia of the facial skeleton and skull. Plast Reconstr Surg 1961;27:489–504.

24. Oakes WJ. Craniosynostosis. In Serafin D, Geargiade NG, editors. Pediatric Plastic Surgery. St. Louis: CV Mosby; 1984; pp. 404–439.

25. Seymour-Dempsey K, Baumgartner JE, Teichgraeber JF, et al. Molding helmet therapy in the management of sagittal synostosis. J Craniofac Surg 2002;13:631–635.

26. Lee RP, Teichgraeber JF, Baumgartner JE, et al. Long-term treatment effectiveness of molding helmet therapy in the correction of posterior deformational plagiocephaly: a five-year follow-up. Cleft Palate Craniofac J 2008;45:240–245.

27. Sinn DP, Ghali GE, Ortega M. Major craniofacial surgery. In Levin DL, Morriss FC, editors. Essentials of Pediatric Intensive Care. New York: Churchill-Livingstone; 1997; pp. 636–643.

28. Arndt EM, Travis F, Lefebvre A, Munro IR. Psychological adjustment of 20 patients with Treacher Collins syndrome before and after reconstructive surgery. Br J Plast Surg 1987;40: 605–609.

29. Barden RC, Ford ME, Jensen AG, et al. Effects of craniofacial deformity in infancy on the quality of mother-infant interaction. Child Dev 1989;60:819–824.

30. Barden RC, Ford ME, Wilhelm W, et al. The physical attractiveness of facially deformed patients before and after craniofacial surgery. Plast Reconstr Surg 1988;82:229–235.

31. Barden RC, Ford ME, Wilhelm W, et al. Emotional and behavioral reactions to facially deformed patients before and after craniofacial surgery. Plast Reconstr Surg 1988;82:409–418.

32. Lafebvre A, Travis F, Arndt EM, Munro IR. A psychiatric profile before and after reconstructive surgery in children with Apert's syndrome. Br J Plast Surg 1986;39:510–513.

33. Arnaud E, Meneses P, Lajeunie E, et al. Postoperative mental and morphological outcome for nonsyndromic brachycephaly. J Craniofac Surg 2002;110:6–12.

34. Warschausky S, Kay JB, Buchman S, et al. Health-related quality of life in children with craniofacial anomalies. J Craniofac Surg 2002;110:409–414.

35. Marchac D. Forehead remolding for craniosynostosis. In Converse JM, McCarthy JG, Wood-Smith D, editors. Symposium on Diagnosis and Treatment of Craniofacial Anomalies. St. Louis: CV Mosby; 1979; p. 323.

36. Edgerton MT, Jane JA, Berry FA, et al. The feasibility of craniofacial osteotomies in infants and young children. Scand J Plast Reconstr Surg 1974;8:164–168.

37. Edgerton MT, Jane JA, Berry FA. Craniofacial osteotomies and reconstruction in infants and young children. Plast Reconstr Surg 1974;54:13–27.

38. McCarthy JG, Epstein F, Sadove M, et al. Early surgery for craniofacial synostosis: an 8-year experience. Plast Reconstr Surg 1984;73:521–533.

39. Whitaker LA, Barlett SP, Schut L, Bruce D. Craniosynostosis: an analysis of the timing, treatment and complication in 164 patients. Plast Reconstr Surg 1987;80:195–212.

SECTION 5

40. Cohen SR, Holmes RE. Immediate cranial vault reconst-ruction with bioresorbable plates following endoscopically assisted sagittal synostectomy. J Craniofac Surg 2002;13:578–584.

41. Pietrzak WS. Critical concepts of absorbable internal fixation. J Craniofac Surg 2000;11:335–341.

42. Pietrzak WS, Kumar M, Eppley BL. The influence of temperature on the degradation rate of lactosorb copolymer. J Craniofac Surg 2003;14:176–183.

43. Ahmad N, Lyles J, Panchal J, Deschamps-Braly J. Outcomes and complications based on experience with resorbable plates in pediatric craniosynostosis patients. J Craniofac Surg 2008;19:855–860.

44. Jane JA, Park TS, Zide BM, et al. Alternative techniques in the treatment of unilateral coronal synostosis. J Neurosurg 1984;61:550–556.

45. Persing JA, Babler WJ, Jane JA, Duckworth PF. Experimental unilateral coronal synostosis in rabbits. Plast Reconstr Surg 1986;77:369–377.

46. David LR, Fisher D, Argenta L. New technique for reconstructing the affected cranium and orbital rim in unicoronal craniosynostosis. J Craniofac Surg 2009;20:194–197.

47. Hoffman HJ, Mohr G. Lateral canthal advancement of the supraorbital margins: a new corrective technique in the treatment of coronal synostosis. J Neurosurg 1976;45:376–381.

48. Marchac D, Renier D, Jones BM. Experience with the "floating forehead." Br J Plast Surg 1988;41:1–15.

49. Greenberg BM, Schneider SJ. Trigonocephaly: surgical considerations and long-term evaluation. J Craniofac Surg 2006;17:528–535.

50. Weinzweig J, Baker SB, Whitaker LA, et al. Delayed cranial vault reconstruction for sagittal synostosis in older children: an algorithm for tailoring the reconstructive approach to the craniofacial deformity. J Craniofac Surg 2002;110:397–408.

Craniofacial Dysostosis Syndromes: Evaluation and Treatment of the Skeletal Deformities

Paul S. Tiwana, DDS, MD, MS, Ramon L. Ruiz, DMD, MD, and Jeffrey C. Posnick, DMD, MD, FRCS(C), FACS

INTRODUCTION

Cranial sutures are a form of bone articulation in which the margins of the bones are connected by a thin layer of fibrous tissue. The cranial vault is composed of six major sutural areas and several minor sutures, which serve two critical functions during the postnatal period. Initially, the sutures allow head deformation during vaginal delivery. Later, during an infant's postnatal development, cranial vault sutures facilitate head expansion to accommodate propulsive brain growth.[1] Only small amounts of pressure (5 mmHg) from the growing brain are required to stimulate bone deposition at the margins of a cranial bone.[2,3] Under normal conditions, the brain volume will triple within the first year of life, and by age 2 years, the cranial capacity is four times that at birth.[4] Normally, closure of the cranial vault sutures occurs earlier than closure of the membranous facial bone sutures, which often remain patent until adulthood.

The term *craniosynostosis* is defined as a premature fusion of a cranial vault suture. With rare exception, this is an intrauterine event. A more accurate description of craniosynostosis may be a *congenital absence* of the cranial vault sutures. The result is fusion of the bones adjacent to the suture and arrested sutural growth of the adjacent bones. The classic theory known as *Virchow's law* states that premature fusion of a cranial vault suture results in limited development of the skull perpendicular to the fused suture and a compensatory "overgrowth" through the sutures that remain open.[5] The result is a dysmorphology with characteristics depending on the sutures affected and potential neurologic consequences related to underlying brain compression. Most forms of craniosynostosis represent nonsyndromic malformations limited to the cranial vault and orbital regions. Management typically requires a combined neurosurgical and craniofacial approach for release of the involved suture and reshaping of the dysmorphic skeletal components. Discussion of the management of nonsyndromic craniosynostosis is beyond the scope of this chapter. *Craniofacial dysostosis (CFD)* is the term applied to syndromal forms of craniosynostosis. These disorders are characterized by sutural involvement that not only includes the cranial vault but also extends into the skull base and midfacial skeletal structures. CFD syndromes have been described by Carpenter, Apert, Crouzon, Saethre-Chotzen, and Pfeiffer.[6] Although the cranial vault and cranial base are thought to be the regions of primary involvement, there is also significant impact on midfacial growth and development.[7,8] In addition to cranial vault dysmorphology, patients with these inherited conditions exhibit a characteristic "total midface" deficiency that is syndrome-specific and must be addressed as part of the staged reconstructive approach.

GENETIC ASPECTS

FGFR-related CFD syndrome includes: *FGFR1*-related craniosynostosis (Pfeiffer's syndrome types 1, 2, and 3); *FGFR2*-related craniosynostosis (Apert's syndrome; Beare-Stevenson syndrome; Crouzon's syndrome; *FGFR2*-related isolated coronal synostosis; Jackson-Weiss syndrome; Pfeiffer's syndrome types 1, 2, and 3); and *FGFR3*-related craniosynostosis, (Crouzon's syndrome with acanthosis nigricans, *FGFR3*-related isolated coronal synostosis, Muenke's syndrome).

The eight disorders considered as part of the *FGFR*-related craniosynostosis spectrum are *Pfeiffer's syndrome, Apert's syndrome, Crouzon's syndrome, Beare-Stevenson syndrome, FGFR2-related isolated coronal synostosis, Jackson-Weiss syndrome, Crouzon's syndrome with acanthosis nigricans,* and *Muenke's syndrome.* All but Muenke's syndrome and *FGFR2*-related isolated coronal synostosis generally present with bicoronal synostosis or cloverleaf skull anomaly.

The diagnosis of Muenke's syndrome (*FGFR3*-related coronal synostosis) is based on identification of a disease-causing mutation in the *FGFR3* gene. The diagnosis of *FGFR2*-related isolated coronal synostosis is based on identification of a disease-causing mutation in the *FGFR2* gene. The diagnosis of the other six *FGFR*-related craniosynostoses is based on clinical findings; however, molecular genetic testing of the *FGFR1, FGFR2,* and *FGFR3* genes may be helpful in establishing the diagnosis of these syndromes in questionable cases.

FGFR-related craniosynostosis is inherited in an autosomal dominant manner. Affected individuals have a 50% chance of passing the mutant gene to each child. Prenatal testing is available; however, its use is limited by poor predictive value. Molecular testing is necessary to establish the diagnosis for two of the disorders, Muenke's syndrome and *FGFR2*-related isolated coronal synostosis. Individuals with Muenke's syndrome may have unilateral coronal synostosis or megalencephaly without craniosynostosis: The accurate diagnosis depends upon identification of a disease-causing mutation in the *FGFR3* gene. *FGFR2*-related isolated coronal synostosis is characterized only by uni- or bicoronal craniosynostosis: The accurate diagnosis depends upon identification of a disease-causing mutation in the *FGFR2* gene.

FUNCTIONAL CONSIDERATIONS

Brain Growth and Intracranial Pressure

If the rapid brain growth that normally occurs during infancy is to proceed unhindered, the cranial vault and base sutures must remain open and expand during phases of rapid growth, resulting in marginal ossification. In craniosynostosis, premature fusion of sutures causes limited and abnormal skeletal expansion in the presence of continued brain growth.

Depending on the number and location of prematurely fused sutures, the growth of the brain may be restricted.[2,9–11] In addition, abnormal cranial vault and midfacial morphology occurs as determined by Virchow's law. If surgical release of the affected sutures and reshaping to restore a more normal intracranial volume and configuration are not performed, decreased cognitive and behavioral function is likely to be the end result.

Elevated intracranial pressure (ICP) is the most serious functional problem associated with premature suture fusion. A "beaten-copper" appearance along the inner table of the cranial vault seen on a plain radiograph or the loss of brain cisternae as observed on a computed tomography (CT) scan may suggest elevated ICP,[12] but these are considered soft radiographic findings.

Intracranial hypertension can be established invasively by means of a burhole craniotomy used to place either an epidural or an intraparenchymal pressure sensor. Increased ICP is most likely to affect individuals with great disparity between brain growth and intracranial capacity and may occur in as many as 42% of untreated children in whom more than one suture is affected.[2,10,13] Unfortunately, there is no absolute agreement on what levels of ICP are normal at any given age in infancy and early childhood.

The clinical signs and symptoms related to elevated ICP may have a slow onset and be difficult to recognize in the pediatric population. Although standardized CT scans allow for indirect measurement of intracranial volume, it is not yet possible to use these studies to make judgments as to who requires craniotomy for decompression.[14,15] Careful neurosurgical and pediatric ophthalmologic evaluation are critical components of the data gathering required to formulate a definitive treatment plan in a patient with craniosynostosis.

Vision

Untreated craniosynostosis with elevated ICP will cause papilledema and eventual optic nerve atrophy, resulting in partial or complete blindness. If the orbits are shallow (exorbitism) and the eyes are proptotic (exophthalmos), as occurs in the CFD syndromes, the cornea may be exposed and abrasions or ulcerations may occur. An eyeball extending outside of a shallow orbit is also at risk of trauma. If the orbits are extremely shallow, herniation of the globe itself may occur, necessitating emergency reduction followed by tarsorrhaphies or urgent orbital decompression.

Some forms of CFD result in a marked degree of orbital hypertelorism, which may compromise visual acuity and restrict binocular vision. Divergent or convergent nonparalytic strabismus or exotropia occurs frequently and should be considered during the diagnostic evaluation. This may be the result of congenital anomalies of the extraocular muscles themselves. Paralytic or nonparalytic unilateral or bilateral upper eyelid ptosis also occurs with greater frequency with CFD than in the general population.

Hydrocephalus

Hydrocephalus affects as many as 10% of patients with a CFD syndrome.[16–19] Although the etiology is often not clear, hydrocephalus may be secondary to a generalized cranial base stenosis with constriction of all the cranial base foramina, which affects the patient's cerebral venous drainage and cerebrospinal fluid (CSF) flow dynamics. Hydrocephalus may be identified with the help of CT or magnetic resonance imaging (MRI) to document progressively enlarging ventricles. Difficulty exists in interpreting ventricular findings as seen on a CT scan especially when the skull and cranial base are brachycephalic. The skeletal dysmorphology seen in a child with severe cranial dysmorphology related to craniosynostosis may translate into an abnormal ventricular shape that is not necessarily related to abnormal CSF flow. Serial imaging and clinical correlation is indicated, and a great deal of clinical judgment is often required in making these assessments.

Effects of Midface Deficiency on Airway

All newborn infants are obligate nasal breathers. Many infants born with a CFD syndrome have moderate to severe hypoplasia of the midface as a component of their malformation. They will have diminished nasal and nasopharyngeal spaces with resulting increased nasal airway resistance (obstruction). The affected child is thus forced to breathe through the mouth. For a newborn infant to ingest food through the mouth requires sucking from a nipple to achieve negative pressure as well as an intact swallowing mechanism. The neonate with severe midface hypoplasia will experience diminished nasal airflow and be unable to accomplish this task and breathe through the nose at the same time.[20–23] Complicating this clinical picture may be an elongated and ptotic palate and enlarged tonsils and adenoids. The compromised infant expends significant energy respiring, and this may push the child into a catabolic state (negative nitrogen balance). Failure to thrive results unless either nasogastric tube feeding is instituted or a feeding gastrostomy is placed. Evaluation by a pediatrician, pediatric otolaryngologist, and feeding specialist with craniofacial experience can help distinguish minor feeding difficulties from those requiring more aggressive treatment.

Sleep apnea of either central or obstructive origin may also be present. If the apnea is found to be secondary to upper airway obstruction based on a formal sleep study, a tracheostomy may be indicated. In rare situations, "early" midface advancement is useful to improve the airway and allow for tracheostomy decannulation. Central apnea may occur from poorly treated intracranial hypertension and other contributing factors. If this is the case, the condition may improve by reducing the ICP to a normal range through cranio-orbital or posterior cranial vault decompression or expansion.

The literature confirms that as many as 50% of children with Apert's, Crouzon's, or Pfeiffer's syndrome develop obstructive sleep apnea (OSA) during the first 6 years of life.[24,25] Documented OSA in a child with CFD is frequently treated with tracheostomy. It may also be treated by adenoidectomy, tonsillectomy, midface advancement, or continuous positive airway pressure (CPAP). If left untreated or ineffectively treated, OSA will result in disabilities ranging from failure to thrive; recurrent upper respiratory infection; cognitive dysfunction; developmental delay; cor pulmonale; or sudden death.[26] Overwhelmingly, the documented midface hypoplasia in many CFD children is a primary cause of OSA. If feasible, effective surgical midface advancement is the preferred biologic treatment approach.

Clinical symptoms of OSA will include heavy snoring, difficulty in awake breathing, observed apnea during sleep, excessive perspiration during sleep, and daytime somnolence. Polysomnography remains the gold standard for diagnosis. In the pediatric population, *apnea,* defined as absence of air flow for more than two breadths, and *hypopnea,* defined as a reduction of greater than or equal to 50% of nasal flow signal amplitude of more than two breadths, defines OSA syndrome. The *apnea-hypopnea index (AHI)* is the number of obstructive apneas in combination with hypopneas (followed by desaturation) per hour. The *oxygenation-desaturation index (ODI)* is the number of desaturations ($\geq$4% decrease with respect to the baseline) per hour. A score of less than 1.0 is considered normal. Definition of the severity of the condition in children includes between 1 and 5 events as mild OSA; 6 to 25 as moderate OSA; and greater than 25 events as severe OSA. In the child with CFD and moderate to severe midface deficiency who is documented to have OSA, neither tonsillectomy nor adenoidectomy generally provides sufficient opening of the upper airway.

Ishii and coworkers[27] used lateral cephalometric radiographs to evaluate the nasopharyngeal airway after Le Fort III advancement in Apert's and Crouzon's syndrome individuals with OSA. They were able to document improvement in the nasopharyngeal airway in the study patients after successful midface advancement surgery.

Arnaud and colleagues[28,29] completed a studies to review respiratory improvement in CFD patients suffering with OSA that underwent monobloc advancement (DO approach). Fourteen of the 16 study patients (88%) showed improvement as measured by oxygen level during sleep. Tracheostomy removal was possible in 4 of 6 study patients. In one of the patients, a tracheostomy was required 6 months after midface advancement due to recurrent severe OSA.

Witherow and colleagues[30] found a significant improvement in OSA in all patients diagnosed with CFD (Apert's, Crouzon's, Pfeiffer's) as documented by polysomnography at 24 months after undergoing monobloc advancement (distraction osteogenesis approach). Before monobloc advancement, 14 of their patients had severe OSA with either tracheostomy or the use of CPAP in place. For the study patients undergoing monobloc advancement, only 43% (6/14) had resolution of their OSA. Unfortunately, 8 of the

14 patients (57%) remained dependent on tracheostomy or CPAP despite the monobloc advancement procedure.

Nelson and associates[31] studied 18 CFD individuals, all presenting with bilateral coronal synostosis and midface deficiency. In 15/18 patients (83%), either tracheostomy or CPAP was required for treatment of OSA before midface advancement. After the midface advancement procedures, 5 of the tracheostomy patients were decannulated, and in 6, CPAP was no longer required (11/15 = 73%). The mean post-surgical follow-up was 3 years.

In the CFD patient undergoing midface advancement, the lack of universal success in the relief of OSA could be for a combination of reasons including inadequate midface advancement, midface relapse after initial advancement, other anatomic factors not addressed by the midface advancement (septum, turbinates, soft palate, tonsils, adenoids, mandible, tracheomalacia), a central sleep apnea component, or inadequate (abnormal) contraction forces of the pharyngeal dilator muscles during sleep. In CFD, not only is the anatomy of the upper airway different for each syndrome, but a wide variation of deformity is also seen within each syndrome. Differences in the soft tissues and the quality of the pharyngeal muscles compared with normal may be attributed to a mutation of the fibroblast growth factor receptor (FGFR).[32] CFD patients with OSA who are nonresponders to an effective midface advancement may have pharyngeal wall collapse due to poor pharyngeal dilator muscle function during sleeping. Whereas a tendency for airway collapse can be overcome through midface advancement, the individual must also have sufficient ability to control/contract (maintain tone) of the pharyngeal muscles while asleep.

It would appear that in some CFD individuals (Apert's, Crouzon's, Pfeiffer's syndromes) despite effective midface advancement (Le Fort III/monobloc/facial bipartition), the long-term dependence on tracheostomy or CPAP for resistant OSA should be anticipated. In patients with persistent OSA despite optimal maxillofacial skeletal morphology, airway collapse due to inadequate pharyngeal muscle tone appears to play a role.

Dentition and Occlusion

The incidence of dental and oral anomalies is higher among children with CFD syndromes than in the general population. In Apert's syndrome in particular, the palate is high and constricted in width. The incidence of isolated cleft palate in patients with Apert's syndrome approaches 30%.[13] Clefting of the secondary palate may be submucous, incomplete, or complete. Confusion has arisen over whether the oral malformations and absence of teeth that are often characteristic of these conditions are a result of congenital or iatrogenic factors (e.g., injury to dental follicles associated with early midface surgery). The midfacial hypoplasia seen in the CFD syndromes often results in limited maxillary alveolar bone to house a full complement of teeth. The result is severe crowding, which often requires serial extractions in order to address the

problem. An Angle class III skeletal relationship in combination with anterior open bite deformity is typical.

Hearing

Hearing deficits are more common among patients with the CFD syndromes than in the general population.[24] In Crouzon's syndrome, conductive hearing deficits are common, and atresia of the external auditory canals may also occur. Otitis media is more common in Apert's syndrome, although the exact incidence is unknown. Middle ear disease may be related to the presence of a cleft palate that results in eustachian tube dysfunction. Congenital fixation of the stapedial footplate is also believed to be frequent. The possibility of significant hearing loss is paramount in importance and should not be overlooked because of preoccupation with other, more easily appreciated craniofacial findings.

Extremity Anomalies

Apert's syndrome results in joint fusion and bony and soft tissue syndactyly of the digits of all four limbs.[24] These Apert-associated extremity deformities are often symmetrical. Partial or complete fusion of the shoulder, elbow, or other joints is common. Broad thumbs, broad great toes, and partial soft tissue syndactyly of the hands may be seen in Pfeiffer's syndrome, but these are variable features. Preaxial polysyndactyly of the feet may also be seen in Carpenter's syndrome.

MORPHOLOGIC CONSIDERATIONS

Examination of the patient's entire craniofacial region should be meticulous and systematic. The skeleton and soft tissues are assessed in a standard way to identify all normal and abnormal anatomy. Specific findings tend to occur in particular malformations, but each patient is unique. The achievement of symmetry and normal proportions and the reconstruction of specific aesthetic units are essential to forming an unobtrusive face in a child born with a CFD syndrome.

Frontoforehead Aesthetic Unit

The frontoforehead region is dysmorphic in an infant with CFD.[25–30] Establishing normal position of the forehead is critical to overall facial symmetry and balance. The forehead may be considered as two separate aesthetic components: the supraorbital ridge–lateral orbital rim region and the superior forehead (Figure 46-1).[31,32] The supraorbital ridge–lateral orbital rim region includes the glabella and supraorbital rim extending inferiorly down each frontozygomatic suture toward the infraorbital rim and posteriorly along each temporoparietal region. The morphology and position of the supraorbital ridge–lateral orbital rim region is a key element of upper facial aesthetics. In a normal forehead, at the level of the frontonasal suture, an angle ranging from 90 to 110 degrees, is formed by the supraorbital ridge and the nasal

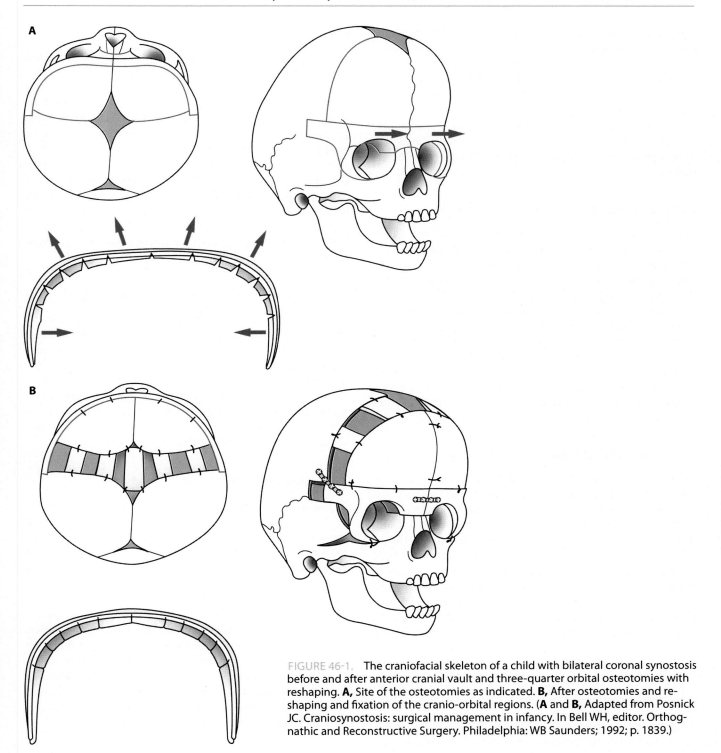

FIGURE 46-1. The craniofacial skeleton of a child with bilateral coronal synostosis before and after anterior cranial vault and three-quarter orbital osteotomies with reshaping. **A,** Site of the osteotomies as indicated. **B,** After osteotomies and reshaping and fixation of the cranio-orbital regions. (**A** and **B,** Adapted from Posnick JC. Craniosynostosis: surgical management in infancy. In Bell WH, editor. Orthognathic and Reconstructive Surgery. Philadelphia: WB Saunders; 1992; p. 1839.)

bones when viewed in profile. In addition, the eyebrows, overlying the supraorbital ridge, should be anterior to the cornea. When the supraorbital ridge is viewed from above, the rim should arc posteriorly to achieve a gentle 90-degree angle at the temporal fossa with a center point of the arc at the level of each frontozygomatic suture. The superior forehead component, approximately 1.0 to 1.5 cm up from the supraorbital rim, should have a gentle posterior curve of about 60 degrees, leveling out at the coronal suture region when seen in profile.

Posterior Cranial Vault Aesthetic Unit

Symmetry, form, and the appropriate intracranial volume of the posterior cranial vault are closely linked. Posterior cranial vault flattening may result from either a unilateral or a bilateral lambdoidal synostosis, which is rare; previous craniectomy with reossification in a dysmorphic flat shape, which is frequent; or postural molding because of repetitive sleep positioning.[33] A short anteriorposterior cephalic length may be misinterpreted as an anterior cranial vault (forehead) problem when the occipitoparietal (posterior) skull represents the primary region of the deformity. Careful examination of the entire cranial vault is essential to defining the dysmorphic region so that appropriate therapy may be carried out.

Orbitonasozygomatic Aesthetic Unit

In CFD syndromes, the orbitonasozygomatic regional deformity is a reflection of the cranial base malformation. For example, in Crouzon's syndrome when bilateral coronal suture synostosis is combined with skull base and midfacial deficiency, the orbitonasozygomatic region will be dysmorphic and consistent with a short (anteroposterior) and wide (transverse) anterior cranial base.[34] In Apert's syndrome, the nasal bones, orbits, and zygomas, like the anterior cranial base, are transversely wide and horizontally short (retruded), resulting in a shallow hyperteloric upper midface (zygomas, orbits, and nose).[34] Advancing the midface without simultaneously addressing the increased transverse width will not adequately correct the dysmorphology.[35]

Maxillary–Nasal Base Aesthetic Unit

In the CFD patient with midface deficiency, the upper anterior face (nasion to maxillary incisor) is vertically short, and there is a lack of horizontal anteroposterior projection of the midface.[36,37] These findings may be confirmed with cephalometric analysis that indicates a sella-nasion angle (SNA) below the mean value and a short upper anterior facial height (nasion to anterior nasal spine). The width of the maxilla in the dentoalveolar region is generally constricted with a high-arched palate. In order to normalize the maxillonasal base region, multidirectional surgical expansion and reshaping are generally required. The maxillary lip-to-tooth relationship and occlusion are normalized through Le Fort I osteotomy and orthodontic treatment as part of the staged reconstruction.

Quantitative Assessment

A quantitative analysis of measurements taken from CT scans, surface anthropometry, cephalometric analysis, and dental casts is critical to data gathering for evaluation of craniofacial deformities.[38–43] This analysis will confirm or refute clinical impressions, aid in the treatment planning of intraoperative skeletal movements and reshaping, and provide a framework for objective assessment of immediate and long-term results. These methods of assessment rely on the measurement of linear distances, angles, and proportions based on accurate, reliable, and reproducible anatomic landmarks found to be useful for patient evaluation.

CT Scan Analysis

The use of CT scans has clarified our appreciation of the dysmorphology of a child born with a craniofacial malformation.[44,45] Accurate standardized points of reference have been identified in the cranio-orbitozygomatic skeleton based on axial CT images.[42,43] Knowledge of differential facial bone growth patterns and normal measurement values can now be used to improve diagnostic accuracy, assist in the staging of reconstruction by understanding growth vectors, and offer the option of making intraoperative measurements that correlate with the preoperative CT scan measurements and ideal dimensions. This information can effectively guide the surgeon in the reconstruction of an individual with a craniofacial malformation and also allows for accurate postoperative reassessment.

Anthropometric Surface Measurements

Cross-sectional studies of the patterns of postnatal facial growth based on anthropometric surface measurements have been carried out in growing white children.[38–41,46] This published material has proved useful in the quantitative evaluation and recognition of discrepancies in postnatal development in the head and face of patients with specific craniofacial syndromes. This is particularly useful when evaluating basic distances, angles, and proportions of the head, face, and orbits in patients affected with CFD syndromes.

Cephalometric Analysis

Cephalometric radiography, first introduced by Broadbent in 1931, has been traditionally used to study the morphology and patterns of growth of the maxillofacial skeleton.[47] The large collection of normative data developed allows clinicians to monitor an individual's facial growth. The interpretation of cephalometric radiographs remains useful in the analysis of facial heights and maxillary, mandibular, and chin positions and their relationships to one another, the cranial base, and the dentition.[30,36,48,49] The lateral cephalometric radiograph offers an accurate view from the midsagittal plane if the facial skeleton being analyzed is relatively symmetrical. Unfortunately, the number of anatomic landmarks that can be identified accurately in the cranio-orbitozygomatic region is limited because of the overlap of structures, which makes predictably locating these anatomic landmarks more difficult.

SURGICAL MANAGEMENT

Historical Perspectives

As early as 1890, Lannelongue[50] and then Lane[51] reported a surgical approach to the treatment of craniosynostosis. Lannelongue's aim was to remove the fused suture (strip craniectomy) in the hopes of controlling the problem of brain compression within a congenitally small cranial vault. By the turn of the century, Harvey Cushing, the most prominent neurosurgeon of his day, suggested that surgical intervention for the problem of craniosynostosis was misdirected and that more attention should instead be given to the schooling of these children. Schillito disagreed with Cushing and enthusiastically supported the concept of surgical intervention to improve the outlook for these children. He believed that the linear "strip" craniectomy of the fused sutures would "release" the skull and allow the cranium to reshape itself and continue to grow in a normal and symmetrical fashion.[52] The strip craniectomy procedures were supposed to allow for a new suture line at the site of the previous synostosis. With the realization that this goal was not biologically feasible, attempts were made to remove portions of the cranial vault surgically and to either leave large open areas or use the removed segments as free grafts to refashion the cranial vault shape. Problems with these methods included uncontrolled postoperative skull molding, re-ossification into dysmorphic configurations, and the occurrence of large residual skull defects.

The concept of simultaneous release of the fused suture combined with more meticulous cranial vault reshaping carried out in infants was initially suggested by Rougerie and coworkers[53] and then refined by Hoffman and Mohr in 1976[54] for children born with unilateral coronal synostosis. Whitaker and colleagues[55] proposed a more formal anterior cranial vault and orbital reshaping procedure for unilateral coronal synostosis in 1977. Marchac and associates[41] published their experience with a "floating forehead" technique for simultaneous unilateral coronal and bilateral coronal suture release and forehead and upper orbital osteotomies with advancement to manage craniosynostosis in infancy. Unfortunately, the "floating forehead" technique resulted in unpredictable re-ossification of the open cranial vault areas. In addition, bitemporal constrictions or bulging and vertex of the skull concavities or bulging were frequent developments as re-ossification occurred. In any case, the hoped for midface growth did not materialize.

In the 1950s, Gillies and Harrison[56] reported experience with an extracranial Le Fort III "type" osteotomy to improve the anterior projection of the midface in an adult with Crouzon's syndrome. The initial Gillies procedure was actually carried out in 1942. He mobilized the midface by a variety of osteotomies preformed through skin excisions directly over each osteotomy site. The midface was mobilized and advanced and intermaxillary fixation (IMF) applied. After removal of the IMF (2 wk after the operation) the metal cast cap (dental) splint was attached to a plaster head cap, which was maintained for 3 weeks. There is no evidence that Gillies and Harrison used any bone grafts in the surgical gaps created. The early enthusiasm for this technique later turned to discouragement when the patient's facial skeleton relapsed to its preoperative status. There was relapse—both at the maxillary incisor level and of the eye proptosis.

Dr. Tessier was aware of Gillies' previous work and the accompanying difficulties. In 1967, Tessier[57] described a new (intracranial–cranial base) approach to the management of Crouzon's syndrome. This work was first presented in France at a meeting in Montpelier in 1966 and the following year at the International Plastic Surgery Meeting in Rome. Tessier's landmark presentations and publications were the beginning of modern craniofacial surgery. To overcome the earlier problems encountered by Gillies and Harrison, Tessier developed an innovative basic surgical approach that included new locations for the Le Fort III osteotomy, a combined intracranial-extracranial (cranial base) approach, use of a coronal (skin) incision to expose the upper facial bones, and use of fresh autogenous bone graft. He also applied an external fixation device to help maintain bony stability until healing had occurred.

In 1971, Tessier[58] described a single-stage frontofacial advancement in which the fronto-orbital bandeau was advanced as a separate element in conjunction with the Le Fort III complex below and the frontal bones above.[57–66] Seven years later, Ortiz-Monasterio and coworkers[67,68] refined the "monobloc" osteotomy to advance the orbits and midface as one unit, combined with frontal bone (anterior cranial vault) repositioning to correct the upper and midface deformity of Crouzon's syndrome. In 1979, Van der Meulen[69] described the "medial fasciotomy" for the correction of midline facial clefting. Van der Meulen split the monobloc osteotomy vertically in the midline, removed central nasal and ethmoid bone, and then moved the two halves of the facial skeleton together for correction of the orbital hypertelorism. To correct the midface dysplasia and associated orbital hypertelorism in Apert's syndrome, Tessier refined the vertical splitting and reshaping of the midline split monobloc segments, thus correcting the midface deformity in three dimensions in a procedure now known as *facial bipartition*. More recently, Posnick and colleagues[70,71] have independently documented the advantages of Tessier's facial bipartition technique for the correction of the Apert upper and midface deformity.

The widespread use of autogenous cranial bone grafting has virtually eliminated the need for rib and hip grafts when bone replacement is required in cranio-orbitozygomatic procedures. This represents another of Tessier's contributions to craniofacial surgery.

In 1968, Luhr[72] introduced the use of small metal (vitalium) plates and screws to stabilize maxillofacial fractures and then osteotomies. In current practice, the use of internal miniplate and microplate and screw (titanium) fixation (of various sizes) is the preferred form of fixation when stability and three-dimensional craniomaxillofacial reconstruction of multiple osteotomized bone segments and grafts are required. In infants and young children, for the stabilization of non–load-bearing osteotomy segments such as the cranial vault stabilization with resorbable materials is now generally preferred. This avoids issues or uncertainty concerning either growth restriction or brain trauma from retained hardware.

More recently, the intraoperative placement of a distraction device as a method of achieving advancement of the midface in patients with severe forms of craniofacial hypoplasia has been added to the surgeon's armamentarium.[47]

If used, distraction osteogenesis is not applied until after successful completion of standard osteotomies and disimpaction in the operating room. The distraction apparatus is anchored to the "stable" skeleton either internally or externally (through a "halo" head frame) and then to the palatal (intraoral) and infraorbital rims or zygomatic buttresses. Advancement of the "total midface" can then proceed. Once adequate (midface) advancement has been accomplished (on an outpatient basis) over a period of several weeks, the patient is generally returned to the operating room for stabilization and final reconstruction. The final reconstruction may require additional segmental osteotomies, bone grafting, or placement of plate and screw fixation. The "distraction approach" to the midface deformity is a labor-intensive, technique-specific, and relatively crude method of accomplishing horizontal advancement with difficulty in controlling the vertical dimension of the midface and without the ability to alter the transverse deformity or deficiency. In our opinion, the current level of distraction technology leaves it an adjunctive rather than a primary technique. It is most useful when the midfacial hypoplasia is severe to the extent that conventional techniques cannot reliably allow the immediate (in the operating room) desired advancement and when complex vertical and transverse reconstruction is not required.

Philosophy Regarding Timing of Intervention

In considering the timing and type of intervention the experienced surgeon will take several biologic realities into account: the natural course of the malformation (i.e., is the dysmorphology associated with Crouzon's syndrome progressively worsening or is it a nonprogressive craniofacial deformity?), the tendency toward growth restriction of an operated bone (aesthetic unit) that has not yet reached maturity (i.e., we know that operating on a palate of a child born with a cleft in infancy will cause scarring and later result in maxillary hypoplasia in a significant percentage of individuals), and the uncertain relationship between the underlying growing viscera (i.e., brain or eyes) and the congenially affected and surgically altered skeleton (i.e., if the cranial vault is not surgically expanded by 1 yr of life in a patient with multiple suture synostosis, will brain compression occur?).

In attempting to limit functional impairment and also achieve long-term ideal facial aesthetics, an essential question the surgeon must ask is, "During the course of craniofacial development, does the operated-on facial skeletal of the child with CFD tend to grow abnormally, resulting in further distortions and dysmorphology or are the initial positive skeletal changes (achieved at operation) maintained during ongoing growth?" Unfortunately, the theory that craniofacial procedures carried out early in infancy will "unlock growth" has not been documented through the scientific method.[57,73,74]

Incision Placement

For exposure of the craniofacial skeleton above the Le Fort I level, the approach used is the coronal (skin) incision. This allows for a relatively camouflaged access to the anterior and posterior cranial vault, orbits, nasal dorsum, zygomas, upper maxilla, pterygoid fossa, and temporomandibular joints. For added cosmetic advantage, placement of the coronal incision more posteriorly on the scalp and with postauricular rather than preauricular extensions is useful. When exposure of the maxilla at the Le Fort I level is required, a circumvestibular maxillary intraoral incision is used. Unless complications occur that warrant unusual exposure, no other incisions are required for managing any aspect of the CFD patient's reconstruction. These incisions (coronal [scalp] and maxillary [circumvestibular]) may be reopened as needed to further complete the patient's staged reconstruction.

Management of Cranial Vault Dead Space

Cranial reshaping in the CFD patient provides space for the compressed brain to expand into. Unfortunately, after anterior cranial vault expansion and monobloc advancement, an immediate extradural (retrofrontal) dead space is combined with the osteotomy-created gap across the skull base (connecting the anterior cranial fossa and the nasal cavity). This combination of factors may complicate the postoperative recovery (e.g., CSF leakage, infection, bone loss, fistula formation). After frontofacial advancement, the nasal cavity–cranial fossa communication is managed by being gentle to the tissues; good hemostasis; effective repair of any dural tears (dural grafting as needed); complete separation of dural and nasal mucosal tissue planes by interposing a combination of bone grafts, tissue sealants, and flaps; avoidance of pressure gradients across the opening while the nasal mucosa is healing; and prevention of "over-" or "under-" shunting (when a shunt is in place). The preferred way to manage the retrofrontal (lobes of the brain) dead space and the gap across the skull base osteotomy site (separating the cranial fossa and nasal cavities) after frontofacial advancement remains controversial but all agree that it is a critical aspect of the reconstruction.

In the CFD patient, relatively rapid (6–8 wk) filling of the surgically expanded intracranial volume by the previously compressed frontal lobes of the brain has been documented after cranio-orbital expansion in infants. It has also been shown to occur after frontofacial advancement in children and young adults when the volume increase remains in a physiologic range. These observations support the conservative management of the retrofrontal dead space in younger patients. More gradual and less complete filling of the space is thought to occur in older children and adults. If so, this may be particularly troublesome when the anterior cranial fossa dead space communicates directly with the nasal cavity (i.e., monobloc advancement, facial bipartition, intracranial Le Fort III) across the (open-gap) skull base interface. When feasible, closing off (sealing) the nasal cavity from the cranial fossa across the skull base osteotomy at the time of operation is preferred. Insertion of a pericranial flap or other fillers can help to separate the cavities. The use of fibrin glue to seal the anterior cranial base provides a temporary separation between the cavities, allowing time for the reepithelialization (healing) of the torn nasal mucosa. To reconstruct the defect across the skull base, (gap) bone grafts of various types have also been used. Until the torn nasal mucosa heals, potential communication between the nasal cavity and the cranial fossa may result in the transfer of air, fluid, bacteria and nasocranial fistula formation. To facilitate nasal mucosa healing and limit a pressure gradient across the communication, postoperative endotracheal intubation may be extended for 3 to 5 days and/or bilateral nasopharyngeal airways may be placed after extubation. The avoidance of positive-pressure ventilation, enforcement of sinus precautions, and restriction of nose blowing further limit reflux of air, fluid, and bacteria (nose to cranial fossa) during the early postoperative period. When anterior cranial vault procedures are performed and aerated frontal sinuses are present, management is by either cranialization or obliteration.

Aside from a learning curve in mastering the technical skills of completing the monobloc osteotomies and disimpaction, the surgical morbidity from these procedures primarily results from a combination of the anticipated retrofrontal dead space, unavoidable tears in the nasal mucosa, and management of nasocranial communication across the skull base gap with the potential for fluid, air, and bacterial contamination. Two benchmark studies clarify these issues.

Posnick and associates[75] studied the issue of retrofrontal dead space, the communication across the skull base, nasal mucosal lacerations, and associated morbidity in a consecutive series of patients ($N = 23$) undergoing either monobloc or facial bipartition osteotomies combined with cranial expansion by a single surgeon (JCP) during a 4-year time frame (1987–1991). The extradural (retrofrontal) dead space was measured from consistent CT scan images at specific postoperative intervals (immediate, 6–8 wk, and 1 yr). The study confirmed the presence of an immediate retrofrontal dead space that generally filled in with the expanding brain/dura by 6 to 8 weeks after surgery. Specific intraoperative measures were taken by the surgeon to close (seal) the nasofrontal communication using flaps, fibrin glue, and Gelfoam. Precautions to prevent a pressure gradient across the communication (repair of dural tears, sinus precautions, and nasal stinting) were meticulously adhered to with the objective of providing time for nasal mucosal healing. The infection rate in this study group was limited to 2 of 23 patients or 9%. In both patients who developed infection, a retrofrontal (extradural) fluid collection with drainage across the residual nasofrontal communication occurred. Both patients healed without major sequela but did require further reconstruction of resorbed portions of the cranial vault.

Wolfe[76] completed a critical analysis of 81 monobloc advancements carried out over a 27-year period. This was a retrospective chart analysis of a series of patients undergoing either monobloc (frontofacial) advancement (MFFA) or facial bipartition (MFFA plus FB). The procedures were carried out at seven different craniofacial centers and included 49 MFFAs and 32 MFFAs plus FBs. This included the techniques of osteotomy followed by placing the osteotomized units in their preferred location in the operating room (classic

approach) and osteotomies carried out followed by distraction (buried versus external). There were significant complications in the distracted (DO) group and fewer in the nondistracted (classic osteotomy) group. Complications included 2 deaths (cardiac arrest in 1 patient and complications arising from hypovolemia in the other). One case was aborted owing to large volume blood loss; there were 3 infections/sequestrations; and 1 CSF leak (no meningitis). The authors concluded that the MMFA or MMFA plus FB provided a superior morphologic result to the Le Fort III advancement. All patients were believed to also require orthognathic surgery. Blood loss and operative time were equivalent for both classic and distraction procedures. The authors concluded that for the majority of patients, the classic approach offered improved morphologic results. The incidence of infection and CSF leaks was not diminished through the use of the distraction approach.

Bradley and coworkers[77] recently completed a single-center retrospective chart review study comparing differences in morbidity in a series of CFD patients undergoing combined cranial vault expansion and monobloc advancement for correction of the upper and middle face deformities/hypoplasia. They describe three different sequential treatment groups over a period of 23 years. Group I patients (1979–1989: $N = 12$) underwent monobloc advancement without any special attention to the retrofrontal dead space or the communication through the skull base between the anterior cranial fossa and the nasal cavity. Group II (1989–1995: $N = 11$) patients underwent varied attempts at closure of the skull base gap with pericranial flaps and fibrin glue. Group III (1995–2002: $N = 24$) patients underwent monobloc osteotomies and disimpaction but without any immediate advancement. An internal distraction device was placed across the osteotomized zygoma on each side. After 7 days, the monobloc and forehead advancement was initiated at 1 mm/day for approximately 2 to 4 weeks. The infection rate for group III patients was significantly lower (2 of 24 patients or 8%) than for those in groups I and II. Neither of the two infections in group III resulted in bone loss. Not surprisingly, the group I patients had the greatest morbidity.

Advancement of the monobloc osteotomy in the CFD patient using the DO technique described by Bradley and coworkers[77] is likely to facilitate early nasal mucosa healing and thereby limit communication of fluid, air, and bacteria across the surgically created skull base gap. By allowing a 1-week delay in the actual advancement, the nasal mucosa may achieve sufficient healing to explain a drop in the infection rate from the 9% described by Posnick and associates[75] to the 8% described by Bradley and coworker's group III patients.

Bradley and coworkers[77] also describe a greater advancement in their group III (DO treatment) patients compared with their groups I and II patients. Confounding variables in their study may explain these differences including greater experience and improved surgical technique by the surgeons in the later years of their study (group III patients) and effect of co-morbidities (e.g., high rate of infection in group I and group II patients that likely increased relapse and limited long-term advancement). More important, no correlation is shown by Bradley and coworkers[77] between a number of millimeters of advancement of the frontofacial osteotomies in the CFD patient and either greater functional gains or enhanced facial aesthetics. In fact, with a monobloc (frontofacial) osteotomy as much aesthetic damage is done by overadvancement (enophthalmos) as by underadvancement (residual eye proptosis). In addition, the achievement of a "normal" occlusion is rarely a treatment objective at the time of monobloc advancement. Accomplishing an ideal occlusion without creating enophthalmos requires a separate Le Fort I osteotomy to differentially advance the maxilla often combined with maxillary segmentation and mandibular (sagittal split) osteotomies. To achieve the most favorable facial balance for the CFD patient, an experienced clinician's aesthetic sense of the preferred morphology and focused technical expertise to alter the skeleton intraoperatively is essential. Several key technical aspects include

1. The ability to remove, segment, and then reshape and stabilize (plates and screws) the anterior cranial vault.
2. The ability to separate the orbits and midface as a unit (monobloc) from the skull base.
3. The ability to further segment the monobloc (at the upper orbits) and reconstruct (with cranial grafts) as needed.
4. The ability to separate the monobloc into halves (facial bipartition) and then alter the two facial halves to achieve the most favorable morphology. This often requires simultaneously increasing the maxillary transverse width and decreasing the upper face width to correct hypertelorism of the orbits, zygomas, nose, and bitemporal regions (e.g., Apert's syndrome). Facial bipartition also provides the ability to correct transverse facial arc of rotation deformities. For example, changing the Apert's syndrome patients' concave facial arc of rotation toward a normal convexity is an essential aspect of the reconstruction.

Any potential advantage of limiting morbidity due to infection across the skull base with the DO technique should be considered in light of limitations to achieve the previously mentioned key technical and aesthetic aspects (points 1–4). Added morbidity with the DO technique occurs: due to pin tract infection/scarring/loosening requiring reapplication; the need for device removal; and dependence on a patient's, family's, and clinician's continued commitment to staying the course for necessary outpatient DO procedures/adjustments to achieve an acceptable result must also be factored into the decision-making process.

When a CFD patient is to undergo intracranial volume expansion as part of the craniofacial procedure and they also require hydrocephalus management, the potential for morbidity increases. Complications may arise from excessive CSF drainage (overshunting). With "overshunting," there is decreased brain volume to fill any surgically created retrofrontal dead space. Frontofacial advancement and/or cranial vault expansion procedures should be carefully staged with

ventriculoperitoneal (VP) shunting procedures. We believe that the presence or absence of a VP shunt is not in itself a major risk factor in the success of a frontofacial advancement procedure. An important aspect is satisfactory physiologic function of the ventricular system. Ultimately, the decision regarding the need for and sequencing of shunting is based on the patient's neurologic findings and the neurosurgeon's judgment. In a patient with a VP shunt in place before the surgery, experienced neurosurgical evaluation including CT scanning of the ventricular system is carried out to confirm physiologic shunt function.

Soft Tissue Management

A layered closure of the coronal incision (galea and skin) optimizes healing and limits scar widening. Resuspension of the midface periosteum to the temporalis fascia in a superior and posterior direction facilitates redraping of the soft tissues. Each lateral canthus should be adequately suspended or reattached in a superoposterior direction to the lateral orbital rim. The use of chromic gut for closure of the scalp skin in children may be used to obviate the need for postoperative suture or staple removal.

CROUZON'S SYNDROME

Crouzon's syndrome is a frequent form of CFD. It is characterized by multiple anomalies of the craniofacial skeleton with an autosomal dominant inheritance pattern. Its manifestations are generally less severe than those of Apert's syndrome and there are no malformations of the extremities. Typically, the cranial vault presentation is premature synostosis of both coronal sutures with a resultant brachycephalic shape to the skull. Cranial vault suture involvement other than coronal may include sagittal, metopic, or lambdoidal, either in isolation or in any combination. The cranial base and upper face sutures are variably involved, resulting in a degree of midface hypoplasia with an Angle class III malocclusion. The orbits are hypoplastic, resulting in a degree of proptosis with additional orbital dystopia that may produce a mild orbital hypertelorism and flatness to the (transverse) arc of rotation of the midface

By clinical examination alone, it may be difficult to accurately separate nonsyndromic bilateral coronal synostosis from Crouzon's syndrome, with its expected midface deficiency. It is now known that Crouzon's syndrome is caused by multiple mutations in the fibroblast growth factor receptor-2 (FGFR2) gene, some of which are identical to those seen in Pfeiffer's and Jackson-Weiss syndromes. It is likely that in the past many of these individuals have been misdiagnosed as having Crouzon's syndrome. The 5% of individuals with Crouzon's syndrome who have acanthosis nigricans (pigmentary changes in the skin fold regions) are said to have Crouzon's syndrome with acanthosis nigricans. It can be present in the neonatal period or appear later. Crouzon's syndrome with acanthosis nigricans has been described with a specific Ala391Glu mutation in *FGFR3*.

Primary Cranio-orbital Decompression: Reshaping in Infancy

The initial treatment for Crouzon's syndrome generally requires bilateral coronal suture release and simultaneous anterior cranial vault and upper orbital osteotomies with reshaping and advancement (see Figure 46-1).[63–66] Our preference is to carry this out when the child is 9 to 11 months of age unless clear signs of increased ICP are identified earlier in life (Figure 46-2). Reshaping of the upper three quarters of the orbital rims and supraorbital ridges is geared toward decreasing the bitemporal and anterior cranial base width,

with simultaneous horizontal advancement to increase the anteroposterior dimension. This also increases the depth of the upper orbits, with some improvement of eye proptosis. The overlying forehead is then reconstructed according to morphologic needs. A degree of overcorrection is preferred at the level of the supraorbital ridge when the procedure is carried out in infancy. In our opinion, by allowing additional growth to occur (waiting until the child is 9–11 mo old), the reconstructed cranial vault and upper orbital shape is better maintained with less need for repeat craniotomy procedures but without risking compression of the underlying brain.

The goals at this stage are to provide increased intracranial space in the anterior cranial vault for the brain; to increase the orbital volume, which allows the eyes to be positioned more

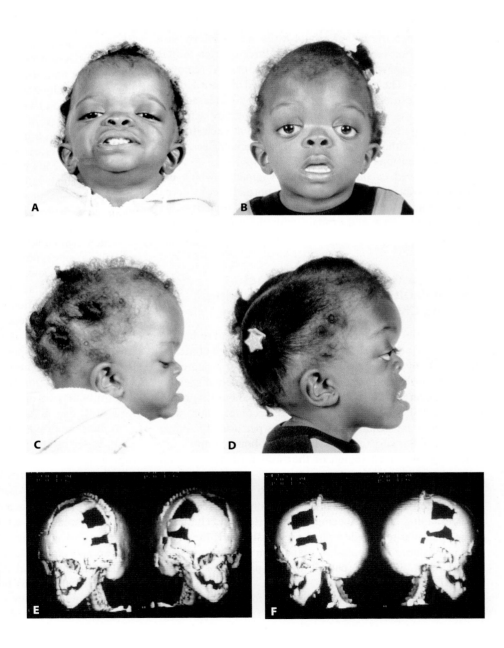

FIGURE 46-2.   An 18-month-old girl with brachycephaly and midface deficiency with a mild degree of papilledema was referred for evaluation. She was found to have bilateral coronal synostosis and midface hypoplasia without extremity anomalies. The diagnosis of Crouzon's syndrome was made. She underwent cranio-orbital reshaping (see Figure 46-1). Several months later, a ventriculoperitoneal shunt was placed for management of hydrocephalus. Further staged reconstruction will include a total midface advancement procedure later in childhood followed by orthodontic treatment and orthognathic surgery in the early teenage years. **A,** Frontal view before surgery. **B,** Frontal view at 3 years of age, 1.5 years after undergoing cranio-orbital decompression and reshaping. **C,** Profile view before surgery. **D,** Profile view at 3 years of age, 1.5 years after undergoing first-stage cranio-orbital decompression and reshaping. **E** and **F,** Three-dimensional computed tomography (CT) scan views of craniofacial skeleton, just 1 week after cranio-orbital reshaping with advancement. (**A–F,** Reproduced with permission from Posnick JC. Crouzon syndrome: evaluation and staging of reconstruction. In Posnick JC, editor. Craniofacial and Maxillofacial Surgery in Children and Young Adults. Philadelphia: WB Saunders; 2000; p. 275.)

normally for better protection from exposure; and to improve the morphology of the forehead and upper orbits.

A postauricular coronal (scalp) incision is made, and the anterior scalp flap is elevated along with the temporalis muscle in the subperiosteal plane. Bilateral circumferential periorbital dissection follows, with detachment of the lateral canthi, but with preservation of the medial canthi and nasolacrimal apparatus to the medial orbital walls. The subperiosteal dissection is continued down the lateral and infraorbital rims to include the anterior aspect of the maxilla and zygomatic buttress. The neurosurgeon then completes the craniotomy to remove the dysmorphic anterior cranial vault. With protection of the frontal and temporal lobes of the brain (remaining anterior to each olfactory bulb), safe direct visualization of the anterior cranial base and orbits is possible at the time of orbital osteotomies.

The orbital osteotomies are then completed across the orbital roof and superior aspect of the medial orbital walls, laterally through the lateral orbital walls and inferiorly just into the inferior orbital fissures. The three-quarter orbital osteotomy units, with their tenon extensions, are removed from the field. The orbital units are reshaped and reinset into a preferred position. Orbital depth is thereby increased, and global proptosis is reduced. Fixation is generally achieved with 28-gauge interosseous wires or suture at each infraorbital rim and with plates and titanium or resorbable screws at the tenon extensions and frontonasal regions.

The removed calvaria is cut into segments, which are placed individually to achieve a more normally configured anterior cranial vault. The goal of reshaping is to narrow the anterior cranial base and orbital width slightly and provide more forward projection and overall normal morphology.

Repeat Craniotomy for Additional Cranial Vault Expansion and Reshaping in Young Children

After the initial suture release, decompression, and reshaping are carried out during infancy, the child is observed clinically at intervals by the craniofacial surgeon, pediatric neurosurgeon, pediatric ophthalmologist, and developmental specialist and undergoes interval CT scanning. Should signs of increased ICP develop, urgent brain decompression with cranial vault expansion and reshaping is performed.[47] When increased ICP is suspected, the location of brain compression influences for which region of the skull further expansion and reshaping is planned.

If the brain compression is judged to be anterior, then further anterior cranial vault and upper orbital osteotomies with reshaping and advancement are carried out. The technique is similar to that described previously.[47,65] If the problem is posterior compression, expansion of the posterior cranial vault, with the patient in the prone position, is required (Figure 46-3).

The "repeat" craniotomy carried out for further decompression and reshaping in the child with Crouzon's syndrome is often complicated by brittle cortical bone (which lacks a diploic space and contains sharp spicules piercing the dura), the presence of previously placed fixation devices in the operative field (e.g., Silastic sheeting, metal clips, stainless steel wires, plates, and screws), and convoluted thin dura compressed against (or herniated into) the inner table of the skull. All of these issues result in a greater potential for dural tears during the calvarectomy than would normally occur during the primary procedure. A greater potential for morbidity should be anticipated when reelevating the scalp flap, dissecting the dura free of the inner table of the skull and cranial base, and then removing the cranial vault bone.

Management of "Total Midface" Deformity in Childhood

The type of osteotomies selected to manage the "total midface" deficiency or deformity and residual cranial vault dysplasia should depend on the extent and location of the presenting dysmorphology rather than on a fixed approach to the midface malformation.[47,53–56,65,66,72,78–82] The selection of a monobloc (with or without additional orbital segmentation), facial bipartition (with or without additional orbital segmental osteotomies), or Le Fort III osteotomy to manage the basic horizontal, transverse, vertical orbital, and upper midface deficiencies or deformities in a patient with Crouzon's syndrome depends on the patient's presenting midface and anterior cranial vault morphology. The observed dysmorphology is dependent on the original malformation, the previous procedures carried out, and the effects of ongoing growth (Figures 46-4 and 46-5).

When evaluating the upper and midface in a child born with Crouzon's syndrome, if the supraorbital ridge is in good position when viewed from the sagittal plane (the depth of the upper orbits is adequate), the midface and forehead have a normal arc of rotation in the transverse plane (not concave), and the root of the nose is of normal width (minimal orbital hypertelorism), there is little need to reconstruct this region (the forehead and upper orbits) any further. In such patients, the basic residual midface deformity is in the lower half of the orbits, zygomatic buttress, and maxilla. If so, the deformity may be effectively managed using an extracranial Le Fort III osteotomy.

If the supraorbital ridges, anterior cranial base, zygomas, nose, lower orbits, and maxilla all remain deficient in the sagittal plane (horizontal retrusion), a monobloc osteotomy is indicated (see Figures 46-4 and 46-5). In these patients, the forehead is generally flat and retruded and will also require reshaping and advancement. If upper midface hypertelorism (increased transverse width) and midface flattening (horizontal retrusion) with loss of the normal facial curvature (concave arc) are also present, the monobloc unit is split vertically in the midline (facial bipartition), a wedge of interorbital (nasal and ethmoidal) bone is removed, and the orbits and zygomas are repositioned medially while the maxilla at the palatal level is widened. The facial bipartition is rarely

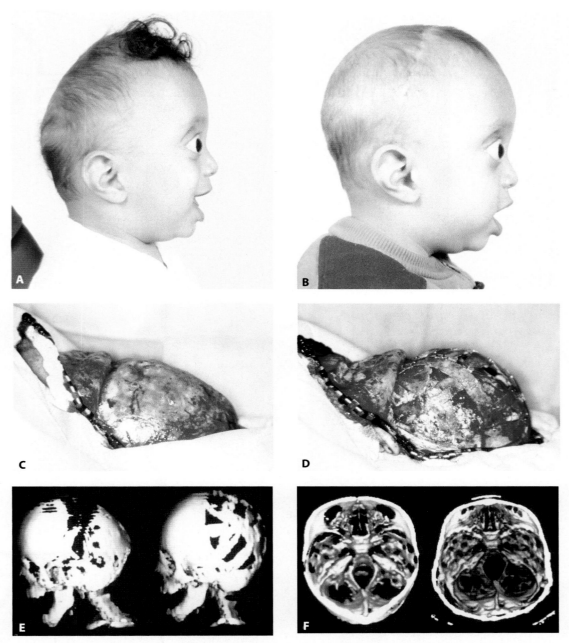

FIGURE 46-3.   A child with Crouzon's syndrome is shown at 10 months of age. His deformities are characterized by mild bilateral coronal and marked bilateral lambdoid synostosis in combination with midface deficiency. He has diminished intracranial volume, resulting in brain compression. The orbits are shallow with resulting eye proptosis, and the midface is deficient with malocclusion. He is shown before and after undergoing posterior cranial vault decompression and reshaping to expand the intracranial volume. He later underwent placement of a ventriculoperitoneal shunt for management of hydrocephalus. He will require a total midface advancement (monobloc) with further anterior cranial vault reshaping after 5 years of age. This will be followed by orthognathic surgery in combination with orthodontic treatment in the teenage years. **A,** Profile view before surgery. **B,** Profile view after posterior cranial vault reconstruction. **C,** Intraoperative lateral view of the cranial vault (patient in prone position) as seen with the posterior scalp flap elevated. **D,** Same intraoperative view after posterior cranial vault decompression, reshaping, and fixation of bone segments with microplates and screws. **E,** Comparison of three-dimensional CT scan views before and after reconstruction. **F,** Comparison of three-dimensional CT scan views of the cranial base before and after reconstruction. (**A–F,** Reproduced with permission from Posnick JC. The craniofacial dysostosis syndromes: secondary management of craniofacial disorders. Clin Plast Surg 1997;24:429.)

required in Crouzon's syndrome, but the monobloc is. When a monobloc or facial bipartition osteotomy is carried out as the "total midface" procedure, additional segmentation of the upper and lateral orbits for reconstruction may also be

required to normalize the morphology of the orbital aesthetic units.[83–88]

For most patients, a surgeon's attempt to simultaneously adjust the orbits and idealize the occlusion using the Le

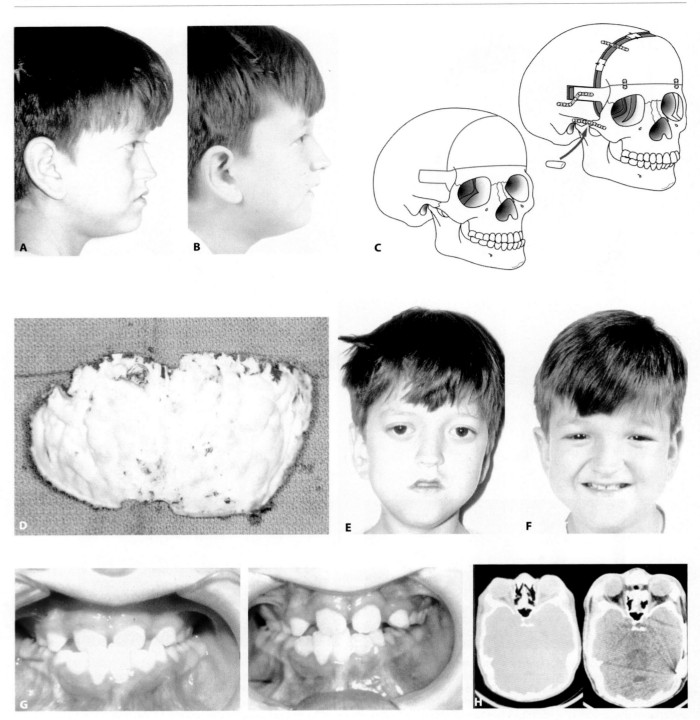

FIGURE 46-4.   A child at 8 years of age with Crouzon's syndrome who underwent a limited first-stage cranio-orbital procedure at 6 weeks of age. He then underwent anterior cranial vault and monobloc (orbits and midface) osteotomies with advancement. **A,** Profile view before the monobloc procedure. **B,** Profile view after reconstruction. **C,** Craniofacial morphology before and after anterior the cranial vault and monobloc osteotomies with advancement as carried out. Osteotomy locations indicated. Stabilization with cranial bone grafts and miniplates and screws. **D,** View of the inner surface of the frontal bones after bifrontal craniotomy. Compression of the brain against the inner table has resulted in resorption of the inner skull. This is an indication of longstanding increased intracranial pressure (ICP). **E,** Frontal view before surgery. **F,** Frontal view after reconstruction. **G,** Occlusal views before and after reconstruction. **H,** Comparison of axial CT slices through the midorbits before and after reconstruction indicates resulting increased intraorbital depth and decreased proptosis achieved. *(Continued)*

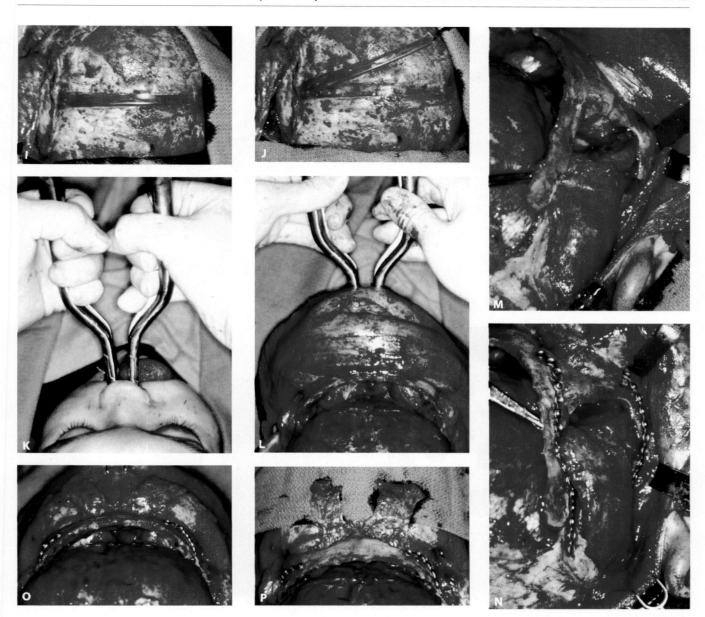

FIGURE 46-4.   *(Continued)* **I,** Intraoperative bird's-eye lateral view of the cranial vault demonstrates Silastic strip that had been placed by the neurosurgeon when the patient was 2 months of age (8 yr earlier). **J,** Removing the Silastic strip along the sphenoid wing region is difficult owing to bone overgrowth. **K,** Intraoperative view of (Rowe) forceps in the nose and mouth after monobloc osteotomy but before disimpaction. **L,** Same view but with the coronal incision turned down, indicating the degree of advancement at the supraorbital ridge level after disimpaction. **M,** Lateral view of the zygomatic arch and tenon extension of the supraorbital rim after monobloc advancement just before miniplate fixation. **N,** Same view after miniplate fixation of the zygomatic arch and tenon extension. **O,** Bird's-eye view of the stabilized monobloc unit after advancement. There is increased intracranial volume (dead space) in the anterior cranial vault for brain expansion. **P,** Same view with elevated pericranial flaps, which will be turned in to close the opening between the nose and the anterior cranial base. (**A, B, D–P,** Reproduced with permission from Posnick JC. Craniofacial dysostosis: management of the midface deformity. In Bell WH, editor. Orthognathic and Reconstructive Surgery. Philadelphia: WB Saunders; 1992; p. 1888; **C,** adapted from Posnick JC. Craniofacial dysostosis: management of the midface deformity. In Bell WH, editor. Orthognathic and Reconstructive Surgery. Philadelphia: WB Saunders; 1992; p. 1888.)

Fort III, monobloc, or facial bipartition osteotomy in isolation, without completing a separate Le Fort I osteotomy, is an error in judgment. The degree of horizontal deficiency observed at the orbits and maxillary dentition is rarely uniform. This further segmentation of the midface complex at the Le Fort I level is required to establish normal proportions.

If a Le Fort I separation of the total midface complex is not carried out and the surgeon attempts to achieve a positive overbite and overjet at the incisor teeth, overadvancement of the orbits with enophthalmos will occur. The Le Fort I osteotomy is generally not performed at the time of the total midface procedure. This will await skeletal maturity and then

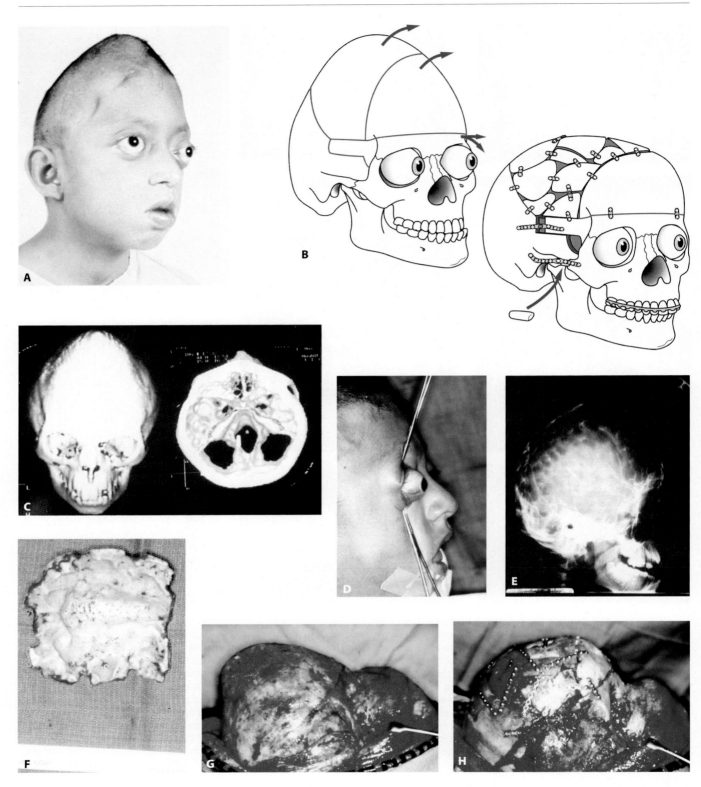

FIGURE 46-5.   A 12-year-old boy with unrepaired Crouzon's syndrome who underwent total cranial vault and monobloc osteotomies with reshaping and advancement. **A,** Oblique view before surgery. **B,** The patient's craniofacial morphology before surgery. Osteotomy locations indicated. A second illustration after the osteotomies were completed with advancement, reshaping, and fixation. **C,** Three-dimensional CT scan views of the cranial vault and cranial base before surgery. **D,** Intraoperative view with forceps placed at the orbital rims indicates the extent of proptosis. **E,** Lateral skull radiograph with "fingerprinting" indicates longstanding increased ICP. **F,** Inner table internal side of the frontal bone indicates compression of the brain against the inner table of the skull. **G,** Intraoperative lateral view of the cranial vault and orbits through the coronal incision before osteotomies. **H,** Same view after osteotomies, reshaping, and stabilization of bone segments with miniplates and screws. *(Continued)*

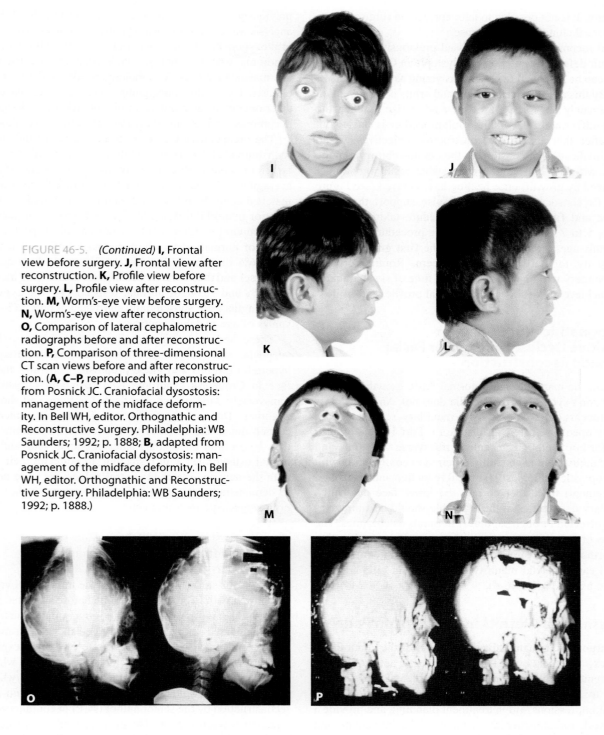

FIGURE 46-5. *(Continued)* **I,** Frontal view before surgery. **J,** Frontal view after reconstruction. **K,** Profile view before surgery. **L,** Profile view after reconstruction. **M,** Worm's-eye view before surgery. **N,** Worm's-eye view after reconstruction. **O,** Comparison of lateral cephalometric radiographs before and after reconstruction. **P,** Comparison of three-dimensional CT scan views before and after reconstruction. (**A, C–P,** reproduced with permission from Posnick JC. Craniofacial dysostosis: management of the midface deformity. In Bell WH, editor. Orthognathic and Reconstructive Surgery. Philadelphia: WB Saunders; 1992; p. 1888; **B,** adapted from Posnick JC. Craniofacial dysostosis: management of the midface deformity. In Bell WH, editor. Orthognathic and Reconstructive Surgery. Philadelphia: WB Saunders; 1992; p. 1888.)

be combined with orthodontic treatment. Until then, an Angle class III malocclusion will remain.

A major aesthetic problem specific to the Le Fort III osteotomy when its indications are less than ideal is the creation of irregular step-offs in the lateral orbital rims. This will occur when even a moderate (Le Fort III) advancement is carried out. These lateral orbital step-offs are unattractive and are visible to the casual observer at conversational distance. Surgical modification performed later is difficult, often with less than

ideal aesthetic results. Another problem with the Le Fort III osteotomy is the difficulty in judging an ideal orbital depth. A frequent result is either residual proptosis or enophthalmos. Simultaneous correction of orbital hypertelorism or correction of a midface arc-of-rotation problem is not possible with the Le Fort III procedure. Excessive lengthening of the nose, accompanied by flattening of the nasofrontal angle, will also occur if the Le Fort III osteotomy is selected when the skeletal morphology favors a monobloc or facial bipartition procedure. It is not possible to later correct the surgically created vertical elongation of the nose.

Final reconstruction, as discussed previously, of the cranial vault deformities and orbital dystopia in Crouzon's syndrome can be managed in patients as young as 5 to 7 years of age.[47] By this age, the cranial vault and orbits normally attain approximately 85% to 90% of their adult size.[43] When the upper midface and final cranial vault procedure is carried out at or after this age, the reconstructive objectives are to approximate adult dimensions in the cranio-orbitozygomatic region, with the expectation of a stable result (no longer influenced by growth) once healing has occurred (see Figure 46-4). Psychosocial considerations also support the upper midface and final cranial vault procedure taking place in patients 5 to 7 years of age. When the procedure is carried out at this age, the child may enter the first grade with an opportunity for satisfactory self-esteem. Routine orthognathic surgery will be necessary at the time of skeletal maturity to achieve an ideal occlusion, facial profile, and smile.

Orthognathic Procedures for Definitive Occlusal and Lower Facial Aesthetic Reconstruction

Although the mandible has a normal basic growth potential in Crouzon's syndrome, the maxilla does not. An Angle class III malocclusion, resulting from maxillary retrusion, with anterior open bite often results. A Le Fort I osteotomy to allow for horizontal advancement, transverse widening, and vertical adjustment is generally required in combination with an osteoplastic genioplasty (vertical reduction and horizontal advancement) to further correct the lower face deformity. Secondary deformities of the mandible should be simultaneously corrected through sagittal split ramus osteotomies. The elective orthognathic surgery is carried out in conjunction with orthodontic treatment planned for completion at the time of early skeletal maturity (~13–15 yr in girls and 15–17 yr in boys) (Figure 46-6).

Assessment of Results in the Crouzon Patient

The purpose of a quantitative assessment of the craniofacial complex, whether by CT scan analysis, anthropometric measurement, cephalometric analysis, or dental model analysis, is to help predict growth patterns, confirm or refute clinical impressions, aid in treatment planning, and provide a framework for objective assessment of the immediate and long-term reconstructive results.

Quantitative Assessment of Presenting Crouzon's Deformity and Surgical Results Based on CT Scan Analysis after First-Stage Cranio-orbital Reconstruction

Waitzman and colleagues[89,90] developed a method of analysis based on CT scan measurements that allows for a more quantitative assessment of the upper and midface skeleton in both the horizontal and the transverse planes than was

previously available. This method of quantitative CT scan analysis was utilized to document the differences in the cranio-orbitozygomatic region between children with Crouzon's syndrome who had not yet undergone reconstruction and age-matched controls. Morphologic results achieved in those children 1 year after undergoing a classic suture release and anterior cranial vault and upper orbital procedure, designed to decompress and reshape these regions, were also evaluated.

The preoperative CT scan measurements of the children with untreated Crouzon's syndrome confirmed a widened anterior cranial vault at 108% of normal and a cranial length averaging only 92% of normal. In comparison with age-matched controls, orbital measurements revealed a widened anterior interorbital width at 122% of normal, an increased intertemporal width at 121% of normal, globe protrusion at 119% of normal, and a short medial orbital wall length at only 86% of normal. The distance between the zygomatic buttresses and the interarch widths were found to be increased at 106% and 103% of normal, respectively. The zygomatic arch lengths were substantially shortened at only 87% of the values of age-matched controls.

These findings confirmed clinical observations of brachycephalic anterior cranial vaults with shallow, frequently hyperteloric orbits and globe proptosis. Generally, the midface in Crouzon's syndrome is horizontally retrusive and transversely wide, which is reflected in wide and shortened zygomas. The same quantitative CT scan assessment was carried out in the children with Crouzon's syndrome more than 1 year after undergoing anterior cranial vault and upper orbital osteotomies with reshaping, to compare their values with the new age-matched control values; we were not able to demonstrate any significant improvement in the cranio-orbitozygomatic measurements.

Quantitative Intracranial Volume Measurements before and after Cranio-orbital Reshaping in Children with Crouzon's Syndrome

In a previous study, we documented the intracranial volumes in children with Crouzon's syndrome before and after cranio-orbital reshaping procedures. The intracranial volumes also were compared with those of an age- and gender-matched cohort, and we also reviewed the rate of cranial expansion with growth.[89,90] The study included 13 children who presented sequentially with Crouzon's syndrome and who subsequently underwent a classic first-stage cranio-orbital reconstruction by the senior author (JCP) in conjunction with a pediatric neurosurgeon. The primary method of osteotomy and bone graft fixation varied (e.g., wires, microplates, miniplates, and screws). The average age at the time of operation was 13 months (range, 6–46 mo). Postoperative clinical follow-up ranged from 12 to 60 months at the time of the study's completion. Of the children with Crouzon's syndrome who were evaluated preoperatively, 12 of 13 had intracranial volume values greater than the mean. When comparing postoperative volumes with the normative data, all 13 maintained volumes at or greater than the mean. Ten of the 13 achieved

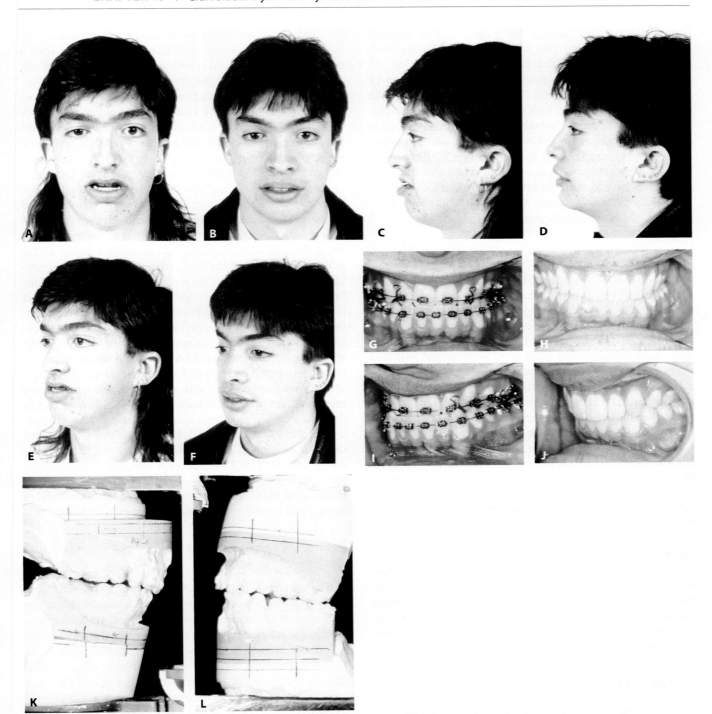

FIGURE 46-6. A 19-year-old boy born with Crouzon's syndrome. When he was 11 years of age, the patient was seen by another surgeon and underwent a Le Fort osteotomy with advancement through an extracranial approach. He presented in his late teenage years with asymmetrical and dystopic orbits, zygomatic hypoplasia, a retrusive upper jaw, an asymmetrical lower jaw, and a long chin. He underwent a combined orthodontic and orthognathic approach, including a Le Fort I osteotomy (horizontal advancement), bilateral sagittal split osteotomies of the mandible (correction of asymmetry), and an osteoplastic genioplasty (vertical reduction and horizontal advancement). Stabilization was accomplished with miniplates and screws. During the same general anesthesia procedure, he underwent a reopening of his coronal (scalp) incision with harvesting of split cranial grafts to recontour and augment the orbits and zygomas. **A,** Frontal view before surgery. **B,** Frontal view after reconstruction. **C,** Profile view before surgery. **D,** Profile view after reconstruction. **E,** Oblique view before surgery. **F,** Oblique view after reconstruction. **G,** Occlusal view before surgery. **H,** Occlusal view after reconstruction. **I,** Oblique occlusal view before surgery. **J,** Oblique occlusal view after reconstruction. **K,** Articulated dental casts before surgery. **L,** Articulated dental casts after model reconstruction. (**A–L,** Reproduced with permission from Posnick JC. Crouzon syndrome: evaluation and staging of reconstruction. In Posnick JC, editor. Craniofacial and Maxillofacial Surgery in Children and Young Adults. Philadelphia: WB Saunders; 2000; pp. 299–300.)

intracranial volumes equal to or greater than 2 standard deviations (SD) above the mean. When reviewing each Crouzon's patient's cranial capacity over time, 5 of the 13 approximated the normal growth curve, whereas 6 of the 13 exceeded it. According to the findings of our study, for the majority of children born with Crouzon's syndrome, the cranial capacity will exceed the mean early in life and expand at a rapid rate in conjunction with cranio-orbital decompression and reconstruction. The biologic explanation for these unexpected findings remains unclear. It should be noted that other researchers have studied the intracranial volume of children born with craniosynostosis. Conflicting data have been reported, and further investigation is needed.

Quantitative Assessment of Presenting Deformity in Children with Crouzon's Syndrome and Surgical Results after Monobloc Osteotomy Based on CT Scan Analysis

In the midchildhood years, a group of children with Crouzon's syndrome were assessed using quantitative CT scan measurements. We found them to have cranial vault lengths averaging only 87% of the age-matched norms. The medial orbital walls were (horizontally) short at 87% of normal, whereas the extent of globe protrusion was excessive at 134% of age-matched norms. The zygomatic arch lengths averaged only 84% of normal. These findings confirmed horizontal (anteroposterior) deficiency of the upper and midface.

After undergoing a monobloc osteotomy (orbits and midface) combined with anterior cranial vault reshaping and advancement carried out through an intracranial approach, the children's' cranio-orbitozygomatic measurements were taken again. The mean cranial length initially achieved (after monobloc osteotomy) was 98%, and at 1 year, it was 92% of the control value. When compared with age-matched controls, the orbital measurements reflected improvement in the midorbital hypertelorism (midinterorbital width was 97% initially after operation and 102% at 1 yr) and orbital proptosis (early after surgery, 86% of values for age-matched normal children; 92% at 1 yr). The medial orbital wall length initially normalized at 101% and later at 97% of normal values. The zygomatic arch length initially corrected at 106% and later to 101% of normal.

APERT'S SYNDROME

Apert's syndrome has previously been classified on the basis of its clinical findings.[91] Postmortem histologic and radiographic studies have confirmed that skeletal deficiencies in the patient with Apert's syndrome result from a cartilage dysplasia at the cranial base, leading to premature fusion of the midline sutures from the occiput to the anterior nasal septum. Molecular genetic studies now clarify that two common mutations account for 98% of Apert's syndrome: P253R and S252W.[92] These mutations occur in the identical location as the *FGFR1* mutation in Pfeiffer's syndrome and the *FGFR3* mutation in Muenke's syndrome. In addition, a component of the syndrome is four-limb complex syndactly of

the hands and feet. Fusion and malformation of other joints, including the elbows and shoulders, often occur. In Apert's syndrome, fused cervical vertebrae (68%), usually C5–6 can occur. Hydrocephalus is less frequent than in Crouzon's syndrome (2% vs. 10%). Occasional internal organ anomalies can occur. The integument (soft tissue envelope) also varies from that in Crouzon's syndrome, with a greater downward slant to the lateral canthi and a distinctive, S-shaped upper eyelid ptosis. The quality of the skin often varies from normal with acne and hyperhidrosis being prominent features.

Apert's syndrome has previously been classified on the basis of its clinical findings.[93,94] Postmortem histologic and radiographic studies suggest that skeletal deficiencies in the patient with Apert's syndrome result from a cartilage dysplasia at the cranial base, leading to premature fusion of the midline sutures from the occiput to the anterior nasal septum.[75,95–98] In addition, a component of the syndrome is four-limb symmetry complex syndactylies of the hands and feet (Figure 46-7). Fusion and malformation of other joints, including the elbows and shoulders, often occur. The soft tissue envelope also varies from that in Crouzon's syndrome, with a greater downward slant to the canthi lateral and a distinctive, S-shaped upper eyelid ptosis. The quality of the skin often varies from normal, with acne and hyperhidrosis being prominent features. Molecular genetic studies now clarify that two common mutations account for 98% of Apert's syndrome: P253R and S252W.[92] These mutations occur in the identical location as the *FGFR1* mutation in Pfeiffer's syndrome and the *FGFR3* mutation in Muenke's syndrome. At the molecular level, one of two *FGFR2* mutations involving amino acids (Ser252Trp and Pro253Arg) have been found to cause Apert's syndrome in nearly all patients studied.[99–104]

Primary Cranio-orbital Decompression: Reshaping in Infancy

The initial craniofacial procedure for Apert's syndrome generally requires bilateral coronal suture release and anterior cranial vault and upper three-quarter orbital osteotomies to expand the anterior cranial vault and reshape the upper orbits and forehead (see Figure 46-1).[105,106] Our preference is to carry this out when the child is 9 to 11 months of age, unless signs of increased ICP are identified earlier in life. The main goals at this stage are to decompress the brain and provide increased space for it in the anterior cranial vault and to increase the orbital volume to decrease globe protrusion. The fronto-orbital surgical technique is similar to that described for Crouzon's syndrome (Figure 46-8).

Further Craniotomy for Additional Cranial Vault Expansion and Reshaping in Young Children

As described for Crouzon's syndrome, after the initial suture release, decompression, and reshaping carried out during infancy, the child is observed clinically at intervals by the

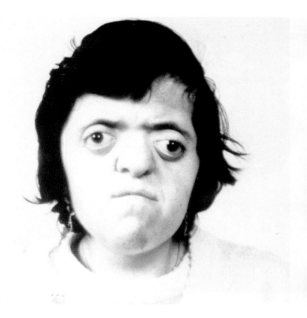

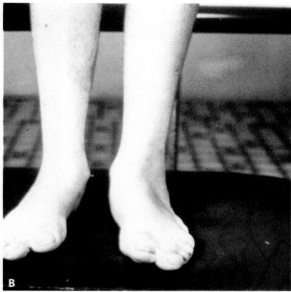

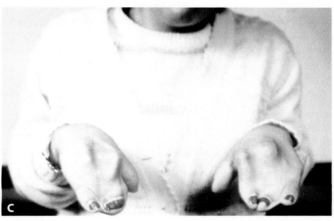

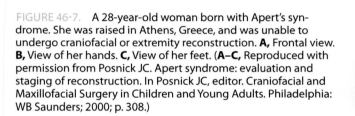

FIGURE 46-7.   A 28-year-old woman born with Apert's syndrome. She was raised in Athens, Greece, and was unable to undergo craniofacial or extremity reconstruction. **A,** Frontal view. **B,** View of her hands. **C,** View of her feet. (**A–C,** Reproduced with permission from Posnick JC. Apert syndrome: evaluation and staging of reconstruction. In Posnick JC, editor. Craniofacial and Maxillofacial Surgery in Children and Young Adults. Philadelphia: WB Saunders; 2000; p. 308.)

craniofacial surgeon, pediatric neurosurgeon, pediatric ophthalmologist, and developmental pediatrician and undergoes interval CT scanning.[63,67,68] Should signs of increased ICP develop, further decompression with reshaping of the cranial vault to expand the intracranial volume is performed (Figure 46-9). In Apert's syndrome, the posterior cranial vault more commonly requires expansion. The technique is similar to that described for Crouzon's syndrome.

Management of the "Total Midface" Deformity in Childhood

In Apert's syndrome, for almost all patients, facial bipartition osteotomies combined with further cranial vault reshaping permit a more complete correction of the abnormal craniofacial skeleton than can be achieved through other midface procedure options (i.e., monobloc or Le Fort III osteotomies). When using the facial bipartition approach, a more normal arc of rotation of the midface complex is achieved with the midline split. This further reduces the stigmata of the preoperative "flat, wide, and retrusive" facial appearance. The facial bipartition also allows the orbits and zygomatic buttresses as units to shift to the midline (correction of hypertelorism) while the maxillary arch is simultaneously widened. Horizontal advancement of the reassembled midface complex is then achieved to normalize the orbital depth and zygomatic length. The forehead is generally flat, tall, and retruded, with a constricting band just above the supraorbital ridge, giving the impression of bitemporal narrowing. Reshaping of the anterior cranial vault is simultaneously carried out (Figure 46-10; see also Figures 46-8 and 46-9). See also Figure 46-9H for preoperative craniofacial morphology and planned and completed osteotomies and reshaping. Note that stabilization was achieved with cranial bone grafts and plate and screw fixation. A Le Fort III osteotomy is virtually never adequate for an ideal correction of the residual upper and midface deformity of Apert's syndrome.[107,108]

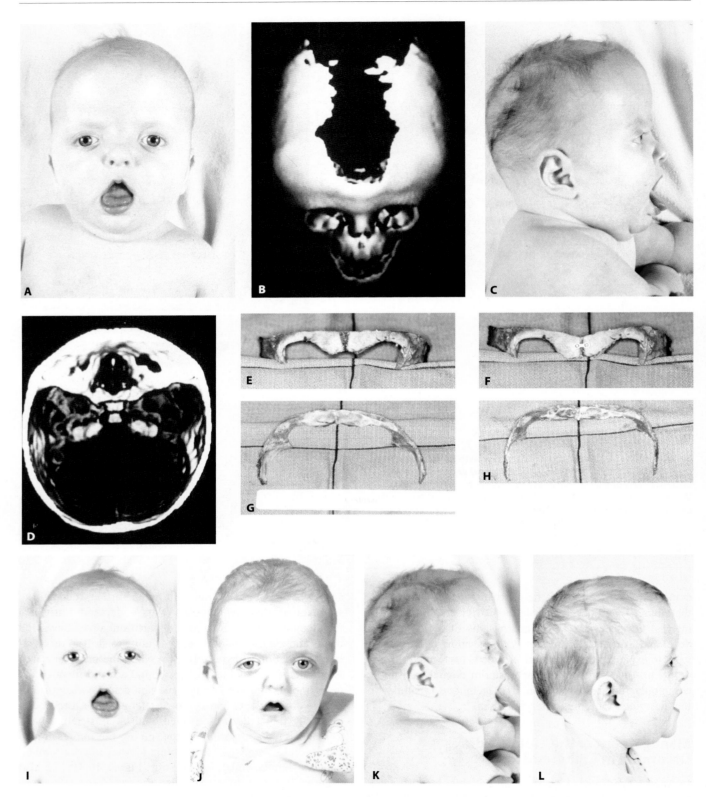

FIGURE 46-8.   A 6-month-old girl with Apert's syndrome underwent anterior cranial vault and three-quarter orbital osteotomies with reshaping as described (see Figure 46-1). **A,** Frontal view before surgery. **B,** Three-dimensional CT scan view of cranial vault before surgery. **C,** Profile view before surgery. **D,** Three-dimensional CT scan view of the cranial base before surgery. **E,** Frontal view of the orbital osteotomy unit before reshaping. **F,** Frontal view of the orbital osteotomy unit after reshaping. **G,** Bird's-eye view of the orbital osteotomy unit before reshaping. **H,** Bird's-eye view of the orbital osteotomy unit after reshaping. **I,** Frontal view before surgery. **J,** Frontal view 1 year later. **K,** Profile view before surgery. **L,** Profile view 1 year later. *(Continued)*

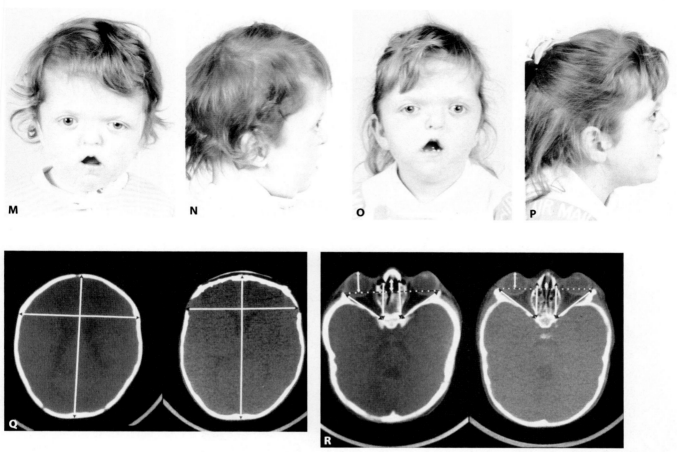

FIGURE 46-8. *(Continued)* **M** and **N,** Frontal and profile views 2 years after reconstruction. **O** and **P,** Frontal and profile views 3 years after first stage cranio-orbital reshaping; further staged reconstruction is required. **Q,** Comparison of standard axial CT slices through the cranial vault before and 1 year after cranio-orbital reshaping. The cranial vault length (cephalic length) has increased from 115 to 158 mm. The anterior cranial vault width (intercoronal distance) has remained stable at 115 mm. **R,** Comparison of standard axial CT slices through the midorbits before and 1 year after reconstruction. Marked globe protrusion of 16 mm has increased to 17 mm 1 year later. The anterior interorbital distance diminished from 29 to 25 mm, which still represented 137% of the age-matched control value. (Magnification of the individual CT scan images was not controlled for.) (**A–R,** Reproduced with permission from Posnick JC, Lin KY, Jhawar BJ, Armstrong D. Apert syndrome: quantitative assessment in presenting deformity and surgical results after first-stage reconstruction by CT scan. Plast Reconstr Surg 1994;93:489–497.)

Orthognathic Procedures for Definitive Occlusal and Lower Facial Aesthetic Reconstruction

The mandible has normal basic growth potential in Apert's syndrome. The extent of maxillary hypoplasia will result in an Angle class III malocclusion with severe anterior open-bite deformity. A Le Fort I osteotomy is required to allow for horizontal advancement, transverse widening, and vertical adjustment in combination with an osteoplastic genioplasty to vertically reduce and horizontally advance the chin, often combined with bilateral sagittal split osteotomies of the mandible. The elective orthognathic surgery is carried out in conjunction with detailed orthodontic treatment planned for completion at the time of early skeletal maturity (~13–15 yr in girls and 15–17 yr in boys).

Assessment of Results in the Apert Patient

Quantitative Assessment of Presenting Apert's Deformity and Surgical Results Based on CT Scan Analysis after First-Stage Cranio-orbital Reconstruction

In a previously published study, we applied a method of quantitative CT scan analysis to document the differences in the cranio-orbitozygomatic region between children with Apert's syndrome who had not been operated on and age-matched controls.[90] We also evaluated the morphologic results achieved in those children 1 year after a classic anterior cranial vault and upper orbital procedure was undertaken, which was designed to decompress the brain and reshape these regions. Eight consecutive infants and young children with Apert's syndrome who underwent a classic cranio-orbital procedure by a craniofacial surgeon (JCP) in

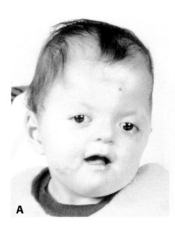

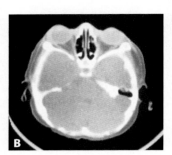

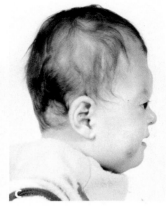

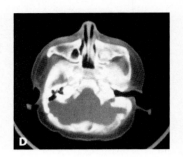

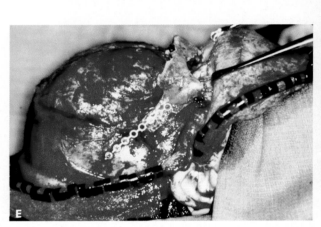

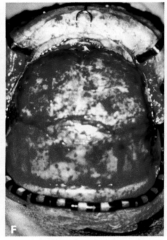

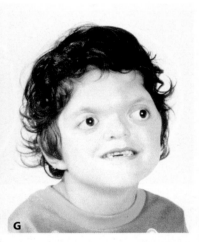

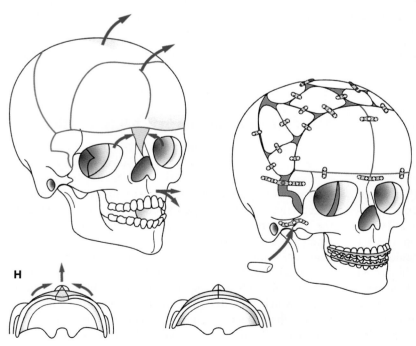

FIGURE 46-9. A child born with Apert's syndrome underwent bilateral "lateral canthal advancement" procedures when she was 6 weeks of age, carried out by the neurosurgeon working independently. At 18 months of age, she returned with turricephaly and a constricted anterior cranial vault requiring further cranio-orbital decompression and reshaping. At 5 years of age, she underwent anterior cranial vault and facial bipartition osteotomies with reshaping. As part of her staged reconstruction, she will require orthognathic surgery and orthodontic treatment planned for the teenage years. **A,** Frontal view at 8 months of age after a lateral canthal advancement procedure with residual deformity. **B,** Axial-sliced CT scan through the midorbits indicates dystopia, hypertelorism, and proptosis. **C,** Lateral view at 8 months of age. **D,** Axial-sliced CT scan through the zygomatic arches indicate midface deficiency.**E** and **F,** Lateral and bird's-eye views of the cranio-orbital region after three-quarter orbital osteotomies and reshaping and anterior advancement. **G,** Frontal view at 5 years of age just before further anterior cranial vault and facial bipartition osteotomies. **H,** Craniofacial morphology with planned and completed osteotomies and reconstruction. *(Continued)*

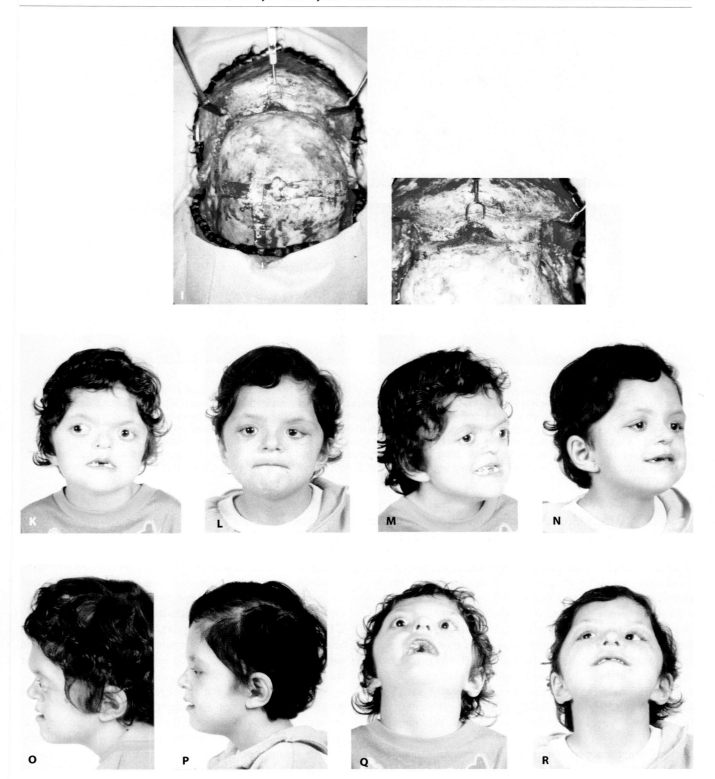

FIGURE 46-9.   *(Continued)* **I** and **J,** Bird's-eye view of the cranial vault and close-up view of the upper orbits after osteotomies with reshaping. **K,** Frontal view before surgery. **L,** Frontal view after facial bipartition reconstruction. **M,** Oblique view before surgery. **N,** Oblique view after reconstruction. **O,** Profile view before surgery. **P,** Profile view after reconstruction. **Q,** Worm's-eye view before surgery. **R,** Worm's-eye view after reconstruction. *(Continued)*

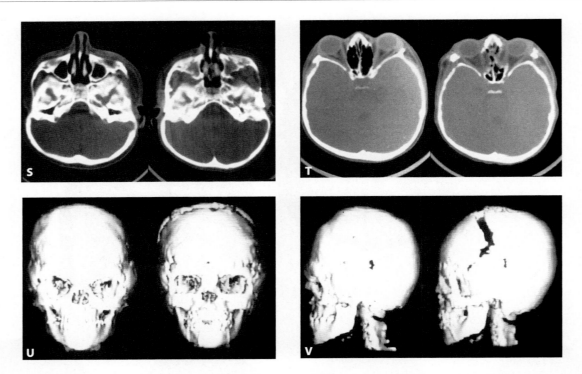

FIGURE 46-9.   *(Continued)* **S,** Comparison of axial-sliced CT scans through the zygomas before and after reconstruction indicates a normalization of zygomatic arch length. **T,** Axial-sliced CT scan views through the midorbits before and after reconstruction indicate correction of orbital hyperteleorism and proptosis. **U** and **V,** Comparison of three-dimensional CT scan views of the craniofacial region before and after reconstruction, including improved morphology of orbits. **A–G** and **I–V,** Reproduced with permission from Posnick JC. Apert syndrome: evaluation and staging of reconstruction. In Posnick JC, editor. Craniofacial and Maxillofacial Surgery in Children and Young Adults. Philadelphia: WB Saunders; 2000; p. 316; **H,** adapted from Posnick JC. Apert syndrome: evaluation and staging of reconstruction. In Posnick JC, editor. Craniofacial and Maxillofacial Surgery in Children and Young Adults. Philadelphia: WB Saunders; 2000; p. 316.)

conjunction with a pediatric neurosurgeon over a 4-year period were reviewed. The series included seven girls and one boy, with an average age at surgery of 12 months (range, 9–23 mo). The average postoperative follow-up period was 34 months (range, 12–48 mo) at the close of the study. Preoperative and postoperative (>1 yr) CT scans were compared with those of age-matched controls. Percentages of normal were then compared for significant differences. All CT scans were reviewed by a consistent neuroradiologist experienced in CT scan measurements. Two of the children had clear evidence of hydrocephalus and required VP shunting before the craniofacial reconstruction procedures (at 3 and 5 mo of age). A third child had mildly increased ventricular size, but clinical correlations did not suggest the need for shunting.

Significant preoperative morphologic findings included a wide anterior cranial vault at 110% of normal, a maximum cranial length that averaged only 90% of normal, a substantially widened anterior interorbital width at 117% of normal, an increased lateral interorbital distance at 112% of normal, and a widened bitemporal width at 122% of normal. Globe protrusion was significant at 121% of normal, and the medial orbital wall length was less than normal at 92%. In the upper midface (zygomatic) region, both the width between the

zygomatic buttresses and the interarch width were found to be increased at 109% of normal, whereas the zygomatic arch lengths were substantially shortened at 79% of normal. The measurements confirmed the clinical observations of brachycephalic, hyperteloric anterior cranial vaults, orbits, and zygomas, accompanied by eye proptosis and midface deficiency. Results of surgical reconstruction, as documented by CT scan measurements (analysis), showed that more than a year after surgery none of the craniofacial measurements had significantly improved ($P < .05$) in comparison with those of the new age-matched controls.

We also reviewed the medical records of this consecutive group of eight children with Apert's syndrome to document any morbidity associated with the cranio-orbital surgery carried out in infancy. There were no infections, wound difficulties, or central nervous system or ophthalmologic sequelae after any of the operations performed. One infant suffered intraoperative cardiac arrest due to intravascular volume depletion; the arrest responded to closed-chest cardiac massage and blood transfusion. The patient was discharged after an unremarkable further recovery. Several years later, she returned and underwent a facial bipartition procedure.

Detailed ophthalmologic examinations were also performed in all infants in the study. Two patients showed fun-

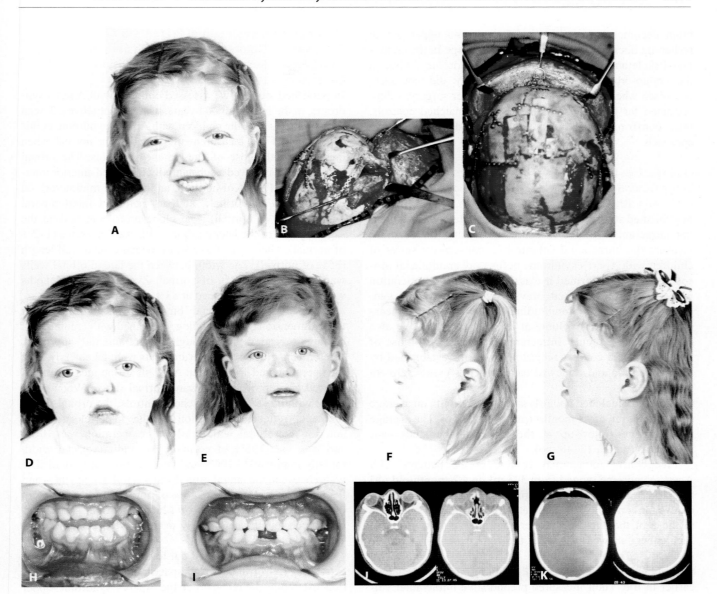

FIGURE 46-10. A 5-year-old girl with Apert's syndrome who underwent decompression and forehead and upper orbital reshaping at 6 months of age. She then presented to us with residual deformity requiring cranial vault and facial bipartition osteotomies with reshaping. She will require orthognathic surgery and orthodontic treatment later in the teenage years to complete her reconstruction. **A,** Frontal view before facial bipartition surgery. **B,** Intraoperative lateral view of the cranial vault and orbits through the coronal incision after reshaping. **C,** Bird's-eye view of the cranial vault after osteotomies and reshaping and fixation of the bone segments. **D,** Frontal view before surgery. **E,** Frontal view 2 years after reconstruction. **F,** Profile view before surgery. **G,** Profile view 2 years after facial bipartition reconstruction. **H,** Occlusal view before surgery. **I,** Occlusal view 6 months after reconstruction. **J,** Comparison of axial-sliced CT scan views through the midorbits before and after reconstruction demonstrates improvement in orbital hypertelorism and orbital depth with diminished eye proptosis. **K,** Standard axial CT scan slices through the cranial vault 1 week after facial bipartition (note dead space in the retrofrontal region), and at 1 year (notice that the initial retrofrontal dead space has been resolved by brain expansion). (**A–K,** Reproduced with permission from Posnick JC. Craniofacial dysostosis: staging of reconstruction and management of the midface deformity. Neurosurg Clin North Am 1991;2:683–702.)

duscopic evidence of increased ICP with papilledema before surgery. Both of these patients had previously undergone limited linear craniectomies. In both patients, the funduscopic examination results normalized by 6 months after the brain decompression and cranio-orbital expansion and reconstruction.

Quantitative measurement of CT scans of the cranio-orbitozygomatic region confirm clinically observed findings in these patients before cranio-orbital surgery in infancy and early childhood to be brachycephalic anterior cranial vaults and upper face hypertelorism (of orbits and zygomas) with eye proptosis and a flat midface. We found that early brain decompression with cranial vault and upper orbital reshaping does not maintain a corrected shape in the cranio-facial skeleton in children with Apert's syndrome. Although the cranio-orbitozygomatic dysmorphology did not seem to worsen when analyzed at least 1 year after surgery, values remained far from those of the new age-matched controls, thus confirming the need for a staged reconstructive approach.

Quantitative Intracranial Volume Measurements before and after Cranio-orbital Reshaping in Children with Apert's Syndrome

In published studies, we applied a proven method for obtaining intracranial volume measurements using CT scans to measure the intracranial volume of a consecutive series of children with Apert's syndrome before any craniofacial procedures.[70] We performed a classic cranio-orbital operation in each child (described previously for Crouzon's syndrome), followed by longitudinal follow-up, and remeasured the intracranial volume at least 1 year later. We also compared our patients' intracranial volumes with those of an age-matched cohort (according to norms established by Lichtenberg[109]) and reviewed each patient's cranial growth velocity.

The study included six girls and two boys with an average age at operation of 12 months (range, 9–23 mo). The average postoperative follow-up at the close of the study was 34 months (range, 12–48 mo).

Preoperative intracranial volume in the patients with Apert's syndrome ranged from 393 mL in a 2-month-old girl to 1715 mL in a 28-month-old girl. Comparison of the preoperative intracranial volume in patients with Apert's syndrome to those of the age- and gender-controlled cohort group of Lichtenberg showed that six of the eight patients had values at least 2 SD above the mean. Interestingly, the other two were infants who underwent VP shunting for hydrocephalus earlier in life. Their measured preoperative intracranial volumes were 2 SD below the mean.

When our patients' postoperative intracranial volumes were compared with those of the Lichtenberg cohort group, all eight achieved values at least 2 SD above the mean. The majority of the measured preoperative and postoperative intracranial volume values of our patients with Apert syndrome followed a growth curve that greatly exceeded the rate expected for normal children. In three of the patients, cranial vault growth velocity seemed to match closely that expected for a normal child, but with a starting point determined by their preoperative values.

Our findings confirmed that untreated patients with Apert's syndrome are generally macrocephalic early in life, that classic cranio-orbital procedures carried out in childhood do not alter this trend, and that continued cranial volume expansion often exceeds the mean. The ability to develop "normal" intracranial volume standards and to identify variations from normal in specific syndromes and in individual patients before and after surgery continues to elude us.

Quantitative Assessment of Presenting Deformity in Children with Apert's Syndrome and Surgical Results after Facial Bipartition Osteotomy Based on CT Scan Analysis

In published studies, we assessed children with Apert's syndrome, in the midchildhood years, using quantitative CT scan measurements.[70] In the children with Apert's syndrome at this age, many of the measurements varied from normal when compared with those of age-matched controls. The orbital measurements showed a substantially increased anterior interorbital width (123% of normal), an increased midinterorbital width (122% of normal), and an increased intertemporal width (126% of normal). The globe protrusion beyond the sagittal plane of the lateral orbital walls was excessive (142% of normal). There was also a short medial orbital wall length (85% of normal). The width between the lateral orbital walls was excessive at 111% of normal. Zygomatic arch lengths were substantially shortened at 83% of normal value.

After undergoing facial bipartition osteotomies with three-dimensional repositioning, combined with cranial vault reshaping carried out through an intracranial approach, assessments of CT scan measurements were taken early after the operation and 1 year later. Analysis of the measurements showed an improvement toward normal range. When compared with those of age-matched controls, the orbital measurements reflected correction of the hypertelorism; the anterior interorbital width early after operation was 106% and later was 105% of normal. The midinterorbital width initially improved to 106% and later to 100% of normal. The width between the lateral orbital walls stabilized at 108% and the intertemporal width at 115% of normal, an improvement over the preoperative value of 126% of normal. The zygomatic arch length was initially overcorrected at 110%, then stabilized at 103% of normal.

Further study was carried out to evaluate the presence of extradural (retrofrontal) dead space after the facial bipartition osteotomy to reconstruct the Apert's syndrome upper and midface deformity. Seven patients with Apert's syndrome (mean age, 8 yr) underwent facial bipartition osteotomies with advancement. Extradural (retrofrontal) dead space was measured from a reproducible axial CT scan slice for each patient at postoperative intervals (1–2 wk, 6–8 wk, and 1 yr). An initial extradural (retrofrontal) dead space was identified early after surgery in each patient, with resolution occurring by the 6- to 8-week postoperative interval through expansion of the dura and frontal lobes of the brain. The dead space was confirmed to be closed in all patients at the 1-year postoperative interval.

We then reviewed the morbidity of the same consecutive series of patients with Apert's syndrome who underwent facial bipartition and cranial vault reshaping through an intracranial approach.[44] Of the seven children with Apert's syndrome, there were no deaths, cardiopulmonary sequelae, or injuries to the brain or eyes. New seizure activity or central nervous system problems did not occur, nor did infection develop in any of the patients after surgery.

PFEIFFER'S SYNDROME

In 1964, Pfeiffer described a syndrome consisting of cranio-synostosis, broad thumbs, broad great toes, and occasionally, partial soft tissue syndactyly of the hands.[110] This syndrome is known to have an autosomal dominant inheritance pattern with complete penetrance documented in all recorded two- and three-generation pedigrees.[69] Variable expressivity of the craniofacial and extremity findings is common (Figures 46-11 and 46-12). Although some authors have found clinical

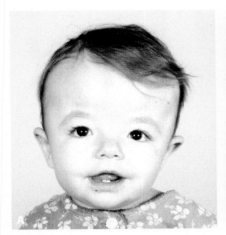
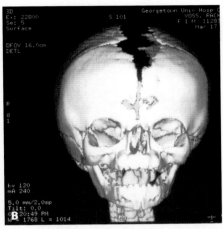
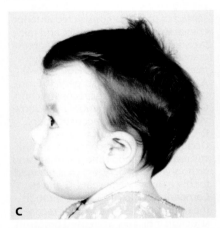
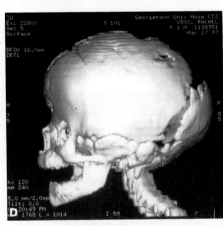
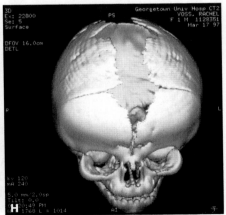
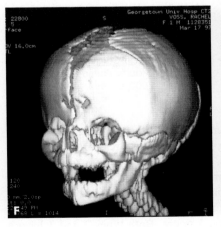
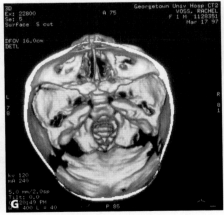
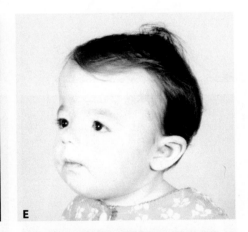

FIGURE 46-11.   A 2-month-old child born with Pfeiffer's syndrome (type 1). She has bilateral coronal synostosis resulting in brachycephaly without suggestion of midface deficiency **A,** Frontal view. **B,** Frontal view of CT scan. **C,** Profile view. **D,** Profile view of CT scan. **E,** Oblique view. **F,** Oblique view of CT scan. **G,** Cranial base view of CT scan. **H,** Craniofacial view of CT scan. (**A–H,** Reproduced with permission from Posnick JC. Pfeiffer syndrome: evaluation and staging of reconstruction. In Posnick JC, editor. Craniofacial and Maxillofacial Surgery in Children and Young Adults. Philadelphia: WB Saunders; 2000; p. 344.)

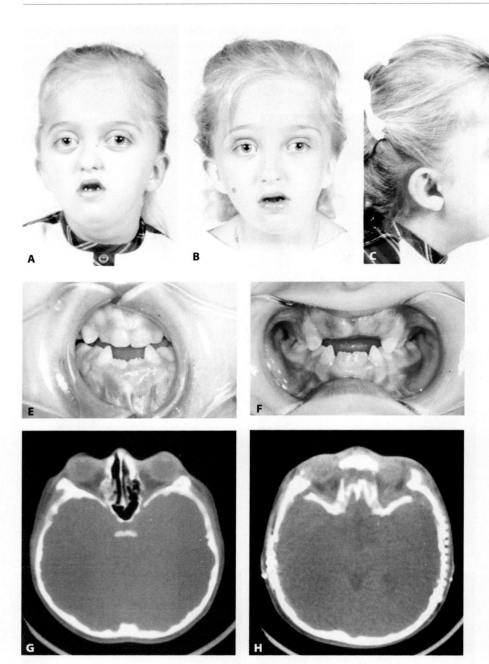

FIGURE 46-12. A 6-year-old girl born with Pfeiffer's syndrome (initially thought to have Crouzon's syndrome). She underwent cranio-orbital decompression early in childhood. She presented to us with a constricted anterior cranial vault, orbital dystopia, and midface deficiency. She underwent anterior cranial vault and monobloc osteotomies with reshaping (see Figure 46-4). **A,** Frontal view before surgery. **B,** Frontal view after monobloc reconstruction. **C,** Profile view before surgery. **D,** Profile view after monobloc reconstruction. **E,** Occlusal view before surgery. **F,** Occlusal view after reconstruction. She still requires orthodontic treatment and orthognathic surgery, which is planned for the early teenage years. **G** and **H,** Comparison of axial CT slices through the midorbits before and after reconstruction indicates decreased proptosis. (**A–H,** Reproduced with permission from Posnick JC. Pfeiffer syndrome: evaluation and staging of reconstruction. In Posnick JC, editor. Craniofacial and Maxillofacial Surgery in Children and Young Adults. Philadelphia: WB Saunders; 2000; p. 349.)

similarities in certain patients with Pfeiffer's syndrome, Crouzon's syndrome, and Jackson-Weiss syndrome, the three disorders are nosologically distinct.[47,111] According to Cohen and Kreiborg,[111] the phenotypes of the three conditions do not correlate well with the known molecular findings.[102] Patients with these three syndromes may have similar or even identical mutations in exon B of *FGFR2,* yet they breed true within families, an observation that is as yet unexplained by the molecular findings.[112–119]

Current thinking suggests that Pfeiffer's syndrome is heterogeneous because it is caused by a single recurring mutation (Pro252Arg) of *FGFR1* and by several different mutations affecting *FGFR2.*[120,121] Cohen and Kreiborg[112] have reviewed the literature and further subgrouped Pfeiffer's syndrome according to clinical features, associated low-frequency anomalies, and outcome. According to Cohen and Kreiborg, type 1 corresponds to the classic Pfeiffer syndrome and is associated with satisfactory prognosis. The type 2 subgroup is associated with the cloverleaf skull anomaly whereas type 3 is not. Both types 2 and 3 have a less favorable outcome, with frequent death in infancy. The type 1 variant frequently presents with bicoronal craniosynostosis and midface involvement. The longitudinal evaluation and staging of reconstruction depend on individual variations but is similar to that described for Crouzon's syndrome.

CARPENTER'S SYNDROME

Carpenter's syndrome is characterized by craniosynostosis often associated with preaxial polysyndactyly of the feet, short fingers with clinodactyly, and variable soft tissue syndactyly, sometimes postaxial plydactyly, and other anomalies such as congenital heart defects, short stature, obesity, and mental deficiency.[24] It was first described by Carpenter in 1901 and was later recognized to be an autosomal recessive syndrome. In general, the reconstructive algorithm described for Crouzon's syndrome can be followed.

SAETHRE-CHOTZEN SYNDROME

Saethre-Chotzen syndrome has an autosomal dominant inheritance pattern with a high degree of penetrance and expressivity.[122,123] Its pattern of malformations may include craniosynostosis, low-set frontal hairline, ptosis of the upper eyelids, facial asymmetry, brachydactyly, partial cutaneous syndactyly, and other skeletal anomalies. As part of the reconstruction, cranio-orbital reshaping will almost certainly be required and is similar to that described for Crouzon's syndrome. Evaluation and management of the total midface deficiency and orthognathic deformities as decribed for Crouzon's syndrome should be followed.

CLOVERLEAF SKULL ANOMALY

Kleeblattschädel anomaly (cloverleaf skull) is a trilobular-shaped skull secondary to craniosynostosis (Figure 46-13).[124,125] The cloverleaf skull anomaly is known to be both

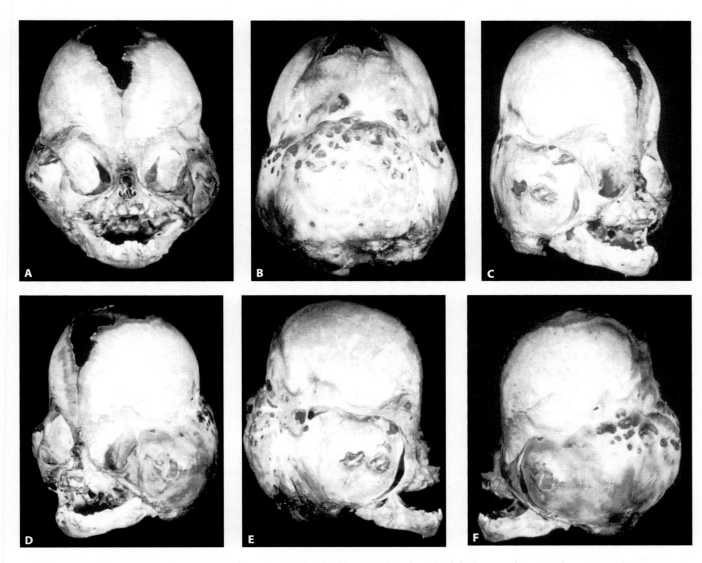

FIGURE 46-13.   The craniofacial skeleton of a 6-month-old child born with a cloverleaf skull anomaly. He underwent tracheostomy and gastrostomy shortly after birth and died of pneumonia before craniofacial reconstruction could be undertaken. **A,** Frontal view. **B,** Posterior view. **C,** Right oblique view. **D,** Left oblique view. **E,** Left profile view. **F,** Right profile view. (**A–F,** Reproduced with permission from Cloverleaf skull anomalies: evaluation and staging of reconstruction. In Posnick JC, editor. Craniofacial and Maxillofacial Surgery in Children and Young Adults. Philadelphia: WB Saunders; 2000; p. 364.)

SECTION 5

etiologically and pathogenetically heterogeneous. This anomaly is also nonspecific: it may occur as an isolated anomaly or together with other anomalies, making up various syndromes (i.e., Apert's, Crouzon's, Carpenter's, Pfeiffer's, and Saethre-Chotzen).[126] The extent and timing of anterior cranial vault or upper orbital, posterior cranial vault, and midface reconstruction will be dependent on individual variation in the presenting deformity. In general, the protocol described for Crouzon's syndrome can be followed.

SUMMARY

Details of the timing and techniques for correction of the varied forms of CFD syndromes differ from center to center. However, an essential element of successful rehabilitation is the delivery of care by committed, experienced, and technically skilled clinicians. The combined expertise of an experienced craniofacial surgeon and pediatric neurosurgeon working together to manage the cranio-orbital malformation and the experienced maxillofacial surgeon and orthodontist working together to manage the orthognathic deformity are essential to achieve maximum function and facial aesthetics for each patient.

Our preferred approach for management of the CFD syndromes is to stage the reconstruction to coincide with facial growth patterns, visceral (brain and eye) function, and psychosocial development. Recognition of the need for a staged reconstruction serves to clarify the objectives of each phase of treatment for the craniofacial surgeon, team, and most important, the patient and patient's family.

By continuing to define our rationale for the timing and extent of surgical intervention and then evaluating both function and aesthetic outcomes, we will further improve the quality of life for the many hundreds of children born with syndromal forms of craniosynostosis. Our objective is to see each individual achieve personal success in life without special regard for the original malformation.

References

1. Cohen MM Jr. Sutural biology and the correlates of craniosynostosis. Am J Med Genet 1993;47:581–616.
2. Renier D. Intracranial pressure in craniosynostosis: Pre- and postoperative recordings. Correlation with functional results. In Persing JA, Jane JA, Edgerton MT, editors. Scientific Foundations and Surgical Treatment of Craniosynostosis. Baltimore: Williams & Wilkins; 1989; pp. 263–269.
3. Gault DT, Renier D, Marchac D, Jones BM. Intracranial pressure and intracranial volume in children with craniosynostosis. Plast Reconstr Surg 1992;90:230–271.
4. Walia HK, Sodhi JS, Gupta BB, et al. Roentgenologic determination of the cranial capacity in the first four years of life. Ind J Radiol 1972;26:250.
5. Virchow R. Uber den cretinismus, nametlich in Franken, under uber pathologische: Schadelformen Verk Phys Med Gessellsch Wurszburg 1851;2:230–271.
6. Turvey TA, Gudeman SK. Nonsyndromic craniosynostosis. In Turvey TA, Vig KWL, Fonseca RJ, editors. Facial Clefts and Craniosynostosis: Principles and Management. Philadelphia: WB Saunders; 1996; pp. 596–629.
7. Moss ML. The pathogenesis of premature cranial synostosis in man. Acta Anat (Basel) 1959;37:351–370.
8. Stewart RE, Dixon G, Cohen A. The pathogenesis of premature craniosynostosis in acrocephalosyndactyly (Apert syndrome): a reconsideration. Plast Reconstr Surg 1977;59:699–703.
9. Pugeaut R. Le Probleme neuro chirurgical des craniostenoses. Cah Med Lyon 1968;44:3343.
10. Renier D, Sainte-Rose C, Marchac D, et al. Intracranial pressure in craniosynostosis. J Neurosurg 1982;57:370.
11. Siddiqi SN, Posnick JC, Buncic R, et al. The detection and management of intracranial hypertension after initial suture release and decompression for craniofacial dysostosis syndromes. Neurosurgery 1995;36:703.
12. Turvey TA, Ruiz RL. Craniosynostosis and craniofacial dysostosis. In Fonseca RJ, Baker SB, Wolford LM, editors. Oral and Maxillofacial Surgery. Philadelphia: WB Saunders; 2000; pp. 195–220.
13. Posnick JC. Craniofacial dysostosis syndromes: a staged reconstructive approach. In Turvey TA, Vig KWL, Fonseca RJ, editors. Facial clefts and Craniosynostosis: Principles and Management. Philadelphia: WB. Saunders; 1996; pp. 630–685.
14. Posnick JC. Quantitative computer tomographic scan analysis: normal values and growth patterns. In Posnick JC, editor. Craniofacial and Maxillofacial Surgery in Children and Young Adults. Philadelphia: WB Saunders; 2000; pp. 36–54.
15. Gault DT, Renier D, Marchac D, et al. Intracranial volume in children with craniosynostosis. J Craniofac Surg 1990;1:1.
16. Golabi M, Edwards MSB, Ousterhout DK. Craniosynostosis and hydrocephalus. Neurosurgery 1987;21:63.
17. Hogan GR, Bauman ML. Hydrocephalus in Apert syndrome. J Pediatr 1971;79:782.
18. Fishman MA, Hogan GR, Dodge PR. The concurrence of hydrocephalus and craniosynostosis. J Neurosurg 1971;34:621.
19. Murovic JA, Posnick JC, Drake JM, et al. Hydrocephalus in Apert syndrome: a retrospective review. Pediatr Neurosurg 1993;19:151–155.
20. Lauritzen C, Lilja J, Jarlstedt J. Airway obstruction and sleep apnea in children with craniofacial anomalies. Plast Reconstr Surg 1986;77:1–6.
21. Guilleminault C. Obstructive sleep apnea syndrome and its treatment in children: areas of agreement and controversy. Pediatr Pulmonol 1987;3:429–436.
22. Moore MH. Upper airway obstruction in the syndromal craniosynostoses. Br J Plast Surg 1993;46:355–362.
23. Drake AF, Sidman JD. Airway management. In Turvey TA, Vig KWL, Fonseca RJ, editors. Facial Clefts and Craniosynostosis: Principles and Management. Philadelphia: WB Saunders; 1996; pp. 174–182.
24. Hoeve HL, Joosten KF, Van den Berg S. Management of obstructive sleep apnea syndrome in children with craniofacial malformation. Int J Pediatr Otorhinolaryngol 1999;49(Suppl 1):S59–S61.
25. Pijpers M, Poels PJP, Vaandrager JM, et al. Undiagnosed obstructive sleep apnea in children with syndromal craniofacial synostosis. J Craniofac Surg 2004;15:670–674.
26. Nixon GM, Brouillette RT. Sleep .8: paediatric obstructive sleep apnoea. Thorax 2005;60:511–516
27. Ishii Kazuhiro, Kaloust S, Ousterhout DK, Vagervik K. Airway changes after Le Fort III osteotomy in craniosynostosis syndromes. J Craniofac Surg 1996;7:363–370.

28. Arnaud E, Marchac D, Renier D. Reduction of morbidity of the frontofacial monobloc advancement in children by the use of internal distraction. Plast Reconstr Surg 2007;120:1009–1026.

29. Mathijssen I, Arnaud E, Marchac D, et al. Respiratory outcome of midface advancement with distraction: a comparison between Le Fort III and frontofacial monobloc. J Craniofac Surg 2006;17:880–882.

30. Witherow H. Functional outcomes in monobloc advancement by distraction using the rigid external distractor device. Plast Reconstr Surg 2008;121:1311–1322.

31. Nelson T, Mulliken J, Padwa B. Effect of midfacial distraction on the obstructed airway in patients with syndromic bilateral coronal synostosis. J Oral Maxillofac Surg 2008;66:2318–2321.

32. Lajeunie E. Mutation screening in patients with syndromic craniosynostoses indicates a limited number of recurrent FGFR2 mutations accounts for severe forms of Pfeiffer syndrome. Eur J Hum Genet 2006;14:289–298.

33. Gorlin RJ, Cohen MM Jr, Levin LS. Syndromes of the Head and Neck. 3rd ed. New York: Oxford University Press; 1990; pp. 524–525.

34. Enlow DH, McNamara JA Jr. The neurocranial basis for facial form and pattern. Angle Orthod 1973;43:256–270.

35. Kreiborg S. Description of a dry skull with Crouzon syndrome. Scand J Plast Reconstr Surg 1982;16:245–253.

36. Marsh JL, Gado M. Surgical anatomy of the craniofacial dysostoses: insights from CT scans. Cleft Palate J 1982;19:212–221.

37. Freide H, Lilja J, Andersson H, Johanson B. Growth of the anterior cranial base after craniotomy in infants with premature synostosis of the coronal suture. Scand J Plast Reconstr Surg 1983;17:99–108.

38. Marsh JL, Vannier MW. The "third" dimension in craniofacial surgery. Plast Reconstr Surg 1983;71:759–767.

39. Kreiborg S. Apert and Crouzon syndromes contrasted. Qualitative craniofacial x-ray findings. J Dent Res 1985;64:203.

40. Marchac D. Radical forehead remodeling for craniosynostosis. Plast Reconstr Surg 1978;62:335–338.

41. Marchac D, Renier D, Jones BM. Experience with the "floating forehead." Br J Plast Surg 1988;41:1–15.

42. Posnick JC. The craniofacial dysostosis syndrome: current reconstructive strategies. Clin Plast Surg 1994;21:585–598.

43. Carr M, Posnick JC, Pron G, Armstrong D. Cranio-orbito-zygomatic measurements from standard CT scans in unoperated Crouzon and Apert infants: comparison with normal controls. Cleft Palate Craniofac J 1992;29:129–136.

44. Posnick JC, Al-Qattan MM, Armstrong D. Monobloc and facial bipartition osteotomies: quantitative assessment of presenting deformity and surgical results based on computed tomography scans. J Oral Maxillofac Surg 1995;53:358–367.

45. Kreiborg S. Crouzon syndrome. A clinical and roentgencephalometric study [thesis (disputats)]. Scand J Plast Reconstr Surg 1981;18(Suppl):198.

46. Posnick JC, Farkas LG. Anthropometric surface measurements in the analysis of craniomaxillofacial deformities: normal values and growth trends. In Posnick JC, editor. Craniofacial and Maxillofacial Surgery in Children and Young Adults. Philadelphia: WB Saunders; 2000; pp. 55–79.

47. Farkas LG, Posnick JC. Growth and development of regional units in the head and face based on anthropometric measurements. Cleft Palate Craniofac J 1992;29:301–302.

48. Farkas LG, Posnick JC, Hreczko T. Anthropometric growth study of the head. Cleft Palate Craniofac J 1992;29:303–307.

49. Farkas LG, Posnick JC, Hreczko T. Growth patterns in the orbital region: a morphometric study. Cleft Palate Craniofac J 1992;29:315–317.

50. Lannelongue M. De la craniectomie dans la microcephalie. Compte Rendu Acad Sci 1890;110:1382.

51. Lane LC. Pioneer craniectomy for relief of mental imbecility due to premature sutural closure and microcephalus. J Am Med Assoc 1892;18:49.

52. McCarthy JG, Epstein FJ, Wood-Smith D. Craniosynostosis. In McCarthy JG, editor. Plastic Surgery. Vol 4. Philadelphia: WB Saunders; 1990; pp. 3013–3053.

53. Rougerie J, Derome P, Anquez L. Craniostenosis et dysmorphies-cranio-faciales: Principes d'une nouvelle technique de traitment et ses resultats. Neurochirurgie 1972;18:429.

54. Hoffman HJ, Mohr G. Lateral canthal advancement of the supraorbital margin: a new corrective technique in the treatment of coronal synostosis. J Neurosurg 1976;45:376.

55. Whitaker LA, Bartlett SP, Schut L, et al. Craniosynostosis: an analysis of the timing, treatment and complications in 164 consecutive patients. Plast Reconstr Surg 1987;80:195.

56. Gillies H, Harrison SH. Operative correction by osteotomy of recessed malar maxillary compound in case of oxycephaly. Br J Plast Surg 1950;3:123.

57. Tessier P. Osteotomies totales de la face: Syndrome de Crouzon, syndrome D'Apert: oxycephalies, scaphocephalies, turricephalies. Ann Chir Plast 1967;12:273.

58. Tessier P. The definitive plastic surgical treatment of the severe facial deformities of craniofacial dysostosis: Crouzon and Apert diseases. Plast Reconstr Surg 1971;48:419.

59. Tessier P. Dysostoses cranio-faciales (syndromes de Crouzon et d'Apert): Osteotomies totales de la face. In Transactions of the Fourth International Congress of Plastic and Reconstructive Surgery. Amsterdam: Mosby; 1969; p. 774.

60. Tessier P. Relationship of craniosynostosis to craniofacial dysostosis and to faciosynostosis: a study with therapeutic implications. Clin Plast Surg 1982;9:531.

61. Tessier P. Autogenous bone grafts taken from the calvarium for facial and cranial applications. Plast Reconstr Surg 1971;48:224.

62. Tessier P. Total osteotomy of the middle third of the face for faciostenosis or for sequelae of the Le Fort III fractures. Plast Reconstr Surg 1971;48:533.

63. Tessier P. Traitement des dysmorphies faciales propres aux dysostoses craniofaciales (DGF), maladies de Crouzon et d'Apert. Neurochirurgie 1971;17:295.

64. Tessier P. Craniofacial surgery in syndromic craniosynostosis: craniosynostosis, diagnosis, evaluation and management. New York: Raven Press; 1986; p. 321.

65. Tessier P. Recent improvement in the treatment of facial and cranial deformities in Crouzon disease and Apert syndrome. In Symposium of Plastic Surgery of the Orbital Region. St. Louis: CV Mosby; 1976; p. 271.

66. Tessier P. The monobloc frontofacial advancement: do the pluses outweigh the minuses? [discussion]. Plast Reconstr Surg 1993;91:988.

67. Ortiz-Monasterio F, Fuente del Campo A, Carillo A. Advancement of the orbits and the midface in one piece, combined with frontal repositioning for the correction of Crouzon syndrome. Plast Reconstr Surg 1978;61:507–516.

68. Ortiz-Monasterio F, Fuente del Campo A. Refinements on the monobloc orbitofacial advancement. In Caronni EP, editor. Craniofacial Surgery. Boston: Little, Brown; 1985; p. 263.

SECTION 5

69. Van der Meulen JC. Medial fasciotomy. Br J Plast Surg 1979; 32:339–342.

70. Posnick JC, Lin KY, Jhawar BJ, Armstrong D. Apert syndrome: quantitative assessment in presenting deformity and surgical results after first-stage reconstruction by CT scan. Plast Reconstr Surg 1994;93:489–497.

71. Posnick JC. Apert syndrome: evaluation and staging of reconstruction. In Posnick JC, editor. Craniofacial and Maxillofacial Surgery in Children and Young Adults. Philadelphia: WB Saunders; 2000; pp. 308–342.

72. Luhr HG. Zur Stabilen osteosynthese bei unterkieferfrakturen. Dtsch Zahnaerztl Z 1968;23:754.

73. McCarthy JG, Epstein FJ, Wood-Smith D. Craniosynostosis. In McCarthy JG, editor. Plastic Surgery. Vol 4. Philadelphia: WB Saunders; 1990; pp. 3013–3053.

74. Gillies H, Harrison SH. Operative correction by osteotomy of recessed malar maxillary compound in case of oxycephaly. Br J Plast Surg 1950;3:123.

75. Posnick JC, Al-Qattan MM, Armstrong D. Monobloc and facial bipartition osteotomies reconstruction of craniofacial malformations: a study of extradural dead space. Plast Reconstr Surg 1996;97:1118.

76. Wolfe SA. Critical analysis of 81 monobloc frontofacial advancements over a 27-year period: should they all be distracted, or not? 2009. Abstract AAPS.

77. Bradley JP, Gabbay JS, Kwan D, et al. Monobloc advancement by distraction osteogenesis decreases morbidity and relapse. Plast Reconstr Surg 2006;118:1585–1597.

78. Farkas LG, Posnick JC, Hreczko T. Growth patterns of the face: a morphometric study. Cleft Palate Craniofac J 1992;29:308–314.

79. Rougerie J, Derome P, Anquez L. Craniostenosis et dysmorphies-cranio-faciales: principes d'une nouvelle technique de traitement et ses resultats. Neurochirurgie 1972;18:429.

80. Hoffman HJ, Mohr G. Lateral canthal advancement of the supraorbital margin: a new corrective technique in the treatment of coronal synostosis. J Neurosurg 1976;45:376.

81. Whitaker LA, Bartlett SP, Schut L, et al. Craniosynostosis: an analysis of the timing, treatment and complications in 164 consecutive patients. Plast Reconstr Surg 1987;80:195.

82. Kaban LB, Conover M, Mulliken J. Midface position after Le-Fort III advancement: a long-term follow-up study. Cleft Palate J 1986;23(Suppl):75–77.

83. Vannier MW, Gado M, Marsh JL. Three-dimensional computer graphics for craniofacial surgical planning and evaluation. Comput Graph 1983;17:263.

84. Vannier MW, Pilgram TK, Marsh JL, et al. Craniosynostosis: diagnostic imaging with three-dimensional CT presentation. AJNR Am J Neuroradiol 1994;15:1861–1869.

85. Kolar JC, Munro IR, Farkas LG. Patterns of dysmorphology in Crouzon syndrome: an anthropometric study. Cleft Palate J 1988;25:235–244.

86. Posnick JC, Ruiz RL. The craniofacial dysostosis syndromes: current surgical thinking and future directions. Cleft Palate Craniofac J 2000;37:433.

87. Kreiborg S, Pruzansky S. Roentgencephalometric and metallic implant studies in Apert syndrome (abstract). Presented at the 50th General Session I.A.D.R. 1972. Las Vegas. 298:120[21].

88. Kreiborg S, Aduss H. Pre and post surgical facial growth in patients with Crouzon and Apert syndromes. Cleft Palate J 1986;23(Suppl):78–90.

89. Waitzman AA, Posnick JC, Armstrong D, Pron GE. Craniofacial skeletal measurements based on computed tomography: part I. Accuracy and reproducibility. Cleft Palate Craniofac J 1992;29:112–117.

90. Waitzman AA, Posnick JC, Armstrong D, Pron GE. Craniofacial skeletal measurements based on computed tomography. Part II. Normal values and growth trends. Cleft Palate Craniofac J 1992;29:118–128.

91. Slaney SF, Oldridge M, Hurst JA, et al. Differential effects of FGFR2 mutations on syndactyly and cleft plate in Apert syndrome. Am J Med Genet 1996;58:923–932.

92. Ferreira JC, Carter SM, Bernstein PS, et al. Second-trimester molecular prenatal diagnosis of sporadic Apert syndrome following suspicious ultrasound findings. Ultrasound Obstet Gynecol 1999;14:426–430.

93. Wolford LM, Cooper RL. Orthognathic surgery in the growing cleft patient and its effect on growth (abstract). Presented at the American Association of Oral and Maxillofacial Surgeons Annual Scientific Sessions. 1987;September; Anaheim, CA: WB Saunders.

94. Wolford LM, Cooper RL, El Deeb M. Orthognathic surgery in the young cleft patient and the effect on growth (abstract). Presented at the American Cleft Palate-Craniofacial Association Annual Meeting. 1990;May; St. Louis.

95. Whitaker LA, Munro IR, Sayler KE, et al. Combined report of problems and complications in 793 craniofacial operations. Plast Reconstr Surg 1979;64:198.

96. David DJ, Cooter RD. Craniofacial infections in 10 years of transcranial surgery. Plast Reconstr Surg 1987;80:213.

97. Marsh JL, Galic M, Vannier MW. Surgical correction of craniofacial dysmorphology of Apert syndrome. Clin Plast Surg 1991;18:251.

98. Saltz R, Sierra D, Feldman D, et al. Experimental and clinical applications of fibrin glue. Plast Reconstr Surg 1991;88:1005.

99. Posnick JC. Craniosynostosis: surgical management in infancy. In Bell WH, editor. Orthognathic and Reconstructive Surgery. Philadelphia: WB Saunders; 1992; p. 1839.

100. Posnick JC. Brachycephaly: bilateral coronal synostosis without midface deficiency. In Posnick JC, editor. Craniofacial and Maxillofacial Surgery in Children and Young Adults. Philadelphia: WB Saunders; 2000; pp. 249–268.

101. Posnick JC. Crouzon syndrome: evaluation and staging of reconstruction. In Posnick JC, editor. Craniofacial and Maxillofacial Surgery in Children and Young Adults. Philadelphia: WB Saunders; 2000; pp. 271–307.

102. Park WJ, Theda C, Maestri NE, et al. Analysis of phenotypic features and FGFR2 mutations in Apert syndrome. Am J Hum Genet 1995;57:321–328.

103. Cohen MM Jr. Transforming growth factor fls and fibroblast growth factors and their receptors: role in sutural biology and craniosynostosis. J Bone Miner Res 1997;12:322–331.

104. Park WJ, Theda C, Maestri NE, et al. Analysis of phenotypic features and FGFR2 mutations in Apert syndrome. Am J Hum Genet 1995;57:321–328.

105. Posnick JC, Goldstein JA, Clokie C. Refinements in pterygomaxillary dissociation for total midface osteotomies: instrumentation, technique and CT scan analysis. Plast Reconstr Surg 1993;91:167–172.

106. Murray JE, Swanson LT. Midface osteotomy and advancement for craniosynostosis. Plast Reconstr Surg 1968;41:299–306.

107. Posnick JC. Craniofacial dysostosis: staging of reconstruction and management of the midface deformity. Neurosurg Clin North Am 1991;2:683–702.

108. Posnick JC. Craniofacial dysostosis: management of the midface deformity. In Bell WH, editor. Orthognathic and Reconstructive Surgery. Philadelphia: WB Saunders; 1992; p. 1888.

109. Vignaud-Pasquier J, Lichtenberg R, Laval-Jeantet M, Larroche JC, Bernard J. Digital Markings on the Skull from Birth to 9 Years. Biol Neonat. 1964;6:250-76.

110. Hogeman KE, Willmar K. On Le Fort III osteotomy for Crouzon disease in children: report of a four year follow-up in one patient. Scand J Plast Reconstr Surg 1974;8:169–172.

111. Cohen MM Jr. An etiologic and nosologic overview of craniosynostosis syndromes. Birth Defects Orig Artic Ser 1975;11:137–189.

112. Cohen MM Jr, Kreiborg S. The central nervous system in the Apert syndrome. Am J Med Genet 1990;35:36–45.

113. Kreiborg S, Prydsoe U, Dahl E, Fogh-Anderson. Calvarium and cranial base in Apert syndrome: an autopsy report. Cleft Palate J 1976;13:296–303.

114. Pfeiffer RA. Dominant Erbliche Akrocephalosyndaktylie. Z Kinderheilkd 1964;90:301–320.

115. Cohen MM Jr, editor. Craniosynostosis: Diagnosis, Evaluation, and Management. New York: Raven Press; 1986.

116. Jabs EW, Li X, Scott AF, et al. Jackson-Weiss and Crouzon syndromes are allelic with mutations in fibroblast growth factor receptor 2. Nat Genet 1994;8:275–9.

117. Cohen MM Jr. Pfeiffer syndrome update, clinical subtypes, and guidelines for differential diagnosis. Am J Med Genet 1993;45:300–307.

118. Lajeunie E, Ma HW, Bonaventure J, et al. FGFR2 mutations in Pfeiffer syndrome. Nat Genet 1995;9:108.

119. Rutland P, Pulley LJ, Reardon W. Identical mutations in the FGFR2 gene cause both Pfeiffer and Crouzon syndrome phenotypes. Nat Genet 1995;9:173–176.

120. Ousterhout DK, Melsen B. Cranial base deformity in Apert syndrome. Plast Reconstr Surg 1982;69:254–263.

121. Kreiborg S, Cohen MM Jr. The infant Apert skull. Neurosurg Clin North Am 1991;2:551–554.

122. Cohen MM Jr, Kreiborg S. Skeletal abnormalities in the Apert syndrome. Am J Med Genet 1993;47:624–632.

123. Paznekas WA, Cunningham ML, Howard TD, et al. Genetic heterogeneity of Saethre-Chotzen syndrome, due to TWIST and FGFR mutations. Am J Hum Genet 1998;62:1370–1380.

124. Cohen MM Jr. Cloverleaf syndrome update. Proc Greenwood Gene Center 1987;6:186–187.

125. Cohen MM Jr. The cloverleaf anomaly: managing extreme cranio-orbito-facio-stenosis (discussion). Plast Reconstr Surg 1993;91:10–14.

126. Cohen MM Jr, Kreiborg S. The growth pattern in the Apert syndrome. Clin Genet 1993;47:617–623.

SECTION 5

Temporomandibular Joint Disease

Anatomy and Pathophysiology of the Temporomandibular Joint

Mark C. Fletcher, DMD, MD, Joseph F. Piecuch, DMD, MD, and Stuart E. Lieblich, DMD

CLASSIFICATION

The temporomandibular joint (TMJ) is a complex structure composed several components including the glenoid fossa of the temporal bone, the condylar head of the mandible, and a specialized dense fibrous connective tissue structure, the articular disk, as well as several ligaments and associated muscles. The TMJ is a specialized joint that can be classified by anatomic type as well as by function.

From an anatomic standpoint, the TMJ is classified as a *diarthrodial joint,* which is a discontinuous articulation of two bones allowing freedom of movement that is dictated by the associated muscles and limited by the associated ligaments.[1] The fibrous connective tissue capsule is well innervated, well vascularized, and tightly attached to the bones at the edges of their articulating surfaces on the medial an lateral aspects of the TMJ. The TMJ is also a *synovial joint,* lined on its inner aspect by a synovial membrane, which

secretes synovial fluid. The fluid acts as a joint lubricant and supplies the metabolic and nutritional needs of the nonvascularized internal joint structures.

From a functional standpoint, the TMJ is classified as a compound joint, composed of four articulating surfaces: the articular facets of the temporal bone (1) and of the mandibular condyle (2) and the superior (3) and inferior (4) surfaces of the articular disk. The articular disk divides the TMJ into two compartments. The lower compartment permits hinge motion or rotation and, hence, is termed *ginglymoid.* The superior compartment permits sliding (or translatory) movements and is, therefore, called *arthrodial.* As a result, the TMJ as a whole can be termed a *ginglymoarthrodial joint.*

BONY STRUCTURES

The articular portion of the temporal bone (Figure 47-1) is composed of three portions. The largest part is the *articular,*

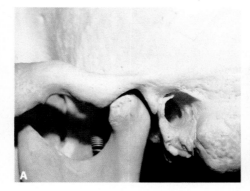
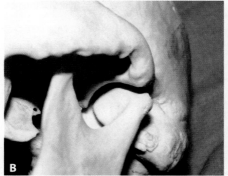
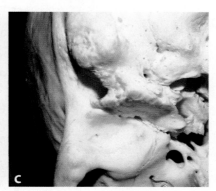

FIGURE 47-1. **A,** The left temporomandibular mandibular joint (TMJ) viewed from the sagittal aspect on a dry skull. **B,** The left TMJ viewed from the oblique/coronal aspect on a dry skull. **C,** The left glenoid fossa and articular eminence.

or *mandibular, fossa,* a concave structure extending from the posterior slope of the articular eminence to the postglenoid tubercle, which is a ridge between the fossa and the external acoustic meatus. The surface of the articular fossa of the temporal bone is very thin and may appear translucent when viewed through a dry skull specimen. As a result, this area is not a major stress-bearing region for the TMJ. The second portion, the *articular eminence,* is a transverse bony prominence that is continuous across the articular surface mediolaterally. The articular eminence is usually thick and serves as a major functional component of the TMJ. The articular eminence is distinguished from the articular tubercle, a non-articulating process on the lateral aspect of the zygomatic root of the temporal bone, which serves as a point of attachment of collateral ligaments. The third portion of the articular surface of the temporal bone is the *preglenoid plane,* a flattened area located anterior to the articular eminence.

The mandible is a U-shaped bone that articulates with the temporal bone by means of the articular surface of the condyles, which are paired structures forming an approximately 145- to 160-degree angle to one another. The mandibular condyle (Figure 47-2) is approximately 15 to 20 mm in transverse width dimension and 8 to 10 mm in an anteroposterior dimension. The condyle tends to be rounded mediolaterally and convex anteroposteriorly. On its medial aspect just below its articular surface is a prominent depression, known as the *pterygoid fovea,* which is the site of insertion of the inferior head of the lateral pterygoid muscle that assists in protrusion of the mandible during condylar translation.

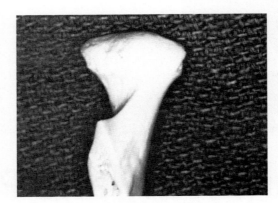

FIGURE 47-2.   The mandibular condyle.

CARTILAGE AND SYNOVIUM

Lining the inner aspect of all synovial joints, including the TMJ, are two types of tissue: *articular cartilage* and *synovium* (Figure 47-3). The space bounded by these two structures is termed the *synovial cavity,* which is bathed in synovial fluid. The articular surfaces of both the temporal bone and the condyle are covered with dense articular fibrocartilage, a fibrous connective tissue. This fibrocartilage covering layer has the capacity to regenerate and to remodel under functional stresses. Deep to the fibrocartilage layer, particularly on the condylar head, is a proliferative zone of cells that may develop into either cartilaginous or osseous tissue, based upon functional loads. Therefore, major changes

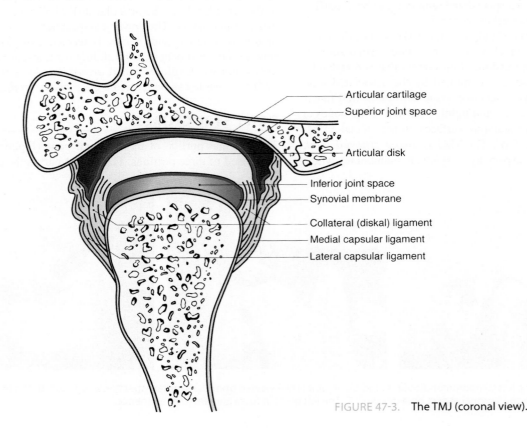

- Articular cartilage
- Superior joint space
- Articular disk
- Inferior joint space
- Synovial membrane
- Collateral (diskal) ligament
- Medial capsular ligament
- Lateral capsular ligament

FIGURE 47-3.   The TMJ (coronal view).

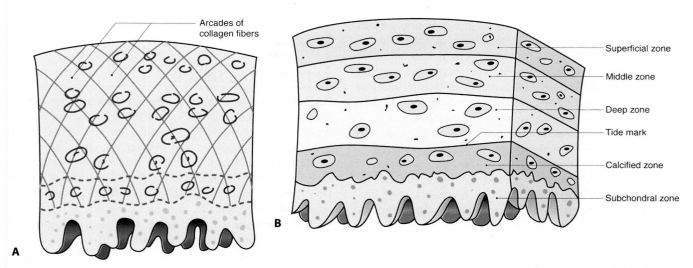

FIGURE 47-4.   The articular cartilage. (Adapted from Albright JA, Brand RA. The scientific basis of orthopedics. 2nd ed. Norwalk, CT: Appleton and Lange; 1987; pp. 373–386.)

in morphology resulting from alterations in joint function are typically seen in this layer.

Articular cartilage is composed of chondrocytes and an intercellular matrix of collagen fibers, water, and a nonfibrous filler material, termed *ground substance.* Chondrocytes are enclosed in otherwise hollow spaces, called *lacunae,* and are arranged in three layers characterized by different cell shapes (Figure 47-4A). The *superficial zone* contains small, flattened cells with their long axes parallel to the surface.[2] In the *middle zone,* the cells are larger, rounded, and oriented in a columnar fashion perpendicular to the surface. The *deep zone* contains the largest cells and is divided by the "tide mark" below which some degree of calcification has occurred. There are few blood vessels in any of these areas, so the cartilage receives nourishment primarily by diffusion from the synovial fluid.

Collagen fibers are arranged in arcades with an interlocking meshwork of fibrils parallel to the articular surface joining together as bundles and descending to their attachment in the calcified cartilage between the tide mark (see Figure 47-4B). Functionally, these arcades provide a framework for interstitial water and ground substance to resist compressive forces encountered during joint loading. Because it is formed by an intramembranous process, the articular cartilage of the TMJ contains a greater proportion of collagen fibers (fibrocartilage) than other synovial joints, which are typically covered instead by hyaline cartilage.

The ground substance contains a variety of plasma proteins, glucose, urea, and salts as well as proteoglycans, which are synthesized by the Golgi apparatus of the chondrocytes. Proteoglycans are macromolecules consisting of a protein core attached to many glycosaminoglycan chains of chondroitin sulfate and keratan sulfate. Proteoglycans play a role in the diffusion of nutrients and metabolic breakdown products. Ground substance permits the entry and release of large quantities of water, an attribute thought to be significant in

giving cartilage its characteristic functional elasticity in response to deformation and loading.

Lining the capsular ligament is the synovial membrane, a thin, smooth, richly innervated vascular tissue without an epithelial lining. Synovial cells appear somewhat undifferentiated and serve both a phagocytic and a secretory role and are thought to be the site of production of hyaluronic acid, a glycosaminoglycan found in synovial fluid. Some synovial cells, particularly those in close approximation to the articular cartilage, are thought to have the capacity to differentiate into chondrocytes. The synovium is capable of rapid and complete regeneration after injury. Recently, synovial cells (as well as chondrocytes and leukocytes) have been the focus of extensive research regarding the production of anabolic and catabolic cytokines within the TMJ.[3]

Synovial fluid is considered an ultrafiltrate of plasma.[2] The fluid contains a high concentration of hyaluronic acid, which is responsible for the fluid's high viscosity (resistance to flow). The proteins found in synovial fluid are identical to plasma proteins; however, synovial fluid has a lower total protein content, with a higher percentage of albumin and a lower percentage of α_2-globulin. Alkaline phosphatase, which may also be present in synovial fluid, is produced by chondrocytes. Leukocytes are also found in synovial fluid, with the cell count being less than 200/mm$_3$ and with less than 25% of these cells being polymorphonuclear leukocytes (PMNs or neutrophils). Only a small amount of synovial fluid, usually less than 2 mL, is present within each healthy functional TMJ.

Functions of the synovial fluid include lubrication of the joint, phagocytosis of particulate debris, and nourishment of the articular cartilage. Joint lubrication is a complex function related to the viscosity of synovial fluid and to the ability of articular cartilage to allow the free passage of water within the pores of its glycosaminoglycan matrix. Application of a loading force to an area of the articular cartilage causes a deformation at that specific location. It has been theorized that water is extruded from the loaded area into the synovial fluid adjacent to the point of contact. The concentration of hyaluronic acid and, therefore, the viscosity of the synovial fluid is greater at the point of maximal load, thus resulting in protection of the articular surfaces. As the load is distributed to adjacent areas, the deformation is transferred as well, whereas the original point of contact regains its shape and thickness through the reabsorption of water from the synovial fluid. The exact mechanisms of fluid balance and flow between the articular cartilage and the synovial fluid are unclear. Nevertheless, the net result is a coefficient of friction for the normally functioning joint of approximately 14 times less than that of a dry joint.

THE ARTICULAR DISK

The articular disk (Figure 47-5) is composed of a dense fibrous connective tissue, and it is nonvascularized and noninnervated; this is an adaptation that allows the disk to resist pressure.[4] Anatomically, the disk can be divided into three general regions as viewed from the lateral perspective: the anterior band, the central intermediate zone, and the posterior band. The thickness of the disk appears to be correlated with the prominence of the eminence, such that proportionally, the anterior band (3, thickest), intermediate zone (1, thinnest), and posterior band (2, middle thickness) have relative thicknesses. The intermediate zone is thinnest and is generally the area of maximum function between the mandibular condyle and the temporal bone. Despite the designation of separate portions of the articular disk, it is in fact a homogeneous tissue and the three bands do not consist of specific anatomic structures. The disk is flexible and adapts to functional demands of the articular surfaces.[5] The articular disk is attached to the capsular ligament anteriorly, posteriorly, medially, and laterally.[6] Some fibers of the superior head of the lateral pterygoid muscle insert on the disk at its anteromedial aspect, serving to stabilize the disk to the mandibular condyle, via the medial and lateral collateral ligaments, during function.

RETRODISKAL TISSUE

Posteriorly, the articular disk blends with a highly vascular, highly innervated structure known as the *retrodiskal tissues*. Anatomically, the retrodiskal tissues are referred to as the *bilaminar zone* (superior and inferior retrodiskal laminae), which is involved in the production of synovial fluid. The superior aspect of the retrodiskal tissue contains elastic fibers and is termed the *superior retrodiskal lamina,* which attaches to the tympanic plate and functions as a restraint to disk displacement in extreme translatory movements.[5] The inferior aspect of the retrodiskal tissue, termed the *inferior retrodiskal lamina,* consists of collagen fibers without elastic tissue and functions to connect the articular disk to the posterior margin of the articular surfaces of the condyle. It is thought to serve as a check ligament to prevent extreme rotation of the disk on the condylar head in rotational movements.

LIGAMENTS

Ligaments associated with the TMJ are composed of collagen and act predominantly as restraints to motion of the condyle and the disk. Three ligaments—collateral, capsular, and temporomandibular ligaments—are considered functional ligaments because they serve as major anatomic components of the joints. Two other ligaments—sphenomandibular and stylomandibular—are considered accessory ligaments because, although they are attached to osseous structures at some distance from the joints, they serve to some degree as passive restraints on mandibular motion.

The collateral (or diskal) ligaments (see Figure 47-3) are short paired structures attaching the disk to the lateral and medial poles of each condyle. Their function is to restrict movement of the disk away from the condyle, thus allowing

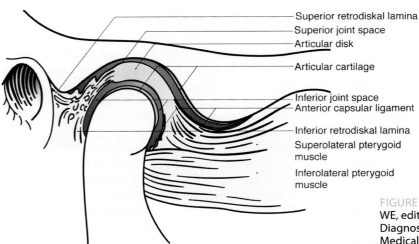

Superior retrodiskal lamina
Superior joint space
Articular disk

Articular cartilage

Inferior joint space
Anterior capsular ligament

Inferior retrodiskal lamina
Superolateral pterygoid muscle
Inferolateral pterygoid muscle

FIGURE 47-5. The TMJ (lateral view). (Adapted from Bell WE, editor. Temporomandibular Disorders: Classification, Diagnosis and Management. 2nd ed. Chicago: Year Book Medical; 1986; pp. 16–62.)

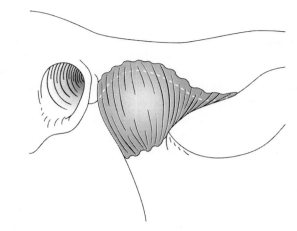

FIGURE 47-6.   The capsular ligament (lateral view).

smooth synchronous motion of the disk-condyle complex. Although the collateral ligaments permit rotation of the condyle with relation to the disk, their tight attachment forces the disk to accompany the condyle through its translatory range of motion.[6]

The capsular ligament (Figures 47-6 and 47-7; see also Figures 47-3 and 47-5) encompasses each joint, attaching superiorly to the temporal bone along the border of the mandibular fossa and eminence and inferiorly to the neck of the condyle along the edge of the articular facet. It surrounds the joint spaces and the disk, attaching anteriorly and posteriorly as well as medially and laterally, where it blends with the collateral ligaments. The function of the capsular ligament is to resist medial, lateral, and inferior forces, thereby holding the joint together. It offers resistance to movement of the joint only in the extreme range of motion. A secondary function of the capsular ligament is to contain the synovial fluid within the superior and inferior joint spaces.

The temporomandibular (lateral) ligaments (see Figure 47-7) are located on the lateral aspect of each TMJ.[5] Unlike the capsular and collateral ligaments, which have medial

and lateral components within each joint, the temporomandibular ligaments are single structures that function in paired fashion with the corresponding ligament on the opposite TMJ. Each temporomandibular ligament can be separated into two distinct portions that have different functions.[6] The outer oblique portion descends from the outer aspect of the articular tubercle of the zygomatic process posteriorly and inferiorly to the outer posterior surface of the condylar neck. It limits the amount of inferior distraction that the condyle may achieve in translatory and rotational movements. The inner horizontal portion also arises from the outer surface of the articular tubercle, just medial to the origin of the outer oblique portion of the ligament, and runs horizontally backward to attach to the lateral pole of the condyle and the posterior aspect of the disk. The function of the inner horizontal portion of the temporomandibular ligament is to limit posterior movement of the condyle, particularly during pivoting movements, such as when the mandible moves laterally in chewing function. This restriction of posterior movement serves to protect the retrodiskal tissue.

The sphenomandibular ligament (Figure 47-8) arises from the spine of the sphenoid bone and descends into the fanlike insertion on the mandibular lingula as well as on the lower portion of the medial side of the condylar neck.[1] The sphenomandibular ligament serves to some degree as a point of rotation during activation of the lateral pterygoid muscle, thereby contributing to translation of the mandible.

The stylomandibular ligament (see Figure 47-8) descends from the styloid process to the posterior border of the angle of the mandible and also blends with the fascia of the medial pterygoid muscle. It functions similarly to the sphenomandibular ligament as a point of rotation and also limits excessive protrusion of the mandible.

VASCULAR SUPPLY AND INNERVATION

The vascular supply of the TMJ arises primarily from branches of the superficial temporal and maxillary arteries posteriorly and the masseteric artery anteriorly. There is a

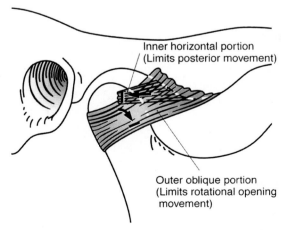

Inner horizontal portion
(Limits posterior movement)

Outer oblique portion
(Limits rotational opening
movement)

FIGURE 47-7.   The TMJ (lateral aspect). (Adapted from Okeson JP, editor. Management of Temporomandibular Disorders and Occlusions. 2nd ed. St. Louis: CV Mosby; 1989; pp. 3–26.)

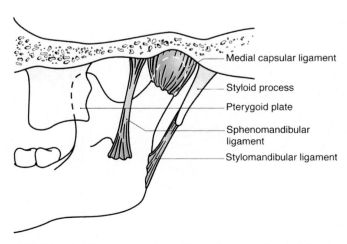

Medial capsular ligament

Styloid process

Pterygoid plate

Sphenomandibular
ligament

Stylomandibular ligament

FIGURE 47-8.   The temporomandibular ligament (medial view).

rich plexus of veins in the posterior aspect of the joint associated with the retrodiskal tissues, which alternately fill and empty with protrusive and retrusive movements, respectively, of the condyle-disk complex and which also function in the production of synovial fluid. The nerve supply to the TMJ is predominantly from branches of the auriculotemporal nerve with anterior contributions from the masseteric nerve and the posterior deep temporal nerve.[1] Many of the nerves providing innervations to the joint appear to be vasomotor and vasosensory, and they may have a role in the production of synovial fluid.

MUSCULATURE

All muscles attached to the mandible influence its movement to some degree. Only the four large muscles that attach to the ramus of the mandible are considered the muscles of mastication; however, a total of 12 muscles actually influence mandibular motion, all of which are bilateral.[1] Muscle pairs may function together for symmetrical movements or unilaterally for asymmetrical movement. For example, contraction of both lateral pterygoid muscles results in protrusion and depression of the mandible without deviation, whereas contraction of one of the lateral pterygoid muscles results in protrusion and opening with deviation to the opposite side.

Muscles influencing mandibular motion may be divided into two groups by anatomic position. Attaching primarily to the ramus and condylar neck of the mandible is the supramandibular muscle group, consisting of the temporalis, masseter, medial pterygoid, and lateral pterygoid muscles. This group functions predominantly as the elevators of the mandible. The lateral pterygoid does have a depressor function as well.[7] Attaching to the body and symphyseal area of the mandible and to the hyoid bone is the inframandibular group, which functions as the depressors of the mandible. The infra-

mandibular group includes the four suprahyoid muscles (digastric, geniohyoid, mylohyoid, and stylohyoid) and the four infrahyoid muscles (sternohyoid, omohyoid, sternothyroid, and thyrohyoid). The suprahyoid muscles attach to both the hyoid bone and the mandible and serve to depress the mandible when the hyoid bone is fixed in place. They also elevate the hyoid bone when the mandible is fixed in place. The infrahyoid muscles serve to fix the hyoid bone during depressive movements of the mandible.

Supramandibular Muscle Group

The temporalis muscle (Figure 47-9) is a large, fan-shaped muscle taking its origin from the temporal fossa and lateral aspect of the skull, including portions of the parietal, temporal, frontal, and sphenoid bones. Its fibers pass between the zygomatic arch and the skull and insert on the mandible at the coronoid process and anterior border of the ascending ramus down to the occlusal surface of the mandible, posterior to the third molar tooth.[1] Viewed coronally, the temporalis muscle has a bipennate character in that fibers arising from the skull insert on the medial aspect of the coronoid process whereas fibers arising laterally from the temporalis fascia insert on the lateral aspect of the coronoid process. In an anteroposterior dimension, the temporalis muscle consists of three portions: the anterior, whose fibers are vertical; the middle, with oblique fibers; and the posterior portion, with semihorizontal fibers passing forward to bend under the zygomatic arch. The function of the temporalis muscle is to elevate the mandible for closure. It is not a power muscle. In addition, contraction of the middle and posterior portions of the temporalis muscle can contribute to retrusive movements of the mandible. To a small degree, unilateral contraction of the temporalis assists in deviation of the mandible to the ipsilateral side.

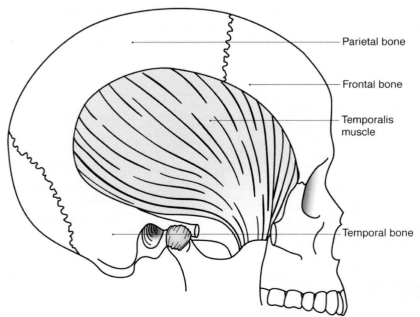

Parietal bone

Frontal bone

Temporalis muscle

Temporal bone

FIGURE 47-9.   The temporalis muscle with zygomatic arch and masseter muscle removed. (Adapted from Clemente CD, editor. Gray's Anatomy of the Human Body. 30th ed. Philadelphia: Lea & Febiger; 1985; p. 451.)

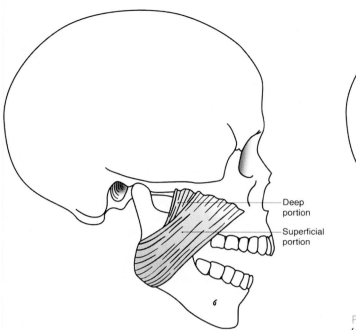

FIGURE 47-10. The masseter muscle.

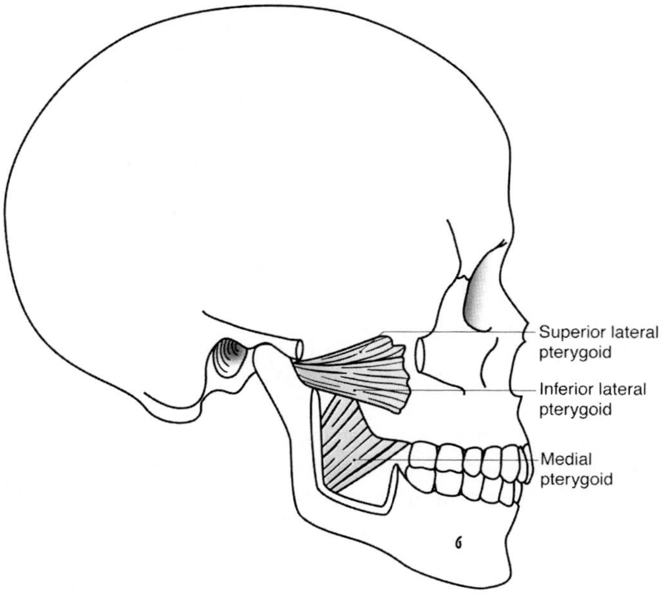

FIGURE 47-11. The medial and lateral pterygoid muscles. (Adapted from Clemente CD, editor. Gray's Anatomy of the Human Body. 30th ed. Philadelphia: Lea & Febiger; 1985; p. 451.)

The masseter muscle (Figure 47-10), a short rectangular muscle taking its origin from the zygomatic arch and inserting on the lateral surface of the mandible, is the most powerful elevator of the mandible and functions to create pressure on the teeth, particularly the molars, in chewing motions. The masseter muscle is composed of two portions, superficial and deep, which are incompletely divided, yet have somewhat different functions. The superficial portion originates from the lower border of the zygomatic bone and the anterior two thirds of the zygomatic arch and passes inferiorly and posteriorly to insert on the angle of the mandible. The deep head originates from the inner surface of the entire zygomatic arch and on the posterior one third of the arch from its lower border. The deep fibers pass vertically to insert on the mandible on its lateral aspect above the insertion of the superficial head. The superficial portion in particular has a multipennate appearance with alternating tendinous plates and fleshy bundles of muscle fibers, which serve to increase the power of the muscle. Both the superficial and the deep portions of the masseter muscle are powerful elevators of the mandible, but they function independently and reciprocally in other movements. Electromyographic studies show that the deep layer of the masseter is always silent during protrusive movements and always active during forced retrusion, whereas the superficial portion is active during protrusion and silent during retrusion.[8] Similarly, the deep masseter is active in ipsilateral movements but does not function in contralateral movements, whereas the superficial masseter is active during contralateral movements but not in ipsilateral movements.

The medial pterygoid muscle (Figure 47-11) is rectangular and takes its origin from the pterygoid fossa and the internal surface of the lateral plate of the pterygoid process, with some fibers arising from the tuberosity of the maxilla and the palatine bone. Its fibers pass inferiorly and insert on the medial surface of the mandible, inferiorly and posteriorly to the lingual. Like the masseter muscle, the medial pterygoid fibers have alternating layers of fleshy and tendinous parts, thereby increasing the power of the muscle. The main function of the medial pterygoid is elevation of the mandible, but it also functions somewhat in unilateral protrusion in a synergism with the lateral pterygoid to promote rotation to the opposite side.

The lateral pterygoid muscle (see Figure 47-11) has two portions that can be considered two functionally distinct muscles. The larger inferior head originates from the lateral surface of the lateral pterygoid plate.[9] Its fibers pass superiorly and outward to fuse with the fibers of the superior head at the neck of the mandibular condyle, inserting into the pterygoid fovea. The superior head originates from the infratemporal surface of the greater sphenoid wing, and its fibers pass inferiorly, posteriorly, and outward to insert in the superior aspect of the pterygoid fovea, the articular capsule, and the articular disk at its medial aspect, as well as to the medial pole of the condyle. Anatomic studies have shown that the majority of the superior head fibers insert into the condyle rather than the disk.

The inferior and superior heads of the lateral pterygoid muscle function independently and reciprocally.[8,10] The primary function of the inferior head is protrusive and contralateral movement. When the bilateral inferior heads function together, the condyle is pulled forward down the articular eminence, with the disk moving passively with the condylar head. This forward movement of the condyle down the

SECTION 6

TABLE 47-1. **Contributions of the Supramandibular Muscles of Mastication to Movements of the Jaw as Confirmed by Electromyography**

Muscles of Mastication	Resultant Jaw Movement
Medial pterygoid	Closure, protrusion
Lateral pterygoid (inferior head)	Protrusion, opening contralateral
Lateral pterygoid (superior head)	Retrusion, closure, ipsilateral
Masseter, superficial layer	Protrusion, closure contralateral
Masseter, deep layer	Retrusion, closure ipsilateral
Temporalis, anterior portion	Closure
Temporalis, posterior portion	Retrusion, closure ipsilateral

inclined plane of the articular eminence also contributes to opening of the oral cavity. When the inferior head functions unilaterally, the resulting medial and protrusive movement of the condyle results in contralateral motion of the mandible. The function of the superior head of the lateral pterygoid muscle is predominantly involved with closing movements of the jaw and with retrusion and ipsilateral movement. A summary of the movements of the lateral pterygoid muscle and the other supramandibular muscles is given in Table 47-1.

Inframandibular Muscle Group

The inframandibular muscles can be subdivided into two groups: the suprahyoids and the infrahyoids. The suprahyoid group consists of the digastric, geniohyoid, mylohyoid, and stylohyoid muscles; lies between the mandible and the hyoid bone; and serves to either raise the hyoid bone, if the mandible is fixed in position by the supramandibular group, or depress the mandible, if the hyoid bone is fixed in position by the infrahyoids. The infrahyoid group, consisting of the sternohyoid, omohyoid, sternothyroid, and thyrohyoid muscles, attaches to the hyoid bone superiorly and to the sternum, clavicle, and scapula inferiorly. This group of muscles can either depress the hyoid bone or hold the hyoid bone in position, relative to the trunk, during opening movements of the mandible.

BIOMECHANICS OF TMJ MOVEMENT

Complex free movements of the mandible are made possible by the relation of four distinct joints that are involved in mandibular movement: the inferior and superior joints—bilaterally. Two types of movement are possible: rotation and translation.

The inferior joints, consisting of the condyle and disk, are responsible for rotation, a hingelike motion. The center of rotation is considered to be along a horizontal axis passing through both condyles.[4,5] In theory, pure hinge motion of approximately 2.5 cm measured at the incisal edges of the anterior teeth is possible. Nevertheless, most mandibular movements are translatory as well, involving a gliding motion between the disk and the temporal fossa, which are the components of the superior joints. The mandible and disk glide

together as a unit because they are held together by the collateral ligaments. The maximum forward and lateral movement of the upper joint in translation is approximately 1.5 cm.

All movements of the mandible, whether symmetrical or asymmetrical, involve close contact of the condyle, disk, and articular eminence. Pure opening, closing, protrusive, and retrusive movements are possible as a result of bilaterally symmetrical action of the musculature. Asymmetrical movements, such as those seen in chewing, are made possible by unilateral movements of the musculature with different amounts of translation and rotation occurring within the joints on either side.

The positioning of the condyle and disk within the fossa, as well as the constant contact between the condyle, disk, and eminence, is maintained by continuous activity of the muscles of mastication, particularly the supramandibular group. The ligaments associated with the TMJ do not move the joint. Although they can be lengthened by movements of muscles, they do not stretch (i.e., do not have an elastic recoil that returns them to a resting position automatically).

Instead, the role of the ligaments is that of a passive restriction of movement at the extreme ranges of motion. During normal function, rotational and translational movements occur simultaneously, permitting the free range of motion necessary in speaking and chewing.

PATHOLOGY OF THE TMJ

The demand for treatment of temporomandibular joint dysfunction (TMJD) is well known. Most studies estimate the prevalence of clinically significant TMJ-related jaw pain to be at least 5% of the general population. Approximately 2% of the general population seeks treatment for a TMJ-related symptom.[11,12] TMJD may be the result of muscular hyperfunction or parafunction and/or underlying primary or secondary degenerative changes within the joint. It is important to note, however, that no single causative factor leading to TMJD has been unequivocally demonstrated in scientifically based studies.[13] Classification of TMJD is separated into nonarticular and articular categories and has been eloquently described by de Bont and colleagues.[13]

Nonarticular disorders include muscle disorders such as myofascial dysfunction, muscle spasm (with splinting, pain, and muscle guarding), and myositis. Articular disorders, often accompanied by internal derangement, include noninflammatory and inflammatory arthropathies, growth disorders, and connective tissue disorders. In diagnosing and treating TMJD, it is helpful to assess patients with the previous classification as a frame of reference Table 47-2. Treatment modalities can vary significantly depending on this classification.

Nonarticular Temporomandibular Disorders

Nonarticular TMJ disorders most commonly manifest as masticatory muscle dysfunction. Approximately one half or more of all TMJDs are forms of masticatory myalgia.[14,15]

TABLE 47-2. **General Classification of Synovial Disorders**

Articular Disorders

Noninflammatory Arthropathies

Primary idiopathic osteoarthrosis
Secondary osteoarthrosis (trauma, prior surgery, avascular necrosis)
Mechanical derangements
Bone and cartilage disorders, with articular manifestations

Inflammatory Arthropathies

Synovitis
Capsulitis
Rheumatoid arthritis
Juvenile rheumatoid arthritis
Seronegative polyarthritis
Ankylosing spondylitis
Psoriatic arthritis
Reactive arthritis (bacterial, viral, fungal)

Growth Disturbances

Non-neoplastic: developmental (hyperplasia, hypoplasia, dysplasia)
Non-neoplastic: acquired (condylolysis)

Neoplasms

Pseudotumors (synovial chondromatosis)
Benign (chondroma, osteotoma)
Malignant (primary, metastatic)

Diffuse Connective Tissue Disorders
Miscellaneous Articular Disorders

Nonarticular Disorders

Muscular Disorders

Muscle spasm (strain)
Myofascial pain and dysfunction
Fibromyalgia
Myotonic dystrophies
Myositis ossificans progressiva
Growth Disturbances

They include such conditions such as acute muscle strain and spasm, myofascial pain and dysfunction (MPD), chronic conditions such as fibromyalgia, and less commonly, myotonic dystrophies and myositis ossificans. They invariably contribute to decreased mandibular range of motion and pain. The important role of the supramandibular and inframandibular muscle groups on mandibular movement and function is evident in these conditions. Other nonarticular disorders include growth disorders affecting TMJ function and miscellaneous factors such as heterotopic bone formation leading to TMJD.

MPD is most commonly related to masseter or temporalis muscle spasm.[16] In addition, it can involve the pterygoids or any combination of the supramandibular or inframandibular muscle groups. Parafunctional habits such as bruxism and jaw clenching are thought to be the main contributors to MPD and have also been found to be causative in acute closed-lock conditions. The literature is replete with various treatment modalities for MPD. Such treatments include occlusal adjustments (for gross discrepancies), night-guard appliances (for joint unloading, jaw repositioning, and occlusal protection), nonsteroidal anti-inflammatory medications, muscle

relaxants, and physical therapy. These treatment modalities, alone or in combination, remain the standard of care for the treatment of nonarticular TMJD, particularly MPD.

Fibromyalgia is a systemic condition marked by poor sleep, generalized pain with absence of localization to joints, and a history of somatization in other organ systems such as irritable bowel syndrome and headaches.[17] It is typically observed in an older population than MPD and has a female predilection. Fibromyalgia is often difficult to differentiate from MPD and is treated in similar fashion; that is, nonsurgically, with anti-inflammatory medications, dietary modifications, home-care techniques, bite appliances, and physical therapy. There appears to be a poorer overall response to the treatment of fibromyalgia when compared with MPD.

Rarely, other nonarticular conditions such as myotonic dystrophy and myositis ossificans progressiva can lead to significant loss of function and pain in the TMJ region. Myotonic dystrophy is a dominantly inherited multisystem disorder that may affect facial muscles in fully developed disease states.[18] This condition may contribute to atrophy and fibrosis of the supramandibular and inframandibular musculature. Clinically, there are a variety of types of myotonic dystrophies. They tend to exert their pathologic effects in similar fashion, sometimes resulting in trismus, loss of function, and pain. Myositis ossificans progressiva is a rare condition resulting in fibrosis of soft tissues after apparent minor trauma. This condition has been reported to affect TMJ function after local trauma, including surgery, and can result in significant loss of mandibular range of motion, trismus, and pain.[19] Soft tissue ossification can sometimes occur after head trauma, severe burns, or neurogenic stimulus. In these cases, heterotopic bone formation is observed and can lead to ankylosis in multiple joints throughout the body including the TMJ.[20]

Articular TMJ Disorders

Noninflammatory articular disorders of the TMJ, the most common of which is osteoarthrosis, are often idiopathic. Osteoarthrosis can manifest as chondromalacia (softening of the cartilage), temporary or permanent disk displacement, degenerative changes within bone and cartilage often with osteophyte formation and remodeling, fibrosis, or any combination of these. Noninflammatory articular disorders may also be secondary to trauma, infection, previous surgery, crystal deposition disorders (gout and pseudogout), avascular necrosis, or structural damage to joint cartilage resulting in disk displacement and/or perforation (Figure 47-12). TMJ disk displacement has been categorized through a widely accepted staging system by Wilkes,[21] using such criteria as severity of displacement and chronicity (Table 47-3).

Noninflammatory arthropathies are distinctly limited in their amount of overt inflammation and may be clinically silent or focal in nature. Alternatively, if the condition becomes more severe, symptoms will ensue. If degenerative changes

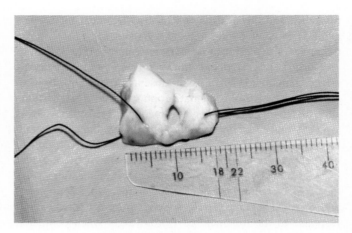

FIGURE 47-12. Perforated disk (Wilkes stage V).

TABLE 47-3. **Wilkes Classification**

Stage I	Early reducing disk displacement
Stage II	Late reducing disk displacement
Stage III	Nonreducing disk displacement: acute/subacute
Stage IV	Nonreducing disk displacement: chronic
Stage V	Nonreducing disk displacement: chronic with osteoarthritis

progress to synovitis, joint effusion (secondary to increased vascular permeability), or capsulitis, it is then considered to have transformed into an inflammatory arthropathy.

Inflammatory arthropathies are primarily due to such conditions as rheumatoid arthritis, juvenile rheumatoid arthritis, ankylosing spondylitis, psoriatic arthritis, or arthritis resulting from infectious causes (see Table 47-2). Secondary causes of inflammatory arthropathies include synovitis, capsulitis, traumatic arthritis, or acute inflamed crystal-induced arthritis, such as gout. As discussed previously, noninflammatory arthropathies can progress to the inflammatory types through increasing concentrations of degradation products within the joint. Degenerative changes resulting in the release of inflammatory mediators have been demonstrated to worsen the degree of tissue destruction and dysfunction within the TMJ. This pathologic inflammatory cascade has been the primary focus of current TMJ research.

Historically, the gross evaluation of disk position and disk integrity has been the mainstay of internal derangement diagnosis and management. More recently, the physiologic activity of synovial cells, chondrocytes, and inflammatory cells in symptomatic joints has been associated with pathogenesis. This fundamental shift in focus has changed the primary treatment approach from open-joint surgery aimed at restoring the functional anatomy of the TMJ to less invasive techniques directed toward lysis of adhesions and intracapsular lavage.[22] TMJ arthrocentesis and arthroscopy are thought to achieve an alteration in the joint milieu favoring a reduction in symptoms and improved joint function.

Open-joint surgery, nonetheless, may still have a role in severe degenerative disease when preoperative criteria are met and surgery is indicated.

Milam and Schmitz[23] have proposed a variety of molecular biologic mechanisms for TMJD. Synovoid cells, chondrocytes, and inflammatory cells in the TMJ produce a physiologic balance between anabolic and catabolic cytokines.[23] Anabolic cytokines such as insulin-like growth factor-I and transforming growth factor-beta are instrumental in the formation of extracellular joint matrix molecules. Collagen, proteoglycans, and glycoproteins are essential in load-bearing joints like the TMJ. Alternatively, catabolic cytokines such as interleukin-1 (IL-1), IL-6, and tumor necrosis factor-alpha (TNF-α) have been identified with the formation of proteases within the TMJ. These proteases (aspartic, cysteine, serine, and metalloproteases, among others) operate at low and neutral pH to exert their pathologic effects leading to degenerative changes.

Oxidative stress, often found associated with pathologic joints, is thought to contribute to free radical formation in the TMJ. The presence of free radicals has been postulated as an amplifying factor in the activation of cytokines, enzymes, neuropeptides, and arachidonic acid metabolites leading to degenerative joint disease.[24] Nitric oxide, a free radical involved in regulating vascular tone, has been observed at higher concentrations in arthritic joints. Nitric oxide has direct effects on prostaglandin synthesis and cyclooxygenase-2 enzymes leading to synovial inflammation and tissue destruction.[25] In a normal functioning joint, a delicate balance is maintained between anabolic and catabolic mechanisms. In symptomatic joints, catabolic processes have been found to exert greater overall effects, thus disrupting the balance between anabolic physiologic maintenance and the negative effects of catabolic cytokines.

TMJ synovial fluid analysis has proved to be an excellent vehicle for evaluating the proposed contribution of cytokines, proteinases, and other catabolites to TMJD. Multiple independent studies support the hypothesis of catabolic imbalance within the joint. Kubota and coworkers[26] demonstrated increased levels of IL-1β, IL-6, and active matrix metalloproteinases in TMJs with internal derangement and osteoarthritis when compared with control samples. This study suggests the presence of elevated concentrations of these cytokines and proteinases serving as potential catabolic markers for cartilage degradation in the human TMJ. Murakami and associates[27] reported high concentrations of chondroitin-4 and chondroitin-6 sulfates compared with hyaluronic acid in the TMJ synovial fluid of patients with internal derangement suggesting glycosaminoglycan components as markers of joint pathology. Israel and colleagues[28] demonstrated the prevalence of synovitis and osteoarthritis through arthroscopic evaluation in symptomatic TMJs. These findings correlated with increased levels of keratan sulfate in the synovial fluid of these joints, suggesting its role as a potential biochemical marker for articular cartilage degradation.[28] Recently, osteoclastogenesis inhibitory factor/osteoprotegerin

(OCIF/OPG), a member of the TNF receptor family, has been studied in synovial fluid samples of TMJD patients.[29] Increased osteoclastic activity has been seen histologically in diseased mandibular condyles. Osteoclast differentiation requires cell-to-cell contact between osteoclast progenitors and bone marrow stromal cells. The presence of OCIF/OPG is thought to inhibit osteoclast differentiation by preventing the cell-to-cell contact needed for such activity. Synovial fluid samples in this study demonstrated decreased amounts of OCIF/OPG in osteoarthritic and internally deranged joints, suggesting its physiologically important function in healthy joints. Although further investigation of synovial fluid components in TMJD is necessary to formulate definitive conclusions, it continues to shed new light on the pathogenesis and treatment of such disorders.

Treatment of patients with internal derangement of the TMJ typically begins with nonsurgical treatment modalities. Bite appliance therapy, diet modifications, nonsteroidal anti-inflammatory medications, muscle relaxants, moist heat or ice, and physical therapy have been found to be efficacious.[30] Surgical intervention is typically employed only after failure of nonsurgical treatment objectives.

A variety of surgical treatment modalities have been used in the treatment of articular TMJD. Arthrocentesis and TMJ arthroscopy have been found to be minimally invasive effective treatments for articular TMJD by decreasing pain and increasing mandibular range of motion. (Surgical techniques for arthroscopy are addressed in Chapter 49). Indications for these modalities include, but are not limited to, acute closed-lock degenerative joint disease accompanied by pain and limited range of motion and joint effusion. Arthrocentesis and arthroscopy have also been reported to be useful in severe, often sudden-onset, closed-lock disease due to an anchored or "stuck disk" phenomenon. This proposed phenomenon involves the disk becoming adherent to the glenoid fossa through increased intra-articular friction, with or without the formation of adhesions within the joint. Lysis of adhesions with joint lavage has been reported efficacious in restoring mandibular range of motion and decreasing pain in these clinical scenarios.[31,32] TMJ arthrocentesis and arthroscopy show promising results using the previously discussed criteria of pain symptoms and mandibular range of motion.[33] Based on the pathophysiology discussed in this chapter, a hypothesis explaining the efficacy of joint lavage relates to a proposed alteration in the biochemical constituents of the joint fluid, thus shifting the balance toward anabolic processes while reducing the amount of active catabolites contained within the joint.[34]

Indications for open arthrotomy include, but are not limited to, joint ankylosis, the need for reconstruction owing to condylar resorption or growth disturbance, history of previous surgery, removal of foreign bodies, neoplasia, trauma, or severe degenerative disease precluding less invasive interventions. (Indications and techniques for open TMJ surgery are addressed more thoroughly in Chapters 51 and Chapter 52). Open-joint surgery is primarily based on restoration of the functional anatomy of the TMJ when less invasive techniques are not feasible or unsuccessful. Data suggest comparable outcomes between open and closed surgery in the TMJ with lower morbidity associated with the latter.[35] Open TMJ surgery remains a viable treatment option at the end of the surgical treatment algorithm. New insight into the pathogenesis of TMJD has opened the door to less invasive (albeit equally effective) treatment options for a large number of TMJD patients.

Infections of the TMJ

Infections of the TMJ are not common. Prompt diagnostic and therapeutic intervention is required when an infection of the TMJ is suspected because joint distention is usually painful and permanent changes in joint function can occur. On examination, patients usually exhibit a posterior open bite on the ipsilateral side as a result of the increased joint fluid. The patient will also maintain a posture toward the contralateral side.[36] The surface overlying an infected joint is often warm, and fluctuance is occasionally felt.

The bacteria causing an infected joint are usually spread through a hematogenous route. The synovium is vascular and lacks a basement membrane, which permits bloodborne bacteria to gain access to the joint space.[37] Joints with underlying arthritic disease tend to be more susceptible to distant infection. Although the source of the bacteria is usually at a distant site, spread from dental infections of maxillary teeth has been reported in which the bacteria are thought to spread through the pterygoid plexus of veins to the joint.[38] Direct innoculation of a joint area after a traumatic injury is also possible. Complications of infections of the TMJ include fistula formation, fibrosis or bony ankylosis, temporal bone osteomyelitis, and intracranial abscess formation.

A thorough history and review of systems aids in the diagnosis of acute infectious arthritis of the TMJ. Active infection in adjacent sites, especially the ipsilateral maxillary molars, should be searched for. Other joints must be assessed to determine whether they are involved. Initially aspiration of the joint should be considered to both relieve the pain from the joint capsular distention and help in the identification of the infecting organism(s). The aspiration is performed by using a 20-gauge or larger needle under sterile conditions. The synovial fluid should be Gram-stained and cultured for both aerobic and anaerobic bacteria. Sedation or general anesthesia may be required for the arthrocentesis.

In sexually active adults, 60% of general acute infectious arthritis is due to *Neisseria gonorrhoeae*.[39] The majority of these patients have a prodrome of malaise, anorexia, headaches, fever, and chills. A few days of migratory arthritis usually precedes the localization of infection in one or two joints. Markowitz and Gerry[40] reported a TMJ involvement rate of 3% in patients with disseminated gonococcal arthritis. In children younger than 2 years, almost 50% of acute infectious arthritis is due to *Haemophilus influenzae*. No reports of TMJ involvement are available. Other gram-positive cocci have been isolated from TMJ infections in all age groups, including staphylococci (particularly in the elderly) and β-hemolytic streptococci. The adherence characteristics of *Staphylococcus aureus* and *N. gonorrhoeae* to synovium account for their prevalence.[41] Thus, the best choice for initial empirical antibiotic therapy for an acute infectious TMJ arthritis is an agent that combines a penicillin with a β-lactamase inhibitor. The combination of ampicillin and sulbactam will cover infections from the staphylococcal and streptococcal groups. Sulbactam, a derivative of penicillin, inactivates bacteria-produced β-lactamase and also has direct bactericidal activity against the *Neisseria* organisms. Therefore, this combination may have an advantage over the combination of a penicillin and clavulanic acid. It should be noted that bacterial resistance has become increasingly more problematic. Reference to up-to-date antibiotic regimens is recommended.

Lyme disease, due to infection with *Borrelia burgdorferi*, has been documented to cause acute infection of the TMJ. The incidence of this is greater in the Northeastern United States where this tick-borne disease is more common and the authors have treated five patients with this disorder. This disorder has been reported even in Slovenia, so it should be considered as part of the differential diagnosis of patients with TMJ disorders.[42] Patients present with acute pain directly in the TMJ region, which may or not be bilateral in distribution. The findings of limitation in opening along with pain on chewing should lead the practitioner to consider this as a cause. Serum titers for antibodies for *B. burgdorferi* become positive in the later phases of this disease and can assist with the diagnosis. Patients may often present with migratory arthritis affecting the large joints such as the knee, but other and multiple joint involvement are reported. Treatment is with a 1-month course of doxycycline or amoxicillin. In more acute or recalitrant cases, a 2-week course of intravenous ceftriaxone is utilized.[43] Cultures of *B. burgdorferi* from joint aspirates have not been documented, but the response to antibiotics along with the findings of antibodies in serum samples lead to the diagnosis.

Effective treatment of other forms of septic arthritis by oral antibiotics has not been well studied; therefore, the parenteral administration of antibiotics should be used initially.[37] Choices include ampicillin and sulbactam (Unasyn) 3 g intravenously (IV) every 6 hours or clindamycin 600 mg IV every 6 hours in penicillin-allergic patients. A third-generation cephalosporin, cefotaxime 6 to 12 g IV per day, could be used for a gram-negative infection in a nonhospitalized patient.[37] Tobramycin 3 mg/kg/day in four doses should be considered to treat a possible presence of *Pseudomonas aeruginosa* in infections that develop in hospitalized or immunocompromised patients.

The duration of treatment depends on the clinical response and the organism isolated. Based on information available for treatment of septic arthritis involving *N. gonorrhoeae*, the patient with a septic TMJ could be placed on oral ampicillin or tetracycline after a 2-week course of intravenous therapy. Reportedly infections involving *S. aureus* and gram-negative bacilli require 4 weeks of total therapy, and 2 to 3 weeks of

therapy is adequate for streptococci and *Haemophilus* species.[44] Thus, it appears that a 30-day total course of antibiotic therapy for acute TMJ infection is appropriate.

In addition to culture and sensitivity testing, the aspirate from the infected joint should be submitted for white blood cell (WBC) count and differential and examined for the presence of crystals and fibrinogen. Fibrinogen is usually present in the synovial fluid of acutely infected joints. Therefore, some of the synovial fluid collected should be placed into a heparinized tube to prevent clotting. It is important to note that ethylenediaminetetraacetic acid (EDTA) interferes with crystal analysis; therefore, synovial fluid should not be placed in tubes containing it. The synovial fluid of an inflamed joint commonly contains greater than 2000 WBC/mm³ (normal < 200 WBC/mm³). Septic joints normally have WBC counts greater than 50,000/mm³. The cells are primarily mononuclear, as opposed to a predominance of PMN cells in infected joint fluid. An exception to this occurs in fungal or mycobacterial joint infections in which the synovial fluid usually contains less than 20,000 WBC/mm³ and shows a greater proportion of mononuclear cells.[45]

Following the institution of antibiotic therapy, lavage of the joint may be useful. Removing the joint fluid containing the products of the inflammation, reducing the bacterial load within the joint, and relieving the joint distention will usually markedly relieve the patient's symptoms and may also decrease the likelihood of spread to the temporal bone. Murakami and workers[38] have reported on the use of the arthroscope for monitoring and treating an acutely infected TMJ.

Following the resolution of an acute TMJ infection, a program must be started to minimize joint disability and to monitor for recurrence of infection. The acute inflammatory process that accompanies an infection can result in the deposition of fibrinogen and other products, which can predispose the joint toward a fibrous or bony ankylosis. Active range of motion exercises are started as soon as possible to prevent intra-articular adhesions. The patient's range of motion should be documented at weekly intervals. If the range of motion is still limited 1 month after the resolution of the infection, a brisement procedure or an arthroscopic procedure to lyse intra-articular adhesions should be considered. However, before this, extracapsular causes of limited opening, such as masseter muscle trismus, need to be differentiated from intracapsular disorders. Intracapsular restrictions are usually accompanied by restriction of lateral excursions to the contralateral side and deviation on opening. Recurrence of joint infection (of all joints) has been reported to occur at a rate of 10.5%.[46] Newman[46] noted that infection recurred as long as 1 year after the initial episode. The patient should be advised of this possibility.

Neoplastic Diseases

Tumors affecting the TMJ area are exceedingly rare. In one review, the authors report a fairly large incidence of 6 patients with TMJ tumors out of 621 patients presenting with initial

TMJD.[47] The tissues from which a neoplasm may arise include the synovium, bone, cartilage, and associated musculature. Neoplasms of this region can present with signs and symptoms similar to those occurring with internal derangement (preauricular pain and dysfunction) and, thus, can result in a delay in the diagnosis. Owing to the proximity of the cranial base, delay in treatment can be detrimental. The clinician should be aware of this when treating temporomandibular disorders, especially if the patient fails to respond to traditional therapy.

Benign Tumors

The most common benign bone tumors of the TMJ include the osteoma and condylar enlargement or condylar hypertrophy. Both present signs related to the increase in size of the condyle, a shift in the mandible to the contralateral side, and an ipsilateral open bite. Often, the range of motion is decreased as the increased size of the condylar head prevents normal translation. Radiographs, including tomograms and computed tomography scans, should be obtained to delineate the extent of the condylar growth and to determine involvement of the glenoid fossa and associated structures. Radionuclide scans should be performed to determine whether the process is still active and bone is being produced. Treatment includes a condylar head resection (partial or complete) for active lesions or a condyloplasty to reduce condylar size and restore the occlusion for nongrowing lesions. Condylar reconstruction is usually not necessary. The disk should be preserved or replaced (if it has been damaged) with a temporalis muscle flap or cartilage graft. Physical therapy is usually required to reduce dysfunction. Postoperative maxillomandibular fixation is not usually necessary, but guiding elastics may be helpful with muscle retraining. An active physical therapy program to reduce joint adhesions prevents permanent restriction of the joint.

Virtually all other benign bone tumors have been reported to occur in the TMJ. These bone tumors behave as they would in other areas of the mandible and, therefore, should be treated in a similar fashion.

Synovial Tumors

Synovial chondromatosis is the most commonly reported neoplasm of the TMJ synovium. Lustman and Zelster[48] reported a series of 50 cases in which the mean age was 47 years. This is in contrast to synovial chondromatosis involving other joints, which is more commonly found in the 20- to 30-year-old age group.[49] Pain and swelling of the preauricular area are the most common initial signs. Depending on the degree of calcification present, radiographs may reveal the presence of loose radiodense bodies within the joint. These loose bodies are formed by metaplastic synovial tissues. Foci of metaplastic synovium detach from the synovial lining and remain viable while suspended in the synovial fluid. While suspended, they form a perichondrium and continue to grow and enlarge. Although the reason is unknown, this process most frequently occurs in the superior joint space. The loose bodies are composed of cartilage containing multinucleated cells. The presence of cellular atypia and hyperchromatism is common, and a careful review of all histologic material removed is necessary to rule out the possibility of chondrosarcoma.

Treatment of synovial chondromatosis involves extirpation of the loose bodies and removal of the synovial lining. Lustman and Zelster[48] reported that a condylectomy was necessary in 13 of 47 cases to gain access to the anteromedial portion of the joint. The condyle itself is not involved and, therefore, should be removed only for access. Recurrence of synovial chondromatosis is quite rare and is thought to be caused by an incomplete excision of the original lesions. No cases of TMJ synovial chondromatosis transforming into chondrosarcoma have been reported, although this has been reported in the knee.[50]

Ganglion Cysts

Ganglion cysts have also been reported to occur in association with the TMJ. These are cystic structures that arise subcutaneously in association with the joint capsule or tendon sheaths. Histologic examination of a ganglion reveals a true cyst, containing a mucinous fluid and hyaluronic acid. These lesions present as a preauricular mass and may produce classic "TMJ symptoms," such as pain and limitation of function. The swelling produced by the ganglion in the preauricular region can be confused with a parotid mass. Surgery is indicated to remove the cyst and recurrences have not been reported.[51]

Malignant Tumors

Malignancies of the TMJ are very rare and are usually the result of direct extensions of primary lesions of adjacent structures. Metastatic disease has been reported to involve the TMJ but is more commonly found in the mandibular angle region. This may be due to the relative paucity of cancellous bone in the condylar head region.[52] The most common lesions to metastasize to the condyle are adenocarcinomas of the breast, kidney, and lungs. As with benign tumors, the early signs of malignant disease of the TMJ are pain and dysfunction. Primary malignancies of the TMJ have been reported as intrinsic tumors of the condylar bone, disk, synovium, and cartilaginous linking. Typically, patients with malignancies of the TMJ are older than the usual internal derangement patient. Patients with a history of preexisting malignant disease must undergo a thorough search for metastasis if TMJ symptoms develop. Radionuclide scans may be useful, although the inflammation from chronic synovitis can result in activity localizing in the condyle.[53] Patients presenting with a fracture of the condyle without a history of trauma should be suspect for the presence of a malignant lesion in the condyle.

Primary TMJ malignancies require aggressive therapy to prevent intracranial extension of the disease. Radiation, surgery, and chemotherapy are all appropriate means of treatment of diseases in this region. Radiation therapy can also be used for palliation in disseminated disease to control pain from the TMJ region and to prevent pathologic fractures.

SECTION 6

References

1. DuBrul EL, editor. Sicher's Oral Anatomy. 7th ed. St. Louis: C.V. Mosby; 1980; pp. 146–161, 174–209.

2. Albright JA, Brand RA. The scientific basis of orthopedics. 2nd ed. Norwalk, CT: Appleton and Lange; 1987; pp. 373–386.

3. Dijkgraaf LC, Milam SB. Osteoarthritis: histopathology and biochemistry of the TMJ. In Piecuch JF, editor. Oral maxillofacial surgery knowledge update. Vol 3. Rosemont, IL: American Association of Oral and Maxillofacial Surgeons; 2001; pp. 5–28.

4. Bell WE, editor. Temporomandibular Disorders: Classification, Diagnosis and Management. 2nd ed. Chicago: Year Book Medical; 1986; pp. 16–62.

5. Okeson JP, editor. Management of Temporomandibular Disorders and Occlusions. 2nd ed. St. Louis: CV Mosby; 1989; pp. 3–26.

6. Rayne J. Functional anatomy of the temporomandibular joint. Br J Oral Maxillofac Surg 1987;25:92–99.

7. Blackwood HJJ. Pathology of the temporomandibular joint. J Am Dent Assoc 1969;79:118.

8. Gay T, Piecuch J. An electromyographic analysis of jaw movements in man. Electromyogr Clin Neurophysiol 1986;26:365–384.

9. Carpentier P, Yung JP, Marguelles-Bonnet R, Meunissier M. Insertions of the lateral pterygoid muscle. J Oral Maxillofac Surg 1988;46:477–482.

10. McNamara JA. The independent functions of the two heads of the lateral pterygoid muscle. Am J Anat 1973;138:197–205.

11. Goulet JP, Lavigne GJ, Lund JP. Jaw pain prevalence among French-speaking Canadians in Quebec and related symptoms of temporomandibular disorders. J Dent Res 1995;74:1738–1744.

12. DeKanter R, Kayser A, Battistuzzi P, et al. Demand and need for treatment of craniomandibular dysfunction in the Dutch adult population. J Dent Res 1992;71:1607–1612.

13. de Bont L, Dijkgraaf L, Stegenga B. Epidemiology and natural progression of articular temporomandibular disorders. Oral Surg Oral Med Oral Pathol Oral Radiol Endod 1997;83:72–76.

14. Marbach JJ, Lipton JA. Treatment of patients with temporomandibular joint and other facial pain by otolaryngologists. Arch Otolaryngol 1982;108:102–107.

15. List T, Dworkin SF, Harrison R, Huggins K. Research diagnostic criteria/temporomandibular disorders: comparing Swedish and U.S. clinics [abstract]. J Dent Res 1996;75(Special Issue):352.

16. Laskin DM. Diagnosis and etiology of myofascial pain and dysfunction. Oral Maxillofac Surg Clin North Am 1995;7:73–78.

17. Demitrack M. Chronic fatigue syndrome and fibromyalgia dilemmas in diagnosis and clinical management. Psychiatr Clin North Am 1998;21:671–692.

18. Kiliardis S, Katsaros C. The effects of myotonic dystrophy and Duchenne muscular dystrophy on the orofacial muscles and dentofacial morphology. Acta Odontol Scand 1998;56:369–374.

19. Steiner M, Gould AR, Kushner GM, et al. Myositis ossificans traumatica of the masseter muscle: review of the literature and report of two additional cases. Oral Surg Oral Med Oral Pathol Oral Radiol Endod 1997;84:703–707.

20. Rubin M, Cozzi G. Heterotopic ossification of the temporomandibular joint in a burn patient. J Oral Maxillofac Surg 1986;44:897–899.

21. Wilkes CH. Internal derangement of the temporomandibular joint pathological variations. Arch Otolaryngol Head Neck Surg 1989;115:469–477.

22. Dolwick MF. Intra-articular disc displacement. Part I: its questionable role in temporomandibular joint pathology. J Oral Maxillofac Surg 1995;53:1069–1072.

23. Milam SB, Schmitz JP. Molecular biology of temporomandibular joint disorders: proposed mechanisms of disease. J Oral Maxillofac Surg 1995;53:1448–1454.

24. Milam SB, Zardeneta G, Schmitz JP. Oxidative stress and degenerative temporomandibular joint disease: a proposed hypothesis. J Oral Maxillofac Surg 1998;56:214–223.

25. Takahashi T, Kondoh T, Ohtani M, et al. Association between arthroscopic diagnosis of osteoarthritis and synovial fluid nitric oxide levels. Oral Surg Oral Med Oral Pathol Oral Radiol Endod 1999;88:129–136.

26. Kubota E, Kubota T, Matsumoto J, et al. Synovial fluid cytokines and proteases as markers of temporomandibular joint disease. J Oral Maxillofac Surg 1998;56:192–198.

27. Murakami KI, Shibata T, Kubota E, Maeda H. Intra-articular levels of prostaglandin E2, hyaluronic acid, and chondroitin-4 and -6 sulfates in the temporomandibular joint synovial fluid of patients with internal derangement. J Oral Maxillofac Surg 1998;56:199–203.

28. Israel HA, Diamond BE, Said-Nejad F, Ratcliffe A. Correlation between arthroscopic diagnosis of osteoarthritis and synovitis of the human temporomandibular joint and keratin sulfate levels in the synovial fluid. J Oral Maxillofac Surg 1997;55:210–217.

29. Kaneyama K, Segami N, Nishimura M, et al. Osteoclastogenesis inhibitory factor/osteoprotegerin in synovial fluid from patients with temporomandibular disorders. Int J Oral Maxillofac Surg 2003;32:404–407.

30. Okeson J. Nonsurgical treatment of internal derangements. Oral Maxillofac Surg Clin North Am 1995;7:63–71.

31. Nitzan D. The process of lubrication impairment and its involvement in temporomandibular joint disc displacement: a theoretical concept. J Oral Maxillofac Surg 2001;59:36–45.

32. Rao VM, Liem MD, Farole A, Razik A. Elusive "stuck" disk in the temporomandibular joint: diagnosis with MR imaging. Radiology 1993;189:823–827.

33. Goudot P, Jaquinet AR, Hugonnet S, et al. Improvement of pain and function after arthroscopy and arthrocentesis of the temporomandibular joint: a comparative study. J Craniomaxillofac Surg 2000;28:39–43.

34. Zardeneta G, Milam SB, Schmitz JP. Elution of proteins by continuous temporomandibular joint arthrocentesis. J Oral Maxillofac Surg 1997;55:709–716.

35. Holmlund AB, Axelsson S, Gynther G. A comparison of diskectomy and arthroscopic lysis and lavage for the treatment of chronic closed-lock of the temporomandibular joint: a randomized outcome study. J Oral Maxillofac Surg 2001;59:972–977.

36. Bounds GA, Hopkins R, Sugar A. Septic arthritis of the temporomandibular joint: a problematic diagnosis. Br J Oral Maxillofac Surg 1987;25:61–67.

37. Simpson ML. Septic arthritis in adults. In Gustilo RB, Grumminger RP, Tsukayama DT, editors. Orthopedic Infection. Philadelphia: WB Saunders; 1900; p. 286.

38. Murakami K, Matsumoto K, Iizuka T. Suppurative arthritis of the temporomandibular joint: report of a case with special reference to arthroscopic observations. J Maxillofac Surg 1984;12:41–45.

39. Parker RH. Acute infectious arthritis. In Schlossberg D, editor. Orthopedic Infection. New York: Springer-Verlag; 1988; pp. 69–75.

40. Markowitz HA, Gerry RG. Temporomandibular joint disease. Oral Surg Oral Med Oral Pathol 1950;3:75–79.
41. Eisenstein BI, Masi AT. Disseminated gonococcal infection and gonococcal arthritis. Semin Arthritis Rheum 1988;10:155–159.
42. Lesnic G, Erdoner D. Temporomandibular joint involvement caused by *Borrelia burgdorferi*. J Craniomaxillofac Surg 2007;35:97–400.
43. Steere AC. Musculoskeletal manifestations of Lyme disease. Am J Med 1995;98(Suppl 1):44S–51S.
44. Smith JW. Infectious arthritis. In Mandell GL, Douglas RG, Bennett JE, editors. Principles and Practice of Infectious Diseases. New York: John Wiley & Sons; 1985; p. 697.
45. Mahowald ML, Messner RP. Chronic infective arthritis. In Schlossberg D, editor. Orthopedic Infection. New York: Springer-Verlag; 1988; pp. 76–95.
46. Newman JH. Review of septic arthritis throughout the antibiotic era. Ann Rheum Dis 1976;35:198–204.
47. Mostafapour S, Furtran N. Tumors and tumorous masses presenting as temporomandibular joint syndrome. Otolaryngol Head Neck Surg 2000;123:459–464.
48. Lustman J, Zelster R. Synovial chondromatosis of the temporomandibular joint. Int J Oral Maxillofac Surg 1989;18:90–94.
49. Orden A, Laskin DM, Leu D. Chronic preauricular swelling. J Oral Maxillofac Surg 1989;47:390–397.
50. King JW, Splut HJ, Fechner RE, Vanderpool DW. Synovial chondrosarcoma of the knee joint. J Bone Joint Surg 1967;49:1389–1396.
51. Copeland M, Douglas B. Ganglions of the temporomandibular joint. Plast Reconstr Surg 1988;69:775–776.
52. Hartman GL, Robertson GR, Sugg WE, et al. Metastatic carcinoma of the mandibular condyle. J Oral Surg 1973;31:716–719.
53. Mizukawa JH, Dolwick MF, Johnson RP, et al. Metastatic breast adenocarcinoma of the mandibular condyle. J Oral Surg 1980;38:448–449.
54. Clemente CD, editor. Gray's Anatomy of the Human Body. 30th ed. Philadelphia: Lea & Febiger; 1985; p. 451.

SECTION 6

Nonsurgical Management of Temporomandibular Disorders

Vasiliki Karlis, DMD, MD, and Robert Glickman, DMD

Temporomandibular disorder (TMD) is the general term used to describe the manifestation of pain and/or dysfunction of the temporomandibular joint (TMJ) and its associated structures. In general, up to 5% of the population is affected by TMD, with significantly more frequent and more severe signs and symptoms appearing in women and older adults.[1,2] The etiology of TMD may include trauma, parafunctional habits, malocclusion, joint overload, arthritides, psychological factors, and chronic nonergonomic positioning of the head and neck. The impact of psychological factors is difficult to determine, but approximately 10% to 20% of patients with TMD also manifest some form of psychiatric illness.[3] Because symptoms of TMD are quite variable and remain exceedingly difficult to attribute exclusively to one or more events (such as the true contribution or extent of involvement of muscles of mastication), the joint itself, or psychological factors, is best understood in terms of interdependence. When a diagnosis of TMD is suspected or confirmed, therapy should be directed toward improvement of function and reduction of pain and discomfort. Sufficient literature is available to suggest that nonsurgical treatment modalities may account for as high as a 74% to 85% favorable response rate in patients with TMD.[4,5] In one study, Suvinen and coworkers[6] reported that 81% of patients showed 50% or greater improvement after conservative physical therapy with a 6-month follow-up period, and the authors attributed the improvement to a possible placebo-type effect. Other sources report significant relief in 30% to 60% of patients when under some form of treatment.[7] In addition, long-term follow-up studies have suggested that almost all patients with TMD will improve over time, regardless of the type of treatment they may receive.[4,8–12] Thus, it appears well established in the literature that the majority of patients with TMD achieve some

relief of symptoms with nonsurgical therapy. The dilemma for the surgeon is compounded by the broad spectrum of results and claims that use a seemingly endless variety of surgical and nonsurgical strategies in the management of TMD. Because the extent or severity of symptoms is apparently unrelated to the specific etiology, and the overwhelming number of symptoms respond to conservative management, the question of whether, and how, to incorporate surgical and nonsurgical treatment into the care of these patients becomes challenging for the oral and maxillofacial surgeon. There are absolute indications in which surgical intervention would be of primary benefit, and the question is whether there is still a role for nonsurgical therapy in these patients, and if so, when and how it should be instituted, as well as the length of treatment. One approach to this dilemma is to consider the concept of nonsurgical versus surgical therapy misleading and incomplete and not evidence-based in the literature. There are many times when it may be inappropriate to consider surgery, and at other times, nonsurgical therapy should precede, and almost always follow, surgical intervention. Therefore, it is essential for the surgeon to have a thorough appreciation of the available techniques and their limitations in order to know when and how to most appropriately manage TMD. The purpose of this chapter is to delineate those nonsurgical treatment modalities that are considered adjunctive to the available surgical options.

TREATMENT CONSIDERATIONS

The primary goal in the treatment of TMD is to alleviate pain and/or mandibular dysfunction. Pain and alteration in function (i.e., mastication and speech) can become quite debilitating, greatly affecting oral health care and diminishing the quality of life for these individuals. Another critical objective relates to patient counseling and education regarding the predisposing factors for TMD. Depending upon the degree of impairment, patients can often be assured that TMD is a benign condition and that clinical improvement may be expected with compliance with appropriate therapeutic recommendations. However, it is prudent, if not incumbent upon the surgeon, to inform patients that complete elimination of symptoms is, in most cases, an unreasonable expectation. Nonsurgical techniques that can decrease unintentional overloading of the masticatory system, eliminate pain, reduce dysfunction, decrease chronicity, and promote healing are essential in all phases of therapy. A patient home care program may prevent further injury and allow for a period of healing. In general, patients can be instructed to limit mandibular function, modify habits, avoid stress, and institute a home exercise program.[8]

Clicking and popping of the TMJ are quite common in TMD as well as in patients with asymptomatic normal TMJs. Internal derangement of the TMJ is difficult to eliminate without surgery and usually recurs; there is inconclusive evidence to suggest whether or not this anatomic abnormality actually presents a problem for the patient, such as accelerated osteoarthritis or the development of TMD. There is considerable support in the literature that joint noise, without pain or dysfunction, requires no intervention or treatment (Table 48-1).

Once the diagnosis of TMD has been established, frequent follow-up appointments are necessary after therapy is initiated in order to determine whether there is any improvement in signs and/or symptoms. Initial results may require reassessment after several weeks of therapy, and further diagnostic procedures may be warranted to rule out vascular, neurologic, neoplastic, psychological, or otolaryngologic abnormalities. TMD is a complex multisystem disorder that is affected by many interacting factors, and strong consideration should be given toward a multidisciplinary diagnostic and treatment approach. The roles of the dentist, physical therapist, orthodontist, neurologist, psychologist/psychiatrist, anesthesiologist, and oral and maxillofacial surgeon cannot be understated and should be key constituents of any facial pain center or TMD team. The precise timing and length of therapy must be determined by the surgeon based upon the severity of clinical symptoms as well as other supporting diagnostic indicators. As with other major joints in the body, clinical suspicions should be directed to rule out pathology, decrease inflammation, allow unimpeded joint motion, and restore range of motion. To accomplish these

goals in a ginglymodiarthrodial joint that is physcially connected to the opposite side, and is intimately involved in oral health and daily stresses of mastication, is indeed a clinical challenge. The remainder of this chapter provides basic guidelines for nonsurgical therapeutic modalities for TMD, and it is not intended to eliminate, or preselect, adjunctive dental or surgical treatment.

NONSURGICAL THERAPY

Diet

A soft diet is is a critical component in the management of TMD in order to allow jaw rest, because this can prevent overloading of the TMJ and decrease muscular hyperactivity. The extent of time that a patient should maintain a soft food diet is dependent upon the severity of the clinical symptoms. Patients should be instructed to divide the foods into smaller pieces and abstain from eating chewy, hard, or crunchy foods, including uncooked vegetables and meats. Intermaxillary fixation is not typically used as a means of jaw rest, although it may be considered in extreme cases. A strict liquid or blenderized diet may be recommended for those patients who manifest severe TMD symptoms (Table 48-2).

Pharmacotherapy

Medications are often prescribed for managing the symptoms associated with TMD, and patients should understand that these medications may not offer a complete cure to their problem but can be a valuable adjunctive aid when prescribed as part of a comprehensive program. With pharmacotherapy, there is always a danger of drug dependency and abuse, particularly with the use of narcotics and tranquilizers. Because many TMD symptoms are periodic, there is a tendency to prescribe medications on an "as-needed," or PRN, philosophy. This type of regimen may provide brief periods of pain relief, but more frequent pain cycles can result in a lower effectiveness of the drugs, with resultant overuse or abuse of these medications.[12–15] The general recommendation for pharmacotherapy is that the medications should be prescribed at regular intervals and for a specific period of time (e.g., four times daily for 3 wk). The clinician must recognize the influence of personality traits in these patients that may contribute to drug dependency or abuse. Other obvious influential factors that must be considered in the choice of drug regimens are co-morbid medical disease, medications and potential interactions, patient age, occupation, and each

TABLE 48-1. **Goals of Nonsurgical Therapy for Temporomandibular Disorder**

Improvement in jaw function
Reduction in facial pain
Patient education and counseling
Provision of referrals for physical therapy, occlusal appliances, if indicated

TABLE 48-2. **Soft Diet Benefits**

Decreased muscular hyperactivity
Decreased loading forces on TMJ
Controlled range of motion with hinge and sliding movements
Full liquid diet with elimination of hard chewy foods
Elimination of gum chewing

TMJ = temporomandibular joint.

patient's attitude toward pharmacotherapy in general. The most common pharmacologic agents used for the management of TMD are analgesics, anti-inflammatory agents, anxiolytic agents, antidepressants, muscle relaxants, antihistamines, and local anesthetics. Analgesics, corticosteroids, and anxiolytics are useful for the treatment of acute pain associated with TMD, whereas anti-inflammatory medications and antidepressants are primarily indicated for chronic pain management. Muscle relaxants, nonsteroidal anti-inflammatory drugs (NSAIDs), and local anesthetics can be used for both acute and chronic pain management.

Analgesics

Analgesic medications are available as either opiate or nonopiate preparations. Nonopiate analgesics (salicylates and acetaminophen) can be added to the anti-inflammatory regimen to assist in pain relief. The salicylates (acetylsalicylic acid [ASA]) are commonly used in TMD and are the benchmark medications to which other analgesics are usually compared. Salicylates are antipyretic, analgesic, and anti-inflammatory. For those patients who cannot take aspirin, a nonacetylated aspirin such as choline magnesium trisali-

cylate, or salsalate, may be effective. As with all salicylates, however, choline magnesium trisalicylate and salsalate should not be prescribed for children or teenagers with chickenpox, influenza, or flu symptoms or exposure. Opioid analgesics (oxycodone, propoxyphene, and hydrocodone) should be prescribed only for moderate to severe pain, and for a limited duration of treatment, owing to the high potential for addiction. These drugs are often administered in conjunction with NSAIDs or acetaminophen-containing drugs (e.g., Vicodin, Lortab, Percocet, or Darvocet). These medications act on opioid receptors in the central nervous system (CNS), producing analgesia and sedation. Because patients can become dependent rapidly on the narcotic analgesics, it is recommended that these drugs not be prescribed for longer than 2 to 3 weeks. Other side effects of this class of medications include constipation secondary to decreased gastrointestinal (GI) motility.

Anti-inflammatory Medications

Two types of anti-inflammatory medications are useful in treating TMD: NSAIDs and corticosteroids (Figure 48-1). Glucocorticoids prevent the release of arachidonic acid, a key

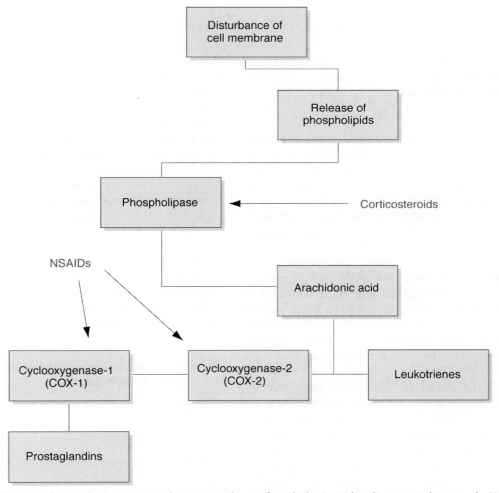

FIGURE 48-1. Arachidonic acid cascade. Corticosteroids prevent release of arachidonic acid and interrupt the cascade. Nonsteroidal anti-inflammatory drugs (NSAIDs) inhibit cyclooxygenase, which inhibits prostaglandin synthesis from arachidonic acid.

SECTION 6

TABLE 48-3. **Commonly Used Nonsteroidal Anti-inflammatory Agents**

Category	Generic	Brand	Half-Life (hr)
Salicylates	Acetylsalicylic acid (aspirin)	Bayer	2.5
	Enteric-coated	Ecotrin	2.5
	Aspirin with buffering agent	Bufferin	2.5
	Aspirin with caffeine	Anacin	2.5
	Diflunisal	Dolobid	8–12
	Choline magnesium trisalicylate	Trilisate	9–17
	Salsalate	Disalcid	16
Propionic acid	Ibuprofen	Motrin, Advil, Nuprin, Rufen	1.8–2.5
	Fenoprofen	Nalfon	2–3
	Suprofen	Suprol	2–4
	Naproxen	Naprosyn	12–15
	Naproxen sodium	Anaprox	12–15
Acetic acid	Indomethacin	Indocin	4.5–6
	Sulindac	Clinoril	7.8 (16.4)*
	Tolmetin	Tolectin	1–1.5
Fenamic acid	Meclofenamate	Meclomen	2 (3.3)*
	Mefenamic acid	Ponstel	2
Pyrazolones	Phenylbutazone	Butazolidin	84
Oxicam	Piroxicam olamine	Feldene	30–86
COX-2 inhibitor	Celecoxib	Celebrex	11–12

COX-2 = cyclooxygenase-2.
*Active metabolite.
Adapted from Syrop SB. Pharmacological therapy. In Kaplan AS, Assael LA, editors. Temporomandibular Disorders—Diagnosis and Treatment. Philadelphia: WB Saunders; 1991; pp. 501–514.

component of the inflammatory cascade, whereas NSAIDs inhibit cyclooxygenase (COX), which inhibits prostaglandin synthesis from arachidonic acid.[16–18]

NSAIDs

The advantages of NSAIDs in TMD management result from their combined analgesic and anti-inflammatory properties (Tables 48-3 and 48-4). NSAIDs may offer relief for patients with synovitis, myositis, capsulitis, symptomatic disk displacement, and osteoarthritis.[19] This form of drug therapy helps to alleviate the inflammation, which thereby causes a decrease in pain perception. Typical side effects of NSAIDs include gastric irritation, allergies, and liver dysfunction. An ideal NSAID would be one that has minimal gastric effects, a quick onset with a long duration of action, low dosage requirements; is tolerated well even at high plasma drug levels; and is low in cost. NSAIDs are divided into seven groups based on their chemical structure: ASA, propionic acids (ibuprofen, naproxen), acetic acids (indomethacin, ketorolac), fenamic acids (meclofenamate), oxicams (piroxicam), and the COX-2 inhibitors (celecoxib [Celebrex] and rofecoxib [Vioxx was removed from the market in 2004]). The most common NSAIDs used are ibuprofen, diclofenac, and naproxen, but because of fewer GI side effects and minimal effect on platelets, COX-2 inhibitors became popular alternatives, although the potential significant cardiovascular effects (increase in thromboxane leading to thrombosis, myocardial infarction, stroke) need to be considered. Several studies have found that COX-2, an important inflammatory mediator, is present in the TMJ synovial tissue and synovial fluid of patients with internal derangement of the TMJ. This suggests that the COX-2 inhibitors may be more effective for TMJ pain and arthralgia than other analgesics.[20,21] A variety of methods may be used to reduce gastric irritation from NSAIDs including the use of enteric coating; use of prodrugs (nabumetone [Relafen]), taking the NSAID with, or after, meals, or in conjunction with antacids; and using gastric protective agents (ranitidine and sucralfate).[22] One typical initial pharmacologic regimen for the patient with TMD may include ibuprofen (Motrin, Advil) 400 to 600 mg orally four times daily (maximum dose, 3200 mg/day), with meals for a period of 3 weeks, with reassessment.

Corticosteroids

Corticosteroids result in the complete blockage of the arachidonic acid cascade, producing a more pronounced anti-inflammatory response than NSAIDs. Systemic steroids are indicated only for short-term therapy (5–7 days) owing to their long-term possible complications, including osteoporo-

TABLE 48-4. **Ideal Nonsteroidal Anti-inflammatory Drug Properties**

Minimal gastrointestinal irritation
Rapid onset
Long duration of action
Lower dosage for effect
Favorable therapeutic index
Well-tolerated at high serum levels
Readily available
Low cost

TABLE 48-5. **Commonly Used Benzodiazepines**

Generic	Brand	Usual Dosage (mg/day)	Elimination (Half-Life [hr])
Alprazolam	Xanax	0.5–1.5 (ddd)	12–15
Chlordiazepoxide	Librium	15–60 (ddd)	5–30
Diazepam	Valium	2–40 (ddd)	20–50
Flurazepam	Dalmane	30 (at bedtime)	47–100
Lorazepam	Ativan	2–6 (ddd)	10–18
Oxazepam	Serax	30–60 (ddd)	5–15
Prazepam	Verstran	20–40 (ddd)	30–100
Temazepam	Restoril	15–30 (at bedtime)	10–20
Triazolam	Halcion	0.25–0.5 (at bedtime)	1.5–5

ddd = divided daily doses
Adapted from Syrop SB. Pharmacological therapy. In Kaplan AS, Assael LA, editors. Temporomandibular Disorders—Diagnosis and Treatment. Philadelphia: WB Saunders; 1991; pp. 501–514.

sis, diabetes, hypertension, electrolyte abnormalities, and clinical Cushing's disease.[23] Steroid preparations have been directly injected into the TMJ in an attempt to decrease inflammation or mediate the inflammatory response (e.g., after arthrocentesis or arthroscopy), but long-term, or excessive, use is associated with condylar hypoplasia through inhibition of chondroblastic activity and increasing loss of calcium in the urine and GI tract.[24]

Anxiolytics

Anxiolytic medications reduce the anxiety, insomnia, and muscle hyperactivity associated with TMD (Tables 48-5 and 48-6). These drugs often help the patient reduce the perception of, or reaction to, stress. Benzodiazepines (e.g., diazepam) decrease anxiety, relax skeletal muscle, and cause sedation and may be preferable owing to their more desirable characteristics (e.g., less associated sedation). The muscle relaxant properties may be used to decrease the effects of bruxism secondary to hyperactivity of muscles of mastication. It is recommended

TABLE 48-6. **Antianxiety Medications: Benzodiazepines**

GABA receptors agonists
5-HT agonists in the amygdala
Useful for anxiety, insomnia, muscle hypertactivity
High abuse potential
Avoid short-acting or high-potency drugs (triazolam, alprazolam, lorazepam)
Taper gradually to avoid withdrawal, rebound anxiety

GABA = γ-aminobutyric acid; 5-HT = 5-hydroxytryptamine (serotonin).

that the benzodiazepines not be used for more than a 2-week period because of the high potential for dependency, although this length of time may be increased up to 3 weeks only at bedtime to control bruxism.[19] Buspar (azaspirode-canedione) is an anxiolytic drug; however, it does not produce either sedation or muscle relaxation, and it may be used to control anxiety in TMD patients without producing drowsiness.

Antihistamines

Antihistamines (promethazine and hydroxyzine) antagonize central and peripheral H_1 receptors and have a sedative effect as well as anxiolytic properties. Antihistamines, unlike the benzodiazepines, do not have the potential for abuse. They can be used more safely in children and the elderly and for the treatment of vertigo and nausea that may accompany TMD.[25]

Antidepressants

Antidepressants that are useful in the management of TMD include monoamine oxidase inhibitors (MAOIs), tricyclic antidepressants (TCAs), and selective serotonin reuptake inhibitors (SSRIs; Tables 48-7 and 48-8). They are prescribed for chronic pain, headaches, sleep disorders, obsessive-compulsive disorders, and central-mediated pain disorders. The relationship between pain and depression is a challenge that often necessitates treatment of both of these clinical entities simultaneously. Depression in the TMD or chronic pain population is greater than in the general population, and studies report that up to 30% of TMD patients have major

TABLE 48-7. **Commonly Used Antidepressants**

Generic	Brand	Dosage (mg/day)	Side Effects
Amitriptyline	Elavil	10–300	High
Desipramine	Norpramin	50–300	Moderate
Doxepin	Sinequan	25–300	High
Imipramine	Tofranil	20–300	Moderate
Nortriptyline	Pamelor, Aventyl	25–150	Moderate
Fluoxetine	Prozac	5–20	Moderate

TABLE 48-8. **Antidepressant Medications**

Tricyclics antidepressants are most commonly used for chronic pain and depression.
MAOIs have many adverse reactions.
SSRIs (fluoxetine [Prozac]) may increase anxiety, bruxism.

MAOIs = monoamine oxidase inhibitors; SSRIs = selective serotonin reuptake inhibitors.

depression at the time of presentation for TMD treatment and up to 74% of patients with chronic TMD have had at least one episode of major depression.[26,27]

MAOIs are not routinely prescribed for TMD owing to the numerous side effects, drug interactions, and dietary restrictions. The benefits of TCAs have been well documented in chronic pain or depression populations and are probably due to analgesic and antidepressant actions. The analgesic properties are independent of the antidepressant effect, which requires higher doses, and it has been shown that low doses of amitriptyline (amitriptyline [Elavil] 10 mg) before sleep can have an analgesic effect on chronic pain but have no relationship to the antidepressant actions that require doses up to 20 times greater.[28] TCAs may also help treat nocturnal bruxism and any sleep disturbance associated with TMD,[29] and the side effects of TCAs are related to anticholinergic activity causing xerostomia, constipation, blurred vision, and urinary retention. SSRIs can also be used for treating the TMD patient with depression. These medications often need to be taken for several months and patients must be counseled appropriately; fluoxetine (Prozac) may, in fact, increase bruxism and anxiety and should be carefully monitored.

Muscle Relaxants

Centrally acting muscle relaxants (cyclobenzaprine, methocarbamol, and carisoprodol) may be used to relax a hyperactive musculature associated with TMD (Tables 48-9 to 48-11). These relaxants may also act as sedatives, and they are commonly combined with the use of NSAIDs. Cyclobenzaprine (Flexeril) has a similar chemical structure to the TCAs and, if given over an extended period of time, will produce antidepressant and sedative actions, as well as the anticholinergic side effects of the TCAs. Central muscle relaxants can be very effective for acute myofascial pain (e.g., secondary to trauma). Baclofen, a peripheral muscle relaxant, has been used in myofascial pain but is most appropriately reserved for severe muscle spasm or neurogenic pain. Botulinum toxin has been used to treat severe bruxism, and by providing muscle relaxation, inflammation of the masseter muscle and TMJ capsule may be reduced.[30,31]

Local Anesthetics

Local anesthetics act on the nerve cell membrane to prevent generation and conduction of impulses (Table 48-12). Local anesthetics can be used as diagnostic blocks intra-articularly and/or intramuscularly to alleviate pain and increase range of motion. For example, local anesthetic injection posterior to the maxillary tuberosity will anesthetize the lateral pterygoid muscles, which if in spasm, will allow maximal protrusion of the mandible without pain. A local anesthetic without vasoconstrictor should be used, because the decrease in blood flow may exacerbate muscular pain. The intrinsic vasodilatory effect of the local anesthesia may improve vascular tissue perfusion and, thereby, further alleviate pain. It has been shown that an intra-articular injection of mepivacaine, along with physiotherapy in patients with TMJ internal derangement (anterior disk displacement), results in pain relief and improved masticatory efficiency.[32]

Physical Therapy

Many factors contribute to limited range of mandibular motion, including muscular pain or spasm, anterior disk displacement (closed lock), pathologic lesions, traumatic injuries (e.g., mandible or zygoma fracture), and bony or fibrous

TABLE 48-9. **Commonly Used Muscle Relaxants**

Generic	Brand	Usual Dosage (mg/day; divided doses)
Carisoprodol	Rela, Soma	1000–1400
Chlorzoxazone	Paraflex, Parafon Forte D.S.C.	750–3000
Meprobamate	Miltown, Equanil	1200–1600
Methocarbamol	Robaxin	1500–4500
Cyclobenzaprine	Flexeril	5–30
Orphenadrine	Norflex, Disipal	150–300
Diazepam	Valium	2–40
Combination Fixed Dosage		
Meprobamate Aspirin	Equagesic	1–2 tablets three or four times daily
Orphenadrine Aspirin Caffeine	Norgesic	1–2 tablets three or four times daily

Adapted from Syrop SB. Pharmacological therapy. In Kaplan AS, Assael LA, editors. Temporomandibular Disorders—Diagnosis and Treatment. Philadelphia: WB Saunders; 1991; pp. 501–514.

TABLE 48-10. **Central Muscle Relaxants**

Central Muscle Relaxants
Carisoprodol (Rela, Soma)
Chlorzoxazone (Paraflex)
Methocarbamol (Robaxin)
Cyclobenzaprine (Flexeril)

Effects
Tranquilizing effects
General sedative effect on central nervous system
No specific neurotransmitter
No effect on skeletal muscle, motor endplate, or nerve fiber

TABLE 48-11. **Peripheral Muscle Relaxants**

Peripheral Muscle Relaxants
Baclofen (lioresal) derivative of GABA that blocks spinal cord contraction; reserved for severe muscle spasm, or neurogenic pain
Botulinum toxin (Botox) is useful for management of oromandibular dystonia

Effects
Block synaptic transmission at neuromuscular junction
Block muscle contraction

GABA = γ-aminobutyric acid.

ankylosis preventing rotatory and/or translational movements of the mandible. It is well known that prolonged jaw immobilization may have deleterious effects on both the TM joints and the facial muscles. Immobilization may cause degenerative cartilagenous and osseous changes to the articulating joint surfaces, significant synovial fluid alterations, and changes to the surrounding tissues. Prolonged reduced jaw motion results in rapid muscle fatigue, muscle weakness, and fibrous tissue contractures. The health and nourishment of the synovium depend upon normal joint function, and synovial fluid generation is reduced, or halted, when the TMJs are immobile. In addition, it has been observed that the synovial fluid of patients with TMD pain and limited jaw motion often contains a variety of inflammatory byproducts demonstrated by synovial fluid analysis (SFA). Kaneyama and colleagues[33] listed a variety of cytokines, such as interleukin (IL)-1β, tumor necrosis factor (TNF)-α, IL-6, and IL-8 in symptomatic TMJs, that were not observed in asymptomatic TMJs. This high level of cytokine activity in SFA is believed to be related to the underlying inflammatory pathogenesis of TMD, because cytokines such as IL-6 and IL-1β may induce the "inflammatory cascade." As a result of the release of selective proteinases, there may be destruction of articular cartilage and underlying osseous destruction. Each cytokine

TABLE 48-12. **Local Anesthetics**

Act on nerve cell membrane to prevent generation and conduction of impulses.
Useful for diagnostic blocks.
Muscular injections to increase range of movement.

TABLE 48-13. **Physical Therapy**

Home Treatment Program (For Mild Acute Symptoms)
Soft diet
Jaw rest (decreased jaw function)
Heat and ice packs
Jaw/tongue posture opening exercises
Lateral jaw movement exercises
Controlled passive jaw motion exercises (Therabite)

Office Treatment (For Reduction of Pain and Inflammation)
Ultrasonography
TENS
Range of motion exercises
Soft tissue manipulation procedures
Trigger point injections
Acupuncture (± electric current or heat applied to acupuncture needles)

TENS = transcutaneous electrical nerve stimulation.

has unique properties that not only affect the surrounding tissues but also aid in the release of other cytokines.[33] As a result, the role of functional mobility on the synovium may be an indeterminate factor in the overall health of the TMJs (Table 48-13).

Exercise Therapy

Physical therapy and exercise are important components of any TMD program. Initial, mild, or acute symptoms can be managed with soft diet, jaw rest, alternating heat and ice packs, jaw/tongue posture opening exercises, lateral jaw movements, and passive stretching exercises. Once again, the precise sequence of exercise therapy is determined on an individual basis as well as the experience of the clinican or physical therapist and is usually based upon the chronicity of the problem, the degree of pain, and the magnitude of limitation of jaw function. Further reduction of pain and inflammation may require an office-based physical therapy program. Ultrasonography, transcutaneous electrical nerve stimulation (TENS), soft tissue manipulation, trigger point injections, iontophoresis, and acupuncture have also been advocated as effective in the management of the TMD patient.

Jaw exercise therapy can be described as passive, active, or isometric. *Passive jaw exercise* allows the patient to manually, or with a device such as Therabite Jaw Motion Rehabilitation System (Atos Medical, Milwaukee, WI), progressively increase interincisal opening (Figure 48-2). Passive jaw exercise has received a great deal of attention, and many authors have reported significant reduction in pain and improvement jaw mobility during the nonsurgical phase of TMD treatment, as well as for the postoperative care after surgical intervention (arthrocentesis, arthrocopsy, or open TMJ surgery).[34–37] Passive jaw exercise is also very effective for patients who experience muscular-associated trismus and myofascial pain and dysfunction (MPD). Jaw exercises should be used with caution or may be contraindicated in patients with severe TMJ disk displacement without reduction owing to the possibility of further damage to the disk or

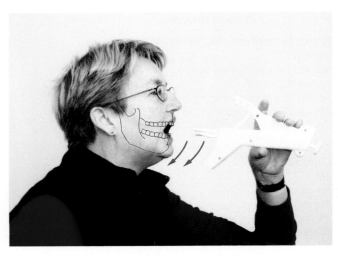

FIGURE 48-2.   Passive jaw exercise device. (TheraBite, Atos Medical, Milwaukee, WI.)

retrodiskal tissues, and the physical therapist should be made aware of any limitations to physiotherapy.

Active jaw exercises, which are initiated by the patient's jaw musculature as opposed to a jaw opening device that allows the muscles to be "passive," may be incorporated into a home therapy program for TMD. One regimen allows the patient to activate, for example, the suprahyoid muscles (geniohyoid, mylohyoid, digastric, and stylohyoid), thereby inactivating the elevators of the jaw (medial pterygoid, masseter, temporalis). This may allow for relaxation of hyperactive muscles of mastication and may assist in increasing maximal interincisal opening. In the active stretch phase, patients are advised to keep their mouth open for several seconds and then relax the muscles. They are instructed to open their mouth until just before they perceive pain, and then to hold for several seconds, and repeat this exercise several times a day, with a gradual increase in the magnitude of mouth opening. An active lateral stretch exercise, which permits the contralateral lateral pterygoid to be stretched, may be accomplished by visualizing the movements in a mirror. In the active protrusion exercise, also performed in front of the mirror, the mandible is protruded forward while stretching the lateral pterygoid muscles bilaterally. All active movements or excursions are maintained for several seconds, and then slowly released, in order to effect a physiologic "stretch" of the muscles.

Isometric exercises have been recommended for patients with severe pain and trismus, and there is no movement during isometrics while the depressor muscles are activated, allowing for relaxation of the opposing elevator musculature (medial pterygoid, masseter, and temporalis). These exercises are typically performed by holding the mandible in a stationary position as the muscles are activated isometrically. The lateral pterygoid muscles may also be exercised in a similar isometric fashion.

Mongini[38] describes a three-stage office technique for mandibular manipulation in patients with pain, decreased mobility, and disk displacement without reduction. Right and left lateral movements are actively initiated by the patient. The patient continues the movement while the clinician applies light pressure in the same direction, and in the last stage of the technique, the mandible is moved to the opposite side with patient assistance.[38] Kurita and associates[39] described a technique of placing one thumb on the last molar on the affected side while the other hand supports the head in the temporal region. The mandible is then moved downward and forward, while the patient is instructed to protrude and move the jaw laterally, and open the mouth while the clinician manipulates the jaw. After this movement, the mandible is manipulated posteriorly so that the condyle is positioned in a posterosuperior position within the glenoid fossa. Only 18% of the patients received significant benefit from the manipulation, and the more advanced the disk displacement the lower the success of the treatment.[39] Yuasa and Kurita[40] suggested that physical therapy, along with administration of NSAIDs (for a 4-wk period), is a more effective way to treat TMJ disk displacement without associated osseous changes. Nevertheless, there is no shortage of recommended jaw exercises, and care must be taken to first do no harm (Table 48-14).

Thermal Agents

Thermal treatment modalities are often incorporated into the management of the patient with TMD. The use of both cold and heat can alleviate muscle pain and play an equal role during jaw stretching and muscle strengthening exercises.[41-43] Heat therapy has been reported to reduce muscle pain by increasing nerve conduction velocity and causing local vasodilation and increased blood flow, thereby clearing out local inflammatory mediators.[43] Superficial heat therapy can be implemented with conductive (gel-type heat packs, paraffin, whirlpool) or radiant (infrared) modalities. The most common types of heat used include a moist hot washcloth, heating pad, or hydrocollator, a pad filled with clay and heated in a water bath to 70°C to 88°C, or a commercially available gel pack that can be used in either a hot or a cold mode. The heat pack chosen is placed on the site (e.g., over the masseter muscle) for 15 to 20 minutes, causing a transient rise in skin temperature to approximately 42°C. The use of a moist, as opposed to dry heat, heating pad (gel pack)

TABLE 48-14. **Manual Physical Therapy**

Soft tissue techniques.
Massage, relaxation, stimulation, release of adhesions, muscle stretching.
Manipulative therapy, cervical spine realignment (chiropractics).
Rapid, passive, short duration, and amplitude thrusting forces to position the TMJ beyond its normal limits.
Patient has no control over treatments.
Pain relief is immediate, but transient.

TMJ = temporomandibular joint.

appears to be an effective modality of treatment for myofascial pain associated with TMD.[44]

Cryotherapy is often used by physical therapists as an aid in muscle stretching exercises in an attempt to increase jaw opening that is limited by muscular pain.[41] The pain perception model described by Melzack and Wall[43] explains why cold therapy stimulates the small myelinated A-delta fibers responsible for thermal discrimination and inhibits pain perception, which is mediated by the small unmyelinated C fibers. A physical therapist typically applies refrigerant sprays superficially on the skin surface in a sweeping motion followed by active stretching of the jaw musculature. Cold therapy should be used with caution because of the potential for increased joint stiffness, muscle contracture, and decreased jaw mobility. Cold can also have analgesic effects when applied immediately after a therapeutic exercise regimen. Ice wrapped in a towel, fluoromethane spray, and reusable ice packs can all be used to deliver cryotherapy to the TMJ and related facial and neck muscles. The "stretch and spray technique," initially described by Modell and Simons,[42] and later modified by Travell and Simons,[41] remains a mainstay of office physiotherapy. The therapist holds the fluoromethane spray approximately 30 to 45 cm from the patient and sprays in a sweeping motion multiple times; this is then followed by active jaw stretching exercises. Possible side effects include superficial skin frostbite and, as mentioned, the potential for increased joint stiffness limiting the jaw exercise regimen. Many physical therapists follow the cryotherapy sprays with moist heat to prevent the jaw muscles from undesirable contracture.

Ultrasonograpy and Phonophoresis

Deep heat may also be delivered by ultrasonography or phonophoresis. The ultrasound machine operates above audible frequency sound waves (0.75–1.0 MHz), which convert to heat while traveling through the soft tissues. The ultrasound probe is applied to the skin using an acoustic conductive gel, then moved slowly over the affected area in small, circular movements. The operator must be careful not to keep the machine in one place for too long as it may cause overheating of the connective tissue, causing structural damage. The deep heat is intended to increase blood perfusion to the area via vasodilation, clearance of inflammatory mediators from the area, decreasing pain and increasing jaw mobility.[45] Reported effects of ultrasound therapy include altered cell membrane permeability, intracellular fluid absorption, decreased collagen viscosity, vasodilation, and analgesia. The beneficial effects to joints include reduced capsular contracture, breakdown of local calcium deposits, and decreased hyaluronic acid viscosity of the joint synovial fluid with improved mobility.[46] Because ultrasonography delivers heat to the deeper soft tissues, it may have some advantages over the superficial heat delivery techniques mentioned previously in managing tendinitis, capsulitis, muscle spasm, and tight, or restricted, ligaments.

Phonophoresis is an application of ultrasound heat therapy that incorporates a pad filled with a steroid or anesthetic cream that is placed over the affected area. As the ultrasound waves are applied, the medications perfuse into the tissues. The most common indication for phonophoresis is synovitis associated with painful jaw hypomobility. Contraindications for the use of ultrasonography and phonophoresis include areas that may have a reduced blood circulation, fluid-filled organs, eyes, radiation therapy sites, and malignant tissues, and ultrasound therapy should be used with caution over active bone growth centers.[47]

Electrical Stimulation (TENS)

TENS has become a viable home therapy option in the management of TMD. The precise mechanism of action is unknown, although it has been suggested that the gate control theory, counterirritation, neurohumoral substance release, and peripheral blockade mechanisms are all involved.[48] TENS uses a low-voltage electrical current that is designed for sensory counterstimulation in painful disorders. It is used in an attempt to decrease muscle pain and hyperactivity and for neuromuscular reeducation.[49,50] TENS units are small and portable, and the electrodes are placed along specific dermatomes or over acupuncture and trigger point sites. The patient can control the settings with variable frequency, amplitude, waveform, width, and pulse modes. Treatment may last for several hours and relies on biofeedback from the patient in the control of the specific delivery of the stimulation. TENS emits an asymmetrical biphasic wave of 100- to 500-msec pulse. The efficacy of TENS for analgesia and muscle relaxation in myofascial pain has been well documented.[51] Electrode placement is contraindicated over the carotid sinus, transcranially, directly over the cervical spine, on a pregnant abdomen, or on patients with demand-type pacemakers.[52]

HIGH-VOLTAGE STIMULATION

High-voltage stimulation units deliver currents of positive and negative polarity with voltages greater than 100 V, which may be administered in a constant, or intermittent, pattern. The positive polarity produces vasoconstriction, whereas the negative polarity produces vasodilation. The positive polarity reduces nerve irritability, and negative polarity enhances nerve conduction and also softens the affected soft tissues, thereby decreasing muscle tension or spasm. Treatment with high-voltage stimulation has been shown to improve jaw mobility and relieve pain intensity in TMD patients.[53] It can also be used for pain relief, reduction of edema, and neuromuscular stimulation.[53]

Iontophoresis

Iontophoresis and phonophoresis are techniques that are capable of enhancing drug penetration through the skin. As mentioned previously, phonophoresis uses ultrasonic waves to transmit molecules of drug through the skin, whereas iontophoresis uses low-level electric current. Iontophoresis transfers ions from a solution through intact skin by passing a direct current between two electrodes.[54] Positive ions are transmitted at the cathode, and negative ions are transmitted at the anode. Examples of negatively ionizing drugs are

SECTION 6

TENS.
Phontophoresis: ultrasound heat drives drugs (steroids, anesthetic crème) into tissues.
Iontophoresis: electric current drives drugs into tissues.
High-volume stimulation (100 V): pumping effects of muscle contraction increase circulation.

TENS = transcutaneous electrical nerve stimulation.

TABLE 48-16. **Behavioral Therapy**

Components of Behavioral Therapy
Patient education in recognition of stress, anxiety, and depression
Relaxation training programs
Biofeedback exercises
Self-hypnosis techniques
Meditation techniques
Cognitive therapy programs

Types of Behavioral Therapy
Psychiatric therapy
Pain clinic management

dexamethasone and methylprednisolone. Other drugs used in iontophoresis include lidocaine and salicylates. Iontophoresis was introduced in treating TMD and postherpetic neuralgia in 1982.[55] It appears to be most effective against inflammation, muscle spasm, and calcium deposits. The deep penetration of the medication also aids in the treatment of severe joint inflammation and pain (Table 48-15).

Trigger Point and Muscle Injections

A trigger point is an area of hyperirritability in a tissue that, when compressed, is locally tender and hypersensitive and results in referred pain and tenderness.[56] The development of trigger points may be due to trauma, sustained contraction or spasm, or acute muscle strain. When a needle penetrates this area, it may cause a twitch response and referred pain.[56] Injection of local anesthetic agents without epinephrine may cause a temporary anesthesia, which enables the clinician to stretch the muscles maximally in the affected area. A vasodilator effect of the local anesthetic may improve vascular perfusion to the area, thereby allowing harmful metabolites or inflammatory mediators, which may induce pain, to be more readily removed by the increased blood flow to the area.

Stress-Reduction Techniques

Relaxation and Biofeedback

Relaxation and stress-reduction techniques for patients with TMD can be very effective treatment modalities. A wide variety of techniques exist, and these typically involve a coordinated sequence of skeletal muscle contracture and release, beginning with the feet and proceeding cranially toward the head and neck region. Patients may also use audiotapes that attempt to train certain synchronized breathing patterns as well as specific relaxation techniques. Biofeedback techniques may incorporate the use of electromyography (EMG) and skin temperature to measure the patient's physiologic function and response to treatment. This information is then conveyed back to the patient by a meter or sound, so that the patient can gauge the level of relaxation, adjust the level of relaxation, and measure progress accordingly.[57] The aim is to achieve psychological self-regulation and to monitor the relationship between muscular tension and pain. In a review of the literature, Crider and Glaros[58] reported 69% of subjects rated their symptoms as improved, or symptom-free, after biofeedback and relaxation treatments, whereas only 35% of patients receiving placebo intervention showed improvement. Furthermore, on follow-up

examination, the patients showed no decline from immediate post-treatment levels of improvement.[58] Scott and Gregg[59] advocate that relaxation techniques and EMG feedback can yield good results, especially in patients who have no clinical depression and have had TMJ pain for only a short period of time. The major limitation of the use of these techniques is the difficulty required to motivate patients with pain to engage in jaw exercise regimens (Table 48-16).

Acupressure and Acupuncture

Acupressure and acupuncture are alternative treatment options that may be implemented along with other treatment modalities during the course of nonsurgical treatment for TMD. Acupuncture uses the relationship between energy flow through meridians, natural elements, and positive and negative life forces. Fine needles are used to reestablish proper energy flow in these areas. There are several theories regarding the mechanism of action of acupuncture and acupressure. The first proposed mechanism is the gate control theory, which states that the needle produces a painless stimulation, causing neuronal gates to close and prevent signal propagation of pain to the spinal cord.[60] Other explanations include the release of endorphins from the pituitary gland, which blocks pain sensation, promotion of alpha waves (associated with stress reduction and relaxation), and rebalancing the electric ion flow pattern, which when disrupted, may elicit pain.[60] There are several different acupressure techniques including Jin Shin (two acupressure points held for 30 sec–5 min), Shiatsu (more rapid techqniue, held for 3–10 sec), reflexology (acupressure on feet, hands, and ears corresponding to areas of the body), Do-In (self-acupressure and breathing exercises), and G-Jo (acupressure for first aid purposes). Some studies have reported favorable results when these techniques are combined with other modalities (e.g., occlusal splint therapy), but overall data are limited,[61,62] and therefore, these alternative therapies may be offered as an adjunct to more conventional well-established therapeutic options for TMD management.

Psychotherapy

In some cases, TMD may be the somatic expression of an underlying psychiatric or psychological disorder such as depression or conversion syndrome.[63,64] The clinician should screen for a personal or familial history of psychiatric disease, physical or sexual abuse, and substance abuse. Anxiety disorders occur much more commonly in patients with chronic pain syndromes.[65] Once a psychiatric component is identified, patients should be referred for psychiatric consultation for adjunctive treatment of these contributing factors. Psychological treatments may include behavioral therapy, cognitive-behavioral therapy, and self-management/support groups. Psychiatric treatments may also include pharmacotherapy along with behavioral therapy. In many cases, the TMD patient may be referred to specialized pain centers for assessment and management, especially when long-term pharmacologic therapy is indicated or when other nonsurgical methods have failed to improve the symptoms and the patient is not a surgical candidate.

Occlusal Appliance Therapy

An occlusal bite appliance is a removable device, usually made of hard acrylic, which is custom fit over the occlusal surfaces of the mandibular or, more commonly, the maxillary teeth. The splint is constructed so that there is bilateral symmetrical posterior occlusal contacts with the teeth of the opposing arch in centric occlusion (flat plane splint), or there may be anterior contacts in lateral and protrusive excursions of the mandible (anterior repositioning splint). The physiologic basis of treatment is not well understood, but the effectiveness of the occlusal splint has been attributed to a decreased loading on the TMJs and reduction of the neuromuscular reflex activitivation. Alleviation of bruxism and MPD may be due to the change in the vertical dimension of occlusion that alters proprioception in the postural position of the mandible.[66–68] There are generally two types of appliances: stabilization, or flat-plane devices, and anterior repositioning splints.

Stabilization (Flat-Plane) Appliance

A stabilization appliance covers all the teeth in one arch, typically the maxilla, and is indicated to relax the muscles of mastication, aid in joint stability, and protect teeth from bruxism (Table 48-17 and Figures 48-3 and 48-4).[68,69] Additional indications for stabilization appliances may include myalgia, inflammation, and retrodiskitis secondary to trauma. Commonly, stabilization devices are used for several weeks after arthrocentesis and arthroscopy procedures

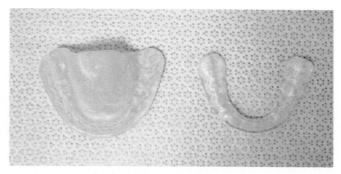

FIGURE 48-3.   Stabilization appliance. Hard acrylic full-coverage occlusal splint.

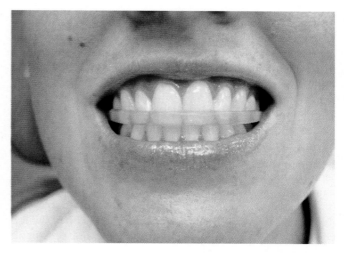

FIGURE 48-4.   Maxillary hard acrylic stabilization appliance does not alter anterior/posterior jaw position.

and after open joint surgery as well. With a stabilization appliance, the condyles are repositioned into the most muscularly stable position, while the teeth have even symmetrical bilateral simultaneous contacts.[70] There must be bilateral equal posterior contacts so that an environment of stable physiologic posture is achievable. Canine guidance may be created during protrusive and lateral excursions, or there may be anterior disocclusion during these jaw movements, depending upon the prexisting occlusal realtionships. As the patient's symptoms improve, the bite splint should be continually adjusted to maintain even contacts bilaterally. Many practicioners often prefer the splint to be fabricated on the maxillary arch because it covers more enamel area, especially with class II or class III patients in whom fabrication of a mandibular appliance can be difficult. The major advantages of a mandibular stabilization appliance, over a maxillary splint, are better speech and less visibility, which may contribute to improved patient compliance with the therapy.[70] The appliance should be worn up to 24 hr/day and may or may not be taken out at mealtimes, because this is the time when masticatory forces and TMJ stresses are at the highest levels. In general, stabilization appliances

TABLE 48-17.   **Occlusal Appliances: Stabilization Appliance**

Hard acrylic flat-plane device
Full coverage maxillary occlusal arch
Worn 24 hr/day (± during meals)
Bilateral even distribution of occlusal forces
Provides stabilization of the TMJ apparatus
Relaxation of masticatory muscles

TMJ = temporomandibular joint.

should be weaned as soon as possible after symptoms improve, or after arthrocentesis or arthroscopy procedures, in order to prevent dental movements and the development of iatrogenic malocclusions.

Major and Nebbe[71] reported effective reduction in headaches and muscle pain using stabilization appliances, but occlusal stabilization appliances have limited value in reducing joint pain. Lundh and coworkers[72] concurred that the stabilization splints have little value in relieving painful disk displacement without reduction. Kai and colleagues[73] reported that after treatment with a stabilization occlusal splint on the maxillary arch, clinical signs and symptoms of nonreducing anteriorly displaced TMJ disks decreased but osteoarthritic radiographic findings increased.

Anterior Repositioning Appliance

The anterior repositioning splint is an interocclusal appliance that guides the mandible into a more anterior position than usual during mandibular protrusion (Table 48-18 and Figures 48-5 and 48-6). The purpose of these appliances is to alter the structural condyle-disk-fossa relationship in an effort to decrease TMJ loading.[74] Indications for this device are primarily anatomic internal disk derangement disorders. The maxillary appliance is preferred, and it is fabricated with a guide ramp that permits gradual anterior repositioning of the mandible.[73] Anterior repositioning appliances are used less frequently because repositioning of the mandible over a period of time can result in irreversible occlusal changes such as posterior open bites, which could require extensive dental restorative and prosthetic rehabilitation.

Occlusal Adjustment

There is a limited role and lack of supporting evidence for occlusal adjustment or selective enamel grinding in the treatment of TMD.[75] The purpose of selective occlusal adjustment is to permanently reposition the dentition into a better occlusal relationship. This is an irreversible process and is most appropriately utilized for acute TMD symptoms that arise from recent dental treatment resulting in overcontoured dental restorations or after orthognathic surgery with isolated areas of occlusal interferences. In these select cases, occlusal equilibration may allow for proper condylar positioning and prevents reflexive muscular problems associated with improper dental interferences.

TABLE 48-18. **Occlusal Appliances: Anterior Repositioning Appliance**

Hard acrylic device.
Maxillary or mandibular occlual coverage splint with anterior inclined plane.
During jaw closure, mandible moves anteriorly.
Useful for anteriorly displaced disk to change condylar position and recapture disk.
Possible need for occlusal equilibration and splint readjustment.

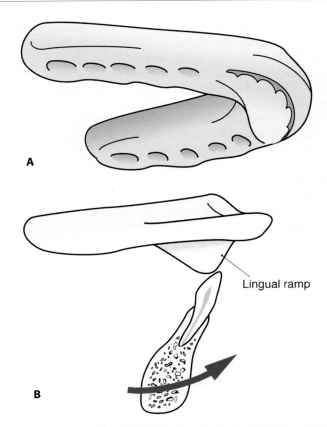

FIGURE 48-5. **A,** Maxillary repositioning appliance. **B,** Lingual ramp engages the mandibular incisors to reposition the lower jaw anteriorly.

Additional Strategies

As mentioned, the concept that nonsurgical therapy is employed solely as an alternative to surgical intervention is flawed, and more accurately, the techniques described should be used whether surgical intevention is indicated or not, in an attempt to resolve the signs and symptoms of TMD. Two clinically relevant examples help to illustrate this philosophy

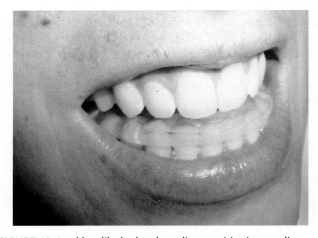

FIGURE 48-6. Mandibular hard acrylic repositioning appliance may alter anterior/posterior jaw position.

of treatment: the use of preemptive analgesia and the prevention of ectopic or heterotopic bone formation.

Preemptive Analgesia

Effective postsurgical pain control begins before the surgery itself, because it is recognized that methods that limit CNS neuronal activation by surgical stimulation may significantly reduce pain in the postsurgical period and may also reduce the possibility of development of some persistent pain syndromes. The term *preemptive analgesia* is used to describe methods that apparently reduce postsurgical pain by protecting the CNS from surgical stimulation. The concept is based upon observations that collectively indicate that nociceptive processing is a highly dynamic process. Nociception, and subsequent pathway sensitization, likely involves de novo protein synthesis and establishment of novel connections made by neurons in the affected pathway.[78-80] The old hypothesis that these pathways are merely static conductors of neural signals generated by noxious stimuli appears to be invalid because we know now that gene transcription is induced in stimulated neuronal populations.[81,82] Some neuropeptides that are translated from these genes may facilitate future neural activities by receptive field expansion or by facilitation of specific interneuronal interactions. The term *neuroplasticity* is often used to refer to the dynamic state of stimulated neural pathways. These, and perhaps other, more ominous changes (i.e., neuronal death from excessive stimulation), may be fundamental to the development of some chronic pain states. Fortunately, these CNS responses may be significantly attenuated by preemptive analgesic techniques.[79,83] From animal and clinical studies, there is evidence that protracted neural responses to painful stimuli can be modified or prevented by the following: (1) neural blockade with local anesthetics,[84-86] (2) administration of opioids,[87-91] (3) administration of *N*-methyl-D-aspartate receptor antagonists (e.g., MK801, ketamine, dextrophan),[92-94] or (4) administration of ketorolac, both a peripheral and a central-acting nonopioid analgesic.[95-97] These agents must be administered *before* noxious stimulation to prevent CNS changes that may be related to the development of postsurgical pain and perhaps persistent pain. It is interesting to note that a general anesthetic state does not prevent neuroplastic changes induced by surgical stimulation, unless the general anesthetic technique employs high-dose opioids or ketamine. Neural impulses from surgical stimulation apparently reach the CNS, evoking sensitization, despite the fact that overt signs of surgical stimulation (e.g., patient movement, elevated heart rate and systemic blood pressure) are blocked by general anesthesia. This stimulus-dependent neural sensitization, characterized by receptive field expansion and the "wind-up" phenomenon,[78,79] has been attributed to postsurgical hyperesthesia and pain. When regional anesthesia is employed as an adjunct to general anesthesia, there is strong evidence that postoperative pain is significantly reduced, and this is consistent with current models of central sensitization and neuroplasticity. However, to ensure that neural activities induced by surgical stimulation are fully blocked, the surgeon must administer regional anesthesia *before* surgical stimulation. If necessary during long procedures, the surgeon should reanesthetize the operative field, and not rely solely on a general anesthetic state for CNS protection. Jebeles and associates[98] studied the effects of preemptive regional anesthesia on postsurgical discomfort associated with tonsillectomy and adenoidectomy performed under general anesthesia. Twenty-two children were given either bupivacaine or saline infiltrations in the peritonsillar regions before surgical stimulation. For this study, postsurgical analgesics were standardized for all subjects and postsurgical pain was assessed over a 10-day period by three dependent measures: constant pain, pain evoked by swallowing a standard volume of water, and the time required to drink 100 mol of water based on the assumption that the rate-limiting factor for this activity is throat pain. All three dependent measures confirmed that subjects given bupivacaine regional anesthesia with general anesthesia experienced significantly less pain over a 10-day postsurgical period than the saline-injected group.[22] Other studies have provided similar evidence that regional anesthesia, provided before surgical stimulation, can significantly reduce pain after craniotomy and bone harvesting from the iliac crest.[99,100] To date, no research has documented the efficacy of preemptive regional anesthesia on postoperative pain, or on the subsequent development of chronic pain, in the operated patient with TMD. Nevertheless, existing evidence strongly suggests that the use of regional anesthesia as an adjunct to general anesthesia will significantly reduce postsurgical pain in this group of patients. Opioids administered *before* surgical stimulation may also reduce postsurgical hyperesthesia believed to be due to central sensitization. For example, isoflurane or isoflurane, and nitrous oxide, administered in a concentration sufficient to suppress cardiovascular responses to surgical stimuli (i.e., minimum alveolar concentration that blocks adrenergic responses [MACBAR]), do not inhibit formalin-induced hyperesthesia.[101] Formalin injected intradermally provides a potent noxious stimulus that results initially in a volley of neural activity that sensitizes central nociceptive neurons in the pathway. This observation reinforces previous studies indicating that general anesthesia alone does not offer protection against central sensitization. However, morphine administered *before* formalin injection significantly reduces postinjection hyperesthesia in this model.[101] In fact, a significant reduction in formalin-induced hyperesthesia was also observed even if morphine was reversed by naloxone shortly after the formalin injection was administered, indicating that even a brief exposure to an opioid before noxious stimulation is sufficient to prevent or significantly reduce stimulation-induced hyperesthesia.[101] Likewise, alfentanil reduces capsaicin-induced hyperalgesia in human subjects, but only if this agent is administered before capsaicin administration.[102] Capsaicin is a vanilloid extracted from chili peppers that is known to selectively stimulate C-fiber neurons expressing the vanilloid receptor (VR-1). Stimulation of C-fiber neurons by capsaicin administration produces receptive field expansion and hyperesthesia by mechanisms that involve central sensitization.[79] Notably, alfentanil did not effectively reduce pain scores, flare response, or secondary hyperalgesia when administered *after* an intradermal injection of capsaicin in these human studies.[102] These studies highlight the fact that as with regional anesthesia, opioids are only optimally effective as modulators of central sensitization and subsequent hyperalgesia if they are administered before surgical stimulation.

Ketorolac is a peripherally and centrally acting nonopioid analgesic that is also an effective preemptive analgesic.[95–97] In a randomized, double-blind trial involving 48 patients undergoing ankle fracture surgery, ketorolac 30 mg administered parenterally before surgical stimulation significantly reduced postsurgical pain relative to the same amount of ketorolac administered after surgical stimulation.[96]

Preemptive analgesia and persistent pain Some preemptive analgesia techniques significantly reduce postsurgical pain, and there is evidence that preemptive analgesia may provide some protection against the development of some chronic pain states. Bach and coworkers[103] reported one of the few investigations designed to assess the impact of preemptive analgesia on the evolution of a chronic pain state. In this clinical study, 25 elderly patients scheduled for a below-the-knee amputation received either treatment with epidural bupivacaine and/or morphine to produce a pain-free state for 3 days before surgery or no pretreatment (control group). All patients subsequently underwent amputation under spinal anesthesia. After 6 months, none of the patients assigned to the presurgery analgesia group experienced phantom limb pain.[103] However, 38% of the subjects who did not receive the presurgical pain treatment had phantom limb pain at the 6-month postamputation period. Furthermore, 27% of these subjects experienced persistent phantom limb pain at the 1-year follow-up period.[103] Based upon this data regarding preemptive analgesia, it is recommended that when feasible, an opioid-based or opioid-supplemented general anesthetic technique be employed for TMJ surgery. Also, a regional anesthetic should be administered to cover the entire surgical field *before* surgical stimulation. During prolonged surgical procedures, the surgical site should be reanesthetized periodically. If there are no contraindications (e.g., bleeding concerns), some consideration can also be given toward ketorolac administration (i.e., 0.5 mg/kg or 30 mg intravenously) *before* surgical stimulation. Finally, postoperative pain should also be well controlled with a combination of regional anesthesia and opioid or ketorolac analgesia in the postoperative period, because these regimens may significantly reduce postsurgical pain, facilitating a shortened convalescence period, and may also protect the patient from CNS responses to surgical stimulation that may be involved in the genesis of some chronic pain syndromes.

NONSURGICAL THERAPY FOR TMJ

PERIARTICULAR ECTOPIC BONE FORMATION

Periarticular ectopic bone formation is viewed as a significant postsurgical complication with a negative impact on functional outcomes in some patients with end-stage TMD. Ectopic bone may form in adjacent native periarticular tissues or in the vicinity of alloplastic materials used to reconstruct the TMJ. In either instance, periarticular ectopic bone formation is viewed as a pathologic entity because it typically restricts normal joint movement and may contribute to chronic facial pain. The pathogenesis of periarticular ectopic bone formation is poorly understood. It has been suggested that displaced osteogenic precursor cells are stimulated to form ectopic bone by inflammatory mediators formed in response to surgical insult.[104] Alternatively, osteoinductive molecules (e.g., bone morphogenetic proteins) may be dispersed into periarticular tissues during surgery, resulting in the stimulation of local pluripotent cells and subsequent ectopic bone synthesis. In addition, other factors, such as genetic influences, sex hormones, systemic disease (e.g., ankylosing spondylitis, Paget's disease), or other local conditions, could also contribute to the formation of ectopic bone in periarticular tissues of the TMJ. Two strategies have been employed to attempt to prevent or minimize periarticular ectopic bone formation in either orthopedic surgery patients or those with TMJ disease. These include low-dose radiation therapy and NSAID therapy.

Low-dose radiation therapy Some clinicians have advocated the use of low-dose radiation to prevent or minimize postsurgical fibro-osseous ankylosis of the TMJ.[105–108] This approach is based on an earlier report indicating that low-dose radiation may be effective at preventing the formation of ectopic bone after hip arthroplasty.[109] For prevention of periarticular ectopic bone formation of the TMJ, fractionated total doses of 10 to 20 Gy have been used. One study reported that 10-Gy dosing was as effective as higher-dose (50-Gy) regimens.[106] Timing appears to be critical for optimum results from low-dose radiation therapy, because it is believed that low-dose radiation therapy elicits its effect on ectopic bone formation by prohibiting the proliferation of pluripotent cells that are precursors to osteoblasts. Therefore, it is recommended that low-dose radiation therapy be initiated within 4 days of surgery to provide optimum suppression of ectopic bone formation. Although there is some concern that early postsurgical radiation may have a detrimental impact on wound healing, one study of the efficacy of a single dose of 600 cGy administered between postsurgical days 2 and 4 (mean, 3.2 days), radiation did not appear to significantly affect wound healing after hip arthroplasty.[110] Radiation therapy was used to prevent ectopic bone formation in the periarticular region of the TMJ in a 53-year-old man[107] who sustained mandible fractures in an automobile accident and subsequently underwent five operations to correct TMJ ankylosis suffered as a complication of his injury. Over an 18-year period, the patient suffered from significant limitation of jaw movement, with reported maximum interincisal movements as low as 6 mm. After his final TMJ arthroplasty, the patient underwent fractionated cobalt radiation therapy consisting of 10 sessions beginning on the first postoperative day, for a total radiation dose of 20 Gy in equal fractions, and at 3-year follow-up, the patient had sustained a maximum interincisal distance of 25.5 mm.[107]

Schwartz and Kagan[108] provided a report describing a similar beneficial effect of fractionated radiation (i.e., 20 Gy in 10 fractions) in a 51-year-old man who experienced a zygomatic-coronoid ankylosis after a depressed fracture of the zygomatic arch. This condition was surgically treated with a 5-mm gap arthroplasty with placement of an intervening sheet of silicone rubber, and postsurgical radiation was initiated 1 week after the operation. At a 19-month follow-up, the patient exhibited a 40-mm maximum interincisal distance, and although the patient initially complained of xerostomia and some loss of facial hair, there was no significant morbidity from this treatment. Experiences with 10 patients suffering from bony ankylosis of the TMJ was reported by Durr and colleagues,[106] consisting of 4 men and 6 women (median age 32.5 yr, range 14–59 yr) with a previous history of TMJ ankylosis who underwent TMJ arthroplasties and immediate postsurgical (within 1–3 days) radiation therapy consisting of 10 to 11.2 Gy in five fractions over a 5-day period. The median follow-up was 19 months (range 7–31 mo). Only 3 patients (30%) were followed for more than 2 years postoperatively, and 40% of these patients experienced some recurrence of ectopic bone formation assessed radiographically. A parotitis was identified in 30% of the patients; however, the radiation therapy did not appear to interfere with healing, and there were no other reported complications.

Reid and Cooke[105] have reported the largest case series to date involving postoperative radiation therapy to manage ectopic bone formation of the TMJ in 14 patients with histories of multiple TMJ surgeries. Each patient underwent TMJ arthroplasty with total joint reconstruction using an alloplastic prosthesis. The majority of these patients received a fractionated 10-Gy radiation dose beginning on the first postoperative day. However, some patients treated early in the series received a fractionated 20-Gy radiation dose. There was a mean follow-up of 4.2 years (range 1–9.6 yr), and the recurrence rate for ectopic bone formation at the 1-year follow-up was 21%. However, long-term follow-up revealed ectopic bone formation in 75% of the patients seen at 5 years and 100% (*n* = 2) of patients examined at the 9-year follow-up (Figure 48-7). Consistent with earlier reports, no significant persistent side effects of radiation therapy were noted.

A major concern with the use of low-dose radiation for the treatment of ectopic bone formation in the TMJ area is the potential for induction of neoplasia. Despite the fact that there have been no reported cases of malignant transformation associated with low-dose radiation therapy used to manage periarticular ectopic bone formation in the TMJ region, this concern seems justified based on a report by Ron and associates,[111] who examined 10,834 patients who had undergone low-dose radiation therapy for the treatment of ringworm infection of the scalp (tinea capitis). All irradiated subjects received treatment (mean radiation dose of 1.5 Gy) before the age of 16 years. Control subjects included 10,834

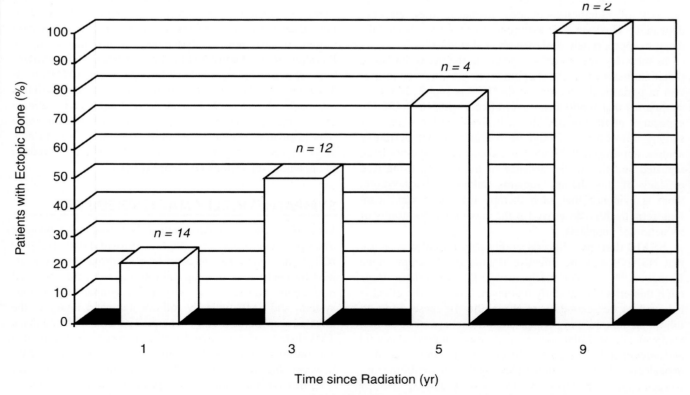

FIGURE 48-7. Recurrence of ectopic bone in patients treated with low-dose radiation. Data adapted from Reid R and Cooke H.[135]

nonirradiated age- and sex-matched individuals not related to the radiated subjects, serving as a general population control, and 5392 nonirradiated siblings of the subjects. The subjects were monitored for up to 33 years for the development of benign and malignant neural tumors. Tumors developed in 73 individuals, 60 among irradiated subjects, 8 in the general population control group, and 5 among siblings of irradiated subjects. Overall, there was a sevenfold increase in neoplasms of the nervous system in individuals who had undergone low-dose radiation therapy. Twenty-four malignant neoplasms were identified in this study, with 18 occurring in irradiated patients, 4 in the general population control group, and 2 in siblings of irradiated subjects. There was a 4.5-fold increase in the incidence of malignant neoplasms in patients who underwent low-dose radiation therapy relative to the control groups. The cumulative risk of developing a neural tumor over a 33-year period was significantly higher in the irradiated group (0.84% ± 0.16%) than in the controls (0.09% ± 0.03%). It should be noted that there was a prolonged latency of tumor occurrence (mean 17.6 yr after radiation exposure). From this study, it appears that the risk of radiation-associated tumors was highest between 15 and 24 years postradiation. This is significant in light of the fact that the longest published follow-up for any case series reporting the effects low-dose radiation therapy for management of ectopic bone formation in the TMJ area is 9 years (only 2 patients).[105] It should be noted that patients receiving radiation therapy for tinea capitis in this study were significantly younger (<16 yr of age) than the TMJ patients reported in the other case series studies; therefore, it is possible that the risk of radiation-associated neoplasia may be age-dependent. However, this assumption has not yet been validated in appropriately designed clinical studies.

In summary, the evidence supporting the use of low-dose radiation therapy to prevent or minimize ectopic bone formation in periarticular regions of the TMJ is supplied by case summaries that report beneficial effects with 10- to 20-Gy exposures in fractionated doses initiated within 4 days of surgery. However, it should be recognized that definitive studies, appropriately blinded and controlled, have not been reported and that in the absence of these studies, the true efficacy of this therapy remains unknown. Furthermore, there is evidence that such therapy may pose significant long-term health risks as well as the uncommon possibility of induction of neoplasia.[141]

NSAID therapy   Several studies have provided evidence that NSAIDs may be effective retardants of ectopic bone formation.[110,112-115] The mechanism(s) by which these drugs elicit this effect is currently unknown; however, the effect is believed to be secondary to the ability of these drugs to inhibit prostanoid, and perhaps leukotriene, synthesis associated with normal inflammatory responses to injury. Kienapfel and coworkers[110] compared the effects of indomethacin, a nonselective COX inhibitor (also capable of inhibiting lipoxygenase), with those of low-dose radiation therapy employed to prevent ectopic bone formation after hip

arthroplasty. For this study, 154 patients scheduled for hip arthroplasty to treat various degenerative arthritides were randomly assigned to one of three groups: (1) low-dose radiation treatment (600 cGy administered as a single dose between postoperative days 2 and 4); (2) indomethacin treatment of 50 mg administered orally twice daily beginning on postoperative day 1 and continuing until postoperative day 42; or (3) control group, with no postoperative radiation or NSAIDs. Patients assigned to the indomethacin treatment group who were either at risk for NSAID-induced GI disease or who developed dyspepsia with the therapy were administered cimetidine 200 mg (H_2 receptor antagonist) concomitantly. All subjects enrolled in the study were assessed clinically and radiographically 18 months after surgery.[110] Ectopic bone formation was significantly inhibited by both treatment conditions relative to the control group, and furthermore, both treatments were found to be equally effective. Surgical wound site secretions were more persistent in the radiated subjects postoperatively, but neither treatment group subsequently exhibited signs of poor wound healing that were significantly different from the controls. The incidence of dyspepsia was higher in the indomethacin-treated group, but GI bleeding was not detected in this group. Other NSAIDs have been used to prevent, or minimize, ectopic bone formation after hip arthroplasty, including ibuprofen, ketorolac, and diclofenac.[112,113,115,145] All of these agents are nonselective COX inhibitors that block COX-1 and COX-2 receptors, and it is not known whether the selective COX-2 inhibitors are effective retardants of ectopic bone formation. To date, there have been no reported studies of NSAID use for the management of ectopic bone formation of the TMJ, so the efficacy of these agents for this specific application remains unclear; however, based upon the orthopedic surgery literature, it may be prudent to consider NSAIDs for patients who are at risk for ectopic bone formation after TMJ surgery. The potential GI and renal complications associated with this approach should not be underestimated, and patients undergoing NSAID therapy to prevent or minimize ectopic bone formation should be properly monitored. If indicated, an H_2 receptor antagonist should be administered to reduce the potential for serious GI complications.

SYMPATHETICALLY MAINTAINED PAIN

Sympathetically maintained pain (SMP), reflex sympathetic dystrophy, causalgia, or *complex regional pain syndrome (CRPS)* are terms used to describe a syndrome(s) characterized by continuous burning pain associated with abnormal nociception affected by activity in the sympathetic nervous system, and SMP typically follows traumatic injury to the affected area. Some multiply operated patients with end-stage TMJ disease with localized tactile or mechanical allodynia and burning pain complaints may be suffering from SMP; however, the incidence of SMP in patients with end-stage TMJ disease is unknown. The typical clinical presentation of SMP may include any of the following signs and symptoms that occur with an incidence of 75% or greater—weakness (95%), pain (93%), altered skin temperature (92%), skin color change (92%), limited range of motion (88%), and hyperesthesia (75%)[116]—whereas less common findings include edema, altered hair growth, tremor, hyperhidrosis, muscle/skin atrophy, and bone resorption.[116]

The mechanism(s) underlying the development of SMP is unknown, but evidence suggests that this condition may result from neuroplastic changes induced by peripheral sensory nerve injury. In animals, the sprouting of sympathetic neurons into sensory dorsal root ganglia has been observed after injury to peripheral sensory nerves, and this sprouting may be induced by a neurotrophic substance, nerve growth factor (NGF), that is released into injured surrounding tissues,[117–121] and a similar response is seen in animals in which NGF is administered intrathecally.[121] These data are consistent with the belief that SMP results from an abnormal sympathetic input to sensory ganglia after peripheral sensory nerve injury that permits the development of physical connections between sympathetic neurons and primary afferent sensory neurons, and this injury may elicit this abnormal response via molecular intermediates, specifically NGF. Clearly, this phenomenon does not occur in all individuals who sustain injuries to peripheral sensory nerves, and further research is needed to investigate this model and to determine risk factors for susceptibility to the development of SMP. Over 25 treatment options for SMP have been reported in the literature,[122] and the most common therapeutic approach has involved the interruption of sympathetic activity via a stellate ganglion anesthetic block. An effective stellate ganglion block may produce protracted pain relief, lasting longer than the duration of anesthetic blockade, although this effect is usually transient. Other pharmacologic interventions (e.g., phentolamine, prazosin, bretylium, guanethidine, calcitonin, nifedipine, gabapentin) as well as surgical sympathectomy have also been used with inconsistent results.[122] With new information concerning the molecular events that may underlie the development of SMP, it is anticipated that more effective therapies will be developed in the future.

MECHANISMS OF FAILURE OF NONSURGICAL THERAPY

Nonsurgical therapy for TMD is composed of a wide variety of management options without consistency and with variable responses reported in the literature. In addition, the diagnosis of TMD is also not based upon strict, univerally accepted criteria, which makes the application of treatment regimens difficult in a heterogenous group of patients. Based upon these factors, nonsurgical therapy as a sole treatment modality, it is very difficult to assess the clinical success or failures of nonsurgical treatment for TMD over time. DeLeeuw and colleagues[76] reported long-lasting satisfactory results for patients treated with nonsurgical therapy for internal derangements and osteoarthrosis with a 30-year follow-up, with persistence of symptoms such as joint noise and

resolution of pain and discomfort. Several possibilities could explain the causes of failure of nonsurgical therapy alone for TMD management including improper data gathering, diagnosis, and treatment planning; lack of patient compliance with treatment recommendations; and difficulties with emotionally debilitated patients or patients with major depression or other significant coexisting morbidities.[77] When significant symptoms persist after 3 to 6 months of nonsurgical therapy, alternative therapies and/or diagnostic modalities should be considered, including radiographic studies (magnetic resonance imaging [MRI]) and possibly TMJ arthrocopic or open joint surgery. In many cases, a critical component of nonsurgical failure is patient noncompliance, because the basic home care modalities require diligence and lack of rapid improvement in symptoms often leads to patient abandonment of the treatment protocol including soft diet, moist heat, the use of NSAIDs, bite splint therapy, and physical therapy. Other possible problems include patients who may experience GI upset and not investigate other pharmacologic options; patients who may not be able to find a dentist to fabricate an occlusal appliance, or the cost of such an appliance may be prohibitive; and patients who may not be able to locate a physical therapist who has experience with the management of TMD. Remember that patients who have had chronic problems with TMD may become easily frustrated when initial nonsurgical modalities fail to result in improvement or if treatment exacerbates their symptoms (e.g., bite splint frequently worsens pain before improvement); patients should be motivated to continue their efforts with nonsurgical treatment, especially because the majority of these patients will never become surgical candidates.

References

1. deBont LGM, Kijkgraaf LC, Stegenga B. Epidemiology and natural progression of articular temporomandibular disorders. Oral Surg Oral Med Oral Pathol Oral Radiol Endod 1997;83: 72–76.
2. Carlsson GE. Epidemiology and treatment needed for temporomandibular disorders. J Orofac Pain 1999;13:232–237.
3. Green CS. Orthodontics and temporomandibular disorders. Dent Clin North Am 1988;32:529–538.
4. Green CS, Laskin DM. Long term evaluation of treatment for myofascial pain dysfunction syndrome: a comparative analysis. J Am Dent Assoc 1983;7:235–238.
5. Okeson JP, Hayes DK. Long-term results of treatment for temporomandibular disorder: an evaluation by patients. J Am Dent Assoc 1986;12:473–478.
6. Suvinen TI, Hanes KR, Reade PC. Outcome of therapy in the conservative management of temporamandibular pain dysfunction disorder. J Oral Rehabil 1997;24:718–724.
7. Gaupp LA, Flinn DE, Weddige RL. Adjunctive treatment techniques. In Tollinson CD, editor. Handbook of Chronic Pain Management. Baltimore: Williams & Wilkins; 1989; p. 174.
8. McNeill C, editor. Temporomandibular Disorders: Guidelines for Classification, Assessment and Management. 2nd ed. Chicago: Quintessence Publishing; 1993.

SECTION 6

9. Mejersjo C, Carlsson GE. Long-term results of treatment for temporomandibular pain-dysfunction. J Prosthet Dent 1983; 49:805–815.

10. Nickerson JW, Boering G. Natural course of osteoarthrosis as it relates to internal derangement of the temporomandibular joint. Oral Maxillofac Surg Clin North Am 1989;1:27–46.

11. Greene CS, Marbach JJ. Epidemiologic studies of mandibular dysfunction: a critical review. J Prosthet Dent 1982;48:184–190.

12. Okeson JP, editor. Management of Temporomandibular Disorders and Occlusion. 2nd ed. St. Louis: CV Mosby; 1989.

13. Fordyce WE, editor. Behavior Methods for Chronic Pain and Illness. St. Louis: CV Mosby; 1976.

14. Black RG. The chronic pain syndrome. Surg Clin North Am 1975;55:999–1011.

15. Fordyce WE. On opioids and treatment targets. Am Pain Soc Bull 1991;1:1–13.

16. Samuelson B. An elucidation of arachadonic acid cascade. Drugs 1987;33(Suppl 1):2–9.

17. Simon LS, Mills JA. Non steroidal anti inflammatory drugs and their mechanism of action. Drugs 1987;33(Suppl 1):18–27.

18. Insel PA. Analgesic-antipyretics and antiinflammatory agents: drugs employed in the treatment of rheumatoid arthritis and gout. In Gilman AG, Rall TW, Nies AS, et al, editors. Goodman and Gillman's the Pharmacological Basis of Therapeutics. 8th ed. New York: Pergamon Press; 1990; pp. 485–521.

19. Syrop S. Pharmacologic management of myofascial pain and dysfunction. Oral Maxillofac Surg Clin North Am 1995;7:87–97.

20. Dimitroulis G, Gremillion HA, Dolwick FM, Walter JH. Temporomandibular disorders. 2. Nonsurgical treatment. Aust Dent J 1995;40:372–376.

21. Yoshida H, Fukumura S, Fujita M, et al. The expression of cyclooxygenase-2 in human temporomandibular joint samples: an immunohistochemical study. J Oral Rehabil 2002;29:1146–1152.

22. Quinn J, Kent J, Moisc A, Lukiw W. Cyclooxygenase-2 in synovial tissue and fluid of dysfunctional temporomandibular joints with internal derangements. J Oral Maxillofac Surg 2000;58:1229–1232.

23. Streeten DHP. Corticosteroid therapy, complication and therapeutic indication. JAMA 1975;232:1046–1059.

24. Cowan J, Moenning JE, Bussard DA. Glucocorticoid therapy for myasthenia gravis resulting in resorption of the mandibular condyles. J Oral Maxillofac Surg 1995;53:1091–1096.

25. Syrop SB. Pharmacological therapy. In Kaplan AS, Assael LA, editors. Temporomandibular Disorders—Diagnosis and Treatment. Philadelphia: WB Saunders; 1991; pp. 501–514.

26. Kinney RK, Gatchel RJ, Ellis E, et al. Major psychological disorders in TMD patients: impactions for successful management. J Am Dent Assoc 1992;123:49–54.

27. Magni G. On the relationship between chronic pain and depression when there is no organic lesion. Pain 1987;31:1–21.

28. Kerrick JM, Fine PG, Lipman AG, Love G. Low-dose amitriptyline as an adjunct to opioids for postoperative orthopedic pain: a placebo controlled trial. Pain 1993;52:325–330.

29. Brown RS, Bottomley WK. The utilization and mechanism of action of tricyclic antidepressants in the treatment of chronic facial pain: a review of the literature. Anesth Prog 1990;37:223–229.

30. Tan E, Janovic J. Treating severe bruxism with botulism toxin. J Am Dent Assoc 2000;131:211–216.

31. Freund B, Schwartz M, Symington JM. Botulism toxin: new treatment for temporomandibular disorders. Br J Oral Maxillofac Surg 2000;38:466–471.

32. Guarda NL, Tito R, Beltrame A. Treatment of temporomandibular joint closed lock using intra-articular injection of mepivacaine with immediate resolution durable in time (six month follow-up) (Italian). Minerva Stomatol 2002;51:21–28.

33. Kaneyama K, Segami N, Nishimura M, et al. Importance of proinflammatory cytokines in synovial fluid from 121 joints with temporomandibular disorders. Br J Oral Maxillofac Surg 2002;418–423.

34. Israel H, Syrop S. The important role of motion in the rehabilitation of patients with mandibular hypomobility: a review of the literature. J Craniomandib Pract 1993;II:298–307.

35. Karlis V, Andreopoulos N, Kinney L, Glickman R. Effectiveness of supervised calibrated exercise therapy on jaw mobility and temporomandibular dysfunction. J Oral Maxillofac Surg 1994;52(8 Suppl 2):147.

36. Sebastian MH, Moffet BC. The effect of continuous passive motion on the temporomandibular joint after surgery. Oral Surg Oral Med Oral Pathol 1989;67:644–653.

37. Maloney G. Effect of a passive jaw motion device on pain and range of motion in TMD patients not responding to flat plane intraoral appliances. J Craniomandib Pract 2002;20:55–56.

38. Mongini F. A modified extraoral technique of mandibular manipulation in disk displacement without reduction. J Craniomandib Pract 1995;13:22–25.

39. Kurita H, Kurashina K, Ohtsuka A. Efficacy of a mandibular manipulation technique in reducing the permanently displaced temporomandibular joint disc. J Oral Maxillofac Surg 1999;57:784–787.

40. Yuasa H, Kurita K. Randomized clinical trial of primary treatment for temporomandibular joint disk displacement without reduction and without osseous changes: a combination of NSAIDs and mouth opening exercise versus no treatment. Oral Surg Oral Med Oral Pathol 2001;91:671–675.

41. Travell JG, Simons DG. Myofascial Pain and Dysfunction: The Trigger Point Manual. Baltimore: Williams & Wilkins; 1983.

42. Modell W, Travell J, Kraus H. Relief of pain by ethyl chloride spray. N Y State J Med 1952;52:1550–1558.

43. Melzack R, Wall P. Pain mechanisms: a new theory. Science 1965;150:971–979.

44. Nelson SJ, Ash MM. An evaluation of a moist heating pad for the treatment of TMJ/muscle pain dysfunction. Cranio 1988;6:355–359.

45. Vanderwindt D, Vanderheijden G, et al. Ultrasound therapy for musculoskeletal disorder: a systemic review. Pain 1999;81:257–271.

46. Ziskin MC, Michlovitz SL. Therapeutic ultrasound. In Michlovitz SL, editor. Thermal Agent in Rehabilitation. Philadelphia: FA Davis; 1990; pp. 141–169.

47. Adler RC, Adachi NY. Physical medicine in the management of myofascial pain and dysfunction: medical management of temporomandibular disorders. Oral Maxillofac Surg Clin North Am 1995;7:99–106.

48. Wolf SL. Neurophysiologic mechanisms in pain modulation: relevance to TENS. In Manheimer JS, Lampe GN, editors. Clinical Transcutaneous Electrical Nerve Stimulation. Philadelphia: FA Davis; 1984; p. 41.

49. Clark GT, Adachi NY, Dornan MR. Physical medicine procedures affect temporomandibular disorders: a review. J Am Dent Assoc 1990;121:151–161.

50. Mohl ND, Ohrbach RK, Crowe HC, Gross AJ. Devices for the diagnosis and treatment of temporomandibular disorders.

Part III. Thermography ultrasound, electrical stimulation and EMG biofeedback. J Prosthet Dent 1990;63:472–477.

51. Gold N, Greene CS, Laskin DM. Transcutaneous electrical nerve stimulation therapy for treatment of myofascial pain dysfunction syndrome. J Dent Res 1983;62:244.

52. Ersek RA. Transcutaneous electrical neurostimulation. Clin Orthop 1977;128:314–324.

53. Eisen AG, Kaufman A, Green CS. Evaluation of physical therapy for MPD syndrome. J Dent Res 1984;63(Special Issue): 344 (abstract 1561).

54. Lark MR, Gangarosa LP. Iontophoresis: an effective modality for the treatment of inflammatory disorders of the temporomandibular joint and myofascial pain. J Craniomandib Pract 1990;8:108–119.

55. Gangarosa LP, Mahan PE. Pharmacologic management of TMJ-MPDS. Ear Nose Throat J 1982;61:670.

56. Gerald MJ. Physical medicine modalities and trigger point injections in the management of temporomandibular disorders and assessing treatment outcome. Oral Surg Oral Med Oral Pathol Oral Radiol Endod 1997;83:118–122.

57. Kaplan AS, Assael LA, editors. Temporomandibular Disorders: Diagnosis and Treatment. Philadelphia: WB Saunders; 1991; pp. 522–525.

58. Crider AB, Glaros AG. A meta-analysis of EMG biofeedback treatment of temporomandibular disorders. J Orofac Pain 1999;13:29–37.

59. Scott DS, Gregg JM. Myofacial pain of the temporomandibular joint: a review of the behavioral-relaxation therapies [review]. Pain 1980;9:231–241.

60. Matsumura WM. Use of acupressure techniques and concepts for nonsurgical management of TMJ disorders. J Gen Orthod 1993;4:5–16.

61. Matsumura TM, Ali NM. Evaluation of acupuncture and occlusal splint therapy in the treatment of temporomandibular joint disorders. Egypt Dent J 1995;41:1227–1232.

62. Berry H, Fernandez L, Bloom B, et al. Clinical study comparing acupuncture, physiotherapy, injection, and oral anti-inflammatory therapy in shoulder cuff lesions. Curr Med Res Opin 1980;7:121–126.

63. Rugh JD. Psychological components of pain. Dent Clin North Am 1987;31:579–594.

64. Moss RA, Adams HE. The assessment of personality, anxiety and depression in mandibular pain dysfunction subjects. J Oral Rehabil 1984;11:233–237.

65. Katon W, Egan K, Miller D. Chronic pain: lifetime psychiatric diagnoses and family history. Am J Psychiatry 1985;142:1156–1160.

66. Okeson JP, Kemper JT, Moody PM. A study of the use of occlusion splints in the treatment of acute and chronic patients with craniomandibular disorders. J Prosthet Dent 1982;48:708–712.

67. Okeson JP, Moody PM, Kemper JT, Haley J. Evaluation of occlusal splint therapy and relaxation procedures in patients with TMJ disorders. J Am Dent Assoc 1983;107:420–424.

68. Clark GT. A critical evaluation of orthopedic interocclusal appliance therapy: design, theory and overall effectiveness. J Am Dent Assoc 1984;108:359–364.

69. Rugh JD, Harlan J. Nocturnal bruxism and temporomandibular disorders. Adv Neurol 1988;49:329–341.

70. Okeson JP. Occlusal appliance therapy. In Duncan LL, editor. Management of Temporomandibular Disorders and Occlusion. 4th ed. Philadelphia: Mosby; 1998; pp. 474–502.

71. Major PW, Nebbe B. Use and effectiveness of splint appliance therapy: review of literature. J Craniomandib Pract 1997; 15:159–166.

72. Lundh H, Per-Lenmart W, Eriksson L, et al. Temporomandibular disk displacement without reduction: treatment with flat occlusal splint versus no treatment. Oral Surg Oral Med Oral Pathol 1992;73:655–658.

73. Kai S, Kai H, Tabata O, et al. Long-term outcomes of nonsurgical treatment in nonreducing anteriorly displaced disk of the temporomandibular joint. Oral Surg Oral Med Oral Pathol 1998;85:258–267.

74. Moloney F, Howard JA. Internal derangements of the temporomandibular joint. III. Anterior repositioning splint therapy. Aust Dent J 1986;31:30–39.

75. Clark GT, Adler RC. A critical evaluation of occlusal therapy. Occlusal adjustment procedures. J Am Dent Assoc 1985;110: 743–750.

76. DeLeeuw R, Boering G, Stegenga B, et al. Symptoms of temporomandibular joint osteoarthrosis and internal derangement 30 years after nonsurgical treatment. J Craniomandib Pract 1995;13:81–88.

77. Abdel-Fattah RA. Considerations before surgical intervention in management of temporomandibular joint disorders. J Craniomandib Pract 1997;15:94–95.

78. Mendell LM, Wall PD. Response of single dorsal cord cells to peripheral cutaneous unmyelinated fibres. Nature 1965;206: 97–99.

79. Woolf CJ, King AE. Dynamic alterations in the cutaneous mechanoreceptive fields of dorsal horn neurons in the rat spinal cord. J Neurosci 1990;10:2717–2726.

80. Owens CM, Zhang D, Willis WD. Changes in the response states of primate spinothalamic tract cells caused by mechanical damage of the skin or activation of descending controls. J Neurophysiol 1992;67:1509–1527.

81. Bereiter DA. Sex differences in brainstem neural activation after injury to the TMJ region. Cells Tissues Organs 2001;169:226–237.

82. Bereiter DA, Bereiter DF. Morphine and NMDA receptor antagonism reduce c-fos expression in spinal trigeminal nucleus produced by acute injury to the TMJ region. Pain 2000;85: 65–77.

83. Woolf CJ, Chong MS. Preemptive analgesia—treating postoperative pain by preventing the establishment of central sensitization. Anesth Analg 1993;77:362–379.

84. Giannoni C, White S, Enneking FK, et al. Ropivacaine with or without clonidine improves pediatric tonsillectomy pain. Arch Otolaryngol Head Neck Surg 2001;127:1265–1270.

85. Goodwin SA. A review of preemptive analgesia. J Perianesth Nurs 1998;13:109–114.

86. Goldstein FJ. Preemptive analgesia: a research review. Medsurg Nurs 1995;4:305–308.

87. Gilron I, Quirion R, Coderre TJ. Pre- versus postformalin effects of ketamine or large-dose alfentanil in the rat: discordance between pain behavior and spinal Fos-like immunoreactivity. Anesth Analg 1999;89:128–135.

88. Kelly DJ, Ahmad M, Brull SJ. Preemptive analgesia I: physiological pathways and pharmacological modalities. Can J Anaesth 2001;48:1000–1010.

89. Kilickan L, Toker K. The effect of preemptive intravenous morphine on postoperative analgesia and surgical stress response. Panminerva Med 2001;43:171–175.

SECTION 6

90. Subramaniam B, Pawar DK, Kashyap L. Pre-emptive analgesia with epidural morphine or morphine and bupivacaine. Anaesth Intensive Care 2000;28:392–398.

91. Chiaretti A, Viola L, Pietrini D, et al. Preemptive analgesia with tramadol and fentanyl in pediatric neurosurgery [discussion]. Childs Nerv Sys 2000;16:93–99.

92. Dickenson AH, Sullivan AF. Evidence for a role of the NMDA receptor in the frequency dependent potentiation of deep rat dorsal horn nociceptive neurones following C fibre stimulation. Neuropharmacology 1987;26:1235–1238.

93. Haley JE, Sullivan AF, Dickenson AH. Evidence for spinal *N*-methyl-D-aspartate receptor involvement in prolonged chemical nociception in the rat. Brain Res 1990;518:218–226.

94. Torrebjork HE, Lundberg LE, LaMotte RH. Central changes in processing of mechanoreceptive input in capsaicin-induced secondary hyperalgesia in humans. J Physiol 1992;448:765–780.

95. Mixter CGR, Hackett TR. Preemptive analgesia in the laparoscopic patient. Surg Endosc 1997;11:351–353.

96. Norman PH, Daley MD, Lindsey RW. Preemptive analgesic effects of ketorolac in ankle fracture surgery [comment]. Anesthesiology 2001;94:599–603.

97. Wittels B, Faure EA, Chavez R, et al. Effective analgesia after bilateral tubal ligation. Anesth Analg 1998;87:619–623.

98. Jebeles JA, Reilly JS, Gutierrez JF, et al. Tonsillectomy and adenoidectomy pain reduction by local bupivacaine infiltration in children. Int J Pediatr Otorhinolaryngol 1993;25:149–154.

99. Honnma T, Imaizumi T, Chiba M, et al. Pre-emptive analgesia for postoperative pain after frontotemporal craniotomy. No Shinkei Geka 2002;30:171–174.

100. Hoard MA, Bill TJ, Campbell RL. Reduction in morbidity after iliac crest bone harvesting: the concept of preemptive analgesia. J Craniomaxillofac Surg 1998;9:448–451.

101. Abram SE, Yaksh TL. Morphine, but not inhalation anesthesia, blocks post-injury facilitation: the role of preemptive suppression of afferent transmission. Anesthesiology 1993;78:713–721.

102. Wallace MS, Braun J, Schulteis G. Postdelivery of alfentanil and ketamine has no effect on intradermal capsaicin-induced pain and hyperalgesia. Clin J Pain 2002;18:373–379.

103. Bach S, Noreng MF, Tjellden NU. Phantom limb pain in amputees during the first 12 months following limb amputation, after preoperative lumbar epidural blockade. Pain 1988;33:297–301.

104. Puzas JE, Miller MD, Rosier RN. Pathologic bone formation. Clin Orthop 1989;245:269–281.

105. Reid R, Cooke H. Postoperative ionizing radiation in the management of heterotopic bone formation in the temporomandibular joint. J Oral Maxillofac Surg 1999;57:900–906.

106. Durr ED, Turlington EG, Foote RL. Radiation treatment of heterotopic bone formation in the temporomandibular joint articulation. Int J Radiat Oncol Biol Phys 1993;27:863–869.

107. Robinson M, Arnet G. Cobalt radiation to prevent reankylosis after repeated surgical failures: report of case. J Oral Surg 1977;35:850–854.

108. Schwartz HC, Kagan AR. Zygomatico-coronoid ankylosis secondary to heterotopic bone formation: combined treatment by surgery and radiation therapy—a case report. J Maxillofac Surg 1979;7:158–161.

109. Coventry MB, Scanlon PW. The use of radiation to discourage ectopic bone. A nine-year study about the hip. J Bone Joint Surg 1981;63:201–208.

110. Kienapfel H, Koller M, Wust A, et al. Prevention of heterotopic bone formation after total hip arthroplasty: a prospective randomised study comparing postoperative radiation therapy with indomethacin. Arch Orthop Trauma Surg 1999;119:296–302.

111. Ron E, Modan B, Boice JD, et al. Tumors of the brain and nervous system after radiotherapy in childhood. N Engl J Med 1988; 319:1033–1039.

112. Elmstedt E, Lindholm TS, Nilsson OS, et al. Effect of ibuprofen on heterotopic ossification after hip replacement. Acta Orthop Scand 1985;56:25–27.

113. Pritchett JW. Ketorolac prophylaxis against heterotopic ossification after hip replacement. Clin Orthop 1995;314:162–165.

114. Sodemann B, Persson PE, Nilsson OS. Prevention of heterotopic ossification by nonsteroid antiinflammatory drugs after total hip arthroplasty. Clin Orthop 1988;237:158–163.

115. Wahlstrom O, Risto O, Djerk K, et al. Heterotopic bone formation prevented by diclofenac. Prospective study of 100 hip arthroplasties. Acta Orthop Scand 1991;62:419–421.

116. Veldman PH, Reynen HM, Arntz IE, et al. Signs and symptoms of reflex sympathetic dystrophy: prospective study of 829 patients. Lancet 1993;342:1012–1016.

117. Jones MG, Munson JB, Thompson SW. A role for nerve growth factor in sympathetic sprouting in rat dorsal root ganglia. Pain 1999;79:21–29.

118. McLachlan EM, Hu P. Axonal sprouts containing calcitonin gene–related peptide and substance P form pericellular baskets around large diameter neurons after sciatic nerve transection in the rat. Neuroscience 1998;84:961–965.

119. Ramer MS, French GD, Bisby MA. Wallerian degeneration is required for both neuropathic pain and sympathetic sprouting into the DRG. Pain 1997;72:71–78.

120. Ramer M, Bisby M. Reduced sympathetic sprouting occurs in dorsal root ganglia after axotomy in mice lacking low-affinity neurotrophin receptor. Neurosci Lett 1997;228:9–12.

121. Woolf CJ. Phenotypic modification of primary sensory neurons: the role of nerve growth factor in the production of persistent pain. Philos Trans R Soc Lond B Biol Sci 1996;351:441–448.

122. Tanelian DL. Reflex sympathetic dystrophy. A reevaluation of the literature. Pain Forum 1996;5:247–256.

Arthroscopy and Arthrocentesis of the Temporomandibular Joint

Joseph McCain, DMD, and Luciano Stroia, DDS

The management of temporomandibular joint (TMJ) disorders from a surgeon's perspective has improved significantly since the advent of arthroscopy. Arthroscopic observations have provided an in vivo examination of the joint. Disk position and quality, texture of articular cartilage, and vascularity and redundancy of synovium can be observed clearly and precisely. Prior to arthroscopy, joint pathology and surgical correction efforts were targeted toward disk displacement, condyle dislocation, and osteoarthrosis with osteophyte formation.

Currently, the emphasis has shifted to the surgical management of the chemistry of joint space inflammation. This refocus of priorities has been successful in reducing joint pain and increasing joint mobility. Structural joint reconstruction is completed secondarily following reduction of pain, when indicated. This chapter offers an arthroscopic cascade in the overall management of the orthopedic TMJ patient.

HISTORY

The first TMJ arthroscopy was performed by Masatoshi Ohnishi in 1974. Murakami and coworkers, Holmund, McCain, Sanders, Koslin, Moses, and others soon followed. This history has been well documented in the literature. Interestingly, arthrocentesis evolved from, rather than preceded, arthroscopy. Lack of proper equipment, poor insurance reimbursement, and good results despite poor arthroscopic technique led surgeons to explore joint lavage and manipulation in lieu of actual more invasive arthroscopic surgery, and positive results have been reported by Nitzan and others.

Currently, there are two tiers of arthroscopic surgeons: those who are capable of single-puncture basic procedures and those who are capable of multiple punctures and triangulation with capability for advanced arthroscopic surgical procedures. Those who perform single-puncture arthroscopy can perform diagnostic and basic interventions. Reconstructive procedures on refractory cases are then managed with open arthrotomy techniques. Advanced arthroscopic procedures may be done with multiple puncture techniques, in lieu of open surgery, by surgeons whose expertise is at a higher level. There still remains the need for open arthroplasty procedures because even advanced arthroscopy has its limitations.

GOALS

As with other surgeries that have converted over the past decade from open to closed, less invasive techniques, the subspecialty of TMJ arthroscopy, has become popular once again. The goals include the ability to establish an accurate diagnosis, restore function, reduce pain, and diminish joint noise with a minimally invasive, safe, effective, and repeatable procedure with acceptable long-term outcomes. In addition, a reduction in the catabolic environment by the preliminary procedures places the joint in an anabolic state. If a reconstructive procedure such as diskopexy does need to be performed after arthroscopy, it is done in a joint space that can better accept the surgical insult with a minimal amount of bleeding or scar formation, thereby yielding a more favorable outcome.

The ability to refine and improve upon current successful open arthroscopic procedures continues to motivate the advanced TMJ arthroscopist.

INDICATIONS

The indications for arthroscopic intervention include patients who have pain and jaw dysfunction not responsive to nonsurgical dental or medical management. The general indications are shown in Table 49-1. The most common presenting clinical signs and symptoms include limited mouth opening (Figure 49-1), painful joint noises, and mandibular dislocation. Other candidates for at least a diagnostic arthroscopy procedure include patients who have persistent preauricular pain and the diagnosis of intra-articular TMJ pathology cannot be ruled out by clinical or imaging examination.

The clinician should formulate a preoperative differential diagnosis. The accepted terminology for articular disorders includes the Wilkes classification system (Table 49-2). This classification is based upon maximum interincisal opening (MIO), joint noise, and radiographic findings.

CONTRAINDICATIONS

The contraindications to arthroscopy and arthrocentesis include bony ankylosis, advanced fibrous ankylosis, ankylosing osteoarthritis, and overlying skin infection.

Bony ankylosis typically requires autogenous or alloplastic joint replacement. Advanced fibrous ankylosis and ankylosing osteoarthritis will only temporarily respond to advanced arthroscopic techniques. These cases respond to open joint débridements, interpositional grafting, or joint replacement. Puncturing through an area of infected skin increases the potential complication of a septic joint postoperatively.

TABLE 49-1. **General Indications for Arthroscopy**

1. Articular disorders (Wilkes classification)
2. Mandibular dislocation
3. Arthralgia
4. Preauricular atypical facial pain

TABLE 49-2. **Wilkes Classification**

I: Clicking without pain
II: Clicking with pain
III: Locking closed without bone changes
IV: Locking with bone changes
V: Crepitation

ADVANTAGES

The advantages of minimally invasive endoscopic interventions in the TMJ area are

1. No significant skin incision or facial scar.
2. Reduced incidence of VII nerve injury.
3. Diagnostic and therapeutic capabilities.

The disadvantages of minimally invasive procedures are

1. Steep learning curve.
2. Cost of equipment.

PATIENT EVALUATION

The evaluation of the TMJ patient can be an arduous task for the clinician. One needs to have a system to access the nature of the problem and its severity. The surgeon must evaluate the need for surgery. A problem-oriented history and physical examination must be completed. This skill must be developed at the risk of burnout and disinterest driving the provider away from participating in the care of these patients. Unfortunately, the characteristic traits of the temporomandibular disorder (TMD) patient, although not misinterpreted, have led to a certain "labeling" of those patients suffering from these disorders or diseases. Notwithstanding the nonmalicious nature of these prejudices, they will significantly diminish the clinician's capability to appropriately diagnose these conditions. TMJ patients come from all walks of life, males and females, young and old, married, widowed, and divorced, those with

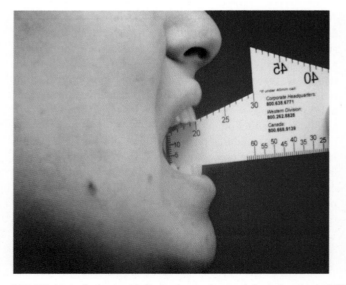
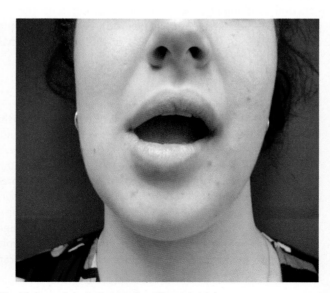

FIGURE 49-1. Patient with limited opening and deviation (right Wilkes III with lateral deviation to the affected side).

children, and those without. Many have the myofascial pain primarily or secondarily to a joint problem, and the astute clinician must be able to discern the clinical differences in order to most appropriately plan for treatment.

McCain TMJ Assessment Standardized Forms

An analogue-driven TMJ practice is recommended. The first document filled out by the patient, after proper introductions and instructions, is the pain and functional analogue (Figure 49-2). This form is completed at the beginning of each visit to monitor progress.

Anamnesis

Chief Complaint
This extremely important step of patient assessment is probably the most easily dismissed area of anamnesis. Over the years, numerous options/windows have been added to a standardized TMJ assessment form, and the list remains fluid, because TMD symptomatology may present with a novel array of complaints that have not yet prompted in-depth explo-

ration by the clinician. As surgeons, our focus of interest is directed more at the orthopedic complaints because they are more likely to require an intervention. However, the patient may report only one, or a variety of, symptoms. 'I can't open my jaw," "My joint clicks and hurts," "I have ear pain," "I have headaches." Whether the otalgia is TMJ referred pain or not is an extremely important step in diagnosis. There are a significant number of patients with tinnitus or other acoustic complaints referred by ear-nose-throat/otorhinolaryngology (ENT/ORL) colleagues to rule out TMD. Some patients can accurately describe the joint noise that has prompted them to seek care (e.g., clicking, popping, grinding, grating). Whereas most patients will describe some form of masticatory dysfunction, some patients will be specific in their description of progressive restriction of mouth opening, transient jaw locking, and so forth, or they will need only a few targeted questions from the examiner in order to help them to delineate their condition.

Parafunction and Associated Causes
The clinician is often tempted to overemphasize parafunctional habits when examining the patient. Masticatory mus-

TO OUR TMJ PATIENTS:

Please take a minute to answers these questions. We ask all of our patients these questions every time they come in. However, in some cases, we feel the answers may not be honest because one of the doctors may be present when you answer. We want a sincere, honest opinion from you because it helps you and those TMJ patients who we will treat in the future, as well as our colleagues who seek to help their patients with arthroscopy.

(Place an "X" at the point along the line which answers the question best).

1-What is your overall level of pain in your jaw joint(s) today?

I ———————————————————— X————————————————————I

most intense   no pain
pain imaginable

2-What is your overall level of jaw function today?

I ———————————————————— X—————————————————————I

can't use   no problems
jaw at all   with jaw use

3-How do you feel now compared to your first visit here?

I ————————————N/A——————————————I————————————————————————I

much wrose   same   much better

Please indicate on the drawings below where you have pain:

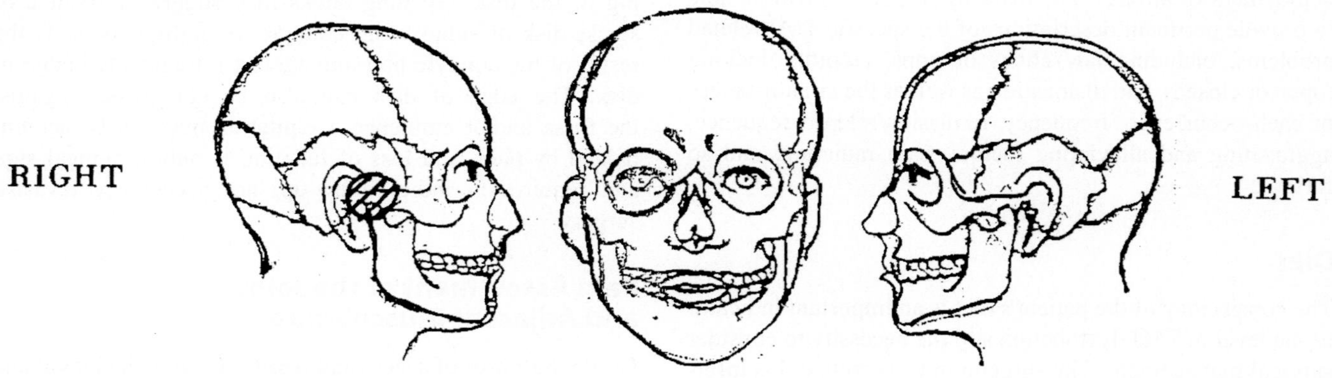

RIGHT   LEFT

FIGURE 49-2.   Functional and pain analog.

culature spasm ("jaw stiffness"), matinal or vesperal, is a common complaint. However, unless the patient admits to vigil bruxing or clenching or the habit is witnessed, parafunction should not be attributed to etiopathogenicity in the particular TMJ condition. Mental or physical stress should definitely be taken into consideration. The surgeon must remain aware of the symbiotic interrelation between parafunction, stress, and the development of TMD.

Analog Scales

The visual analogue scale (VAS) provides a real sense of the acuteness and urgency of the patient's perception of the problem. Remember that arthrocentesis and arthroscopy are elective procedures, so every patient must have insight into her or his condition and be motivated enough to improve her or his present status. The condition should be severe enough for the surgeon to believe it can be ameliorated or suppressed with surgical intervention. Preventive goals are secondary motivators.

History

A pertinent documentation of events should take place in accordance with patient's narrative description of the disease progression. The association between traumatic events and various TMJ conditions cannot be overemphasized. Whether direct (when the mandible has been involved primarily) or indirect (e.g., after a dental appointment, extractions, endodontic treatment, oral surgical procedures, endotracheal intubation maneuvers), the patient may not correlate the events with this specific condition. The clinician should not indiscriminately dismiss minor indirect trauma as a factor in triggering TMD. An interesting fact is that the patient may omit reporting even direct trauma events to the jaw if they occurred in the distant past. The surgeon's keen sense of observation should allow documentation of even small facial cicatricial marks, especially in the inconspicuous submento-submandibular area from prior chin trauma. When a history of motor vehicle accident (MVA) has been established, additional information may be gained from the details of the event (e.g., restrained vs. unrestrained, driver vs. passenger, deployment of airbag). The majority of patients will be able to provide pertinent descriptions of the specific TMJ-related problems, including jaw clicks or pops, crepitus, locking (open or closed), and dislocation as well as the circumstances of each occurrence, frequency, remission/relapse sequence, aggravating and alleviating factors, pain radiation, and so forth.

Diet

The consistency of the patient's diet is an important indicator of the level of TMJ dysfunction and the necessity to consider surgical management. The surgeon must correlate this information with the analogue scales.

Treatment

All prior attempts to treat the TMJ condition both medically and surgically should be recorded. A previous ENT/ORL or neurologic evaluation will, in most instances, provide the surgeon the results of acoustic-vestibular or neuropathic pain workups, helping the specialist to "zero-in" on the TMJ workup of the condition. It is important to know whether the entire spectrum of conservative treatment has been exhausted. The surgeon must ascertain whether the noninvasive therapy (e.g., Boering modifications, orthotics, over-the-counter [OTC]/prescription medications) or surgical treatment has been appropriate and evaluate the outcomes of these treatments and, additionally, the compliance of the patient with these previous regimens.

PHYSICAL EXAMINATION

Mouth Opening and Range of Motion

The physical examination should be problem-focused and brief, but pertinent. Ask the patient to open the mouth and observe the velocity of opening and measure the MIO. A rapid opening to 40 mm is not a very exciting finding for the surgeon in order to motivate a patient toward the operating table, unless you are assessing an undiagnosed facial pain syndrome. A patient who opens to 30 mm then catches and clicks to gain further opening certainly should get the attention of the surgeon. Regardless of their subtlety, lateral deviations should be measured and noted in the record. Complete documentation of range of motion (ROM) in lateral excursive movements and during jaw protrusion follows next. The lack of translation of the condyle may imply a non-reducing disk. Condyle subluxation or dislocation may be palpated in the preauricular region or within the external auditory canal.

Joint Noise

A correlation must be made next between the ROM and associated joint noise/noises. Joint sounds may be audible and/or palpable. Reciprocal clicking may reflect a recapturing of the disk. Opening clicks may suggest a fixated, or stuck, disk or subluxating condyle. A grating sound is the result of the condyle pressing against a fragmented edge of disk. The edge of disk can also be compressed against the fossa and/or eminence. Crepitation may not be accompanied by pain, and loss of function is only a clinical sign and requires periodic follow-up, not necessarily invasive surgery.

Pain Assessment of the Joint and Adjacent Musculature

For the purposes of access and feasibility, only the lateral and posterior poles of the condyle are palpated. Pain at the lateral pole may indicate synovitis, osteoarthritis, joint effusion, or disk dislocation. The latter is best elucidated by palpating superiorly on the neck of the condyle, posterior and slightly inferior to the prominent lateral pole itself. This particular area of the posterolateral pole of the condyle is the site of the attachment of the disk to the lateral capsule and condylar neck. Both acutely and chronically inflamed disk dislocations may provoke a pain response upon palpation. Intrameatal pain suggests a posterior capsule retrodiskal inflammatory process. Both lateral capsular and endaural joint tenderness to palpation are common findings in TMD. The closed-lock patients will invariably demonstrate a "soft tissue crepitance" in at least a portion of their range of normal mouth motion. This bruit is caused by the bilaminar retrodiskal tissues rolled between the condyle and the eminence. Reciprocal, mediolateral, and late opening clicks, although less frequent, may still be encountered. The muscular examination is limited to the superior portion of the anterior margin of masseter muscle and the insertion of the temporalis tendon on the coronoid process. These particular elevator muscles of the mandible provide the most precise information regarding myofascial pain dysfunction syndrome (MPD) and are most likely to be involved with that process. All clinical findings should be recorded on the checklist form (Figure 49-3).

Joint Locking or Dislocation

Mahan's Sign

The most important pathognomonic sign is the "Mahan sign," named after Parker Mahan who described this sign in 1990 (Figure 49-4). The working condyle is loaded by biting on blades with the contralateral canines. If positive with elicitation of pain, there is generally an orthopedic problem in the joint. The sign is usually positive in Wilkes II, III, and IV patients. Some Wilkes II patients will not be positive and that affects the choice of intervention. Noninflamed (negative Mahan's sign) Wilkes II patients may be managed better with diskopexy, and Mahan-positive Wilkes II patients are managed with nonsurgical interventions before diskopexy.

The reason that Wilkes V patients will not have a positive Mahan sign is because the condyle will traverse the perforation and not compress the retrodiskal tissues. Wilkes V patients, however, will have the second important pathognomonic sign, crepitation.

Head, Eyes, Ears, Nose, and Throat

Examination of the head, eyes, ear, nose, and throat (HEENT) is performed next, with special focus on the external ear examination, facial symmetry, and dentoskeletal classification. Also, the Ellis occlusal class, dental interferences during function, and evidence of occlusal wear should be noted.

Panoramic Radiograph

The Panorex is then evaluated with a focus on the condyles and joint spaces. Maintenance of the oval morphology is considered normal. Flattening of the head, loss of cortical detail, osteosclerosis, osteophyte formation, narrowing of the joint space, and subcortical cysts are important bone changes to factor into the Wilkes classification.

Magnetic Resonance Imaging

On occasion, the patient may present with a copy of MRI results, as a part of a pertinent referral from another clinician. Whereas the surgeon should become familiar with the radiology interpretation of the study, the arthroscopist should "re-read" the MRI and interpret it according to his or her clinical and surgical experience. In the most stable relationship, the rather thick posterior band of the disk occupies the greatest concavity of the glenoid fossae (Figure 49-5). Henceforth, a closed-mouth MRI view showing the posterior band in the 10:30 to 11:00 position should be read as abnormal. Preoperative changes on the MRI mandate close consideration of surgical detail and postoperative physical therapy. As long as the disk itself is salvageable, disk form should not preclude disk suturing and/or stabilization. The open-mouth view MRI (Figure 49-6) will give the practitioner the most accurate perspective of the disk position with function (i.e., recapture of the disk in the case of disk displacement), especially in cases that correlate with reciprocal or double clicking on physical examination. Although T1-weighted open- and closed-mouth MRI views are paramount for confirming the clinical diagnosis, the T2-weighted images more accurately reflect an associated inflammatory component of the joint disease, such as the presence of joint effusion (Figure 49-7). This completes the patient assessment.

Etiology

The etiologic factors are organized into five categories/classes.

   I. Parafunction (direct microtrauma, associated MPD). The effects of psychological stress may cause the masticatory system to spasm, thus compressing and disrupting normal joint articulation. Bruxism and clenching inflict repetitive and abnormal overloading of the joint and muscular system, causing spasm and muscle pain to develop with intermittent clicking.

   II. Dentofacial deformities and nalocclusions (direct microtrauma). Articular dysfunction occurs from disharmonious motion between the maxillary and the mandibular arches. The most common patient in this category is the one with vertical maxillary excess (VME) in combination with mandible retrognathia/hypoplasia. A majority of internal derangements may be caused by various components of mandibular retrusion. A class I

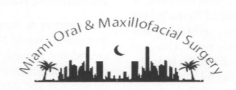

T.M.J CONSULTATION

NAME: JANE DOE

AGE: 24

GENDER: Female

MARITAL STATUS:
SIGNIFICANT OTHER
PARTNER
WIDOWED
MARRIED
DIVORCED
SINGLE.

CHILDREN:
NONE
ONE
TWO
THREE
FOUR
MORE THAN FOUR.

OCCUPATION:
RETIRED
BUSINESS
OTHER
STUDENT
ADMINISTRATION
HEALTHCARE
LAWYER
EDUCATION
SALES
LAW ENFORCEMENT.

MEDICAL HISTORY INFORMATION IS COMPLETED, REVIEWED AND INCLUDED IN THE PATIENT'S CHART.

CHIEF COMPLAINT:
PAIN
JOINT NOISE
MIGRAINE
GRINDING
TINNITUS
OTALGIA
RESTRICTED RAMGE OF MOTION
MASTICATORY DYSFUNCTION
DISLOCATION
CLICKING
MUSCLE SORENESS
OTHER
TRANSIENT LOCKING.

HISTORY:

BRUXISM:
PM JAW STIFFNESS
PATIENT HAS A HISTORY OF BRUXISM
PATIENT HAS NO HISTORY OF BRUXISM.
WITNESSED
AM JAW STIFFNESS.

STRESS:
YES
NO.

CLENCHING:
YES
NO.

ANALOGS
LEFT
RIGHT.

TRAUMA:
INDIRECT
DIRECT
NONE.

MVA:
NO
YES
DATE:
SEATBELT
DRIVER
PASSENGER.

JAW CLICK:
RIGHT NO
RIGHT YES
LEFT YES
LEFT NO.

CREPITUS:
LEFT YES
RIGHT NO
RIGHT YES
LEFT NO.

LOCK:
LEFT YES
RIGHT YES
RIGHT NO
LEFT NO
YES
NO
RIGHT
LEFT.

DISLOCATION:
RIGHT YES
RIGHT NO
LEFT NO
LEFT YES
NO
YES
RIGHT
LEFT.

DIET:
REGULAR
REGULAR COMPROMISED
SOFT
LIQUID.

TREATMENT:
DIET
OTC MEDS
RX MEDS
ORTHOTIC
SURGERY
NEUROLOGIC EVAL
ENT EVAL
OTHER
NONE.

VERTICAL OPENING:
.

PHYSICAL EXAM

ROM:
LL:NTB
PR:JTB
LL: PB
PR:NTB
RL:PB
RL:JTB
RL:NTB
LL: JTB
PR:PB.

JOINT NOISE

CLICK:
RIGHT YES
LEFT YES
LEFT NO
RIGHT NO
YES
NO
RIGHT
LEFT.

CREPITUS
LEFT YES
LEFT NO
RIGHT NO
RIGHT YES
YES
NO
RIGHT
LEFT.

PAIN:
NO
IM RIGHT NO
IM RIGHT YES
MASSETER RIGHT NO
MASSETER LEFT NO
IM LEFT YES
PALPATION CONDYLE LP LEFT NO
PALPATION CONDYLE LP RIGHT NO
MASSETER RIGHT YES
PALPATION CONDYLE LP LEFT YES
MASSETER LEFT YES
IM LEFT NO
PALPATION CONDYLE LP RIGHT YES.

LOCK:
RIGHT YES
RIGHT NO
LEFT NO
LEFT YES
YES
NO
RIGHT
LEFT.

DISLOCATION:
RIGHT NO
LEFT NO
LEFT YES
RIGHT YES
YES
NO
RIGHT
LEFT.

MAHAN DIRECT:
RIGHT YES
LEFT NO
LEFT YES
RIGHT NO
YES
NO
RIGHT
LEFT.

MAHAN INDIRECT:
RIGHT YES
LEFT NO
RIGHT NO
LEFT YES
YES
NO
RIGHT
LEFT.

EARS:
NOT EXAMINED
NORMAL
ABNORMAL.

FACE:
SYMMETRICAL
ASYMETRICAL
MANDIBLE LEFT
MANDIBLE RIGHT.

SKELETAL CLASS:
I
II
III.

HEENT:
OTHERWISE NORMAL.

OCCLUSION:
I
II
III.

INTERFERENCES:
NONE
(LEFT) BALANCING
(LEFT) WORKING
(LEFT) PROTRUSIVE
(RIGHT) BALANCING
(RIGHT) WORKING
(RIGHT) PROTRUSIVE
(PROTRUSION) RIGHT
(PROTRUSION) LEFT
(PROTRUSION) ANTERIOR.

WEAR:
SEVERE
MODERATE
MILD
NORMAL
NONE.

IMAGING:

PANOREX:
WISDOM TEETH YES, WISDOM TEETH
NO, ANTIGONIAL NOTCHING, INFERIOR
BORDER SCALLOPING, RIGHT, NORMAL,
OSTEOARTHRITIS, 1, 2, 3, <u>LEFT</u>, NORMAL,
OSTEOARTHRITIS, 1, 2, and 3.
MRI :
EFFUSION
DISC SIGNAL CHANGES
NORMAL
RIGHT
DISC DISPLACEMENT WITH REDUCTION
DISC DISPLACEMENT WITHOUT REDUC-
TION
OSTEOARTHRITIS
LEFT
NORMAL
DISC DISPLACEMENT WITH REDUCTION
DISC DISPLACEMENT WITHOUT REDUC-
TION
OSTEOARTHRITIS.

ETIOLOGY:
V RHEUMATOID ARTHRITIS/OTHER GEN-
ERAL
IV INDIRECT TRAUMA
III DIRECT TRAUMA
II OCCLUSAL (DENTO-SKELETO-FACIAL
CONGENITAL/AQUIRED MALFORMATIONS)
I PARAFUNCTION

DIAGNOSIS:
OSTEOARTHRITIS RIGHT
OTALGIA
ANKYLOSIS
ANKYLOSIS O.A
OSTEOARTHRITIS LEFT
ARTHRALGIA
HEADACHE
RIGHT WILKES I
LEFT WILKES V
RIGHT WILKES II
RIGHT WILKES III
RIGHT WILKES IV
RIGHT WILKES V
LEFT WILKES I
LEFT WILKES II
LEFT WILKES III
LEFT WILKES IV
RIGHT
NORMAL
MPD
DISLOCATION
INTERNAL JOINT DERRANGEMENT
LEFT
NORMAL
MPD
DISLOCATION
INTERNAL JOINT DERRANGEMENT .

ENTRY LEVEL:
(IV) MEDICAL
(III) SURGICAL
(II) ORTHOTIC
(I) BOERING
(V) NONE.

MEDICATIONS:
MEDROL DOSE PACK
FLEXARIL 10 MG ADVISED
NAPROSYN 375 MG ADVISED.

DISCUSSION:
THE FOLLOWING TREATMENT HAS BEEN
RECOMMENDED.

FIGURE 49-3.   The McCain TMJ Assessment Standardized Form.

SECTION 6

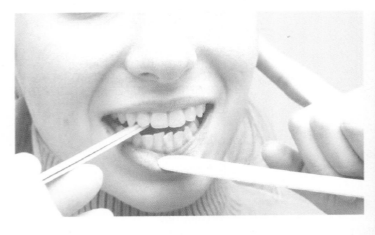
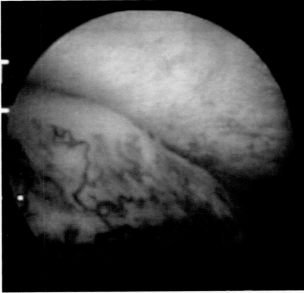

FIGURE 49-4. Mahan's sign. Patient and arthroscopic view.

occlusion in some patients may, however, exhibit vertical maxillary deficiency (VMD), causing early loss of posterior dentition with subsequent posterior or vertical collapse and bite closure. In this case, the dysfunction is the result of the collapse of the vertical dimension, with a direct microtrauma effect on the joint over an extended time.

III. Direct macrotrauma. Direct trauma involves an acute direct trauma to the mandible with or without fracture. Most of the time, patients can specifically recall the event because their TMJ problems developed immediately after the event. In some situations of direct trauma to the mandible, there are no immediate effects on the joint. However, as years progress, the classic symptoma-

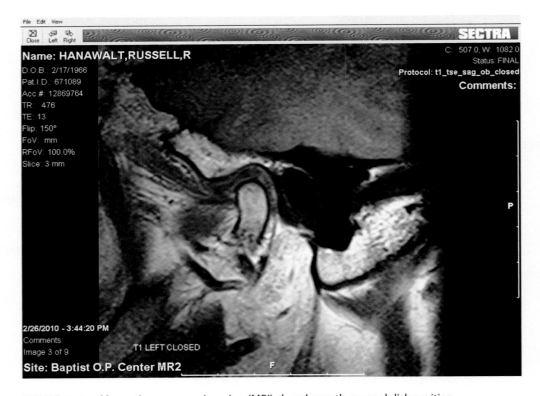

FIGURE 49-5. Magnetic resonance imaging (MRI) closed-mouth–normal disk position

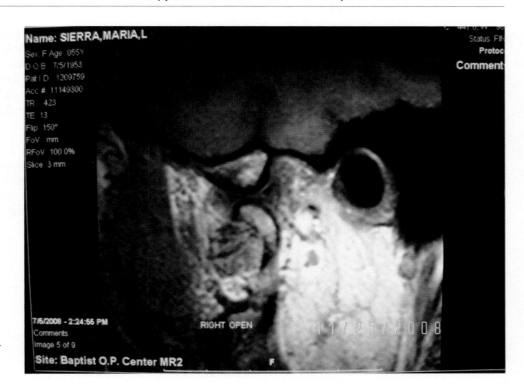

FIGURE 49-6. MRI open-mouth–normal disk position or disk recapture.

tology develops in the joint and no other finding of anamnesis indicates any other etiologic factor.

IV. **Indirect macrotrauma.** These are patients reporting injuries of the acceleration-deceleration type phenomenon, followed by progressive symptoms consisting of muscle splinting that advances to arthralgia and joint noise.

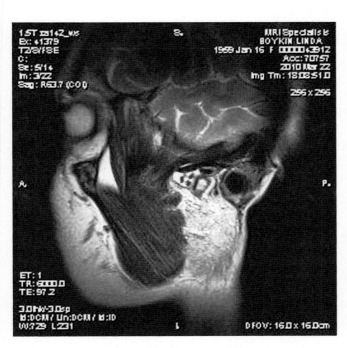

FIGURE 49-7. T2 weighted MRI—joint effusions.

V. **Systemic disease.** Most of the diseases with TMJ involvement fall into the categories of rheumatoid arthritis (RA), systemic lupus erythematosus (SLE), and benign or malignant tumors, although the latter two are rather infrequent occurrences.

Diagnosis

In most cases, the patient will present without prior advanced imaging; however, a comprehensive history and clinical examination will allow a diagnosis to be formulated, and an MRI is indicated only if the clinical examination is equivocal. A diagnostic staging should be made for each patient according to the Wilkes classification system.

Discussion

The conclusion of the TMJ consultation form is the formulation of an initial treatment plan. A few remarks are in order after the completion of the standardized form. If the TMJ anamnesis examination is performed correctly, it will definitely elucidate the necessary information about the patient. This can be achieved only by developing an accurate, concise, and repeatable technique for collection of data. A complete TMJ workup (including diagnosis and initial treatment plan) could be completed in 15 to 30 minutes, using standardized forms and clinical experience.

SECTION 6

Rapid TMJ Assessment

As the clinician becomes more experienced, more accurate and more comfortable with all the rigors of the TMJ examination, the assessment procedures can be expedited. Eventually, the TMJ surgeon performs the same rapid TMJ assessment for the initial assessment of a new patient as well as for the follow-up patients. This rapid assessment helps the surgeon to conduct a problem-focused assessment using a standardized form (see Figure 49-3), thus further increasing the speed of evaluation. The TMJ follow-up form (Figure 49-8) gives the practitioner all the pertinent information with regard to the patient's condition, progress, future course of action, and follow-up. As a quick review, the clinician should assess ROM of the mandible in all excursions, while listening/auscultating and palpating the joints, periarticular structures, the masseter and temporalis muscles as previously described. Also, a check should be performed for Mahan's sign, and all findings should be correlated with those from previous visits.

ARTHROCENTESIS

In 1991, Nitzan and Dolwick identified a unique clinical situation of closed lock of the TMJ that could not be explained by conventional methods of diagnosis of the

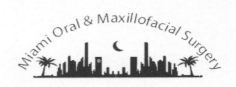

PATIENT NAME: JANE DOE
TODAYS DATE: July 21, 2010
PATIENT ID: 23066

S/P:
STEROID INJECTION
MEDICAL MANAGEMENT
BOERING
ORTHOTIC
DISCOPEXY SCREW
DISCOPEXY SUTURE
EMINECTOMY
PHYSICAL THERAPY
OFFICE ARTHRSCOPY
DISCOPEXY
DEBRIDMENT
SILASTIC PULL OUT
HOSPITAL LYSIS AND LAVAGE
TOTAL JOINT
CHRISTENSEN FOSSA
CONTRACTURE

MEDICATIONS:
ULTRAM
OTC
STEROIDS
ELAVIL
NO
NARCOTICS
NON NSAIDS
MUSCLE RELAXANT
NON STERIODAL
OTHER
YES.

DIET:
REGULAR:
SOFT.

ANALOGS:

LEFT
RIGHT

MIO:

MAHAN DIRECT:
RIGHT YES
LEFT NO
RIGHT NO
LEFT YES

JOINT NOISE:
LEFT YES
LEFT NO
RIGHT NO
RIGHT YES.

MUSCLE PAIN:
LEFT YES
LEFT NO
RIGHT NO
RIGHT YES.

JOINT PAIN:
LEFT YES
LEFT NO
RIGHT NO
RIGHT YES.

OCCLUSION:
UNSTABLE
STABLE.

FIGURE 49-8. The McCain TMJ Follow-up Standardized Form.

disease process. Prior to their description, Murakami in 1986 identified the ability to recapture a persistently displaced anterior disk displacement with a single-puncture technique to accomplish a pumping action and the use of hydraulic pressure in the superior joint space. It was Nitzan and Dolwick, however, who questioned the usual mechanisms of development of disk displacement and identified a condition of severe, limited mouth opening (<30 mm) without translation, no joint noise, that could occur at any age, was not a result of macrotrauma, was unrelated to disk shape or position, was unresponsive to nonsurgical TMJ therapy, and was responsive to the technique of joint pressure lysis and lavage (arthrocentesis). They were convinced that this condition was different from classic disk displacement. The lack of condylar translation was attributed to adherence of the disk to the fossa due to a "vacuum" or "suction-cup" effect of the convex disk pressed against the anterior slope of the glenoid fossa, and this situation is more likely to occur in joints with decreased synovial fluid volume and increased viscosity. Several studies showed the efficacy of dual-puncture arthrocentesis in relieving "disk adhesion" (the stuck disk) with acute painful limited opening and allowing a rapid improvement in mouth opening and decrease in pain. It is important to consider performing the procedure early after the onset of symptoms (<3 mo) and consideration of the use of bite splint therapy postoperatively to unload the joint space. Whereas corticosteroids have been used routinely in the joint space after the arthrocentesis procedure, several studies have indicated that the use of sodium hyaluronate may have better short- and long-term benefits. Over the years, studies have shown comparable results of arthroscopy and arthrocentesis primarily due to the lysis and lavage portion of the technique, resulting in clearance of inflammatory mediators and relief of a vacuum effect in the joint space. It has been concluded that arthrocentesis could be considered as an intervening treatment between nonsurgical management and arthroscopy, especially in cases that could be identified as disk adhesion with acute onset of symptoms. The procedure is relatively simple to perform in office with a low cost and minimal chance of complications (fluid extravasation into soft tissues, transient facial nerve weakness) and potentially high benefit if it can resolve the clinical symptoms. Of course, the major benefits of arthroscopy over arthrocentesis include direct visualization of the joint space and the ability to perform a variety of invasive procedures as described in detail in this chapter, whereas arthrocentesis does little to address the specific etiology of the disk problem or prevent recurrence. Whereas treatment decisions must be individualized in each patient, arthrocentesis should be considered before more invasive techniques.

The Arthroscope

The arthroscope is a specific endoscope designed to extend the eye of the arthroscopist to the tip of the instrument, inside the intra-articular space.

Optical Characteristics

FIELD OF VIEW

The field of view (FOV) of the arthroscope is the included angle drawn from the tip of the scope to the extreme edges of the field or object space. When the scope is used in a fluid medium, the FOV angle is approximately 40% less than the one measured in the air with the same arthroscope (Figure 49-9).

DIRECTION OF VIEW

The direction of view is the angle projected between the normal axis of the arthroscope and a line through the center of the image viewed through the arthroscope. Direction and FOV are the most common angles used in the description of the arthroscope. In order to determine the extreme edge of field of a scope, add the direction of view angle plus half the FOV angle. The sum of the two numbers equals the extreme angle from the axis that can be seen (see Figure 49-9).

APPARENT FOV

The apparent FOV is the included angle drawn from the observer's eye to the extreme edges of the field or object space.

Optical Parameters

STIGMATISM OF THE IMAGE

This parameter refers to focusing a joint in the field identically to a joint in the apparent field. Lack of stigmatism is indicative of either design or manufacturing flaws in the arthroscope.

DISTORTION

This parameter correlates with a straight line in the image. The "shop-terms" "pin-cushion" or "barrel" distortion refer to the sides of a square symmetrically situated in the FOV that has the very sides curved inward or outward, respectively. Unless significant, distortion is of no consequence in endoscopy.

CHROMATIC CORRECTION

Images may be displaced axially as a function of wavelength or color or may be different sizes as a function of color. The chromatic correction of an instrument is much more critical for photography than for visual use. As far as the TMJ arthroscopy is concerned, white-balancing the scope before intra-articular introduction will address the chromatic correction.

VIGNETTING

Vignetting translates into a defect stemmed in the optical design, manufacturing, or misalignment caused by bending or displacement of the optical elements. It results in a loss of brightness of the peripheral area of the image, secondary to light obstruction by mounts, stops, or element cells. On occasion, vignetting may present as an oval rather than a round FOV.

TRANSMISSION

Each surface of an optical system reflects a fraction of the incidence of the luminous ray beam; and each element

SECTION 6

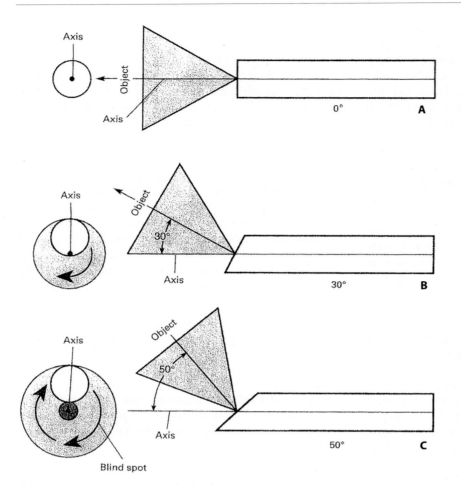

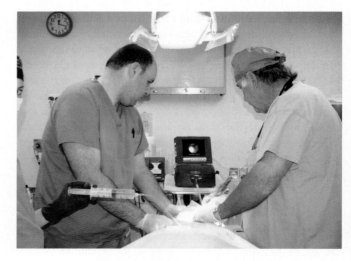

FIGURE 49-9.   Direction of view of three arthroscopes, each with a field of view angle of 60 degrees and an effective field of view (left of each scope) if the arthroscope is rotated 360 degrees about its axis. **A,** The 0-degree scope: the field of view remains the size of the diameter of the scope as it is rotated. **B,** The 30-degree scope: the field of view is greater with this scope as it is rotated. **C,** The 50 degree scope: the field of view is even greater; however, the offset is such that a blind spot *(black circle)* exists as the endoscope is rotated.

of the optical system will absorb a certain fraction. The effectiveness of transmission of an endoscopic system is approximately 90%.

VEILING GLARE

Image-forming light reflected by each surface is, in turn, re-reflected, in part, by all surfaces preceding it in the system. Some of this light, together with a small amount scattered by each surface due to imperfections in polish and debris on the surfaces, reduces the contrast in the image and the ability of the endoscopist to resolve fine detail.

Technology of Video Arthroscopy

The video camera is routinely used in TMJ arthroscopy for viewing the surgical field indirectly on a monitor. The advantages of its use are better operative field sterility (less action in and around the operative field), surgeon comfort, and most important, a high-quality image magnified on the monitor, enhancing visibility and engagement of the entire surgical team (Figure 49-10). It is invaluable in the evaluation of intra-articular pathology by both surgeon and assistant as well as a teaching modality. Recorded media allows for review of surgical findings during the postsurgical visit. The patient can now be educated by virtual means regarding her

or his joint disease process. Also, the medicolegal record-keeping is very accurate. The disadvantage of the entire system is, obviously, pecuniary. The sophisticated miniaturized video camera, high-resolution monitors, as well as the quality recording equipment necessary for video arthroscopy may be rather expensive. In addition, this quite

FIGURE 49-10.   Temporomandibular joint (TMJ) arthroscopy.

complicated equipment requires basic understanding of electronics and video electronics in order to set up and operate appropriately.

A video camera is composed of a lens system that receives the image from the arthroscope and focuses the image on a light-sensitive electronic device that translates this image into an electronic signal. The core of the camera is a silicon wafer with discrete light-sensing elements called *pixels*. The pixels have the ability to translate color and light intensity into electronic signals that, in turn, can be recorded from the camera on a DVD, displayed on a TV monitor, and/or processed into a still image.

The chip sensor determines the quality of the image and specifications of the video camera. The numbers and size of pixels correspond directly to the detail of image reproduction (camera resolution). Out of the charged couple device (CCD) and metal oxide semiconductor (MOS) pixels, only the CCDs are at present used, because their high color sensitivity, color rendition capabilities, and broad dynamic range for various light intensities has permitted a significant reduction of the video camera size while increasing the number of pixels.

A camera produces color by selectively filtering certain pixels on the sensor for one specific color. Electronic signals for red, green, and blue are produced separately. Red, green, and blue, or the complementary colors magenta, yellow, and cyan, can be either added or subtracted to produce any single color. Masks of these colors, in either a striped or a mosaic pattern, filter the individual pixels. These filtered pixels are electrically sampled and the actual color is determined. The latest advancements in technology have permitted the use of a different method of color determination that employs a prism system within the camera, which separates the colors, then directs them to three separate sensors. Despite an increase in the quality of the image, this system was, until recently, technique prohibitive because it promoted an increase in the size of the camera.

Specifications

The quality of the image produced is a factor of several camera specifications, including horizontal and vertical resolution, minimum light sensitivity, color sensitivity, and signal-to-noise ratio. Other factors such as type of signal produced, scanning systems, and color systems also influence the characteristics of the image and its ability to be used with other equipment.

Resolution is the degree of picture detail that can be perceived and is comparable with good vision, allowing the surgeon to visualize more detail or to discern more features. A video image is composed of a series of lines, both horizontal and vertical, scanned in the camera and drawn by the monitor to produce the image. The initial factor in determining the resolution capabilities of the video camera is the actual number of pixels in the camera. Subsequently, resolution is determined by the ability of the electronic equipment to transmit, record, or reproduce the picture elements. The

least sensitive piece of equipment in the system will, finally, determine the observed resolution. In general, the camera should be the least sensitive part in the circuit.

The size of the arthroscopic image is determined by the optics of the scope and lens system on the camera magnifying the image focused on the sensor in the camera. Cameras used for smaller size scopes have a greater lens magnification system in order to adequately enlarge the image. If the image is too reduced on the sensor, the camera's resolution will be underemployed.

The *alignment* and *ability* of the camera to accurately reproduce color are set by the manufacturer. Adjustments in the electronic interpretation of color are imminent due to the variations in the light sources used to illuminate the joint. White light is made of all spectral colors. Certain light sources will emit more blue or yellow light, thus influencing the appearance of joint structures and color of the image. When viewing a white object illuminated by different light sources, the signal from the camera is adjusted to equalize the red, green, and blue electronic signals using the "white balance" settings. Most cameras white-balance automatically or with minimal operator intervention.

A *color temperature* of 5000°K is ideal for accurate color reproduction and corresponds most closely to natural daylight illumination. Further adjustment for color may also be made on the monitor if necessary. A color pattern can be generated by the camera, whereas color reproduction can be altered on the monitor using brightness, tint, and hue adjustments.

The *scanning system* is the means by which the video image is assembled from information provided by the sensors.

The TMJ arthroscopy requires a cold white bright light source to adequately illuminate the joint cavity. The light source must be variable in intensity to adjust for changes in illumination requirements for different parts of the joint. This has been accomplished by controlling the quantity of light delivered at the light source with a variable iris aperture, via an autosensing light source that determines the strength of the video signal and increases or decreases the iris aperture accordingly, thus controlling the quantity of light delivered to the light cable. The arthroscopic system also employs an automatic gain control system of the video signal that leaves the light intensity constant and varies the strength of the video signal proportional to the required illumination.

Light sensitivity is the degree to which the camera determines an image in low-light situations. It measured in lux. The *signal-to-noise ratio* is a measure of the video signal to the background electronic noise. A larger ratio denotes a better, clearer picture. It is measured in decibels.

On Point System

One of the developments in technology of the later years is the On Point system (Biomet, Jacksonville, FL) (Figure 49-11). This diagnostic arthroscopy system uses a 1.2-mm, 0° scope. The high-quality resolution and portable surgical

SECTION 6

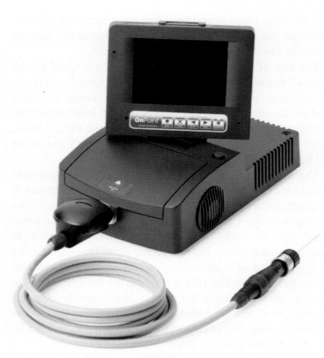

FIGURE 49-11. The On Point System (Biomet).

unit make this operation amenable to the outpatient setting, with significant cost savings for the patient. The armamentarium includes an ergonomic handpiece containing a camera and light source, enabled to capture still images and record videos. The all-digital imaging platform includes a 6.4-inch LCD monitor that combines the performance of the Xenon Fiber Optic Light Source (delivering a 175-W illumination performance) and the High-Resolution Camera System (480-line digital camera) to deliver the image. The 1.2-mm disposable scope is the size of an 18-gauge needle. The other instruments included are a single-use cannula, trocar, obturator, and cannula plug (Figure 49-12). The cannula has an outside diameter of 1.9 mm and a Luer port on the body to connect an irrigation source. The port also permits intra-articular injection.

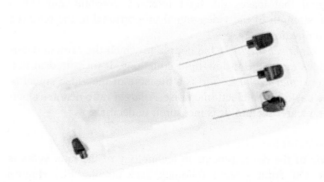

FIGURE 49-12. Sterile single-use instruments: trocar, cannula, obturator, cannula-plug.

Smith-Nephew System

The data acquired by the 560 Series 3-CCD High Definition Camera (HD 1080i) (Figure 49-13) are conveyed to the CCU via high-speed digital-interface. The image data is processed and converted into HDTV images, which are displayed on flat-panel HD monitors. A 1.9-mm-diameter 30-degree scope, with a 75-degree FOV angle and a 65-mm working length, is connected to the camera head. The scope J-locks into a 2.0-mm cannula with flowport. The cannula is versatile for the 2.0-mm short trocar as well as the 2.0-mm short obturator with a conical tip.

Armamentarium

Hand Instrumentation

CANNULAS

The delivery system facilitates not only passing of hand instruments into the joint but also irrigation and maintenance of joint insufflation. The markings on the cannula begin at 15 mm from the tip and continue in 5-mm increments (Figure 49-14). Similar cannulas must be used in double-puncture arthroscopy to allow for the interchanging of instruments and scope between portals. The 1.7-mm-diameter hand instruments leave a 0.3-mm space for irrigation outflow. All instruments are marked in 5-mm increments. For larger-diameter instruments (i.e., 2.7 mm), this author has designed a switch-stick, facilitating the interchange between the 2.0- and the 3.0-mm-diameter cannulas.

PROBES

The **straight probe** is the most basic arthroscopic hand instrument. It is used for palpation, severing adhesions, and mobilization/temporary immobilization of tissue (i.e., disk). The **hooked probe** is similar to the latter except for a small terminal hook. It is the preferred instrument for palpation in cases of chondromalacia. The typical use of this probe is to elevate the anterior aspect of the disk after anterior releasing procedures and to complete the dissection of the disk from capsule and pterygoid muscle. The hooked probe is also preferred in difficult cases of disk reduction, with lax/redundant retrodiskal tissue, where a straight probe may lacerate the structure. Hooking of the oblique protuberance before disk reduction enables reduction without herniation of tissue (Figure 49-15).

BIOPSY FORCEPS

The serrated type (Figure 49-16) has cupped beaks and is used for small biopsy samples and for the débridement of pathologic or fragmented tissues. The basket type (Figure 49-17) harvests mostly full-thickness biopsy specimens (i.e., synovial tissue).

The French no. 5 myringotomy suction tip will evacuate clots or heme during arthroscopy (Figure 49-18). The 2.0-mm cannula easily accommodates this suction.

MENISCUS MENDER

This packaged set consists of straight and curved spinal needles with stylet and a suture loop used to snare the suture

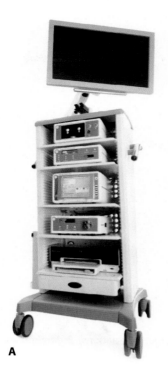
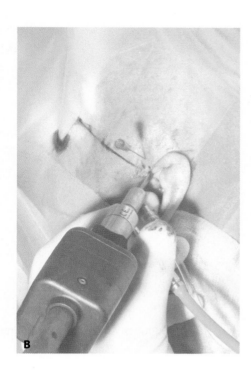

FIGURE 49-13. **A** and **B,** The Smith-Nephew System 560 Series 3-CCD.

once passed through the needle (Figure 49-19). While in the process of designing a less invasive replica of Meniscus Mender I and II, this author uses, for most situations, a 22-gauge needle to pass the suture for diskopexy procedures.

Other Hand Instruments

In the advent of the latest advancements in motorized, electrical, but most of all, laser technology, a number of hand instruments have become obsolete. The suction punch, bone rasps, curettes, banana blades, forked blades, sickles,

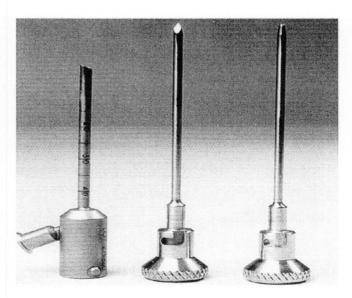

FIGURE 49-14. **Left to right,** Scored cannula, sharp trocar, blunt obturator with J-locking system.

and others are only rarely used and in very specific situations. Two instruments in this category should, however, never be missing from the arthroscopist's arsenal: the obturator and the **golden retriever** (Figure 49-20). The latter is an invaluable magnetized instrument specialized in the apprehension and delivery of intra-articular broken instruments.

Motorized Instruments

The unique concept of motorized shavers and abraders enables suctioning of the arthroscopic field while cutting and removing tissue in an efficient manner. Four factors are paramount for these instruments to function efficiently: (1) the design of the cutting blade, (2) the pressure balance between the suction and the continuous irrigation fluid, (3) the revolution speed (rpm) of the instrument, and (4) the type of tissue that the surgeon is attempting to cut. This author has discovered that the ultimate parameters of efficiency for the shaver are reached at the lower spectrum rpm-range speed. After developing a refined intra-articular tactile sense for the instrument, the author has noticed that the most efficient "shaving" occurs with a repeated pistoning motion.

Shavers

The larger of the two shavers in use at present, 2.9 mm in diameter, is used for more aggressive arthroscopic arthroplasty. A 2.9-mm-diameter suction punch may become necessary with the use of this shaver. For the sake of maintaining the procedures in the least invasive manner, this author has, lately, used only the 1.9-mm shaver.

SECTION 6

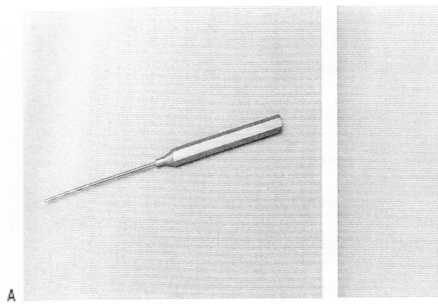

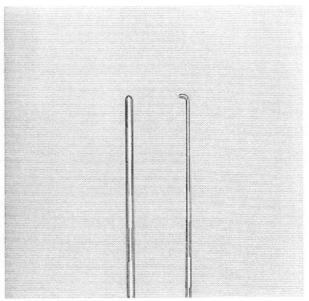

FIGURE 49-15.   Probes. **A,** Straight probe (5-mm-increment gradations). **B,** Straight and hooked probes (active ends).

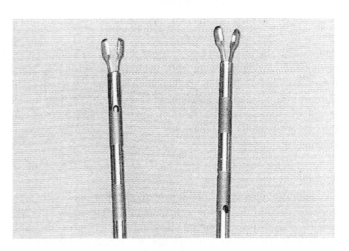

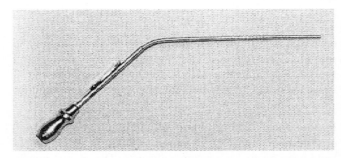

FIGURE 49-18.   French no. 5 myringotomy suction tip.

FIGURE 49-16.   Nonserrated and serrated biopsy forceps.

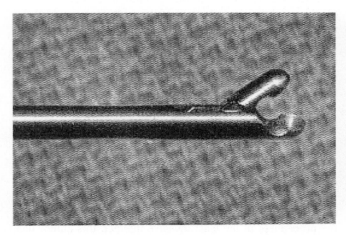

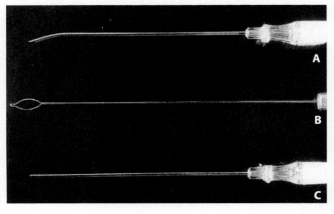

FIGURE 49-17.   Basket biopsy forceps.

FIGURE 49-19.   Meniscus mender set. **A,** Curved needle with stylet. **B,** Suture loop/snare. **C,** Straight needle

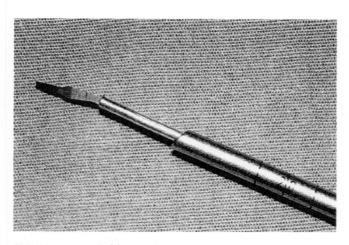

FIGURE 49-20.   Golden retriever.

WHISKER SHAVER

The one disadvantage of this shaver is its ability to generate intra-articular iatrogeny if not controlled appropriately. It can scuff articular surfaces and cause cartilaginous defects transfixiant to the subjacent osseous structures. The instrument has been so profiled that the articular surfaces are completely protected from the cutting portion of the active part (Figure 49-21). The perforations in the external sleeve of the instrument promote a suction effect on the soft tissue that the inner blade cuts next. The whisker shaver has been designed for the débridement of fine fragmented fibrocartilage from articular surfaces, small fibrous adhesions, or small fragments of the disk periphery. It may remove fibrotic or dessicated synovial tissue; however, its use on intact/vascular synovium is discouraged.

FULL-RADIUS SHAVER

Available in 1.9 and 2.9 mm diameters, it is a more aggressive instrument designed to resect tissue of an even more

fibrotic consistency, such as fibrous bands, adhesions, large areas of dessicated synovium, and fragmented edges of meniscus.

ABRADERS

These bone drills (the round and barrel-shaped abraders) are used to decorticate the osseous structures and create pinpoint areas of microhemorrhage in order to promote cartilaginous regeneration.

Electrosurgery

Electrosurgery is the use of high-frequency electric current to facilitate a tissue change. The human body's electrolyte composition makes it a conductor of electricity. During electrocautery, alternating current is passed to the surgical electrode probe in the form of heat. The manner in which the tissue responds to the electrothermal energy depends on the waveform of the current, the power at the electrode tip, the time of exposure at the electric tip, and cooling of tissue with blood circulation. The waveform determines the type of current used. The continuous sinusoidal waveform is used for the cutting mode, because it, mechanically, disrupts cells. The attenuated/"dampened" waveform, eventually oscillating down to resting potential, is used for the coagulating mode.

The McCain monopolar and bipolar electrocautery probes (Figure 49-22) are all insulated with the exception of the tips of the instruments. The safer, more rigid probes have the ability to manipulate tissue while delivering the electrical energy. In order not to compromise the insulation of the probes, the recommended settings of the generator should not be exceeded. Whereas common settings, based on clinical experience, exist for each tip, the individual settings may change. The intro-/extromission of the electrocautery probe at the working cannula is a very deliberate motion. Abrasion of insulation, in the process, should be avoided at all costs because it can expose another potentially active area on the

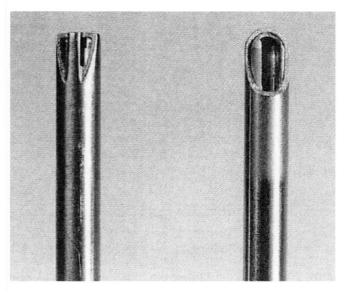

FIGURE 49-21.   Whisker and full-radius shavers.

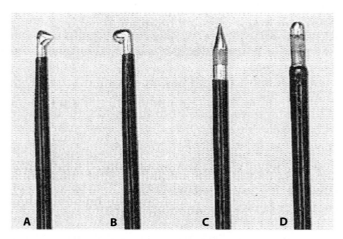

FIGURE 49-22.   McCain monopolar and bipolar probes. **A,** Monopolar sharp hook. **B,** Monopolar blunt hook. **C,** Bipolar sharp hook. **D,** Bipolar blunt hook.

SECTION 6

tip of the instrument. In this particular situation, an area of the joint can be iatrogenically injured while outside the arthroscopic FOV.

A grounding pad should be used at all times. It should self-adhere to the skin. If a grounding discontinuity occurs, the entire system shuts down. The thousands of arthroscopic procedures performed by this author, such as posterior synovial pouch cauterization, electrosurgical anterior release (McCain technique), electrosurgical synovectomy, and electrocautery for hemostasis, have afforded the experience necessary to understand the effects of electrocautery on intra-articular temperature. Extensive intra-articular thermocoupling studies have enabled the author to elaborate an irrigation protocol for these procedures. Except for the case of monopolar cautery, in which the irrigating agent is sterile water, all other procedures will undergo irrigation with lactated Ringer's solution. The reason behind using sterile water (theoretically, the safest, nonconducting medium) only for monopolar procedures stems in the hyposmolar absorption and lack of support for proteoglycan synthesis that will, eventually, translate in chondrocytomegaly. This phenomenon would very likely occur in the case of intra-articular tissues that have sustained injury and, subsequently, would maintain a higher rate of matrix synthesis than normal tissue.

Laser

Laser (light amplification by stimulated emission of radiation) technology transmits energy in the form of light beam. The laser beam is columnated, equally spaced apart and coherent in the same time and space. Laser energy is delivered in a continuous or a pulsated wave. The wavelength of a particular laser determines the physical properties of a laser in the clinical use setting.

Carbon Dioxide Laser

Laser energy in the far infrared spectrum (CO_2 laser) is avidly absorbed by water. Because tissues have a high water content, the CO_2 laser energy is readily absorbed within the superficial layer of tissue with a very localized tissue effect. However, owing to the very long wavelength, this laser cannot be passed through a flexible quartz fiber without undergoing distortion.

Holmium:Yttrium-Aluminum-Garnet Laser

This laser's wavelength is 2140 nm, making it somewhat similar to the CO_2 laser with regards to its high hydroabsorbability. The holmium laser, however, has a limited depth of penetration (0.3–0.5 mm), making it very useful intra-articularly. In this author's hands, this laser variety is the most versatile for arthroscopic techniques on the TMJ, such as anterior release, synovectomy, posterior scarification, and débridement of fibrocartilage. The small size of the delivery tip facilitates excellent access in limited spaces, while its metal encasement prevents the breakage of this quartz fiber. To this date, the holmium:yttrium-aluminum-garnet

(Ho:YAG) laser is considered the most safe and effective modality for intra-articular TMJ delivery of energy.

Portals of Entry and Danger Zones

Fossa Portal

This puncture site has to be situated inside a 20-mm-diameter circle centered over the glenoid fossa (Figure 49-23A). The osseous boundaries of this circle are the apex of the articular eminence anteriorly, the middle of the acoustic meatus posteriorly, the posterior portion of the temporal fossa at the anterior segment of the supramastoid crest of the temporal squama, and finally, the posterosuperior border of the ramus at condylar neck level inferiorly. The superficial correspondent of the posterior osseous landmark is the middle of the tragus, because it is situated 5 mm anterior to the tragal apex and 5 mm posterior to the anterior wall of the osseous external auditory canal. This author's observations have placed the peak of the cartilaginous wall of the meatus at the exact level of the posterior aspect of the TMJ capsule. The neurovascular bundle (auriculotemporal nerve, superficial temporal vein and artery) is, in 80% of cases, 5 to 8 mm anterior to the midportion of the tragus. Within the limits of the glenoid fossa circular trough, the anatomic structures are, from lateral to medial, dermis, subcutaneous tissue, superficial parotid fascia, superior and posterior parotid lobule, auriculotemporal nerve, superficial temporal vein, and superficial temporal artery (see Figure 49-23B).

Anterior Eminence Portal

For teaching visualizing purposes, the same 20-mm-diameter circle can be superimposed over the anterior eminence region in the same fashion as for the fossa portal (Figure 49-24A). The boundaries for this circle are the zygomatic process of the temporal arch anteriorly, the apex of the articular eminence of the zygomatic process of the temporal bone posteriorly, the temporal fossa superiorly, and the mandibular sigmoid notch inferiorly. The anatomic structures at this site are, from lateral to medial, the tegument, the superficial parotid fascia, the superoanterior parotid gland lobule, the deep parotid fascia, and the most posterior point of intersection of the frontal branch of the facial nerve, the masseter, the masseteric nerve, artery, and vein, the anterolateral aspect of the TMJ capsule, and the lateral pterygoid (see Figure 49-24B). Measuring from the midportion of the tragus anteriorly, the frontal branch of the facial would be found ranging 13 to 40 mm with a mean of 20 to 25 mm. The zygomatic orbital branch lies anterior to the frontal branch.

Danger Zones

Before proceeding with the fossa puncture, then the diagnostic sweep, the surgeon must be cognizant of the "danger zones" and proximity of vital structures associated with this procedure. The three "danger zones" are the dura mater and temporal lobe situated immediately cranial to the glenoid fossa, with a thickness of 0.5 to 1.5 mm (Figure 49-25); the

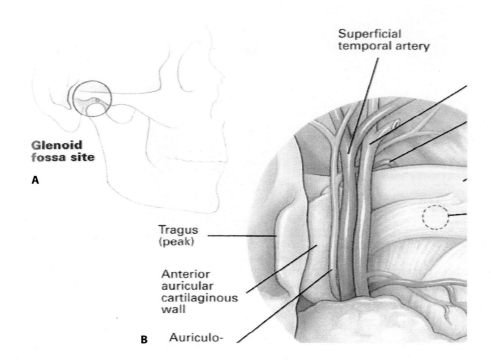

FIGURE 49-23.   Fossa portal. **A,** Lateral view of the glenoid puncture site with the most important adjacent structures. **B,** Coronal view of the TMJ (lateral-to-medial) with the adjacent anatomic structures.

tympanum ossicles, and middle ear; and the entire length of the medial aspect of the capsule represented by the lateral pterygoid. The vital structures that have to be given special consideration are the mandibular division of the trigeminus, especially the lingual and inferior alveolar branches, the ATN and the internal maxillary artery together with all the small branches supplying the capsule (Figure 49-26).

Internal Arthroscopic Anatomy

Posterior Recess

The first structure encountered upon entering the joint is the synovium. The synovial membrane is mesenchymal in origin and a continuation of the cambium layer of the periosteum. Similar to other joints, the TMJ synovium covers the capsule and periarticular disk tissues, with the exception of the

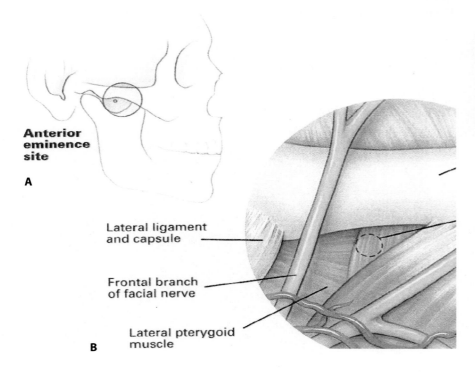

FIGURE 49-24.   Anterior eminence portal. **A,** Eminence puncture site with the adjacent structures. **B,** Coronal view at the level of the articular eminence (lateral-to-medial) with the adjacent anatomic structures.

SECTION 6

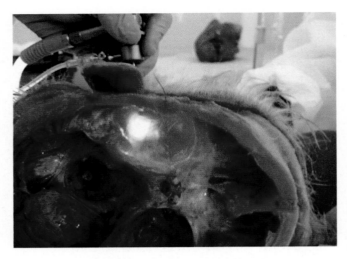

FIGURE 49-25. Danger zones. Meticulous cadaver middle cranial fossa dissection reveals the proximity of the articular glenoid fossa to the temporal lobe dura mater. Courtesy of Gary Warburton, DDS, MD

articular surfaces of the cartilages. The synovial lining is grayish with a translucent background and soft in consistency. The normal synovium has a mild amount of capillary proliferation, diffuse throughout the lining. With the condyle in a forward position (Figure 49-27), the synovium of the posterior pouch lies flat and tight over the retrodiskal tissue. The oblique protuberance is a classic structure of the posterior pouch. With condyle forward, the oblique protuberance is a fibroelastic band that protrudes into the retrodiskal tissue. It is located two thirds medial from lateral to medial into the joint. With the condyle seated, the synovium "buckles and ruffles" like an accordion being closed (Figure 49-28). The synovial tissue attaches from the back portion of the disk. The posterior band of disk running over the retrodiskal tissue

attaches to the posterior aspect of the of the glenoid fossa at approximately midportion or the superior one third of the glenoid posterior wall of the glenoid fossa. The medial synovial drape appears normally as a gray, translucent synovial lining. Very distinct striae run superior to inferior, defining the medial synovium. It serves as another classic landmark in the arthroscopic examination. In the background of the medial aspect of the drape, the pterygoid shadow reflects with a red/purple tinge.

Intermediate Zone

In the middle of the joint, the fibrocartilage of the glenoid fossa is visible, thin, white, and not very reflective. Anterior to the glenoid fossa and along the back slope of the articular eminence, the fibrocartilage becomes whiter and more reflective of light and also takes on a classic appearance of striae formation that runs anterior to posterior. Changing the angle of view inferiorly, with the condyle forward, part of the disk can be seen as milky white, highly reflective of light, and without striations. With the condyle forward, the disk completely covers the condyle. The clear junction between the synovium and the posterior band of the disk is represented by a red-white line where the capillary proliferation stops and the disk begins. A U-shaped depression or flexure between the synovial juncture and the posterior band of the disk can be observed. With the condyle seated, the disk covers the condyle and the flexure deepens significantly to the normal anatomic position of the disk. Toward the most lateral depth of the joint are the articular eminence and the trough within the eminence where the disk moves with the condylar translation.

Anterior Recess

In the anterior pouch, the anterior slope of the articular eminence is evident. The fibrocartilage and anterior band of the

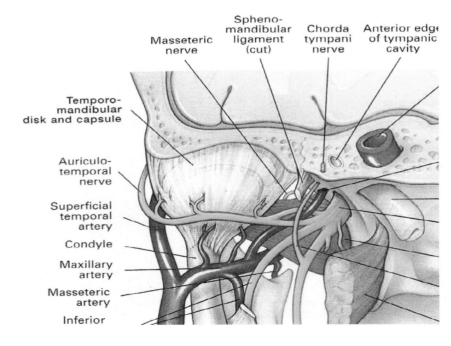

FIGURE 49-26. Posteroinferior view of the TMJ. Entry portals and reports with adjacent anatomic structures.

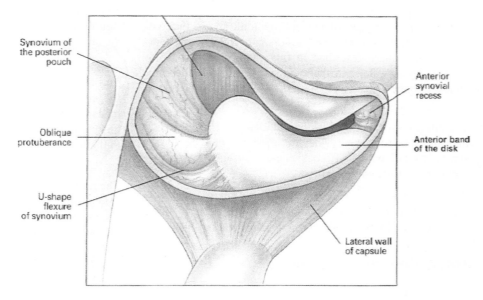

FIGURE 49-27.   Intra-articular structures of the TMJ with the condyle held in the forward position (lateral view).

disk are both white, reflective, and without striae. The synovium is tightly attached and has a gray, translucent background with mild capillary proliferation widely dispersed throughout. The synovium is also attached tightly to the anterior aspect of the ascending aspect of the articular eminence. Looking medially, the continuation of the medial synovial drape can be seen. The vertical striae of the drape are nonexistent, and the background consistency is deep purple secondary to the reflection of the pterygoid muscle fibers, much closer in this area. The lateral synovium is not tightly bound down but maintains the same color as the medial synovium.

The posteroanterior trough on the medial aspect of the joint is where the synovium descends off the medial synovial drape and then attaches to the disk in the same fashion as the medial trough.

Inferior Joint Space Anatomy

With the exception of very specific situations, such as existing disk perforation permitting the inferior joint space exploration without inducing any additional surgical trauma to the joint, this author does not advocate routine inferior joint space arthroscopic exploration.

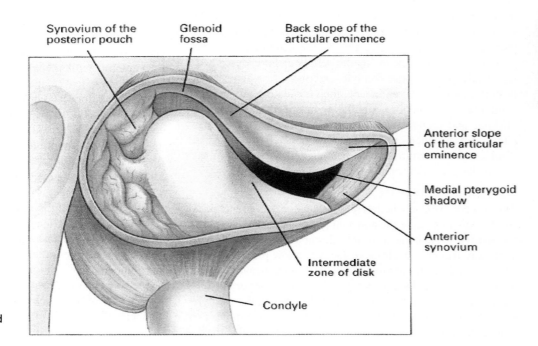

FIGURE 49-28.   Intra-articular structures of the TMJ with the condyle seated into the glenoid fossa (lateral view).

SECTION 6

POSTERIOR RECESS

In the posterior pouch of the inferior joint space, the synovium is similar in appearance, color, and capillary proliferation as previously described in this chapter. However, the consistency is softer and the synovium is not as adherently attached to the capsule.

INTERMEDIATE ZONE

The inferior aspect of the disk has a more grayish appearance than the superior aspect. The striae are absent. The disk is similarly reflective. The fibrocartilage is glistening white and highly reflective, without striae.

ANTERIOR RECESS

The synovial tissue has identical consistency. It is more attached to and less mobile onto the subjacent capsule.

TMJ Arthroscopic Technique

Immediate Preoperative Steps

EXAMINATION UNDER ANESTHESIA

The importance of this initial step of the procedure is paramount. It provides the surgeon with valuable information both pre- and postoperative. The preoperative examination ascertains joint mobility, articular bruits, and most important, the degree of difficulty of the upcoming punctures. Once the anesthesiologist administers the muscle relaxant, all myofascial factors related to condylar motion or disk function are eliminated. The clinician should be aware of the conditions that do not affect the mandibular range of motion independent of muscular tonus (e.g., advanced muscle fibrosis, extra-articular osseous impingements such as coronoid hyperplasia, Eagle's syndrome). Each joint is palpated separately. Normally, the condyle should subluxate the articular eminence. An inconsistent but common finding in patients with non-reducing disk derangements is the absence of this normal eminence subluxation. The postoperative dictation needs to include this particular observation pertaining to the examination under anesthesia. Bruits have to be elicited and described. By firmly pressing the condyle anterosuperior against the posterior slope of the eminence, then translating moving the condyle in all excursions, simulating mastication mechanics, clicking and crepitus can easily be achieved. A "seating-click," for instance, is used to describe a reducing disk displacement situation, when it is elicited during examination under general anesthesia.

PALPATION OF TMJ ANATOMY

The surgeon palpates the lateral joint anatomy in preparation for the puncture while the assistant manipulates the jaw. With the condyle seated, the assistant's thumb rolls into the buccal fold away from the occlusal surfaces to allow proper seating of the condyle in maximum occlusal intercuspation. The areas to be palpated are the superficial temporal artery preauricular (puncture must be anterior to the artery), the condyle in back-and-forth and side-to-side motion of mandible, the zygomatic process of the temporal, particularly the maximum concavity of the glenoid fossa (the soft tissue depression for the fossa portal puncture is located in this area), and the articular eminence with the condyle seated.

MARKING THE FOSSA PORTAL PUNCTURE SITE

The Holmlund-Helsing line is drawn with marker between the lateral canthus and the apex of tragus. A marking point is made at about the midportion of the external tragus. From this point, approximately 10 mm anterior and 2 mm inferior to the line, the maximum concavity of the fossa is located.

INSUFFLATION

The purpose for distention of the joint in this particular case is to expand the target area. In this process, 3 mL 0.5% bupivacaine in a 3-mL syringe with a 25-gauge, $1^1/_2$-inch needle are used. A vasoconstrictor should not be used because it could mask a correct diagnostic evaluation of engorgement of capillaries or reperfusion hypoxia phenomenon reflecting synovitis. From a caudolateral position, the needle penetrates the tegument in the preauricular crease, approximately 10 mm inferior to the Holmlund-Helsing line, at the junction of the tragus and pina. The needle is aimed at the central portion of the back slope of the eminence. Bone is contacted with the tip of the needle. The average joint will take approximately 3 mL. A plunger rebound greater than 0.5 mL indicates sufficient insufflation. Adequate joint distention is indicated by the amount of pressure on the plunger. Stenosed or fibrotic joints will typically take less fluid and the pressure required to insufflate the joint is increased ("early rebound"). Hypermobile joints or joints with disk perforations without adhesions may require more fluid.

Operative Steps

FOSSA PUNCTURE

The puncture is placed at maximum concavity of the glenoid fossa. The cannula is held in the right hand for a right joint puncture or in the left hand for a left joint puncture. The index controls the tip, and the palm of the hand controls the base of the cannula. With the condyle forward, the pollicis of the nondominant hand palpates the stable zygomatic process corresponding to the maximum concavity of the glenoid fossa immediately caudal. The trocar penetrates the skin with a rotational motion. This puncture is performed in a deliberate and careful fashion, attempting one pass through the lateral capsule into the joint space. Multiple lacerations of the capsule from multiple attempts cause problems with extravasation during the course of the operation. The trocar is then advanced until contact is felt with the osseous structure superiorly. The instrument is never to be passed straight through the capsule without locating the bone. The trocar is used almost in the same fashion as a periosteal elevator after it perforates the temporalis and the periosteum at the level of the zygomatic bone (Figure 49-29). The zygomatic arch is felt between the pollicis of the nondominant hand and the index finger of the dominant hand. The trocar then steps off the ledge (Figure 49-30). The distance from the tegument surface to the ledge varies between 5 and 10 mm. If this dis-

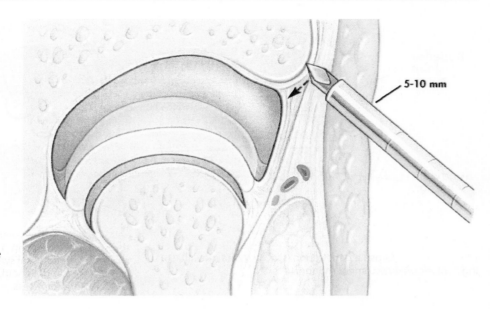

FIGURE 49-29. Cannula and trocar are advanced to the inferolateral aspect of the zygoma, then inferiorly stepped off the osseous ledge.

section is not accomplished properly, there is a high probability of invading the posterolateral subsynovial tissue. The trocar is then rotated until a slight pop is felt (Figure 49-31). It is then inserted approximately 10 to 15 mm. In the resting position, the cannula should be angled anterosuperiorly. A posterior or straight angulation could result in the laceration of the cartilaginous anterior wall of the external auditory meatus and, possibly, the perforation of the tympanic membrane and violation of the middle ear. Upon removal of trocar from the cannula, the reflux of fluid confirms perforation of the capsule. A blunt obturator is inserted and locked into the cannula. The cannula is then angled toward the open joint space. The middle portion of the cannula should, at this point, lever off the lateral aspect of the lateral margin of the glenoid fossa. The cannula should not be inserted more than 20 to 25 mm from tegument to the center of the joint (Figure 49-32). Before inserting the scope, the surgeon backwashes the joint

in order to remove all blood and synovial fluid. The backwashing is continued until the return fluid is clear. The scope can be inserted next. The image on the monitor will confirm correct entry into the joint space. The image may not be very clear due to the absence of outflow.

OUTFLOW NEEDLE PUNCTURE

With the mandible protruded, the scope is directed to the center of the fossa area of the joint. The assistant insufflates the joint with 2 to 3 mL of fluid in order to maintain joint distention. The purpose of the outflow needle is to establish a patent irrigation needle and, at the same time, maintain the joint adequately distended for intra-articular instrumentation. A 22-gauge, $1^{1}/_{2}$-inch needle is inserted approximately 5 mm anterior and 5 mm inferior to the fossa puncture site, under joint insufflation. Irrigation system should now be patent. An improvement in the quality of the image should be apparent.

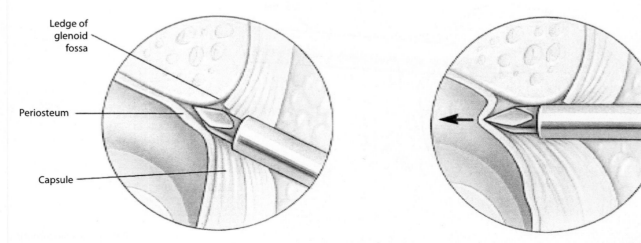

Ledge of glenoid fossa

Periosteum

Capsule

FIGURE 49-30. Cannula and trocar rotated through the capsule. Instrumentation maintains continuous osseous contact throughout this part of the procedure.

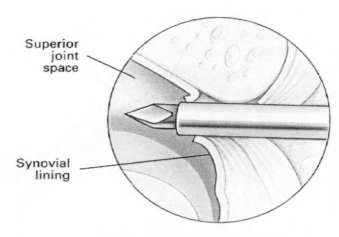

FIGURE 49-31. Capsule penetration (strictly transsynovial) using a rotation/advancement motion.

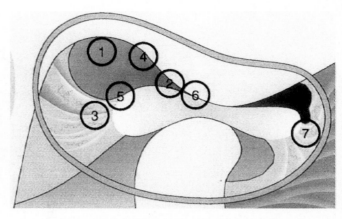

FIGURE 49-33. The seven points of interest of the TMJ arthroscopic examination. **1.** Medial synovial drape. **2.** Pterygoid shadow. **3.** Retrodiskal synovium. **4.** Posterior slope of the articular eminence and glenoid fossa. **5.** Articular disk. **6.** Intermediate zone. **7.** Anterior recess.

The system is switched next to continuous irrigation from the lactated Ringer's solution hanging bag.

DIAGNOSTIC SWEEP (SEVEN POINTS OF INTEREST OF TMJ ARTHROSCOPIC EXAMINATION)

Seven anatomic areas are examined during the sweep: medial synovial drape, pterygoid shadow, retrodiskal synovium (where the oblique protuberance, the retrodiskal synovial tissue attached to the posterior glenoid process, and the lateral recess of the retrodiskal synovial tissue have to be closely inspected), posterior slope of the articular eminence and glenoid fossa, articular disk, intermediate zone, anterior recess (with special consideration for the disk-synovial crease, the midportion, the medioanterior corner and the lateroanterior corner) (Figure 49-33). Losing orientation inside the joint, even for a short time can be a very frustrating experience for

the novice arthroscopist. Adding to the obstacles of inexperience, intra-articular pathology can deepen the confusion. The easiest method of preventing this occurrence is for the operator to be comfortable with the four classic intra-articular anatomic landmarks: medial synovial drape with its distinct superior-to-inferior striae, oblique protuberance of the retrodiskal synovium, posterior slope of the articular eminence with distinct anterior-to-posterior striae and anterior disk-synovial crease, and juncture of anterior synovium and anterior band of disk, which is the area for placement of a second or working cannula.

Area 1. Medial synovial drape (Figure 49-34) In many situations, the surgeon will run into one of the classic landmarks, typically, the oblique protuberance or the posterior slope of the articular eminence. The drape can be reached by

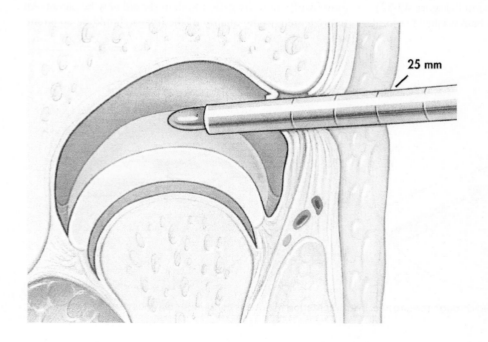

25 mm

FIGURE 49-32. Cannula advancement to the open intra-articular space to the 25-mm mark.

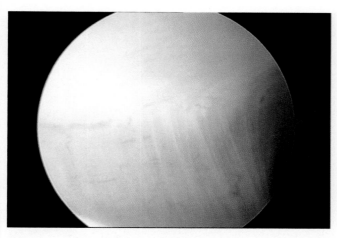

FIGURE 49-34.   Medial synovial drape (normal arthroscopic appearance).

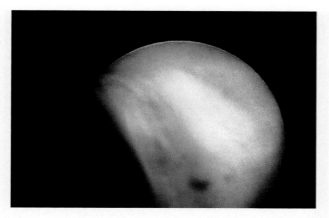

FIGURE 49-36.   Petechial synovitis at the medial synovial drape.

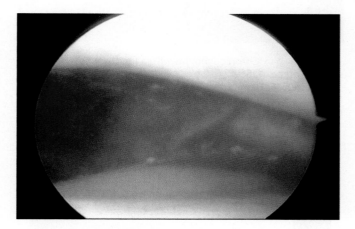

FIGURE 49-37.   Medial synovial drape erythema.

swiveling and pistoning the arthroscope until the drape becomes visible. This particular articular entity represents one of the most important barometers of TMJ synovitis. In acute inflammatory states, capillary proliferation with hyperemia of the medial synovial drape is increased (Figure 49-35). In addition, erythematous patches (petechiae) may be seen on the drape (Figure 49-36), or the entire drape may have an erythematous appearance (Figure 49-37). Occasionally, an in-bulging or prolapsing of the drape into the joint space occurs. Adhesive phenomena can also be seen (Figure 49-38). In chronic synovitis, the drape has a fibrotic or whitish appearance (Figure 49-39).

Area 2. Pterygoid shadow This second area to be examined will be reached by swiveling the scope anteriorly and pistoning medially until the shadow comes into view. A medial trough leads from the medial synovial drape anterior to the pterygoid shadow. The normal-appearing pterygoid shadow has a purple tinge attributed to the superior head of the lateral pterygoid subjacent to the synovial lining (Figure 49-40). Also, an obvious, well-delineated color difference is present between the drape and the shadow. During pathologic states, the pterygoid shadow takes on the appearance of marked erythema and marked hypervascularization and becomes quite thin (Figure 49-41). The synovial lining can

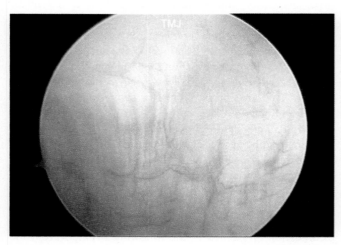

FIGURE 49-35.   Acute synovitis with capillary proliferation and hyperemia at the medial synovial drape.

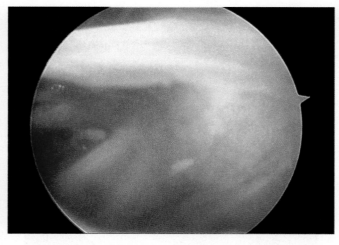

FIGURE 49-38.   Adhesive phenomenon and acute synovitis at the medial synovial drape.

SECTION 6

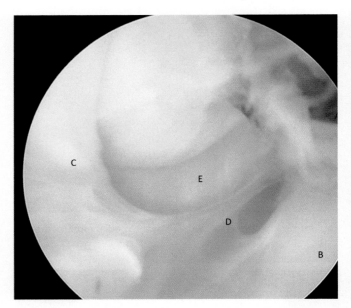

FIGURE 49-39. Chronic synovitis with a fibrotic medial synovial drape. **A,** Scuff (1–2 o'clock). **B,** Posterior band of disk (4–5 o'clock). **C,** Fibrotic retrodiskal synovium (7–11 o'clock). **D,** Horizontal adherence (band) from retrodiskal tissue across the medial synovial drape. **E,** Fibrotic medial synovial drape.

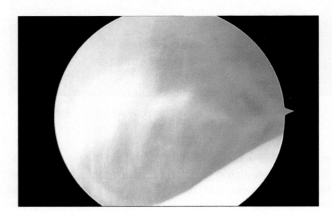

FIGURE 49-40. Pterygoid shadow (normal arthroscopic appearance).

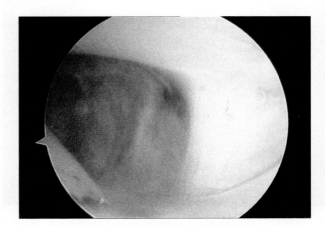

FIGURE 49-41. Erythema at the pterygoid shadow.

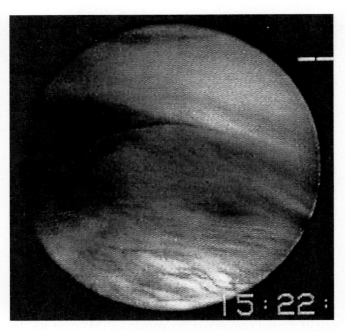

FIGURE 49-42. Intra-articular prolapse/herniation of the lateral pterygoid secondary to erosion/perforation of inflamed synovial lining at area no. 2.

thin to the extent at which it causes a perforation of this area and herniation of the pterygoid muscle directly into the anteromedial aspect of the superior joint space (Figure 49-42).

Area 3. Retrodiskal synovium This third area to be examined is reached by backtracking the initial path of the scope. Once the medial synovial drape is visible, the scope is pistoned-out (lateral) and swiveled minimally to bring into view both anterior and posterior components of the retrodiskal synovium (Figure 49-43). The arthroscopically normal retrodiskal synovium with pertaining structures have been previously described. In inflammatory pathologic states, the synovial tissue takes on the appearance of increased hypervascularity and erythema along with a redundant pattern.

Zone 1: Oblique protuberance: This area is visualized by pistoning-out the scope. It is located about one third of the way lateral from the drape (Figure 49-44).

Zone 2: Retrodiskal tissue attached to posterior glenoid process: This area takes a superior swivel of the scope to visualize (Figure 49-45).

Zone 3: Lateral recess of the retrodiskal synovial tissue: This area can be accessed by pistoning-out from the oblique protuberance (see Figure 49-45). In this zone as well, the pathologic states induce a hyperemic or petechial appearance of synovium (Figure 49-46).

Area 4. Posterior slope of the articular eminence and glenoid fossa This fourth area of the intra-articular examination is reached in the following manner. From the lateral recess the scope is pistoned-out until the periphery of the capsule is visible. From there, the scope is advanced so

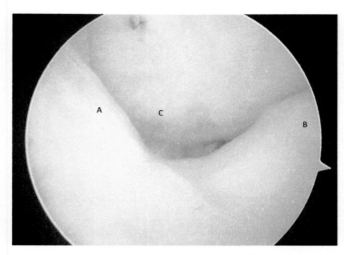

FIGURE 49-44. Oblique protuberance. **A,** Oblique protuberance. **B,** Articular disk. **C,** Articular tubercle.

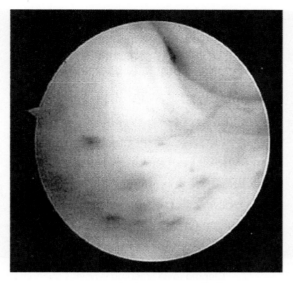

FIGURE 49-46. Petechial synovitis in the lateral recess.

that the capsular fragmentation is no longer visible. To examine the fibrocartilage of the back slope of the eminence, the scope is pistoned-in to the most medial aspect of the articular eminence then slowly pistoned-out, backtracking the last travel path. The fibrocartilage of this area has a distinct, classic white and highly reflective appearance with anteroposterior striae within the fibrocartilage (Figure 49-47). As it tapers toward the glenoid fossa, the fibrocartilage becomes darker (more brownish) and thinner. The arthroscopist has to give special consideration to this area because it is the most prone to iatrogenic injury (scuffing) during intra-articular scope manipulation. The fibrocartilage over the bulk of the posterior slope of the articular eminence is significantly thicker compared with the glenoid fossa. The pathology occurring often in this area is various stages of

chondromalacia. This important entity is discussed in detail later in this chapter. To complete the examination of this area, the scope is swiveled superiorly and posteriorly. From that position, pistoning-out to the joint periphery will permit visualization of the glenoid fossa. Normal fibrocartilage over the glenoid fossa is thin, white, and without striae. When destruction (thinning) of the fibrocartilage is advanced, the underlying bone appears slightly yellow or brownish. In inflammatory states, creeping of the synovial tissue can be observed in the glenoid fossa (Figure 49-48) and the posterior slope of the eminence (Figure 49-49).

Area 5. Articular disk When the examination of the glenoid fossa is complete, the scope should be at the extreme periphery of the joint and in position to examine the fifth area. From this posterolateral position, the posterior band of disk is located. The posterior band should always be visible in the posterior recess. With the condyle forward, the inspection proceeds in an anterior and inferior direction from

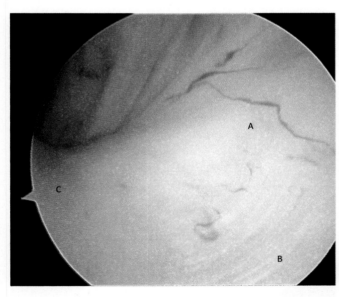

FIGURE 49-45. Retrodiskal tissue. **A,** Retrodiskal tissue of the left TMJ. **B,** Lateral recess of retrodiskal tissue. **C,** Posterior edge of disk.

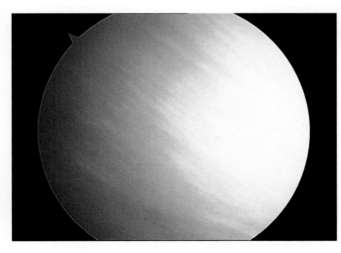

FIGURE 49-47. Posterior slope of the articular eminence.

SECTION 6

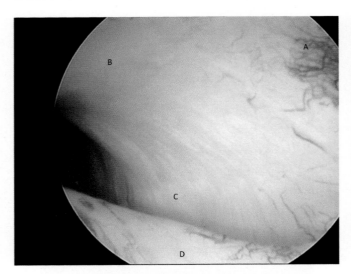

FIGURE 49-48. Glenoid fossa creeping synovitis phenomenon. **A,** Creeping synovitis at the fossa. **B,** Posterior slope of the eminence fibrocartilage of normal aspect. **C,** Medial synovial drape. **D,** Retrodiskal tissue with synovitis.

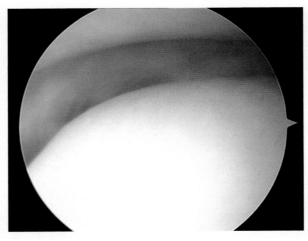

FIGURE 49-50. Normal articular disk.

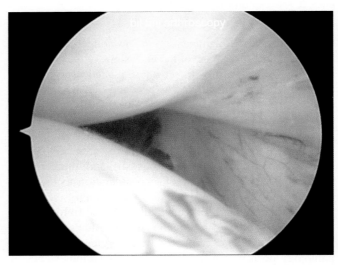

FIGURE 49-51. Posterior band of disk creeping synovitis phenomenon (at 6 o'clock). Less prevalent creeping synovitis at the drape and fossa is noted in the same image.

this peripheral position. The normal disk anatomy has been previously described (Figure 49-50). In pathologic states, the synovium creeps onto the surface of the disk (Figure 49-51). Fragmentation of the disk surface (Figure 49-52) is usually an indication that a perforation of the disk is either imminent or present (Figure 49-53). In cases of disk perforation, the inferior joint space can be examined by introducing the scope through the perforation into the inferior joint space.

Joint dynamics and disk mobility: The next step of the diagnostic sweep is to examine dynamics and mobility from the posterolateral position. The scope needs to be at the most peripheral posterolateral position, almost exiting the joint space. If the operator does not ensure the appropriate position of the scope in this instance, damage to the retrodiskal tissues and the disk may occur along with scuffing of the

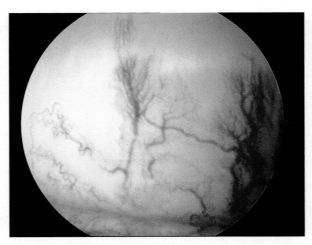

FIGURE 49-49. Creeping synovitis phenomenon on the fibrocartilage of the posterior slope of the articular eminence.

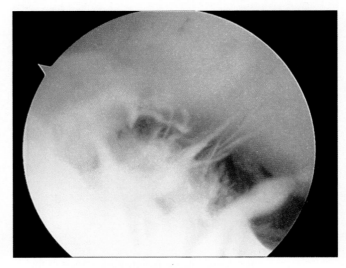

FIGURE 49-52. Disk surface fragmentation (leading to perforation).

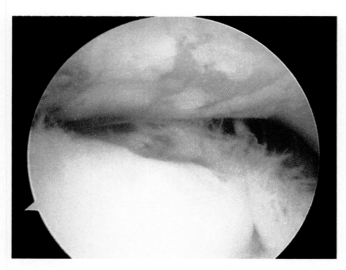

FIGURE 49-53.   Disk perforation (also note the denuded osseous structure on the posterior slope of the eminence and fossa, consistent with stage IV chondromalacia).

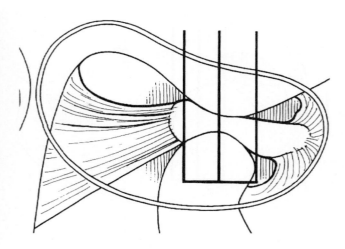

FIGURE 49-54.   Condyle forward with 100% roofing.

glenoid fossa and the back slope of the eminence. At this stage in the operation, the assistant manipulates the condyle in a seated position in a reciprocal fashion, together with the surgeon. Observation of disk mobility between the fossa and the disk can now be ascertained and disk mobility between the condyle and the disk can be inferred. In nonpathologic states, the disk should glide smoothly along the articular eminence in a fluid movement, without any anteroposterior or mediolateral erratic movements. If an erratic movement is noted in the anteroposterior direction with a simultaneous audible or palpable clicking phenomenon, then a reducing disk is the most likely situation.

Arthroscopic assessment of disk position: This is possible whether or not the disk is in a normal position. In normal arthroscopic anatomy, the posterior band of the disk lies adjacent to the back slope of the fibrocartilage of the articular eminence and the glenoid fossa when the condyle is in the forward and seated positions, respectively. To indentify the reducing disk, arthroscopic observation is performed first with the condyle forward. In the seated position, the retrodiskal synovium comes into view. The non-reducing disk is determined arthroscopically by observing the roofing of the disk with the condyle forward. In non-roofing situations, the disk is not reducing.

Roofing: This concept was developed to evaluate the covering of the articular disk over the condyle when the condyle is either forward or seated. An attempt is made to specifically grade the amount of displacement by arthroscopic observation of the disk. The first observation of roofing is made with the condyle forward (Figures 49-54 to 49-56). When viewed in physiologic disk position, with the condyle 100% roofed by the disk, the posterior band of the disk can be seen lying adjacent to the posterior slope of the articular eminence, thus giving a white-on-white appearance. The disk flexure with its U-shape is prominent; the retrodiskal synovial tissue appears

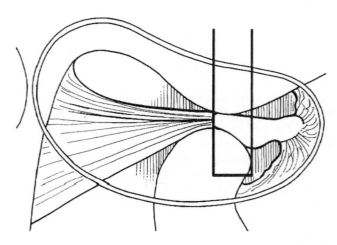

FIGURE 49-55.   Condyle forward with 50% roofing secondary to anterior disk displacement.

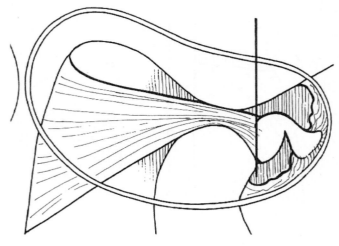

FIGURE 49-56.   Condyle forward with no roofing (0%) secondary to complete disk dislocation.

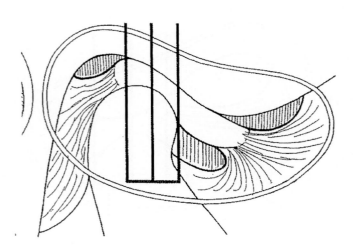

FIGURE 49-57.   Condyle seated with 100% roofing.

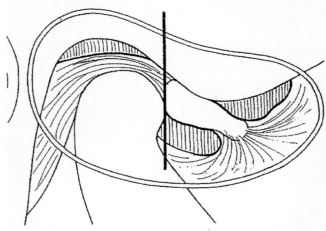

FIGURE 49-59.   Condyle seated with 0% roofing (complete disk displacement).

normal, without hypervascularity. The second observation of roofing is made with the condyle seated (Figures 49-57 to 49-59). This assessment describes the degree of displacement in reducing the disk. Gradations of roofing are ascertained by the arthroscopic view of the posterior band of disk as it abuts the midportion of the glenoid fossa and the articular eminence. In nonpathologic states, with the condyle 100% roofed, the posterior band of the disk abuts at approximately the midportion of the glenoid fossa or just at the beginning of the back slope of the articular eminence. When evaluating the degree of roofing with the condyle seated, occasionally there are some technical difficulties. In certain instances, the condyle cannot be completely seated into the glenoid fossa because it is obstructed by the tip of the arthroscope, notwithstanding the capsular peripheral position of the scope. In abnormal situations of disk displacement and marked redundant retrodiskal synovium, the arthroscopic view quickly becomes obstructed by the redundant synovium, even though the condyle is seated and the position of

the scope maintained. These factors are valuable diagnostic indicators that disk displacement in the seated position is occurring.

Area 6. Intermediate zone In order to examine this sixth area, with condyle forward, the scope is pistoned to facilitate placement at approximately 1 mm away from the interface between the juncture of the articular eminence and the articular disk. From this 11 to 1 o'clock position, the scope contours the path of the articular eminence. In normality, this area should have a complete white-on-white appearance, with the fibrocartilage, cranial, white and the disk, caudal, also white (Figure 49-60). The scope is swiveled, first anteriorly, contouring down the articular eminence, then laterally, positioning it in the lateral synovial trough while observing the intermediate zone. With the condyle forward, the scope is pistoned and swiveled anteriorly as far as permitted. With disk displacement without reduction, it is paramount to note when disk tissue is first observed. The degree of roofing can be assessed by comparing the white

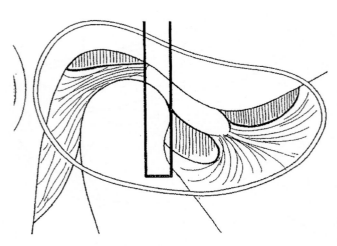

FIGURE 49-58.   Condyle seated with 50% roofing (anterior disk displacement).

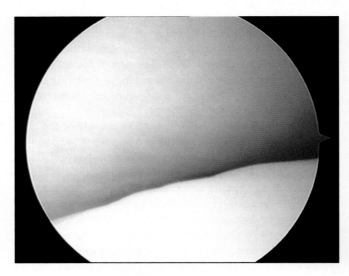

FIGURE 49-60.   Intermediate zone.

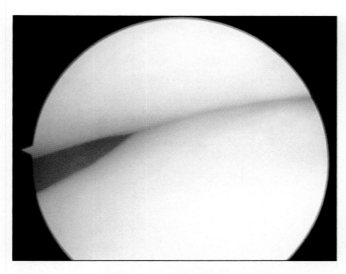

FIGURE 49-61.   Anterior triangle of the intermediate zone and anterior recess.

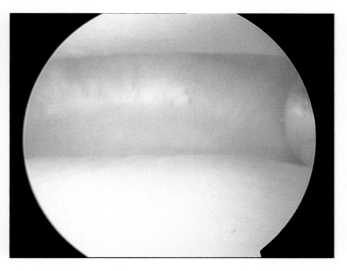

FIGURE 49-63.   Anterior recess anterior limit (note puncture bubble at 3 o'clock).

fibrocartilage, cranial, and the red retrodiskal synovium, caudal. The scope is then pistoned as far anterior as permitted to the apex of the articular eminence. When the arthroscope cannot be negotiated any more anterior, the condyle is seated. A triangle reflecting an open space and pathway to the anterior recess should be visualized. The triangle is limited by the apex of the anterior slope of the articular eminence, the articular disk inferiorly, and the beginning of the anterior synovium anteriorly (Figures 49-61 and 49-62). Seating the condyle and pistoning the scope into the anterior recess must be precisely coordinated.

Area 7. Anterior recess This seventh area is the last one to be examined. Examination can only begin after the condyle is seated and the anterior triangle identified. The arthroscope is pistoned directly into the anterior recess until the midportion of the anterior synovium is visible. At this point, by swiveling and pistoning the scope slightly posteriorly

as well as inferiorly, the anterior disk-synovial crease is identified. The crease is examined by following it to the terminal medial point, the most extreme medioanterior corner of the crease and the pterygoid shadow (Figure 49-63). The scope is then pistoned-out along the synovial crease to the periphery of the capsule. At the lateral and anterior limit, the juncture between the anterior disk-synovial crease and the lateral synovial capsule can be viewed. In pathosis, the vascularity of the anterior synovial pouch increases and all characteristics of inflammation of synovium are present. Occasionally, synovial redundancy and synovial plicae (Figure 49-64) are also present. Creeping of synovium onto the articular eminence can also be seen. The disk below in the anterior recess may appear "buckled," with the anterior band becoming prominent (Figure 49-65).

Manipulation under anesthesia: A slight increase in the level of sedation will be necessary for this step of the

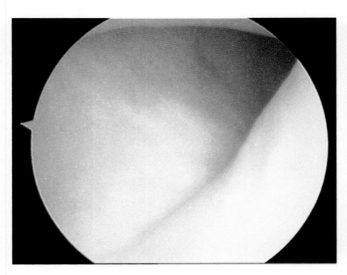

FIGURE 49-62.   Anterior triangle (close up).

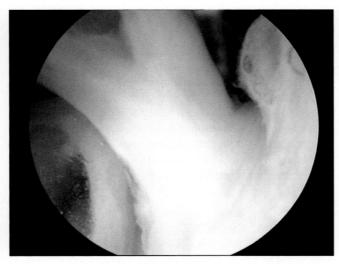

FIGURE 49-64.   Fibrous bands/adhesions.

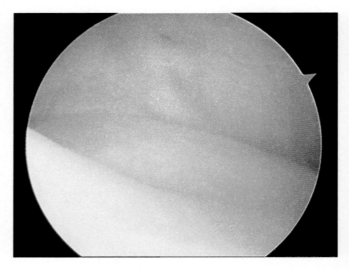

FIGURE 49-65.   Anteromedial disk displacement/"buckled" disk.

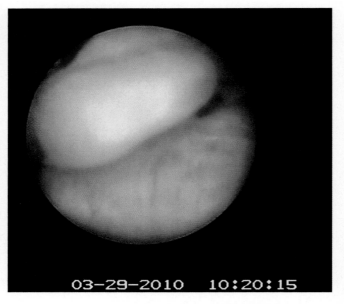

FIGURE 49-66.   Villonodular synovitis (On Point Biomet).

procedure for most patients. A relatively cooperative patient is preferred. Unassisted first, then assisted maximal MIO are performed. When the patient fails to open at least 35 to 40 mm, the surgeon executes a very gentle "pry bar" assisting in the achievement of an acceptable MIO. This manipulation not only provides the initial step in the patient's postoperative rehabilitation/physical therapy (PT) but also represents a prediction factor for the postoperative course of the case. One of the pertinent observations we have made over the years is that, in cases of Wilkes III and IV, pain at the end-range of opening is a high predictive factor for diskopexy. In other words, notwithstanding the reversal of these patients to "no clicking" or a Wilkes I, these particular entities usually relapse to a stage II, III or II to IV, making disk repositioning/diskopexy a necessity as the next step of the arthroscopic cascade.

Intra-articular Pathology

Before continuing with the description of surgical therapeutic arthroscopic techniques, a review of intra-articular pathology entities is necessary to correlate with the diagnostic findings.

Synovitis

The acute form consists of acute inflammation with dilated superficial capillaries without hyperemia in the early stages, progressively increasing hyperemia in the early stages, and total obliteration of the superficial vascularity in the most severe stages. For clinical description purposes, it has been staged 1 to 4, with 2 and 3 for the intermediate stage. The chronic form is characterized by synovial hyperplasia with increasing proliferation of tissue folds, particularly in the retrodiskal area.

Fibrosis

Intra-articular hemorrhage results in the formation of a fibrin scaffold for the fibroblasts to migrate upon and produce fibrous adhesions. In addition, pseudodigit villous proliferations are frequently present. Fibrosis can present as fibrous adhesions or total synovial fibrosis.

Villonodular Synovitis

This entity consists of diffuse pigmented multiple nodular villi, which can involve the entire synovium (Figure 49-66). Typically, it occurs after prolonged inflammation stages, most commonly seen in conjunction with osteoarthritis.

Synovial Chondromatosis

This rare disease of the synovial membrane presents with multiple osteocartilaginous bodies attached to the synovium and others floating freely in the joint space. This rare entity deserves to be documented with the appropriate imagery: Panorex (Figure 49-67), computed tomography (CT) views (Figures 49-68 and 49-69), three-dimensional reconstruction images (Figures 49-70 and 49-71), and arthroscopic images of the three stages of the disease (Figures 49-72 to 49-74).

Rheumatoid Arthritis

RA is a systemic disease of undetermined etiology. It is considered an autoimmune disease with a rheumatoid antibody factor, anti-immunoglobulin G (IgG), present in 85% to 90% of patients. From a TMJ perspective, it is characterized by

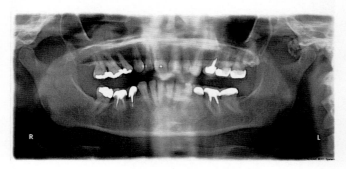

FIGURE 49-67.   Synovial chondromatosis (Panorex view).

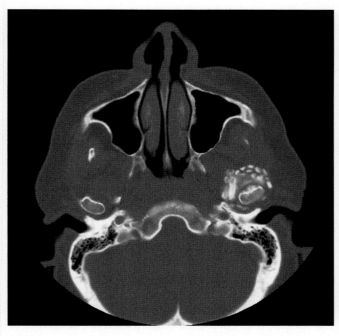

FIGURE 49-68.   Synovial chondromatosis (axial computed tomography [CT]).

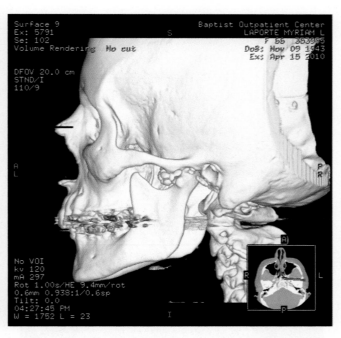

FIGURE 49-70.   Synovial chondromatosis (three-dimensional recon, lateral view).

synovial hypervascularity with elongated villous lesions and aggregates of lymphocytes, as well as dilated capillaries. More than 50% of the RA patients have TMJ involvement.

PSEUDOGOUT/CHONDROCALCINOSIS

As opposed to gout, where the crystals are deposited in the synovium, synovial villi, fibrillated and fragmented fibrocartilage (chondromalacia grade III), chondrocalcinosis

is characterized by calcium pyrophosphate crystals in the synovium with an unaltered articular cartilage.

JOINT STENOSIS

In cases of synovitis without any disk or cartilage pathology, some joint stenosis accompanies the condition along with generalized capsulitis. This will cause a restriction of the ROM of the joint. Small intrasynovial adhesions are not

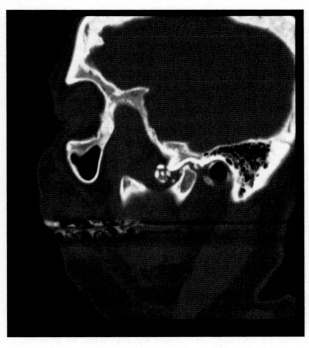

FIGURE 49-69.   Synovial chondromatosis (lateral CT).

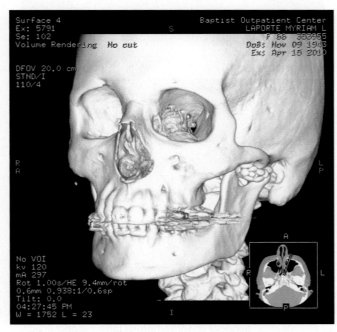

FIGURE 49-71.   Synovial chondromatosis (three-dimensional Recon, half profile view).

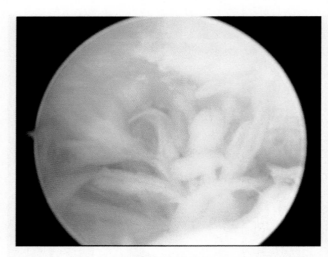

FIGURE 49-72.   Synovial chondromatosis (arthroscopic image, stage I of the disease).

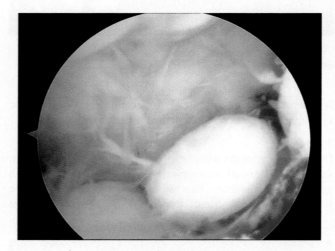

FIGURE 49-73.   Synovial chondromatosis (arthroscopic image, stage II before loose body).

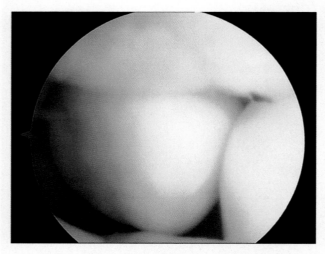

FIGURE 49-74.   Synovial chondromatosis (arthroscopic image, stage III loose bodies, in this particular situation completely obturating the articular space).

likely to restrict joint motion; however, the combination of these adhesions, alteration of synovial fluid mechanics, and generalized capsulitis and stenosis will restrict condylar motion from both a functional and a pain standpoint. In this author's experience, adhesive synovitis is most commonly diagnosed in the anterior recess, with the posterior recess being the second most common area. Less frequent, lateral recess adhesions are identified, whereas medial wall and medial trough adhesions are rather infrequent. It is important to mention that lateral adhesions cannot be determined without an arthroscopy. Characteristically, patients with lateral adhesions present with limited opening status posttrauma, essentially negative disk mechanic problems, and negative arthritic changes in the joint. During the diagnostic sweep, when the arthroscope is contoured toward the front, the mechanical blockage is encountered, which prohibits the scope's advancement. This obstacle is a fibrotic adhesion in the lateral recess that most often begins to occur at approximately the peak or anterior portion of the articular eminence. This fibrous and synovial adhesive phenomenon restricts translation. At this point, the scope should not be levered or forced any farther. On the monitor, a partial eclipse of the normal arthroscopic view is visible, indicating bending of the arthroscope, with imminent risk of dislodging the lens. After appropriate documentation of the problem, the procedure should be discontinued and, pending symptomatology, the joint should be arthroscopically reentered in the operating room with a double- or multiple-puncture procedure.

ARTICULAR DYSFUNCTION

From an arthroscopic perspective, the discussion revolves around reducing and non-reducing disks. In the situation of a reducing disk, the posterior band of the disk is visible and accessible for suturing when the condyle is in the forward position. In the non-reducing disk, no posterior band is seen with the condyle forward. Also, the entire anterior band may be obscured with fibrosis. Obviously, the cases of chronic disk dislocation associated with fibrosis and pseudowall formation will obliterate the disk-synovial crease.

OSTEOARTHRITIS

The studies of Boering and Rasmussen seem to support the idea of a natural process of joint aging. Whether this process occurs slowly or rapidly, the operative procedures to treat this condition are limited by joint size, stenosis, and pathologic state, not to mention the technical limitations of the surgeon and instrumentation. One of the typical arthroscopic findings when dealing with this particular entity is articular cartilage degeneration that can be observed along the posterior slope and peak of the articular eminence. A brief discussion of chondromalacia at the same time with the classification of this pathognomonic finding follows.

Chondromalacia Grading

Grade I: Softening of Cartilage

Softening of cartilage is caused by digestion of proteoglycan collagenases from injured chondrocites. Clinically, the

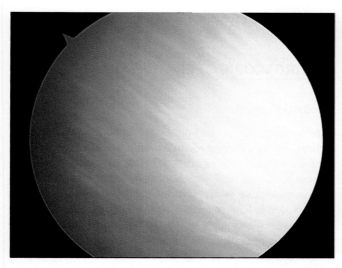

FIGURE 49-75. Normal appearance of the posterior slope of the eminence (chondromalacia stage 0) of the right TMJ.

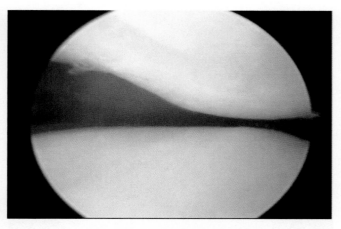

FIGURE 49-77. Chondromalacia stage II (furrowing) of the right TMJ (note the "opacification" of the posterior slope cartilage and furrowing/incipient fibrillation between 10 and 11 o'clock).

cartilage turns opaque white, as opposed to a tannish normal (Figure 49-75) appearance. The difference is quite subtle; however, palpation of the articular cartilage, very gently with the scope, will determine its compressibility and friability, as well as the dimpling or pitting effect of this edematous tissue, evident mostly on the posterior slope of the eminence (Figure 49-76).

Grade II: Furrowing

Furrowing is the result of disruption of some of the deep-zone collagen fibrils at the calcified and noncalcified cartilage attachment and hydrated swelling of the proteoglycan-depleted areas along the fibrils in the TMJ (Figure 49-77).

Grade III: Fibrillation and Ulceration

Fibrillation and ulceration are caused by rupture of the deeper collagen fibrils from their calcified and noncalcified cartilage attachment and then the disruption of the parallel articular surface fibrils. These disruptions result in fibrillar

strands of degenerating cartilage that can be observed hanging from the posterior slope and peak of the articular eminence when suspended in the Ringer's lactate arthroscopic medium (Figure 49-78).

Grade IV: Crater Formation and Subchondral Bone Exposure

Crater formation and subchondral bone exposure are a result of a progressive breakdown of the deep and superficial fibrils followed by a breakdown of the intermediate cartilage fibrils (Figure 49-79).

Arthrofibrosis

We chose to describe this condition separately from the "fibrosis" discussed previously for the severity of this condition and its association with the severe hypomobility of Wilkes stage IV and V. It also represents one of the most

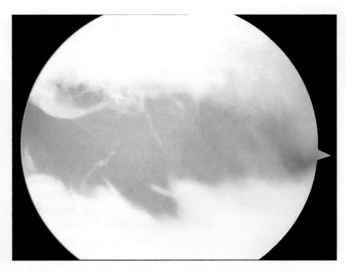

FIGURE 49-78. Chondromalacia stage III (fibrillation and ulceration) of the right TMJ (note also typical presentation of disk perforation inferior to and opposing the area of chondromalacia).

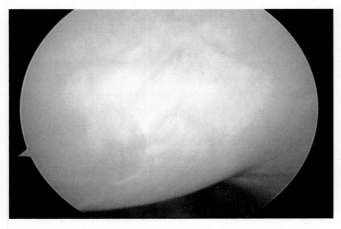

FIGURE 49-76. Chondromalacia stage I of the left TMJ.

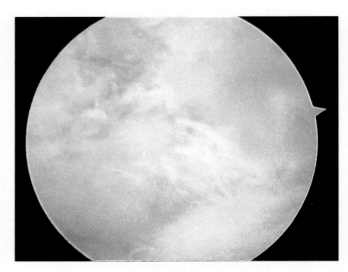

FIGURE 49-79. Chondromalacia stage IV (crater formation and subchondral osseous structure exposure).

difficult surgical challenges for the TMJ arthroscopist. Correlation with clinical findings compels us to reiterate that severe trismus in the presence of good excursive joint motion should prompt the surgeon in diagnosing an extra-articular condition. Hence, the focus should be more on myotomy/fasciotomy procedures, followed by aggressive physical therapy and counseling. The patient with intra-articular degeneration and hypomobility presents typically with minimal opening, minimal excursive motion, and focal joint pain. Documentation of baseline interincisal opening should be done under sedation/anesthesia immediately before the procedure. The entire diagnostic arthroscopy for this particular entity becomes very different from what we have presented earlier. Particular consideration in puncturing into the hypomobile joint has to increase the awareness of the surgeon. Frequently, the greatest concavity of the glenoid fossa is less evident, whereas the condyle becomes difficult to palpate, particularly if the lateral pole is degenerated or absent. Also, insufflation of the superior joint compartment is made difficult by the inability to palpate the lateral capsular wall distention and the absence or reduced capability of ascertaining plunger rebound. These are typical signs of joint stenosis and intra-articular fibrosis or, more concisely, arthrofibrosis. The diagnostic sweep is attempted. However, a "white-out" of fibrillar tissue makes visualization of structures very difficult. A lysis maneuver is performed blindly to increase the working space. During this initial sweep, it is paramount that the contours of the fossa and eminence are palpated at all times. The joint is again backwashed and the scope reinserted. The glenoid fossa and eminence should be visible at this point. Sometimes, the condyle is visible as well. As previously described, the next step of the diagnostic sweep is the positioning of the scope medial into the joint to identify the medial synovial drape. Extreme caution should be exercised so as not to violate this structure and venture too medially, where the internal maxillary artery as well as other vital

structures could be found. This complication can be avoided by continuous awareness of cannula depth.

ARTHROSCOPIC OPERATIVE PROCEDURES

Second Puncture

The variations in second-puncture site and technique are dictated by the anterior recess volume and condition of the joint. Conditions such as synovitis, disk displacement with or without reduction, and osteoarthritis will present with a normal or reasonable (increased or slightly decreased) anterior pouch volume. The second puncture (Figure 49-80) is performed with the condyle seated in the fossa. The irrigation needle is removed, then the puncture site is located according to the triangulation principles. The vectors of instrument orientation create an equilateral triangle, facilitating a repeatable and safe pattern of placement for the second punctures. The depth of the arthroscope can be assessed on the cannula. A second measuring cannula is positioned flat against the tegument with the tip (0-mm marking) contiguous with the scope at the point of entry (skin) and continuous (in a straight line) with the plane of the arthroscope. The depth of scope penetration is now translated to the cannula. Depending on the angle formed by the arthroscope and the tegument, 1 to 3 mm can be added to the previous measurement. The site for the second puncture has now been established. The ideal position of the working cannula is directly parallel to the disk-synovial crease in the anterior recess in order to facilitate the operative procedures. In a fashion similar to the fossa puncture, the assistant insufflates the joint with 2 mL of irrigation fluid. The trocar/cannula penetrates perpendicular to the tegument, then continues in the very same direction, ensuring the appropriate geometry and orientation of triangulation described previously. The tendency to direct the cannula posteriorly has to be avoided. The trocar is rotated through the skin and advanced transfixiant to the osseous structure. The attempted point of contact is the juncture between the anterior aspect of the anterior slope of the articular eminence and the continuation of the zygoma. As opposed to the fossa puncture, no vigorous dissection of the periosteum is performed at this level. The frontal ramus of the temporofacial division of cranial nerve VII crosses the anterior aspect of the eminence in close proximity to the second puncture site. Only the tip of the trocar should touch the subjacent cortical plate. Next, the trocar/cannula is rotated through the capsule and synovium. The trocar is observed on the monitor entering the joint space. Once intra-articular, the trocar is removed and drainage of the irrigating fluid is noted through the cannula. The assistant stabilizes the working cannula while the surgeon proceeds with instrumentation. In the case of fibrosis or advanced arthrosis, the anterior recess is very difficult to negotiate. The scope will be maneuvered as far as possible during the diagnostic sweep. When the arthroscope cannot be advanced or laterally positioned any further and the condyle has been seated, the

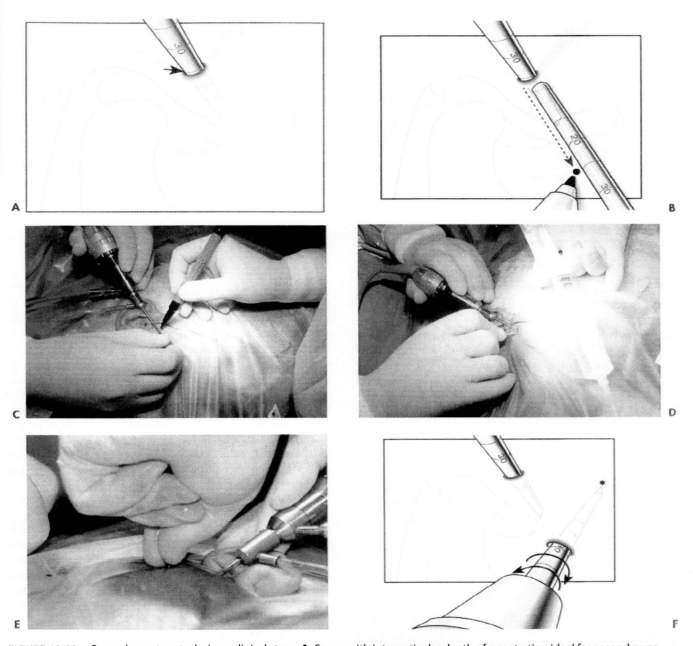

FIGURE 49-80.   Second puncture technique clinical steps. **A,** Scope with intra-articular depth of penetration ideal for second puncture. **B,** Vector/triangulation system and utilization of measurements. **C,** Marking the second puncture site. **D,** Trocar/cannula at the second puncture site, ready for puncture. **E,** Trocar/cannula perpendicular to the skin. **F,** Osseous landmark for second puncture (target area).

second puncture is placed at the most anterolateral aspect permitted by the pathology of that particular joint. The joints with advanced arthrofibrosis, stenosis, or fibrous ankylosis present a distorted intra-articular anatomy. Henceforth, the second puncture is placed in the most open area of the joint. When no open space can be visualized arthroscopically, confirmation of the arthroscopic cannula in the superior joint space is confirmed by palpation. Once the cannula position is confirmed, the scope is removed and the obturator inserted. With the blunt obturator, a blind lysis maneuver is performed

until osseous contact is perceived (Figure 49-81). This will create the opening necessary for the placement of the second puncture.

Lysis and Lavage

Although there are still practitioners performing the traditional lysis and lavage procedure (Figure 49-82) with a certain degree of success, the limitations of the procedure are obvious.

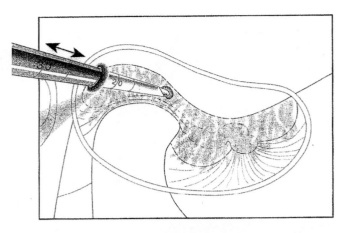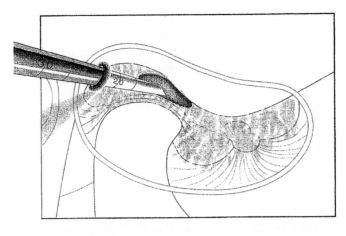

FIGURE 49-81.   Blind lysis maneuver technique.

In addition to the diagnostic lysis and lavage, the double-puncture arthroscopic lysis and lavage emphasizes more on the lytic aspect. Utilizing a straight probe, the pouches and recesses of the superior joint space can be directly manipulated. The lysis procedure is designed to distend all pouches and recesses along the capsule in order to give the physical therapist a head start in postoperative joint manipulation.

Anterior and Posterior Recess Adhesions

The sequential lysis of adhesions in the superior joint space follows an anterior-to-posterior pattern, avoiding repeated motion of instrumentation from the back to the front of the joint, increasing the risk of unnecessary articular surface scuffing. The lysis maneuvers with a probe under direct arthroscopic visualization are performed according to the triangulation techniques. The purpose of the procedure is to restore the volume and architecture of the joint. The probe is first placed in the most medial aspect of the joint and then swept laterally along the disk-synovial junction with an infer-

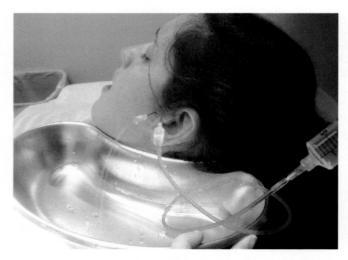

FIGURE 49-82.   Traditional arthrocentesis.

oanterior maneuver. Then, by sweeping medially-to-laterally along the articular eminence, a superoanterior maneuver is executed to complete the lysis (Figure 49-83). These maneuvers are repeated until an adequate recess volume is restored. In many instances, the anterior recess lysis is followed by posterior recess lysis. Under direct observation, the probe and the scope are translated back into the posterior pouch. Upon release of lateral adhesions, a marked increase in the ROM of the condyle occurs immediately. There is one critical observation this author has made over thousands of procedures performed. Medial wall synovitis is, in many instances, related to the inflammation of the insertion of the superior belly of the lateral pterygoid, causing myalgia, restricted ROM of the mandible, and pain.

Lateral Recess Adhesions

Lateral adhesions can be identified only during the diagnostic arthroscopic examination. Typically, the patients with lateral adhesions present with posttraumatic restricted ROM, essentially negative disk mechanical problems, and negative arthritic changes. During the diagnostic sweep, when the scope is contoured toward the front, the mechanical obstruction encountered will prohibit the advancement of the arthroscope. This blocking fibrotic adhesion in the lateral recess is part of an adhesive phenomenon that restricts translation. In most cases, it occurs at the peak or anterior portion of the articular eminence. A partial eclipse of the arthroscopic view will become apparent on the monitor, indicative of bending of the arthroscope. Excessive bending of the instrument can break or dislodge the lens, rendering the scope unusable. In order to access this particular pathology, the second puncture is positioned at the posterior limit of the adhesion. When a blunt probe lysis does not suffice, a small motorized whisker shaver will perform a débridement of fragments of adhesions from the joint. If necessary, bipolar electrocautery or laser will execute the lysis of more resilient fragments. If this particular articular area is not given the appropriate consideration, there is an increased likelihood of postoperative crepitation during function. The

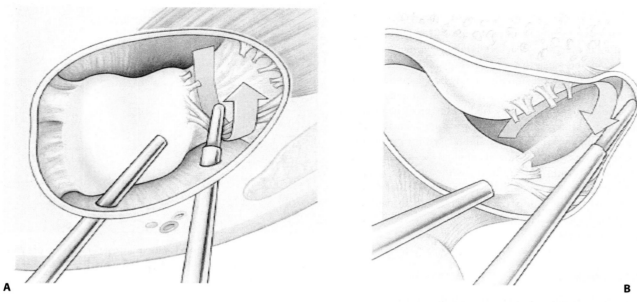

FIGURE 49-83. Anterior recess lysis maneuver. **A,** Medial-to-lateral sweep (axial view). **B,** Second medial-to-lateral sweep (superoanterior motion) (sagittal view).

release of lateral adhesions facilitates an immediate increase in the ROM.

Intra-articular Medications

Steroids

Before the advent of arthroscopy, intra-articular steroids were injected via blind technique. The double-puncture arthroscopic technique, however, has made possible the injection of medications specifically targeting various anatomic articular sites. Although this author has a tremendous amount of firsthand experience with the use of intra-articular steroids, he does not advocate their routine administration. In the past, some beneficial results have been shown in cases of marked synovitis and/or marked redundancy, particularly in stage III and IV medial wall synovitis. This author's experience and research support the theory that medial wall synovitis is related to inflammation of the insertion of the superior head of the lateral pterygoid, which, in turn, causes restricted opening pain. The benefit of the steroid injection is the reduction of muscular irritation and spasm, thus decreasing joint pain with function. The technique employs a 3-mL syringe with a 25-gauge spinal needle to inject a combination of 1 mL of 2 mg/mL dexamethasone and 1 mL of 6 mg/mL betamethasone.

Botulinum Toxin A

The positive therapeutic effect of botulinum toxin type A (Botox) on functional disorders and symptomatology in connection with the treatment of cervical dystonia is very well documented. The later studies of von Lindern, Israel, Mendes, and others have explored local injection of Botox as treatment method for chronic facial pain associated

with hyperactivity of the masticatory muscles, with very promising outcomes. We are currently conducting a study on the efficacy of arthroscopically assisted direct injection of Botox into the superior head of the lateral pterygoid at the pterygoid shadow.

Hyaluronic Acid

This polysaccharide of the glucosaminoglycans family is a component of many extracellular tissues including synovial fluid and cartilage. It is a product of the articular chondro- and synoviocytes. The concept behind TMJ injection of hyaluronate is the stimulation of the endogenous synthesis of hyaluronic acid by the exogenous hyaluronic acid. Hyalgan is a 500- to 730-kDa molecular weight fraction of highly purified avian sodium hyaluronate buffered (pH 6.8–7.5) in physiologic saline. This author believes hyaluronate to be an excellent intra-articular lubricating agent that facilitates navigation while minimizing iatrogenic intra-articular injury (scuffing).

Débridement

There are instances when adhesions cannot be overcome with the probe or the breaking of adhesions results in fragments tenaciously attached to the walls. A motorized whisker shaver is then used to débride these fragments. Sometimes, it is necessary to use an alternating sequence of whisker shaver and bipolar electrocautery to first desiccate and then remove some of the more resilient fragments. In the absence of the débridement, there is a high chance of postoperative crepitation in the area.

Synovectomy

The most effective technique of reduction of redundant synovium is bipolar electrocautery. Redundant synovium most often occurs in the posterior pouch, especially after disk reduction procedures. Occasionally, it may be encountered in the anterior recess. Hypervascularity and redundancy can effectively be reduced by means of bipolar electrocautery. The McCain-Leibinger bipolar electrocautery easily fits through a 2.0-mm working cannula and is used for synovium reduction purposes. The synovial clinical response is a change in color from bright red to off-white or even a light brown. On occasion, the synovial tissue cauterized and desiccated fragments fail to vaporize with bipolar electrocautery. For these situations, the Ho:YAG laser will effectively perform the synovectomy.

Anterior Release

Conditions such as chronic disk dislocation, fibrosis, adhesive bands, or pseudowall formation can obliterate the disk-synovial crease. Using a blunt probe, a lysis procedure is performed, if necessary, in the anterior recess until the entire disk-synovial crease can be visualized from medial to lateral. Just before commencing the release, the disk-synovial crease is confirmed with a hook probe. If the crease is not properly identified, iatrogenic disk perforation may occur during the anterior release procedure. If the anteroposterior disk dimension appears adequate and a relatively normal disk shape is ascertained, the release starts in the medial one half of the disk-synovial crease (Figure 49-84). Using an Ho:YAG laser, the synovial capsule is incised just anterior and parallel to the anterior margin of the disk (Figure 49-85). The surgeon observes the muscle fibers inserting into the disk and capsule. Dissection should be performed to a depth no greater than 5 mm or until the anterior band is freely mobile and without tethering (Figure 49-86). Caution must be observed

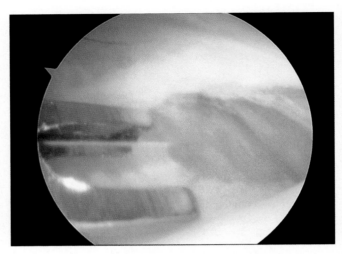

FIGURE 49-85. Anterior release (holmium laser incision of synovial capsule just anterior and parallel to the margin of the disk).

when making the myotomy at the most anteromedial corner. When the anteromedial synovial drape is incised at the junction with the disk (Figure 49-87), an artery, approximately 1 to 2 mm in diameter, is usually found directly subjacent to the junction. Arthroscopically, it appears as a white tubular structure. If this vessel is inadvertently incised, copious intraarticular hemorrhaging will occur. This vessel cannot be cauterized or tied off by any current means. To tamponade the bleeder, all instruments must be removed and constant lateral pressure maintained on the joint for 5 minutes by the clock, while the condyle is held in a forward and contralateral position. The puncture techniques are then repeated and the joint is lavaged and suctioned free of clots. No further releasing is done in that area and the release is completed laterally. Identification of this artery will avoid this problem and the myotomy can be carefully completed around the artery. The other potential bleeding points encountered in the

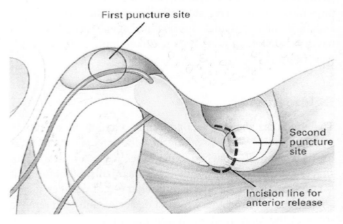

FIGURE 49-84. Anterior release along the entire medial-to-lateral extent of the anterior recess, 1 to 2 mm anterior to the anterior band of disk *(dotted line)*.

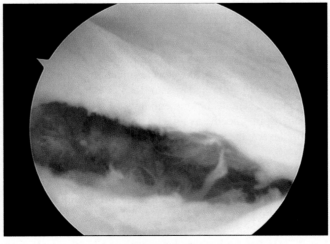

FIGURE 49-86. Anterior release (dissection 5 mm deep, completely freeing the anterior band of the disk).

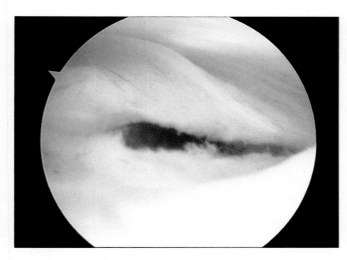

FIGURE 49-87.   Anterior release (completed).

lateral pterygoid can be relatively easily controlled with bipolar cautery. The lateral one third to two thirds of the anterior release may be performed more expediently with less concern for hemorrhage. One of the concerns with an excessively deep anterior release is that of avascular necrosis that has been documented on postoperative MRIs. The most plausible explanation for this complication is that the fibers inserting in the pterygoid fovea (of the condyle) have been transected, causing subsequent venous congestion in the condylar head and, ultimately, changes on the MRI. In light of these observations, this author surmises that the myotomy should be confined to a depth of 5 mm, to only release the superior head insertion. Probing to assess anterior band mobility should be routinely performed during the anterior release. Obviously, the message here is to always err on the conservative side.

Disk Reduction

Once the anterior release is achieved, the disk reduced in the anatomic position. To begin the reduction, the blunt probe is introduced and passed posteriorly by contouring the intermediate zone. Simultaneously, the condyle is distracted anteriorly and to the contralateral side. Once the probe is positioned in the posterolateral recess, the retrodiskal tissues are depressed in a posteroinferior direction. Disk reduction should be felt by the surgeon and confirmed arthroscopically. The disk is held in reduced position with the probe and the working cannula, while the scope is retracted to a lateral position. Then the probe pressure is released in order to ascertain passive reduction/positioning of the disk in the anatomic position.

Posterior Scarification/Cauterization

Once the disk reduction is achieved, an increased amount of redundant synovium is noted in the retrodiskal flexure. Even with minor disk repositioning procedures and less evidence

of redundancy of posterior synovium, in the absence of diskopexy, this procedure should be performed. Special consideration should be given to this step in the APS procedure. Postoperative MRIs have shown thickening of the retrodiskal tissue in a number of cases. This author's extensive experience has confirmed the most plausible theory explaining this occurrence as a certitude. It is mostly the inadequate ablation and, to a much lesser extent, the hypertrophic scar that cause the postoperative redundancy of the retrodiskal tissue. Typically, a "reefing" phenomenon occurs, in which the retrodiskal tissue is bunched up and needs to be reduced in bulk with bipolar cautery. If not, this fairly large amount of tissue can fibrose during healing. During postoperative settling, the disk may then be displaced by this potential fibrotic mass. Retrodiskal ablation should, therefore, be performed until a normal-shaped retrodiskal flexure is sculpted (Figure 49-88 and 49-89). The inflamed synovium is cauterized and the areas of excess tissue bulk ablated with bipolar cautery, laser, or both. Deep electrocautery of the oblique protuberance should then be performed. An examination of the anterior and posterior pouches is then completed.

Disk Function

Before making the decision to exit the TMJ, joint mechanics have to be reascertained. If disk reduction is inadequate or clicking is noted, the anterior release is revisited with the blunt probe. If tethering is observed, it is most likely in the medial muscle insertion area or in the most lateral extent of the crease. Once the anterior release is extended, disk function is rechecked. If clicking persists or the disk position does not present satisfactory stability, the diskopexy procedure needs to be seriously contemplated.

Arthroscopic Diskopexy

This procedure was developed with the thought that restoration of functional intra-articular anatomy, especially in

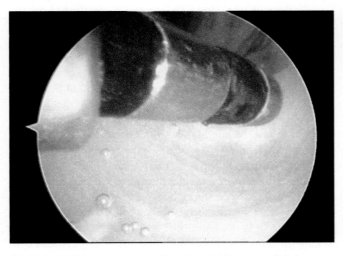

FIGURE 49-88.   Posterior scarification (bipolar retrodiskal ablation).

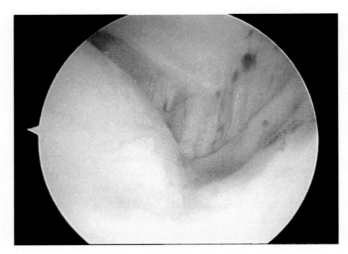

FIGURE 49-89. Appropriate contouring of retrodiskal tissue (after ablation).

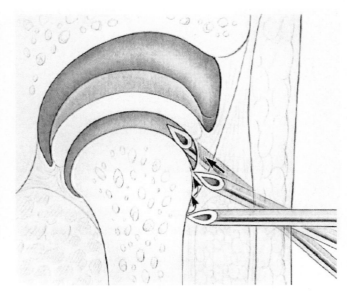

FIGURE 49-90. Technique of placement of the suture passing needle.

arthroscopic fashion, is the best treatment alternative for managing articular dysfunction. This author believes that symptomatic internal derangements have to be restored to a normal condyle-disk relationship, arresting the natural course of osteoarthritis. With this in mind, the diskopexy is performed to achieve and maintain this end point. This technique addresses both the reducing and the non-reducing disk.

Diskopexy for the Reducing Disk
PLACEMENT OF THE SUTURE PASSING NEEDLE
Since it is visible, the surgeon scans the posterior band of the disk in order to identify the ideal area in the disk for placement of suture. The best place is at the junction between the middle and the medial thirds of the disk. From this point, the arthroscope is swiveled into the lateral recess in preparation for suture passing, while the assistant maintains the condyle in a forward position. The vector technique is applied to determine the exact point of entry of the suture passing needle through the skin. The scope is positioned in the lateral recess directly lateral to the posterior band of the disk. This location will correlate with the lateral pole of the condyle. The depth of the scope is noted, then using an empty cannula, this distance is marked off on the skin at this point. The suture passing needle enters the skin at this point. A 20- gauge $1\frac{1}{4}$-inch needle threaded with a single no. 1 polydioxanone suture is passed perpendicular to the skin and advanced until the lateral pole of the condyle is felt with the needle. The needle-tip is then "walked" superiorly until it slides off the head of the condyle (Figure 49-90). An upward bulging of the posterior band will be noted at the point where the needle is passing through the disk. The suture passing needle is redirected to engage the desired amount of posterior band tissue (a 2- to 3-mm bite of disk fibrocartilage). The needle tip is then advanced and observed in the greatest concavity of the fossa. This area provides the greatest accessibility for suture retrieval.

PLACEMENT OF THE SUTURE CATCHING NEEDLE
This needle is passed percutaneous from the preauricular skin crease at the level of the pinna. This particular instrument is called Meniscus Mender II and is provided with an interchangeable obturator and a lasso-type suture retriever. Once it enters the skin, the mender is advanced anteromedially and toward the maximum concavity of the glenoid fossa. As it enters the superior joint space, particular consideration is given to avoiding disk incorporation as the mender passes. The scope is fixed on the greatest concavity of the glenoid fossa, and once the mender is visualized, it is positioned in close proximity to the suture passing needle (Figure 49-91). At this point, the obturator is removed and the retriever is inserted. The lasso portion is slipped over the 20-gauge needle and the needle is advanced slightly (Figure 49-92). The suture is advanced through the passing needle and retrieved with the lasso (Figures 49-93 and 49-94). The suture passing needle and the meniscus mender are removed, leaving the two free ends of the suture exiting the skin. The scope is also removed.

RETROGRADE PASSING OF THE ANTERIOR SUTURE END
With a no. 11 blade, two small incisions (~5 mm each) are placed in the preauricular skin crease, away from each other, extending superiorly from the suture exit point. Using a fine straight hemostat, a blunt dissection is performed adjacent to the suture ends and along the tragal cartilage, down to the joint capsule. The anterior suture end must now be passed posteriorly for final tying. Using a no. 3 half-circle, tapered, French spring-eye needle, the anterior suture (lower end) is passed back down its needle tract to the capsule. The suture needle is then redirected posterosuperiorly along the extracapsular fatty tissue. The tip should emerge in the center of the superior blunt dissection wound and is retrieved with an

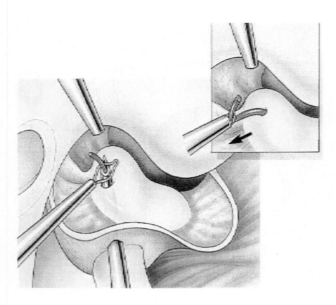

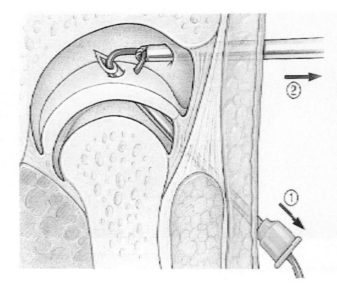

FIGURE 49-91. Suture diskopexy technique.

Adson. The passing of the needle through the middle of both blunt dissections is a very deliberate move, avoiding any impingement on epidermal or dermal tissue layers. If impingement occurs, a dimple in the skin will be noted and a less ideal disk traction results. This may also lead to frontal branch impingement. The suture is tied down in the extracapsular fatty tissue (Figure 49-95). A "surgeon's knot" is used to prevent slippage when cinching the knot down. Once the knot has been cinched down for the first time, the condyle is seated by the assistant and the knot is cinched again. Additional ties are placed in the suture and the suture is trimmed at the knot. The skin incisions are closed with 6-0 nylon or 5-0 fast gut, one interrupted suture per incision.

Diskopexy for the Non-reducing Disk

In this situation, with the condyle forward, the posterior band is not visible. This is a double-puncture technique. After performing the anterior release, posterior cauterization, and disk reduction in the same fashion described previously, the operator can proceed with the diskopexy. Here are the fine points of this procedure in the non-reducing disk. First, the disk is held in the reduced position with the working cannula and probe, with the scope pistoned laterally. In preparation for suturing, the surgeon hands the assistant the blunt probe. The assistant firmly stabilizes the disk in the reduced position. The scope is carefully swiveled laterally from the desired disk suturing point to the lateral recess. In general, this will locate the FOV over the lateral pole area, the work-

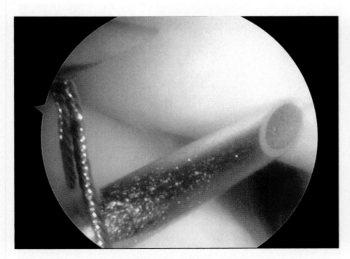

FIGURE 49-92. Placement of the suture passing needle in diskopexy (suture passing needle engaged by snare/lasso).

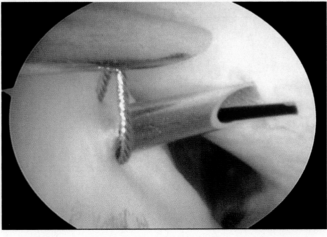

FIGURE 49-93. Intra-articular positioning of suture passing needle with protruding suture engaged by lasso.

SECTION 6

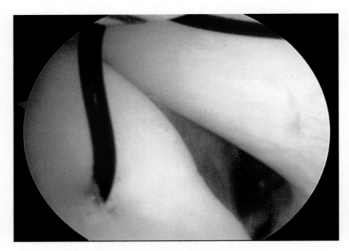

FIGURE 49-94.   Suture apprehended into the meniscus mender/suture catching needle.

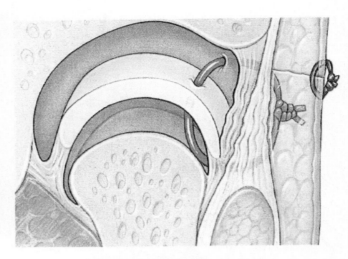

FIGURE 49-95.   Suture diskopexy closure.

ing cannula occupying the lower portion of this field. The suture is passed as previously described. Once the suture passes through the disk, the assistant takes charge of the scope and the reduction probe while the surgeon retrieves the suture with the meniscus mender. All the other steps of the procedure are performed as described previously. Despite some limitations, such as inferior joint space adhesions or anchored disk phenomenon, the arthroscopic surgical techniques for disk repositioning and fixation are predictably repeatable.

ARTHROSCOPIC RIGID DISK FIXATION

The normal anatomic picture of an articular disk is that of a lateral pole ligament and posterior capsule of the inferior joint space acting similarly to a shock cord on an aircraft carrier. The concept for arthroscopic rigid disk fixation origi-

nates in the Walker procedure, designed specifically to repair these ligaments. Essentially, the procedure calls for creating an anchor or a cavity at the posterolateral pole of the condyle to facilitate rigid or semirigid fixation of the disk to the condyle. The author has pioneered the arthroscopic technique for rigid disk fixation, involving three different products: the Osteomed 2-mm cannulated screw, the Linvatec bicortical "smart-nail," and the Inion screw. Regardless of the device employed, this three-puncture technique places the third cannula in the preauricular crease, targeting the disk condyle assembly at the lateral pole of the condyle (Figures 49-96 to 49-102). The technique exhibits several advantages that call for serious consideration. First, it promotes significantly increased stability, especially long term. Second, it allows immediate aggressive postoperative stage II to IV physiotherapy, significantly reducing the incidence of hemarthrosis,

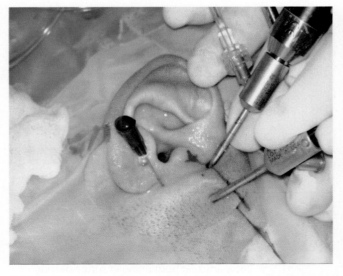

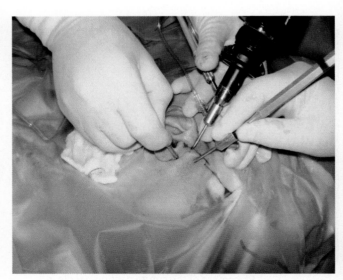

FIGURE 49-96.   Condyle sounding with 20-gauge needle and third puncture.

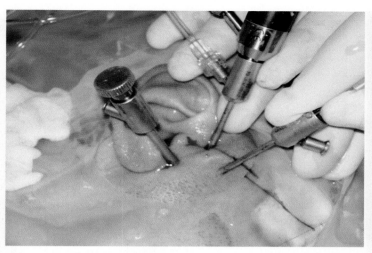

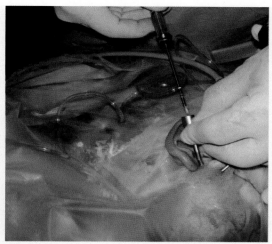

FIGURE 49-97.   Third cannula placement and fixation device cannular intromission.

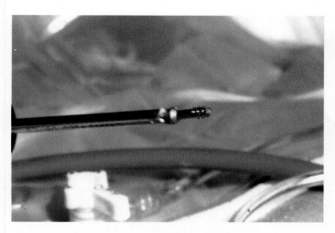

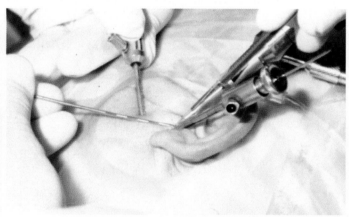

FIGURE 49-98.   Fixation device delivery close-up.

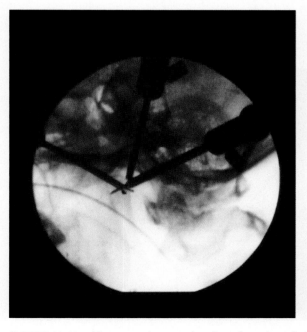

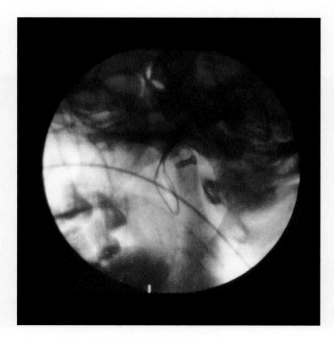

FIGURE 49-99.   Fluoroscopic control and confirmation of placement and position of the disk fixation device.

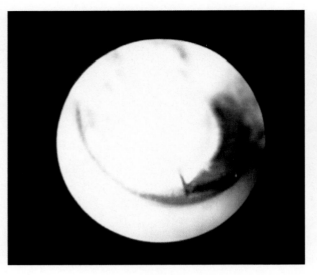
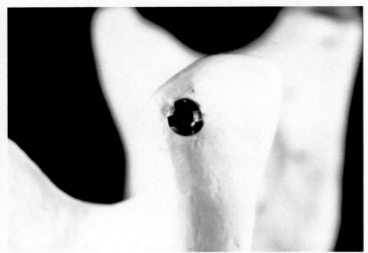

FIGURE 49-100. Target area for placement of the disk fixation device.

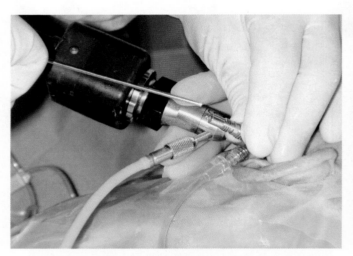
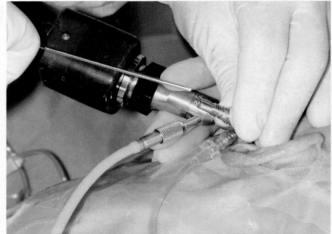

FIGURE 49-101. Delivery of the fixation device.

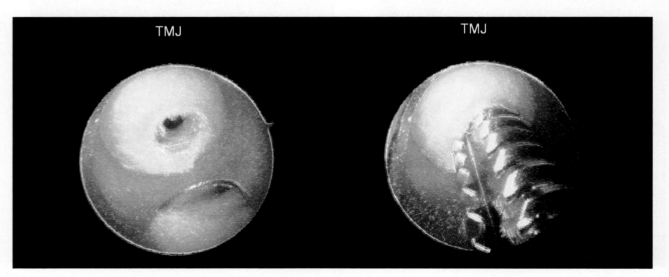

FIGURE 49-102. Arthroscopic view of rigid fixation.

with subsequent arthrofibrosis. Last, but by no means least, this much more user-friendly technique prevents the infamous nerve injury, because there is no suture passing over the nerve. Also, there is considerable decrease in the levels of postoperative pain. The rigid fixation technique resulted almost consistently in postoperative malocclusion. In the majority of situations, resolution was achieved between 2 weeks and 2 months. Unfortunately, a small number of cases with irretractable malocclusion had to undergo open diskectomy. Wilkes IV cases, with insufficient intra-articular space to accommodate the malformed disk, were eventually incapable of returning spontaneously to preoperative occlusion and had to be treated as described earlier. The "smart nail," extrapolated from orthopedic surgical technique, turned out to be rather sizable for our purposes, in many instances, transfixating the condyle. Finally, the Inion screw, on occasion, demonstrated significant cavitation defects in some of the cases associated with severe synovitis. Although not completely insurmountable, these inadequacies have led this author into revisiting and refining the, thought obsolete, semirigid, suture diskopexy technique described previously. The rigid disk fixation, however, remains a solid option for all Wilkes II and III situations, in which adequate disk shape and joint volume are still present.

Osteoarthritis Management

Obviously, the purpose of developing these techniques is to provide avenues of therapy for TMJ cartilage destruction and severe synovitis. In order for the treatment goals to be achieved, a multidisciplinary approach is necessary, to include stress counseling, PT, and orthotic therapy to reduce joint overloading. The advent of TMJ diagnostic and operative arthroscopy provides the surgeon with the means to prevent the advanced degeneration of articular cartilage and osseous resorption secondary to advanced osteoarthritis. The final consensus emphasizes that the definitive surgical treatment of these pathologic entities is ultimately decided and finalized at the time of surgery, using TMJ examination under anesthesia, followed by arthroscopic diagnostic sweep. The latter is the decisive factor in determining the final choice of treatment.

Retrodiskal Perforations

Identification and documentation of the retrodiskal perforation should exist from the previous diagnostic arthroscopy. This time, the surgeon performs a short diagnostic sweep and, without further delay, using the vector technique previously described, establishes a second portal in the anterior recess. A blunt probe will, next, ascertain the disk quality and mobility. The anterior disk-synovial juncture is identified with a hook probe. The blunt probe and scope are then swiveled into the posterior recess. The perforation is measured and, if visible, the condyle is palpated. A whisker shaver may be now employed for removal of any "crab-meat" type of cartilage degeneration on the periphery of the perforation, which will permit better assessment of the size and shape of perforation. This also allows for better visualization of the condyle. Now is the time to make all the MRI and arthro-

scopic finding correlations. If feasible, the anterior release is performed, followed by disk reduction and diskopexy. The suturing technique in this particular situation is modified from the one presented previously in the incorporation of the perforation into the retrodiskal flexure. Sometimes this is not practically achievable with just one suture. Additional anterolateral releasing is indicated together with placement of additional sutures, up to a total of two or three. If, despite all attempts, the perforation is not completely closed, an assessment of the size and position of the residual perforation has to be performed. In the absence of crepitation and osseous contact in the fully seated condyle position, the goal of an interposed soft tissue pad has been met, much like the case of the autogenous dermal graft, temporalis muscle flap graft, conchal graft, or lyophilized/freeze-dried dura graft.

Central Perforations

The goal of managing the large central perforation does not focus so much on restoring the normal functional anatomy as on rather achieving a balance between the loading forces sustained by the condyle, the remainder of disk, and the glenoid fossa. No diskopexy should be attempted for these cases. Efforts are directed at decreasing crepitation, smoothing bone-to-bone contact while improving joint mobility if indicated. Meniscectomy is reduced only to the diseased portions or the ones impinging on condylar motion. The first step is débridement of all advanced degenerative fibrocartilage by means of bipolar/monopolar cautery or laser instrumentation. The margins of the disk perforation are trimmed while the degenerative changes of grade III and IV chondromalacia are removed from the eminence. The joint is then lavaged and the joint mechanics are observed arthroscopically. Particular consideration is given to the bone-to-bone contact areas. Wherever these are noticed, abrasion arthroplasty is performed. Once the area to be reduced is identified, the condyle is translated well past the apex of the articular eminence while the assistant pivots the mandible to the contralateral side, thus increasing the space between the impinging surfaces to allow access for instrumentation. The area is adjusted and blended into the medial and lateral aspects as well as the posterior slope of the eminence into the normal contour of the fossa. The maneuver is repeated until the crepitation is removed or significantly reduced. Osteophytes on the medial aspect of the apex of the eminence are osteoplasticized. Not all medial osseous prominences are removed, because they sometimes provide useful meniscus loadbearing area. High condylar osteoplasty transperforation may sometimes be necessary. The procedure is terminated once osseous impingement is relieved and crepitation abolished/reduced. Irretractable clicking or clicking developed postarthroplasty is usually a consequence of anterior and/or anteromedial meniscus perforation. This author manages this problem by trimming the margins of the perforation with a suction punch or by means of laser instrumentation. In the rare instances in which the anterolateral aspects of a perforation need to be adjusted an interchanging of the straight- and side-firing laser tips will be necessary.

ARTHROFIBROSIS

With the invaluable information provided by the diagnostic arthroscopy at hand, the surgeon proceeds with a short diagnostic sweep, assessing also any changes in the status of joint stenosis and/or refibrosis of the areas that were previously opened by the lysis and lavage. After assessment of the medial sulcus, the scope is pistoned laterally and swiveled through the intermediate zone into the anterior recess. In most instances, this will not be possible for the same reasons (impingement or "white out"). Using the vector triangulation technique, the second puncture establishes the anterior recess portal. The Ho:YAG laser is used for the débridement of the joint. This maneuver is carefully advanced into the anterior recess by contouring along the eminence. As the débridement proceeds anteriorly and more joint space is opened, a third puncture may be necessary to gain adequate access for the procedure. The scope can be switched into the second-puncture portal. The limiting factor for the débridement is a normal anterior recess volume. Evidence may reveal that there is no residual disk present. Osteoplasty of the condylar head is performed in the same fashion as described earlier. Indiscriminate arthrectomy should be discouraged and surfaces with normal aspect fibrocartilage and/or synovium should not be violated. The arthrectomy procedure is terminated when a notable improvement in excursive motion is reached. The interincisal opening is reassessed and documented. In bilateral cases, the procedure follows the same pattern in the contralateral joint. The interincisal opening is always documented at the end of the procedure

POSTOPERATIVE PATIENT MANAGEMENT

General Anesthesia Considerations

The concept of patient management implemented immediately after termination of the surgical procedure. Irrespective of the type of arthroscopic procedure performed, the postarthroscopic surgeon's guidance of the anesthesia team is a necessity, not a recommendation. Reversal of anesthesia stages (refer to American Society of Anesthesiologists [ASA] classification) to consciousness has to be a much more deliberate and controlled process. The classic low stage II/stage I extubation procedure, with the patient following commands of "eyes open" and "deep breath," followed by extromission of the nasoendotracheal (NET) tube, does not necessarily apply to the TMJ arthroscopic patient. The spastic perimandibular musculature contractions secondary to the gag reflex have to be avoided, especially in patients who have undergone suture diskopexies or posterior scarification procedures. Extubation in a semi-obtunded patient is the ideal in these clinical situations. To ensure uneventful extubation, the surgeon passes a nasogastric tube and suctions all existent gastroesophagopharyngeal contents or secretions at the end of surgical procedure. This author has taken the time to get oral and maxillofacial surgery (OMS) residents very proficient with this elementary procedure by implementing its performance

with every single operated case by the OMS team. Unfortunately, open airway general anesthesia is more in the comfort zone of the OMS than most of the medical anesthesiologists. This particular request for the anesthesia team may not have a positive response in most hospitals at this point, for more than the previously mentioned reason. Longer awakening time/minimal alveolar concentration would be necessary, encroaching on operating room turnover times that are already "stretched" in many hospital environments. There are, definitely, a few remarks to be made with regards to our foreign colleagues who are performing TMJ arthroscopic surgery under intravenous sedation and local anesthesia.

Analgesia/Pain Management

This author advocates administration of toradol 30mg both intravenously and intramuscularly before extubation, for the purpose of smooth transition from general anesthesia to intravenous or oral. analgesia. A regimen of oral toradol, if tolerated, is instituted for the next 5 to 7 days, with class III narcotic analgesics for breakthrough pain, in the majority of cases. In the immense majority of cases, we have been very successful in managing postoperative discomfort with this regimen.

Anti-inflammatory Management

Regardless of the positive effects of toradol administered by the previously mentioned protocol, our patients are receiving tapered doses of intravenous/oral steroids for the next 18 to 24 hours postoperatively. On occasion, the patient diagnosed with osteoarthritis may be prescribed a longer (up to 4 wk) regimen of nonsteroidal anti-inflammatory drugs (NSAIDs).

Antibiotics

Notwithstanding minimal invasive character of TMJ arthroscopic procedures and impeccable surgical technique, since the inception of routine postoperative antibiotics, our rate of postoperative infection has been 0%. Every patient is bridged from intravenous to oral cephalexin (Keflex) for no more than 8 to 10 days, in the absence of intolerance or allergic reactions.

Diet

The full liquid diet is advanced to a strictly soft diet in a very gradual fashion. The expected transitional malocclusion, usually with posterior inocclusion, is a period of intra-articular settling that has to occur in an undisturbed environment. This critical postoperative transition to norm-occlusion cannot be encroached upon by an accelerated return to function or parafunction. The importance of an appropriate orthotic for this postoperative period cannot be overemphasized. The description of the occlusal splint falls beyond the scope of this chapter. It is sufficient to emphasize that this author prefers to fabricate soft splints with appropriate anterior guidance to be inserted regularly qhs.

Stage	Goal	Exercises
I	Maintain mobility and strength	1. Limited active vertical opening, right and left excursion and protrusion 2. Isometrics in neutral
II	Increase range of motion	1. Active assisted exercises (guided by hand) to opening 2. Left and/or right side excursion 3. Protrusion
III	Smooth active range of motion without deviation or asymmetry	1. Feel for deviation in rotation, translation, and protrusion 2. Correct deviations in rotation, translation, and protrusion through isotonic resistance 3. Create smooth movement through isometrics 4. Create smooth motion with resistance throughout the range through active correction
IV	Progressively load	1. Opening and closing 2. Side excursion 3. Protrusion

FIGURE 49-103.   Rehabilitation stages, goals, and exercises.

POSTOPERATIVE REHABILITATION

Routine referral to a physical therapist is not recommended. There are specific situations in which the patient benefits from the help of the therapist, mainly cases that have a very slow progress, no progress at all, or the opposite. The table in Figure 49-103 addresses the stages of rehabilitation, specific objectives, and exercises.

Stage I Physiotherapy

In most instances, patients start stage I rehabilitation on postoperative day 1. The exceptions are the cases with significant loss of ROM, where stretching must be initiated immediately, hence stage II rehabilitation, and at the opposite end of the spectrum, patients who have undergone posterior contracture as treatment for dislocation, in whom mandibular hypomobility is advisable for the immediate postoperative recovery. Nevertheless, most patients are discouraged in developing hypomobility habits to prevent the inherent cicatricial tissue formation. Stage I rehabilitation focuses on reducing discomfort, pain, spasms, and inflammation (mainly swelling). Stage I exercises consist of limited ROM exercises and gentle isometrics. The entire physiotherapy is performed in a slow and comfortable fashion, short of any sharp pain. Typically, regardless of the results of postoperative manipulation under anesthesia, the patients will only hinge-open 10 to 20 mm (one fingerwidth). The target of stage I PT is for the patient to open two finger widths (30–35 mm). The following exercises are performed in series of 10 each four times a day. With apex lingue contiguous with the anterior palate at all times, the patient will vertically open as permitted by tongue length. Patients are educated to feel the rotation of the joint, avoiding excessive translation. Lateral excursion exercises are performed with a finger on the incisor teeth and moving jaw tooth-to-tooth. Protrusion exercises involve only lining up of the anterior dentition. One way to characterize excursion exercises in stage I is "just-to-border" ROM. Isometrics are accomplished by gentle resistance to the elevators and depressors of the mandible in all excursions, with tongue in the palate and slight inocclusion. Stage I PT is performed for at least 2 weeks postoperatively.

Stage II Physiotherapy

The obvious goal of stage II PT is to increase ROM with stretching exercises, using intraoral manipulation. The joint is stretched into rotation, translation, protrusion, lateral excursion, and longitudinal distraction, in order to prevent development of adhesions and/or muscle rigidity/shortening. PT stage II follows the same basic philosophy and frequency as described for stage I. Patients should feel stretching and some discomfort, short of sharp pain or ripping sensation. The following are time-tested PT exercises allowing the patient to maintain and increase ROM. The "contract-relax" is an opening exercise consisting of attempting maximal intermaxillary opening while using a hand to resist opening and closing isometrically and then opening a little farther. In the "hook-pull," another opening exercise, the patient hooks the index around the menton attempting maximal MIO, and then giving a gentle pull. The most effective opening exercise is the "pry-bar." The patient places each pollicis on the incisal margins of the anterior maxillary dentition and each index or middle finger on the antagonist mandibular dentition. The MIO is gently increased by assisting the end motion (prying the mouth open). To increase the ROM of excursions, the exercises described for stage I are performed in a "past borders" fashion. The unilateral surgery cases require more patient education in performing the PT assignments, because stretching a joint past the point of restriction, especially in the opposite direction dictated by the contralateral working condyle, has a certain learning curve from the patient's perspective.

Stage III Physiotherapy

Stage III PT consists of muscle reeducation. The patient is assessed for asymmetry or interruptions in motion, overstretching, and/or inappropriate movement patterns. Because stage II has already addressed the possible ROM problems, adequate joint mobility should be present. Nevertheless, the patients continue with the entire gamut of earlier stages of PT, while making neuromuscular progress in order to ensure maintenance of ROM. Patients learn to correct vertical opening, protrusion, and lateral excursion movements with the goal of fostering appropriate function. Correction of asymmetries is achieved by increased perception of "internal cues" (correction of restrictions and deviations using fingers and tongue as guides). Visual input (mirrors) is discouraged. Opening deviations are corrected by opening to the point of deviation/excessive translation and using a hand on the contralateral side to resist the incorrect motion. Once initial correction is achieved, the tongue takes over by inserting the apex into the palate and controlling vertical opening without deviation. Also, isometric and isotonic exercises are performed opposite the deviation, at the particular point in the ROM at which the deviation occurs.

Stage IV Physiotherapy

The goal of stage IV PT is to progressively strengthen the mastication musculature until *restitutio ad integrum* (return of full functional ROM and premorbid diet) is reached. Isotonic and isometric exercises are performed throughout the entire ROM. Close monitoring of the patient will prevent development of synovitis and myositis. Prevention of injury by loading in the extremes of motion is implemented. Advancement of diet is also monitored closely in order to prevent an accelerated detrimental progress.

Diagnosis-oriented PT Intervention

MPD

The end point of PT should consist of regaining full painless ROM and significantly raising the sensitivity threshold of the "trigger-zones," while slowly progressing the patient through stages I to IV. Case-oriented injury prevention, neuromuscular relaxation, corporeal mechanics, and stress management to reduce abnormal mechanics to the myofascial system are implemented. Appropriate function of the entire stomatognathic system is ensured.

Maxillomandibular Deformities

While the patients progress through the four stages of PT, the scope of intervention consists of treating the myositis and TMJ dysfunction at the same time with maintenance of uncomplicated PT.

Direct and Indirect Macrotrauma

Whether involving fractures or not, PT for these patients is progressively taken through all stages, with the mind-set of limiting cicatricial and, most important, fibrotic changes that could potentially result in decreased ROM with or without pain.

Hypomobility/Fibrosis

After manipulation under general anesthesia at the end of the surgical procedure, stage I PT is initiated immediately in order to maintain ROM and mobility. Stage II requires aggressive management. Patients are stretched vigorously, short of eliciting severe pain. During stages III and IV, patients progress to normal function via muscle reeducation and strengthening.

Hypermobility

Patients remain in a conservative stage I for at least 2 to 3 weeks. Overstretching is to be avoided. Stage II is also performed in a conservative fashion with emphasis on avoiding overstretching. The focus of stage III is to maintain the patient within, and not beyond, his or her functional ROM. During stage IV, the emphasis is on strength training and progressive joint loading, advancing diet to the premorbid state.

Myositis

PT is performed in conjunction with anti-inflammatory medications and cryotherapy.

Synovitis, chondromalacia and osteoarthritis

Stages I to IV PT with concomitant anti-inflammatory treatment is implemented.

Articular Disk Disorder

These patients require only a short stage I protocol. If any disk repositioning or diskopexy was performed, stage I is maintained for 2 weeks postoperatively. Then stages II to IV follow in a conventional fashion.

COMPLICATIONS OF TMJ ARTHROSCOPIC SURGERY

Damage to Cranial Nerve VII and Facial Palsy/Atony

When approaching the TMJ for a glenoid fossa portal puncture, the frontotemporal branch of the facial nerve should be anteriorly, whereas for an eminence/working portal puncture, it is located posteriorly. However, the zygomatic branch may be in jeopardy as well. In this author's experience, paresis of the frontotemporal branch occurs in less than 1% of procedures (reaching a high of 0.73% in the early days of arthroscopy). Invariably, these patients had undergone open arthrotomy before the minimally invasive procedure. This is suggestive of scarring of the preauricular tissues, causing an added amount of pressure on the nerve branches from joint distention, resulting in palsy of the frontotemporal and zygomatic facial rami. It becomes manifest as an atony of the orbicularis oculi and the frontal division of the occipitofrontalis, translated in the partial ability to elevate the eyebrow and to completely occlude the superior palpebral, both in the immediate postoperative period. A definite diagnosis is made 24 hours postoperatively. Typically, the duration of signs varies between 1 week and 6 months. An additional mechanism of injury for cranial nerve VII with this procedure is the extravasation phenomenon with/without hematoma formation. Misplacement of the irrigating cannula or overpressure joint lavage can force solutions beyond the confines of the capsule into the adjacent tissues. The immense undisputed majority of incidents involving cranial nerve VII are compressive in nature (equivalent to neurapraxia described by Seddon and Sutherland) in which injuries include both mechanical deforming forces and ischemic factors. Upon injury, first, there is an increased vascular permeability resulting in subperineural and endoneural edema, leading to connective tissue changes including perineural and epineural thickening, followed by localized nerve fiber changes, in which some patients function normally whereas others exhibit segmental demyelinization. As the magnitude and the duration of compression increases, wallerian degeneration becomes apparent. The peripheral fascicles and nerve fibers are affected primarily, whereas more centrally located fascicles and nerve fibers may be spared. Should axonotmesis and/or neurotmesis occur during puncture, the only factor obstructing nerve regeneration would be cicatricial tissue, which competes with the axonal cone growth to bridge the gap. In this author's experience, cranial nerve VII injuries have a good prognosis for *restitutio ad integrum* of function.

Damage to the Collaterals of Cranial Nerve V (Auriculotemporal, Lingual, or Inferior Alveolar Paresthesia)

The ATN along with the superficial temporal artery and vein are posterior but in proximity to the fossa puncture site. Our present experience has revealed that hemorrhage is uncommon, and if encountered, it is not significant and is stopped with direct pressure. Postoperative anesthesia around the entry sites is a common occurrence that spontaneously resolves within 2 weeks. No hyper- or dysesthesia has been reported. Rotation of the trocar cannula while penetrating the portal sites permits the bypass of important vital structures as well as puncture into the intracapsular space with minimal resistance. This complication stems in a placement too far posterior of the fossa portal as a consequence of operator concern for cranial nerve VII damage. When the lingual nerve is concerned, the most immediate proximity to the mandibular condyle report comes from Johansson. On an extensive cadaver study, the mandibular nerve was dissected running vertically from foramen ovale at approximately 10 mm inferior to the foramen. It then divided into the inferior alveolar and lingual rami, with the later passing 3.5 mm medial to the condyle. The nerve can be injured if the operator is not very cognizant of the intra-articular anatomy and perforates the drape at a distance of more than 35 mm from the tegument. Another possibility is the medial extravasation of irrigation fluid secondary to medial capsular perforation without a correct irrigation system, involving also the inferior alveolar nerve. Hyperesthesia of the infraorbital nerve is associated with long operative time, excessive volumes of irrigation fluid, and extravasation of irrigant into the medial tissues. The condition is self-limiting because the fluid is resorbed into the lymphatic and venous systems. Extravasation is prevented by careful puncture technique, observation of the surgical site, gentle pressure to irrigation, and a patent inflow/outflow system.

Damage to Cranial Nerve VIII and Vestibulocochlear Dysfunction

Tympanic membrane perforation and ossicles disruption in the middle ear has been reported, including otitis media with subsequent hypoacousia. The mechanism of entry into the middle ear is through either the osseous or soft tissue external auditory meatus. If the tympanic membrane is perforated and the ossicles appear in the view field, immediate cessation of procedure and intraoperative ENT/ORL consultation is warranted. The ossicles have a classic melted-wax appearance. If no manipulation is performed, the incidence of permanent disruption of ossicles is low and the complication will be limited to the tympanic membrane. Small perforations in the anterior or inferior portions of the tympanum typically cause minimal hearing loss and heal uneventfully, without sequelae. Posterior tympanum injuries may dislocate the ossicles and potentially result in more significant loss of hearing. All perforations involving more than 30% of the tympanum surface or the posterior portion of it should be managed by an ORL. Postoperative complaints of severe hearing loss and/or vertigo alert the surgeon for a possible middle ear injury and an ORL/ENT referral should not be delayed. Laceration of the external auditory meatus occurs by transfixion of the canal with the arthroscope at the junction of tragus and osseous meatus. Minor hemorrhage is controlled with bipolar cautery, while the external auditory meatus is treated with hydrocortisone suspension drops for up to 2 weeks. If granulation tissue develops at the osseous/cartilaginous junction, bipolar cautery is employed. Baldursson and Blackmer have suggested the existence of a correlation between specific sensorineural hearing loss, with a predictable decrease in hearing levels at the 1000- to 2000-Hz range, and TMJ dysfunction and/or parafunction. In this author's experience, all patients regained normal hearing levels within 2 months postoperatively. This confirms the fact that arthroscopy does not affect hearing levels if no direct trauma to the middle ear has occurred. Close consideration of the detail of not advancing the scope past 20 to 25 mm without accurately checking its position will prevent the occurrence of this complication.

Scuffing of Fibrocartilage

The cartilage covering the eminence and fossa is most prone to iatrogeny, the most common arthroscopic complication. At the time of insufflation, the needle point is directed toward the posterior slope of the eminence, making contact with the fibrocartilage. Also, examination sweeps of the joint cavity, involving translation of arthroscope along with cannula, could also release pieces of cartilage into the superior joint space. If scuffing becomes significant, it impairs visibility during arthroscopic procedures to the point of misdiagnosis of chondromalacia by the inexperienced arthroscopist.

Damage to the Maxillary Artery/ Collaterals with or without Formation of Arteriovenous Fistula

As it courses medial to the condylar neck, the artery was found immediately lateral to the lateral pterygoid in two thirds of reviewed cases. This author has encountered this complication, resulting in one isolated case of left pterygoid arteriovenous fistula (AVF).

Damage to the Superficial Temporal Vessels with or without Formation of AVF

Whether profuse or not, all cases of hemorrhage from the superficial temporal artery and vein intimately related to the posterior aspect of the joint capsule were managed uneventfully by applying controlled pressure. Other authors have reported the formation of an AVF. Typically, the patient complains of a constant "hissing"/"whishing" sound over the operated TMJ. The fistulectomy and subsequent emboliation of the superficial temporal artery were uneventful.

Perforation of the Glenoid Fossa

As previously discussed under "Danger Areas," this complication can be consistently avoided by directing the instruments toward the tubercle and away from the fossa. Most violations of the middle cranial fossa will result in cerebrospinal fluid leaks that resolve spontaneously. Should the leak persist in the wound or through the incision, a pressure dressing is applied and the patient is hospitalized with head elevation. Persistence of leak after 48 hours mandates neurosurgical consult and lumbar subarachnoid drain placement. Head CT with bone windows is obtained to document the site. Surgical dural neuroraphy is very uncommon.

Damage to the Disk

Repairs of the meniscus result in a fibrous tissue seal of the surfaces as seen arthroscopically. Core biopsies have shown minimal tissue reaction at the area of repair, consisting of fibrous cell repair with sparse vasculature. There is minimal collagen formation at the repair state and no collagen penetration or angioproliferation into the substance of the repaired meniscus. All needle punctures are filled in and smooth with the meniscus surface 12 weeks postoperatively. Exposed non-resorbable sutures are covered with translucent fibrous tissue. The cellular response to meniscal tears stems in four potential sources: the adjacent synovium, the capsule vascularity, the intra-articular microhemorrhage, and the free synovial cells. The adjacent synovium contributes angioblastic and cellular tissue for peripheral meniscal tears. The synovium proliferates in the area and migrates over the disk in a similar way to the pannus noticed on articular cartilage defects. Tears in the lateral one third of the meniscus have abundant vascularity for hemorrhage and angioblastic prolif-

eration. The avascular portion of disk presents fibrous tissue healing response 4 to 6 weeks postoperatively.

Hemarthrosis

Hemarthrosis is a consequence of laceration of the superficial temporal artery and vein and severely inflamed synovium/retrodiskal tissue upon entry, as well as laceration of the pterygoid artery during myotomy for anterior release procedures. Hemorrhage can be significant enough to cause abortion of procedure. When pressure irrigation cannot tamponade the hemorrhage (despite some clearing of the surgical field), the joint remains congested, prolonging the healing, increasing postoperative discomfort, and extending recovery time. While the intra-articular coagulum organizes, it increases the risk of formation of adhesive bands and scarring, reflected clinically in fibrous ankylosis. This results in limited range of motion of the mandible in all excursions (vertical, protrusive, and lateral). Interincisal opening will be less than 35 mm, while the lateral and protrusive movements are in excess of 6 mm. This author uses the following protocol for stopping excessive hemorrhage:

1. The pressure in the irrigation bag is increased.
2. A small amount of Healon (0.5 mL) is injected intra-articularly.
3. Cautery/laser is applied to the bleeding area.
4. Using a $3^1/_2$-inch spinal needle on a 3-mL syringe, passed through the cannula into the affected area, a small amount of local anesthetic with vasoconstrictor is administered directly into the bleeding site.
5. De novo insufflation of the joint with local anesthetic, transcannula (2% lidocaine 1/100,000 epinephrine) should tamponade the hemorrhage.
6. The entire joint is insufflated under pressure, with irrigation fluid while all cannulas are obturated for 5 minutes for the hydrostatic pressure to achieve tamponade of the site.
7. Should all previous measures be unsuccessful, all the instruments are removed from the joint and direct palmar or digital external pressure is applied for 5 minutes by the clock. For added pressure, the condyle is seated in the fossa, particularly if the source of bleeding is located in the posterior pouch. If the source is in the anterior pouch, the mandible is manipulated to a protrusive position. The instruments are then reinserted in their original portals and the condition of the joint is reassessed.
8. A no. 4 catheter balloon is inserted through the working portal and inflated with normal saline. It is left in place for 5 minutes, then deflated, and the joint is reassessed.
9. If all measures were rendered unsuccessful, the joint is approached via open technique.

Infection

Infection is quasi-infrequent as a consequence of proper sterilization, sterile operating environment, forgiving high vascular tissues, antibiotherapy, and high-volume irrigation. The presentation is with erythematous puncture sites with surrounding edematous halos 3 to 5 days postoperatively. Administration of a cephalosporin for 7 days resolves the problem. This author now uses a standard protocol for all arthroscopic cases. Preoperative cephalosporin (with the alternative for erythromycin in penicillin-allergic patients) is administered at recommended doses. The intravenous antibiotics are continued while in-patient status is maintained (usually 24 hr). Oral antibiotics are continued for 7 days.

Noninfectious Postoperative Effusions

Noninfections postoperative effusions present with preauricular edema, with a higher level of tenderness to palpation than normally encountered postoperatively. The patients were managed with soft diet, joint rest, and application of heat over the affected area. NSAIDs were prescribed as needed. Uneventful, complete resolution of symptoms was evident at 4 weeks postoperatively. If an effusion is persistent after 6 weeks, it can be aspirated. If that fails, steroid injection is administered as the last nonsurgical modality. Caution should be exercised to avoid misdiagnosis of this condition, because some effusions develop a few weeks/months after the surgery. Those are an indication of progression of degenerative disease.

Instrument Failure/Loose Bodies

Instrument failure can be attributed to manufacturing defects, misuse, and wear of parts of the instrument itself, all potentially leading to breakage. Backup instruments, including the arthroscope, are mandatory while performing arthroscopy. All instruments with flexible parts should be tested by the surgeon before introduction in the joint (including On Point scope, trocar/cannula, scissors, biopsy forceps). Application of excessive force, extreme bending of the scope, especially when negotiating access to the most anterolateral aspect of the superior joint compartment to determine the site for the second puncture, can cause damage or breakage to the optical system and need for replacement or repair. The "golden rules" include never force/power-move an instrument; use ferromagnetic instruments; always have a "golden retriever" available; avoid force in removing the instruments; and confirm that every movable instrument is closed before removal. In the case of such an inadvertent event occurrence, this author has established a standard protocol. The following steps are to be followed:

1. Stop the procedure, while maintaining the position of the arthroscope and working cannulas.
2. Keep the instrument or foreign body in view.
3. Check the inflow bags to confirm sufficient irrigation fluid remains in order for the joint to be maintained distended at all times.
4. Record and measure the depth of the instrument with a scored cannula.

5. Have adequate removal instruments available, including extras.
6. Adjust inflow to ensure optimal visibility.
7. Take a radiograph of the joint if the instrument cannot be located arthroscopically.
8. Consider fluoroscopic assistance.
9. Remove the fragment/object.
10. When using a grabber, tips may not fit in the working cannula upon removal. It may be desirable to step-up the working cannula to a 3-mm diameter, using a "switch stick," and then perform the retrieval maneuvers. If the instrument cannot be retrieved, the next arthroscopic attempt should be made in the early postoperative phase (10 days to no longer than 6 wk postoperative). Should this second attempt fail, the doctor and the patient must review all possible outcomes associated with leaving the foreign body as is. The possibility/likelihood of future osteoarthritis or foreign body reaction must be very well understood by the patient.

CONCLUSIONS

This chapter contains rather overwhelming information for the reader, whether a resident training in our specialty or a seasoned specialist. One of the points we have, time and time again, made over the years is that training in this particular aspect of our specialty is inadequate. Henceforth, it is not our intention to dissuade the oral surgeon from pursuing training in this particular aspect of our specialty, but the contrary. By writing this chapter, we hope to make the readership aware of how underrated this subspecialty is in reality.

Throughout our formation as maxillofacial surgeons we have self-trained to give particular consideration to minute detail. This author has designed the office arthroscopy procedure banking on this particular trait of character of the OMS. It is one of the products of almost 30 years of experience in the field of arthroscopy. The surgical procedure has been refined and simplified to prevent the surgeon from thinking the arthroscopy is complicated and inefficient. Whereas the advanced arthroscopist does need to possess not only skill but also a certain personality to develop the interest in perfecting her or his knowledge and technique, the office-based arthroscopy is designed in such a manner that makes it feasible and predictable in the hands of all OMSs. As mentioned earlier in the chapter, the lysis and lavage procedure will resolve the acute TMJ-related symptomatology in 65% to 70% of patients. Performed arthroscopically, this procedure provides valuable visual information and makes the surgeon comfortable with basic arthroscopic maneuvers. We feel most surgeons will develop the interest to make the progression to advanced arthroscopy once confident at this level.

The second major point we are making at the end of this chapter is the importance of the arthroscopic cascade. This concept is also a product of this author's vast experience. The results of treating TMJ disorders based on this concept have shown impressive percentages of success. These results have been published numerous times over the past few years. The predictability of achieving success in the arthroscopic treatment of Wilkes stages I to V disease dramatically decreased the necessity for traditional/"open-joint" surgery. Although many reputed academicians of OMS will retort by showing numbers revealing success with open technique, ultimately culminating with a total joint replacement, we should bear in mind that, as successful as it may be, the final treatment (i.e., total joint) is the end point of TMJ surgical therapy. It is the strong belief of this author that the TMJ surgeon should not indiscriminately stampede to the final treatment. One of the characters that brought Clint Eastwood to stardom, inspector Harry Callahan a.k.a. "Dirty Harry," often used to state that "A man's gotta know his limitations!" As TMJ surgeons, we need to accept the idea that we are managing an existing problem and not curing a disease. Notwithstanding the tremendous results and improvement in the quality of life of the patient after total joint replacement, these devices have major limitations that fall out of the purpose of discussion of this chapter. The arthroscopic cascade stems in these very premises. It will postpone the end point procedure, in most instances, indefinitely.

We close the circle of conclusions for the chapter with a pleonasm, exactly where we started. As difficult as TMJ arthroscopy seems, attention to detail and strict adherence to the steps and stages of arthroscopic technique will make the surgeon not only successful but also comfortable and confident. We are overemphasizing this concept because, as opposed to traditional surgical technique, any minor deviations from the arthroscopic surgical technique will result in less than desirable outcomes or complications.

Ending on a positive note, this very reasonable approach to the orthopedic management of TMJ-related problems has a very high rate of acceptance and satisfaction with patients. Because the progress of the science and technology is virtually unstoppable, the discipline of TMJ arthroscopy will continue to evolve. This author is committed to the advancement of technology by directing a number of manufacturers in specifically decreasing the size of instruments, making them more accurate, more multitasking, and more suited to minimally invasive TMJ arthroscopic surgery.

Suggested Readings

Carls FR, Engelke W, Locher MC, Sailer HF. Complications following arthroscopy of the temporomandibular joint: analysis covering a 10-year period (451 arthroscopies). J Craniomaxillofac Surg 1996;24:12–15.

Dimitroulis G. The role of surgery in the management of disorders of the temporomandibular joint: a critical review of the literature. Part 1 [review]. Int J Oral Maxillofac Surg 2005;34: 107–113.

Dimitroulis G. The role of surgery in the management of disorders of the temporomandibular joint: a critical review of the literature. Part 2 [review]. Int J Oral Maxillofac Surg 2005;34:231–237.

Dolwick MF. Temporomandibular joint surgery for internal derangement. [review] Dent Clin North Am 2007;51:195–208, vii–viii.

Hosaka H, Murakami K, Goto K, Iizuka T. Outcome of arthrocentesis for temporomandibular joint with closed lock at 3 years follow-up. Oral Surg Oral Med Oral Pathol Oral Radiol Endod 1996;82:501–504.

Kaneyama K, Segami N, Sato J, et al. Outcomes of 152 temporomandibular joints following arthroscopic anterolateral capsular release by holmium: YAG laser or electrocautery. Oral Surg Oral Med Oral Pathol Oral Radiol Endod 2004;97:546–551; discussion 552.

McCain JP. Complications of TMJ arthroscopy. J Oral Maxillofac Surg 1988;46:256.

McCain JP. Principles and Practice of Temporomandibular Joint Arthroscopy. St. Louis: Mosby; 1996.

Murakami K, Segami N, Okamoto M, et al. Outcome of arthroscopic surgery for internal derangement of the temporomandibular joint: long-term results covering 10 years. J Craniomaxillofac Surg 2000;28:264–271.

Sanders B. Arthroscopic surgery of the temporomandibular joint: treatment of internal derangement with persistent closed lock. Oral Surg Oral Med Oral Pathol 1986;62:361–372.

White RD. Arthroscopy of the temporomandibular joint: technique and operative images. Atlas Oral Maxillofac Surg Clin North Am 2003;11:129–144.

Wilk BR, McCain JP. Rehabilitation of the temporomandibular joint after arthroscopic surgery [review]. Oral Surg Oral Med Oral Pathol 1992;73:531–536.

50
CHAPTER

Internal Derangement of the Temporomandibular Joint

Luis G. Vega, DDS, Florencio Monje Gil, MD, and Rajesh Gutta, BDS, MS

With a multifactorial etiology and poorly understood pathophysiology, the surgical management of temporomandibular joint (TMJ) disorders is one of the most controversial and challenging topics in oral and maxillofacial surgery. Without randomized clinical trials comparing treatment options for TMJ disease including surgical treatment, medical management, and no treatment, the true value of surgery in the management of TMJ disorders may never be established conclusively. Albeit, the literature on TMJ surgery is considered suboptimal, the results cannot be ignored, and current recommendations for TMJ surgery must rely on the best available evidence.[1]

The term *TMJ internal derangement* was adopted to classify any pathologic entity that interfered with the smooth function of the TMJ. Movement disturbances in which the articular disc plays a central role are referred to as TMJ disc derangements. Although they are viewed as a separate category of intra-articular conditions, some authors suggest that disc derangements and osteoarthritis are intimately related since much of their clinical courses overlap.[2–4]

Historically, clinicians have recognized that surgery for disc derangements should be reserved for patients with pain or dysfunction that is severe, disabling, and is refractory to nonsurgical management. These conditions still form the basic indications for TMJ surgery. However, the approach to open joint surgery for TMJ disc derangements has undergone a complete metamorphosis as a result of the research and clinical results of TMJ arthrocentesis and arthroscopy. At one time, only a handful of surgeons professed the viability of function with a displaced disc and argued against surgical repositioning of the disc. Today the philosophy is reversed, and the majority of surgeons recognize that a disc derangement does not imply an ipso facto need for open joint surgery. Furthermore, the presence of persistent symptoms in light of disc derangement does not imply that surgical correction is necessary or imminent. Surgery is indicated only if the mechanical obstruction is felt to be the primary etiology of the patient's symptoms.

This chapter discusses the pathophysiology and possible etiologic factors of TMJ disc displacement. The chapter also describes the clinical examination and imaging assessment, as well as the indications and goals for surgical intervention. A brief discussion of surgical anatomic considerations is followed by a description of the classic surgical approaches to the TMJ. Finally, a review of the most common surgical techniques for TMJ disc derangements and their clinical outcomes is also presented.

PATHOPHYSIOLOGY

Clinical course

TMJ disc derangement is a commonly found condition in which the disc is usually displaced from its normal anatomical position. Several stages of progression have been identified wherein not only the disc position, but also its configuration, is altered. The belief that TMJ disc displacements follow a progressive course is based on retrospective and cross-sectional studies.[5,6] For a disc to become displaced, the functional capability of the associated TMJ ligaments must be compromised by deterioration, elongation, or detachment.[7] Once the disc is displaced, the absence of a normal anatomic relationship between the disc, condyle, and fossa has been identified as the most important factor in the initiation of disc deformation.[8] Studies have demonstrated that reducing disc derangements have a greater tendency to progress to nonreducing disc derangements when the posterior band of the disc shows significant plastic deformation as well as a gradual flattening of the eminence.[9,10] Yet studies have also shown that disc displacements can remain constant over the years[6,7,11,12]. Other studies have demonstrated that in the vast majority of patients with disc displacement, the signs and symptoms gradually resolved regardless of the type of treatment.[13–16] Thus a disc displacement with reduction does not necessarily progress to disc displacement without reduction.

Etiologic factors

Many etiologic factors have been proposed to explain the occurrence of disc derangement including *trauma, joint laxity, bruxism, and changes in the joint lubrication system.*

Trauma

Trauma is probably the most common cause of disc derangement, and this includes acute injury such as blunt trauma to the jaws or whiplash injury, or chronic trauma such as habits bruxism, or occlusal trauma. The traumatic event, or series of events, usually results in soft tissue injury that elongates, tears, or detaches ligaments and disc attachments. Additionally, the traumatic arthritis that may follow produces intra-articular bleeding that can result in fibrosis and adhesions, or hyperplastic tissue leading to pain and dysfunction.[17]

Joint Laxity

Laxity of the joint ligaments, with hypermobility, have been associated with disc derangements.[18] However, the prevalence of joint laxity does not parallel the higher presence of disc derangements. Due to the female predominance of this condition, it has been suggested that hormonal factors may also play a role in the development of disc derangements.[19,20]

Bruxism

Bruxism has been implicated due to the compressive overloading that stimulates production of highly reactive oxidative radicals that destroy hyaluronic acid, collagen, and proteoglycans.[21]

Altered Joint Lubrication System

Although the exact mechanism of joint lubrication is still unknown, it has been suggested that it is primarily dependent upon the synovial fluid. Synovial fluid provides the nutritional and metabolic needs for the articular tissues of the joint. It has been theorized that regardless of the etiologic factor, disc derangement seems to be associated with an increased intra-articular friction preventing the smooth gliding of the joint.[22]

Two major components have been identified as responsible for free joint movement: surface-active phospholipids and hyaluronic acid. Surface-active phospholipids are major boundary lubricants protecting the articular surfaces.[23]

Hyaluronic acid, a high molecular weight mucopolysaccharide, forms a film that keeps the articular surfaces separated and prevents friction. It additionally plays an indirect role in joint lubrication by adhering to surface-active phospholipids protecting them against uncontrolled degradation by phospholipase A_2.[24] Joint function remains normal until its adaptive capacity is compromised.[25] Once it is compromised, joint overloading generates a hypoxia-reperfusion cycle that induces the release of free-oxygen radicals that degrade hyaluronic acid, causing a marked decrease in synovial fluid viscosity. Moreover the lack of hyaluronic acid allows the phospholipase A_2 to lyse surface-active phospholipids further jeopardizing the lubrication system. The absence of lubrication will lead to increased adhesiveness, friction, shear and rupture of articular surfaces.[26]

DIAGNOSIS

Clinical Diagnosis

The diagnosis of TMJ disc derangement is achieved predominantly through a thorough clinical examination. A large segment of the general population has only minimal signs and symptoms associated with disc derangements. Careful recording of the chief complaint and history of present illness is imperative, with attention being paid to the details of onset and duration of facial pain and joint noise, timing of symptoms of facial tightness, inability to open or close the mouth, and distribution of headaches. The mere coexistence of muscle dysfunction and a disc derangement does not imply a causal relationship. Concomitant sources of pain need to be identified and consultations are obtained with other medical and dental specialty services including neurology, otolaryngology, psychology, rheumatology, internal medicine, and/or general dentistry, as required. The history of previous surgical and nonsurgical treatment is equally important since the literature suggests that the likelihood of improvement in function and pain management decreases after multiple surgical procedures.[27] Imaging of the joint is performed after a thorough physical examination indicates the need for further information. When a diagnostic dilemma exists, a magnetic resonance imaging (MRI) is usually required to elucidate the clinical presentation. No pain and/or dysfunction are identical to one another, and consequently, cookbook approaches to the diagnosis and surgical management of TMJ disc derangements should not be used. Furthermore, in the surgical decision-making process the surgeon should not take into consideration only the specific diagnosis, but also the patient's perception of the problem, the effect on activities of daily living, and the patient's overall psyche.

TMJ disc derangements can be classified into four clinical settings: disc *incoordination, disc displacement with reduction, disc displacement without reduction, and anchored-disc phenomenon.* Qualifying descriptors are sometimes included, such as the direction of disc displacement, degree of disc displacement, and presence of a disc perforation. Unfortunately, these large diagnostic rubrics fail to identify the finer stages of the disease process. Disc morphology and severity of displacement are only gross indicators of the disease process. Although more complicated classifications such as the Wilkes classification do exist, the treatments applied to the diagnostic categories have been diverse, rendering specific boilerplate recommendations unadvisable.

Joint Incoordination

Joint incoordination represents the earliest indication of an increase in the frictional properties of the joint. The patients may describe the need to perform a special maneuver with the mandible to achieve a normal opening, or they may describe an annoying terminal jolting sensation associated with mandibular closing. Usually there is no pain, but when present, it is typically not chronic and appears to be related to the instability of the condyle-disc relationship. Most of these cases demonstrate a reducing disc displacement, in which the disc represents a mechanical obstacle and the condyle is not permanently restricted in its range of motion.

Disc Displacement With Reduction

Disc displacement with reduction represents a category in which the articular disc has usually moved in an anteromedial position following the shape of the condyle and anterior slope of the glenoid fossa as well as the influence of the lateral pterygoid muscle. Posterior, medial and lateral displacements can also occur.[28] Reduction refers to the ability of the condyle to negotiate around the disc, with the ability of the disc to assume a normal position in relation to the condyle and glenoid fossa. Normally in these patients, mouth opening is accompanied by a clicking or popping sound that is produced as the condyle passes over the posterior portion of the disc and it returns to a normal position. Clicks are typically reciprocal, occurring both during mouth opening and during mouth closing. The point in the opening cycle where the click occurs (early, middle, late) may correlate with the degree of ligament damage and disc displacement. Patients may be asymptomatic except for the popping or clicking sound, and if the condition is unilateral, the mandible may deviate to the affected side on mouth opening. MRI studies have estimated that the prevalence of disc displacement with reduction in asymptomatic individuals is approximately 30%.[29,30] When the condition is symptomatic, patients complain of localized preauricular pain particularly while joint loading (function). In late stages of the disease, patients could also suffer from intermittent locking, headaches, and myofascial pain that are associated with chronic parafunction of the joint.

Disc Displacement Without Reduction

In disc displacement without reduction, mouth opening becomes limited as the mandibular condyle fails to pass over the posterior band of the articular disc. In symptomatic patients, the overloading and stretching of the highly innervated retrodiscal tissue elicits pain at the affected joint on forced mouth opening and loading. Mandibular deviation to the affected side can be observed in unilateral cases. In some patients, a prior history of clicking or popping that involves the affected joint, or disc displacement with reduction, may precede the condition of a non-reducing disc. Patients often complain of muscle dysfunction secondary to efforts to achieve a normal mouth opening by deviating or deflecting the mandible in order to negotiate over the disc displacement. In the absence of pain, many patients are able to tolerate the restriction in mouth opening, that may gradually improve over several months to years with stretching of the retrodiscal tissues.

Anchored Disc Phenomenon

The anchored disc phenomenon, or acute disc displacement without reduction, is characterized by a sudden, severe and persistent limited mouth opening that is considerably more decreased than disc displacement without reduction (10-30mm). Since the disc is not anatomically displaced, the highly innervated retrodiscal tissue is not compressed, and pain is only experienced when the patient attempts forced mouth opening. Research has suggested that a suction-cup effect occurs, in which the disc is adherent to the articular eminence due to a vacuum effect in the joint space, and well as the presence of increased joint viscosity.[26]

Other Conditions

While establishing a diagnosis of internal derangement of the TMJ, clinicians must be aware of other conditions that could mimic the signs and symptoms to TMJ disc derangement such as joint sounds, limitation of mouth opening, and facial pain. Intra-articular causes include synovial chondromatosis, pigmented villinodular synovitis, various forms of arthritis, and primary and secondary neoplasms involving the TMJ. Extra-articular conditions include pathologies such as myofascial pain, myositis, scleroderma, masticatory muscle fibrosis, hypertrophy of the coronoid process, depressed zygomatic arch fracture, parotid gland pathology, and intraoral and lateral pharyngeal tumors.

Imaging Diagnosis

Although studies have shown that TMJ arthrography has a higher diagnostic value than computer tomography (CT) scans and magnetic resonance imaging (MRI) in the diagnosis of TMJ disc derangements, it has the disadvantage of being an invasive imaging modality that currently is rarely performed.[31]

Magnetic resonance imaging (MRI) has become the study of choice when evaluating TMJ disc derangements. The standard imaging protocol consists of oblique sagittal and coronal images of the TMJ that are obtained perpendicular and parallel to the long axis of the mandibular condyle, obtained in the open- and closed-mouth positions of the mandible. Disc position and morphology as well as bony structures are clearly visualized on closed-mouth and open-mouth MRI images. Open-mouth images are used to evaluate the function of the disc and condyle, in which the disc position is compared to the closed-mouth images, and to differentiate disc displacement with reduction from disc displacement without reduction. Additionally T1- and T2-weighted MRI studies may be required to delineate intra-articular fluid accumulation, interstitial synovial inflammation, and overall disc morphology.

In the incoordination phase of TMJ disease, the MRI may be normal. Conversely, a closed-mouth sagittal view of disc displacement with reduction will usually demonstrate a disc with varying degrees of displacement and possible deformation. Upon mouth opening, a TMJ click or pop may occur, and the MRI will show the disc back in the normal relationship to the condyle (Figure 50-1). In the case of a disc displacement without reduction, the disc is located in a position more anterior than in patients with disc displacement with reduction. However, the disc remains displaced in the open mouth position (Figure 50-2). With an increasing displacement of the disc, the retrodiscal tissue comes into contact with the condyle and sustains increasing joint loading. The loading results in decreased vascularity of the retrodiscal tissue. With the reduction in retrodiscal tissue vascularity, this tissue transforms into a fibrous band, or a pseudodisc. MRI

of chronically displaced retrodiscal tissues demonstrates a signal intensity of the tissue that resembles the disc itself. In fact, radiologists may inaccurately describe a disc fragmentation because only a portion of the displaced disc may display its original signal intensity. The remainder, due to alterations in the glycoprotein distribution and hence the attraction of water, demonstrate a moderate signal intensity. Adhesions or disc perforations associated with disc displacement without reduction cannot be definitively identified on an MRI. However, the evolution of new technologies may allow their visualization in the future.[32] In the case of a MRI of an anchored disc phenomenon, the disc is either in a normal or displaced position, but does not change position from the closed to the open mouth position. Again, on T2-weighted MRI images, inflammatory fluid or increased vascularity appears as a high intensity signal (Figure 50-3).

INDICATIONS, GOALS AND OUTCOMES ASSESSMENT

The American Association of Oral and Maxillofacial Surgeons (AAOMS) initially developed criteria and guidelines

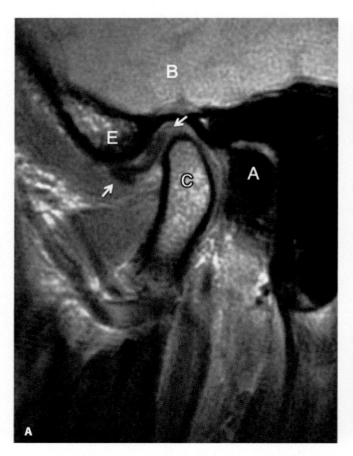 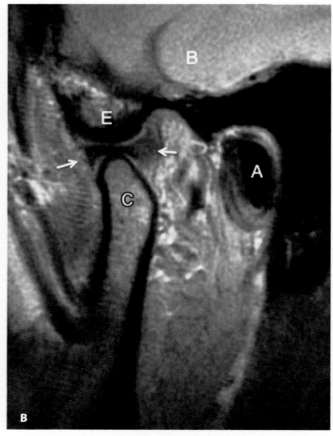

FIGURE 50-1. MRI disc displacement with reduction. **A,** Oblique sagittal view in closed-mouth position showing a partially displaced articular disc (arrows). Note the loss of the normal biconcave (bow-tie) disc morphology. **B,** Oblique sagittal view in open-mouth position showing normalization of the disc morphology and position. (arrows). (A auditory canal, B brain, C condyle, E eminence)

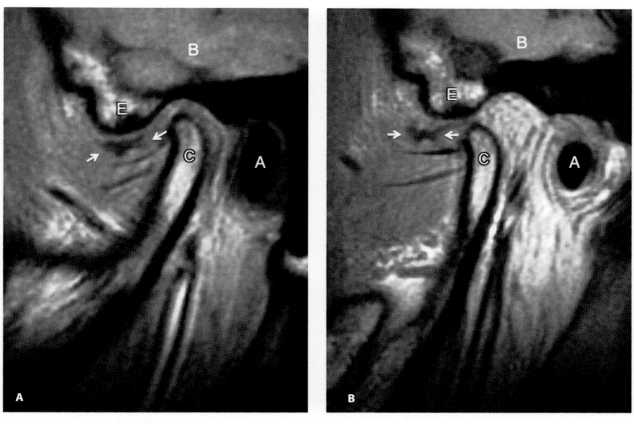

FIGURE 50-2. MRI disc displacement without reduction. **A,** Oblique sagittal view in a closed-mouth position showing a complete displaced articular disc (arrows). **B,** Oblique sagittal view in open-mouth position showing lack of normalization of the disc position. (arrows). (A auditory canal, B brain, C condyle, E eminence)

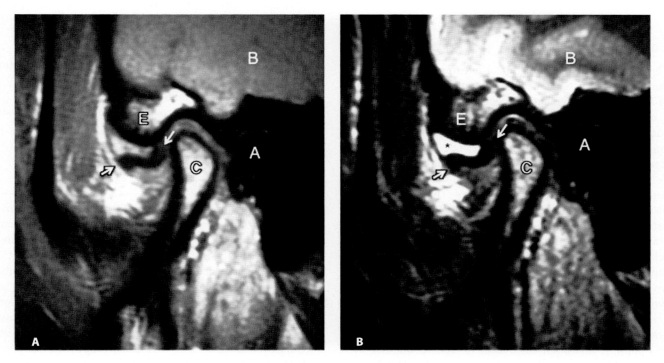

FIGURE 50-3. MRI disc disc placement with joint effusion. **A,** T1 weighted MRI in closed-mouth position showing a displaced articular disc. (arrows) **B,** Same view as a T2 weighted MRI, showing a superior joint space effusion (*). (A auditory canal, B brain, C condyle, E eminence)

for TMJ disc surgery in 1984.[33] The standards were established through a comprehensive literature review and surgeon consensus opinion. Subsequent documents have been updated and further established the indications, goals, and outcome assessment for TMJ surgery. The AAOMS Parameters of Care 2007 (ParCare07) is the latest of such documents.[34]

Indications

Surgical intervention for TMJ disc derangements is indicated only when nonsurgical therapy has been ineffective and pain and/or dysfunction are moderate to severe. Surgery is not indicated for preventive reasons in patients without pain and with satisfactory function.

The AAOMS ParCare 07[34] established the indications for surgical therapy for TMJ disc derangements as a combination of the following factors:

1. Moderate-to-severe pain
   a. Localized TMJ pain
   b. Preauricular pain
   c. Referred pain (e.g. otalgia)
2. Dysfunction that is disabling and characterized by any of the following:
   a. Restricted range of motion
   b. Excessive range of motion
   c. Joint noises
   d. Abnormal masticatory function
3. Imaging evidence of disc derangement
4. Arthroscopic evidence of disc derangement

Goals

The general goals of any surgical intervention are to return the patient to function and/or form. In the case of the surgery of TMJ disc derangements, the goal is to return the patient to a regular diet, with some limitations, and to establish an adequate functional range of motion. However, risk factors and potential complications may preclude the complete restoration of form and function. Each patient complaint must be analyzed individually, and specific outcomes must be determined for each surgical procedure. The goals for TMJ disc derangement surgical procedures should include preservation of articular tissue to permit normalization and regeneration of synovium, and a restoration of the articular relations allowing the joint structures to adapt and function through an adequate range of motion. Joint function may be asymptomatic and satisfactory in the presence of various types of disc derangement. Thus, surgically returning a displaced disc to the ideal position found in a healthy joint may not be appropriate for each individual patient. To illustrate this point, it would not be prudent to reposition a disc in a joint in which the articular tissue is so severely damaged that it is incapable of healing; in this situation, removing the disc is recommended.

Specific therapeutic goals for surgery of TMJ disc displacement established by AAOMS ParCare 07[34] include:

1. Relief or reduction of TMJ pain
2. Limited period of disability
3. Improved range of jaw motion and/or function
4. Elimination or reduction of noise in the joint
5. Appropriate understanding by patient of treatment options and acceptance of treatment plan
6. Appropriate understanding and acceptance by the patient of favorable outcomes and known risk and complications

Outcomes assessment

Folowing any surgical intervention, the surgeon should evaluate the patient response to therapy including whether the patient feels there has been a total eradication, significant reduction, or minimal reduction of the initial complaints, or no change or worsening of the condition. Studies on TMJ surgery contain a wide range of definitions of surgical success criteria, or symptom improvement.[35] It is unreasonable for the surgeon to evaluate the results of an operation on the basis of attainment of a normal mouth opening. Many patients are quite satisfied with a reduction in their mouth opening, as long as their facial pain is relieved. Efforts to standardize clinical outcomes and criteria for success have been reported in the literature.[36]

Favorable therapeutic outcomes established by AAOMS ParCare 07[34] include:

1. A level of pain that is of little or no concern to the patient, preferably measure objectively (e.g. visual analog scale)
2. Improved mandibular function that is compatible with mastication, deglutition, speech, and oral hygiene
3. A stable occlusion
4. Acceptable clinical appearance (e.g., absence of motor deficits, absence of hypertrophic scar formation, etc.)
5. Limited period of disability
6. Patient acceptance of procedure and understanding of outcomes

NONSURGICAL AND MINIMALLY INVASIVE SURGERY

Nonsurgical therapies such as nonsteroidal anti-inflammatory drugs, muscle relaxants, soft diet, moist heat, physical therapy, splint therapy, and behavioral therapy are, in the vast majority of the cases, the first line of nonsurgical treatment in the management of TMJ disc derangements. Surgery should be considered only when the dysfunction or pain could not be corrected to a level of patient satisfaction by nonsurgical modalities. The role of minimally invasive procedures such as TMJ arthrocentesis and arthroscopy in the surgical management of TMJ disc derangements has been well identified in the literature[37]. Both nonsurgical therapies and minimally invasive TMJ surgery are discussed in greater detail in other chapters of this text.

OPEN JOINT SURGERY

According to a meta-analysis on surgical treatment for TMJ disc derangement, open joint surgery treatments appear to provide some benefit to patients refractory to nonsurgical therapies.[37] Multiple open joint surgical procedures have also been described in the literature for the management of TMJ disc derangements. They include *disc repositioning, disc repair, discectomy, and discectomy with disc replacement.* Studies have suggested that success rates with these types of procedures are similar to more conservative procedures such as TMJ arthrocentesis, arthroscopy, and even modified condylotomy.[38-41] Still, some surgeons have advocated open joint procedures as first-line treatment for TMJ disc derangements.[42-44] According to Dimitroulis[1], three main controversies exist in open joint surgery:

1. The role of disc repositioning in light of the results of TMJ arthrocentesis and arthroscopic lysis and lavage.
2. The necessity for disc replacement after discectomy.
3. Use of alloplastic TMJ replacement for end-stage TMJ disease.

Surgical anatomy

Fascial Layers

Anterior to the auricle, the auricularis anterior and superior muscles overlie the superficial temporalis fascia and the temporalis fascia. These muscles are incised in the classic preauricular and endaural approaches. The fascia superficial to the muscles is thin and a dull white color. This layer is confluent with the galea aponeurotica above and the parotideomasseteric fascia below. The temporalis fascia is a tough fibrous connective tissue layer, substantially thicker than the overlying superficial fascia. It is stark white and extends from the superior temporal line of the temporal bone to the zygomatic arch. The deep surface furnishes one of the origins of the temporalis muscle. Inferiorly, at a variable distance, the fascia splits into two well-defined layers (Figure 50-4). The outer layer attaches to the lateral margin of the superior border of the zygomatic arch, and the inner layer to the medial margin. A small quantity of fat, the zygomatico-orbital branch of the temporal artery, and zygomaticotemporal branch of the maxillary nerve are located between the fascial layers in this area. The splitting of the fascial layers is most noticeable at the level of the zygomatic arch. Posteriorly, superior to the glenoid fossa, the separation is not as well defined (Figure 50-5).

Facial Nerve (Main Trunk and Frontal Branch)

Numerous authors have studied the anatomic relations of the facial nerve to determine clinically applicable landmarks for its main trunk, the temporofacial division, and the temporal branches. Al-Kayat and Bramley[45] noted that the facial nerve bifurcated into temporofacial and cervicofacial components within 2.3 cm (range 1.5 - 2.8 cm) inferior to the lowest concavity of the bony external auditory canal and within 3.0 cm

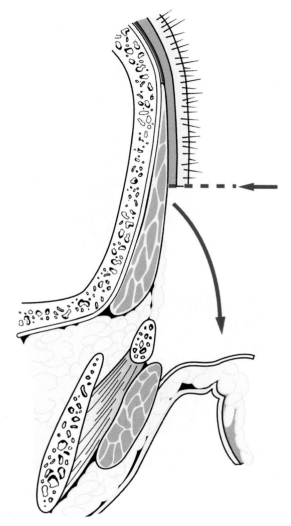

FIGURE 50-4. Coronal section at the level of the zygomatic arch. Two well-defined layers of temporalis fascia are noted (arrows).

(range 2.4 - 3.5 cm) in an inferoposterior direction from the postglenoid tubercle. The temporal nerve branches lie closest to the joint and are the most commonly injured branches during surgery. These nerves are located in a condensation of superficial fascia, temporalis fascia, and periosteum as they cross the zygomatic arch. The most posterior temporal branches lie anteriorly to the postglenoid tubercle. Their location was measured as 2.0 cm (range 0.8 - 3.5 cm) from the anterior margin of the bony external auditory canal (Figure 50-6). Using a high-resolution MRI and the same landmarks as Al-Kayat and Bramley, Miloro and colleagues[46] found that the temporal branch is in a slightly less vulnerable position during a preauricular approach with a mean distance of 2.12 cm (range 1.7 - 2.5cm). Thus, the two potential sources of facial nerve injury are dissection anterior to the posterior glenoid tubercle where the temporal branches cross the arch, and aggressive retraction at the inferior margin of the flap where the main trunk and temporofacial division are located.

SECTION 6

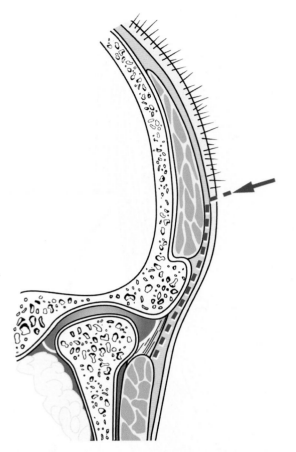

FIGURE 50-5. Coronal section at the level of the glenoid fossa. The splitting of the temporalis fascia is not as well-defined (broken line).

Auriculotemporal Nerve

The auriculotemporal nerve represents the first branch of the third division of the trigeminal nerve (V_3) after exiting the skull through the foramen ovale. It runs medial to lateral behind the neck of the mandibular condyle to give the sensitivity of the skin of the temporal and preauricular region, the external auditory canal and tympanic membrane. The other branch of this nerve descends to innervate the TMJ capsule and it also enters the joint in a posterolateral fashion to innervate the retrodiscal tissues. Damage to this branch is inevitable during a classic open TMJ surgery but rarely gives clinical problems.

Superficial Temporal Vessels

The superficial temporal artery (STA) is one of the terminal branches of the external carotid artery. It normally runs with the superficial temporal vein posterior to the condylar neck approximately 2mm anterior to external auditory canal. Before it crosses the posterior portion of the zygomatic arch, the STA gives rise to the transverse facial artery that runs in an anterior direction. Then it continues all the way to the temporal fossa where it divides into two branches: frontal and parietal. The superficial temporal vessels are typically located in the superficial fascia below the auricularis anterior muscle. The vessels are often visible, invested in the superficial fascia without incising the muscle. The superficial temporal vein lies posterior to the artery and the auriculotemporal nerve immediately behind the vessels.

Internal Maxillary Artery

The internal maxillary artery, or maxillary artery, emerges from the external carotid artery deep and posterior to the

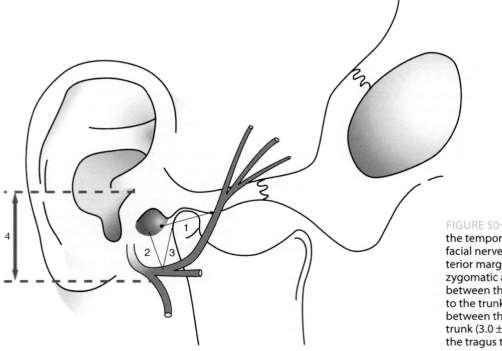

FIGURE 50-6. Landmarks for the location of the temporal branches and main trunk of the facial nerve: (1) the distance between the anterior margin concavity of the meatus to the zygomatic arch (2.0 ± 0.5 cm); (2) the distance between the inferior margin of the meatus to the trunk (2.3 ± 0.28 cm); (3) the distance between the postglenoid tubercle to the main trunk (3.0 ± 0.31 cm); (4) the distance from the tragus to the facial nerve trunk is variable.

mandible at the level of the sigmoid notch. The internal maxillary artery crosses laterally to the external pterygoid muscle in 50% of the cases and medially to the muscle in the other 50%. Additionally according to Turvey and Fonseca[47] the internal maxillary artery exits the infratemporal fossa 2.5 cm above the pterygomaxillary fissure. Injury to this vessel could create a considerable hemorrhage especially in cases that require osteotomy of the condylar neck.

Surgical approaches

The classical surgical approaches to the TMJ may be classified as preauricular, endaural, and postauricular. The choice of approach is usually a matter of surgeon preference and is based on his or her ability and surgical experience. Cosmetic considerations may also influence the choice of surgical approach.

Preauricular Approach

Historically, a myriad of preauricular incisions have been proposed. Many of the earlier designs afforded good access but increased the risk of facial nerve injury and compromised esthetics. The preauricular incisions used today are essentially modifications of the Blair curvilinear or inverted-L incision.[48] This approach has become the favorite chosen by most oral and maxillofacial surgeons. The technique consists of an incision commencing from within the temporal hairline and extending inferiorly into a preauricular crease immediately anterior to the auricle. The exact length and decision to incorporate an anterior temporal extension are governed largely by the nature of the surgical procedure. For some surgeons, the approach for discectomy requires a smaller incision than that for discoplasty. The incision is approximately 3 to 4 cm in length and consists of two limbs: a small superior curved limb (1–2 cm) and an inferior vertical limb anterior to the tragus (variable distance approximately 1–2 cm) (Figure 50-7). The junction of these limbs is the site of attachment of the superior aspect of the helix to the temporal tissue. The extent of the superior limb of the preauricular incision is dictated by the amount of access required, which may not be determined until the dissection has reached the lateral TMJ ligament and capsule. The incision is usually not extended as inferiorly as the lobule of the ear.

The incision should be placed posteriorly to the superficial temporal vessels and auriculotemporal nerve and within a preauricular crease. The skin and subcutaneous tissues are incised the length of the entire incision. The deeper dissection is begun in the temporal region by sharply dissecting progressively through the auricularis anterior and superficial fascial layers to the stark white temporalis fascia (Figure 50-8). A retractor is placed on the anterior flap, and tension is applied in a forward direction. The dissection over the zygomatic arch is addressed. The anatomic layers in this region are usually not clearly defined. There is a condensation of tissues consisting variably of the auricularis interior, superficial fascia, temporalis fascia, periosteum, and occasionally cartilage.

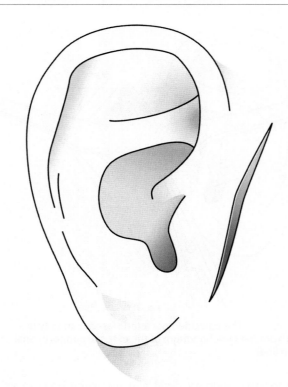

FIGURE 50-7.   The preauricular incision

This tissue is incised to the level of fibrous connective tissue. A retractor is placed in the incision opposite the tragus, and forward traction is applied to the flap. This results in the definition of a cleft between the perichondrium and cartilage

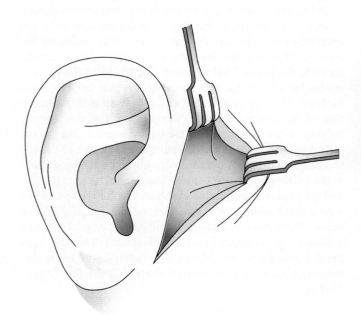

FIGURE 50-8.   The preauricular incision has been carried sharply through the skin, subcutaneous tissue, superficial temporal fascia, auricularis anterior and superior, and outer layers of the temporal fascia. The flap is reflected anteroinferiorly, revealing the inner layer of the temporal fascia.

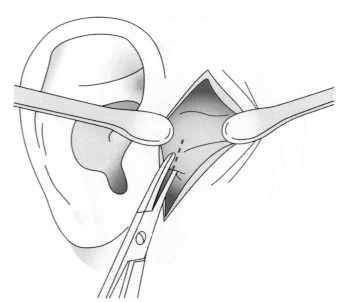

FIGURE 50-9. The parotideomasseteric fascia is sharply dissected from the perichondrium of the external auditory canal (broken line).

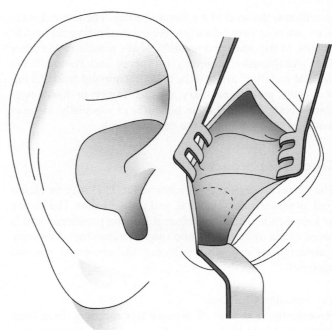

FIGURE 50-10. Retraction is accomplished by using a self-retaining retractor positioned between the external auditory canal and flap and a right-angle retractor at the interior portion of the flap. The condyle (dotted line) is noted under the lateral TMJ ligament and/or simply the lateral capsule depending on the depth of the reflection.

of the external auditory canal and the parotideomasseteric fascia. The perichondrium is followed medially with sharp dissection (Figure 50-9). Care should be exercised not to proceed perpendicularly to the skin surface, as the external auditory canal inclines anteromedially at approximately 45° to the surface. The dissection is continued along the outer surface of the external auditory canal until the lateral TMJ ligament is reached.

When the condyle and its overlying temporomandibular ligament are palpated, the flap is reflected inferiorly and anteriorly forward with a combination of sharp and blunt dissections. Scissors may be used to cut some fascial attachments to the lateral TMJ ligament. The blades of the scissors are held parallel to the ligament to ensure that the joint is not violated. The flap is reflected as far forward as the midportion of the anterior tubercle. The surgeon can now see the bulging of the lateral pole of the condyle under cover of the lateral ligament and capsule. Gentle manipulation of the jaw to cause movement of the condyle helps to orient the surgeon to the location of the joint space. The deep surface of the flap and the tissues overlying the zygomatic arch may be touched with a nerve stimulator to ascertain the location of the facial nerve. Retraction is accomplished using a self-retaining retractor (eg, Weitlaner or a Dolwick-Reich) placed between the flap and the perichondrium. A small right-angled retractor may be placed at the inferior portion of the flap (Figure 50-10).

Endaural Approach

Rongetti described a modification of Lempert's endaural approach to the mastoid process for surgical improvement of otosclerosis, for approaching the TMJ.[49,50] The endaural incisions employed today is simply a cosmetic modification of the preauricular approach in which the skin incision is incorporated over the prominence of the tragus itself (Figure 50-11). The access obtained is equal to that achieved through the preauricular approach. Disadvantages include the potential for perichondritis and an esthetic compromise if tragal projection is lost or significant iatrogenic cartilage damage occurs.

Postauricular Approach

In the postauricular approach the incision is made posterior to the ear and involves the sectioning of the external auditory meatus.[51] Excellent posterolateral joint space and condylar exposure is afforded with this technique. The flap, once reflected, contains the entire auricle and superficial lobe of the parotid gland. A perimeatal approach combining the preauricular and postauricular incisions has also been described.[52,53]

Preoperative considerations for this approach were described by Walters and Geist[54] and include:

1. History of normal scar formation
2. Healthy auditory system with no infection
3. Normal width of the external auditory canal
4. No TMJ infection
5. Medically-compromised patient unable to tolerate long operative period

The incision in the postauricular approach begins near the superior aspect of the external pinna and is extended to the tip of the mastoid process. The superior portion may be extended obliquely into the hairline for additional exposure.

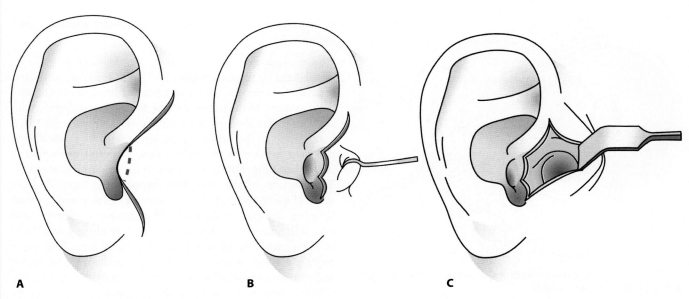

FIGURE 50-11. **A–C,** Endaural approach.

The incision is made 3 to 5 mm parallel and posterior to the postauricular flexure (Figure 50-12). The dissection is performed through the posterior auricular muscle to the level of the mastoid fascia, which is contiguous with the temporalis fascia. A combination of blunt and sharp dissections is used to isolate the cartilaginous portion of the external auditory canal. A blunt instrument is placed in the external auditory canal to assist in the transection of the external auditory canal. The transection may be partial or complete, depending on the need for exposure. The incision should leave 3 to 4 mm of cartilage on the medial aspect to permit adequate reapproximation of the canal (Figure 50-13). This technique helps to prevent meatal, or external auditory canal (EAC), stenosis. The incision is carried through the outer layer of the temporalis fascia, continuing inferiorly, reflecting the parotideomasseteric fascia off the zygomatic arch and lateral TMJ ligament (Figure 50-14). A self-retaining retractor is used to maintain exposure. The advantages of the postauricular approach lie in the predictability of the anatomic exposure as well as the cosmetic superiority and the low risk of facial nerve injury. Dissection to the joint is rapid with minimal bleeding. The approach offers an alternative for a patient who has had previous procedures in this region. This approach

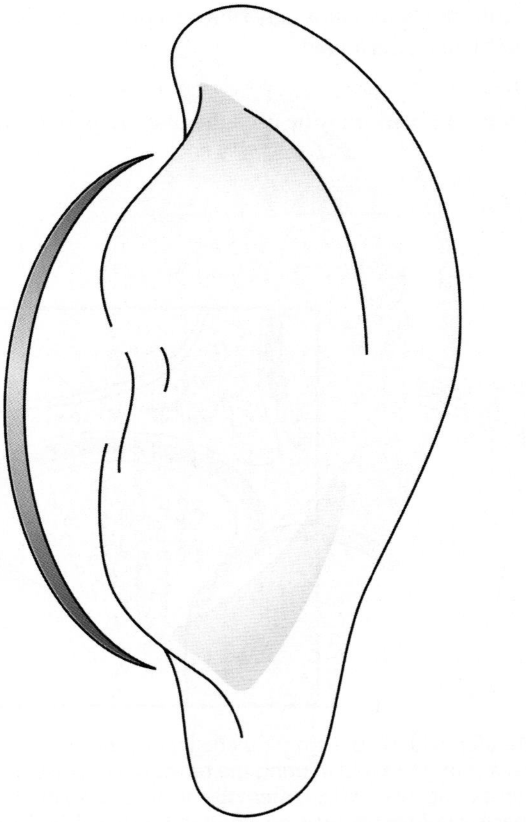

FIGURE 50-12. Postauricular approach. The incision is placed 3 to 5 mm parallel and posterior to the postauricular flexure.

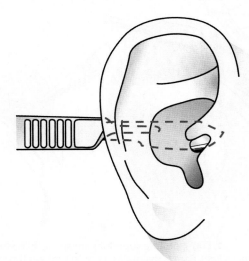

FIGURE 50-13. The external auditory canal is sectioned, leaving 3 to 4 mm of cartilage on the medial aspect to assist reapproximation of the canal.

SECTION 6

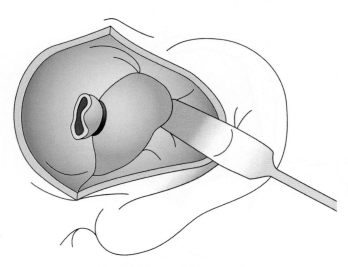

FIGURE 50-14.   The external auditory canal has been sectioned and the flap retracted forward.

may not be desirable in the patient susceptible to keloid formation, owing to the potential for a keloid to develop in the meatus. Meatal atresia has been reported with this technique, but can be avoided with the use of moldable ear canal plugs left in place for an extended period of time to prevent EAC scarring and narrowing. The risk of facial nerve injury is reduced, but not eliminated. Paresthesia in the area of the posterior aspect of the auricle usually occurs and may last for 3 to 4 months.

Capsular Incisions

Once the capsule has been identified, access to the articular surfaces (superior and inferior joint spaces) can be obtained by a great variety of incisions. The most commonly used include:

HORIZONTAL INCISION OVER THE LATERAL RIM OF THE GLENOID FOSSA

The lateral ligament, capsule, and periosteum are reflected inferiorly en masse. Discal or posterior attachment connections, or both, to the lateral capsule are dissected sharply with scissors to the level of the condylar neck (Figure 50-15A). Insufflation of the superior joint space with local anesthesia can help to identify the entry point. Posterior dissection is performed diligently to avoid severing the retrodiscal tissue. This portion of the dissection exposes the superior joint space (Figure 50-15B). A Freer septum elevator may be used to define and explore the space. The posterior attachment and disc attachments are then severed sharply at the lateral pole of the condyle from within the developed flap. The Freer septum elevator is used to reflect the posterior attachment and disc superiorly off the head of the condyle to expose the inferior joint space. A periosteal elevator may be used to stretch the capsule and lateral ligament flap outward to form a pocket (Figure 50-15C).

There is a risk of reflecting the fibrous connective tissue that lines the glenoid fossa when this approach is used (Figure 50-16A). The surgeon may form the incorrect assumption that he or she is stripping adhesions from the temporal bone while defining the space. The result may be a partial or total synovectomy of the superior joint space. Prearthrotomy arthroscopic examinations have alerted clinicians to this error. The ability of the pathologic joint to regenerate this synovium and fibrous connective tissue layer has not been determined.

HORIZONTAL INCISION BELOW THE LATERAL RIM OF THE GLENOID FOSSA

A no. 11 blade may be used to puncture into the superior joint

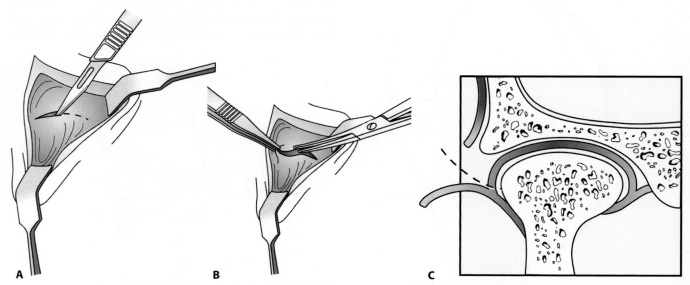

A   B   C

FIGURE 50-15.   **A,** Entry into the superior joint space following its distention with fluid. A no. 11 blade incises the lateral capsule and ligament *(broken line)*. Care is maintained not to prolong the incision posteriorly to avoid injuring the retrodiscal tissues. **B,** The incision is prolonged posteriorly using baby metzenbaum scissors. **C,** The horizontal capsular and ligament flap is developed inferiorly and the discal insertions sharply dissected *(broken line)*. The inferior joint space is defined by incising along the superolateral aspect of the condyle. A Freer septum elevator is used to define the joint spaces.

space at the level of the lateral discocapsular sulcus (Figure 50-16B). The opening is then lengthened anteriorly and posteriorly using sharp-pointed scissors. A dissection technique, similar to that described in the foregoing approach, is used to define the superior joint space. A dissection is then carried inferiorly removing the attachment of the capsule to the disc and exposing the inferior joint space. There is less risk of injury to the retrodiscal tissue with this approach; the risk to the fibrocartilage is also reduced.

HORIZONTAL INCISIONS ABOVE AND BELOW THE DISC

The horizontal approach above and below the disc (Figure 50-16C) leaves some of the capsule and ligament attached to the disc or remodeled retrodiscal tissue.

T-SHAPED INCISION

A horizontal incision may be joined by a vertical incision that extents over the capsule insertion over the lateral condyle to create a T-shaped incision over the midportion of the glenoid fossa (Figure 50-16D).

Wound closure

Closure of the capsule is often difficult to obtain following open surgical joint procedures. Support for the lateral liga-

ment can be obtained by raising a temporalis muscle and fascia flap, about 2 cm in length, pedicled inferiorly, and rotated inferiorly over the lateral rim of the glenoid fossa and sutured to the lateral capsular tissue. The pedicle stabilizes the flap but has not been shown to contain nutrient vessels. Closure of the capsule and ligament after disc repositioning lends stability to the discorrhaphy but may not critical to the success of the discectomy.

Surgical Procedures

Disc repositioning

The goal of disc-repositioning procedures is to relocate the disc to the normal condyle-disc-fossa relationship. The repositioned disc facilitates movement of the condyle previously blocked by the displaced disc, provides joint stabilization, and improves articular cartilage nutrition and lubrication. Moreover, the workload of the masticatory muscles is reduced when the obstructing disc is repositioned. The literature appears to support the successful application of disc repositioning surgery in 80-95% of cases[55,56] (Table 50-1). However the role of disc repositioning surgery has significantly diminished with the success of less invasive procedures, as well as the reported

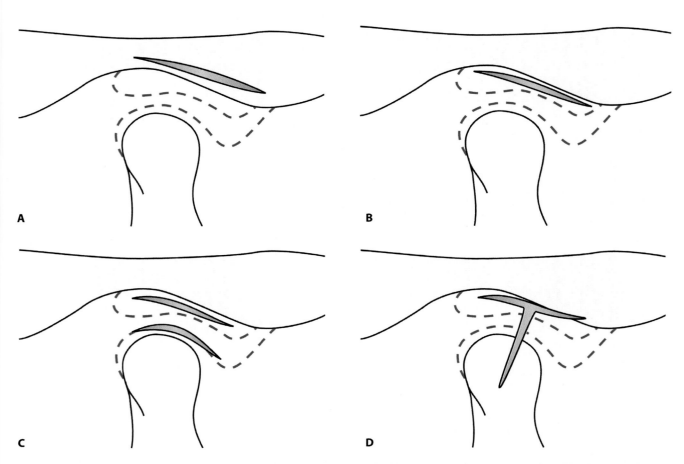

FIGURE 50-16. Capsular incision designs: **A,** horizontal incision over the lateral rim of the glenoid fossa; **B,** horizontal incision below the lateral rim of the glenoid fossa; **C,** horizontal incisions above and below the disc; **D,** T-shaped incision. The lateral pole of the condyle and lateral aspect of the remodeled posterior attachment (*broken lines*) are illustrated.

TABLE 50-1.   **Selective Studies In TMJ Disc Repositioning Surgery**

Author	Year	Type of study	Procedure	Patients/Joints	Follow-up	Results
Diskoplasty						
Dolwick[1]	1983	Retrospective Case Series	Diskoplasty	50 pts /54jts	12-60m	94% success
Dolwick et al[2]	1990	Retrospective Case Series	Diskoplasty	152pts/155jts	6m-8yrs	70-80% improvement
Anderson et al[3]	1991	Retrospective Case Series	Diskoplasty	33pts/39jts	8-35m	77% pain free
Montgomery et al[4]	1992	Retrospective Case Series	Diskoplasty	51pts/74jts	6m-6yrs	65% pain-free / 78% improved jaw motion
Zeitler et al[5]	1993	Retrospective Comparative Study	Diskoplasty	24pts	25m	83%
Kuwahara et al[6]	1994	Retrospective Comparative Study	Diskoplasty	90pts	12m	92% improvement
Abramowicz et al[7]	2010	Retrospective Case Series	Diskoplasty	18pts/36jts	20yrs	94% improvement quality of life
Diskoplasty & eminectomy						
Hall[8]	1984	Retrospective Case Series	Diskoplasty & eminectomy	20jts	18m	65% pain –free
Weinberg[9]	1984	Retrospective Case Series	Diskoplasty & eminectomy	33pt/40jts	44m	89% better
Dolwick et al[10]	1985	Retrospective Case Series	Diskoplasty & eminectomy	68pts/78jts	18-60m	55% excellent / 35% good
Kertens et al[11]	1989	Retrospective Case Series	Diskoplasty & eminectomy	25pts	14-29m	87% felt better
Trumpy et al[12]	1995	Retrospective comparative study	Diskoplasty & eminectomy	13pts	74-91m	77% improvement
Baldwin et al[13]	2004	Retrospective Case Series	Diskoplasty & eminectomy	92pts/119jts	44m	49% asymptomatic / 19% improved
Meniscocondylar plication						
Weinberg et al[14]	1987	Retrospective Case Series	Meniscocondylar plication	84pt/89jts	6-24m	91% improvement
Vazquez-Delgado et al[15]	2004	Retrospective Case Series	Meniscocondylar plication	20pts/29jts	51.2m	75% success
Diskoplasty & high condylotomy						
Benson et al[16]	1985	Retrospective comparative study	Diskoplasty & high condylotomy	60pts	6-48m	88% improved
Walker et al[17]	1987	Retrospective Case Series	Diskoplasty & high condylotomy	50pts/65jts	4-24monts	100% success
Griffts et al[18]	2007	Retrospective Case Series	Diskoplasty & high condylotomy	117pts/154jts	1-16yrs	86% success
Others						
McCarty et al[19]	1979	Retrospective Case Series	Diskoplasty & arthroplasty	327jts	6yrs	94% success
Mercuri et al.[20]	1982	Retrospective Case Series	Diskoplasty, arthroplasty & eminectomy	13pts	45m	87% success
Wolford[21]	1997	Retrospective Case Series	Disk reposition & mini anchor	43pts/78jts	2yrs	91% success
Kondoh et al[22]	2003	Retrospective Case Series	Disk reshaping	11pts/11jts	5yrs	91% success

1. Dolwick MF. Surgical management. In: Helms CA, Katzberg RW, Dolwick MF (eds). Internal derangements of the temporomandibular joint. San Francisco: Radiology research and education foundation. 1983:167–91.
2. Dolwick MF, Nitzan DW. TMJ disk surgery: 8-year follow-up evaluation. Fortschr Kiefer Gesichtschir. 1990;35:162–3.
3. Anderson DM, Sinclair PM, McBride KM. A clinical evaluation of temporomandibular joint disk plication surgery. Am J Orthod Dentofacial Orthop 1991;100:156–62.
4. Montgomery MT, Gordon SM, Van Sickels JE, Harms SE. Changes in signs and symptoms following temporomandibular joint disc repositioning surgery. J Oral Maxillofac Surg. 1992;50:320–8.
5. Zeitler D, Porter BA: A retrospective study comparing arthroscopic surgery with arthrotomy and disc repositioning. In: Clark G, Sanders B, Bertolami C (eds): Advances in Diagnostic and Surgical Arthroscopy of the Temporomandibular Joint.Philadelphia, PA, Saunders, 1993, p 47.
6. Kuwahara T, Bessette RW, Maruyama T. A retrospective study on the clinical results of temporomandibular joint surgery. Cranio 1994; 12:179–83
7. Abramowicz S, Dolwick MF. 20-year follow-up study of disc repositioning surgery for temporomandibular joint internal derangement. J Oral Maxillofac Surg. 2010;68:239–42.
8. Hall MB. Meniscoplasty of the displaced temporomandibular joint meniscus without violating the inferior joint space. J Oral Maxillofac Surg. 1984;42:788–92.
9. Weinberg S. Eminectomy and meniscorhaphy for internal derangements of the temporomandibular joint. Rationale and operative technique. Oral Surg Oral Med Oral Pathol 1984;57:241–249.
10. Dolwick MF, Sanders B. TMJ internal derangement and arthrosis: surgical atlas. CV Mosby, St. Louis 1985; p321.
11. Kerstens HC, Tuinzing DB, Van Der Kwast WA. Eminectomy and discoplasty for correction of the displaced temporomandibular joint disc. J Oral Maxillofacial Surg 1989;47:150–4.
12. Trumpy IG, Lyberg T. Surgical treatment of internal derangement of the temporomandibular joint: long-term evaluation of three techniques. J Oral Maxillofac Surg. 1995;53:740–6.
13. Baldwin AJ, Cooper JC. Eminectomy and plication of the posterior disc attachment following arthrotomy for temporomandibular joint internal derangement. J Craniomaxillofac Surg 2004:32:354–9
14. Weinberg S, Cousens G. Meniscocondylar plication: a modified operation for surgical repositioning of the ectopic temporomandibular joint meniscus. Rationale and operative technique. Oral Surg Oral Med Oral Pathol. 1987:63:393–402.
15. Vázquez-Delgado E, Valmaseda-Castellón E, Vázquez-Rodríguez E, Gay-Escoda C. Long-term results of functional open surgery for the treatment of internal derangement of the temporomandibular joint. Br J Oral Maxillofac Surg 2004;42:142–8.
16. Benson BJ, Keith DA Patient response to surgical and nonsurgical treatment for internal derangement of the temporomandibular joint. J Oral Maxillofac Surg1985;43:770–7.
17. Walker RV, Kalamchi S. A surgical technique for management of internal derangements of the temporomandibular joint. J Oral Maxillofac Surg 1987; 45;299–305.
18. Griffitts TM, Collins CP, Collins PC, Bernie OR. Walker repair of the temporomandibular joint: a retrospective evaluation of 117 patients. J Oral Maxillofac Surg 2007;65:1958–62
19. McCarty WL, Farrar WB. Surgery for internal derangements of the temporomandibular joint. J Prosthet Dent. 1979;42:191–6.
20. Mercuri LG, Campbell RL, Shamaskin RG. Intra-articular meniscus dysfunction surgery. A preliminary report. Oral Surg Oral Med Oral Pathol. 1982 Dec;54(6):613–21.
21. Wolford LM. Temporomandibular joint devices: treatment factors and outcomes. Oral Surg Oral Med Oral Pathol Oral Radiol Endod. 1997;83:143–9.
22. Kondoh T, Hamada Y, Kamei K, Seto K. Simple disc reshaping surgery for internal derangement of the temporomandibular joint: 5-year follow-up results. J Oral Maxillofac Surg. 2003;61:41–8

SECTION 6

success of discectomy without replacement.

There are two main indications for disc-repositioning procedures:

1. Patients with painful anterior disc displacement with reduction that has not responded to nonsurgical and minimally invasive procedures
2. Patients with anterior disc displacement without reduction with persistent pain and limited mouth opening that has not responded to nonsurgical and minimally invasive procedures

Absolute contraindications of the procedure include: infection in the surgical site and uncontrolled psychogenic disease. Relative contraindications involve medically compromised patients, lack of signs and symptoms of intra-articular disease, psychiatric disorders, and the possibility of solving the problem using minimally invasive techniques.[57]

Disc repositioning can be accomplished by either of the following techniques: a partial-thickness excision in which the superior lamina of the retrodiscal tissue and posterior attachment are removed, without violation of the inferior joint space, and the lateroposterior tissues are reapproximated[58] (Figure 50-17); or full-thickness excision in which a wedge-shaped portion of the posterior attachment is removed and the lateroposterior tissues are approximated[59] (Figure 50-18); or full-thickness excision of a wedge-shaped portion of the posterior attachment with stabilization of the disc with mini-anchors[60].

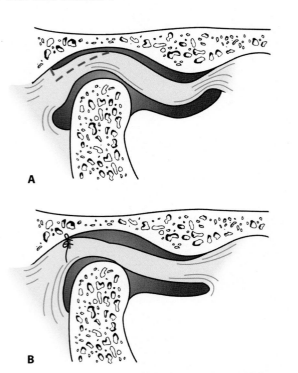

FIGURE 50-17. Disc repositioning achieved through a partial-thickness excision of the superior lamina of the retrodiscal tissue. The inferior joint space is not violated. **A,** Outline of a partial-thickness excision of the superior lamina. **B,** Excision is closed, resulting in posterior repositioning of the disc.

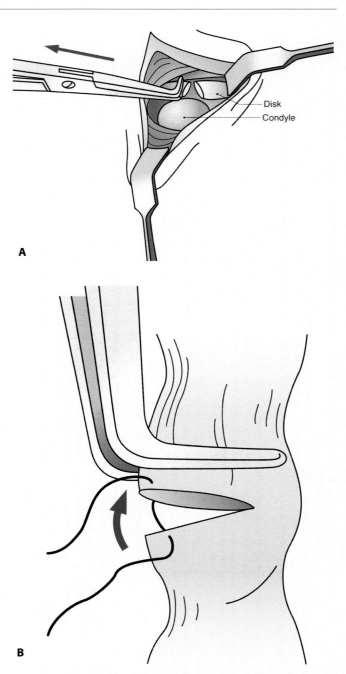

FIGURE 50-18. Disc repositioning achieved through a full-thickness excision of the posterior attachment. Retention of disc position is through sutures placed on posterior and lateral margins. **A,** A clamp has been placed over the posterior attachment. The arrow represents the direction of pull of the clamp to complete the incision and reveal the condylar surface. **B,** View from above demonstrating the wedge-shaped resection (arrow indicates the direction of closure).

The chances of a successful disc repositioning procedure increase if the disc has: 1) minimal displacement, 2) near-normal length, 3) near-normal anatomic structure. When the disc displaces, the pathologic changes are not seen uniformly throughout the entire lateromedial extent of the joint. It is believed that a variable decrease in the vascularity of

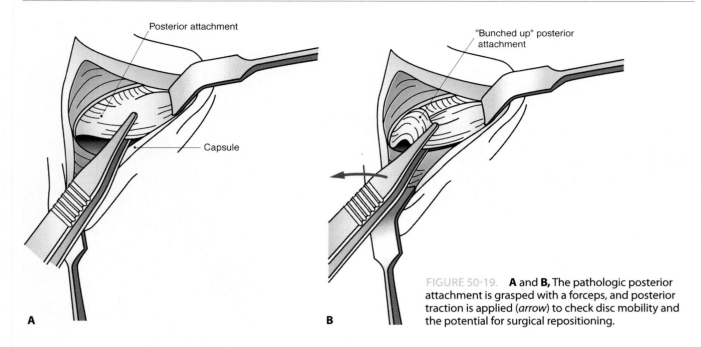

SECTION 6

FIGURE 50-19. **A** and **B,** The pathologic posterior attachment is grasped with a forceps, and posterior traction is applied (*arrow*) to check disc mobility and the potential for surgical repositioning.

the remodeled posterior attachment occurs with an increasing duration of disc displacement and load. The disc-repositioning techniques thus involve a repair in the pathologic retrodiscal tissue with a variable degree of vascularity. The primary source of nourishment to the repositioned disc appears to be through the synovium on the medial aspect of the disc and posterior recesses of the joint spaces. Thus, a critical aspect of the successful surgical repair in the retrodiscal tissue appears to be the rapid migration of synoviocytes to the area of the surgical repair. In general, the limiting factor to disc repositioning is the degree of lateral disc atrophy or resorption. Despite severe lateral atrophy, the most medial aspect of the disc may have a normal length and shape.

DISC REPOSITIONING AND DISCOPLASTY

Deformation of the disc in all planes is an important feature to recognize when planning a repositioning procedure. When a bulge-shaped disc is of appropriate length and can be repositioned, a discoplasty may be performed to minimize the change in the occlusion. In addition, removal of the posterior attachment overlying the condyle is intended to remove a source of localized inflammation.

The surgical technique for disc repositioning with discoplasty includes the exposure of the articular surfaces with any of the previously discussed surgical approaches. Once the capsule has been incised, joint distention for better visualization can be achieved by manual manipulation or placement of Wilkes retractor. A Freer elevator can be used to sweep gently across the top of the disc. Access to the medial aspect of the joint is greatly improved when the anterior attachment is released, permitting the surgeon to draw the disc outward posterolaterally while it remains pedicled to the medial attachment. The disc is then inspected for deformities, perforations. Disc mobility is evaluated by applying traction

with a forceps (Figure 50-19). Typically, the medially displaced disc must be rotated posterolaterally to achieve a correct condyle-disc-fossa relation; therefore, a greater amount of tissue is plicated or excised laterally rather than medially. A DeBakey bulldog vascular clamp is inserted to the medial limit of the posterior attachment and guided posteriorly as far as possible in the glenoid fossa (Figure 50-20). The clamp greatly assists in the control of hemorrhage from the retrodiscal tissue, stabilization of the posterior attachment during tissue excision, and stabilization of the posterior attachment during suturing.[61] The design of the instrument minimizes tissue damage. A wedge of remodeled posterior attachment is excised, leaving a 1 mm margin anterior to the beaks of the clamp. This permits suturing of the disc to the retrodiscal tissue without removal of the clamp. Range of

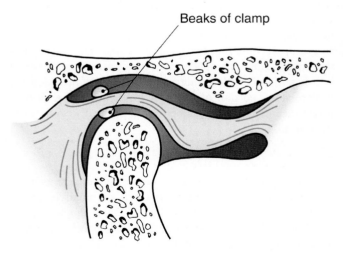

FIGURE 50-20. Positioning of the beaks of the DeBakey clamp on retrodiscal tissue

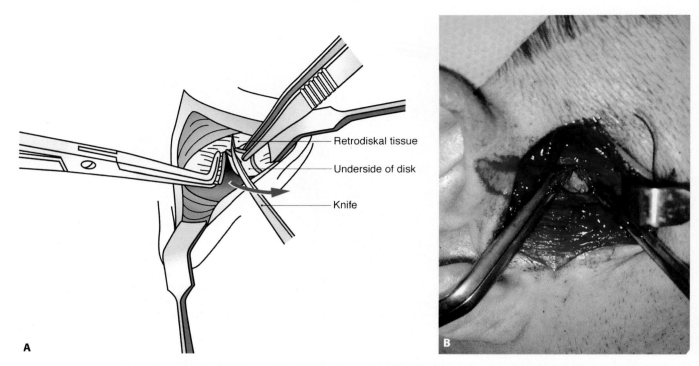

— Retrodiskal tissue

— Underside of disk

— Knife

A

B

FIGURE 50-21. **A,** Discoplasty is performed following wedge resection of the pathologic posterior attachment. The disc is slightly evened, and an arthroscopic orthopedic knife is used to sculpt the inferior surface of the bulge-shaped disc. **B,** The DeBakey vascular clamp is in place. Note the protruding edge of the posterior attachment used for reapproximation to the disc and lateral capsule.

motion is then verified. Tissue forceps are used to stabilize and slightly evert the disc so that the inferior surface may be sculpted (Figure 50-21). The tissue is closed with nonresorbable suture (Figure 50-22). Once the disc has been sutured into its new position, its lateral rim is sutured to the lateral capsule ligament.

In a study by Montgomery and colleagues, postoperative MRIs demonstrated an unchanged disc position in 86% of patients 2 years after TMJ disc repositioning surgery.[62] Some authors have advocated the use of mini-anchors (Mitek) for better stabilization of the disc in a more physiologic position with success rates reported between 82-91%.[63–65] Long-term studies are required to further determine the stability of the technique as well as the best moment to be applied. The surgical procedure for placement of mini-anchors establishes that once the disc is properly reduced, the mini-anchor, which is a metal insert with a suture attached to it, is placed in the posterolateral portion of condylar head. The suture is then used to secure the lateral and posterior of the disc to the condylar head.

Disc Repositioning and Arthroplasty

Several authors have advocated combining a disc repositioning procedure with an arthroplasty of the condyle or the articular eminence.[66–70] Arthroplasty reduces the amount of posterolateral repositioning required and therefore permits an easier repositioning of an atrophic disc (Figure 50-23).

A 2 to 4 mm condylar/eminence arthroplasty procedure can be performed with rotary or hand instruments. Hand instruments such as fine chisels are preferable to avoid heat generation (Figure 50-24). Bone files should be used judiciously because, once the compact bony layer is interrupted, the trabeculae of bone can be easily and rapidly removed. A periosteal elevator may be used to burnish sharp edges. Care should be exercised not to exaggerate the arthroplasty in the lateral condylar regions while accessing the medial condylar region. In some cases an arthroplasty of the eminence is essentially a lateral tuberculectomy for access and decompression of the anterior recess of the superior joint space (Figure 50-25). Disc repositioning is then performed through the plication or excision technique. The capsule is closed in the customary fashion. Intermaxillary fixation or training elastics are used for 1 to 3 weeks to allow muscular adaptation and dental compensations to occur. The current trend, however, is to avoid removal of any normal articular bone since the postoperative healing phase already involves some loss of bone substance, which may be additive and result in occlusal disturbances. In addition, postoperative bleeding from cut bone surfaces into the joint can result in fibrous adhesions of the disc or fibrous/bony ankylosis of the joint.

Disc Repair

Perforations rarely occur within the disc proper but rather within the lateral third of the remodeled posterior attachment.[71] When the disc is perforated, it may be secondary to a developmental rather than a pathologic process. Small perforations (1-3mm) can be treated with primary closure. The atrophic displaced disc is repositioned posteriorly to only a

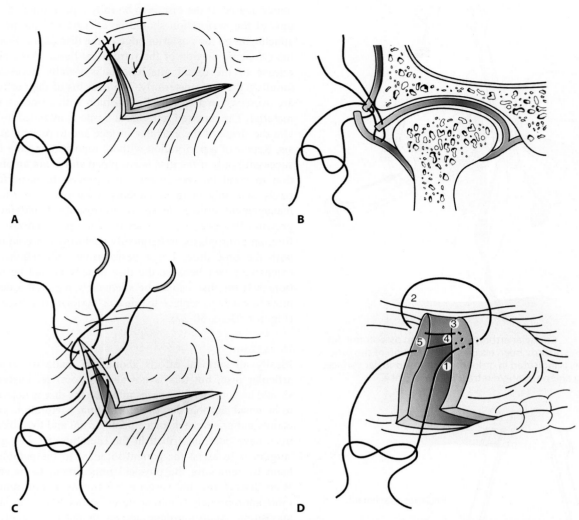

FIGURE 50-22. Disc reapproximation: **A,** simple posterior and lateral sutures; B, layered closure of the superior and inferior lamina; **C,** figure-of-8 closure; **D,** the order of passage of the figure-of-8 suture labeled 1 to 5.

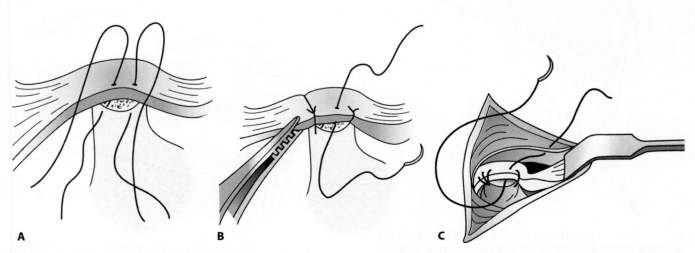

FIGURE 50-23. **A–C,** Disc repositioning with arthroplasty according to Walker and Kalamchi. The disc is sutured to the condyle stump. Adapted from Walker RV and Kalamchi S[67]

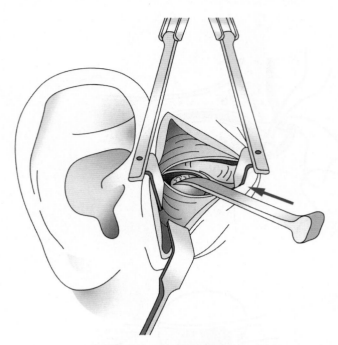

FIGURE 50-24.   Condylar arthroplasty using an osteotome. An osteophyte has already been excised. The direction of the osteotome (*arrow*) is indicated in order to skim the condylar surface. Self-retaining and right-angle retractors are in place.

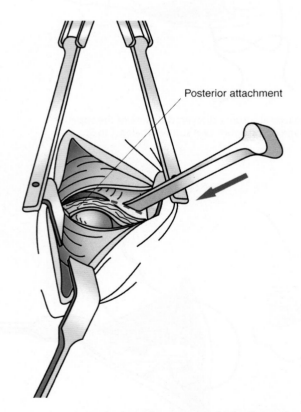

FIGURE 50-25.   Lateral tuberculectomy may be performed to acquire access to the anterior glenoid and eminence regions (*broken line* indicates bone to be excised and *arrow* indicates direction of osteotome).

minor degree. If the disc is to be fully repositioned, the margins of the perforation should be excised and the posterior attachment on the posterior edge of the disc approximated to the tympanic portion of the retrodiscal tissue. Anterolateral release of the discal attachments is usually necessary to mobilize the disc posteriorly. The margins of the perforation are oversewn in a straight-line fashion with a nonresorbable material. The repaired retrodiscal tissue is intended to maintain the shape of the articular surface and to prevent ankylosis. Repair of a perforation without repositioning the disc is successful only if the disc is atrophied and is not an obstruction to condylar movement. This procedure is performed rarely and only in those patients refractory to nonsurgical management, arthrocentesis, or arthroscopy. Condylar overgrowth often occurs in the areas of the perforations; therefore, an arthroplasty is frequently performed in conjunction with the procedure. Large perforations will require more extensive repair because the disc usually cannot be repositioned. If the disc cannot be adequately repaired a decision must be made to replace the disc or performed a discectomy (Figures 50-26, 50-27).

Discectomy

Ideally all surgical efforts should be made to retain the articular disc, but this is not always possible. Discectomy should be considered in cases in which the disc is determined to be unsalvageable due to deformation, perforation, calcification and/or severe displacement. Partial and total discectomies have been described in the literature.[72,73] The goal of surgery is to assist the patient to adapt to the pathology at hand by removing the physical impediment to movement. With discectomy, the surgeon transforms a joint into what more appropriately would be described as two bones in close apposition. Adult cartilage derives its nutrients solely from synovial fluid. The prolonged contact of bony surfaces following discectomy may interfere with diffusion of nutrients from the synovial fluid. The decreased diffusion of nutrients

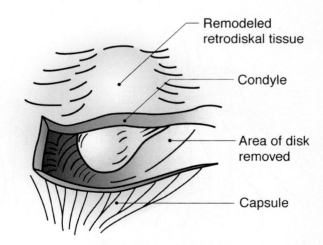

Remodeled retrodiskal tissue

Condyle

Area of disk removed

Capsule

FIGURE 50-26.   For repair of a large perforation, a partial discectomy is performed first. A portion of the disc and the retrodiscal tissue may be retained.

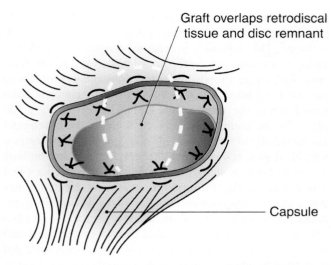

FIGURE 50-27. A dermal graft covers the surgically created perforation. The edges of the graft overlay the disc, retrodiscal tissue, and lateral capsule to assist in suturing.

to cartilage may result in the eventual resorption of noncalcified cartilage. As a result, several adaptive changes rapidly occur. Agerberg and Lundberg[74] described radiographical erosion of the articular surfaces of the operated and nonoperated joints. They also concluded that the remodeling process is due to altered joint loading after discectomy but stabilization occurred after 2 years. They used the term *remodeling* and not osteoarthrosis to describe the radiographic changes because the osseous changes occurred in the absence of symptoms. The bony changes appear similar to those that are observed longitudinally with chronic disc displacement, suggestive of the same mechanism. The rate of remodeling, however, is accelerated in the post-discectomy state.

After a discectomy some masticatory muscle and joint tenderness can be expected for a variable period, extending from several weeks to months. The patient at first favors mastication on the operated side. Later, when healing is advanced, mastication is performed on the nonoperated side. An opening deviation of as much as 8 to 9 mm may occur toward the operated side. Hypermobility of the nonoperated joint may develop or increase after discectomy. Limitation of mandibular movement on the operated side appears to be responsible for the hypermobility. Physical therapy greatly assists the control of the ipsilateral deviation and hence contralateral hypermobility. Patients often report an alteration in their bite, although rarely as a major complaint. The thicker the retrodiscal tissue removed, the greater is the anticipated change in occlusion. The sensation of an altered bite usually resolves within a week to several months and occlusal equilibration is rarely indicated.

There is considerable variation in the ability of each patient and joint to adapt to the postdiscectomy state. Individual factors, such as inclination of the eminence, state of preoperative symptoms, loss of molar support, and amount of postoperative remodeling, seem to play a substantial role.

The mechanism of pain relief and improvement in function over the long-term following discectomy is still unknown. However long-term follow up studies on TMJ discectomies have shown complete resolution in pain and dysfunction in almost all the patients reviewed[75–79]. (Table 50-2)

TABLE 50-2. Selective Studies in TMJ Discectomy

Author	Year	Type of study	Patients/Joints	Follow-up	Results
Brown et al[1]	1980	Retrospective Case Series	214pts	15yrs	85% improvement
Takaku et al[2]	1994	Retrospective Case Series	39pts	20yrs	95% improvement
Kuwahara et al[3]	1994	Retrospective Comparative Study	74pts	1yr	95% improvement
Trumpy et al[4]	1995	Retrospective Comparative Study	17pts	6–7.5yrs	94% improvement
Windmark et al[5]	1997	Retrospective Case Series	16ts	2yrs	88% improvement
Holmlund et al[6]	2001	Prospective Randomized Comparative Study	72pts	1yr	83% improvement
Eriksson et al[7]	2001	Retrospective Case Series	64pts	5yrs	85% good results
Bjørnland et al[8]	2003	Retrospective Case Series	24pts	10yrs	79% no pain
Nyberg et al[9]	2004	Retrospective Case Series	15pts	5yrs	87% successful
Miloro et al[10]	2010	Retrospective Case Series	24pts	2–60m	83% sucessful

1. Brown WA. Internal derangement of the temporomandibular joint: review of 214 patients following meniscectomy. Can J Surg 1980;23:30–2.
2. Takaku S, Toyoda T. Long term evaluation of discectomy of the temporomandibular joint. J Oral Maxillofac Surg 1994; 52:722–726.
3. Kuwahara T, Bessette RW, Maruyama T. A retrospective study on the clinical results of temporomandibular joint surgery. Cranio 1994; 12:179–83
4. Trumpy IG, Lyberg T. Surgical treatment of internal derangement of the temporomandibular joint: long-term evaluation of three techniques. J Oral Maxillofac Surg. 1995;53:740–6.
5. Widmark G, Dahlström L, Kahnberg KE, Lindvall AM. Diskectomy in temporomandibular joints with internal derangement: a follow-up study. Oral Surg Oral Med Oral Pathol Oral Radiol Endod. 1997;83(3):314–320.
6. Holmlund AB, Axelsson S, Gynther GW. A comparison of discectomy and arthroscopic lysis and lavage for the treatment of chronic closed lock of the temporomandibular joint: a randomized outcome study. J Oral Maxillofac Surg 2001;59:972–7.
7. Eriksson L, Westesson PL. Discectomy as an effective treatment for painful temporomandibular joint internal derangement: a 5-year clinical and radiographic follow-up. J Oral Maxillofac Surg. 2001;59:750–8.
8. Bjørnland T, Larheim TA. Discectomy of the temporomandibular joint: 3-year follow-up as a predictor of the 10-year outcome. J Oral Maxillofac Surg. 2003;61:55–60.
9. Nyberg J, Adell R, Svensson B. Temporomandibular joint discectomy for treatment of unilateral internal derangements—a 5 year follow-up evaluation. Int J Oral Maxillofac Surg. 2004;33:8–12.
10. Miloro M, Henriksen B. Discectomy as the primary surgical option for internal derangement of the temporomandibular joint. J Oral Maxillofac Surg 2010;68:782–9.

SECTION 6

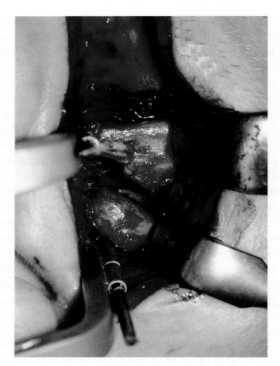

FIGURE 50-28.   The Wilkes retractor allows an increased area of maneuverability within the joint space. As it retracts the condyle moves in an anterior and inferior direction. Note the better visualization of medial remanents of the disc.

During discectomy without replacement, once the capsule has been incised, joint distention for better visualization can be achieved by manual manipulation or placement of Wilkes retractor (Figure 50-28). Disc extirpation is facilitated when the disc is severed from its anterior and lateral attachments and then retracted laterally and posteriorly to complete the incisions. This approach permits the surgeon to verify the ability of the disc to be repositioned posteriorly before excision. With severe atrophy of the disc, substantial resistance to posterolateral traction is noted. A hemostatic clamp is positioned across the anterior attachment to serve as a guide plane for the knife, which is used to sever the attachment lateromedially. As the posterior attachment demonstrates a variable degree of vascularity changes, the DeBakey bulldog vascular clamp or straight mosquito clamp may be applied here before severing the posterior attachment. Next, a hemostat is used to apply outward traction to the tissue to be extirpated. A meniscus knife is used to sever the medial attachments. When the remodeled posterior attachment and disc are extirpated, the retrodiscal tissue is electrocauterized to control bleeding. Care is taken not to disrupt the fibrous connective tissue lining of the fossa and condyle. The morphology of the condyle and glenoid fossa often prevents excision in one piece. Incomplete excision of the posterior attachment over the lateral pole of the condyle may account for some cases of failure with discectomy. With the disc and posterior attachment removed, mandibular range of motion is checked. Joint noises, characterized as snappings, may indicate a disc remnant. Disc remnants are usually located on the medial aspect of the joint cavity. (Figure 50-29) The surgeon should remove all disc remnants that appear to impede movement.

Disc Replacement

Despite the reported success of long-term studies of TMJ discectomy, there is a perception among surgeons that disc

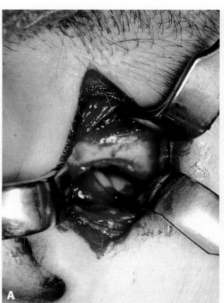
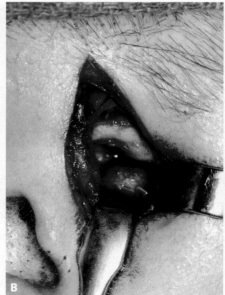
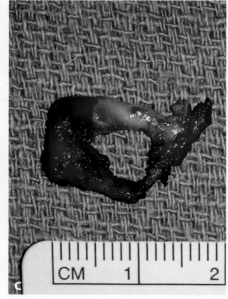

FIGURE 50-29.   Discectomy without disk replacement. **A,** Large perforation through the articular disc. The top of the condylar head can be seen through the disc perforation. **B,** Postdiscectomy view of the joint with the condyle free of mechanical interferences. **C,** Surgical specimen.

replacement is required to help prevent or reduce the significant osseous remodeling, intra-articular adhesions, and recurrent pain that is seen following discectomy alone. An interpositional material was believed to decrease joint noises by dissipating loading forces on the osseous surfaces. The effectiveness of routine interpositional materials and grafts to reduce adhesions, protect the articular surfaces, and diminish pain and postdiscectomy joint noise has not been substantiated by the literature, as long-term results of discectomy alone are far superior to short-term discectomy with grafts and disc preservation procedures.[80–82]

The popularity of alloplastic for TMJ disc displacement materials suffered considerably after the experience with silastic[83] and teflon-proplast.[84] Both materials while enduring continuous loading by the mandibular condyle suffered fragmentation, migration, foreign body giant cell reactions, and recurrent joint symptoms.[85] The recognition of these limitations led to the abandonment of the permanent placement of both materials.[86] The use of silastic as a temporary disc replacement material is not supported by the literature.[87–88] However, it is currently used as a temporary spacer to prevent TMJ ankylosis, for a 6 to 12-week period of waiting for the fabrication of a CAD-CAM generated custom permanent alloplastic TMJ prosthesis. Additionally the vitallium alloy (cobalt, chromium, molybdenum) fossa-eminence prosthesis is another alloplastic material used after a discectomy that has reported in the literature with moderate success.[89–93] (Figure 50-30)

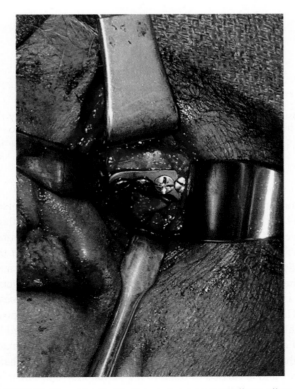

FIGURE 50-30.   Alloplastic disc replacement. Vitallium alloy (cobalt, chromium, molybdenum) fossa-eminence prosthesis.

The debacle of silastic and teflon-proplast created an increased use of autogenous grafts.[94] Most autogenous grafts have been used to replace failed alloplastic implants, which means there are few reports of autogenous grafts placed at the time of the discectomy. In a critical review of interpositional grafts, Dimitroulis[95] suggests that the criteria for the ideal interpositional material used to replace the articular disc after discectomy should include:

1. Long term safety
2. Adequate bulk
3. Good handling properties
4. Easy to procure
5. Abundantly available
6. Survives the intrajoint environment
7. Facilitates normal joint function
8. Prevents bone formation and joint ankylosis
9. Protects condyle from severe remodeling

TEMPORALIS MUSCLE/FASCIA FLAP

The temporalis muscle/fascia is the most popular interpositional material for reasons of close proximity and ease of use. The flap may be pedicled in a variety of ways. Advantages of this technique over a free graft include its stability, owing to its connection at the base, its availability at the same surgical site, and its lack of cosmetic, and functional morbidity. The disadvantages include flap necrosis, fibrosis and similar to other TMJ surgical procedures is the risk of postoperative decreased interincisal opening.

Feinberg and Larsen described a technique which a temporalis muscle flap is develop that includes the temporalis fascia and the underlying pericranium from the most inferior horizontally oriented fibers of the temporalis muscle. The flap is based anteriorly off the coronoid process and passed anteriorly around the zygomatic arch in the TMJ that pedicled the posterior temporalis muscle fibers anteriorly. The muscle is then sutured to the retrodiscal tissues.[96,97] (Figure 50-31). Studies have reported that the muscle maintains its viability with some fibrosis.[96,98]

A procedure in which the muscle is placed over the zygomatic arch has also been described.[99] (Figure 50-32), The shape and size of the flap is outlined by incising posteriorly near the postglenoid spine of the joint through temporalis fascia muscle and periosteum. This incision is extended superiorly near the temporal line. Subperiosteal dissection elevates the amount of flap needed from the temporal bone. A transverse incision is made at the superior portion anteriorly to create a 3 cm–wide flap. The width should be greater than the anteroposterior coverage desired in the joint to allow flap contraction. An anterior incision is made parallel to the posterior incision. The superior aspect of the anterior incision is carried to bone in this thin area of the temporalis. Inferiorly, as the arch is approached, the muscle thickens; therefore, the dissections are not carried completely through muscle to bone. Blunt dissection is carried inferiorly to a point just medial to the arch to permit adequate mobility of the flap. Branches of the temporal artery found in this area are pre-served if possible. The

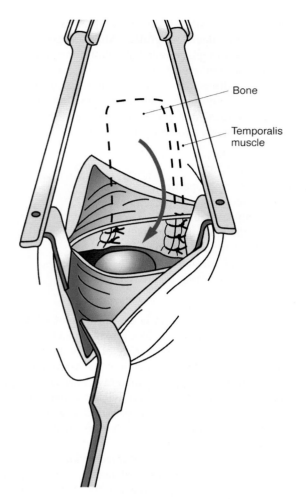

FIGURE 50-31.   Disc replacement using temporalis mucle/fascial graft (*broken line*) pedicled from above the glenoid fossa and rotated inward (*arrow*). Lateral, anterior, and posterior sutures hold the graft in place.

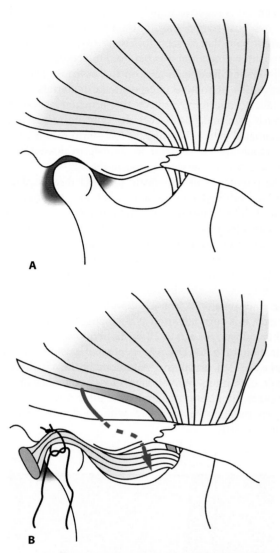

FIGURE 50-32.   **A** and **B,** Disc replacement using temporalis muscle/fascial graft pedicled anteriorly and rotated anteriorly and inferiorly around (beneath) the posterior root of the zygomatic arch (*arrow*). The graft is sutured to the retrodiscal tissues.

length of the flap is usually 5 cm. The flap is fully reflected off the bone, and resorbable interrupted sutures are placed in several areas on the edge of the flap through fascia, muscle, and the periosteum to keep the layers from separating. Holes are drilled in the bone of the lateral lip of the glenoid fossa posteriorly and anteriorly before placement of the flap into the joint. One suture is placed through bone anteriorly near the eminence, and a second posterior suture is placed near the postglenoid spine. Two additional sutures hold the medial edge to anterior and posterior medial tissues. These medial sutures are sometimes difficult or impossible to secure, and the sutures through lateral bone are usually adequate to hold the flap in place. A cosmetic temporal defect may result depending on the thickness of tissue harvested.

The results from numerous clinical studies show a high success rate with the use of a variety of techniques involving temporalis muscle flaps of varying sizes and shapes, based either inferiorly or anteriorly.[96,99–102] A meta-analysis of the literature from 1965 to 2001 calculated mean success rate of 91.4% for the temporalis muscle flap.[82]

EAR CARTILAGE

Autogenous conchal cartilage has been described and praised as TMJ disc replacement by several authors.[103–107] Cartilage harvested from the cavum conchae results in minimal esthetic compromise and the graft can be tailored to fit the condyle or glenoid fossa. Notably, the quality and thickness of the aural cartilage is variable. In some cases an iatrogenic tear in the cartilage may occur during the harvesting process.

The procedure to obtain chondral cartilage as interpositional material for TMJ reconstruction has been described by Hall and Link.[105] A 3 to 4 cm postauricular incision is made on the ear a few millimeters lateral to the auriculocephalic sulcus and is carried through to the perichondrium. The middle division of the posterior auricular artery may be encountered and ligated or cauterized. A careful supraperichondral dissection with a fine dissecting scissors exposes the surface of the cartilage. A scalpel is used to cut through the cartilage in the shape of the desired amount of graft, usually 1.5 by 2.5 cm. It is important not to extend to the rim of the antihelix to avoid permanent deformity of the ear. Subperichondral dissection between the skin of the bowl and cartilage permits the cartilage to be removed without tearing it or perforating the skin. The ear is packed with gauze or other material to maintain the shape of the bowl and to apply pressure to the skin. The pressure pack is maintained for 48 hours.

Although mean success rates of 82.4% have been published with auricular graft as disc replacement[82], other studies have shown their tendency to fragment, proliferate and result in fibrous ankylosis with progressive mouth opening limitation.[108–110]

Dermal Fat Graft

Georgiade originally reported the use of dermal fat graft for surgical correction of TMJ dysfunction.[111] Only a few clinical studies published on the use of dermis grafts for disc repair[112] and disc replacement material in the TMJ.[113] Dimitroulis showed 35 joints in 29 patients that demonstrated dermis grafts were effective in reducing joint sounds, but the author conceded that dermis grafts were difficult to anchor and failed to prevent regressive remodeling of the condyle.[114]

The dermal graft may be harvested from the buttock, upper lateral thigh, groin, or the inner aspect of the upper extremity.[112,115] An elliptic wedge of epidermis and underlying dermis is harvested. The donor site wound is closed primarily and occlusive dressing placed. The underlying surface of the dermis must be defatted before being the graft is implanted. The defatted graft is trimmed and sutured to the retrodiscal tissue and the anterior and lateral capsular attachments. Unfortunately, in some cases, anchoring is difficult and the graft is simply inserted as space filler.

Abdominal dermis-fat graft

Dimitroulis published the first description of abdominal dermis-fat graft as disc replacement after TMJ discectomy.[116] The greatest advantage of this type of graft is its ability to be easily sculptured to fit precisely into any size cavity. Several studies by Dimitroulis and collegues have demonstrated that abdominal dermis-fat is a promising graft material that satisfies most, but not all the criteria for an ideal interpositional graft following discectomy.[95,116–120] They showed, in a quality of life study, that although discectomy was largely responsible for the resolution of joint pain and dysfunction, abdominal dermis-fat was a safe procedure and helps promote smooth, pain-free joint function.[118] While their studies have been largely positive, there are still concerns as dermis-fat graft is not always successful, as it fails to protect the condyle from further degeneration in one-third of cases and the ultimate fate of a joint replacement in 7% of cases.[119–120]

Tissue engineered TMJ disc

The rapidly growing technologies of tissue engineering will provide in the future alternatives for TMJ disc replacement.[121–123] Tissue engineered articular discs are at the nascent phase of development but the real challenge will come when researchers try to anchor the newly developed disc to the surrounding articular structures without compromising the normal function of the joint.

Modified mandibular condylotomy

Modified mandibular condylotomy is an extra-articular surgical procedure that differs from other TMJ disc derangement procedures, as it does not directly involve the articular surfaces. Essentially, the procedure consists of an intraoral vertical ramus osteotmy in which the medial pterygoid muscle is partially detached to allow for 3 to 4 mm of condylar sag. Ideally, the downward position of the condylar segment increases the joint space, reducing the load on the retrodiscal tissue and relieving the pain and dysfunction[124] The extra-articular nature of the procedure explains the observation that a joint will not be made worse by a modified condylotomy[125] The procedure carries low morbidity and significant complications are rare. It has the disadvantage that requires a brief period of maxillomandibular fixation (MMF) followed by several weeks of training elastics. The principal indication for modified mandibular condylotomy is the management of pain and mechanical symptoms in patients who have disc displacement with reduction (79-94% successful)[126–128] or patients who recently progressed to disc displacement without reduction (82% successful)[129]. Still, regardless of the stage of disc derangement, the increase of the joint space unloads of the retrodiscal tissues and articular surfaces, as well as relieves mechanical interferences. Thus, contrasting intra-articular procedures, no surgical joint pain occurs and joint pain is relief nearly immediate.[130] Absolute contraindication of the procedure includes uncontrolled bruxism and relative contraindications involve risk factors for occlusal disturbances after surgery. Two interesting facts about modified mandibular condylotomy are: 1) it is claimed that it can result in a more normal disc-condyle relationship[128] and 2) it seems to positively affect the progression of the disease.[131]

The surgical technique to perform a modified condylotomy includes the standard instrumentation for an intraoral vertical ramus osteotomy. Once arch bars are placed and local anesthesia is given, a standard incision is made over the external oblique ridge. Periosteum is elevated from the whole lateral ramus to identify important landmarks for the osteotomy that include the sigmoid notch, the mandibular angle and the posterior border of the mandibular ramus. Visualization is greatly facilitated with the use of endoscopy. Although the classical description of this procedure calls for the identification of the ante-lingula to avoid damage to the inferior alveolar nerve, Aziz and colleagues demonstrated complete concordance of the position of the lingula and antelingula in only 11.1% of the specimens studied.[132] In an anatomic study of the position of the mandibular foramen in relation to the LeVasseur-Merrill retractor, da Fontoura and colleagues[133] showed that the mandibular foramen was located within 7 mm of the posterior edge of the mandible in only 3.3% of the rami. When properly placed, the LeVasseur-Merrill

SECTION 6

retractor was effective in avoiding the inferior alveolar nerve in 98.9% of the analyzed rami. The osteotomy is carried out in the central portion of the ramus using a 7mm angled oscillating saw against the LaVasseur-Merrill retractor. The inferior limb of the osteotomy is done through the inferior border of the mandible to allow for the desired condylar sag and better control of the condylar segment. The superior portion of the osteotomy is directed towards the sigmoid notch, with care to avoid excesive soft tissue trauma. Once the osteotomy is completed MMF is established and condylar sag is estimated mobilizing the segment and evaluating the step between the tip of the condylar segment and the inferior border. Medial pterygoid muscle is detached from the distal end of the condylar segment using a periosteal elevator to achieve 3-4 mm of condylar sag. Wire or plate fixation of the osteotomized segments is not necessary except in the cases of excessive condylar after excessive stripping of the medial pterygoid muscle or in cases in which condylar segment mobility is inadequate after previous TMJ surgical procedures. Finally if necessary, the tip of the condylar segment can be trimmed to avoid palpation. Immediate postoperative imaging is obtained to corroborate the correct position and the sag of the condylar segment. (Figure 50-33) Postoperatively after unilateral modified condylotomy, MMF is maintained for approximately 1 week, followed by 5 weeks of training elastics (single class II canine region on the operated side and single vertical on the nonoperated side). Bilateral cases will require 2 to 3 weeks of MMF follow by 3 to 4 weeks of training elastics (bilateral class II canine region).

Complications of this procedure include: bleeding, excessive condylar sag, fracture of the condylar segment, injury to the inferior alveolar nerve (1-8%), infection (1-2%), and malocclusion (22%). Three potential complications of modified condylotomy that may require reoperation are: excessive condylar sag with condylar dislocation, malocclusion, and fracture of the condylar segment.[134]

Postoperative Management

After surgery a combination of physical, pharmacological, and splint therapies are normally employed postoperatively to achieve an acceptable postoperative pain and range of motion. The positive role of physical therapy in recovery after TMJ surgery has been reported in the literature.[135–136] It is important to weigh the contribution of masticatory muscle myalgia to the patient's chief complaint. Although joint surgery can relieve the joint pain, in many cases it may be ineffectual in controlling muscle discomfort. Nonsurgical management of the muscle disorders must continue in many patients after surgery for TMJ disc derangements. Joint surgery does not restore the joint to its prepathologic state. The patient should understand that biting force may be reduced and jaw fatigue may become apparent with heavy meals or long conversations. After primary surgery (i.e., no previous TMJ surgery), one should strive for the following passive range-of-motion parameters: maximum interincisal opening of 35 to 40 mm, lateral excursive movements of 4 to 6 mm,

and protrusive excursive movements of 4 to 6 mm. However, success should not be measured by the attainment of a finite measurement. A patient's overall success should be measured by the eradication or diminution of the preoperative complaints. Surgery is rarely performed to correct purely functional complaints. Elimination of pain during function is usually the predominant concern for the patient, who is willing to accept some compromise in degree of opening and lateral excursions.

Postoperative outcomes may be influenced by several factors, including concomitant facial pain from other sources, degenerative bony changes, advanced morphologic changes in the disc, perforation of the posterior attachment, poorly controlled parafunctional habits, malocclusion, psychological overlay, previous TMJ surgery, history of facial nerve paralysis or orofacial numbness, history of infection, or systemic diseases affecting the muscles, ligaments, or bone[34].

Splint therapy should be used to maintain a stable occlusal relation in the immediate postoperative phase. This is particularly important after disc repositioning. The appliance is frequently adjusted as the edema resolves and disc tissues heal. Splint therapy is routinely used as well when a large parafunctional component is present. The patient should be able to return to a normal mechanical diet with minimal dietary restrictions. Joint sounds may develop or persist, but the asymptomatic sounds should be of minimal concern to the patient.

The clinician must balance the desire to rapidly and actively restore a normal range of motion with the capacity of the joint and facial muscles to adapt. Some latitude must be maintained on the part of the clinician in dealing with a patient's rehabilitation schedule. Care should be exercised in the rehabilitative process of the patient with bilateral joint disease whose operation was unilateral. Diet restrictions are important. Excessive lateral excursive movements to the ipsilateral side may contribute to the exacerbation of contralateral symptoms. There is no cookbook recipe to postoperative management of these patients. Some patients, regardless of the procedure, achieve an acceptable range of motion within 7 to 14 days, with minimal effort on their part. Others need to follow a strict physical therapy regimen. The devices such as Therabyte (Actos Medical) or Dynasplint (Dynasplint) are routinely used as part of the patient's physical therapy. Additionally the help of a physical therapist may sometimes be enlisted to regain joint mobility, especially when patient cooperation with a home exercise program is questionable. In general, some light passive opening and protrusion stretching exercises are prescribed four times a day beginning 5 days postoperatively. With disc repair procedures the physical therapy exercises should be more gradual. Patients should be maintained on a full liquid to soft diet for the first 2 post-operative weeks. Heat may be applied before and after exercises to improve comfort.

Complications

As with all surgical procedures, TMJ disc surgery is not exempt from potential complications. Complications after

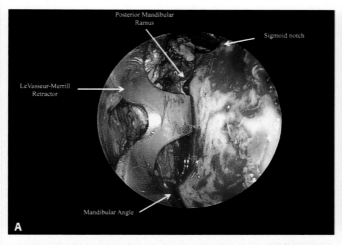

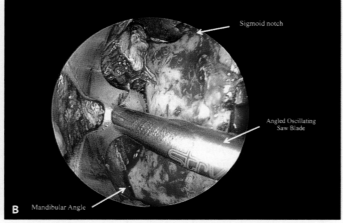

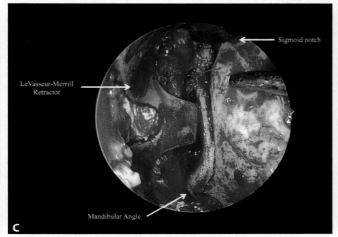

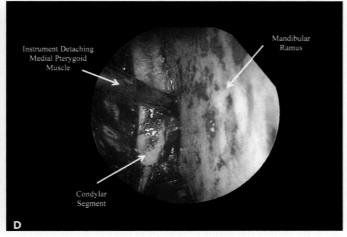

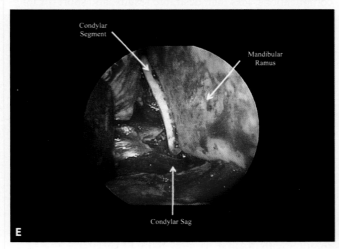

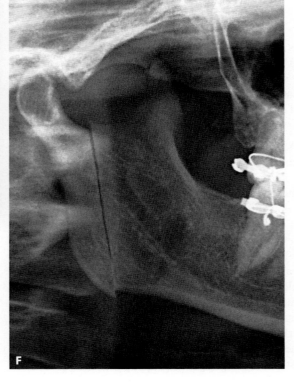

FIGURE 50-33.   Endoscopically assisted modified condylotomy. **A,** Complete exposure of the lateral ramus and placement of the LeVasseur-Merrill retractor. Note the identification the landmarks: sigmoid notch, posterior ramus and mandibular angle. **B,** Angled oscillating saw blade in proper position against the LeVassuer-Merrill retractor. **C,** Osteotomy completed. **D,** Detachment of medial pterygoid muscle. **E,** Condylar sag with the amount of downward displacement of the condylar segment. **F,** Postoperative x-ray

TMJ disc surgery can be divided in: *perioperative and long-term surgical complications.*[137–138]

Perioperative complications

VASCULAR INJURY AND HEMORRHAGE

Hemorrhage from the retrodiscal tissue may interfere with performance of the disc repair. Temporary control may be obtained with seating of the condyle in the glenoid fossa. Electrocautery, injection of epinephrine, or application of hemostatic agents while maintaining the mandible in the closed position may be necessary.

Hemorrhage from the internal maxillary artery can be problematic and difficult to control. Usually the bleeding can be controlled with pressure and vascular clips. Control via selective embolization has also been described in the literature.[139]

NEUROLOGIC INJURY

The incidence of facial nerve transient neuropraxia after open joint surgery ranges from 1-25%; it is generally limited to the temporal branch and usually resolves in 3 to 6 months.[137] It is also more frequent on patients with previous open joint surgery. Rarely, the zygomatic branches and, even more rarely, the entire temporofacial division may be injured. Injury to the chorda tympani from aggressive condylar retraction in the medial aspect of the fossa may occur rarely as well. Neuropraxia of the inferior alveolar and, less commonly, the lingual nerves may result from clamp placement for joint manipulation.

Auriculotemporal nerve syndrome (Frey's syndrome or gustatory sweating) has been reported after the dissection of the joint.[140] It is the result of auriculotemporal nerve damage with reinervation of the eccrine sweat glands by parasympathetic salivary fibers.

INFECTION

Infections rarely occur. Normally they are superficial wound infections in which microorganisms cultured may originate from the skin or external auditory meatus flora. To avoid contamination ear packing is avoided as it frequently becomes dislodged during surgery. In addition, the ear is not suctioned during surgery.

OTOLOGIC COMPLICATIONS

The proximity of the TMJ to the ear increases the risk for potential damage. Lacerations of the external auditory canal (EAC) usually occur at the junction with the bony portion of the canal due to the anteromedial inclination of the canal. If a laceration occurs packing the EAC with iodoform gauze for 5-7 days will be enough to prevent stenosis. Alternatively antibiotic-hydrocortisone otic drops can be used to prevent infection and aid healing. Although rare, an aural-TMJ fistula may develop as long-term complication of EAC laceration.

Perforation of the tympanic membrane occurs when an instrument is inadvertently passed through the membrane. Small perforations in the anterior or inferior portion of the membrane result in minimal hearing loss. Larger and injuries to the posterior region may cause hearing loss due to possible

ossicle disruption. If perforation is noted, otolaryngologist consultation is warranted. Auriculitis and external otitis are more likely to occur with the postauricular and endaural approaches. Treatment consists of pain control, cleaning of the EAC, and antibiotic-hydrocortisone otic drops.

Long-term complications

MALOCCLUSION

Significant occlusal changes can be found in some cases after aggressive open joint surgery was performed.

Correction may require the services of orthodontist and/or prosthodontist and even further surgery like orthognathic surgery or total TMJ replacements.

Ankylosis

Fibrous ankylosis can form between the disc and the articular eminence if hemoarthrosis develops. Lack of patient compliance with postoperative physical therapy can also develop fibrous ankylosis. Bony ankylosis is more common after discectomy with poor postoperative physical therapy; with heterotopic bone formation and it can also be seen in the multiple-operated patient.

Reoperations

Unfortunately, TMJ surgeries are not always successful, and the patient's preoperative symptoms persist or may even increase after surgery. There are many potential pitfalls that can occur during any phase of the treatment that can lead to complications, less than desirable results, and short- or long-term failures. Establishing the possible causes of the unsatisfactory outcome is paramount in the reoperation planning process. Multiple causative factors have been described in the literature[134] and include:

1. Misdiagnosis of the original pathology
2. Patient selection
3. Inappropriate procedure
4. Surgeon's experience
5. Complications
6. Systemic disease
7. Improper postoperative care

When contemplating surgical failure and the necessity for reoperation, the surgeon must take into account all the different variables of the disease process to select the best surgical solution with the highest probability of success.

SUMMARY

Remarkably good success has been reported with several TMJ disc procedures, which differ in their fundamental approach to the problem and their aggressiveness. Open surgical approaches to TMJ disc derangements are now relegated to a tertiary line of care following nonsurgical therapy and arthrocentesis/arthroscopy for most conditions. They do, however, have a clear indication for certain mechanical conditions directly attributed to a disc obstruction.

As we increase our understanding of the pathology, open joint surgical procedures are being performed for specific well-defined conditions. However, the new TMJ surgeon will never quite appreciate the experience that comes with performance of arthrotomy procedures. Arthroscopy developed as a consequence of this experience. Now, as we regress with progress, arthrocentesis with and without steroid injection, a procedure performed by many surgeons, years before the pathology of the joint was even elucidated, has become a mainstay for treatment. This treatment alone has significantly reduced the need to intervene via arthrotomy.

References

1. Dimitroulis G. The role of surgery in the management of disorders of the temporomandibular joint: a critical review of the literature. Part 2. Int J Oral Maxillofac Surg 2005;34: 231–7.

2. Stengenga B. Osteoarthritis of the temporomandibular joint organ and its relationship to disc displacement. J Orofac Pain 2001;15:193–205.

3. Dimitroulis G. The prevalence of osteoarthrosis in cases of advanced internal derangement of the temporomandibular joint: a clinical, surgical and histological study. Int J Oral Maxillofac Surg 2005;34:345–9.

4. Sylvester DC, Exss E, Marholz C, Millas R, Moncada G. Association between disc position and degenerative bone changes of the temporomandibular joints: an imaging study in subjects with TMD. Cranio 2011;29:117–26.

5. Lundh H, Westesson P, Kopp S. A three-year follow-up of patients with reciprocal temporomandibular clicking. Oral Surg Oral Med Oral Pathol Oral Radiol Endod 1985;60:131–6.

6. de Leeuw, Boering G, Stegenga B, de Bont LG. Clinical signs of TMJ osteoarthrosis and internal derangement 30 years after nonsurgical treatment. J Orofac Pain 1994;8:18–24.

7. Stegenga B, de Bont L. TMJ Disc Derangements. In: Laskin D, Greene C, Hylander W, editors. Temporomandibular disorders: an evidence-based approach to diagnosis and treatment. 1st Edition Hanover Park (IL): Quintessence Publishing Co.; 2006. p 125–136.

8. Hamada Y, Kondoh T, Sekiya H, Seto K. Morphologic changes in the unloaded temporomandibular joint after mandibulectomy. J Oral Maxillofac Surg 2003;61:437–41.

9. Westesson PL, Lundh H. Arthrographic and clinical characteristics of patients with disc displacement who progressed to closed lock during a six-month period. Oral Surg Oral Med Oral Pathol Oral Radiol Endod 1989;67:654–7.

10. Ren YF, Isberg A, Westesson PL. Steepness of the articular eminence in the temporomandibular joint: tomographic comparison between asymptomatic volunteers with normal disc position and patients with disc displacement. Oral Surg Oral Med Oral Pathol Oral Radiol Endod 1995;80:258–66.

11. Wänman A, Agerberg G. Temporomandibular joint sounds in adolescents: a longitudinal study. Oral Surg Oral Med Oral Pathol Oral Radiol Endod 1990;69:2–9.

12. Könönen M, Waltimo A, Nyström M. Does clicking in adolescence lead to painful temporomandibular joint locking? Lancet 1996;347:1080–1.

13. Sato S, Goto S, Kawamura H, Motegi K. The natural course of nonreducing disc displacement of the TMJ: relationship of clinical findings at initial visit to outcome after 12 months without treatment. J Orofac Pain 1997;11:315–20.

14. Sato S, Kawamura H, Nagasaka H, Motegi K. The natural course of anterior disc displacement without reduction in the temporomandibular joint: follow-up at 6, 12, and 18 months. J Oral Maxillofac Surg 1997;55:234–9.

15. Kurita K, Westesson PL, Yuasa H, Toyoma M, Machida J, Ogi N. Natural course of untreated symptomatic temporomandibular joint disc displacement without reduction. J Dent Res 1998;77:361–5.

16. Minakuchi H, Kuboki T, Matsuka Y, Maekawa K, Yantani H, Yamasita A. Randomized controlled evaluation of nonsurgical treatments for temporomandibular joint anterior disc displacement without reduction. J Dent Res 2001;80:924–8.

17. Isberg A, Isacsson G, Johansson AS, Larson O. Hyperplastic soft tissue formation in the temporomandibular joint associated with internal derangement. Oral Surg Oral Med Oral Pathol Oral Radiol Endod 1986;61:32–8.

18. Johansson AS, Isberg A. The anterosuperior insertion of the temporomandibular joint capsule and condylar mobility in joints with and without internal derangement: a double-contrast arhtrotomographic investigation. J Oral Maxillofac Surg 1991;49:1142–8.

19. Isberg A, Hágglund M, Paesani D. The effect of age and gender on the onset of symptomatic temporomandibular joint displacement. Oral Surg Oral Med Oral Pathol Oral Radiol Endod 1998;85:252–76.

20. LeResche L. Epidemiology of temporomandibular disorders: implications for the investigation of etiologic factors. Crit Rev Oral Biol Med 1997;8:291–305.

21. Milam SB, Zardeneta G, Schmitz JP. Oxidative stress and degenerative temporomandibular joint disease: a proposed hypothesis. J Oral Maxillofac Surg 1998;56:214–23.

22. Nitzan DW. The process of lubrication impairment and its involvement in temporomandibular joint disc displacement: a theoretical concept. J Oral Maxillofac Surg 2001;59:36–45.

23. Hills BA. Synovial surfactant and the hydrophobic articular surface. J Rheumatol 1996;23:1323–5.

24. Nitzan DW, Nitzan U, Dan P, Yedgar S. The role of hyaluronic acid in protecting surface-active phospholipids from lysis by exogenous phospholipase A_2. Rheumatology (Oxford) 2001;40: 336–40.

25. Milam SB, Schmitz JP. Molecular biology of temporomandibular joint disorders: proposed mechanisms of disease. J Oral Maxillofac Surg 1995; 53:1448–54.

26. Nitzan DW. Arthrocentesis - incentives for using this minimally invasive approach for temporomandibular disorders. Oral Maxillofac Surg Clin North Am 2006;18:311–28.

27. Bradrick J, Indresano A. Failure rates or repetitive temporomandibular joint surgical procedures. J Oral Maxillofac Surg 1992;50(Suppl 3):145.

28. Leidberg J, Westesson PL, Kurita K. Sideways and rotational displacement of the temporomandibular joint disc: diagnosis by arthrography and correlation to cryosectional morphology. Oral Surg Oral Med Oral Pathol Oral Radiol Endod 1990;69: 757–63.

29. Kircos LT, Ortendahl DA, Mark AS, Arakawa M. Magnetic resonance imaging of the TMJ disc in asymptomatic volunteers. J Oral Maxillofac Surg 1987:45:397–401.

SECTION 6

30. Katzberg RW, Westesson PL, Tallents RH, Drake CM. Anatomic disorders of the temporomandibular joint disc in asymptomatic subjects. J Oral Maxillofac Surg. 1996;54:147–53

31. Liedberg J, Panmekiate S, Petersson A, Rohlin M. Evidence-based evaluation of three imaging methods for the temporomandibular disc. Dentomaxillofac Radiol 1996;25:234–41.

32. Iwasaki H, Kubo H, Harada M, Nishitani H. Temporomandibular joint and 3.0T pseudodynamic magnetic resonance imaging. Part 1: evaluation of condylar and disc dysfunction. Dentomaxillofac Radiol. 2010 Dec;39(8):475–85.

33. American Association of Oral and Maxillofacial Surgeons. 1984 criteria for TMJ meniscus surgery. Chicago;1984.

34. American Association of Oral and Maxillofacial Surgeons. Parameters of care: clinical practice guidelines for oral and maxillofacial surgery (AAOMS ParCare07). Chicago; 2007.

35. Kropmans TJ, Dijkstra PU, Stegenga B, de Bont LG. Therapeutic outcome assessment in permanent temporomandibular joint disc displacement. J Oral Rehabil 1999;26:357–63.

36. Holmlund AB. Surgery for TMJ internal derangement. Evaluation of treatment outcome and criteria for success. Int J Oral Maxillofac Surg 1993;22:75–7.

37. Reston JT, Turkelson CM. Meta-analysis of surgical treatments for temporomandibular articular disorders. J Oral Maxillofac Surg 2003;61:3–10

38. Holmlund AB, Axelsson S, Gynther GW. A comparison of discectomy and arthroscopic lysis and lavage for the treatment of chronic closed lock of the temporomandibular joint: a randomized outcome study. J Oral Maxillofac Surg 2001;59:972–7.

39. Hall HD, Indresano AT, Kirk WS, Dietrich MS. Prospective multicenter comparison of 4 temporomandibular joint operations. J Oral Maxillofac Surg 2005;63:1174–9.

40. Ng CH, Lai JB, Victor F, Yeo JF. Temporomandibular articular disorders can be alleviated with surgery. Evid Based Dent 2005;6:48–50.

41. Undt G, Murakami KI, Rasse M, Ewers R. Open versus arthroscopic surgery for internal derangement of the temporomandibular joint: a retrospective study comparing two centres' results using the Jaw Pain and Function Questionnaire. J Craniomaxillofac Surg 2006;34:234–41.

42. Kirk WS, Kirk BS. A biomechanical basis for primary arthroplasty of the temporomandibular joint. Oral Maxillofac Surg Clin North Am 2006;18:345–68.

43. Holmlund A. Disc derangements of the temporomandibular joint. A tissue-based characterization and implications for surgical treatment. Int J Oral Maxillofac Surg 2007;36:571–6.

44. Miloro M, Henriksen B. Discectomy as the primary surgical option for internal derangement of the temporomandibular joint. J Oral Maxillofac Surg 2010;68:782–9.

45. Al-Kayat A, Bramley P. A modified pre-auricular approach to the temporomandibular joint and malar arch. Br J Oral Surg 1979;17:91–103.

46. Miloro M, Redlinger S, Pennington DM, Kolodge T. In situ location of the temporal branch of the facial nerve. J Oral Maxillofac Surg 2007;65:2466–9.

47. Turvey T, Fonseca R. The anatomy of the internal maxillary artery in the pterigopalatal fossa: its relationship to maxillary surgery. J Oral Maxillofac Surg 1980;38:92–5.

48. Blair VP. Operative treatment of ankylosis of the mandible. South Surg Gynecol 1914;26:436–65.

49. Rongetti JR. Meniscectomy—a new approach to the temporomandibular joint. Arch Otolaryngol 1954; 60:566–72.

50. Lempert J. Improvement of hearing in cases of otosclerosis. Arch Otolaryngol 1938; 28:818–23.

51. Alexander RW, James RB. Postauricular approach for surgery of the temporomandibular articulation. J Oral Surg 1985;33: 346–500.

52. Dolwick MF, Kretzschmar DP. Morbidity associated with the preauricular and perimeatal approaches to the temporomandibular joint. J Oral Maxillofac Surg 1982;40:699–700.

53. Eggleston DJ. The perimeatal exposure of the condyle. J Oral Surg 1978;36:369–71.

54. Walters PJ, Geist ET. Correction of TMJ internal derangements by postauricular approach. J Oral Maxillofac Surg 1983;41:616–8.

55. Dolwick MF. Disc preservation surgery for the treatment of internal derangements of the temporomandibular joint. J Oral Maxillofac Surg 2001;59:1047–50.

56. Abramowicz S, Dolwick MF. 20-year follow-up study of disc repositioning surgery for temporomandibular joint internal derangement. J Oral Maxillofac Surg. 2010;68:239–42.

57. Serrano H, Monje F. Técnicas de plicatura discal o discopexia. In: Diagnóstico y tratamiento de la patología de la articulación temporomandibular. 1era Edición. Madrid, Spain: Ripano S.A.;2009. p453–72.

58. Hall MB. Meniscoplasty of the displaced temporomandibular joint meniscus without violating the inferior joint space. J Oral Maxillofac Surg. 1984;42:788–92.

59. Dolwick MF, Sanders B. TMJ internal derangement and arthrosis: surgical atlas. CV Mosby, St. Louis 1985; p321.

60. Wolford LM. Temporomandibular joint devices: treatment factors and outcomes. Oral Surg Oral Med Oral Pathol Oral Radiol Endod. 1997;83:143–9.

61. Saunderson SR, Dolwick MR. Increased hemostasis in temporomandibular joint surgery with the DeBakey clamp. J Oral Maxillofac Surg 1983;91:271–2.

62. Montgomery MT, Gordon SM, Van Sickels JE, Harms SE. Changes in signs and symptoms following temporomandibular joint disc repositioning surgery. J Oral Maxillofac Surg. 1992 Apr;50:320–8.

63. Mehra P, Wolford LM. The Mitek mini anchor for TMJ disc repositioning: surgical technique and results. Int J Oral Maxillofac Surg. 2001;30:497–503.

64. Salmeron JL, Borja A, Llopis P, Verdaguer JJ, Lopez de Atalaya J. Tempomandibular discopexy with Mitek mini anchor. J Craniomaxillofac Surg 1996;24:99.

65. Zhang S, Liu X, Yang X, Yang C, Chen M, Haddad MS, Chen Z. Temporomandibular joint disc repositioning using bone anchors: an immediate postsurgical evaluation by magnetic resonance imaging. BMC Musculoskelet Disord 2010;11:262.

66. Weinberg S, Cousens C. Meniscocondylar plication: a modified operation for surgical repositioning of the ectopic temporomandibular joint meniscus. Oral Surg 1987;63:393–402

67. Walker RV, Kalamchi S. A surgical technique for management of internal derangements of the temporomandibular joint. J Oral Maxillofac Surg 1987; 45:299–305.

68. Vázquez-Delgado E, Valmaseda-Castellón E, Vázquez-Rodríguez E, Gay-Escoda C. Long-term results of functional open surgery for the treatment of internal derangement of the temporomandibular joint. Br J Oral Maxillofac Surg 2004;42: 142–8.

69. Baldwin AJ, Cooper JC. Eminectomy and plication of the posterior disc attachment following arthrotomy for temporoman-

dibular joint internal derangement. J Craniomaxillofac Surg 2004;32:354–9

70. Griffitts TM, Collins CP, Collins PC, Bernie OR. Walker repair of the temporomandibular joint: a retrospective evaluation of 117 patients. J Oral Maxillofac Surg 2007;65:1958–62

71. Isaacson A, Isberg A, Johansson AS, Larson O. Internal derangement of the temporomandibular joint: radiographic and histologic changes associated with severe pain. J Oral Maxillofac Surg 1986;44:771–8.

72. Eriksson L, Westesson PL. Discectomy in the treatment of anterior disc displacement of the temporomandibular joint. A clinical and radiological one-year follow-up study. J Prosthet Dent 1986;55:106–16.

73. Hall HD. Meniscectomy for damaged discs of the temporomandibular joint. South Med J 1985;78:569–72.

74. Agerberg C, Lundberg M. Changes in the temporomandibular joint after surgical treatment. A radiologic follow-up study. Oral Surg 1971;32:865–75.

75. Silver CML. Long-term results of meniscectomy of the temporomandibular joint. J. Craniomandib. Pract. 1984;3:46–9.

76. Eriksson L, Westesson P-L. Long-term evaluation of menisectomy of the temporomandibular joint. J. Oral Maxillofac. Surg. 1985;43:263–6.

77. Tolvanen M, Oikarinen VJ, Wolf J. A 30 year follow-up study of temporomandibular joint menisectomies: a report of 5 patients. Br. J. Oral Maxillofac. Surg. 1988;26:311–3.

78. Takaku S, Toyoda T. Long-term evaluation of discectomy of the temporomandibular joint. J. Oral Maxillofac. Surg. 1994;52:722–6.

79. Bjørnland T, Larheim TA. Discectomy of the temporomandibular joint: 3-year follow-up as a predictor of the 10-year outcome. J Oral Maxillofac Surg. 2003;61:55–60.

80. Takaku S, Sano T, Yoshida M. Long-term magnetic resonance imaging after temporomandibular joint discectomy without replacement. J. Oral Maxillofac. Surg. 2000;58:739–45.

81. McKenna SJ. Discectomy for the treatment of internal derangements of the temporomandibular joint. J. Oral Maxillofac. Surg. 2001;59:1051–6.

82. Kramer A, Lee JJ, Beirne OR. Meta-analysis of TMJ discectomy with or without autogenous/alloplastic interpositional materials: comparative analysis of function outcome. J Oral Maxillofac Surg 2004;62 (suppl):49

83. Westesson PL, Eriksson L, Lindstrom C. Destructive lesions of the mandibular condyle following discectomy with temporary silicone implant. J. Oral Maxillofac. Surg. 1989;47:1290–3.

84. Wagner JD, Mosby EL. Assessment of Proplast-Teflon disc replacements. J. Oral Maxillofac. Surg. 1990;48:1140.

85. Dolwick MF, Aufdemorte TB. Silicone induced foreign body reaction and lymphadenopathy after temporomandibular joint arthroplasty. Oral Surg. Oral Med. Oral Pathol. 1985;59:449–52.

86. Recommendationss for management of patients with temporomandibular joint implants. J Oral Maxillofac Surg 1993;51;1164–72.

87. Eriksson L, Westesson PL. Temporomandibular joint discectomy: no positive effect of temporary silicone implant in a 5-year follow-up. Oral Surg Oral Med Oral Pathol 1992;74:259–72.

88. Fricton JR, Look JO, Schiffman E, Swift J. Long-term study of temporomandibular joint surgery with alloplastic implants compared with nonimplant surgery and nonsurgical rehabilitation for painful temporomandibular joint disc displacement J Oral Maxillofac Surg. 2002 Dec;60:1400–11.

89. Christensen RW. Mandibular joint arthrosis corrected by the insertion of a cast Vitallium glenoid fossa prosthesis: a new technique. Report of a case. Oral Surg Oral Med Pathol 1964;17:712–22.

90. Chase DC, Hudson JW, Gerard DA, Russell R, Chambers K, Curry J, Latta J, Christensen R. The Christensen prosthesis. A retrospective clinical study. Oral Surg Oral Med Oral Pathol Oral Radiol Endod. 1995;80:273–8.

91. McLeod NM, Saeed NR, Hensher R. Internal derangement of the temporomandibular joint treated by discectomy and hemiarthroplasty with a Christensen fossa-eminence prosthesis. Br J Oral Maxillofac Surg. 2001;39:63–6.

92. Park J, Keller EE, Reid KI. Surgical management of advanced degenerative arthritis of temporomandibular joint with metal fossa-eminence hemijoint replacement prosthesis: an 8-year retrospective pilot study. J Oral Maxillofac Surg. 2004;62:320–8.

93. Baltali E, Keller EE. Surgical management of advanced osteoarthritis of the temporomandibular joint with metal fossa-eminence hemijoint replacement: 10-year retrospective study. J Oral Maxillofac Surg. 2008;66:1847–55.

94. MacIntosh RB. The use of autogenous tissues for temporomandibular joint reconstruction. J Oral Maxillofac Surg 2000;58: 63–9.

95. Dimitroulis G. A critical review of interpositional grafts following temporomandibular joint discectomy with an overview of the dermis-fat graft. Int J Oral Maxillofac Surg. 2011;40:561–8.

96. Feinberg SE, Larsen PE. The use of a pedicled temporalis muscle-pericranial flap for replacement of the TMJ disc: preliminary report. J Oral Maxillofac Surg. 1989;47:142–6.

97. Edwards SP, Feinberg SE. The temporalis muscle flap in contemporary oral and maxillofacial surgery. Oral Maxillofac Surg Clin North Am. 2003;15(4):513–35.

98. Umeda H, Kaban LB, Pogrel MA, Stern M. Long-term viability of the temporalis musle/fascia flap used for tempormandibular joint. J Oral Maxillofac Surgery, 1993;51:530–3.

99. Albert T, Merrill R. Temporalis myofascial flap. Oral Maxillofac Surg Clin N Am 1989;1(341–349.

100. Pogrel MA, Kaban LB. The role of a temporalis fascia and muscle flap in temporomandibular joint surgery. J Oral Maxillofac Surg. 1990;48:14–9.

101. Kearns GJ, Perrott DH, Kaban LB. A protocol for the management of failed alloplastic temporomandibular joint disc implants. J Oral Maxillofac Surg. 1995;53:1240–9.

102. Smith JA, Sandler NA, Ozaki WH, Braun TW. Subjective and objective assessment of the temporalis myofascial flap in previously operated temporomandibular joints. J Oral Maxillofac Surg. 1999;57:1065–7.

103. Witsenberg B, Freihofer HP. Replacement of the pathological temporomandibular articular disc using autogenous cartilage of the external ear. Int J Oral Surg 1984;13:401–5.

104. Ioannides C, Freihofer HPM. Replacement of the damaged inter-articular disc of the TMJ. J Craniomandib Pract 1988;16:273–6.

105. Hall HD, Link JL. Discectomy alone and with ear cartilage interposition grafts in joint reconstruction Oral Maxillofac Clin North Am 1989;1:329–40.

106. Matukas VJ, Lachner J. The use of autologous auricular cartilage for temporomandibular joint disc replacement. A preliminary report. J Oral Maxillofac Surg 1990;48:348–353.

107. Svensson B, Wennerblom K, Adell R. Auricular cartilage grafting in arthroplasty of the temporomandibular joint: a retrospective clinical follow-up. Oral Surg Oral Med Oral Pathol Oral Radiol Endod. 2010;109:e1–7.

108. Dimitroulis G, Lee DK, Dolwick MF. Autogenous ear cartilage grafts for treatment of advanced temporomandibular joint disease. Ann Roy Australas Coll Dent Surg 2004;17: 87–92.

109. Sandler NA, MacMillan C, Buckley MJ, Barnes L. Histological and histochemical changes in failed auricular cartilage grafts used for a temporomandibular joint disc replacement. J Oral Maxillofac Surg 1997;55:1014–9.

110. Yih WY, M. Zysset M, R.G. Merrill RG. Histological study of the fate of autogenous auricular cartilage grafts in the human temporomandibular joint. J Oral Maxillofac Surg. 1992;56:964–7.

111. Georgiade N. The surgical correction of temporomandibular joint dysfunction by means of autogenous dermal grafts. Plast Reconstr Surg. 1962;30:68–73.

112. Tucker MR. Dermal graft harvest technique for use in temporomandibular joint disc repair J Oral Maxillofac Surg. 1989;47:1116–21.

113. Meyer RA The autogenous dermal graft in temporomandibular disc surgery. J Oral Maxillofac Surg. 1988;46:948–952.

114. Dimitroulis G, The use of dermis grafts after discectomy for internal derangement of the temporomandibular joint. J Oral Maxillofac Surg. 2005;63:173–8.

115. Steinberg MJ, Hohn FI. Procurement of dermal graft from the suprapubic or inguinal fold region with primary linear closure. J Oral Maxillofac Surg 1994;52:813–6.

116. Dimitroulis G. The use of dermis grafts after discectomy for internal derangement of the temporomandibular joint. J Oral Maxillofac Surg. 2005;63:173–8.

117. Dimitroulis G, Trost N, Morrison W. The radiological fate of dermis-fat grafts in the human temporomandibular joint using magnetic resonance imaging. Int J Oral Maxillofac Surg. 2008;37:249–54.

118. Dimitroulis G, McCullough M, Morrison W. Quality of life survey of patients prior to and following temporomandibular joint discectomy. J Oral Maxillofac Surg. 2010;68:101–6.

119. Dimitroulis G. Condylar morphology after temporomandibular joint discectomy with interpositional abdominal dermis-fat graft. J Oral Maxillofac Surg. 2011;69:439–46.

120. Dimitroulis G. Macroscopic and histological analysis of abdominal dermis-fat graft retrieved from human temporomandibular joints. J Oral Maxillofac Surg. DOI:10.1016/j.joms.2011.01.048.

121. Almarza AJ, Athanasiou KA. Seeding techniques and scaffolding choice for tissue engineering of the temporomandibular joint disc. Tissue Eng 2004:10:1787–91.

122. Allen KD, Athanasiou KA. Tissue engineering of the TMJ disc: a review. Tissue Eng 2006:12:1183–96.

123. Naujoks C, Meyer U, Wiesmann HP, Jäsche-Meyer J, Hohoff A, Depprich R, Handschel Principles of cartilage tissue engineering in TMJ reconstruction. Head Face Med. 2008 Feb 25;4:3.

124. Nickerson JW, Veaco NS. Condylotomy in surgery of the temporomandibular joint. Oral Maxillofacial Surg Clin N Am 1989;1:303–27

125. Hall HD. The condylotomy procedure. Atlas Oral Maxillofac Clin North Am 1996;4:93–106.

126. Hall HD, Navarro EZ, Gibbs SJ. One- and three-year prospective outcome study of modified condylotomy for treatment of reducing disc displacement. J Oral Maxillofac Surg 2000;58:7–17

127. Upton et al. The treatment of temporomandibular joint internal derangements using a modified open condylotomy: a preliminary report. J Oral Maxillofac Surg 1991;49:578–83

128. Werther JR, Hall HD, Gibbs SJ. Disc position before and after modified condylotomy in 80 symptomatic temporomandibular joints. Oral Surg Oral Med Oral Pathol Oral Radiol Endod 1995;79:668–79.

129. Hall HD, Navarro EZ, Gibbs SJ. Prospective study of modified condylotomy for treatment of nonreducing disc displacement. Oral Surg Oral Med Oral Pathol Oral Radiol Endod 2000;89:147–58.

130. McKenna SJ. Modified mandibular condylotomy. Oral Maxillofac Surg Clin North Am 2006;18:369–81.

131. McKenna SJ, Cornella F, Gibbs SJ. Long-term follow-up of modified condylotomy for internal derangement of the temporomandibular joint. Oral Surg Oral Med Oral Pathol Oral Radiol Endod 1996;81:509–15.

132. Aziz SR, Dorfman BJ, Ziccardi VB, Janal M. Accuracy of using the antilingula as a sole determinant of vertical ramusvosteotomy position. J Oral Maxillofac Surg. 2007 May;65:859–62.

133. da Fontoura RA, Vasconcellos HA, Campos AE. Morphologic basis for the intraoral vertical ramus os- teotomy: anatomic and radiographic localization of the mandibular foramen. J Oral Maxillofac Surg 2002;60:660–5

134. Vega LG, Gutta R, Louis P. Reoperative temporomandibular joint surgery. Oral Maxillofac Surg Clin North Am. 2011;23:119–32

135. Austin BD, Shupe SM. The role of physical therapy in recovery after temporomandibular joint surgery. J Oral Maxillofac Surg. 1993 May;51:495–8.

136. Oh DW, Kim KS, Lee GW. The effect of physiotherapy on post-temporomandibular joint surgery patients. J Oral Rehabil. 2002 May;29:441–6.

137. Dolwick F, Armstrong J. Complications of temporomandibular joint surgery. In: Kaban L, Pogrel A, Perrot D, editors. Complications in oral and maxillofacial surgery. 1st edition. Philadelphia: WB Saunders; 1997. p. 89–103.

138. Moreno C, Gonzalez R, Monje F. Complicaciones en cirugía de la articulación temporomandibular. In: Diagnóstico y tratamiento de la patología de la articulación temporomandibular. 1era Edición. Madrid, Spain: Ripano S.A.;2009. p811–825.

139. Peoples JR 3rd, Herbosa EG, Dion J. Management of internal maxillary artery hemorrhage from temporomandibular joint surgery via selective embolization. J Oral Maxillofac Surg. 1988;46:1005–7.

140. Kryshtalskyj B, Weinberg S. An assessment for auriculotemporal syndrome following temporomandibular joint surgery through the preauricular approach. J Oral Maxillofac Surg. 1989;47:3–6.

Hypomobility and Hypermobility Disorders of the Temporomandibular Joint

Meredith August, DMD, MD, Maria J. Troulis, DDS, MSc, and Leonard B. Kaban, DMD, MD

HYPOMOBILITY

Etiology

The etiology of mandibular hypomobility is varied, and successful treatment requires an understanding of the underlying disorder. Trauma is the most commonly identified cause, followed by infection (odontogenic, otitis media, and mastoiditis). Various systemic disease states have been associated with hypomobility, including ankylosing spondylitis, rheumatoid arthritis, and other collagen vascular diseases such as scleroderma. Iatrogenic causes have also been identified and include the sequelae of high-dose radiation involving the muscles of mastication, craniotomy procedures, and uncommonly, orthognathic surgery. Internal temporomandibular joint (TMJ) derangements may also lead to chronic hypomobility problems. Traumatic perinatal events and neuromuscular conditions can result in hypomobility in infancy. In general terms, *congenital ankylosis* is defined as limited interincisal opening noted at birth with no known causative factor. Table 51-1 lists the etiologic factors associated with mandibular hypomobility.

Classification

Various classification schemes have been proposed to describe hypomobility.[1–3]

Trismus is most commonly found in conjunction with spasm of the muscles of mastication. It can be secondary to myofascial pain dysfunction, infection, trauma, tumors, and various medications as well as psychiatric and neurologic factors. Ankylosis may be classified according to location (intra-articular vs. extra-articular), type of tissue involved (bony, fibrous, or mixed), and extent of fusion (complete vs. incomplete). True ankylosis is caused by either fibrous or bony fusion of the structures contained within the TMJ capsule and, in its most severe state, is characterized by a bony union of the condyle to the glenoid fossa. True ankylosis has been further classified into subtypes depending on the anatomic positioning of the condyle and the extent of bridging bone. Topazian[4] proposed a three-stage classification to grade complete ankylosis as follows: stage I, ankylotic bone limited to the condylar process; stage II, ankylotic bone extending to the sigmoid notch; and stage III, ankylotic bone extending to the coronoid process. Other classification schemes have also been proposed.[5] However, the utility of these designations in terms of treatment planning is questionable. So-called false ankylosis (pseudoankylosis), in contrast, describes limited mobility based on extra-articular factors such as fibrosis, mechanical obstruction (e.g., zygomatic arch fracture), muscle spasm, or other pathologies.

Clinical Presentation

Patients with fibrous or bony ankylosis present with restricted mandibular motion and, depending on the patient's age and the condition's etiology, may have an abnormality in mandibular size and shape. Unilateral pathology in children may result in significant problems with lower facial symmetry. A shortened ramus on the affected side is usually accompanied

TABLE 51-1. **Etiologic Factors Associated with Hypomobility of the Mandible**

Trismus
Odontogenic: myofascial pain, malocclusion, erupting teeth
Infection: pterygomandibular, lateral pharyngeal, temporal
Trauma: fracture of the mandible, muscle contusion
Tumors: nasopharyngeal tumors, tumors that invade jaw muscles
Psychologic: hysteric trismus
Pharmacologic: phenothiazines
Neurologic: tetanus

Pseudoankylosis
Depressed zygomatic arch fracture
Fracture dislocation of the condyle
Adhesions of the coronoid process
Hypertrophy of the coronoid process
Fibrosis of the temporalis muscle
Myositis ossificans
Scar contracture after thermal injury
Tumor of the condyle or coronoid process

True Ankylosis
Trauma: intracapsular fracture (child), medial displaced condylar fracture (adult), obstetric trauma, intracapsular fibrosis
Infection: otitis media, suppurative arthritis
Inflammation: rheumatoid arthritis, Still's disease, ankylosing spondylitis, Marie-Strümpell disease, psoriatic arthritis
Surgical: postoperative complications of temporomandibular joint or orthognathic surgery

by a prominent antegonial notch noted on radiographs. Such unilateral mandibular growth disturbances have secondary effects on the maxillary occlusal plane and midfacial structures (pyriform rims and bony orbits).

Ankylosis in adults is characterized by limited jaw opening and decreased translation, but the morphologic characteristics found in the growing patient are frequently absent. Loss of condylar structure and mandibular angle prominence is seen in cases caused by rheumatologic disease, specifically scleroderma. An associated anterior open bite is frequently noted with the loss of ramus/condyle height (Figure 51-1).

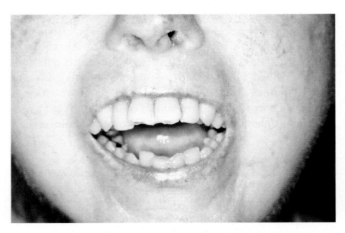

FIGURE 51-1. Patient with systemic sclerosis (scleroderma) demonstrating a limitation in jaw opening and skin changes characterized by perioral furrows and telangiectasia.

Unilateral cases with a traumatic etiology may result in malocclusion and ipsilateral dental prematurities. A physical examination is helpful in identifying whether the process is bilateral or unilateral and may be suggestive of the etiology.

Imaging Assessment

In addition to the clinical examination, radiographic assessment is critical in evaluating and treating patients with hypomobility disorders. Plain radiographs are limited in delineating the true extent of the deformity. What can be identified with these studies are the presence or absence of a TMJ space, obvious bony abnormalities in the region of the joint, and coronoid hyperplasia. Sanders and colleagues[6] have reported that conventional radiographs underestimate the extent of bony ankylosis and give little information about the anatomy medial to the condyle. The use of computed tomography (CT) scans (including axial, coronal, and sagittal views with three-dimensional reconstruction) is helpful in fully defining the extent of ankylosis as well as the relationship of the ankylotic mass to important anatomic structures, especially at the skull base (pterygoid plates, carotid canal, jugular foramen, and foramen spinosum) (Figure 51-2).[7,8] Often in post-traumatic cases. the distance between the maxillary artery and the medial pole of the condyle is reduced—a contrast CT helps to determine this distance. Fusion of the ankylotic mass to the base of the skull can also be appreciated on CT scans. Because adequate treatment requires the removal of the mass in toto, knowledge of this anatomy preoperatively is critical to surgical planning and long-term success.

Magnetic resonance imaging (MRI) has had a great impact on TMJ evaluation, especially regarding the delineation of meniscal position. Diagnosis of fibrous ankylosis is possible with the use of MRI, but the CT scan is superior in demonstrating bony pathology.[9]

Post-traumatic Hypomobility

Trauma is the most common cause of bony and fibrous ankylosis as reported by multiple authors.[10–12] It is hypothesized that the formation of an intra-articular hematoma with subsequent scarring and new bone formation is the common precipitant. Most often, a medially displaced fracture dislocation of the condyle is found. Subsequent hypomobility is of particular concern in growing children in whom the development of hypomobility can have significant impact on facial growth (Figure 51-3). In addition, resultant hypomobility can lead to speech impairment, difficulty with chewing, poor oral hygiene, limited access to dental care, and possible airway compromise. In large reviews of pediatric facial fractures, the condylar and subcondylar regions were involved in more than 40% of cases.[13,14] In many cases, a direct blow to the chin with transmission of the impact force to the condyles resulted in the fracture. Prolonged immobilization, secondary to treatment with maxillomandibular fixation, splinting, or mechanical obstruction, can lead to subsequent ankylosis.

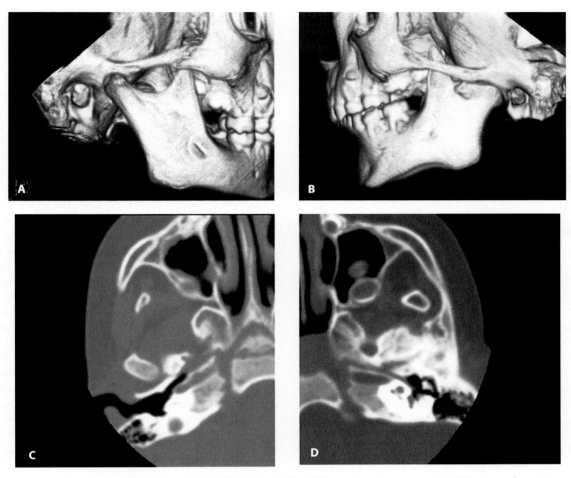

FIGURE 51-2. Three-dimensional (**A** and **B**) and axial (**C** and **D**) computed tomography (CT) scans of a patient with extensive bony ankylosis of the left temporomandibular joint. **A** and **C,** Note the comparison with the unaffected right side. **B** and **D,** Coronoid hyperplasia is also seen on the affected left side.

Extra-articular ankylosis can also occur with coronoid fractures and fractures of the zygomatic arch. In both cases, the resultant hematoma may calcify, resulting in a fusion of the coronoid process to the zygomatic arch.

Myositis ossificans traumatica (MOT), or fibrodysplasia ossificans circumscripta, is generally associated with a traumatic event or repeated episodes of minor trauma and can result in mandibular hypomobility.[15,16] The precise mechanism remains to be elucidated but appears to involve fibrous metaplasia and subsequent ossification of both soft tissues and muscle after bleeding and myonecrosis. Histologically, both mature and woven bone can be noted (sometimes in distinct zones), and both osteoblasts and osteocytes are abundant. MOT is characterized by soft tissue ectopic ossifications and is relatively uncommon in the head and neck regions. Of all reported cases involving the muscles of mastication, the masseter is most commonly affected. MOT involving the medial pterygoid muscle and secondary to local anesthesia injections has also been reported.[17] Diagnosis is confirmed by identification of calcifications within the muscles of mastication on CT scans (Figure 51-4). Minimal response is found with physical therapy and stretching exercises; consequently, surgical treatment is often undertaken to remove the ectopic bone. Other treatment modalities include acetic acid iontophoresis, magnesium therapy, and the use of etidronate sodium.[18,19] Because repeated relapses and refractory cases are common, the use of multiple treatment modalities may be associated with the best outcome.

Postinfectious Hypomobility

A TMJ infection resulting in hypomobility is most commonly the result of contiguous spread from an odontogenic infection, otitis media, or mastoiditis.[20,21] In the era of aggressive antibiotic treatment of infection, such reported cases are now relatively uncommon. Hematogenous spread of infection has also been reported in association with disease states such as tuberculosis, gonorrhea, and scarlet fever.

Various case series describe deep fascial space infections manifesting themselves as hypomobility and often being misdiagnosed at initial presentation.[22,23] Odontogenic infection is commonly associated with trismus. In such cases, associated symptoms (fever, dysphagia) are likely present, and CT scanning is invaluable in determining a diagnosis and

SECTION 6

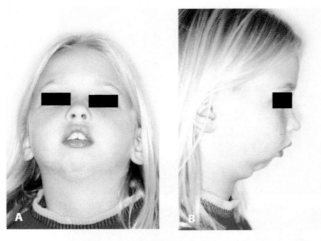

FIGURE 51-3.   **A** and **B,** Evident mandibular growth disturbance is noted in this child who has had bilateral condylar fractures. Note the submental scar secondary to a laceration sustained at the time of the bony injury.

in treatment planning. Medial pterygoid abscess formation or fibrosis secondary to hematoma organization can be precipitated by an inferior alveolar nerve block or posterior superior alveolar block. A history of recent dental treatment should suggest this possibility; the use of CT imaging can help delineate the anatomy of the masticator and pharyngeal spaces.

Mass lesions (both benign and malignant) can also result in mandibular hypomobility. Squamous cell carcinoma of the tongue base or tonsillar pillar is often accompanied by trismus. Masses involving the mandibular condyle invariably

affect range of motion and need to be included in the differential diagnosis of hypomobility.

Hypomobility after Radiation Therapy

Mandibular hypomobility is a common sequela of the treatment of head and neck malignancies (Figure 51-5). The resultant fibromyositis caused by radiation therapy may exacerbate the postsurgical problems caused by large ablative procedures.[24] Goldstein and coworkers[25] reviewed the effects of tumoricidal radiation therapy on restricted mandibular opening and found a linear dose-related effect. Mandibular dysfunction increased as the dose to the pterygoid muscles increased. The authors reported diminution in opening with doses as low as 15 Gy. Pow and associates reported that 30% of patients treated for nasopharyngeal carcinoma with high-dose radiation therapy had significant trismus compared with age-matched nonradiated control subjects.[26] Radiation therapy for primary tumors of the retromolar trigone was associated with a 12% incidence of long-term trismus. This association, compounded by resultant xerostomia, severely compromises the ability of these patients to maintain oral health.

The efficacy of early interventional physical therapy has been described. Buchbinder and colleagues[27] compared the outcome of unassisted exercise, mechanically assisted exercise with the use of tongue blades, and use of the Therabite System in radiated patients. All patients presented with an interincisal opening of less than 30 mm. The response to each therapy was recorded every 2 weeks over a 10-week period.

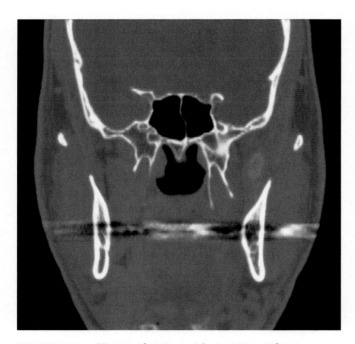

FIGURE 51-4.   CT scan of patient with myositis ossificans traumatica demonstrates a focus of calcification within the medial pterygoid muscle on the left side.

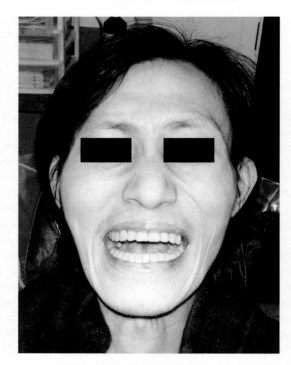

FIGURE 51-5.   Patient with a history of high-dose radiation therapy and subsequent reirradiation for recurrence of nasopharyngeal carcinoma. Note the severe temporal atrophy and the limitation in opening.

All groups showed improvement over the first 4 weeks, but the group using a mechanical exercising device (i.e., Therabite System) continued to demonstrate an improvement of maximal interincisal opening (MIO) over the full 10-week period that was significantly greater than that of the other two groups.

Postcraniotomy Hypomobility

Mandibular hypomobility after intracranial surgical procedures is an uncommon yet reported phenomenon.[28,29] Mechanistically, this problem is secondary to neurosurgical procedures performed through the temporal bone requiring an incision of the temporalis muscle. Subsequent fibrosis of the muscle may then result in limited opening, which is best treated with coronoid resection followed by vigorous physical therapy. The incidence of this problem is not known, but a review by Kawaguchi and coworkers[30] reported limited mouth opening in as many as 33% of patients undergoing frontotemporal craniotomy procedures. Although most are self-limiting, persistent hypomobility can severely compromise subsequent airway and anesthesia management in these patients and needs to be recognized. The maximal opening is not improved with the use of muscle relaxants or local or general anesthesia. Patients who have undergone skull base surgery may also manifest severe hypomobility postoperatively. If such surgery requires the dissection of the temporalis muscle inferior to the zygoma, pseudoankylosis of the mandible may be encountered.

Inflammatory and Rheumatologic Causes

Ankylosing spondylitis (Bekhterev's disease) is a chronic and progressive inflammatory condition most commonly affecting the sacroiliac joints and the spine. The male-to-female ratio of incidence is reported to be 2.4:1, and the severity and extension of the disease in male patients is found to be more severe. TMJ involvement in ankylosing spondylitis has been reported in between 1% and 22% of affected individuals and can include severe bony deformation and ankylosis.[31,32] The most commonly reported radiographic findings in the condyle and glenoid fossa region include flattening, erosions, sclerosis, osteophytes, subcortical cysts, and bony erosion at the insertion of the masseter (angle of the jaw) and temporalis muscles (coronoid process). One large prospective study evaluating 50 patients with ankylosing spondylitis did not show any correlation between the bony severity noted in the cervical spine and TMJ abnormalities.[33] These authors reported a 22% incidence of TMJ involvement, either clinical or radiographic. Because the majority of patients reported no pain or limitation in function, the radiographic findings included in this study may well have represented early changes in the disease process.

TMJ involvement in rheumatoid arthritis follows the same destructive path as do other joints. Generally, the severity of

joint dysfunction is correlated with the stage of rheumatoid arthritis. Radiographically, the most common findings in the condylar region are sclerosis (75%), erosion (50%), and flattening (30%).[34] These bony changes commonly result in progressive malocclusion secondary to the loss of ramus/condyle height and subsequent apertognathia. Juvenile rheumatoid arthritis is chronic arthritis diagnosed in childhood before the age of 16 years. It is estimated that greater than 60% of patients with juvenile rheumatoid arthritis manifest TMJ involvement.[35] However, multiple authors point out that despite radiographic and morphologic changes in the joint, a minority of affected children (generally < 25%) report pain with function.[36,37] Svensson and associates[38] report that restricted mouth opening was a more common finding. The duration of active disease and a history of pain with function correlate positively with progressive TMJ dysfunction. With active disease in growing children, abnormalities in facial growth, mandibular hypoplasia, and hypomobility are common problems (Figure 51-6).

Scleroderma (progressive systemic sclerosis) is a disorder of unknown etiology affecting multiple organ systems and characterized by abundant fibrosis of the skin, blood vessels, and visceral organs. It is believed that abnormalities in small blood vessels result in the progressive thickening and fibrotic changes noted in affected tissues, particularly those of the gastrointestinal tract, heart, lung, and kidney as well as diffuse skin involvement. Mandibular movement can become severely limited in affected individuals secondary to facial

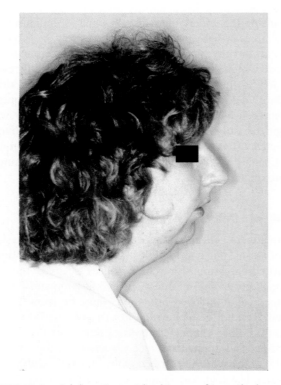

FIGURE 51-6. Adult patient with a history of juvenile rheumatoid arthritis affecting the temporomandibular joints and resulting in a mandibular growth disturbance and hypomobility.

skin fibrosis and atrophy of the muscles of mastication (particularly the masseter and medial pterygoid muscles).[39] Bony changes in the mandible are also reported and include severe resorption of the angles, condyles, and coronoid processes (osteolysis).[40] The bony lesions are believed to be of ischemic origin but may be exacerbated by the tightness of the tissue in the region of the mandibular angles causing pressure resorption as well. In addition to the severe limitation in jaw movement, the small mouth orifice and progressive malocclusion make oral function and access to dental care problematic for these patients.

Hypomobility after Orthognathic Surgery

Hypomobility after orthognathic surgery has been reported by multiple authors and appears to be most commonly associated with the bilateral sagittal split osteotomy.[41,42] This postoperative limited opening has been commonly attributed to muscle atrophy and soft tissue scar formation. Atrophic muscular changes seem to be exacerbated by prolonged use of maxillomandibular fixation, and the advent of rigid internal fixation appears to have limited this problem. Intra-articular pathology (edema, hemorrhage) as well as condylar torque may also result in hypomobility. In such cases, rigid internal fixation may predispose to this problem. Van Sickels and colleagues[43] have hypothesized that condylar torque at the time of the bilateral sagittal split osteotomy may cause impingement of the condyle against the disk, causing a mechanical impediment to opening.

Management of hypomobility after orthognathic surgery depends on the underlying cause. Trauma to the muscles of mastication is best managed postoperatively by vigorous physical therapy protocols. Those patients who fail to improve within the first 3 months need to be carefully evaluated for an intra-articular source of the problem. Edema, bleeding, and fibrosis within the joint space can frequently be managed by arthrocentesis procedures, especially when recognized early. If a mechanical obstruction to opening is suspected, CT is a helpful diagnostic aid. Condylar torque is best treated by reoperation with appropriate positioning of the proximal segment.[44]

General Treatment Considerations

The treatment goal for all hypomobility states is the restoration of normal and comfortable jaw motion and prevention of disease progression. Reversible causes such as muscular hyperactivity or spasm, infectious and inflammatory causes, and medication-induced limitations must be identified and treated. Restoration of function in cases of ankylosis can be difficult. Proper treatment requires excision of the involved structures and immediate reconstruction. Many operative techniques have been described in the literature, with varying and often less than satisfactory results. As mentioned previously, understanding the etiology and anatomy of the problem is critical and can be greatly aided with CT.

The gap arthroplasty is a procedure that creates a new area of articulation distal to the fused TMJ and ankylotic segment.[45,46] Advocates of this procedure describe its simplicity. However, the creation of a pseudoarticulation significantly shortens the ramus height, and the procedure is associated with a high degree of reported reankylosis. Development of postoperative malocclusion and a decreased range of motion are the most common problems associated with this procedure as reported by Rajgopal and coworkers.[47] Because of these limitations, the use of the gap arthroplasty to treat ankylosis has been largely abandoned.

TMJ ankylosis is more commonly treated with complete excision of the ankylotic mass and, if required, by subsequent joint reconstruction. Our protocol for the treatment of ankylosis follows that documented by Kaban and associates,[48] a sequential protocol for the treatment of TMJ ankylosis that is based on aggressive resection of the ankylotic mass. Wide intraoperative exposure is required, and special attention is directed to the medial aspect of the joint to ensure that bony, fibrous, and granulation tissue are completely removed. In addition to this aggressive resection of the bony and fibrous mass, dissection and stripping of the temporalis, masseter, and medial pterygoid muscles followed by ipsilateral coronoidectomy are performed in all cases through the same incision. Longstanding ankylosis frequently results in muscle fibrosis and coronoid hyperplasia. After this resection is completed, the MIO is measured. If it is found to be less than 35 mm, a contralateral coronoidectomy is performed via an intraoral approach to attain the desired level of opening. Because complete resection of the ankylotic mass frequently results in substantial loss of ramus height, subsequent reconstruction must address this fact and attempt to restore occlusion as well as function. Commonly, a temporalis fascia flap and costochondral graft are employed to both line the glenoid fossa and create ramus height. The patient is placed into maxillomandibular fixation after the reconstruction, and the teeth are placed into a prefabricated occlusal splint. Fixation is maintained for approximately 10 days, and after release, a strict protocol of physiotherapy is employed. Overall results have been excellent with this approach. After 1 year, MIO was maintained at greater than 35 mm in all 18 patients included in the report. Furthermore, absence of pain with function was reported in all but 2 patients (Figure 51-7).[48]

Recently, the Kaban protocol[49] has been modified to substitute ramus/condyle reconstruction using distraction osteogenesis, when possible, instead of costochondral grafting. This protocol has the major advantage of eliminating the donor site operation and allowing for immediate vigorous TMJ mobilization. The surgical procedure for the release of the ankylosis is identical to that described previously. After the release, the jaw is mobilized and the glenoid fossa lined with a temporalis myofascial flap if the native disk is unavailable. The remaining mandibular stump is reshaped to create a narrow and rounded top. A corticotomy is created distally, leaving sufficient bone to serve as a transport disk. The distraction device is secured, the corticotomy completed, and

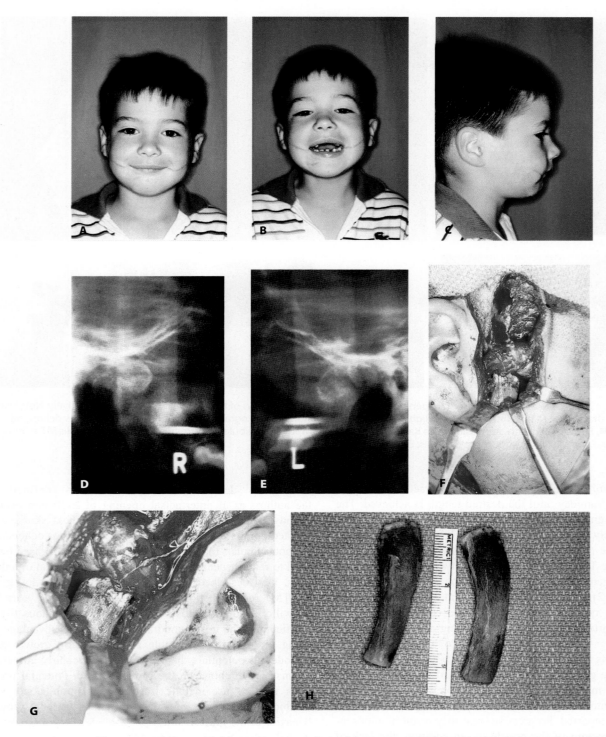

FIGURE 51-7. Three-year-old boy with bilateral bony ankylosis after a motor vehicle accident that also produced bilateral lacerations of the commissures. Frontal photograph **(A)**, frontal maximal incisal opening (MIO; **B)**, and lateral photograph **(C)**. Note the limited opening. Right **(D)** and left **(E)** panoramic views of the ankylotic masses of the temporomandibular joints (TMJs). Right **(F)** and left **(G)** TMJs exposed after the dissection was completed. **H**, Harvested costochondral grafts with 1- to 2-mm cartilaginous caps. *(continued)*

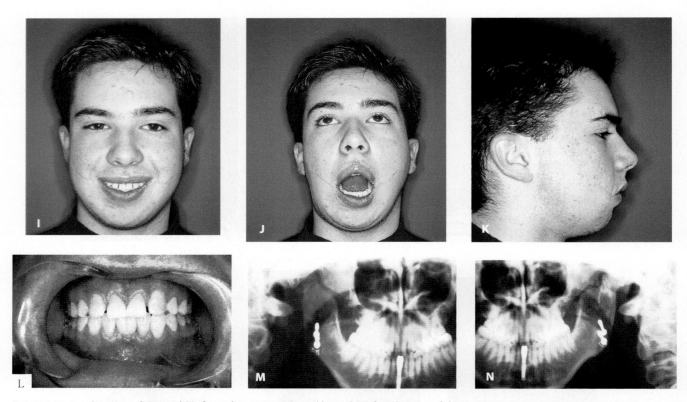

FIGURE 51-7. *(continued)* Frontal **(I)**, frontal opening **(J)**, and lateral **(K)** facial views of the patient 11 years postoperatively. Note maintenance of the normal MIO. **L,** Intraoral views. Right **(M)** and left **(N)** panoramic radiographs show remodeling of the costochondral grafts. (**A–M,** Reproduced with permission from Kaban LB. Acquired temporomandibular deformities. In Kaban LB, Troulis MJ, editors. Pediatric Oral and Maxillofacial Surgery. St. Louis: Elsevier; 2004; pp. 361–365.)

the mobility of the segments tested. Distraction then proceeds at 1 mm/day until the desired length is achieved. The patient begins a program of active jaw motion exercises immediately postoperatively (Figure 51-8).

The use of total joint prostheses has an interesting history in the TMJ. Advocates describe two major advantages over autogenous reconstruction: (1) the absence of a donor site and (2) the ability of the patient to return to function more quickly. However, multiple complications have been reported—some with devastating consequences for patients.[50–52] Foreign body reaction to any alloplast may occur. In its most severe form, extensive bony erosion in the area of the glenoid fossa has been found. Fragmentation of alloplastic material secondary to function with a migration of particles into contiguous tissue and regional lymph nodes has also been reported. Progressive wear may result in a loosening and fracture of the prosthesis. In addition, the lack of growth potential precludes the use of these joint replacement systems in young children. Recurrent ankylosis after prosthesis placement has also been reported, with periprosthetic calcifications most commonly seen in younger patients.

TMJ reconstruction with a variety of autogenous tissues has been described. When the extent of bony resection does not severely shorten ramus height, autogenous interpositional grafts may be employed. These include skin, temporal muscle, cartilage, and fascia. A review by Chossegros and

colleagues[53] demonstrated superior results (defined by the authors as an interincisal opening of ≥ 30 mm over a follow-up period of 3 yr) using full-thickness skin grafts and temporalis muscle. Various bone grafts (costochondral, sternoclavicular, iliac crest, and metatarsal head) have been used to reconstruct ramus height after the resection of ankylosis. First described in the 1920s, the costochondral graft for TMJ reconstruction was popularized in later years by Poswillo[54] and MacIntosh and Henny.[55] Autogenous tissue (particularly the costochondral graft) has the advantage of being biologically acceptable and possessing growth and remodeling potentials that make it a particularly attractive reconstructive choice in the growing child. Potential problems with its use include fracture, resorption, donor site morbidity, recurrence of ankylosis, and a variable growth behavior of the graft in situ.

Complications Associated with Treatment

Various complications have been reported secondary to the treatment of ankylosis. Dolwick and Armstrong[56] caution that a severe limitation of opening can make the palpation of landmarks difficult and increases the surgical risks. The aggressive bony removal and recontouring that is often required can increase the risk of development of an aural-TMJ fistula if the tympanic plate is displaced posteriorly. In

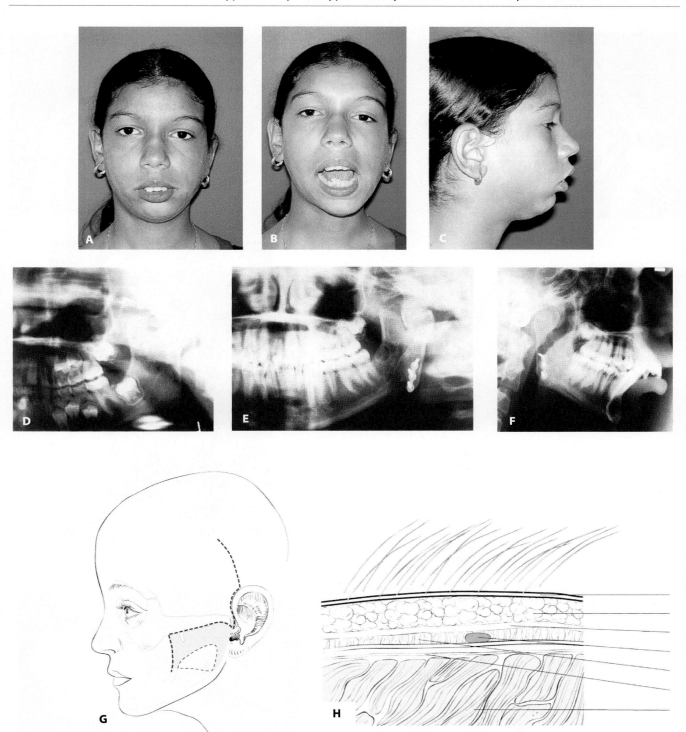

FIGURE 51-8. Thirteen-year-old female with recurrent ankylosis of the left TMJ secondary to trauma sustained in a motor vehicle accident. Frontal **(A),** frontal at MIO **(B),** and lateral facial **(C)** photographs of a teenage female with recurrent ankylosis of the left TMJ. **D,** Panoramic radiograph before the first operation demonstrates bony ankylosis of the left TMJ. **E,** Panoramic radiograph after the patient developed reankylosis. She had had a condylectomy and coronoidotomy at another institution. The TMJ was reconstructed with a costochondral graft. There was no soft tissue lining in the joint. **F,** Lateral cephalogram documents the mandibular retrognathism. **G,** Diagram of the operative plan; the ankylosis release is carried out via a preauricular incision (outlined in *dashed blue line*). Excision of the ankylotic mass and coronoidectomy is shown by the *shaded area*. **H,** Diagram of the layers of the scalp. *(continued)*

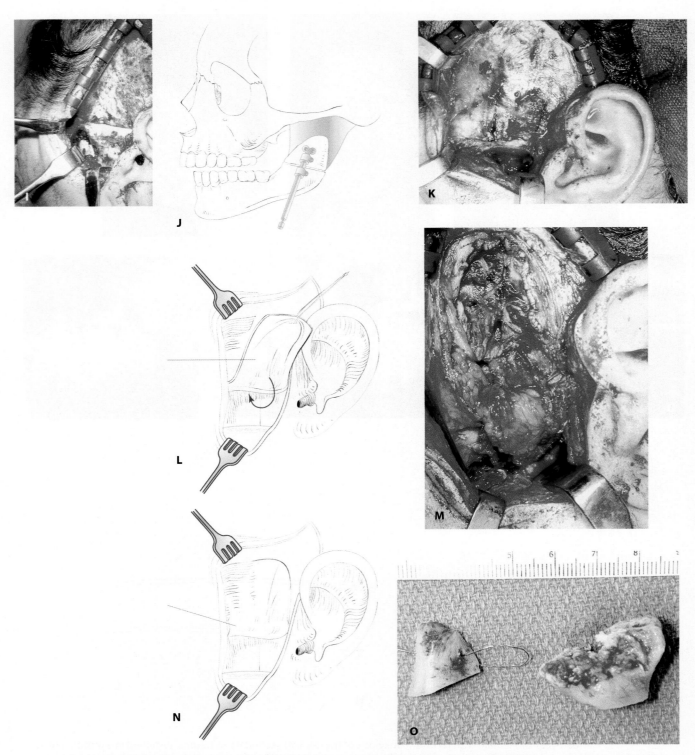

FIGURE 51-8. *(continued)* **I,** Intraoperative view after dissection was completed. Note the bony ankylotic mass and the coronoid process with obliteration of the sigmoid notch. **J,** Diagram of the bone removed *(shaded area)* and the proposed reconstruction using a distraction device (Synthes Maxillofacial, Paoli, PA) instead of a costochondral graft. **K,** Temporalis flap is outlined with malachite green. The flap is dissected and rotated over the arch **(L)** and sutured in place **(M** and **N). O,** Specimen: ankylotic mass and coronoid process. *(continued)*

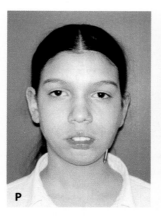
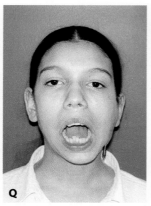
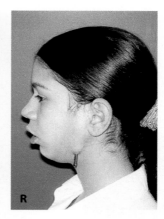
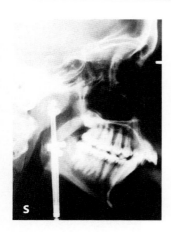

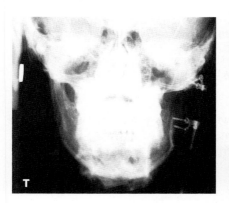
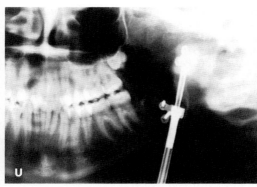
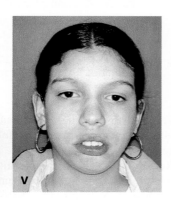

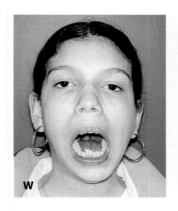
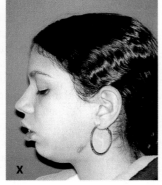
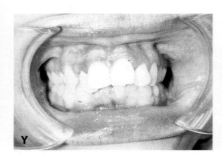
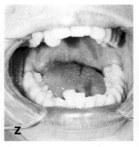

FIGURE 51-8. *(continued)* Frontal **(P),** frontal opening **(Q),** and lateral **(R)** photographs at end distraction. The patient was mobilized and started on physical therapy immediately postoperatively. She was comfortable because there was no donor site operation and no period of maxillomandibular fixation. Lateral **(S)** and anteroposterior (AP; **T)** designated as cephalogram and panoramic radiograph **(U)** at the end of distraction osteogenesis demonstrate the lengthened mandibular ramus. Frontal **(V),** frontal opening **(W),** and lateral **(X)** photographs 1 year after completion of treatment. The patient maintained her TMJ motion and will be beginning presurgical ortho-dontic treatment to correct her preexisting malocclusion. Open **(Y)** and closed **(Z)** intraoral views with the patient opening 39 mm at 1 year. *(continued)*

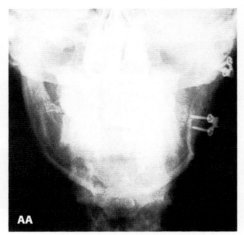
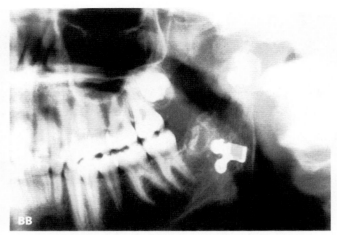

FIGURE 51-8. *(continued)* AP cephalogram **(AA)** and panoramic radiograph **(BB)** at 1 year. The ramus lengthening is demonstrated by the space between the retained footplates. (**A–F, I, K, M,** and **O–BB,** Reproduced with permission from Kaban LB. Acquired temporomandibular deformities. In Kaban LB, Troulis MJ, editors. Pediatric Oral and Maxillofacial Surgery. St. Louis: Elsevier; 2004; pp. 354–357; **G, H, J, L,** and **N,** adapted from Kaban LB. Acquired temporomandibular deformities. In Kaban LB, Troulis MJ, editors. Pediatric Oral and Maxillofacial Surgery. St. Louis: Elsevier; 2004; pp. 354–357.)

addition, stenosis of the external auditory meatus and subsequent hearing impairment may follow tympanic plate displacement.

Recurrent ankylosis may result from inadequate initial treatment. It most commonly occurs on the medial aspect of the condyle where surgical access is most difficult. Such maneuvers as the postoperative use of nonsteroidal anti-inflammatory drugs and vigorous physical therapy limit problems with recurrent hypomobility.[57,58]

In pediatric patients treated for ankylosis, the expected outcome may be less sanguine.[59] The improvement in interincisal opening, despite strict adherence to the previoously discussed treatment protocol and compliance with physical therapy regimens, is often significantly less than 35 mm. Posnik and Goldstein[60] reviewed the outcome of nine children and demonstrated a mean MIO of 24.8 mm in unilateral cases and 17.5 mm in bilateral cases measured an average of 2 years postoperatively. The authors caution that improvement in bilateral congenital cases is particularly problematic and may be confounded by the associated neuromuscular and atrophic changes found in these patients.

Peripheral nerve injuries are possible sequelae of all TMJ operations, with the upper branches of the facial nerve being the most vulnerable. Parotid gland injury with subsequent sialocele and fistula formation has also been reported.

As previously described, the costochondral graft is the most commonly used autogenous material for TMJ reconstruction. However, its growth pattern can be unpredictable. Linear overgrowth with the subsequent development of asymmetry and malocclusion has been reported by multiple authors.[61,62] The frequency is more common in the growing patient. Munro and coworkers[61] reported 2 of 22 cases of considerable linear overgrowth with resultant chin deviation and development of a class III malocclusion. Perrott and associates[62] reported 3 of 26 cases of lateral bony overgrowth

(tumor-like overgrowth), with an evident preauricular fullness and subsequent limitation of opening. However, no cases of linear overgrowth were found in that series of patients.

Postoperative Physical Therapy

Patients with hypomobility disorders require aggressive physical therapy programs, often in conjunction with surgical treatment, to maintain a functional MIO. Various rehabilitation programs have been described in the literature, and approaches include unassisted exercise, tongueblade and finger-stretch exercises, manual exercisers, and mechanically assisted mandibular motion devices (Figure 51-9). Manipulation under general anesthesia may also be required in refractory or recurrent cases. Most authors agree that the duration of physical therapy should be prolonged well after a desired MIO is achieved to prevent subsequent relapse.[63]

HYPERMOBILITY

Classification

Mandibular subluxation occurs when there is a momentary inability to close the mouth from a maximally open position. It is defined as a self-reducing partial dislocation of the TMJ, during which the condyle passes anterior to the articular eminence. In distinction, dislocation may be considered a long-lasting inability to close the mouth. Subluxation of the condyle may be an early feature of TMJ pathology in a subset of patients. It is often associated with an abnormally wide opening while eating or yawning. Extended periods of mouth opening (e.g., during dental treatment or endotracheal anesthesia) may also precipitate subluxation. Subluxation

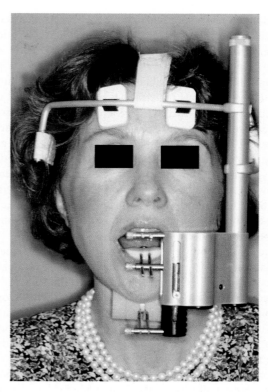

FIGURE 51-9.   A continuous passive motion device used in the postoperative management of hypomobility.

may occur secondary to acute trauma or after a seizure and is also associated with systemic diseases such as Ehlers-Danlos syndrome and Parkinson's disease.

Etiology

TMJ dislocation is defined as an internal derangement characterized by a condylar position anterior and superior to the articular eminence that is not self-reducing. Recurrent dislocation is a relatively unusual problem. Much like subluxation, the etiology is varied. It is observed most frequently in patients with neurologic and connective tissue disorders, those with TMJ dysfunction, and those being treated with phenothiazines and other neuroleptic agents (Table 51-2).

Extrinsic trauma, especially that sustained while the mouth is open, may result in dislocation. Wide opening of any type as well as capsular laxity may be etiologic. Muscular problems secondary to medication use or neurologic disorders may be associated. The problem may be unilateral or bilateral, and patients generally present with associated muscle spasm and pain.

Treatment Considerations

In the absence of pain, subluxation requires no specific treatment because it is self-reduced by the patient. When associated with wide mouth opening, conscious efforts to avoid this are usually successful at preventing recurrent subluxation. Patients are advised to modify their diets, and

TABLE 51-2. **Causes of Hypermobility**

Intrinsic Trauma: Overextension Iinjury
Yawning
Vomiting
Wide biting
Seizure disorder

Extrinsic Trauma
Trauma: flexion-extension injury to the mandible, intubation with general anesthesia, endoscopy, dental extractions, forceful hyperextension

Connective Tissue Disorders
Hypermobility syndromes, Ehlers-Danlos syndrome, Marfan syndrome

Miscellaneous Causes
Internal derangement, dyssynchronous muscle function, contralateral intra-articular obstruction, lost vertical dimension, occlusal discrepancies

Psychogenic
Habitual dislocation, tardive dyskinesia

Drug-Induced
Phenothiazines

dental treatment is done over multiple shorter appointments. The use of bite blocks during procedures can also be helpful. In cases in which extreme laxity in the joint results in continued problems, surgical intervention may be warranted.

Reduction of mandibular dislocation should be done precipitously before muscle spasm becomes severe and makes the procedure more difficult. Reduction is accomplished by pressing the mandible downward and then backward to relocate the condyle within the glenoid fossa (Figure 51-10).

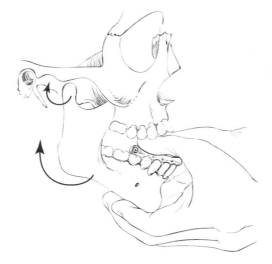

FIGURE 51-10.   Bimanual mandibular manipulation in a downward-posterior direction to disengage the condyle from its open-locked position posterior to the articular eminence. (Adapted from Rotskoff KS. Management of hypomobility and hypermobility disorders of the temporomandibular joint. In Peterson LJ, Indresano AT, Marciani RD, Roser SM, editors. Principles of Oral and Maxillofacial Surgery. Vol 3. Philadelphia: JB Lippincott; 1992; p. 2009.)

SECTION 6

In acute cases, this can generally be accomplished without the use of anesthesia. In cases of prolonged or chronic dislocation, the use of muscle relaxants and analgesics may be required. If reduction cannot be thus achieved, general anesthesia may be required. After reduction, the mandible should be immobilized for several days to allow for capsular repair, muscle rest, and prevention of recurrence.[64,65]

Chronic dislocation usually requires a more interventional approach. The use of various sclerosing agents has been described in the past. However, caustic agents can result in progressive damage to other joint structures, and multiple reports of misapplications and complications have resulted in the abandonment of this technique. Surgical treatments of various types are reported. Identification of etiology is important when considering surgical correction. In cases of extreme joint laxity, mechanical tightening may be indicated. Plication procedures involve fastening the condyle to a fixed structure to maintain its position within the glenoid fossa. Certain authors advocate the creation of a mechanical impediment to translation by altering the conformation of the articular eminence. Procedures targeting a decrease in muscle pull can also be effective.

Plication procedures are aimed at limiting mandibular motion and may be accomplished in various ways. Removal of redundant capsular tissue (Figure 51-11) is a relatively simple method for addressing laxity, and a review by Mac-Farlane[66] reported excellent long-term results. Plication of the condyle to the temporal bone and of the coronoid process to the zygomatic arch have also been described. Multiple materials have been used for plication procedures, including both resorbable and nonresorbable sutures and wire. Mini-plates and surgical anchors have also been used in both the lateral pole of the condyle and the posterior roof of the zygomatic arch. Wolford and colleagues[67] have described the

threading of heavy suture material between the eyelets of the surgical anchors, thereby preventing condylar dislocation.

Mechanical impediments to condylar translation effectively deepen the glenoid fossa. Bone and cartilage grafts (cranial, iliac crest, rib, tibial) have been used for this purpose. Nonautogenous material has also been onlayed to the articular eminence. In 1943, LeClerc and Girald[68] described a procedure for inferior displacement of the zygomatic arch to prevent translation (Figure 51-12). Access was gained through an extended preauricular incision, and dissection of the zygomatic arch was performed. An oblique osteotomy downward and forward then allowed the arch to be moved inferiorly. Chossegros and colleagues[53] reported excellent success using this technique in 36 patients with chronic and recurrent dislocation.

The eminectomy procedure was first introduced by Myrhaug in 1951[69] as a treatment for chronic and habitual dislocation of the condyle. In addition to the standard open eminectomy, reports describing the use of the arthroscope for this purpose have more recently appeared in the literature.[70] Both procedures involve the removal of a portion of the articular tubercle and eminence to allow the condyle to move freely.

Concerns regarding the use of the eminectomy procedure include hypermobility of the joint with further damage to contiguous tissues; significant and often bothersome TMJ noise (clicking and crepitation) with function; and the potential for facial nerve injury, recurrent dislocation, and inadvertent temporal lobe exposure (anatomic variant).[71]

Reported success rates of surgery to treat dislocation vary considerably. Recurrent dislocation after standard eminectomy procedures ranges from 7% to 33%.[72-74] Patients with significant ligamentous laxity or predisposing conditions (e.g., seizure disorders) are prone to recurrent problems.

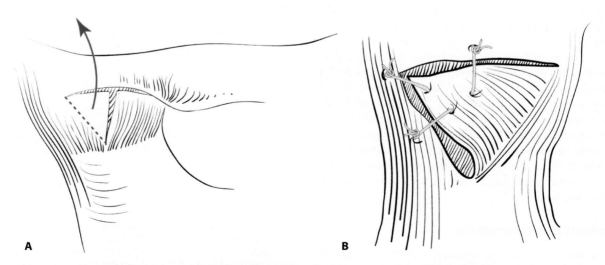

A   **B**

FIGURE 51-11. Capsular plication. The exposed lateral capsule is incised (**A**) and sutured back on itself (**B**) to tighten and limit capsular laxity. (**A** and **B,** Adapted from Rotskoff KS. Management of hypomobility and hypermobility disorders of the temporomandibular joint. In Peterson LJ, Indresano AT, Marciani RD, Roser SM, editors. Principles of Oral and Maxillofacial Surgery. Vol 3. Philadelphia: JB Lippincott; 1992; p. 2010.)

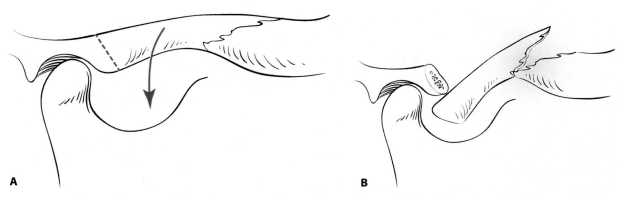

A

B

FIGURE 51-12. LeClerc procedure. **A,** An oblique cut using a fissure bur is created anterior to the articular eminence to decrease the frequency of condylar dislocation by obstructing the path of condylar movement. **B,** The osteotomized segments of the articular eminence are made to overlap one another. (**A** and **B,** Adapted from Rotskoff KS. Management of hypomobility and hypermobility disorders of the temporomandibular joint. In Peterson LJ, Indresano AT, Marciani RD, Roser SM, editors. Principles of Oral and Maxillofacial Surgery. Vol 3. Philadelphia: JB Lippincott; 1992; p. 2010.)

Arthroscopic eminectomy, owing to technical limitations, prevents the complete removal of the medial aspect of the eminence. The consequence of this in terms of recurrence remains to be elucidated.[72,73]

If muscular hyperactivity is associated with chronic recurrent dislocation, removal of the insertion of the lateral pterygoid muscle (lateral pterygoid myotomy) may be an effective treatment. Bowman has reported good success with this procedure,[74] but subsequent animal studies have shown lateral pterygoid electromyographic activity returning to baseline several months after the procedure.[75] However, the long-term efficacy often attributed to this procedure may be secondary to scarring anterior to the joint capsule, thereby limiting condylar excursion.[76]

The injection of botulinum toxin type A into the lateral pterygoid muscles has also been proposed as a treatment for chronic and recurrent dislocation of the mandible. Ziegler and coworkers[77] reviewed 21 patients treated in this fashion. Injections were given on a 3-month basis with only 2 of 21 patients suffering further dislocations. No adverse side effects were reported in this series. Botulinum toxin type A has an associated latency of 1 week, and its duration of action is between 2 and 3 months. Injections should not be done more often than every 12 weeks to avoid the development of antibodies. An injection dose of between 10 and 50 U into the targeted muscle is usually sufficient.

Clark[78] reviewed the use of botulinum toxin for the treatment of mandibular motor disorders, as well as for the treatment of facial spasm, and expanded on the potential side effects of such treatment. Although local side effects are unusual, the two most common problems encountered were alterations in salivary consistency and an inadvertent weakness of swallowing, speech, and facial muscles. These complications were more commonly reported with lateral pterygoid, soft palate, and tongue injections and were found to be dose-dependent.

SUMMARY

This chapter summarizes the spectrum of mobility problems that can affect the TMJ and contiguous structures. The varied etiologic factors associated with hypo- and hypermobility have been reviewed; an understanding of the etiology in each particular case is imperative for appropriate treatment to be rendered. Fortunately, improved imaging techniques, including three-dimensional CT, can be invaluable adjuncts to the history and physical examination. In cases of ankylosis, the extent and nature of the problem is best appreciated with these CT images. Altered anatomy and the extent of bony bridging can be assessed preoperatively. In addition to operative intervention, long-term success in the management of ankylosis requires aggressive physical therapy programs and longitudinal follow-up.

Hypermobility (both subluxation and dislocation) is similarly reviewed. Again, understanding the causative factors (ligamentous laxity, shallow eminentia, muscular hyperactivity) helps one to focus the treatment planning and to minimize problems with recurrence.

References

1. Aggarwal S, Mukhopakhyay S, Berry M, Bhargava S. Bony ankylosis of the temporomandibular joint: a computed tomographic study. Oral Surg Oral Med Oral Pathol 1990;69:128–132.
2. Chandra P, Dave PK. Temporomandibular joint ankylosis. Prog Clin Biol Res 1985;187:449–458.
3. El-Mofty S. Ankylosis of the temporomandibular joint. Oral Surg Oral Med Oral Pathol 1972;33:650–660.
4. Topazian RG. Etiology of ankylosis of the temporomandibular joint: analysis of 44 cases. J Oral Surg 1964;22:227–233.
5. Adekeye EO. Ankylosis of the mandible: analysis of 76 cases. J Oral Maxillofac Surg 1983;41:442–449.
6. Sanders R, MacEwan CJ, McCulloch AS. The value of skull radiography in ophthalmology. Acta Radiol 1994;35:429–433.

SECTION 6

7. El-Hakim IE, Metwalli SA. Imaging of temporomandibular joint ankylosis. A new radiographic classification. Dentomaxillofac Radiol 2002;31:19–23.

8. de Bont LG, van der Kuijl B, Stegenga B, et al. Computed tomography in the differential diagnosis of temporomandibular joint disorders. Int J Oral Maxillofac Surg 1993;22:200–209.

9. Roberts D, Schenck J, Joseph P. Temporomandibular joint: magnetic resonance imaging. Radiology 1985;154:829–830.

10. Chidzonga MM. Temporomandibular joint ankylosis: review of thirty-two cases. Br J Oral Maxillofac Surg 1999;37:123–126.

11. de Burgh JE. Post-traumatic disorders of the jaw joint. Ann R Coll Surg Engl 1982;64:29–36.

12. Guralnick WC, Kaban LB. Surgical treatment of mandibular hypomobility. J Oral Surg 1976;34:343–348.

13. Marianowski R, Martins CC, Potard G, et al. Mandibular fractures in children—long-term results. Int J Pediatr Otorhinolaryngol 2003;67:25–30.

14. Zachariades N, Papavassiliou D, Koumoura F. Fractures of the facial skeleton in children. J Craniomaxillofac Surg 1990;18: 151–153.

15. Aoki T, Naito H, Ota Y, Shiiki K. Myositis ossificans traumatica of the masticatory muscles: review of the literature and report of a case. J Oral Maxillofac Surg 2002;60:1083–1088.

16. Parkash H, Goyal M. Myositis ossificans of the medial pterygoid muscle. A cause for temporomandibular joint ankylosis. Oral Surg Oral Med Oral Pathol 1992;73:27–28.

17. Luchetti W, Cohen RB, Hahr GV, et al. Severe restriction in jaw movement after routine injection of local anesthetic in patients who have fibrodysplasia ossificans progressiva. Oral Surg Oral Med Oral Pathol Oral Radiol Endod 1996;81:21–25.

18. Wieder DL. Treatment of myositis ossificans with acetic acid iontophoresis. Phys Ther 1992;72:133–137.

19. Steidl L, Ditmar R. Treatment of soft tissue calcifications with magnesium. Acta Univ Palacki Olomuc Fac Med 1991;130:273–287.

20. Faerber TH, Ennis RL, Allen GA. Temporomandibular joint ankylosis following mastoiditis: report of a case. J Oral Maxillofac Surg 1990;48:866–870.

21. Hadlock TA, Ferraro NF, Rahbar R. Acute mastoiditis with temporomandibular joint effusion. Otolaryngol Head Neck Surg 2001;125:111–112.

22. Cohen SG, Quinn PD. Facial trismus and myofascial pain associated with infectious and malignant disease. Oral Surg Oral Med Oral Pathol 1988;65:538–544.

23. Leighty SM, Spach DH, Myall RW, Burns JL. Septic arthritis of the temporomandibular joint: review of the literature and report of two cases in children. Int J Oral Maxillofac Surg 1993;22:292–297.

24. Huang CJ, Chao KS, Tsai J, et al. Cancer of the retromolar trigone: long-term radiation therapy outcome. Head Neck 2001;23:758–763.

25. Goldstein M, Maxymiw WG, Cummings BJ, Wood RE. The effects of antitumor irradiation on mandibular opening and mobility: a prospective study of 58 patients. Oral Surg Oral Med Oral Pathol Oral Radiol Endod 1999;88:365–373.

26. Pow EH, McMillan AS, Leung WK, et al. Oral health condition in southern Chinese after radiotherapy for nasopharyngeal carcinoma: extent and nature of the problem. Oral Dis 2003;9:196–202.

27. Buchbinder D, Currivan RB, Kaplan AJ, Urken ML. Mobilization regimens for the prevention of jaw hypomobility in the radiated patient: a comparison of three techniques. J Oral Maxillofac Surg 1993;51:863–867.

28. Hollins RR, Moyer DJ, Tu HK. Pseudoankylosis of the mandible after temporal bone attached craniotomy. Neurosurgery 1988; 22:137–139.

29. Nitzan DW, Azaz B, Constantini S. Severe limitation in mouth opening following transtemporal neurosurgical procedures: diagnosis, treatment, and prevention. J Neurosurg 1992;76: 623–625.

30. Kawaguchi M, Sakamoto T, Furuya H, et al. Pseudoankylosis of the mandible after supratentorial craniotomy. Anesth Analg 1996;83:731–734.

31. Resnick D. Temporomandibular joint involvement in ankylosing spondylitis. Radiology 1974;112:587–591.

32. Ramos-Remus C, Major P, Gomez-Vargas A, et al. Temporomandibular joint osseous morphology in a consecutive sample of ankylosing spondylitis patients. Ann Rheum Dis 1997;56:103–107.

33. Locher MC, Felder M, Sailer HF. Involvement of the temporomandibular joints in ankylosing spondylitis (Bechterew's disease). J Craniomaxillofac Surg 1996;24:205–213.

34. Voog U, Alstergren P, Eliasson S, et al. Inflammatory mediators and radiographic changes in temporomandibular joints of patients with rheumatoid arthritis. Acta Odontol Scand 2003;61:57–64.

35. Bakke M, Zak M, Jensen BL, et al. Orofacial pain, jaw function and temporomandibular disorders in women with a history of juvenile chronic arthritis or persistent juvenile chronic arthritis. Oral Surg Oral Med Oral Pathol Oral Radiol Endod 2001;92:406–414.

36. Larheim TA, Hoyeraal HM, Stabrun AE, Haanaes HR. The temporomandibular joint in juvenile rheumatoid arthritis. Radiographic changes related to clinical and laboratory parameters in 100 children. Scand J Rheumatol 1982;11:5–12.

37. Olson L, Eckerdal O, Hallonsten AL, et al. Craniomandibular function in juvenile chronic arthritis. A clinical and radiographic study. Swed Dent J 1991;15:71–83.

38. Svensson B, Larsson A, Adell R. The mandibular condyle in the juvenile chronic arthritis patients with mandibular hypoplasia. Int J Oral Maxillofac Surg 2001;30:300–305.

39. Seifert MH, Steigerwald JC, Cliff MM. Bone resorption of the mandible in progressive systemic sclerosis. Arthritis Rheum 1975;18:507–512.

40. Haers PE, Sailer HF. Mandibular resorption due to systemic sclerosis. Case report of surgical correction of a secondary open bite deformity. Int J Oral Maxillofac Surg 1995;24:261–267.

41. Hori M, Okaue M, Hasegawa M, et al. Worsening of pre-existing TMJ dysfunction following sagittal split osteotomy: a study of three cases. J Oral Sci 1999;41:133–139.

42. Feinerman DM, Piecuch JF. Long-term effects of orthognathic surgery on the temporomandibular joint. Comparison of rigid and nonrigid methods. Int J Oral Maxillofac Surg 1995;24:268–272.

43. Van Sickels JE, Tiner BD, Alder ME. Condylar torque as a possible cause of hypomobility after sagittal split osteotomy: report of three cases. J Oral Maxillofac Surg 1997;55: 398–402.

44. Sanders B, Kaminishi R, Buoncristiani R, Davis C. Arthroscopic surgery for treatment of temporomandibular joint hypomobility after mandibular sagittal osteotomy. Oral Surg Oral Med Oral Pathol 1990;69:539–541.

45. Roychoudhury A, Parkash H, Trikha A. Functional restoration by gap arthroplasty in temporomandibular joint ankylosis: a report of 50 cases. Oral Surg Oral Med Oral Pathol Oral Radiol Endod 1999;87:166–169.

46. Sawhney CP. Bony ankylosis of the temporomandibular joint: follow-up of 70 patients treated with arthroplasty and acrylic spacer interposition. Plast Reconstr Surg 1986;77:29–40.

47. Rajgopal A, Banerji PK, Batura V, Sural A. Temporomandibular ankylosis. A report of 15 cases. J Oral Maxillofac Surg 1983;11:37–41.

48. Kaban LB, Perrott DH, Fisher K. A protocol for management of temporomandibular joint ankylosis. J Oral Maxillofac Surg 1990; 48:1145–151.

49. Kaban LB. Acquired temporomandibular deformities. In Kaban LB, Troulis MJ, editors. Pediatric Oral and Maxillofacial Surgery. St. Louis: Elsevier; 2004; pp. 353–355.

50. Mercuri LG. The use of alloplastic protheses for temporomandibular joint reconstruction. J Oral Maxillofac Surg 2000;58:70–75.

51. Kent JN, Misiek DJ. Controversies in disc and condyle replacement for partial and total temporomandibular joint reconstruction. In Worthington P, Evans JR, editors. Controversies in Oral and Maxillofacial Surgery. Philadelphia: WB Saunders; 1994; pp. 397–435.

52. Henry CH, Wolford LM. Treatment outcomes for temporomandibular joint reconstruction after Proplast-Teflon implant failure. J Oral Maxillofac Surg 1993;51:352–358.

53. Chossegros C, Guyot L, Cheynet F, et al. Comparison of different materials for interposition arthroplasty in treatment of temporomandibular joint ankylosis surgery: long-term follow-up in 25 cases. Br J Oral Maxillofac Surg 1997;35:157–160.

54. Poswillo DE. Biological temporomandibular joint reconstruction. Annu Meet Am Inst Oral Biol 1975;3:72–82.

55. MacIntosh RB, Henny FA. A spectrum of applications of autogenous costochondral grafts. J Maxillofac Surg 1977;5:257–267.

56. Dolwick MF, Armstrong JW. Complications of temporomandibular joint surgery. In Kaban LB, Pogrel MA, Perrott DH, editors. Complications in Oral and Maxillofacial Surgery. Philadelphia: WB Saunders; 1997; pp. 89–103.

57. Topazian RG. Comparison of gap and interpositional arthroplasty in the treatment of TMJ ankylosis. J Oral Surg 1966;24:405–409.

58. Padgett GC, Robinson DW, Stephenson KL. Ankylosis of the temporomandibular joint. Surgery 1948;24:426–432.

59. Oji C. Fractures of the facial skeleton in children: a survey of patients under the age of 11 years. J Craniomaxillofac Surg 1998;26:322–325.

60. Posnick JC, Goldstein JA. Surgical management of temporomandibular joint ankylosis in the pediatric population. Plast Reconstr Surg 1993;91:791–798.

61. Munro IR, Phillips JH, Griffin G. Growth after construction of the temporomandibular joint in children with hemifacial microsomia. Cleft Palate J 1989;26:303–311.

62. Perrott DH, Umeda H, Kaban LB. Costochondral graft construction/reconstruction of the ramus/condyle unit: long-term follow-up. Int J Oral Maxillofac Surg 1994;23:321–328.

63. Friedman MH, Weisberg J, Weber FL. Postsurgical temporomandibular joint hypomobility. Rehabilitation technique. Oral Surg Oral Med Oral Pathol 1993;75:24–28.

64. Caminiti MF, Weinberg S. Chronic mandibular dislocation: the role of non-surgical and surgical treatment. J Can Dent Assoc 1998;64:484–491.

65. Hoard MA, Tadje JP, Gampper TJ, Edlich RF. Traumatic chronic TMJ dislocation: report of an unusual case and discussion of management. J Craniomaxillofac Trauma 1998;4:44–47.

66. MacFarlane WI. Recurrent dislocation of the mandible: treatment of seven cases by a simple surgical method. Br J Oral Surg 1977;14:227–229.

67. Wolford LM, Pitta MC, Mehra P. Mitek anchors for treatment of chronic mandibular dislocation. Oral Surg Oral Med Oral Pathol Oral Radiol Endod 2001;92:495–498.

68. LeClerc G, Girald G. Un nouveau procede de butee dans le traitment chirurgical de la luxation recidivante de la manchoire inferieure. Mem Acad Chir (Paris) 1943;69:457–459.

69. Myrhaug H. A new method of operation for habitual dislocation of the mandible—review of former methods of treatment. Acta Odontol Scand 1951;9:247–261.

70. Sato J, Segami N, Nishimura M, et al. Clinical evaluation of arthroscopic eminoplasty for habitual dislocation of the temporomandibular joint: comparative study with conventional open eminectomy. Oral Surg Oral Med Oral Pathol Oral Radiol Endod 2003;95:390–395.

71. Undt G, Kermer C, Rasse M. Treatment of recurrent mandibular dislocation, part II: eminectomy. Int J Oral Maxillofac Surg 1997;26:98–102.

72. Westwood RM, Fox GL, Tilson HB. Eminectomy for the treatment of recurrent temporomandibular joint dislocation. J Oral Surg 1975;33:774–779.

73. Courtemanche AD, Son-Hing QR. Eminectomy for chronic recurring subluxation of the temporomandibular joint. Ann Plast Surg 1979;3:22–25.

74. Miller GA, Murphy EJ. External pterygoid myotomy for recurrent mandibular dislocation. Review of the literature and report of a case. Oral Surg Oral Med Oral Pathol 1976;42:705–716.

75. Burke RH, McNamara JA Jr. Electromyography after lateral pterygoid myotomy in monkeys. J Oral Surg 1979;37:630–636.

76. Sindet-Pedersen S. Intraoral myotomy of the lateral pterygoid muscle for treatment of recurrent dislocation of the mandibular condyle. J Oral Maxillofac Surg 1988;46:445–449.

77. Ziegler CM, Haag C, Muhling J. Treatment of recurrent temporomandibular joint dislocation with intramuscular botulinum toxin injection. Clin Oral Investig 2003;7:52–55.

78. Clark GT. The management of oromandibular motor disorders and facial spasms with injections of botulinum toxin. Phys Med Rehabil Clin North Am 2003;14:727–748.

SECTION 6

End-Stage Temporomandibular Joint Disease

Louis G. Mercuri, DDS, MS

INTRODUCTION

End-stage disease represents the worst condition or disease state of an organ system, at which point in time, the organ is functioning minimally or not at all. Systemic examples include end-stage renal disease, in which the kidneys have essentially shut down and the patient requires dialysis or renal transplantation in order to accomplish the essential roles of the kidney; and end-stage cardiac disease, in which the heart is functioning very poorly with minimal cardiac output and a compromised ejection fraction, and may need mechanical support (e.g., left ventricular assist device) or cardiac transplantation in order for the patient to survive, considering the vital role of the cardiovascular system. When applying the term *end-stage* to the functional joints of the human body, *end-stage joint disease* indicates a joint that is so negatively affected architecturally by disease or injury that severe functional impairment is the final result for the patient. As with all other joints in the body, the temporomandibular joint (TMJ) is affected by any and all of the end-stage joint diseases (Table 52-1). These disease processes may result from developmental disorders (Figure 52-1), neoplasia (Figure 52-2), trauma, arthritic disease (Figures 52-3 and 52-4), failed prior joint surgery (Figure 52-5), or fibrous or bony ankylosis (Figure 52-6). Regardless of the etiology of the end-stage disorder, it should be noted that the goals of any reconstructive joint surgery include improvement of mandibular function and form; reduction of further suffering and disability; containment of excessive treatment and cost; and prevention of further morbidity (Table 52-2).[1]

Reconstruction of the TMJ presents many unique problems as opposed to other joints because of the integral and complex roles this specific joint plays in establishing and maintaining proper form and function within the stomatog-

TABLE 52-1. Indications for Total Joint Replacement

Developmental Disorders
Condylar agenesis
Condylar hyperplasia
Condylar hypoplasia

Neoplasia
Benign
Osteoma
Chondroma
Osteochondroma
Malignant
Osteosarcoma
Chondrosarcoma

Arthritic Disease
High inflammatory
Low inflammatory

Trauma
Fracture
Intracapsular
Extracapsular
Multiple Prior Surgical Procedures

Ankylosis
Fibrous ankylosis
Bony ankylosis

nathic and upper respiratory and digestive systems. The TMJ not only provides a secondary growth center for the mandible in the prepubertal phases but also is of primary importance to the functions of mastication, speech, airway support, and deglutition in both child and adulthood. At present, there are three accepted management modalities available to

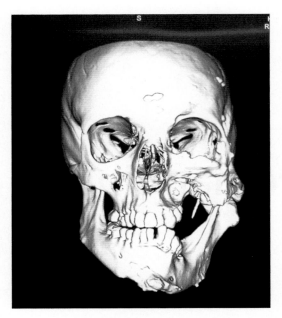

FIGURE 52-1.   Developmental anomaly (cystic hygroma treated in a child with left facial anomalies with temporomandibular joint [TMJ] ankylosis). (Courtesy of Michael Bowler, Newcastle, New South Wales, Australia.)

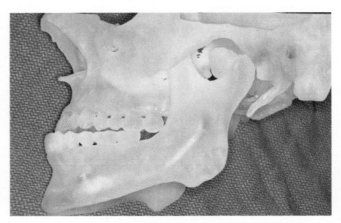

FIGURE 52-2.   Pathology stereolithography (SLA model) with osteoma of the left condyle.

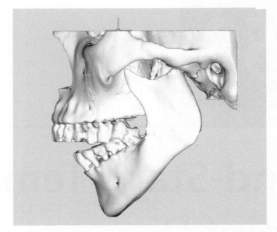

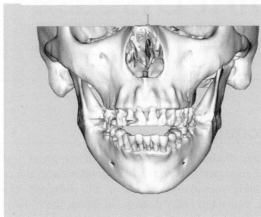

FIGURE 52-3.   High inflammatory arthritic disease (rheumatoid arthritis).

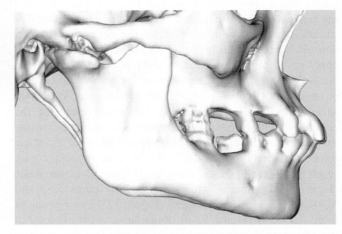

FIGURE 52-4.   Low inflammatory arthritic disease (degenerative joint disease, osteoarthritis) with flattening of the condylar head, loss of joint space, and osteophyte formation.

reconstructive TMJ surgeons for total temporomandibular joint reconstruction (TJR) including autogenous bone grafting, alloplastic replacement, and transport distraction osteogenesis techniques. Bioengineered TMJ devices are currently being investigated and may provide a viable option for the future. This chapter addresses the management of end-stage TMJ disease considering all four of these treatment modalities, presents an evidence-based literature review for each, and provides a suggested algorithm based on those reviews from which the reconstructive surgeon may determine which alternative provides the most appropriate management option as a TMJ salvage procedure in order to provide acceptable facial form and joint function in each individual clinical case scenario.

AUTOGENOUS BONE GRAFTING

Classically, end-stage TMJ disorders have been managed with the use of autogenous bone and soft tissue grafting (Tables 52-3 and 52-4). The costochondral graft has been the

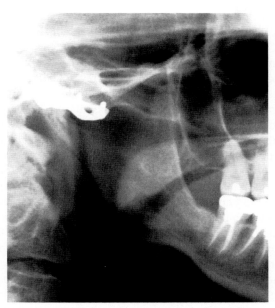

FIGURE 52-5.   Progressive loss of condylar architecture after placement of a fossa-eminence device in a patient with degenerative joint disease.

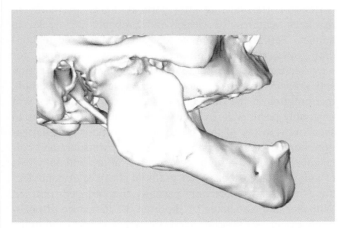

FIGURE 52-6.   Ankylosis after trauma and failed gap arthroplasty with a temporalis myofascial flap.

TABLE 52-2. **Goals of Temporomandibular Joint Reconstruction**

Improvement in mandibular function and form
Reduction of further suffering and disability
Containment of excessive treatment and cost
Prevention of further patient morbidity

most frequently recommended autogenous bone for the reconstruction of the TMJ owing to its ease of adaptation to the recipient site, its gross anatomic similarity to the mandibular condyle, the reported low morbidity rate at the donor site, and its "growth potential"[2-7] (Figure 52-7). In theory, costochondral autogenous grafting will "grow with the patient"; however, often this so-called growth potential has

TABLE 52-3. **Autogenous Bone Grafting Total Joint Replacement Options**

Costochondral (rib) graft
Sternoclavicular joint
Calvarium
Iliac crest
Fibula
Second, fourth, or fifth metatarsophalangeal joint

TABLE 52-4. **History of Autogenous Total Joint Replacement**

1860—Temporalis flap (Verneuil)
1914—Autogenous fat (Murphy)
1953—Sternoclavicular joint (Steinhardt)
1957—Dermis (Georgiade)
1967—Metatarsophalangeal joint (Glahn)
1973—Auricular cartilage (Perko)
1975—Fascia lata (Narang)
1981—Costochondral graft (Ware & Brown)

been shown to be unpredictable or may result in ankylosis due to graft and/or fixation failure; or the poor results may be related to the expected noncompliance of the young patient with essential postreconstruction physical therapy.[2,8-21] Several studies have questioned the necessity for using a cartilaginous graft to restore and maintain mandibular growth.[22,23] Long-term reports of mandibular growth in children whose TMJs were reconstructed with costochondral grafts revealed that excessive growth on the treated side occurred in 54% of the 72 cases examined, and equal growth with the opposite side occurred in only 38% of the cases.[20,24-28] Further, Peltomäki and coworkers,[29-31] in an investigation of mandibular growth after costochondral grafting, supported previous

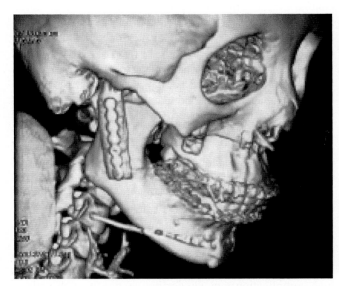

FIGURE 52-7.   Costochondral graft fixated to the right mandible with a bone plate and screws.

experiments with regards to the inability of the graft to adapt to the growth velocity of the new environment. Cole and colleagues[32] recommend the use of a composite costochondral–iliac crest technique to resolve the issue of the flexibility of growing patient ribs. They states that "although graft instability and resorption seems to affect adults much more frequently, we believe the limited, sometimes overly malleable costochondral material harvested in pediatric cases leads to an unacceptably high rate of failure." The authors conclude, "in the adult population where costochondral grafts for the TMJ are decidedly unpredictable, this modification may also be advantageous." Peltomäki and coworkers[29] studied the growth of the mandible in the marmoset animal model after costochondral grafting with emphasis on the required amount of cartilage to be included in the graft. These investigators found that depending on the amount of cartilage in the unilateral costochondral graft, the mandible is shifted toward the unoperated side. This occurs during the entire period of growth, which indicated to them a strong hormonal influence. These authors concluded that these results supported previous experiments with regard to adaptability[2,3,30,31] in that costochondral grafts do not seem to adapt to the growth velocity of the new environment. Poswillo[3] had reported this adaptability in young monkeys; however, the animals used in his experiments had essentially ceased their craniofacial growth. Ellis and associates[22] compared the use of sternoclavicular grafts with costochondral grafts in the monkey and concluded that these grafts behaved similarly with regard to growth/overgrowth, suggesting that in growing individuals, maintenance of biomechanical architecture and reasonably normal function may be more important than the nature of the autogenous graft used for condylar replacement. Further, these investigators recommended retaining as little cartilage as possible to prevent overgrowth when replacing the mandibular condyle with a costochondral graft in growing individuals. Although contour overgrowth with deviation of the chin to the contralateral side was reported as a significant aesthetic problem, Perrott and coworkers[25] state that they documented contour overgrowth of the articulating surface of only "a small group" of growing and nongrowing patients. Despite the fact that these patients did not develop malocclusions, they developed decreased mandibular range of motion, as has been reported by other investigators.[20,21] MacIntosh[7] states that the chief disadvantages of costochondral grafting are their unpredictable growth, particularly in childhood and adolescent application, and the potential for reankylosis when used to treat cases of ankylosis. Saeed and Kent[33] retrospectively reviewed 76 costochondral grafts (57 patients) after a mean of 53 months (range 24–161 mo). They reported that in patients with no previous TMJ surgery, "arthritic disease" or congenital deformity, the costochondral graft performed well. However, they concluded that a preoperative diagnosis of ankylosis was associated with a high complication rate, suggesting caution in such patients using the autogenous costochondral graft.

With increasing patient age, adult ribs become mainly cortical bone and, therefore, contain very little cancellous bone. Consequently, when transplanted to the mandible, ribs are free grafts that rely on the ability of the local tissues to provide the optimal conditions for revascularization and, ultimately, the graft's survival and function. As with any bone grafting technique, it is important not only that the receptor site support revascularization and promote osteogenesis but also that stable fixation is provided over this period to allow incorporation of the donor bone into the host site. The vascularity of the recipient site will be adversely affected by the scar tissue that invariably develops from previous surgery, thus compromising the vascularity and ultimate success of the autogenous costochondral free graft. It has been reported that capillaries can penetrate a maximum thickness of 180 to 220 μm of tissue, whereas scar tissue surrounding previously operated bone averages 440 μm in thickness. This may account for the clinical observation that free autogenous tissue grafts, such as cartilage, costochondral, and sternoclavicular grafts, often fail in cases of multiply operated patients or those with extreme anatomic architectural discrepancies resulting from pathology.[34] Reitzik[35] reported that in an analogous situation to autogenous costochondral grafting, cortex-to-cortex healing after vertical ramus osteotomy in monkeys requires 20 weeks and probably 25 weeks in humans. Typically, in patients reconstructed with costochondral grafts, maxillomandibular fixation is maintained for only 4 to 6 weeks in order to return the mandible to function and prevent ankylosis. Despite screw and plate fixation, micromotion at the donor-host interface in such cases will invariably occur with early mandibular function resulting in shear movements of the graft, leading to poor vascularization, nonunion, and/or potential failure.[36] Matsuura and colleagues[37] reported a high incidence of failure and ankylosis of autogenous costochondral grafts in sheep after condylectomy if the jaws were only partially immobilized. Further, Whitaker and associates[38-40] reported the incidence of pneumothorax in 149 rib graft harvest patients as 5.3% and in the next 151 such patients as 18%. They reported pneumothorax in 20% to 30% of the 793 patients they studied.[40] James and Irvine[41] reported an incidence of postoperative donor site chest wound infection after rib harvest of 14.6%.

TRANSPORT DISTRACTION OSTEOGENESIS

The use of transport distraction osteogenesis, which induces new bone formation along the vector of movement without the use of a bone graft, has been employed as a reconstruction option for a variety of mandibular defects, including condylar reconstruction.[42-44] The techniques described include a vertical ramus-type osteotomy of the mandible after correction of the indication for TJR (e.g., gap arthroplasty for ankylosis). After the ramus osteotomy (or corticotomy), a distraction device is placed with a vertical vector to move the proximal segment of the mandible toward the glenoid fossa (Figure 52-8). This form of reconstruction

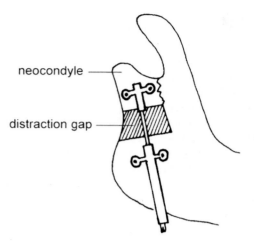

FIGURE 52-8. Transport distraction osteogenesis in an animal study. (Adapted from Zhu S, et al. Biomechanical properties of the condyle created by osteodistraction. J Dent Res 2008;87:490–494).

takes advantage of the fibrocartilagenous cap that forms on the advancing front of the distracted bone heading toward the fossa, thereby creating a "cartilage cap" on the newly formed condyle, which may function more normally than a pseudoarthrosis (Figure 52-9). Stucki-McCormick and coworkers[45,46] reported the application of transport distraction osteogenesis to reconstruct the mandibular condyle in two patients as well as in the animal model. Cavaliere and Buchman[47] reported using similar methods to manage hemifacial microsomia patients with 1- and 2-year follow-up, respectively. The long-term growth potential for the use of this modality in the reconstruction of prepubescent cases also has yet to be determined. In 1992, McCarthy and colleagues[42] developed the technique for mandibular elongation in patients with hemifacial microsomia and Nager's syndrome. Since then, distraction osteogenesis has been used for craniofacial lengthening,[48–50] bifocal distraction for repair of mandibular defects,[51,52] mandibular widening,[53] and increasing alveolar height.[54] Pensler and associates in 1995[55] reported a case of a

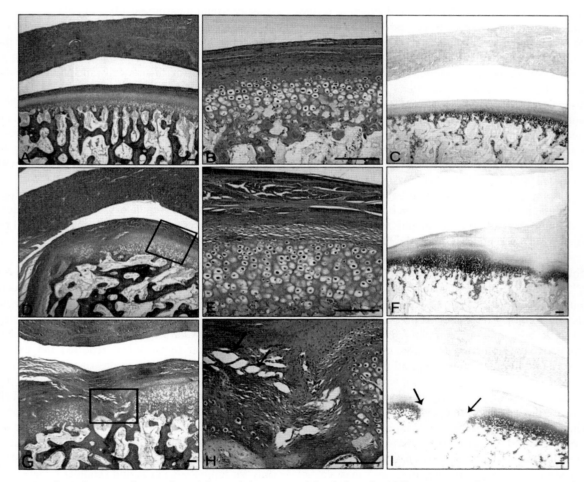

FIGURE 52-9. Histologic features of normal condyles and the neocondyles (**left** and **middle,** Masson trichrome staining; **right,** toluidine blue staining). **A–C,** A normal condyle showing the normal structures. **D** and **G,** The newly formed fibrocartilage covering the upper surface of the neocondyle. **E** and **H,** High-power views of the boxed areas in **D** and **G.** Lacunae can be observed *(arrow).* **F** and **I,** Uneven distribution and complete discontinuity *(between two arrows)* of the cartilaginous matrix were detected by toluidine blue staining. *Scale bar* represents 200 μm. (**A–I,** Adapted from Zhu S, et al. Biomechanical properties of the condyle created by osteodistraction. J Dent Res 2008;87:490–494.)

$5\frac{1}{2}$-year-old with micrognathia and TMJ ankylosis treated with distraction osteogenesis. Diner and coworkers in 1997[56] reported on a series of nine children with mandibular hypoplasia caused by TMJ ankylosis treated with distraction osteogenesis. Also in 1997, Acero-Sanz[57] and colleagues reported the use of distraction osteogenesis in the management of a 2-year-old with bilateral TMJ hypoplasia. In 1999, Dean and Alamillos[58] and Papageorge and Apostolidis[59] reported the management of TMJ ankylosis in growing patients utilizing simultaneous distraction osteogenesis and TMJ arthroplasty. These studies stress that experience with this technique in the management of childhood ankylosis and long-term follow-up are important, but according to Moss and Rankow's functional matrix theory,[60] with the association of distraction osteogenesis and TMJ arthroplasty, the conditions for normal mandibular growth should develop properly. In 2000, Yonehara and associates[61] reported a case of an 11-year-old boy with bilateral TMJ ankylosis and resultant severe micrognathia managed with bilateral distraction osteogenesis. They describe the greatest advantage of distraction osteogenesis as the gradual distraction of the soft tissues as well as the hard tissues associated with the mandible. Yoon and Kim in 2002[62] reported good results after more than 2 years follow-up after the use of intraoral distraction osteogenesis in a growing and an adult patient with mandibular asymmetry and unilateral TMJ bony ankylosis. Molina and Ortiz-Monteserio[63] and Ortiz Monasterio and coworkers[64] state that many cases of hemifacial microsomia treated in infancy will require a second course of distraction osteogenesis or formal orthognathic surgery later in life to maintain the position of the mandible. However, in cases associated with mandibular hypoplasia as the result of TMJ ankylosis, the etiology is traumatic, rather than developmental, in nature; therefore, correction of function of the associated bone and soft tissues should result in normal mandibular growth potential based on the functional matrix theory.[60] A further demonstration of Moss and Rankow's theory may be inferred from a report by Nitzan and colleagues.[65] They report on the management of four patients (three female, one male; ages 9–48 yr) with type III TMJ ankylosis in whom they freed the ankylosis and retained the displaced disk and condyle complex only, followed by aggressive active physiotherapy to restore mandibular function. After 15- to 60-month follow-up, all patients had significantly improved mandibular function and the 9-year-old with preoperative facial asymmetry demonstrated complete symmetrical growth 5 years after surgery. In the other growing patients, 15 months postoperative, improved facial symmetry was reported. Despite the short-term promising clinical results, the histomorphologic changes in the associated joint structures (i.e., cartilage, disk, and masticatory musculature) have not been elucidated completely. Experimental studies with rabbits and monkeys addressing this issue have appeared in the literature.[66,67] Based on their animal experiments, Zhu and associates[68] list several potential advantages of mandibular condyle reconstruction using

transport distraction over conventional autogenous bone grafting: (1) avoidance of donor site morbidity; (2) the rigid distraction device allows for immediate postoperative physical therapy, which allows for the formation of a pseudoarthrosis and prevents ankylosis; and (3) the risk of bone graft necrosis and resorption is greatly reduced compared with nonvascularized free-bone grafts (i.e., costochondral) because the transported bone in this technique retains its internal muscle and periosteal blood supply. However, these experimental studies were carried out in animals with normal TMJs and extrapolation of these data to patients with compromised TMJ anatomy due to pathology or multiple prior surgeries remains a question and concern when utilizing this technique.

BIOENGINEERED TISSUE FOR TJR

Mandibular condyle tissue engineering has been proposed recently to address the current limitations of both autogenous and alloplastic reconstruction options.[69] A tissue engineering strategy would incorporate a biodegradable scaffold delivering biologic substances such as cells, genes, and/or proteins to regenerate the bone/cartilage tissues of the mandibular condyle. Tissue engineering could be applied to regenerate localized defects or, theoretically, the entire articulating condylar surface. Implementation could take one of three approaches: (1) ex vivo growth of tissue on the scaffold/biologic composite in a bioreactor before implantation on the mandible; (2) implantation of the scaffold/biologic composite at secondary surgical site before implantation on the mandible; and (3) direct implantation at the mandible site.[69] Whereas this modality holds the potential to revolutionize the TMJ reconstruction in the future, many biologic, physiologic, mechanical, regulatory, and ethical issues must be tested and addressed before it becomes a clinical reality.

ALLOPLASTIC TJR

In order to avoid the donor site morbidity of autogenous bone grafting, alloplastic TJR has become an acceptable alternative to autogenous grafting (Table 52-5 and Table 52-6). In 1960, Sir John Charnley, the father of orthopedic low-friction alloplastic joint replacement, reported the use of a total alloplastic prosthetic hip reconstruction system utilizing a titanium-backed ultrahigh-molecular-weight polyethylene acetabular cup articulating with a chromium-cobalt femoral head attached to a titanium femoral shaft component that was cemented into place with polymethylmethacrylate (PMMA).[70] Modifications of this device with the same materials, now without the cement, have become the gold standard not only for hip but also knee and shoulder replacement devices in orthopedic surgery.[71] The modern practice of reconstructive orthopedic surgery would be unthinkable without the use of alloplastic joint replacements. All implanted alloplastic devices (dental implants, orthopedic, and TMJ prostheses) depend on the principle of osseointegration of

TABLE 52-5. **Comparison of Autogenous and Alloplastic Total Joint Replacement**

Autogenous	Alloplastic
Biocompatible	Biocompatible
Donor site	No donor site
Ankylosis potential	Low ankylosis (heterotopic bone)
Longevity	May require revision/replacement
Young patient with growth potential	Adult patient with growth completion
Lack of growth or overgrowth	Mechanical wear

TABLE 52-7. **Relative Contraindications to Alloplastic Total Joint Replacement**

Systemic
Incomplete facial bone growth (child)
Advanced medical-surgical risk
Uncontrolled systemic disease
Psychological instability

Local, Regional
Insufficient hard and soft tissues to support the implants
Active or recent infection (local or systemic)
Allergy to prosthetic materials (rare)
Uncontrolled parafunctional oral habit

the components for their ultimate stability and longevity. *Osseointegration* implies the direct incorporation of the implant by the bone without the preliminary phase of fibrous tissue ingrowth. The requirements for osseointegration are essentially the same as for primary fracture healing—the transmission of forces from the implant to the bone and vice versa must occur without relative motion or without intermittent loading.[72] Therefore, just as with a dental implant, the most important principle in total joint alloplastic reconstruction is primary stability of the device components from the moment of their implantation. In orthopedic surgery, total joint alloplastic devices can be initially stabilized by press fitting or cementation into the cancellous shaft of the host long bone. Unfortunately, in the case of the TMJ, the anatomy of the mandible and the nonlinear architecture of temporal glenoid fossa do not provide such options. Therefore, screw fixation of both the fossa and the ramus/condyle components of all TMJ alloplastic devices must be utilized for initial fixation and stabilization. Compounding the stability problems in the TMJ region is the fact that most patients presenting with indications for total TMJ alloplastic reconstruction have fossa and/or ramus anatomy distortion as a result of end-stage disease. There may be local and/or systemic relative contraindications to alloplastic TJR (Table 52-7).

TABLE 52-6. **Advantages and Disadvantages of Alloplastic Total Joint Replacement**

Advantages
Rigid fixation allows immediate postoperative physical therapy.
No donor site morbidity.
Decreased surgical time (vs. autogenous bone).
Mimics normal anatomy (CAD/CAM or patient-fitted TJR).
Maintenance of stable occlusion (no remodeling).
Can correct apertognathia, retrognathia without potential for relapse.

Disadvantages
Device cost.
Material wear and/or failure (screw loosening, fracture).
Possible heterotopic bone formation (ankylosis).
Possible need for revision and/or replacement.
Size and design limitations (stock devices).
No growth potential.

CAD/CAM = computer-aided_design/computer-aided_manufacturing;
TJR = total joint replacement.

History of Alloplastic TMJ Reconstruction

Alfred Stille[73] said "Medicine, like all knowledge, has a past as well as a present and a future, and . . . in that past is the soil out of which improvement must grow." Therefore, a look back is important to the understanding of the use of alloplastic materials in joint reconstruction. The citations made in this section are intended to show that many surgeons in the past found a need for alloplastic TMJ reconstruction in particularly difficult clinical situations. Further, it provides an archive of the materials and methods used in these cases (Table 52-8). Typically, the materials used in these devices mirrored their introduction into industry and medicine. It must be noted that in many instances, the reports of the use of these materials were of single cases and their follow-up was typically 1 year or less with the only criterion for success being that the patient could open the mouth.

Before 1980, alloplastic joint replacement or resurfacing (hemiarthroplasty/partial joint replacement) was performed mainly in cases of ankylosis, after ablative surgery, trauma, or in severe joint disease. After the mid- to late 1980s, partial and total TMJ devices were also being used to manage failed nonsurgical and surgical TMJ patients. In 1840, John Murray Carnochan[74] was credited with the idea of interposing material between the surfaces of a diseased joint. He reported an attempt to mobilize a patient's ankylosed TMJ by placing a small block of wood between the raw bony surfaces of the residual mandible after creating a gap at the neck of the condyle. In 1890, a German surgeon, Gluck[75] reported total joint arthroplasties using ivory prosthetic TMJ and hip joints that he stabilized with cement made of colophony, pumice, and gypsum. Risdon in 1933[76] reported the treatment of an ankylosis of the TMJ by interposing gold foil between the bony surfaces after a gap was created. Eggers in 1946[77] and Goodsell in 1947[78] reported the use of tantalum foil in cases of TMJ ankylosis. In 1951, Castigliano and Gross[79] and Kleitsch[80] resurfaced the bone in TMJ ankylosis cases with vitallium. In 1952, Smith and Robinson[81] reported hemiarthroplasty for ankylosis using stainless steel. In 1955, Ueno and coworkers[82] reported experimental and clinical results with zirconium in TMJ ankylosis. In 1960, Henry[83] described replacement of an ankylosed TMJ with prosthesis

TABLE 52-8. **History of Alloplastic Total Joint Replacement**

1840—Wood (Carnochan)
1890—Ivory (Gluck)
1934—Gold foil (Risdon)
1946—Tantalum foil over condyle (Eggers)
1947—Tantalum foil (Goodsell)
1951—Vitallium (Castigliano & Kleitsch)
1952—Stainless steel (Smith)
1955—Zirconium (Ueno)
1957—Stainless steel fossa (Robinson)
1963—Vitallium fossa (Christensen)
1964—Tantalum foil/PT (Hellinger)
1968—Silastic sponge fossa (Robinson)
1970—Mesh/PMMA (Corgill & Hahn)
1971—Vitallium/Silastic fossa (Morgan)
1972—Gold custom (Taurus)
1974—Proplast-coated ticonium (Hinds)
1974—PMMA (Wallace)
1974—Cr-Co fossa and condyle with PMMA head (Kiehn)
1974—Vitallium condyle, Proplast I fossa (Hinds & Kent)
1976—Stainless steel ramus and condyle reconstruction plate (Spiessl)
1976—Vitallium-acrylic condylar prosthesis (Robinson)
1977—Corgill-Hahn prosthesis (Seymour)
1977—Charnley intramedullary orthopedic pin, PMMA cement (Silver)
1978—Cr-Co fossa and condyle with PMMA head (Kummona)
1982—Three-dimensional THORP design (Raveh)
1983—Vitek, Kent I fossa, Cr-Co ramus and condyle (Kent)
1984—Hip joint prosthetic design (Flot & Chassagne)
1984—Delrin condyle with Cr-Co ramus, Cr-Co/Silastic fossa (House & Morgan)
1985—Cr-Co ramus and fossa, PMMA condyle, PMMA cement (Sonnenburg)
1986—VK I (20% success) and VK II (80% success) (Kent)
1987—Delrin (Boyne)
1988/95—CAD/CAM (Techmedica/TMJ Concepts), CP-Ti backed UHMWPE custom fossa, Cr-Co-Mb condyle, 6Al/4V Ti custom ramus (Mercuri/Wolford)
1990—Ceramics (Szabo)
1990—CP-Ti backed UHMWPE fossa, Cr-Co condyle, 6Al/4V Ti ramus (Sonnenburg)
1993—Titanium/Cr-Co-Mo (Falkenstrom)
1994—Osteomed, UHMWPE fossa, PMMA cement, Cr-Co condyle, 6Al/4V Ti ramus (McBride)
1995—Cr-Co fossa and ramus, PMMA condyle (stock) (Chase)
1999—TMJ Concepts (Mercuri)
2000—Groningen device (van Loon & DeBont)
2006—Biomet/Lorenz device (Quinn)

CAD/CAM = computer-aided_design/computer-aided_manufacturing; PMMA = polymethylmethacrylate; PT = ; THORP = titanium-coated hollow screw and reconstruction plate; TMJ = temporomandibular joint; UHMWPE = ultrahigh-molecular-weight polyethylene.

and Robinson[84] reported correction of a TMJ ankylosis by creating an artificial stainless steel fossa. In 1963,[85] 1964,[86] and 1970,[87] Christensen reported resurfacing of the glenoid fossa with a thin vitallium fossa-eminence prosthesis in cases of TMJ ankylosis. He added a ramus-condyle component with a PMMA head and a vitallium ramal component to create a total TMJ prosthesis. Chase and colleagues in 1995[88] reported on the results of the use of both devices. In 1996, a chromium-cobalt condylar head was offered as an option to the PMMA. Garrett and associates[89] reported the use of a custom modification of the standard Christensen total alloplastic TMJ prosthesis for use in multiply operated patients. Small and coworkers[90] experimented with the use of Teflon and Silastic in mandibular reconstruction and in 1964 reported that Teflon seemed more adaptable to restoration of large mandibular resections whereas Silastic seemed better suited for replacement of the condyle. In 1968, Robinson[91] reported on the use of Silastic in a case of TMJ ankylosis as an interpositional material; other reports of the use of Silastic for partial TMJ reconstruction soon followed.[92–98] Hellinger, also in 1964,[99] reported the use of tantalum foil in such cases and was the first to stress the importance of physical therapy in the rehabilitation of these patients. Hahn and Corgill in 1970[100] first reported the use of ramus-condyle hemiarthroplasty prosthesis for the treatment of ankylosis. The condylar component was fashioned from dental PMMA. The ramus component was stainless steel wire mesh. In 1971,[101] 1975,[102] and 1977,[103] Morgan and colleagues presented another form of fossa resurfacing device that consisted of a vitallium eminence prosthesis and a Silastic fossa component. They added a variation of the Hahn and Corgill ramus-condyle component with a polyoxymethylene (Delrin) condyle to make a total joint prosthesis. In 1984, House and associates[104] reported the results of the use of the Morgan devices. In 1992, Morgan[105] reviewed the development of alloplastic materials for TMJ prostheses with an emphasis on his prostheses described previously. In 1972, Taurus and coworkers[106] first reported the use of a custom-made cast gold ramus-condyle hemiarticulation in reconstruction of a TMJ.

Hinds and colleagues in 1972[107] reported the use of a Proplast-Teflon–coated vitallium ramus-condyle component for hemiarticulation reconstruction of the TMJ. Kent and associates in 1983[108–110] reported the use of a Dacron/Proplast-Teflon (VK-I) and later still a Dacron/Proplast-Teflon/ultrahigh-molecular-weight polyethylene (UHMWPE) (VK-II) fossa. The ramus-condyle and fossa components were then reported as used as a total alloplastic TMJ reconstruction prosthetic device. Kent and associates in 1993[111] long-term follow-ups.

In 1974, Kiehn and coworkers[112] applied the principles used in total hip reconstruction to the TMJ, utilizing a vitallium mandibular fossa plate reinforced on its temporal side with PMMA and a vitallium-modified Cargill-Hahn ramus/condyle prosthesis. In 1978, the same authors[113] presented a follow-up of 27 patients who had undergone total TMJ reconstruction using the same prostheses previously described for the treatment of ankylosis, arthritis, neoplasm, infection, or refractory pain. They reported 23 successful cases over a 1- to 3-year period of follow-up, success being defined by the authors as the ability to open the mouth to eat without pain.[113–117] In 1978, Kammoona[118] essentially reproduced the work of Kiehn and coworkers in 6 monkeys. After 9 to 10 months of function, half failed due to condylar component failure. Microscopically, there was a minimum of inflammatory cells, no evidence of infection, and well-organized granulation tissue and collagen fibers with fibrous tissue beneath the cement and the condylar component. Reaction to the bone cement appeared good. Collagen fibers ran parallel to the implant. The bone in the surrounding area was vital and healthy, and in some areas, the fibrous tissue had turned to bone. Microradiographs demonstrated tolerance of the metallic joint and bone cement, with incorporation by healthy granulation tissue, collagen fibers, and new bone to such an extent as to justify complete biologic acceptance of the implant by the natural tissue. This was the second report of animal studies with alloplastic TMJ devices after Ueno and coworkers.[82] In 1985[119] and again in 1990,[120] Sonnenburg and Sonnenburg reported the use of a total TMJ device that consisted of a chromium-cobalt-molybdenum ramus-condyle component that articulated against an UHMWPE fossa. This mimicked the materials and geometry used in the design of alloplastic joint prostheses by orthopedic surgeons.

From 1990 to 1995, others reported on the development and use of alloplastic partial and total TMJ reconstruction prostheses. The indications for their use ranged from ankylosis to reconstruction after ablative surgery for disease and/or trauma to the multiply operated failed TMJ patient.[121–131] Mercuri and colleagues in 1995[132] reported on preliminary results with the use of a patient-fitted computer-aided_design/computer-aided_manufacturing (CAD/CAM) total alloplastic TMJ reconstruction prosthesis in a prospective limited clinical study. The ramus component of this prosthesis was titanium, and the condylar component chromium-cobalt-molybdenum and the fossa component titanium were backed with UHMWPE. This was followed by further long-term results indicating the safety and effectiveness of TJR for the TMJ using this device.[133,134]

At present, there are three U.S. Food and Drug administration (FDA)–sanctioned TMJ prosthetic systems available for implantation, the pre-1976 Amendment Christensen stock as well as the Christensen/Garrett custom devices (TMJ Implant, Inc., Golden, CO) (Figure 52-10); the 1999 FDA-approved

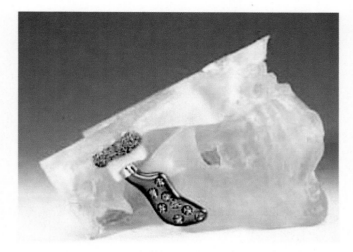

FIGURE 52-11.   TMJ Concepts (Ventura, CA) patient-fitted TMJ TJR device.

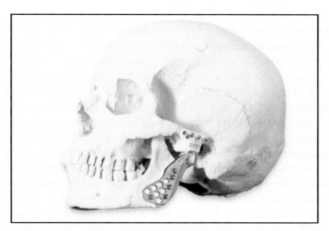

FIGURE 52-12.   Biomet-Microfixation (Jacksonville, FL) stock TMJ TJR device.

TMJ Concepts patient-fitted device (TMJ Concepts [previously Techmedica], Ventura, CA) (Figure 52-11); and the 2006 FDA-approved Biomet Microfixation total joint stock device (Jacksonville, FL) (Figure 52-12).

TMJ Implants, Inc., also manufactures a hemiarthroplasty fossa-eminence device, originally designed to manage TMJ ankylosis, that has been utilized as a disk substitute in the recent past. Hemiarthroplasty, a metallic-bearing surface articulating with normal articular cartilage, is frequently utilized in orthopedic surgery for fractures of the hip and shoulder in geriatric patients. The surgery can be quite successful in such cases in which functional demands are low; however, over time, the metallic component against the articular cartilage causes cartilage wear and may cause pain, requiring total joint replacement. For this reason, hemiarthroplasty is generally not performed in young patients or in patients with preexisting degenerative joint disease[135,136] (see Figure 52-5).

Although some surgeons have also advocated partial joint replacement utilizing only the condylar component, it is best to

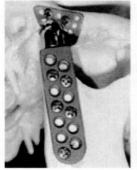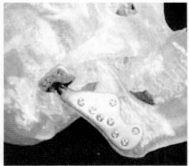

FIGURE 52-10.   TMJ, Inc. (Golden, CO) stock and custom TMJ total joint replacement (TJR) devices.

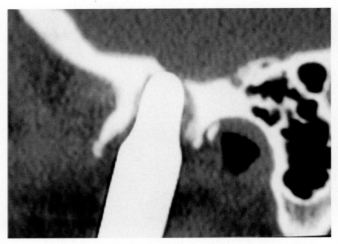

FIGURE 52-13. Erosion of the condyle from a hemiarthroplasty procedure into the middle cranial fossa and development of heterotopic bone.

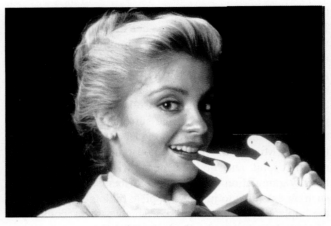

FIGURE 52-14. Postoperative home physical therapy using a commercially available jaw exercising device.

perform a total joint replacement. Lindqvist and associates in 1992[127] and Westermark and coworkers in 2006[137] found that in cases of condylar element replacement alone, there was severe erosion of the fossa with significant heterotopic bone formation. (Figure 52-13). Stock or "off-the-shelf" joint replacement devices must be bent to fit or shimmed with bone and/or PMMA cement or the precious host bone must be recontoured to develop some reasonable host-to-bone interface. All such maneuvers can lead to component material fatigue or overload, promoting early failure with functional loading. More significantly, these manipulations can lead to "stock" component micromotion that will interfere with osseointegration. Micromotion leads to the formation of a fibrous connective tissue interface between the altered component and the host bone, resulting in early loosening of that component and potential early catastrophic or certain premature device failure in the future. In addition, there are patient-fitted or custom-made devices that are designed and manufactured for each specific anatomic situation, can conform to any unique anatomic situation, and require no alteration or supplementation to achieve initial implantation stability. Because the components interface precisely with the host bone, the screw fixation secures the components to the host bone, mitigating micromotion and maximizing the opportunity for osseointegration of the components and fixation screws.

In 2003, Wolford and colleagues[138] compared two of the available TMJ TJR systems in 45 patients, including TMJ Implants (23 patients) and TMJ Concepts (22 patients). The average number of previous surgeries was 3.9 for the TMJ Implants patients and 2.6 for the TMJ Concepts patients, and the average follow-up period was 2 to 3 years. It was determined that TMJ Concepts had statistically significant improved outcomes compared with the TMJ Implants group in terms of postsurgical maximum interincisal opening, pain, jaw function, and diet. It was noted that both groups showed good skeletal and occlusal stability over the follow-up period.

Returning the joint(s) and muscles of mastication to function as soon as possible postoperatively enhances healing and decreases the development of intra-articular scar tissue that will compromise mandibular range of motion.[139] One of the biggest advantages of alloplastic over autogenous TMJ replacement is the ability to start active physical therapy immediately postoperatively utilizing any of the commercially available jaw exercising devices (Figure 52-14).

When calculating cost of a procedure or device, it is important that not only is the cost of the device considered but also all factors associated with its placement, including overall treatment time and patient morbidity. The major advantages of alloplastic over autogenous TMJ reconstruction is that there is no need for a second surgical site with the potential of increasing morbidity and the expensive intraoperative and postoperative hospital time is greatly decreased.

Finally, the concern often raised that any alloplastic devices when utilized in the TMJ will result in the same scenario as Proplast-Teflon/silicone rubber are unfounded and unsubstantiated in a growing body of literature.[132–134,140–147]

In conclusion, this chapter discussed the management of end-stage TMJ disease employing the management options of autogenous tissue, alloplastic materials, osseodistraction, and bioengineered tissue. It also presented an evidence-based literature review for each of these modalities from which the reconstructive surgeon may determine which alternative provides the best management option for regaining and maintaining savaged TMJ function and facial form in the face of end-stage disease for each individual case. Table 52-9 provides a useful resource when considering clinical options for TJR based upon the specific indication for surgery. It should be kept in mind that, in general, TJR may be considered a "salvage" procedure for end-stage TMJ disease and that "success" may need to be qualified especially in the multiply operated patient with chronic facial pain. The quality of life in these patients remains poor and possible revision procedures may be necessary in the life-long management of this patient group.

TABLE 52-9. **Options for Total Joint Replacement Based upon End-Stage Disease**

	Bone Grafting	Distraction	Bioengineered	Alloplastic
Developmental	+++	++	+++	+*
Neoplastic	+++	+	++	+++
Traumatic	+++	++	+++	+++
Arthritic	+†	+	+	+++
Multiple Failed Surgery	+	+	+	+++
Ankylosis	+	++	+	+++

*Mercuri LG, Swift JQ. Considerations for the use of alloplastic temporomandibular joint replacement in the growing patient. J Oral Maxillofac Surg 2009;67:1979–1990.
†Juvenile rheumatoid arthritis: Svensson B. On costochondral grafts replacing mandibular condyles in juvenile chronic arthritis: a clinical, histologic and experimental study. Goteborg, Sweden: Orebro, 2000.

References

1. Mercuri LG. The use of alloplastic prostheses for temporomandibular joint reconstruction. Oral Maxillofac Surg 2000;58:70–75.
2. Ware WH, Taylor RC. Cartilaginous growth centers transplanted to replace mandibular condyles in monkeys. J Oral Surg 1966;24:33–43.
3. Poswillo DE. Experimental reconstruction of the mandibular joint. Int J Oral Surg 1974;3:400–411.
4. Poswillo DE. Biological reconstruction of the mandibular condyle. Br J Oral Maxillofac Surg 1987;25:100–104.
5. Ware WH, Brown SL. Growth center transplantation to replace mandibular condyles. J Maxillofac Surg 1981;9:50–58.
6. MacIntosh RB. Current spectrum of costochondral grafting. In Bell WH, editor. Surgical Correction of Dentofacial Deformities: New Concepts. Vol 3. Philadelphia: WB Saunders; 1985; pp. 355–410.
7. MacIntosh RB. The use of autogenous tissue in temporomandibular joint reconstruction. J Oral Maxillofac Surg 2000;58:63–69.
8. MacIntosh RB, Henny FA. A spectrum of application of autogenous costochondral grafts. J Oral Maxillofac Surg 1977;5:257–267.
9. Tasanen A, Leikomma H. Ankylosis of the TMJ of a child. Int J Oral Surg 1977,6:95–99.
10. Smith BR, Wolford LM. Long-term growth in costochondral grafts in children [abstract]. Presented at the 67th Annual Scientific Session of the American Association of Oral and Maxillofacial Surgeons. 1985;September 13–15; Washington, DC
11. Obeid G, Gutterman SA, Connole PW. Costochondral grafting in condylar replacement and mandibular reconstruction. J Oral Maxillofac Surg 1988;48:177–182.
12. Ware WH. Growth center transplantation in TMJ surgery. In Walker RV, editor. Transactions of the Third Congress of the International Association of Oral and Maxillofacial Surgeons; 1970; pp. 148–157.
13. Marx RE, Kretzschmar DP. Autogenous costochondral grafting in growing children. Curr Adv Oral Surg 1983;4:124–132.
14. Heffez L, Doku C. The Goldenhar syndrome: diagnosis and early surgical management. Oral Surg 1984;58:2–9.
15. Politis C, Jossion E, Bossuyt M. The use of costochondral grafts in arthroplasty of the temporomandibular joint. J Craniomaxillofac Surg 1987;15:345–356.
16. Lindqvist C, Jokinen J, Paukku P, et al. Adaptation of autogenous costochondral grafts used for temporomandibular joint reconstruction. J Oral Maxillofac Surg 1988;46:465–470.
17. Munro IR, Phillips JH, Griffin G. Growth after construction of the temporomandibular joint in children with hemifacial microsomia. Cleft Palate J 1989;26:303–311.
18. Peltomäki T, Isotupa K. The costochondral graft: a solution or a source of facial asymmetry in growing children? A case report. Proc Finn Dent Soc 1991;87:167–176.
19. Fukuta K, Jackson IT, Topf JS. Facial lawn mower injury treated by a vascularized costochondral graft. J Oral Maxillofac Surg 1992;50:194–198.
20. Guyuron B, Lasa CI. Unpredictable growth pattern of costochondral graft. Plast Reconstr Surg 1992;90:880–886.
21. Link JO, Hoffman DC, Laskin DM. Hyperplasia of a costochondral graft. J Oral Maxillofac Surg 1993;51:1392–1394.
22. Ellis E, Schneiderman ED, Carlson DS. Growth of the mandible after replacement of the mandibular condyle: an experimental investigation in *Macaca mulatta*. J Oral Maxillofac Surg 2002;60:1461–1470.
23. Guyot L, Richard O, Layoun W, et al. Long-term radiological findings following reconstruction of the condyle with fibular free flaps. J Craniomaxillofac Surg 2004;32:98–102.
24. Marx RE. The science and art of reconstructing the jaws and temporomandibular joints. In Bell WH, editor. Modern Practice in Orthognathic and Reconstructive Surgery. Vol 2. Philadelphia: WB Saunders; 1992; pp. 1448–1461.
25. Perrot DH, Umeda H, Kaban LB. Costochondral graft/reconstruction of the condyle/ramus unit: Long-term follow-up. Int J Oral Maxillofac Surg 1994;23:321–328.
26. Svensson A, Adell R. Costochondral grafts to replace mandibular condyles in juvenile chronic arthritis patients: long-term effects on facial growth. J Craniomaxillofac Surg 1998;26:275–283.
27. Ross RB. Costochondral grafts replacing the mandibular condyle. Cleft Palate Craniofac J 1999;36:334–339.
28. Wen-Ching K, Huang C-S, Chen Y-R: Temporomandibular joint reconstruction in children using costochondral grafts. J Oral Maxillofac Surg 1999;57:789–796.
29. Peltomäki T, Vähätalo K, Rönning O. The effect of a unilateral costochondral graft on the growth of the marmoset mandible. J Oral Maxillofac Surg 2002;60:1307–1314.
30. Peltomäki T, Rönning O. Interrelationship between size and tissue-separating potential of costochondral transplants. Eur J Orthod 1991;13:459–465.
31. Peltomäki T. Growth of a costochondral graft in the rat temporomandibular joint. J Oral Maxillofac Surg 1992;50:851–857.
32. Cole P, Crawford MH, Hollier LH, et al. The composite costochondral-iliac crest bone graft: a novel techniques for TMJ reconstruction. J Oral Maxillofac Surg 2008;66:1299–1301.

33. Saeed NR, Kent JN. A retrospective study of the costochondral graft in TMJ reconstruction. Int J Oral Maxillofac Surg 2003;32:606–609.

34. Mercuri LG. Alloplastic temporomandibular joint reconstruction. Oral Surg 1998;85:631–637.

35. Reitzik M. Cortex-to-cortex healing after mandibular osteotomy. J Oral Maxillofac Surg 1983;41:658–663.

36. Lienau J, Schell H, Duda G. Initial vascularization and tissue differentiation are influenced by fixation stability. J Orthopaed Res 2005;23:639–645.

37. Matsuura H, Miyamoto H, Ishimura J, et al. Effect of partial immobilization on reconstruction of ankylosis of the temporomandibular joint with autogenous costochondral graft. Br J Oral Maxillofac Surg 2001;39:196–203.

38. Whitaker LA, Monroe IR, Jackson IR, et al. Problems in craniofacial surgery. J Oral Maxillofac Surg 1976;4:131–136.

39. Whitaker LA, Zins J, Reichman J. Bone graft donor site considerations in craniofacial reconstruction. Abstracts of the Fourth Congress of the European Association for Maxillofacial Surgery; 1978; p. 66.

40. Whitaker LA, Munro IR, Salyer KE, et al. Combined report of problems and complications in 793 craniofacial operations. Plast Reconstr Surg 1979;64:198–203.

41. James DR, Irvine GH. Autogenous rib grafts in maxillofacial surgery. J Maxillofac Surg 1983;11:201–203.

42. McCarthy JG, Schreiber JS, Karp N, et. al. Lengthening of the human mandible by gradual distraction. Plast Reconstr Surg 1992;89:1–8.

43. Molina F, Monasterio FO. Mandibular elongation and remodeling by distraction: farewell major osteotomies. Plast Reconstr Surg 1995;96:825–831.

44. Perrott DH, Berger R, Vargervik k, et al. Use of a skeletal distraction device to widen the mandible: a case report. J Oral Maxillofac Surg 1993;51:435–439.

45. Stucki-McCormick SU. Reconstruction of the mandibular condyle using transport distraction osteogenesis. J Craniofac Surg 1997;8:48–52.

46. Stucki-McCormick SU, Fox RM, Mizrahi RD. Reconstruction of a neocondyle using transport distraction osteogenesis. Semin Orthod 1999;5:59–63.

47. Cavaliere CM, Buchman SR. Mandibular distraction in the absence of an ascending ramus and condyle. J Craniofac Surg 2002;13:527–532.

48. Block MS, Brister GD. Use of distraction osteogenesis for maxillary advancement: preliminary results. J Oral Maxillofac Surg 1994;52:282–286.

49. Chin M, Toth BA. Distraction osteogenesis in maxillofacial surgery using internal devices. Review of five cases. J Oral Maxillofac Surg 1996;54:45–53.

50. Polley JW, Figueroa A. Management of severe maxillary deficiency in childhood and adolescence through distraction osteogenesis with an external, adjustable, rigid distraction device. J Craniofac Surg 1997;8:181–185.

51. Block MS, Otten J, Mclauren D, et al. Bifocal distraction osteogenesis for mandibular defect healing. Case reports. J Oral Maxillofac Surg 1996;54:1365–1370.

52. Annino DJ, Goguen LA, Karmody CS. Distraction osteogenesis for reconstruction of mandibular symphyseal defects. Arch Otolaryngol Head Neck Surg 1994;120:911–916.

53. Bell WH, Harper RP, Gonzalez M, et al. Distraction osteogenesis to widen the mandible. Br J Oral Maxillofac Surg 1997;35:11–19.

54. Block MS, Chang A, Crawford C. Mandibular alveolar ridge augmentation in the dog using distraction osteogenesis. J Oral Maxillofac Surg 1996;54:310–314.

55. Pensler JM, Goldberg DP, Lindell B, et al. Skeletal distraction of the hypoplastic mandible. Ann Plast Surg 1995;34:130–136.

56. Diner PA, Kollar E, Martinez H, et al. Submerged intraoral device for mandibular lengthening. J Craniomaxillofac Surg 1997;25:116–123.

57. Acero-Sanz J, Calderón J, Verdaguer F, et al. Distracción mandibular en un caso de hipoplasia mandibular neonatal asociado a anquilosis temporomandibular. Rev Esp Cir Oral y Maxilofac 1997;19(Suppl I):52.

58. Dean A, Alamillos F. Mandibular distraction in temporomandibular joint ankylosis. Plast Reconstr Surg 1999;104:2021–2031.

59. Papageorge MB, Apostolidis C. Simultaneous mandibular distraction and arthroplasty in a patient with temporomandibular joint ankylosis and mandibular hypoplasia. J Oral Maxillofac Surg 1999;57:328–333.

60. Moss ML, Rankow RM. The role of the functional matrix in mandibular growth. Angle Orthod 1968;38:95–103.

61. Yanehara Y, Takato T, Susami T, et al. Correction of micrognathia attributable to ankylosis of the temporomandibular joint using a gradual distraction technique: case report. J Oral Maxillofac Surg 2000;58:1415–1418.

62. Yoon HJ, Kim HG. Intraoral mandibular distraction osteogenesis in facial asymmetry patients with unilateral temporomandibular joint ankylosis. Int J Oral Maxillofac Surg 2002;31:544–548.

63. Molina F, Ortiz Monteserio F. Mandibular elongation and remodeling by distraction. Plast Reconstr Surg 1995;96:825–832.

64. Ortiz Monesterio F, Molina F, Andrade L, et al. Simultaneous mandibular and maxillary distraction in hemifacial microsomia in adults: Avoiding occlusion disasters. Plast Reconstr Surg 1996;100:852–860.

65. Nitzan DW, Bar-Ziv J, Shteyer A. Surgical management of temporomandibular joint ankylosis type III by retaining the displaced condyle and disc. J Oral Maxillofac Surg 1998;56:1133–1138.

66. Hikiji H, Takato T, Matsumoto S, et al. Experimental study of reconstruction of the temporomandibular joint using bone transport technique. J Oral Maxillofac Surg 2000;58:1270–1276.

67. Zhu S, Hu J, Li J, et. al. Reconstruction of mandibular condyle by transport distraction osteogenesis: experimental study in Rhesus monkey. J Oral Maxillofac Surg 2006;64:1487–1492.

68. Abukawa H, Terai H, Hannouche D, et al Formation of a mandibular condyle in vitro by tissue engineering. J Oral Maxillofac Surg 2003;61:94–100.

69. Zouhary KJ, Feinberg SE. Regeneration of the mandibular condyle in minipigs. J Oral Maxillofac Surg 2006;64:565–566.

70. Swanson SAV, Freeman MAR, editors. The Scientific Basis of Joint Replacement. New York: Wiley & Sons; 1977.

71. Petty W, editor. Total Joint Replacement. Philadelphia: WB Saunders; 1991.

72. Branemark PI, Hansson HA, Adell R. Osseointegrated implants in the treatment of the edentulous jaw: experience from a ten year period. Scand Plast Reconstr Surg 1977;16:1–132.

73. Stille A. Med News 1884;44:443.

74. Carnochan JM. Mobilizing a patient's ankylosed jaw by placing a block of wood between the raw bony surfaces after resection. Arch Med 1860;2:284.

75. Gluck T. Referat Uber die Durch das Moderne Chirurgische Experiment Gewonnenen Positiven Resultate, Betreffenddie Naht

und den Ersatz von Defecten Hoerer Gewebe, Sowie Uber die Verwerthung Resorbirbarer und Bebendiger Tampons in der Chirgurie. Arch Klin Chir 1891;4:186.

76. Risdon F. Ankylosis of the temporomandibular joint. J Am Dent Assoc 1933;21:1933–1937.

77. Eggers GWN. Arthroplasty of the temporomandibular joint in children with interpositional tantalum foil. J Bone Joint Surg 1946;28:603–606.

78. Goodsell JO. Tantalum in temporomandibular joint arthroplasty: report of case. J Oral Surg 1947;5:41–45.

79. Castigliano SG, Gross PP. Immediate prosthesis following radical resection in advanced primary malignant neoplasm of the mandible. J Oral Surg 1951;9:31–38.

80. Kleitch WP. Vitallium reconstruction of a hemimandible and temporomandibular joint. Plast Reconstr Surg 1951;7:244–253.

81. Smith AE, Robinson M. A new surgical procedure in bilateral reconstruction of condyles utilizing iliac crest bone grafts and creating new joints by means of non-electric metal: a preliminary report. Plast Reconstr Surg 1952;9:393–410.

82. Ueno T, Miura I, Kohno H. The use of zirconium metal plate in arthroplasty of temporomandibular joint ankylosis. Bull Tokyo Med Dent Soc 1955; 2:137–139.

83. Henry TC. Prosthetic restoration of the left temporomandibular joint in a case of partial ankylosis. Transactions of the 2nd Congress of the International Society of Plastic Surgeons. London: Livingstone; 1960; p. 159.

84. Robinson M. Temporomandibular joint ankylosis corrected by creating a false stainless steel fossa. J So Calif 1960;6:186–190.

85. Christensen RW. The correction of mandibular ankylosis by arthroplasty and insertion of a cast vitallium glenoid fossa. Am J Orthop 1963;48:16–24.

86. Christensen RW. Mandibular joint arthrosis corrected by insertion of cast vitallium glenoid fossa prosthesis. Oral Surg 1964;17:712–722.

87. Christiansen RW. Arthroplastic Implantation of the TMJ, Oral Implantology. Springfield, IL: Charles C. Thomas; 1970; pp. 284–298.

88. Chase DC, Hudson JW, Gerard DA, et al. The Christensen prosthesis. Oral Surg 1995;80:273–278.

89. Garrett WR, Abbey PA, Christensen RW. Temporomandibular joint reconstruction with a custom total temporomandibular joint prosthesis: use in the multiply operated patient. In Szabo Z, Lewis JE, Fantini GA, Savalgi RS, editors. Surgical Technology International VI. San Francisco: University Medical Press; 1997; pp. 347–354.

90. Small IA; Brown S, Kobernick SD. Teflon and Silastic for mandibular replacement: experimental studies and reports of cases. J Oral Surg 1964;22:37–41.

91. Robinson M. Temporomandibular joint ankylosis corrected by creating a false Silastic sponge fossa. J So Calif Dent Assoc 1968;36:14–16.

92. Hansen WC, Deshazo BW. Silastic reconstruction of temporomandibular joint meniscus. Plast Reconstr Surg 1969;43:388–391.

93. Rast WC, Waldrep AC, Irley WC. Bilateral temporomandibular joint arthroplasty. J Oral Surg 1969;27:871–874.

94. Wukelich S, Marshall J, Walden R, et al. Use of a Silastic testicular implant in reconstruction of the temporomandibular joint of a 5-year-old child. Oral Surg 1971;32:4–9.

95. Cook HP: Teflon implantation in temporomandibular arthroplasty. Oral Surg 1972;33:706–716.

96. Hartwell SW, Hall MD. Mandibular condylectomy with silastic rubber replacement. Plast Reconst Surg 1974;53:440–444.

97. Howe DJ. Preformed Silastic temporomandibular joint implant. J Oral Surg 1979;37:59.

98. Cope MR, Moos KF, Hammersley N. The compressible silicone rubber prosthesis in temporomandibular joint disease. Br J Oral Maxillofac Surg 1993;31:376–384

99. Hellinger MJ. Bony ankylosis of the temporomandibular joint. Oral Surg 1964;18:293–302.

100. Hahn GW, Corgill DA. Surgical implant replacement of the fractured displaced mandibular condyle: report of three cases. J Oral Surg 1970;28:898–901.

101. Morgan DH. Dysfunction, pain, tinnitus, vertigo corrected by mandibular joint surgery. J So Cal Dent Assoc 1971;39:505.

102. Morgan DH. Surgical correction of temporomandibular joint arthritis. J Oral Surg 1975;33:766–773.

103. Morgan DH, Hall WP, Vamvas SJ, editors. Diseases of the Temporomandibular Apparatus. A Multidisciplinary Approach. St. Louis: CV Mosby; 1977; pp. 318–324.

104. House LR, Morgan DH, Hall WP, Vamvas SJ. Temporomandibular joint surgery. Report of a 14-year joint implant study. Laryngoscope 1984;94:537–538.

105. Morgan DH. Development of alloplastic materials for temporomandibular joint prosthesis: a historical perspective with clinical illustrations. J Craniomand Pract 1992;10:192–204.

106. Tauras SP, Jordan JE, Keen RR. Temporomandibular joint ankylosis corrected with a gold prosthesis. J Oral Surg 1972; 30:767–773.

107. Hinds EC, Homsy CA, Kent JN, Use of biocompatible interface for compatible interface for combining tissues and prostheses in oral surgery. In Kay LW, editor. Transactions of the IVth International Conference on Oral Surgery. Copenhagen: Munksgaard; 1972; pp. 210–216.

108. Hinds EC, Homsy CA, Kent JN. Use of a biocompatible interface for binding tissues and prosthesis in temporomandibular joint surgery. Oral Surg 1974;38:512–519.

109. Kent JN, Misiek DJ, Akin RK, et al. Temporomandibular joint condylar prosthesis: a ten year report. J Oral Maxillofac Surg 1983;41:245–254.

110. Kent JN, Block MS, Homsy CA, et al. Experience with a polymer glenoid fossa prosthesis for partial or total temporomandibular joint reconstruction. J Oral Maxillofac Surg 1986;44:520–533.

111. Kent JN, Block MS, Halpern J, Fontenot MG. Long-term results on VK partial and total temporomandibular joint systems. J Long-term Effects Med Imp 1993;3:29–40.

112. Kiehn CL, DesPrez JD, Converse CF. A new procedure for total temporomandibular joint replacement: case report. Plast Reconstr Surg 1974;53:221–226.

113. Kiehn CL, DesPrez JD, Converse CF. Total prosthetic replacement of the temporomandibular joint. Ann Plast Surg 1979;2:5–15.

114. Kameros J, Himmelfarb R. Treatment of TMJ ankylosis with methyl methacrylate interpositional arthroplasty. J Oral Surg 1975;33:282–291.

115. Spiessl B, Schmoker R, Mathys R. Treatment of ankylosis of the mandible. In Spiessl B, editor. New Concepts in Maxillofacial Bone Surgery. Vol 1. New York: Springer; 1976.

116. Silver CM, Motamed M, Carlotti E. Arthroplasty of the temporomandibular joint with the use of a vitallium condyle prosthesis: report of three cases. J Oral Surg 1977;35:909–914.

SECTION 6

117. Seymour RL, Bray TE, Irby WB. Replacement of condylar process. J Oral Surg 1977;35:405–408.

118. Kummoona R. Functional rehabilitation of ankylosed temporomandibular joints. Oral Surg 1978;46:495–505.

119. Sonnenburg S, Sonnenburg M. Total condylar prosthesis for alloplastic jaw articulation replacement. J Craniomaxillofac Surg 1985;13:131–135.

120. Sonnenburg M, Sonnenburg S. Development and clinical application of the total temporomandibular joint (T.M.J.) endoprosthesis. Rev Stomatol Chir Maxillofac 1990;91:165–169.

121. Raveh J, Sutter F, Hellum S. Surgical procedures for reconstruction of the lower jaw using the titanium-coated hollow-screw reconstruction plate system: bridging defects. Otolaryngol Clin North Am 1987;20:535–558.

122. Boyne PJ, Matthews FR, Stringer DE. TMJ bone remodeling after polyoxymethylene condylar replacement. Int J Oral Maxillofac Implant 1987;2:29–33.

123. Hellum S, Olofsson J. Titanium-coated hollow screw and reconstruction plate system (THORP) in mandibular reconstruction. J Craniomaxillofac Surg 1988;16:173–183.

124. Szabo G, Barabas J, Matrai J. Application of compact aluminum oxide ceramic implants in maxillofacial surgery. J Oral Maxillofac Surg 1990;48:354–361.

125. Westermark AH, Sindet-Pedersen S, Boyne PJ. Bony ankylosis of the temporomandibular joint: case report of a child treated with Delrin condylar implants. J Oral Maxillofac Surg 1990;48:861–865.

126. Chassagne JF, Flot F, Stricker M, et al. Prosthese totale intermediaire d'articulation temporo-mandibulaire. Rev Stomatol Chir Maxillofac 1990;91:423–429.

127. Lindqvist C, Soderholm AL, Hallikainen D, Sjovall L. Erosion and heterotopic bone formation after alloplastic temporomandibular joint reconstruction. J Oral Maxillofac Surg 1992;50:942–949.

128. McAfee KA, Quinn PD. Total temporomandibular joint reconstruction with Delrin titanium implant. J Craniofac Surg 1992;3:160–163.

129. Henry CH, Wolford LM. Treatment outcomes for temporomandibular joint reconstruction after Proplast-Teflon implant failure. J Oral Maxillofac Surg 1993;51:352–358.

130. McBride KL. Total temporomandibular joint reconstruction. In: Worthington P, Evans Jr, editors. Controversies in Oral and Maxillofacial Surgery. Philadelphia: WB Saunders: 1994; 381–396.

131. VanLoon JP, DeBont LGM, Boering G. Evaluation of temporomandibular joint prostheses: review of the literature from 1946–1994 and implications for future designs. J Oral Maxillofac Surg 1995;53:984–996.

132. Mercuri LG, Wolford LM, Sanders B, et al. Custom CAD/CAM total temporomandibular joint reconstruction system: preliminary multicenter report. J Oral Maxillofac Surg 1995;53:106–115.

133. Mercuri LG, Wolford LM, Sanders B, et al. Long-term follow-up of the CAD/CAM patient-fitted total temporomandibular joint reconstruction system. J Oral Maxillofac Surg 2002;60:1440–1448.

134. Mercuri LG, Edibam NR, Giobbie-Hurder A. 14-year follow-up of a patient fitted total temporomandibular joint reconstruction system. J Oral Maxillofac Surg 2007;65:1140–1148.

135. Beckenbaugh RD, Tressler HA, Johnson EW Jr. Results of hemiarthroplasty of the hip using a cemented femoral prosthesis. A review of 109 cases with average follow-up of 36 months. Mayo Clin Proc 1977;52:349–353.

136. Petrera P, Rubash HE. Revision total hip arthroplasty: the acetabular component. Am Acad Orthop Surg 1995;3:15–21.

137. Westermark A, Koppel D, Leiggener C. Condylar replacement alone is not sufficient for prosthetic reconstruction of the temporomandibular joint. Int J Oral Maxillofac Surg. 2006;35:488–492.

138. Wolford LM, Dingworth DJ, Talwar RM, et al. Comparison of 2 temporomandibular joint prosthesis systems. J Oral Maxillofac Surg 2003;61:685–690.

139. Salter RB, editor. Continuous Passive Motion. Baltimore: Williams & Wilkins; 1993.

140. Henry CH, Wolford LM. Treatment outcomes for temporomandibular joint reconstruction after Proplast-Teflon implant failure. J Oral Maxillofac Surg 1993;51:352–358.

141. Wolford LM, Cottrell DA, Henry CH. Temporomandibular joint reconstruction of the complex patient with the Techmedica custom-made total joint prosthesis. J Oral Maxillofac Surg 1994;52:2–10.

142. Mercuri LG. Subjective and objective outcomes in patients reconstructed with a custom-fitted alloplastic temporomandibular joint prosthesis. J Oral Maxillofac Surg 1999;57:1427–1430.

143. Donlon WC, editor. Total temporomandibular joint reconstruction. In Oral and Maxillofacial Surgery Clinics of North America. Vol 12. Philadelphia: WB Saunders; 2000.

144. Mercuri LG. Alloplastic vs. autogenous temporomandibular joint reconstruction. In Indresano AT, Haug RH, editors. Oral and Maxillofacial Surgery Clinics of North America. Philadelphia: Elsevier; 2006; Vol 18, No. 3: pp. 399–411.

145. Mercuri LG, Alcheikh Ali F, Woolson R. Outcomes of total alloplastic replacement with peri-articular autogenous fat grafting for management of re-ankylosis of the temporomandibular joint. J Oral Maxillofac Surg 2008;66:1794–1703.

146. Mercuri LG: Temporomandibular joint reconstruction. In Fonseca R, editor: Oral and Maxillofacial Surgery. Philadelphia: Elsevier; 2008; pp. 945–960.

147. Mercuri LG. Temporomandibular joint reconstruction. Alpha Omegan 2009;102:51–54.

Orthognathic Surgery

Craniofacial Growth and Development

Peter M. Spalding, DDS, MS, MS

The goal of this chapter is to provide a review of the current understanding of prenatal and postnatal craniofacial growth and its relevance for clinical orthognathic and craniofacial treatment. Although there clearly is awareness of the importance of genetic and environmental influences on craniofacial growth and development, the control and precise biologic mechanisms are not well understood and continue to be fertile areas of investigation. This chapter reviews human morphogenesis, prenatal and postnatal growth and development, the factors that influence these phases of growth and development, and the orthopedic and orthodontic clinical considerations that will determine whether surgical intervention will be necessary to achieve optimum cosmetic and functional craniofacial treatment outcomes.

PRENATAL CRANIOFACIAL DEVELOPMENT

Human prenatal development can be divided simply into the embryonic period, from fertilization through the 8th week of development, and the fetal period, continuing from the 9th to the 40th week at birth. The embryonic period is characterized by new tissue differentiation and organogenesis, whereas the fetal period is distinguished by growth and expansion of the basic structures already formed.

During the first few days after the formation of the single-cell zygote at conception, four mitotic divisions occur to form the 16-cell morula. After entering the uterus, the morula develops into a 100-cell blastocyst consisting of an outer (trophoblast) and inner (embryoblast) cell mass. The trophoblast further differentiates to form the placenta and other peripheral embryonic structures, whereas the embryoblast differentiates into the future embryo. At the end of the first week, the blastocyst adheres to the uterine endometrium to begin implantation. During the second week, the embryoblast forms a bilaminar disk composed of two germ layers: the ectoderm, forming the amniotic cavity floor; and the endoderm, lying beneath and forming the yolk sac floor. Later, the ectoderm will form a variety of epidermal structures including dental enamel, oral mucosa, and nasal epithelia. The endoderm will later form the pharyngeal epithelium. By the end of the second week, the endoderm develops a thickened area called the *prechordal plate,* located at the cranial end of the bilaminar disk, that prefaces the development of the head (Figure 53-1).

Embryonic Period

Germ Layer Formation

Craniofacial embryogenesis begins during the third week of gestation, when gastrulation and neurulation occur. *Gastrulation* is the process whereby the bilaminar disk is converted into a trilaminar one with the appearance of the third germ layer, the mesoderm, forming between the other two from ectodermal cell proliferation and differentiation in the caudal area of the disk. The prominence created from this proliferation forms a craniocaudal midline furrow termed the *primitive streak.* Cell proliferation and differentiation of the cranial end of the primitive streak form the notochord around which the axial skeleton will form.

Neural Tube Formation

Neurulation, occurring at the same time as gastrulation during the third week and continuing through the fourth week, is a process that results in the formation of the neural tube, the primordium of the central nervous system (CNS). Neurulation is characterized by development of the neural

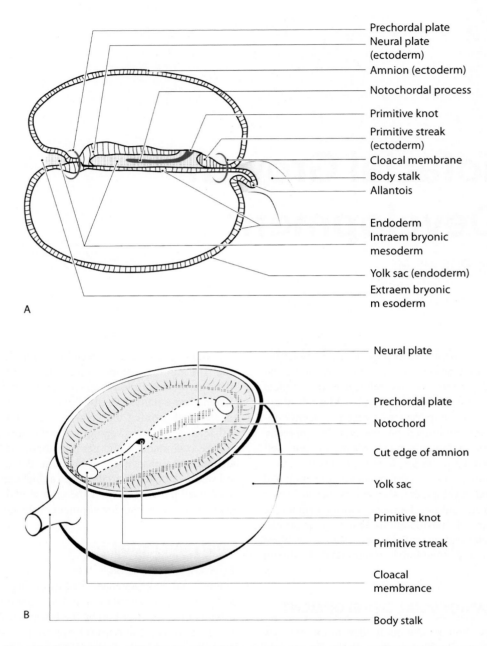

FIGURE 53-1. Embryo, 14 days old. **A,** Longitudinal section shows amnion *(top)* and yolk sac *(bottom)*. **B,** Dorsal surface view with the amnion cover removed, shows embryonic disk. Adapted from Sperber G. Craniofacial development. Hamilton (ON): BC Decker Inc; 2001. pp. 19 and 20.

plate from the ectoderm overlying the notochord. As the neural plate grows caudally toward the primitive streak, the lateral edges of the neural plate rise up to create neural folds, forming the neural groove between them. Mesoderm on either side of the groove develops into paired blocks of tissue called *somites* (ultimately 48 somite pairs will develop). In the fourth week, the neural folds begin to fuse at the midline in the central part of the embryo, at the level of the fourth to fifth somite, to form the neural tube (Figure 53-2). The neural tube continues to form toward the cranial and caudal ends, completing caudal formation by the time about 20 somite pairs are present. The anterior portion of the neural tube develops into the forebrain, midbrain, and hindbrain. After neural tube closure is complete on day 28, the two hemispheres of the brain begin development, increasing in size to eventually cover the roof of the brainstem. The otic, optic, and olfactory placodes develop in association with the forebrain neuroectoderm.

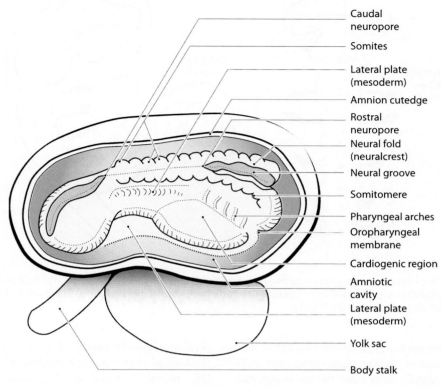

Caudal neuropore
Somites
Lateral plate (mesoderm)
Amnion cutedge
Rostral neuropore
Neural fold (neuralcrest)
Neural groove
Somitomere
Pharyngeal arches
Oropharyngeal membrane
Cardiogenic region
Amniotic cavity
Lateral plate (mesoderm)
Yolk sac
Body stalk

FIGURE 53-2.   Longitudinal section of amnion in a 23-day-old embryo shows fusion of the neural folds and initial formation of somites. Adapted from Sperber G. Craniofacial development. Hamilton (ON): BC Decker Inc; 2001. p. 21.

The Cranial Neural Crest

The neural crest is a multipotential cell population derived from the lateral edges of the neural plate during the fourth week of embryonic life. It was first described in 1868 as a band of cells between the surface epithelium and the neural tube in chicken embryos that appears at the dorsolateral edge of the closing neural folds along nearly the entire length of vertebrate neuraxis.[1] This is the line usually termed the *neural plate border* where the surface ectodermal epithelium functionally splits into two areas, the neuroectoderm or neural plate, which forms the neural tube and completely invaginates into the embryonic body, and the body surface epithelium that becomes the epidermis. Cell fate tracing experiments have revealed that neural crest cells originate from the dorsal surface of the neural tube by delamination from the epithelium and migrate extensively in a proper sequence over extensive distances through the embryo, developing into a wide variety of differentiated cell types at multiple distant sites (Figures 53-3 and 53-4).[2]

Neural crest cell differentiation occurs along multiple distinctive pathways and its contribution to the formation of a specific tissue or organ has generated considerable interest in developmental biology.[3,4] Progress has been made toward our understanding of how this important population of pluripotent cells is initially established in the early embryo and how

genetic and epigenetic mechanisms mediate their subsequent lineage segregation, differentiation, and final contribution to a particular phenotype.[5–7]

Neural crest cells migrate ventrolaterally as they populate the pharyngeal (or branchial) arches. Each pharyngeal arch is delineated by discrete swellings that are produced by the proliferative activity of these crest cells. These ectodermally derived cells contribute extensively to the formation of mesenchymal structures in the head and neck as they migrate. All of the skeletal and connective tissue of the face, with the exception of dental enamel, is derived from neural crest cells, whereas skeletal and connective tissue of the trunk is mesodermal in origin. Cell labeling studies have demonstrated that neuroectoderm cells of rhombomeres 1–3 in the forming posterior midbrain and anterior hindbrain transform into cranial neural crest cells that migrate into the first pharyngeal arch and thereafter reside within the maxillary and mandibular prominences.[3,8,9] The migration of these rhombencephalic crest cells may be regulated by growth factor signaling pathways and their downstream transcription factors before they become committed to several different phenotypes, including progenitor tooth mesenchymal cells, osteoblasts, chondroblasts, and cranial nerve ganglia of the first pharyngeal arch.[4,6,10–12] Several studies provide strong supportive evidence that the cranial neural crest cells are developmentally

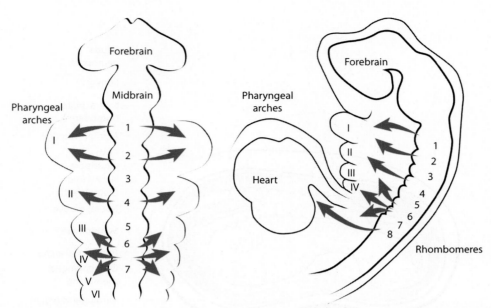

FIGURE 53-3. Illustration of neural crest migration pathways from rhombomeres 1 through 7 to pharyngeal arches I through VI, from dorsal **(left)** and lateral **(right)** views. Adapted from Sperber GH. Pathogenesis and morphogenesis of craniofacial developmental anomalies. Ann Acad Med Singapore 1999; 28:708–13.

modifiable with their fate not being predetermined before they reach their final destination. Rather, these progenitor cells must be instructed by signals from other tissues to generate craniofacial skeletal elements of appropriate shape and size. Tissues that provide the instructive signaling for cranial neural crest fate specification include, but are not limited to, the isthmic organizer behind the midbrain region, cranial placode, and the pharyngeal arch ectoderm and endoderm.[13–15] Transforming growth factor-beta (TGF-β) signaling has been shown to be critical in specifying neural crest cell differentiation.[16]

Our understanding of the migration and differentiation pathways of neural crest cells during embryogenesis have

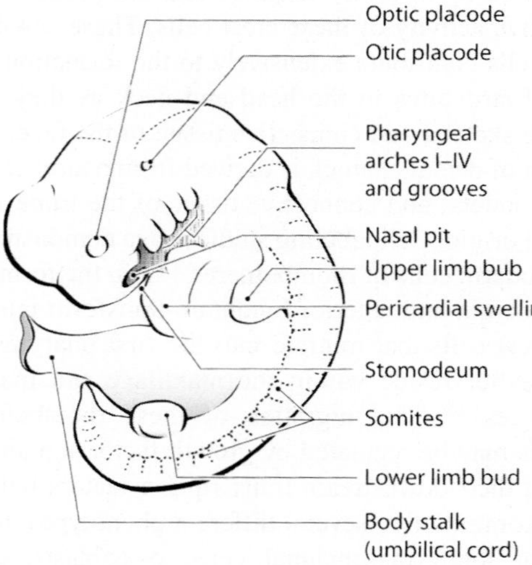

Optic placode
Otic placode

Pharyngeal arches I–IV and grooves

Nasal pit
Upper limb bub
Pericardial swelling

Stomodeum

Somites

Lower limb bud

Body stalk (umbilical cord)

FIGURE 53-4. Lateral view of a 31-day-old embryo shows somites along the back and development of the pharyngeal arches and limb buds. Adapted from Sperber G. Craniofacial development. Hamilton (ON): BC Decker Inc; 2001. p. 24.

been signifcantly advanced by cell lineage studies using chick-quail chimeras,[4] cell labeling with a vital dye such as DiI,[9] neural crest cell–specific antibodies,[17] and retroviral-mediated gene transfer.[18] However, a comprehensive cell lineage analysis of mammalian neural crest cells that follow their complete differentiation ultimately into a particular phenotype has been historically precluded by the lack of a genetic marker permitting these cells to be indefinitely followed. Fortunately, a two-component genetic system for indelibly marking the progeny of neural crest cells has significantly improved our ability to analyze the fate of the cranial neural crest during normal as well as abnormal craniofacial embryogenesis.[19–21] This genetic system utilizes expression of the proto-oncogene *Wnt1* as a marker, following *cre* expression restricted to the precursors of the neural crest.[22] An additional benefit of this genetic system has been its ability to integrate the analysis of the fate and function of mammalian neural crest with mouse molecular genetics, which has helped to clarify the molecular mechanism of neural crest–related congenital malformations.[23]

Facial Prominences and Formation of the Face

Facial formation occurs between the fourth and the eighth week of gestation. Early facial development is remarkably similar between different vertebrate species. In mice, cranial neural crest cells start to migrate soon after gastrulation, and the entire delamination takes place between the stages of 3 to 16 somites.[24] During the fourth week of gestation, neural crest cells selectively migrate to form four bilaterally paired pharyngeal arches on the ventral external surface of the embryo that will give rise to most of the head and neck structures. Pharyngeal arch identity, similar to other repetitive structures (somites, vertebrae, limb parts), is determined by expression of a unique combination of homeobox genes that determine when particular groups of genes are expressed during embryologic development.[12,25,26] The subepithelial mass of the first pharyngeal arch is populated by neural crest cells delaminating from the midbrain to the rhombomere 2 that do not show homeobox expression.[24,27] This represents an exception from other pharyngeal arches expressing *Hox* (a subgroup of homeobox) genes and may be a result of distinct regulation of the corresponding neural crest by the isthmus.[4,15,28] Following immigration of neural crest cells, the first pharyngeal arch consists of the ectodermal epithelium of the stomodeum (future oral cavity), the primitive gut endoderm beyond the pharyngeal membrane, surface ectodermal epithelium (future skin) and ectomesenchyme,[19,29] and a small portion of central mesenchymal core, probably derived from the original mesodermal cells of the first pharyngeal arch.[24]

Five facial prominences (primordia or processes) form from the first pair of pharyngeal arches that include the single median frontonasal prominence and the paired maxillary and the paired mandibular prominences that form the superior, inferior, and lateral boundaries of the stomodeum or primitive oral cavity. These facial prominences, each of whose outgrowth is composed of different neural crest cells and regulated by different genes, are covered by a thin epithelium derived from the ectoderm.[30] The mesenchcyme is composed primarily of the neural crest whereas the core of the facial prominences contains some mesodermal cells.[24] The final shape of the embryonic face is believed to be defined by the differential proliferation of the facial prominences.[31] Following the development of appropriate form and size, the facial prominences merge with adjacent prominences when the epithelium between them breaks down, followed by invasion of the mesenchyme and coalescence of the adjoining prominences (Figure 53-5).[32] Shortly after neural crest cell migration, the paired mandibular prominences merge in the midline to form the chin and lower lip. At the same time, the ectoderm of the frontonasal prominences forms two thickened epithelial regions, the nasal placodes, which

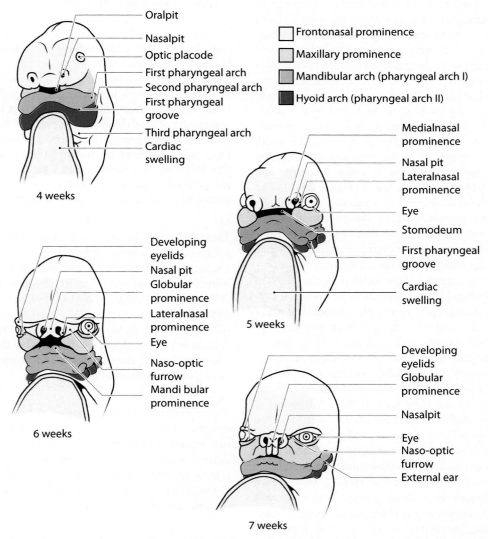

FIGURE 53-5. Frontal view of the developing face in 4-, 5-, 6-, and 7-week-old embryos shows merging of the facial prominences (primordia or processes). Adapted from Sperber G. Craniofacial development, Hamilton (ON): BC Decker Inc; 2001. p. 32.

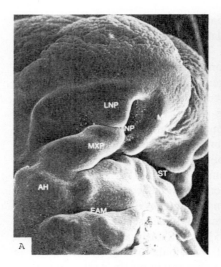 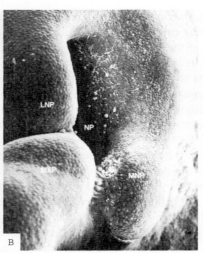

FIGURE 53-6. Scanning electron micrograph of a 41-day-old human embryo. **A,** Craniofacial region. AH = right auricular hillock; EAM = right external acoustic meatus; LNP = right lateral nasal prominence; MDP = mandibular prominence; MNP = right medial nasal prominence; MXP = right maxillary prominence; NP = right nasal pit; ST = left side of stomodeum. **B,** Enlarged view shows epithelial bridges between the merging MXP) and the MNP). Failure of the prominences to merge together with the LNP results in cleft of the lip. (**A** and **B,** Reproduced with permission from Hinrichsen K. The early development of morphology and patterns of the face in the human embryo. In: Advances in anatomy, embryology and cell biology. Vol. 98. New York: Springer-Verlag; 1985.)

subsequently curl outward to give rise to the medial and lateral nasal prominences. The medial nasal prominences grow further, moving toward each other and eventually merge in the midline (globular prominence) early in the sixth week to form the central part of the upper lip and the primary palate. There still is some controversy regarding the origin of the central part of the upper lip, which some believe is of frontonasal prominence origin.[21] The maxillary prominences move medially as well, merging with the lateral and medial nasal prominences during the sixth week, to complete formation of the upper lip. At this same time, the maxillary and mandibular prominences merge laterally, determining the width of the mouth. Merging of facial prominences requires disintegration of surface epithelia in order to permit the underlying mesenchymal cells to unite (Figure 53-6). The groove between the prominences is gradually filled out by proliferation of the mesenchyme so that the prominences appear to merge. Facial clefting is a result of failure of epithelial disintegration and lack of merging. Facial prominence growth and merging is dependent on ectodermal-mesenchymal interactions that appear to be regulated by the secreted protein sonic hedgehog (*SHH*).[30] Mutations in *SHH* that prevent its signaling during early neural plate patterning cause midline defects that range from hypotelorism and cleft lip/palate to holoprosencephaly and cyclopia.[33] There also is evidence that adequate epidermal growth factor receptor signaling is necessary for sufficient secretion of matrix metalloproteinases for normal facial development.[34] From 5 weeks' gestation to the early part of the fetal period at 9 weeks, there is medial migration of the eyes, assisted by frontal and temporal lobe expansion and greater proliferation of the lateral facial regions relative to the central face, resulting in facial expansion and interocular reduction.

The nasal placodes that formed at about 5 weeks each are separated inferiorly by a nasal groove. With continued proliferation of mesenchyme, the placodes submerge to form the nasal pits, the precursors to the anterior nares. As the nasal pits continue to submerge with the proliferating mesenchyme, they are eventually separated from the stomo-

todeum by only a thin oronasal membrane. This membrane will rupture at the beginning of the seventh week, forming a continuous nasal and oral cavity.

Genetic Analysis of Craniofacial Development

Our fundamental understanding of normal and abnormal human craniofacial development has been enormously advanced by gene targeting in mice in which more than 90 knockout mutants have been created to date. Although this large number reflects both the genetic and the morphogenetic complexity of head development, many of these malformations cluster into a few groups that can be characterized by the age of onset and the pattern of malformations observed in humans. The following is a summary of what is known at present of the genetics of the major human craniofacial malformations gained from homozygous knockout mouse studies.[35]

MIDLINE DEFECTS OR CRANIAL TRUNCATIONS

These defects initiate at mouse embryonic days 7 to 8 and are occasionally accompanied by laterality defects, with mutants frequently being resorbed before birth. Some examples include mice that are null for *Hesx1* (homeobox gene expressed in embryonic stem cells), *Lhx1* (LIM homeobox protein 1), *Otx2* (orthodenticle homologue 2), *Pcsk6* (proprotein convertase subtilisin/kexin type 6), *SHH,* and *Sil* (Tal1 interrupting locus). A number of these genes are expressed in the anterior visceral endoderm, which may act as an independent head organizer during early mammalian development.

NEURAL TUBE DEFECTS

These defects initiate at mouse embryonic day 8 and are designated as *exencephaly* when they are present in the cranial region. Examples of this rapidly increasing number of defects being identified include mice that are null for *Cart1* (cartilage homeoprotein 1), *Pax3* (paired box gene 3), *Tcfap2a* (transcription factor AP-2, α), and *Twist, Gli3* (GLI-Kruppel family member 3).

NEURAL CREST DEFECTS

These defects influence neural crest specification, migration, proliferation, and epithelial-mesenchymal induction. This is a notably large group that includes many members of the *Dlx* (distal-less), *Msx* (Msh-like) and *Prrx* (paired-related) homeodomain families, as well as *Gsc* (goosecoid), *Pax3*, and elements of the endothelial pathway. An unusual case is a homozygous knockout of *Hoxa2* (normally expressed in the second pharyngeal arch), which produces a homeotic respecification into first archlike structures. Clefts of the secondary palate frequently occur with this group, as an outcome of disturbed facial structural anatomic relationships.

SENSORY ORGAN DEFECTS

These defects include mice that are null for *Pax2, Pax6, Chx10* (ceh-10 homeodomain homologue), *Chrd* (chordin), *Rax* (retina and anterior neural fold homeobox), and *Bmp7* (bone morphogenetic protein 7). They exhibit sensory organ defects typically affecting the ear or eye.

ISOLATED CLEFTS OF THE SECONDARY PALATE

Although these defects are rare, they occur in the absence of other abnormalities in the *Jag2* (Jagged 2), *Lhx8*, and *Tgfβ3* (TGF-β3) knockout mice. These palatal clefts occur by different mechanisms, with the palatal shelves failing to elevate in *Jag2–/–* mice, whereas correctly positioned palatal shelves fail to fuse in *Tgfβ3–/–* mice.

SKELETAL DIFFERENTIATION DEFECTS

These defects of skeletal differentiation include mice that are null for *Runx2* (runt-related transcription factor 2), which is a master regulator of osteoblast and extracellular matrix differentiation such as *Col2a1* and *Col11a1* (collagens), *Crtl1* (cartilage link protein 1), and *Hspg2* (perlecan).

Some notable examples of orthologous gene mutations associated with craniofacial malformations in mice or humans include *SHH*, a signalling molecule that produces cyclopia and absent limbs in mice and holoprosencephaly in humans; *DHCR7*, an enzyme that produces growth and motor retardation in mice and Smith-Lemli-Opitz syndrome in humans; *TCOF1*, a nucleolar protein that produces multiple abnormalities in mice and Treacher Collins syndrome in humans; *EYA1*, a nuclear protein that produces a middle ear abnormality in mice and branchio-otorenal syndrome in humans; *TP63*, a transcription factor that produces a generalized epithelial defect in mice and ectrodactyly, ectodermal dysplasia, and cleft lip/palate in humans; *COL11A1*, a structural protein that produces a generalized cartilage defect in mice and Stickler and Marshall syndromes in humans; fibroblast growth factor receptor 1 *(FGFR1)*, a signal transduction that produces craniosynostosis in mice and Pfeiffer syndrome in humans; and *ALX4*, a transcription factor that produces polydactyly in mice and parietal foramina in humans.[35]

There is a progressively rapid increase in the identification of a known genetic map location or molecular basis for many human craniofacial malformations. Some selected examples include achondroplasia, from *FGFR3* gene at chromosome location 4p16.3; Apert syndrome, from *FGFR2* gene at 10q26; cleft lip/palate-ectodermal dysplasia syndrome from gene *PVRL1* at 11q23-q24; isolated cleft palate at chromosome location 2q32; X-linked cleft palate at Xq21.3; cleidocranial dysplasia from gene *RUNX2* at 6p21; Crouzon syndrome with acanthosis nigricans from gene *FGFR3* at 4p16.3; Crouzon syndrome and Jackson-Weiss syndrome from gene *FGFR2* at 10q26; isolated dental anomalies from gene *RUNX2* at 6p21; dentogenesis imperfecta from gene *DSPP* at 4q21; DiGeorge syndrome from gene *TBX1* at 22q11; anhydrotic ectodermal dysplasia from gene *ED1* at Xq12-q13.1; hemifacial microsomia at 14q32; holoprosencephaly-1 at 21q22.3; holoprosencephaly-2 from gene *SIX3* at 2p21; holoprosencephaly-3 from gene *SHH* at 7q36; holoprosencephaly-4 from gene *TGIF* at 18p11.3; holoprosencephaly-5 from gene *ZIC2* at 13q32; oligodontia from gene *PAX9* at 14q12-q13; oral-facial-digital syndrome 1 from gene *OFD1* at Xp22.3-p22.2; orofacial cleft-1 at 6p24.3; orofacial cleft-2 at 2p13; otopalatodigital sydrome, type I at Xq28; Pfeiffer syndrome from gene *FGFR1* at 8p11.2-p11.1; Pfeiffer syndrome from gene *FGFR2* at 10q26; Stickler syndrome, type I from gene *COL2A1* at 12q13.11-q13.2; Stickler syndrome, type II from gene *COL11A1* at 1p21; Stickler syndrome, type III from gene *COL11A2* at 6p21.3; Treacher Collins syndrome from gene *TCOF1* at 5q32-q33.1; Van der Woude syndrome at 1q32; and velocardiofacial syndrome at 22q11.[35] This is only a partial list of a constantly growing number of craniofacial malformations in which the genetic or molecular basis is being identified.

Formation of Neurocranium and Viscerocranium

Formation of the craniofacial bones begins with development of the cartilaginous and membranous precursors to the neurocranium and viscerocranium during the latter part of the fifth week of gestation (Figure 53-7). Major signaling pathways control skeletal patterning and are mediated by *Wnt* signaling proteins (Wnts), hedgehogs (SHH), bone morphogenetic proteins (BMPs), fibroblast growth factors (FGFs), and Notch/Delt.[36] The membranous neurocranium (desmocranium) that will give rise to the flat bones of the calvaria is connective tissue derived from the paraxial mesoderm and neural crest. The cartilaginous neurocranium (chondrocranium) that will form the cranial base is cartilage from neural crest origin. Cartilage maturation occurs in a caudal-rostral sequence. The membranous viscerocranium that will give rise to the maxilla, zygomatic bone, squamous temporal bone, and mandible is derived from the neural crest. The cartilaginous viscerocranium that will form the middle ear ossicles, styloid process of the temporal bone, hyoid bone, and laryngeal cartilages is from neural crest ectoderm. Endochondral ossification centers occur in the cartilaginous components and intramembranous ossification sites form in the membranous components of the neurocranium and viscerocranium. Osteoblast differentiation with the onset of mineralization results from a rapid angiogenic process with vascular ingrowth closely surrounding the centers and sites of ossification. The earliest ossification of the craniofacial bones begins in the seventh and eighth weeks of gestation. There are eventually 110 ossification centers, nearly all of

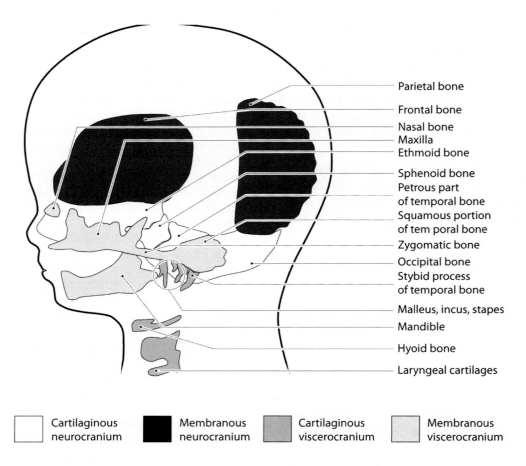

Parietal bone
Frontal bone
Nasal bone
Maxilla
Ethmoid bone
Sphenoid bone
Petrous part
of temporal bone
Squamous portion
of tem poral bone
Zygomatic bone
Occipital bone
Stybid process
of temporal bone
Malleus, incus, stapes
Mandible
Hyoid bone
Laryngeal cartilages

Cartilaginous
neurocranium

Membranous
neurocranium

Cartilaginous
viscerocranium

Membranous
viscerocranium

FIGURE 53-7.   Lateral view of a 20-week-old embryo illustrates initial development of the cartilaginous and membranous neurocranium and viscerocranium. Adapted from Moore KL, Persaud TVN. The developing human: clinically oriented embryology. 5th ed. Philadelphia (PA): W.B. Saunders; 1993. p. 361.

which appear between 6 and 12 weeks' gestation, that develop in the embryo to form 45 bones at birth, which ultimately form 22 bones in the adult.

Ossification

The onset of ossification generally follows the chronologic sequence of mandible, maxilla, palatine, cranial base, and cranium, with intramembranous sites usually preceding endochondral centers.[37] Intramembranous ossification of the mandible begins in the mental foramen region at 6 weeks of gestation lateral to Meckel's cartilage. The secondary mandibular condylar cartilage forms at 10 weeks' gestation as a separate endochondral condensation, adjacent to but independent of Meckel's cartilage and separated from the intramembranous the body of the mandible. Endochondral ossification of the mandibular condylar cartilage does not begin until 15 weeks. Maxillary intramembranous ossification begins in the area of the infraorbital foramen lateral to the nasal capsule. This ossification progresses anteriorly and posteriorly from this region. The vertical portion of the palatine bone then begins intramembranous ossification in the region of the palatine nerve, followed by ossification of the

anterior, then the posterior borders of the incisive foramen, spreading through the hard palate from the canine area. Following ossification of the main portion of the mandible and maxilla, during the sixth week of gestation, endochondral ossification of the cranial base occurs in the midline from the foramen magnum to the nasal bone, and intramembranous ossification occurs laterally. Finally, intramembranous ossification of the cranial bones follows.

Final Tissue Differentiation

Interaction between pharyngeal endoderm and neural crest tissue, followed by oral ectoderm proliferation, produces identifiable odontogenic tissue by the end of 4 weeks' gestation. There are four origin sites of odontogenic epithelium for both the maxillary and the mandibular arches, appearing at the end of 5 weeks' gestation. The primary anterior and first molar tooth germs appear at 6 weeks' gestation, followed by development of the primary second molar germs at 7 weeks. Apposition of bone on the alveolar margins of the maxilla and mandible in the presence of developing tooth germs forms the initial alveolar processes.

One of the last orofacial structures to reach completion at the end of the embryonic period is the secondary palate, developing from the paired lateral palatine shelves of the maxilla. These shelves are oriented vertically with the tongue interposed, but the tongue and floor of the oral cavity descend as the nasal chambers expand laterally and inferiorly (Figure 53-8). As this occurs, the palatal shelves become elongated and elevate medially toward each other, beginning fusion at the end of the eighth week and completing in the ninth week of gestation. There is evidence that TGF-β3 is intimately involved in regulating secondary palatal fusion by mediating the breakdown of the midline epithelial seam before fusion.[38]

Fetal Period

The fetal period begins during the ninth week, at 60 days' gestation, lasting until birth at 40 weeks, and overall

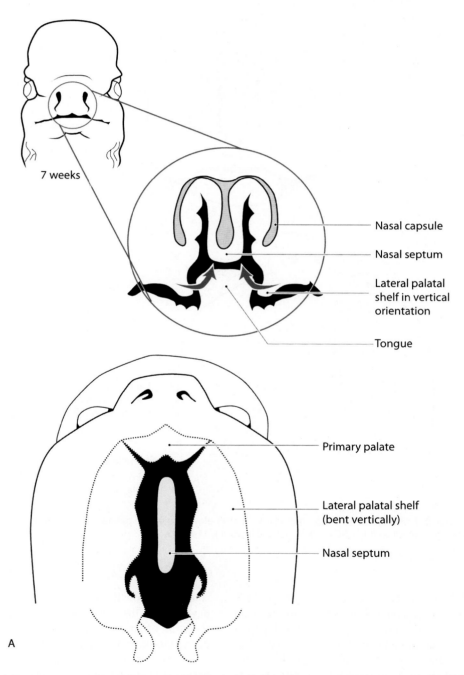

FIGURE 53-8. Frontal view of face, coronal section of stomodeum, and inferior view of palate in 7- and 12-week-old embryos. **A,** Embryo at 7 weeks shows the palatal shelves oriented vertically. *(Continued)*

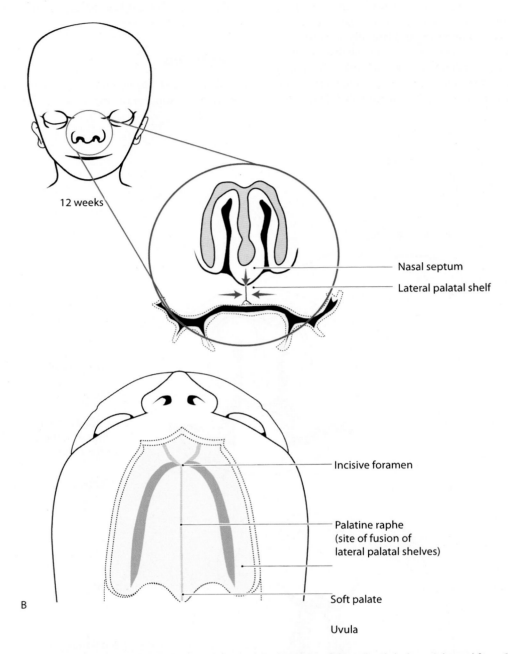

12 weeks

Nasal septum

Lateral palatal shelf

Incisive foramen

Palatine raphe
(site of fusion of
lateral palatal shelves)

Soft palate

B

Uvula

FIGURE 53-8. *(Continued)* **B,** Embryo at 12 weeks shows fusion after elevation of the palatal shelves. Adapted from Sperber G. Craniofacial development. Hamilton (ON): BC Decker Inc; 2001. pp. 41, 114, 116.

somatic growth follows a cephalocaudal growth gradient (Figure 53-9). There is a prenatal growth spurt between 20 and 30 weeks' gestation with the peak growth velocity at 27 to 28 weeks being approximately 2.5 cm per week. The prenatal spurt in weight is slightly later at 30 to 40 weeks' gestation with a peak at 34 to 36 weeks.[39] The rate steadily decreases during the last trimester and continues to decline after birth until adulthood, with two exceptions. The first is a

small "midgrowth" spurt that occurs in many children at 6 to 8 years old that has been attributed to increased adrenal secretion of androgenic hormones. The second is a dramatic endocrine-mediated "pubertal growth" spurt during adolescence. Growth of the craniofacial complex during the fetal period is characterized by a constant rate during the second trimester. The craniofacial skeletal components increase more in the anteroposterior dimension than in the vertical or

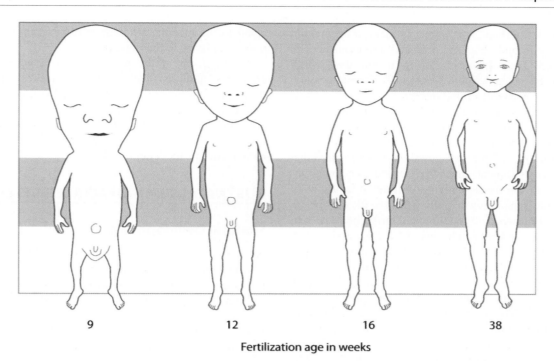

9   12   16   38

Fertilization age in weeks

FIGURE 53-9. Changes in fetal body proportions with all stages drawn to same total height. At the start of the fetal period, the head is half the length of the fetus, and by birth, it is one quarter the length. Adapted from Moore KL, Persaud TVN. The developing human: clinically oriented embryology. 5th ed. Philadelphia (PA): W.B. Saunders; 1993. p. 97.

transverse, with the exception of the mandible, which increases more in the transverse dimension in order to maintain appropriate articulation.[40]

During the fetal period, the neurocranium undergoes precocious development relative to the viscerocranium with earlier brain and neurocranial bone vault growth than facial and masticatory portions of the skull. This results in an early proportional predominance of the neurocranium over the face that only reduces to an 8:1 proportion by birth. The brain nearly doubles in size from 4 months' gestation to birth, achieving about 25% of its adult dimension. The formation and maintenance of cranial sutures are regulated by tissue interactions with the underlying dura mater as the brain develops.[41] A number of growth factors have been identified that regulate cranial bone growth and suture fusion, including TGF-β1, TGF-β2, TGF-β3, BMP-2, BMP-7, FGF-4, insulin-like growth factor-I (IGF-I), and SHH.[42,43] Transcription factors MSX2 and TWIST also play a role in suture development, binding to target effector genes to determine their expression.[44] The cranial vault elements are developed at the boundary between cranial neural crest– and mesoderm-derived tissue. The frontal bones are derived from neural crest, whereas the parietal and occipital bones are of mesoderm origin.[21] This results in the coronal, sagittal, and lambdoid sutures occurring at the neural crest–mesoderm interface. The metopic suture is the only human cranial suture not formed between neural crest and mesoderm, being entirely of neural crest origin. Mandibular morphogenesis is tightly controlled by BMP and FGF signaling in the ectoderm.[45] The eyeballs grow concurrently with the early brain growth,

increasing facial expansion and separating the neural and facial skeletons to increase skull height. The cranial base growth parallels the rapid growth of the cranial vault during the fetal period. The anterior cranial base grows sevenfold whereas the posterior cranial base increases fivefold. The intraethmoidal and intrasphenoidal synchondroses close before birth.

The ossification centers that begin the formation of the facial bones late in the embryonic period at 6 to 8 weeks enlarge during the early fetal period until most of the bones have developed into a definitive shape by 14 weeks. At this time, they begin to remodel as they continue to grow by intramembranous and/or endochondral ossification. Mandibular condylar cartilage appears relatively late at 10 weeks, well after the embryonic period when a rudimentary mandible already is present.[46] This secondary cartilage may serve as an intrinsic center of growth at this stage, in contrast to its later growth that is predominantly extrinsically determined. The anterior aspects of the maxilla, mandible, and zygoma of the fetal and early postnatal face undergo osseous deposition at this time. This early anterior deposition is necessary to permit adequate osseous mass for the developing tooth buds of the primary and permanent dentitions. Although the tooth germs start to develop as early as 6 weeks' gestation, the onset of dental mineralization does not begin until ossification has occurred. The maxilla demonstrates a rapid height increase associated with dental development.[47] Once the primary teeth have erupted, the anterior aspect of the maxilla undergoes resorption rather than deposition to produce the descent of the maxilla with continued growth. Meanwhile,

SECTION 7

the posterior, infraorbital, and lingual surfaces of the maxilla are depository in both fetal and postnatal development. The fetal temporal bone grows faster in height than width whereas the lateral and inferior margins of the zygomatic bone grow faster than its orbital margin.[47]

The paranasal sinuses, including the maxillary, sphenoidal, frontal, and ethmoidal, start developing at the beginning of the fetal period. Pneumatization begins first with the maxillary sinus, starting at 5 months' gestation. It is proposed that a septomaxillary ligament, attached to the sides and anteroinferior border of the nasal septum and inserted in the nasal spine, transmits septal growth, pulling the maxilla downward. Between the 10th week of gestation and birth, the nasal septum increases its vertical height sevenfold. The nasal septum growth, together with neural growth and facial sutural growth, transposes the maxilla inferiorly and anteriorly. The frontomaxillary, frontonasal, frontozygomatic, frontoethmoidal, and ethmoidomaxillary sutures grow predominantly in a vertical direction. The temporozygomatic and nasomaxillary sutures contribute most of the anteroposterior change. The intermaxillary and zygomaticomaxillary sutures provide most of the transverse expansion of the face. Overall, the middle and lower thirds of the face develop primarily in a downward and slightly forward direction away from the cranial base owing to brain development, maxillary and palatine sutural growth, and possibly nasal septum growth.

Although the midsagittal part of the middle face consists entirely of nasal septal cartilage during the fetal period, ossification leaves only a small anterior part of this cartilage remaining postnatally. Currently, there is controversy regarding the role of the nasal septum in postnatal facial growth. Some believe it is limited to a compensatory and biomechanical role, and others believe it serves a more extensive role, particularly in promoting vertical maxillary growth.

Although the mandible is larger than the maxilla during the embryonic period, the mandible approximates the size of the maxilla within the first month of the fetal period. The three secondary cartilages of the mandible do not appear until the 10th and 14th weeks of gestation, forming on the lateral and superior aspects of the condylar processes. This secondary type of cartilage differs morphologically from epiphyseal and synchondrosal cartilage.[48] Two of these secondary cartilages forming at the mental protuberance and the coronoid process ossify before birth, leaving only the cartilage on the condylar head as a site of postnatal mandibular endochondral growth. This cartilage never undergoes complete ossification, providing a means for absorbing functional forces and retaining growth potential throughout life. Between the 13th and the 20th weeks of gestation, the mandible lags behind the maxilla again while there is a transition from Meckel's cartilage to condylar cartilage as the primary growth site. During the third trimester, there is a significant deepening of the corpus in association with the developing dentition. The mandibular ramus growth rate is greater than the growth rate of the mandibular body during this time.[49] At the time of birth, the mandible usually is equal in size

again to the maxilla, although it often is in a retrognathic position relative to the maxilla.

Development of the permanent tooth germs begins at 16 weeks' gestation, with the first permanent molar germs developing posteriorly from the dental lamina followed by the permanent anterior tooth germs emerging from the lingual side of the primary enamel organs. At birth, the primary tooth crowns are still not completely calcified, as the first permanent molars begin to calcify.

POSTNATAL CRANIOFACIAL DEVELOPMENT

Skeletal Development

An area of craniofacial growth can be differentiated as a growth center or growth site. A *growth center* is where there is primarily intrinsic genetic growth control with a minimal environmental or functional role. Although a *growth site* also is controlled to some extent by genetic programming, it is more vulnerable to extrinsic growth control, being dependent more on the functional influence of the surrounding tissues. Cranial base synchondroses, where endochondral ossification of primary cartilage occurs, represent growth centers. The role of the cartilaginous nasal septum as a growth center or site remains controversial. There is a clearer understanding that the endochondral growth of the secondary cartilage of the mandibular condyles acts as a growth site, being greatly influenced by mandibular and soft tissue function. Areas of membranous bone growth resulting from sutural or periosteal ossification are primarily growth sites and represent the bulk of the remaining craniofacial complex. There are exceptions, such as craniosynostosis, that can be due to an underlying genetic cause. Membranous ossification by sutural and periosteal remodeling is essentially the only type of craniofacial bone growth that occurs after adolescence and throughout adulthood.

Development and completion of craniofacial growth follow the overall somatic cephalocaudal growth gradient throughout prenatal and postnatal growth, with cranial vault growth completing before the cranial base, followed by the nasomaxilla and finishing with the mandible. During postnatal growth, the neurocranium continues to develop ahead of the viscerocranium (Figure 53-10). It increases from about 30% of its ultimate adult size at the time of birth to 50% by 6 months of age, 75% by 2 years of age, and nearly 90% by 3 years of age. By 5 years of age, the orbits have reached nearly 80% of their adult size.[50] This is why a child of this age appears to have a disproportionately large cranium and eyes. After birth, the neurocranium increases about five times in size, whereas the viscerocranium increases about 10 times. There is also a difference in the amount of postnatal increase in the three dimensions, with the vertical increasing by about 200%, the anteroposterior by somewhat less, and the transverse by the least at approximately 75%. By 10 years of age, the neurocranial growth is nearly 95% complete, whereas facial growth is only about 60% complete.

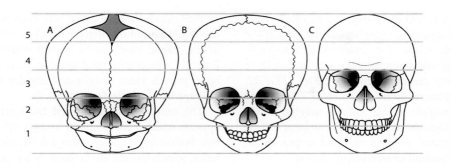

FIGURE 53-10.   Changes in postnatal skull proportions with all stages enlarged to the same skull height and oriented in Frankfort horizontal plane with skull height divided into fifths. **A,** Neonate, showing the viscerocranium representing one fifth of the total height. Three-year-old **(B)** and adult **(C)** show the proportional increase in height of the viscerocranium relative to the neurocranium. Adapted from Sarnat BG. Normal and abnormal craniofacial growth. Some experimental and clinical considerations. Angle Orthod 1983;53:263.

The craniofacial complex can be divided conveniently into four primary units: the cranial vault, the cranial base, the nasomaxilla, and the mandible. Each of these units has its growth regulated to some extent by both intrinsic and extrinsic controls. Our understanding of postnatal craniofacial growth has developed in part from cross-sectional anatomic and histologic studies of human cadavers and skeletal material. What has been particularly helpful in supplementing this material is a number of North American longitudinal craniofacial growth records and longitudinal implant (used for stable reference points) studies that were gathered from the 1940s to the mid-1960s before radiation hygiene and human subject research standards became more stringent.[51]

Cranial Vault

At birth, the cranial bones are separated by sutures with fontanelles where the corners of the bones meet, permitting compression of the skull during the birthing process (Figure 53-11). Postnatal bone growth results in narrowing of the sutures with all of the fontanelles closing within the first 2 years. In the absence of any intrinsic growth potential in the sutures, the pressures exerted by the developing brain determine the size and shape of the cranium. As the brain expands, the internal pressure creates tension across the connective tissue of the sutures and compression against the cranial bones, resulting in intramembranous bone growth by suture and surface apposition. Modeling of the cranial bones to a flatter shape is necessary to adapt to the expanding surface of the brain. This occurs primarily from endocranial resorption and ectocranial apposition. Although suture apposition plays a larger role than surface apposition in overall cranial vault capacity, the postnatal shape primarily is determined by extrinsic factors.

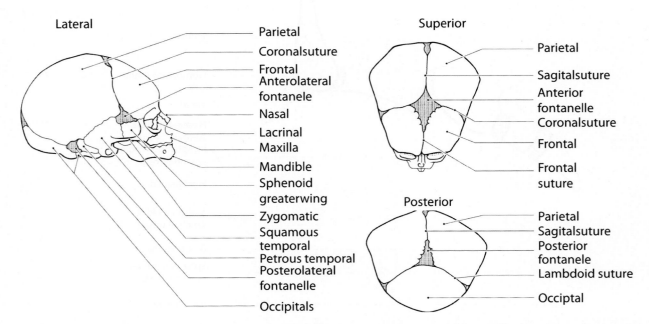

FIGURE 53-11.   Fontanelles and sutures of the neonatal skull. Adapted from Sperber G. Craniofacial development. Hamilton (ON): BC Decker Inc; 2001. p. 84.

The premature fusion (craniosynostosis) of one cranial suture may not cause a significant functional effect but, if left untreated, will distort the shape of the cranium. Craniosynostosis is often caused by dominant mutations in one of three fibroblast growth factor receptor genes (*FGFR*1, *FGFR2, and FGFR3*) or in the transcription factor *TWIST.*[52] Untreated premature fusion of multiple cranial sutures may adversely affect neurologic development as well. Early surgical release during the first 2 postnatal years is required to prevent or minimize cranial deformation or neurologic deficit.

By 6 to 7 years of age, the inner table of the cranial bones becomes stable due to the cessation of cerebral growth. However, the outer table continues to model in response to extracranial muscular forces. The temporal muscles tend to laterally compress the cranium, forming temporal sulci and zygomatic arches. The lateral and posterior cervical muscles insert primarily on the squamous part of the temporal and occipital bones, influencing their shape. Even after attainment of the adult form, the cranial bones continue to thicken during adulthood.

Cranial Base

Compared with the other craniofacial units, the shape of the cranial base is relatively stable during growth, due likely to its greater intrinsic growth potential. Perhaps more than any other craniofacial area, growth of the cranial base is genetically predetermined in the midline by endochondral bone growth at the synchodroses and influenced the least by functional matrices.[53,54] However, prenatal brain growth may provide a minor extrinsic influence, causing some flattening

of the cranial base, because this does not occur with anencephaly. In addition, there is evidence that chondral growth of the cranial base can be altered with mechanical forces.[55] Lateral to the cranial base midline, there is intramembranous bone growth from sutures and surface remodeling that are affected by extrinsic factors.

The cranial base is formed from primary cartilage that appears underneath the brain in the sixth week of embryonic life. Following initial osseous calcification during the eighth week, synchodroses are created by the residual cartilage and continue the endochondral bone formation, pushing the cranial base bones apart centrally while sutures more laterally produce intramembranous bone growth. The anterior cranial base matures earlier than the posterior cranial base, with the posterior intraoccipital synchondroses closing during the second and third years postnatally and the anterior intraoccipital synchondroses closing at 3 to 4 years of age (Figure 53-12). The sphenoethmoidal synchondrosis closes at about 6 years of age. Although the spheno-occipital synchondrosis is not a main growth site before birth, it provides the greatest contribution to cranial base growth postnatally, delaying fusion until adolescence. The prolonged postnatal growth period of the spheno-occipital synchondrosis permits posterior growth of the maxilla to provide adequate bone for the developing posterior permanent teeth and adequate space for the nasopharynx. In addition to endochondral bone growth in the midline, intramembranous remodeling of the cranial base occurs, including apposition on the basioccipital bone and anterior margin of the foramen magnum, resulting in continued lengthening of the posterior cranial base even

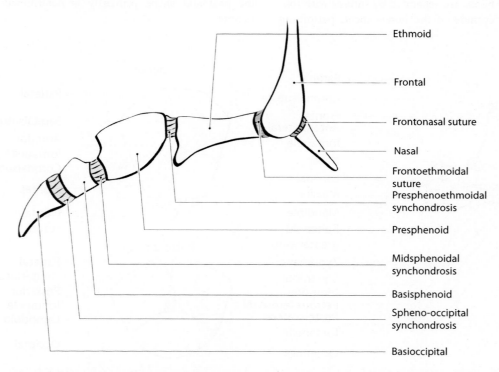

Ethmoid

Frontal

Frontonasal suture

Nasal

Frontoethmoidal suture
Presphenoethmoidal synchondrosis

Presphenoid

Midsphenoidal synchondrosis

Basisphenoid

Spheno-occipital synchondrosis

Basioccipital

FIGURE 53-12. Midsagittal neonatal cranial base shows sutures and synchondroses. Adapted from Mooney MP, Siegel MI. Understanding craniofacial anomalies: the etiopathogenesis of craniosynostoses and facial clefting. New York (NY): Wiley-Liss, Inc.; 2002.

after adolescence. Enlargement of the sella turcica continues postnatally, with the anterior wall stabilizing at about 6 years of age and the posterior wall continuing to resorb until late adolescence.

Failure of normal endochondral bone growth in the cranial base is manifested in achondroplasia, caused from a mutation in FGFR3 gene, that usually results in midface deficiency associated with a class III malocclusion (Figure 53-13). Premature fusion of multiple sutures lateral to the cranial base midline may occur with some congenital malformations that also result in midface deficiency, such as craniofacial dysostosis (Crouzon syndrome) or acrocephalosyndactyly (Apert syndrome) both of which are caused from a mutation in the *FGFR2* gene (Figure 53-14).

Nasomaxilla

The prenatal precocity of neurocranial growth relative to the face becomes less predominant postnatally. Nevertheless, considerable postnatal displacement of the nasomaxilla downward and forward occurs owing to continued growth of the brain and cranial base. This inferior and anterior maxillary transposition is augmented by the sutural growth between the cranial base and the maxilla and growth of the nasal septum. After birth, the vertical growth of the maxilla continues with contributions from the frontomaxillary, frontonasal, frontozygomatic, frontoethmoidal, ethmoidomaxillary sutures, and possibly, the nasal septum (Figure 53-15). The vertical descent of the maxilla is further increased by modeling with resorption on the nasal surfaces and the simultaneous apposition on the oral surfaces. The zygomas are repositioned down and forward with resorption on their internal surfaces and apposition on their external surfaces. Anteroposterior growth continues with temporozygomatic and nasomaxillary sutural growth and transverse growth from intermaxillary and zygomaticomaxillary sutures. The resulting downward and forward translation displaces

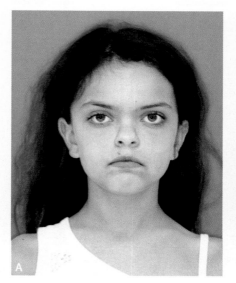
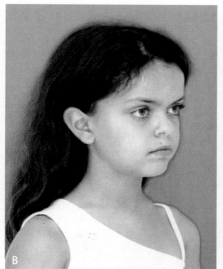
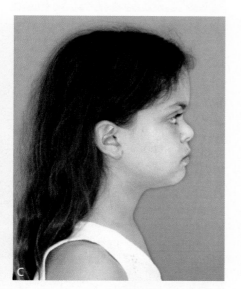
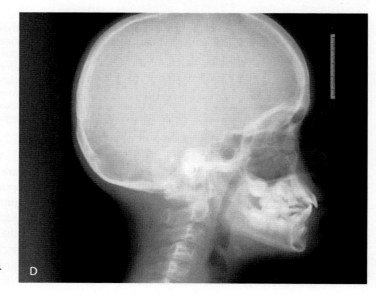

FIGURE 53-13.   A 10-year and 3-month-old female with achondroplasia, characterized by short stature and midface deficiency from failure of normal primary cartilage growth. The severity of the skeletal discrepancy from the deficient cranial base growth usually results in class III malocclusion but is not present here. **A,** Frontal view. **B,** Three-quarter view. **C,** Profile view. **D,** Lateral cephalometric radiograph.

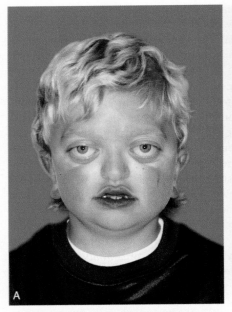
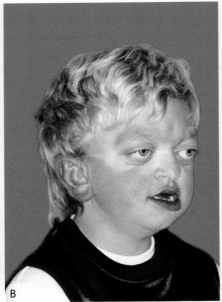
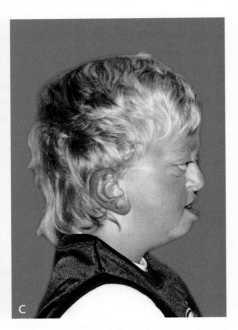

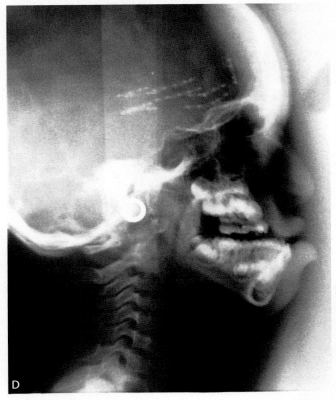

FIGURE 53-14. A 7-year and 1-month-old male with craniofacial dysostosis (Crouzon syndrome), characterized by midface deficiency from multiple premature suture synostoses and abnormal cranial base growth. This can result in significant optic and nasal airway functional issues as well as intracranial pressure and a class III malocclusion. This patient had a frontal bone advancement at 14 months old to relieve intracranial pressure. **A,** Frontal view. **B,** Three-quarter view. **C,** Profile view. **D,** Lateral cephalometric radiograph.

adjacent bones and permits adequate space for the developing nasopharynx and appositional growth at the posterior aspect of the maxilla and maxillary tuberosities to provide additional posterior alveolar space for the development and eruption of the maxillary molars. Following the postnatal growth of the facial sutures, they serve as sites of fibrous union where some remodeling still can take place. In fact, a number of cranial and facial sutures are interdigitated but still not fused even beyond 50 years of age.

Growth determinants for postnatal nasomaxillary growth are not well understood and include a variety of intrinsic and extrinsic factors. Passive displacement secondary to genetic intrinsic brain and cranial base growth and, perhaps, nasal septal growth guidance are the most significant influences on the downward and forward movements of the maxilla after birth until about the seventh postnatal year when most neural growth is complete. From that age through adolescence, these influences dramatically decrease, accounting for about

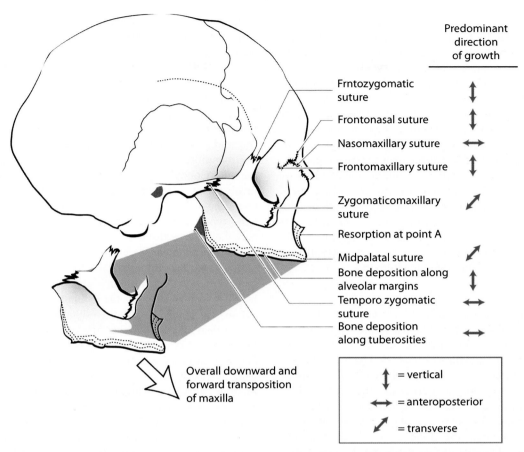

Predominant direction of growth

Frntozygomatic suture

Frontonasal suture

Nasomaxillary suture

Frontomaxillary suture

Zygomaticomaxillary suture

Resorption at point A

Midpalatal suture

Bone deposition along alveolar margins

Temporo zygomatic suture

Bone deposition along tuberosities

Overall downward and forward transposition of maxilla

= vertical

= anteroposterior

= transverse

FIGURE 53-15. Nasomaxillary intramembranous growth at various sites, resulting in an overall downward and forward transposition of the maxilla relative to the cranial base. Adapted from Sperber G. Craniofacial development. Hamilton (ON): BC Decker Inc; 2001. p. 107.

one third of forward maxillary movement, as intramembranous epigenetic extrinsic sutural growth and surface modeling predominate. Maxillary growth also depends to a great extent on various functional matrices. In addition to the effect of brain growth on the maxillary position, there is the influence of eyeball growth and their functional movement on the size and shape of the orbits, the influence of respiration on the nasal cavity, the influence of oral function in determining tuberosity, palatal and alveolar development, and the surrounding facial soft tissues, all of which contribute functional roles in determining the extent of sutural growth and modeling of the nasomaxilla.[56]

Although the mode of nasomaxillary growth is predominantly intramembranous from sutural growth and surface remodeling, some endochondral bone growth takes place in the nasal septum, made up of secondary cartilage. As mentioned previously, the growth mechanism is mostly the nasomaxilla being pushed from behind by the brain and cranial base growth until about age 7, when a different mechanism begins to predominate whereby the nasomaxilla is pulled forward by soft tissue and probably to a small extent from nasal cartilage growth with concomitant growth of circummaxillary sutures. Significant modeling must occur in order to maintain the general shape of the maxilla as it is displaced

downward. As mentioned previously, resorption of the nasal side of the maxilla, providing nasal cavity enlargement, occurs concomitantly with apposition on the oral side, resulting in descent of the maxilla. This descent, together with variable amounts of dental eruption, is reflected as external rotation of the maxilla. The maxilla undergoes a modest and variable amount of internal rotation as it remodels that can result in slight forward or backward rotation but usually is equal to the external rotation, resulting in a zero net rotational change. However, the cumulative rotation may be significant in individuals with short or long face types.[57]

Although secondary pneumatization of the maxillary sinus begins prenatally, it does not occur for the other paranasal sinuses until after birth (first 2 postnatal years for ethmoidal and frontal sinuses and the 6–7 postnatal years for sphenoidal sinuses). The vertical growth of the maxillary alveolar process is rapid during dental eruption, surpassing the vertical descent of the palate threefold. This alveolar development provides a large contribution to the depth and width of the palate and vertical height of the face. Considerable resorption of the anterior surface of the maxilla minimizes the overall forward displacement of the maxilla by about 25% and creates a deeper supra-alveolar concavity while increasing the relative prominence of the anterior nasal

SECTION 7

spine. Transverse growth occurs by lateral displacement of the maxillary bodies by means of the midpalatal suture and bone resorption on the lateral borders of the nasal cavity. Transverse development of the maxillary alveolar process continues with buccal eruption of the posterior teeth. Growth of the midpalatal suture ends after the first 2 postnatal years, but the suture remains patent until late adolescence, with fusion usually not being complete until the third decade.

Preadolescent and adolescent nasal growth increases on average at a rate about 25% greater than maxillary growth. The mechanism of nasal growth is a combination of an endochondral component from the nasal cartilage and an intramembranous component from sutural growth behind the nose. Although the nasal bone grows up until about age 10 with frontonasal sutural apposition and modeling, interstitial nasal cartilage growth continues increasing the overall size beyond adolescence and throughout adulthood.

Mandible

The mandible has the most delayed growth and the most postnatal growth of all the facial bones. Although usually in a retrognathic position relative to the maxilla at birth, rapid postnatal growth corrects this discrepancy. The right and left bodies of the mandible are still separate at birth, uniting at the midline mental symphysis during the first year of life. There are no intrinsic centers of mandibular growth. The primary sites of mandibular postnatal growth are the endochondral apposition occurring at the condylar cartilages and extensive intramembranous surface modeling. This modeling includes, but is not limited to, apposition on the posterior and lateral aspects of the rami and the posterior alveolar ridges as well as resorption of the anterior surface of the condyles, the anterior contours of the rami, and the inner surface of the mandibular bodies (Figure 53-16). The accentuation of

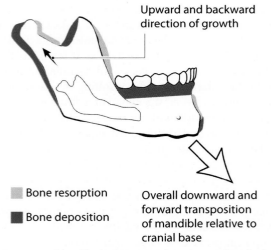

Upward and backward direction of growth

■ Bone resorption
■ Bone deposition

Overall downward and forward transposition of mandible relative to cranial base

FIGURE 53-16. Mandibular intramembranous and endochondral growth, resulting in an overall downward and forward transposition of mandible relative to cranial base. An outline of the fetal mandible is superimposed on the adult mandible for size and shape comparison. Adapted from Sperber G. Craniofacial development. Hamilton (ON): BC Decker Inc; 2001. p. 130.

chin prominence that typically occurs results primarily from facial resorption between the chin and the base of the mandibular alveolus rather than apposition on the chin itself. The growth of the condylar cartilage contributes most of the total ramus height, whereas growth of alveolar bone contributes aproximately 60% to the mandibular body height.[58] Proliferation of condylar cartilage, in response to growth and function of muscles and adjacent soft tissue, results in superior and posterior growth of the condylar heads, displacing the mandible downward and forward in concert with the maxilla. Condylar growth appears to involve the sequential involvement of transcription factor SOX9, expressed by chondrocytes, which regulates the synthesis of type II collagen, type X collagen secreted as matrix, and vascular endothelial growth factor secreted to regulate the neovascularization of the cartilage.[59]

At birth, the inclination of the mandibular condyles is more horizontal, resulting in a greater increase in length than height. During childhood, the inclination becomes more vertical so that condylar growth results in a greater increase in height than length. However, there is great variability in this inclination within the general population, influencing the degree to which the mandibular growth is expressed in a forward anteriorly rotating, as opposed to downward posteriorly rotating, direction. Simultaneous modeling of the inferior mandibular border with resorption at the gonial angle and minimal apposition of the anterior aspect of the lower border tends to reduce the effect of this rotation on facial morphology. The final rotational position of the mandible with growth is a result of the combined influences of external mandibular rotation from downward nasomaxillary growth and dental eruption and the internal mandibular rotation from compensatory modeling. Internal mandibular rotation is variable but is typically 15 degrees whereas external mandibular rotation averages 11 to 12 degrees, producing an overall forward rotation of 3 to 4 degrees.[57,60] This overall rotation tends to decrease with greater internal rotation in individuals with short faces, resulting in a deep anterior overbite. With the long face individual, the internal rotation is decreased or even backward internal rotation may occur, often resulting in an anterior open bite and mandibular deficiency.

The mandible has its greatest postnatal growth velocity in the first 6 months after birth with the greatest change in mandibular length, followed by ramus height, then corpus length.[61] Although minimal maxillary growth occurs after approximately 10 years of age, mandibular growth continues longer, to the end of adolescent growth. This differential growth, typically characterized by a peak in the rate of mandibular growth at puberty, usually results in the final correction of the mandibular position relative to the maxilla. Longitudinal growth studies have demonstrated that there are a substantial number of individuals, more commonly females, who demonstrate an early acceleration in mandibular growth that can occur during preadolescence.[62] This "juvenile" acceleration may equal or even exceed the later acceleration during puberty.

If the cranial base is the craniofacial skeletal unit whose growth is least determined by extrinsic epigenetic or environmental factors, the mandible is the opposite extreme with its growth highly dependent on the postnatal functional demands placed on it. It has a great capacity to adapt to mandibular displacement and accommodate to lingual and labial soft tissue, resting postural and active muscular function, and mastication. The condylar inclination, dictating the type of mandibular growth rotation, is determined by these pulling secondary functional influences. The relevant functional matrices include the lateral pterygoid attached to the condylar neck, the growth and function of the tongue, the masticatory muscles attached to the buccal and lingual aspects and to the coronoid process, and the facial soft tissue and musculature, all influencing the ultimate size and shape of the mandible. For this reason, the mandible, more than any other part of the craniofacial complex, may have a low intrinsic growth poten-

tial that is significantly increased and regulated in response to extrinsic functional demand. This mandibular growth dependence on function is clearly reflected in clinical conditions in which mandibular growth has been restricted from persistent unilateral or bilateral limited mandibular function owing to a congenital disorder, postnatal trauma, or pathology. It is just as evident in clinical conditions in which mandibular growth is enhanced in the presence of a postnatal pathology in which persistant lingual soft tissue affects the size or resting position of the tongue or a pituitary adenoma increases skeletal and soft tissue growth (Figures 53-17 and 53-18).

Dental Development

The alveolar processes contribute a great portion of the vertical height of the lower face. Their development is entirely dependent on the presence and eruption of the primary and

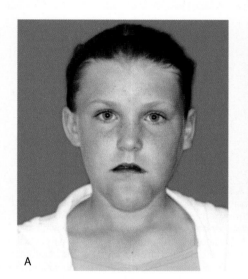

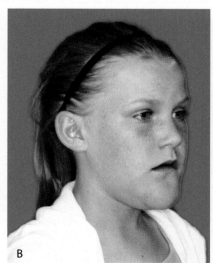

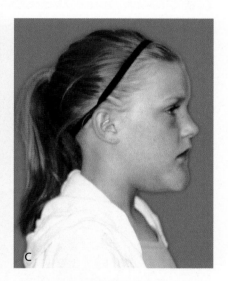

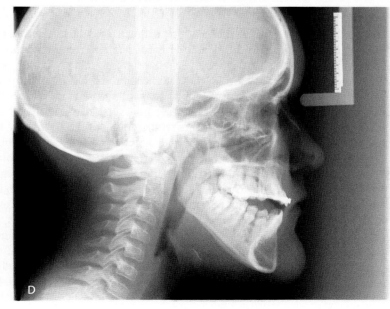

FIGURE 53-17.   A 10-year and 4-month-old female with a lymphatic malformation of the floor of the mouth and tongue, with an elevated and enlarged tongue, creating a class III malocclusion with mandibular prognathism, anterior and posterior open bites, and an expanded mandibular arch from the lingual soft tissue mass and additional mandibular condylar growth. **A,** Frontal view. **B,** Three-quarter view. **C,** Profile view. **D,** Lateral cephalometric radiograph.

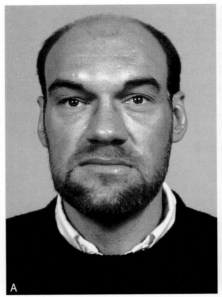
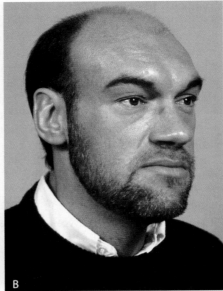
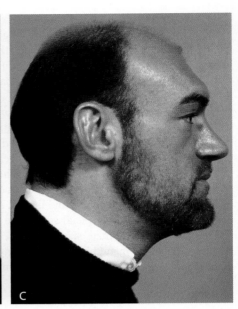

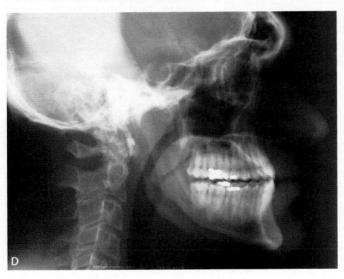

FIGURE 53-18. A 33-year and 3-month-old male with acromegaly (adult hyperpituitarism), with mandibular prognathism and coarse facial features from additional intramembranous and mandibular condylar endochondral skeletal growth as well as soft tissue growth. This condition results in a class III malocclusion and an expanded mandibular arch from tongue and mandibular condylar growth. **A,** Frontal view. **B,** Three-quarter view. **C,** Profile view. **D,** Lateral cephalometric radiograph.

permanent dentition. Just as vertical appositional alveolar growth accompanies vertical dental eruption, transverse apposition complements transverse dental eruption. This minor contribution to the transverse dimension of the alveolar processes continues until about 7 years of age, with eruption of the permanent incisors. Further transverse dentoalveolar growth is minimal, occurring with eruption of the premolars and canines. Facial growth and the concomitant increase in the size of the jaws occur posteriorly, creating additional space for the dentition only in the molar region.

Eruption of the maxillary teeth enhances the vertical dimension of the maxilla with posterior development of the maxillary tuberosities to accommodate the development and eruption of the maxillary posterior teeth. In the mandible, progressive resorption of the anterior ramal surfaces and apposition of the posterior ramal surfaces provide alveolar space for the sequential development and eruption of the mandibular posterior teeth. Eruption of the mandibular teeth

enhances the vertical growth of the mandible and also contributes to the height of the face. However, compensatory condylar growth and internal mandibular rotational modeling must occur to prevent the mandible from rotating posteriorly as the maxilla grows downward and the dentition erupts. Dental emergence into the oral cavity begins at approximately the sixth postnatal month, and the primary dentition is established by 2.5 years of age. The primary incisors begin to exfoliate at 6 to 7 years of age, and the permanent dentition begins to emerge with eruption of the mandibular incisors and first molars. The permanent dentition is established by 12 to 14 years of age except for the eruption of the third molars, contributing to the vertical dimension of the lower face during adolescent growth.

The anteroposterior eruption of the permanent incisors is affected by the facial growth pattern.[63a] Individuals with class III facial growth tend to have minimal anterior and some distal mandibular dental eruption, whereas class II facial growth results in greater anterior mandibular dental eruption to compensate for the underlying anteroposterior skeletal discrepancies. Short facial growth pattern tends to promote anterior mandibular rotation with increased incisor uprighting and deepening of the anterior overbite, whereas long facial growth pattern results in posterior mandibular rotation with increased incisor protrusion and opening of the anterior overbite.[63]

Facial Development

The growth of the facial soft tissue follows the underlying facial bones but is not directly correlated with bone growth. Facial soft tissue is thicker relative to the underlying skeletal tissue in the young child owing to subcutaneous fat. This is one of the reasons it is more challenging to assess potential underlying skeletal discrepancies in the young child based only on a clinical appraisal. The thicker soft tissue envelope, together with the relative retrognathic position of the mandible, creates a more convex profile in infancy and early childhood. Lip thickness increases until it reaches a maximum at the end of the pubertal growth spurt, then decreases in late teens and adulthood.[64,65] These later changes, combined with continued forward nasal growth as well as anterior mandibular and chin projection, leave the lips with a more retrusive appearance and the nose and chin with a more prominent appearance. These changes usually create a flatter facial profile in older adolescents and adults. This tendency is even greater on average in males than females, owing to less subcutaneous fat, combined with more nasal cartilage growth and anterior mandibular and chin projection in males.

The facial soft tissue also follows the cephalocaudal growth gradient, with the soft tissue of the lower face growing more in magnitude and duration than the upper face. Before adolescence, vertical lip growth lags behind skeletal jaw growth, resulting in lack of resting lip apposition. During and after pubertal growth, vertical lip growth increases proportional to the underlying vertical skeletal growth, creating a more likely chance of resting lip apposition in adults.[66]

There is significant growth in the length and prominence of the nose during adolescence, influencing the facial balance between the nose, the lips, and the chin.[67] In fact, the vertical nasal growth is much greater than anteroposterior or transverse nasal growth. Nasal growth during adolescence is primarily limited to cartilage and soft tissue because the nasal bone usually has completed growth before puberty. The nasal shape often changes before adolescence, with the upper nasal dorsum developing superiorly and anteriorly, and the lower nasal dorsum more often following the lower facial growth pattern. In other words, individuals who have a more anterior and superior rotational pattern of lower face growth will exhibit a similar rotation of the lower nasal dorsum. There is some evidence that skeletal class II jaw relationships usually demonstrate a more prominent nasal bridge and convex dorsum than balanced jaw relationships.[68]

The upper third of the face grows the most rapidly early in life owing to brain growth and achieves its ultimate size earliest, finishing most growth by 12 years of age. Orbital height already reaches 55% of its adult height at birth and 94% by 7 years of age.[69] The middle and lower thirds of the face are less affected by brain growth, growing more slowly and for a longer time. Most of the middle third growth is completed later during puberty, with the lower third of the face continuing to grow beyond puberty into adulthood.

In addition to this vertical sequential growth gradient, craniofacial growth does not take place at an equal rate in the three planes of space. Facial growth follows a sequence in which transverse growth finishes first, followed by anteroposterior and finally vertical growth, although all three continue to some extent during adulthood.[70] The face reflects the early transverse neural expansion of the cranium, the early fusion of the mandibular symphysis, and the early growth cessation of the midpalatal suture during the first few years of life. The width of both jaws, including the dental arches, is largely completed before adolescent growth, with the exception of dental arches achieving greater width posteriorly owing to continued increase in jaw length. This presents clinically as a disproportionately wide face relative to the height in the infant and young child. Both jaws continue to grow in length and height throughout pubertal growth. As the maxilla and mandible displace and grow downward and forward, the anteroposterior and vertical growth begin to take proportionately greater roles. The growth rate of the maxilla slows down after approximately 10 years of age and, together with anterior maxillary resorption, reduces the relative anterior projection of the midface. The maxillary length reaches maturity before the upper facial height, which is followed by mandibular length and finally ramus height.[71] The somewhat retrognathic position of the mandible at birth usually is corrected early in postnatal life. The mandible grows for a longer duration than the maxilla, typically undergoing a growth spurt at puberty. Anteroposterior growth is accompanied and then followed by vertical facial growth, primarily in the mandible, often continuing well beyond puberty, even into the third and fourth decades.

There are gender differences in facial growth, with males characteristically having volume changes of greater magnitude than females. Females have much less nasal growth on average, with many not even exhibiting a pubertal nasal growth spurt, in contrast to males who characteristically have a nasal growth spurt throughout puberty. Females have earlier soft tissue growth that follows their earlier puberty and they have greater lip thickness at all ages. The flattening of the facial profile during adolescence is less dramatic in females, owing in part to their fuller lips and less prominent noses but also owing to females having less forward mandibular growth projection and chin growth. Females have on average more late vertical maxillary growth than males. If mandibular growth is not matching these late maxillary changes, the mandible translates downward and backward, resulting in a more convex profile. Not only are male facial volume changes on average greater in magnitude, but the duration of the changes is longer and there is more predominance of volume increase in the lower third of the face.[72] Males are on average more likely to have late mandibular growth that may be beneficial in improving a maxillary protrusion or mandibular retrusion but is disadvantageous when a mandibular prognathism or maxillary retrusion is present before late growth.

Growth and Facial Changes during Adulthood

There has been awareness since the late 19th century that human growth continues beyond adolescence, at least until the fourth or fifth decade of life.[73] Nevertheless, investigators in the mid-20th century were surprised to find that facial growth continues into the sixth decade of life.[74] Later, it was found that the craniofacial complex models throughout adulthood, with thickening of the frontal region of the cranium and a symmetrical modest increase in the size of the cranium, cranial base, maxilla, and mandible.[75,76]

In the late 20th century and early 21st century, a number of longitudinal craniofacial growth studies have examined changes during adulthood.[77–84] Evaluation of the serial cephalometric radiographs in these studies revealed that craniofacial growth continues in all three dimensions, similar to the growth pattern and changes seen during adolescence, but of a much lesser magnitude and rate. Vertical increases are more prominent than anteroposterior changes with the least changes in width. The cephalocaudal gradient continues with more mandibular than maxillary changes. There is evidence of continued jaw rotation and dental eruption with the vertical changes. Females grow less and their craniofacial growth is expressed more vertically with posterior mandibular rotation and an increased mandibular plane angle, whereas males tend to grow with anterior mandibular rotation during adulthood, thereby straightening their profile and decreasing the mandibular plane angle (Figure 53-19).

It appears that there is a subtle growth acceleration in females during their 20s that may be attributable to the endocrine influence of their first pregnancy. Late mandibular incisor crowding usually develops as these incisors are positioned distally relative to the mandible owing to late mandibular growth. Accompanying the skeletal changes throughout adulthood, dental arches continue to change as well with decreasing arch width and depth, further increasing mandibular incisor irregularity.[85]

Facial soft tissue changes during adulthood are much larger in magnitude than changes in hard tissue. Typical lip changes during adulthood include less prominence with decreased thickness, thinning of the vermilion and flattening of its contour (more so in the upper than the lower lip), increased upper lip vertical length, and less prominence of the philtral columns. Male lips continue to appear more retrusive with age, whereas female lips generally do not become as retrusive and their lower lip thickness tends to slightly increase. The lips become positioned more inferiorly, resulting in less vertical display of maxillary incisors, more vertical display of mandibular incisors, and less lip separa-

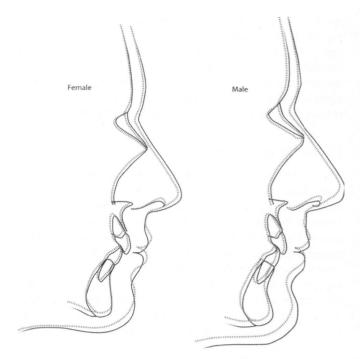

Female   Male

FIGURE 53-19. Composite lateral cephalometric views of female and male show mean longitudinal growth changes from young adult (*broken line* at mean age 17) to middle age adult (*solid line* at mean age 47–51). Note continued downward and forward skeletal and soft tissue growth with relative flattening of the lips. Adapted from Behrents RG Growth in the aging craniofacial skeleton. Craniofacial growth monograph series. Ann Arbor (MI): Center for Human Growth and Development, University of Michigan; 1985.

tion with age.[86] Glabella moves forward and downward. The nose and ears continue to increase in size in all dimensions, with the nasal tip and columella dropping inferiorly to create a more acute nasolabial angle, with all these features occurring to a greater extent in males. There is deepening of the nasolabial folds with jowling developing and the oral commissures tend to sag inferiorly with the loss of elasticity.[87] Males tend to exhibit more chin prominence owing to continued soft tissue increase. The cervicomental angle usually becomes more obtuse from sagging soft tissue that is accentuated with submental fat deposition.[88]

It is clear that while the great preponderance of craniofacial growth subsides after the completion of sexual maturity at the end of adolescence, growth continues on a small scale in all three planes throughout adulthood, following the adolescent pattern. Essentially, craniofacial growth must be viewed as an ongoing process throughout life with postadolescent transverse growth being minimal, followed by anteroposterior growth, with vertical growth being the greatest during adulthood.[70] Our improved understanding of the aging face should compel orthodontists and surgeons to carefully consider their treatment procedures in terms of their future cosmetic effects on the aging face. It is wise to attempt to increase dental and skeletal volume to tighten the facial soft tissue when possible. Any treatment that deepens nasolabial folds or decreases lower face height, lip projection, or vertical maxillary incisor display should be avoided. If any of these adverse changes are unavoidable in order to achieve an acceptable dental occlusion, secondary soft tissue cosmetic procedures may ultimately be considered.

The biologic regulator mechanism for initiating and directing craniofacial growth and dental eruption timing, pattern, and rate remains a poorly understood phenomenon. It is clear that it is a complex mechanism, influenced by an intricate interaction of genetic, epigenetic, and local environmental factors.

FACTORS INFLUENCING CRANIOFACIAL GROWTH

Craniofacial growth is a complex process influenced by both prenatal and postnatal genetic, epigenetic, and environmental factors. The principal influence on craniofacial growth and morphogenesis is one of multifactorial genetic control. However, the interaction of this genetic control with environmental factors is a complex one, and it is usually impossible to accurately differentiate between these influences.

Prenatal Factors

Prenatal defects of craniofacial development can be classified conveniently into three categories: (1) malformation—a morphologic defect of an organ, part of an organ, or larger region of the body resulting from an intrinsically abnormal developmental process, which is intrinsically determined owing to the genome or a teratogen, and occurs during the embryonic period; (2) deformation—an abnormal form, shape, or position of a part of the body caused by mechanical forces, which is influenced directly by the fetal environment; and (3) disruption—a morphologic defect of an organ, part of an organ, or a larger region of the body resulting from the extrinsic breakdown of, or an interference with, an originally normal developmental process, which also occurs during the fetal period and may result from intrauterine pressure as well, but can be of metabolic, vascular, and/or teratogenic origin.[89]

Genetic

Craniofacial malformations arise from disturbance in morphogenesis as early as the germ layer formation to the final formation of organ systems at the end of the embryonic period. Four to 8 weeks' gestation is a particularly critical time because this is the period when neural crest migration is at its most active, the facial prominences and dental laminae are forming, and neurovascular bundles are being generated before facial bone ossification. Malformations are caused from chromosome abnormalities or single-gene mutations or are multifactorial (genetic and/or teratogenic) in origin. Growth retardation, premature death, and mental retardation seem to be more frequent in autosomal recessive or X-linked syndromes.[90] Craniofacial malformations range from acephaly to mild facial defects such as a microform cleft or notching of the lip. Cranial malformations include premature or

delayed fusion of the cranial sutures due to mutations in FGFR1, FGFR2 and FGFR3 and the transcription factor MSX2 associated with syndromes such as trisomy 21 and cleidocraniodysostosis or with simply a deformation craniosynostosis.[52,91] Cranial base malformations usually are related to malformations that affect primary cartilage growth such as achondroplasia (see Figure 53-13) or in combination with premature fusion of facial and cranial sutures as with Apert, Crouzon, and Pfeiffer syndromes (see Figure 53-14).[92] Many facial malformations originate from a deficiency, incomplete migration, or failure in cytodifferentiation of neural crest tissue during embryogenesis.[93] The result is a failure in normal formation of the skeletal and connective tissue portions of the facial prominences. Nasomaxillary malformations include deficiencies and/or absence of facial bones that occur in ectodermal dysplasia or mandibulofacial dysostosis, as well as facial clefts that are associated with over 250 syndromes. The most common craniofacial malformation is unilateral cleft lip, affecting 1 in 700 to 800 births. Malformations that affect the mandible range from the rare absence (agnathia) to various forms of micrognathia, associated with a number of syndromes, such as mandibulofacial dysostosis (Treacher Collins syndrome) or Turner syndrome, to macrognathia, associated with hyperpituitarism or hemifacial hypertrophy.

Two more common chromosomal disorders that result in growth retardation are Down syndrome and Turner syndrome, both of which are characterized by short stature and brachycephaly. The protruding resting tongue typical of Down syndrome usually results in an anterior open bite, whereas a narrow, high-arched palate often is seen with Turner syndrome. Triple X syndrome is characterized by overall small craniofacial dimensions.[94] The Russell-Silver syndrome is a chromosomal disorder characterized by poor fetal and postnatal growth and small triangular facies. Other syndromes associated with prenatal growth retardation include Bloom syndrome, de Lange syndrome, leprechaunism (mutations of the insulin receptor gene), Ellis-van Creveld syndrome, Aarskog syndrome, Rubenstein-Taybi syndrome, Perheentupa syndrome, Dubowitz syndrome, and Johanson Blizzard syndrome.[95]

Single-gene disorders that result in fetal overgrowth include Sotos syndrome, Weaver syndrome, and Beckwith-Wiedemann syndrome. Sotos syndrome includes craniofacial features of macrocephaly, dolichocephaly, a prominent forehead, hypertelorism, prominent ears, high-arched palate, and mandibular prognathism. The Beckwith-Wiedemann syndrome, an example of uniparental disomy, is associated with excessive somatic and specific organ growth (e.g., macroglossia) apparently caused by excess IGF-II. In spite of the overgrowth with these disorders that extends from the fetal period into early childhood, both lead to early epiphyseal fusion, resulting in adult short stature. Klinefelter syndrome (XXY) is a chromosomal disorder that leads to postnatal extended growth from pubertal failure, resulting in tall adult stature.

Another example of a single-gene growth disorder is achondroplasia (see Figure 53-13), the most common form of human dwarfism, which is autosomal dominant with complete penetrance, involving mutations in the *FGFR3* gene. Because the primary cartilage of the cranial base synchondroses is affected, and not the secondary cartilage of the mandibular condyles, midfacial hypoplasia resulting in a class III skeletal discrepancy is the usual facial outcome. A single-gene disorder that leads to postnatal overgrowth resulting in tall adult stature is Marfan syndrome.

It is fortunate that embryologic defects are relatively rare in spite of the extensive number of possibilities. It is estimated that the number of children who have an embryologic disturbance as the major contributing factor to their malocclusion is less than 1%.[96]

There appears to be more evolutionary gene conservation for mammalian organ systems, including humans. The coding genomes vary little between mammals with humans differing by less than 2% with chimpanzees and only 25% with mice.[97,98] There only are subtle differences in the shape and size of human organ systems because appreciable differences can compromise optimal organ function. In contrast, facial characteristics seem to be characterized by more diversity owing to genetic, epigenetic, and environmental factors. Facial structures certainly need to be present and in proper location for proper function, but there can be significant facial morphology variability without impairing function. No two faces are alike, and this variability may be more necessary in humans than other animals owing to the human dependence on vision, more than other senses, to identify one another.

Environmental

Prenatal environmental growth factors are those not directly determined by the genome, including cytoplasmic and extracellular contents in the embryo or fetus and the placenta, influenced by the mother and her interaction with the external environment. Some of these environmental factors may be internal (such as focal embryonic hemorrhages) or external (from maternal malnutrition, metabolic factors, and disease, or exposure to pollutants, chemicals, drugs, infectious agents, or radiation) and may impair normal growth or act as teratogens during either the embryonic or the fetal period if the maternal exposure is large or frequent enough (Figure 53-20).

Cytomegalovirus and rubella are examples of pathogens that can cause microcephaly, hydrocephaly, and microphthalmia. Glucocorticoids, phenytoin, ethyl alcohol, tobacco

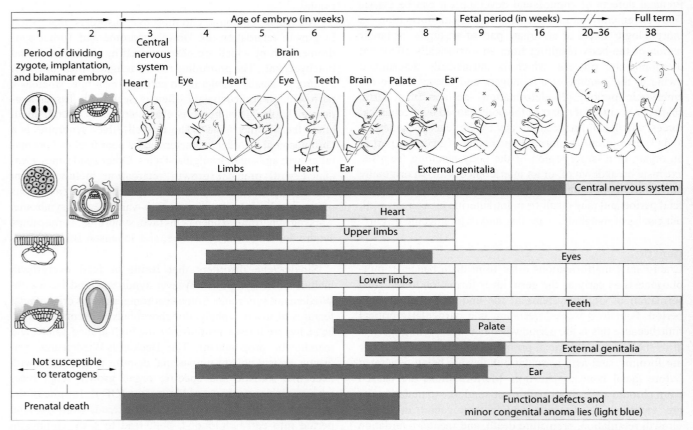

FIGURE 53-20. Teratogen susceptibility during periods of prenatal human development. During the first 2 weeks' gestation, damage from teratogen results in death of the conceptus, or damages only a few cells, allowing recovery by the embryo to develop without birth defects. *Dark blue* indicates highly sensitive periods when major defects may be produced (e.g., amelia, absence of limbs). *Light blue* indicates less sensitive time periods when minor defects may be produced (e.g., hypoplastic thumbs). Adapted from Moore KL, Persaud TVN. The developing human: clinically oriented embryology. 5th ed. Philadelphia (PA): W.B. Saunders Co.; 1973. p. 156.

smoke, aspirin, and retinoic acid (a vitamin A metabolite) are examples of an ever-increasing number of substances that are being identified as teratogens, causing cleft lip and palate as well as other craniofacial anomalies.[99] Fetal alchohol syndrome, characterized in part by maxillary and midface deficiency, has been diagnosed with disturbing frequency, now estimated at 1 in 750 births in the United States.[100] Teratogens have distinct mechanisms of action and are selective to certain target cells, but the severity of the resulting malformation is variable. It is speculated that the range of phenotypic effects caused by a teratogen is due to factors that include the concentration or method of delivery, the timing and duration of exposure, variations in susceptibility, and synergistic interactions among teratogenic compounds.[101] Even in the absence of any detectable malformations, serious long-term physical and mental development can result from drug intake during pregnancy.

When the fetal period begins during 9 weeks' gestation, environmental factors can still have a profound growth effect on the developing fetus. Maternal malnutrition adversely affects fetal growth.[102] Maternal diet composition is relevant, with a high-protein diet being associated with increased linear fetal growth and a high-fat diet linked to an increased birth weight. Maternal consumption of alcohol, recreational drugs, or tobacco all have an important negative influence on growth in utero as well as during the first year of life.[103-105] Even maternal exposure to passive tobacco smoke reduces fetal growth.[106] Frequent high maternal noise exposure has been shown to adversely affect prenatal growth, perhaps related to the stress imposed.[107] Maternal pathology such as rubella can cause a prenatal growth deficit with no long-term recovery.[108]

Intrauterine pressures can result in deformations or disruptions. Intrauterine restrictions can result in mild to severe deformations that can present as mild facial or cranial asymmetry. Some isolated forms of craniosynostosis, causing cranial deformations such as plagiocephaly, may be caused from intrauterine mechanical factors.[109] These deformations may resolve after birth with catch-up growth but usually require orthopedic or surgical intervention during infancy. Another deformation is the Robin sequence whereby retrognathia from posterior restraint of the mandible forces the developing tongue into a posterior position, often acting as a mechanical obstruction that prevents elevation of the palatal shelves, resulting in an isolated cleft palate. Severely affected newborns can have airway compromise that has been more recently treated by advancing the deficient mandible with distraction osteogenesis to avoid the need for a tracheostomy. A disruption is a typically more serious anomaly than a deformation, from the standpoint of both treatment and future growth, because it presents as a morphologic and functional defect that requires surgical repair. An example of a disruption is when a strand of torn amnion or amniotic band is swallowed by the fetus, resulting in a facial cleft that is not located at a site of embryonic fusion. There can be congenital absence of mandibular elevator muscles from unknown causes, resulting in growth deficiency affecting both the maxilla and the mandible on the affected side.

The hormonal regulation of fetal growth is not well understood. Fetal androgens appear to be growth promoters. At midgestation, the level of gonadotropin is similar to pubertal levels.[110] Although there is some evidence that estrogen promotes fetal bone development, there are also data that suggest that it inhibits fetal growth.[111,112] There is a marked and progressive increase in prolactin during late gestation. Before 12 weeks' gestation, maternal hypothyroidism can have long-term deleterious effects on hearing and intelligence, but neither maternal nor fetal hypothyroidism has an appreciable effect on fetal length or weight. However, when both conditions are present, linear growth is still unaffected but there is incomplete pulmonary, cardiovascular, and skeletal maturation.[113] Although poorly understood, insulin appears to have an important role in regulation and promotion of fetal growth. Maternal diabetes increases fetal length and weight, whereas fetal insulin deficiency results in decreased length and weight at birth.[114]

Although growth hormone (GH) is essential for postnatal growth, growth in utero and probably in the first 2 years of life is largely GH-independent.[115] Nevertheless IGF-I and -II play important roles in determining fetal growth, but the specific nature of these roles are not well understood. IGF-II is important in supporting fetal growth during early gestation, whereas IGF-I has a greater role during later gestation and especially in postnatal life.[116] The fetal roles of growth factors such as nerve, epidermal, and platelet-derived growth factors also remain unclear. Other fetal growth factors include hematopoietic growth factors, FGFs, vascular endothelial growth factor, and members of the TGF-β family.[117]

The placenta functions as an additional endocrine organ, providing a secondary source of hypothalamic, pituitary, adrenal, and gonadal hormones and growth factors.[118] Placental GH and lactogen can alter the production of maternal IGF-I.[116] Maternal IGF-I in turn affects placental nutrient transport, increasing fetal growth.[119] Lactogen regulates maternal glucose, amino acid, and lipid metabolism, facilitating nutrient transport to the fetus. Disruption of placental GH or lactogen production can occur from vascular disease, infection, or intrinsic placental abnormalities, impairing fetal growth.[120]

Postnatal Factors

The size of infants in the first months of life is more related to the prenatal environment than is parental height. If prenatal factors caused only mild growth attenuation and it occurred during the last trimester, postnatal catch-up growth is feasible.

Genetic

Heritability appears to have an effect on somatic growth, from a greater to lesser extent in the following order: skeletal length, skeletal breadth, weight, circumference, and skin folds.

By the same token, skeletal tissues respond less to changes in the nutritional environment than do soft tissues.[121] The timing and pace of postnatal maturation are also genetically controlled to a large degree. The extent to which heredity is the cause of postnatal growth that results in jaw discrepancies is controversial.[122] Whereas it appears that there is a substantial genetic component to skeletal characteristics, it apparently is low for dental characteristics.[123,124] There is evidence that malocclusions have shown modest increases in prevalence for the last millennium, with more significant increases during the last 150 years.[125,126] Contrary to the popular belief that greater ethnic and racial diversity are principally responsible for the prevalence of jaw discrepancies, population diversity results in only a modest additive effect with no significant increase in severe problems.[127] Some U.S. data support specific malocclusions being more prevalent in certain racial groups.[128] More extensive international epidemiologic studies are needed to properly characterize racial differences and confirm empirical convictions such as the greater prevalence of maxillary deficiency in East Asian populations. Perhaps two thirds of anteroposterior and vertical facial variation is genetically determined.[124,129,130] Genetic influence does play an important role in skeletal class III growth and excessive vertical facial growth.[131,132] There appears to be at least five autosomal dominant phenotypic subtypes of class III with genetic linkage to at least five loci that suggest a common upstream genetic element for both maxillary deficiency and mandibular prognathism.[133,134] GH receptor gene has been associated with mandibular height.[135] Overall, it is speculated that the majority of human facial skeletal variation is due to the genetic component, with the remaining due to environmental influence.[129,136,137] Functional forces have a crucial influence in altering craniofacial bone growth, and it is apparent that gene expression can be modified by muscular and soft tissue forces, representing epigenetic influences.[138,139] Although genetic influence is important, the membranous viscerocranium is determined to a great extent by functional influences, with these extrinsic factors having the greatest control over mandibular growth.

Environmental and Epigenetic

A multitude of postnatal environmental factors interact with genetic control mechanisms, including functional, traumatic, endocrine, nutritional, pathologic, psychological, cultural, and climatic or seasonal factors.

The functional environment is determined by neuromuscular behavior necessary for survival such as respiration, mastication, deglutition, speech, and posture. However, it is clear that functional influences at rest (i.e., postural activity or the presence of a pathologic mass) are the important determinants of craniofacial growth, not transient muscle contractions and mandibular movement.[140] Chronic pressure alters regional skeletal growth and may be used to improve or correct some craniofacial deformities.[141] Habitual behavior such as non-nutritive sucking and other oral or postural habits can exert such pressure if it is present with great enough frequency and duration, usually at least 4 to 6 hr/day.[142,143]

Mastication limited to one side for sufficient duration can cause asymmetrical mandibular growth.[144] There is some evidence that diet consistency has an effect on mandibular morphology.[145,146] It has been popular to attribute changes in craniofacial dimensions from early to modern human civilizations to dietary changes from a coarse to a refined diet, but this relationship remains unclear. Certainly, it is apparent that more recent diet alterations in contemporary societies have reduced functional jaw demands, but it is not clear whether this change is accelerating the evolutionary trend toward reduced jaw size. The extent of masticatory muscular and dental development can modify the morphology of skeletal superstructures, including the temporal fossae and sagittal crests, the zygomatic arches, the lateral pterygoid plates, the angular and coronoid processes and rami of the mandible, and parts of the temporomandibular joints.[147] The size and function of masticatory muscles have been correlated with facial morphology, but the location of muscle attachments is probably more important in determining bone shape than the amount of activity.[148–150] Other studies have demonstrated an atrophic effect from muscle denervation.[151,152] However, it also is clear that external craniofacial bone growth nevertheless can occur in the absence of any muscle function.[153,154]

Growth deficiency due to neuromuscular deficits can occur in muscle weakness conditions such as muscular dystrophy. The difficulty in returning function to the area makes such conditions particularly resistant to treatment. However, if the muscle is normal, it appears that the normal force range of masticatory muscular function in the general population does not significantly affect facial growth.[155] Long-term impairment of nasal breathing historically has been viewed as a cause of long face deformity, but this assumption continues to be controversial.[156] Although there is some evidence that there is a change in posture with total nasal obstruction,[157] long-term presence of this condition is extremely rare in humans. There is less disagreement about a relationship between nasal obstruction and facial deformity than there is with the extent and duration of mouth breathing necessary to cause a deformity.[158]

Postnatal surgery during infancy for congenital malformations such as cleft lip and palate introduces scarring that is responsible for some midfacial growth attenuation. Typical surgery to close palatal clefts requires that mucoperiosteal flaps be raised and moved medially and posteriorly. This results in denuded bony areas that will heal with the formation of scar tissue bands of variable size and elasticity. This scar tissue usually connects across the maxilla and includes the palatal bones and possibly the pterygoid plates. It is thought that the presence of this scar tissue during postnatal growth compromises midfacial growth.[159,160] The longer postnatal surgery can be delayed, the less growth is affected. There is some evidence demonstrating brain morphology and neuropsychologic differences in nonsyndromic children affected by clefts.[161,162]

Natal or postnatal trauma to the craniofacial complex can modify growth if there is limitation of blood supply or mechanical constriction due to scarring. Extensive midfacial trauma can cause midface growth deficiency as a result of the loss of intrinsic nasal septal growth or from a structural collapse that prevents normal morphologic expression of growth.[163] Trauma that results in scarring across circummaxillary sutures is rare and usually results in a unilateral growth deficit. Untreated burns of the head and neck can cause significant craniofacial dysmorphology.[164] Neurologic damage may lead to muscle paralysis that can alter craniofacial form due to decreased muscle function. There should be caution when considering early craniofacial reconstructive surgery, because the surgery itself may produce additional scarring that can exacerbate the growth attenuation. There is no evidence that the use of rigid plate fixation for trauma reconstruction causes restrictive growth effects in addition to the trauma alone.[165]

Mandibular condylar neck fracture is not uncommon in young children owing to the fragility of this area and the common occurrence of blows to the chin. These fractures almost invariably result in anterior displacement and resorption of the condylar head, yet regeneration of the condylar process and subsequent normal mandibular growth is common. (Lund, 1974) In 15% to 20%, however, there is some reduction in growth on the affected side, the severity usually related to the amount of soft tissue trauma and scarring, and likely is the most common cause of mandibular asymmetry in children.[166,167] With trauma involving the mandible, mandibular function must be maintained, in selective cases requiring physical therapy and the use of a functional appliance. As long as mandibular ankylosis is prevented, surgical open reduction should be avoided when treating condylar fractures in children.[168]

Endocrine disturbances originating from pathology or the environment are among the most potent regulators of postnatal growth. Mandibular growth is reduced by sex hormone deficiency.[169] The primary growth-promoting hormone, GH, is secreted by the pituitary and regulated by somatostatin and GH-releasing hormone release from the hypothalamus. Studies have demonstrated increased GH secretion throughout the day and night in the newborn. However, IGF-I levels are lower at birth and gradually increase during childhood and into adolescence, indicating an early immaturity in the feedback loop. Although the growth process in utero and in the first months after birth is more nutritionally dependent than GH-dependent, this changes during the first year of life, with full GH dependence attained during the second year. GH has been shown to have a direct stimulatory effect on cartilage growth, whereas IGF-I acts as a secondary stimulatory effector.[170]

GH has an important endocrine influence on modulating the size and relationships of the craniofacial structures.[171] GH-deficient children have excess subcutaneous fat and overall delayed facial and cranial base development, resulting in infantile, but proportional, facies. Dental development is delayed as well but to a much lesser degree than facial or somatic growth. In contrast, the craniofacial growth is disproportionate in an autosomal recessive condition known as Laron syndrome in which there is IGF-I deficiency in spite of increased serum GH levels.[172] There is a normal calvarium with small facial bones, resulting in the forehead appearing large and prominent relative to the small recessed face.[173] This suggests that some areas of the face are more directly affected by GH than by IGF-I. GH supplementation in GH-deficient children accelerates catch-up craniofacial growth.[174]

GH excess, usually a consequence of a pituitary adenoma, results in gigantism if it occurs before the end of adolescence and presents with overall larger craniofacial dimensions with coarser facial features. Acromegaly is the outcome if the GH excess is produced after adolescence, characterized by increased periosteal bone that includes cranial thickening, increased size of the frontal sinuses, prominent supraorbital ridges, and nasal enlargement as well as an enlarged tongue and renewed mandibular condylar cartilage growth, leading to mandibular prognathism and a broader mandibular arch (see Figure 53-18). Late mandibular growth also occurs in hemimandibular hypertrophy, a unilateral condition with an unknown cause that most commonly affects females after pubertal growth.

Hypothyroidism will decrease GH release and results in delayed bone and dental development.[175] The craniofacial outcome of this deficiency differs from GH deficiency primarily by the smaller cranium. Anabolic steroids increase craniofacial growth but may lead to excessive anterior maxillary growth in high doses.[176] Testosterone, GH, and IGF-I accelerate endochondral and intramembranous craniofacial skeletal growth as well as statural height. Estrogen appears to decrease endochondral growth.[177,178]

Although glucocorticoid production is necessary for normal growth, glucocorticoid therapy in the prepubertal child must be carefully managed to avoid its inhibitory effect on GH and IGF-I production, resulting in short stature.[179] Although there are no clinical studies indicating the effect on craniofacial growth, animal model studies have suggested a retarding effect on mandibular condylar cartilage growth and acceleration in dental eruption.[180,181]

Poor nutrition, hygiene, and health adversely affect growth. Insufficient caloric and protein intake is the most common cause of growth failure worldwide.[182] Growth deficiency from malnutrition is proportional to the severity of the nutritional deficit. Malnutrition is associated with increased GH but decreased production of IGF-I, reallocating calories from anabolic to survival requirements.[183] It is estimated that 55% of the morphologic variation of the cranium is due to nutritional factors.[184] Because of the early rapid growth of the brain, the cranium is affected more by infant malnutrition than the rest of the craniofacial complex. The size of the neurocranium decreases in rats subjected to malnutrition.[185] A diet deficient in calcium and vitamin D results in cranial dimensional changes in rats.[186] It is thought that maternal vitamin A deficiency alters endocrine function that causes a disturbance in chondrogenesis, reducing the cranial base.[187]

SECTION 7

Nasomaxillary hypoplasia in humans can be related to maternal vitamin K deficiency, since this condition induced in rats causes limited nasal septal cartilage growth.[188] Protein malnutrition in rats decreases the length of the skull relative to the width.[189,190] Voluntary undernutrition has become more common during adolescence, especially with females trying to decrease weight for athletics and those with anxiety about being overweight. This may develop into extreme eating disorders such as anorexia or bulimia nervosa, which may result in impaired growth, delayed puberty, and osteopenia.[191] Obesity has been associated with larger maxillary and mandibular dimensions as well as bimaxillary prognathism.[192] Improved nutrition is considered the primary reason for a phenomenon termed the *secular trend* that has resulted in progressively increased growth rate and attainment of stature and earlier sexual maturation, particularly in industrialized cultures. The secular growth trend has had special relevance for the timing of orthopedic and surgical treatment for craniofacial skeletal discrepancies, resulting in earlier average intervention. There also is evidence that craniofacial skeletal proportions are becoming progressively taller and narrower during the last century.[193] Chronic disease such as congenital heart disease, malabsorption syndrome (e.g., chronic inflammatory disease, cystic fibrosis, celiac disease), chronic renal or liver disease, chronic anemia, inborn errors of metabolism, chronic infections (e.g., tuberculosis, acquired immunodeficiency syndrome), severe asthma, or other chronic pulmonary disease can adversely affect growth.[194] There are a variety of mechanisms causing the growth deficits from these conditions, including reduced nutritional intake, metabolic disbalance, hypoxia, chronic metabolic acidosis protein loss, and often the treatment for the pathology itself.[39] Medications that limit potential growth include chronic adrenal steroid therapy (used for asthma, nephritic syndrome, lupus, and other chronic diseases) and cytostatics (for cancer treatment). Irradiation of the head and face for childhood cancer can result in severe hypoplasia of soft and hard tissues.[195,196] If cranial irradiation is required in cases of leukemia and tumors of the CNS, hypothalamic function can be damaged, affecting the release of hypothalamic and pituitary hormones, notably GH.

Muscle dysfunction can adversely affect craniofacial growth through chronic excessive contraction or loss of function. Untreated torticollis results in facial asymmetry from growth restriction on the side affected by excessive contraction of neck muscles.[197] Loss of tonic muscle contraction experienced in muscular dystrophy and other muscle weakness conditions or due to congenital or post-traumatic CNS disturbance often results in an open mouth posture that leads to increased vertical eruption of posterior teeth, increased face height, and altered mandibular form and position. However, differences in biting forces in otherwise healthy individuals do not appear to make a difference in vertical facial form.[155]

Chronic psychological trauma, emotional deprivation, or psychosocial stress can have a profound effect on somatic growth, causing a functional and reversible GH deficiency, often mimicking growth disorders that are caused from endocrine or nutritional deficiencies.[198]

Cultural and seasonal factors can affect the rate of physical growth. Children in an urban environment tend to mature faster than those from rural settings, particularly in preindustrial societies. Physical growth tends to be more rapid in the spring and summer than in the fall and winter. Additional minor factors have been shown to have a significant influence on postnatal growth and development. These include climate, altitude, exposure to environmental pollutants, and noise.[199,200] Future research will increase our understanding of the role that these and other yet unidentified environmental factors play in altering human genetic growth potential.

In summary, most individuals with severe craniofacial skeletal discrepancies who do not have identifiable congenital malformations likely have a combination of genetic, epigenetic, and environmental determinants influencing their skeletal growth. Our knowledge of the genetic determinants will certainly make rapid progress with the identification of the human genome and advanced genetic diagnostic techniques. The progress of our knowledge of the environmental determinants and their interaction with the genetic control mechanisms will undoubtedly be more delayed and challenging to attain.

ORTHODONTIC, ORTHOPEDIC, AND ORTHOGNATHIC CLINICAL CONSIDERATIONS

Craniofacial Growth Assessment

An evaluation of physical development is needed when considering whether craniofacial orthopedic treatment or orthognathic surgery is indicated for an adolescent. There is a tendency to orthopedically treat females too late owing to a secular trend characterized by progressively earlier sexual maturation and adolescent growth, often before complete eruption of the permanent dentition. Correspondingly, there can be a tendency to orthopedically and surgically treat males too soon because they begin puberty on average 2 years later and continue adolescent craniofacial growth longer, often years after eruption of the permanent dentition. It is well recognized that orthognathic surgery will have a minimal effect on an individual's pattern of craniofacial growth, underscoring the importance of surgical correction of undesirable growth after it has occurred rather than expecting growth to be redirected while it is occurring. Instability of orthopedic as well as orthognathic surgical treatment usually has much more to do with post-treatment growth than surgical relapse.

One indicator for physical growth is skeletal maturation, which historically has been determined with a hand and wrist radiograph. This image provides a view of 30 bones with a predictable ossification sequence and still is considered the assessment standard for skeletal development. A somewhat less accurate, but acceptable, alternative, using standardized lateral cephalometric radiographs to assess vertebral maturation, is being utilized more recently by orthodontists and oral and maxillofacial surgeons because it precludes the need for an additional radiograph.[201,202] It is important that the orthodontist and surgeon not rely solely on this variable to predict the likelihood of adequate remaining jaw growth for successful orthopedic treatment or minimal jaw growth for successful orthognathic surgical treatment. Although it may provide some idea of growth potential, it certainly cannot accurately predict the magnitude, timing, or direction of remaining growth.[203–205] There is some hope that saliva or blood samples may provide future reliable indicators for the timing, intensity, and end of pubertal growth.[206] Superimposition of serial lateral cephalometric radiographs remains the most reliable current method for demonstrating minimal remaining adolescent craniofacial growth. Even with assurance from cephalometric radiographs that adolescent growth is complete, orthodontists and surgeons need to appreciate that the craniofacial growth pattern exhibited before and during adolescence will continue to some extent after orthognathic surgery long into adult life, leading to some return of previous jaw discrepancies in certain individuals, particularly those who have a growth pattern characterized by vertical excess, mandibular excess, or asymmetry.

Orthopedic Treatment for Growth Modification

A harmonious aesthetic facial appearance and balanced dentoskeletal segments facilitating a functional occlusion are both goals that orthodontists and oral maxillofacial surgeons work to achieve by means of orthodontic treatment combined with orthognathic surgery. However, before a surgical correction is contemplated in a growing patient, a determination should be made as to whether the patient is a candidate for orthopedic treatment that may modify craniofacial growth to improve the skeletal imbalance to a favorable aesthetic and functional outcome without the need for orthognathic surgery. It is well known that craniofacial orthopedic devices can generate forces that cause stress in sutures capable of modifying suture growth.[207] As indicated earlier in the chapter, almost 50% of the total cumulative growth of the midface and mandible remains when a child is entering adolescence, making it possible to have an orthopedic treatment effect on the jaws before adolescent growth is completed.

In spite of over a century of clinical experience with orthopedic facial appliances, it remains controversial as to what extent craniofacial skeletal growth can be predictably and permanently modified by orthopedic treatment. Although consensus exists that there is an important genetic influence on the outcome of craniofacial growth, there is a wide range of views regarding the amount in which postnatal factors, particularly orthopedic treatment, influence this outcome. Views vary from the belief that orthopedic alteration of jaw relationships is predictable and stable to the contrasting opinion that skeletal growth is primarily determined genetically and cannot be significantly altered long-term by orthopedic

treatment. The current consensus based on our best basic and clinical data is that clinically significant craniofacial orthopedic treatment is possible, depending on the type of orthopedic treatment, the patient compliance, and the extent of skeletal growth during and after active treatment. The best outcome of craniofacial orthopedic treatment occurs when there is only mild to moderate skeletal discrepancies in patients with short or average face height and mild to moderate dental crowding. The poorest outcome is in individuals with more severe jaw discrepancies, a long lower face height, and moderate to severe dental crowding. It is essential that orthodontists and surgeons bear in mind that dental compensation for the skeletal discrepancies is inevitable and some degree of facial aesthetic compromise may be a part of craniofacial orthopedic treatment. It has been proposed that the typical range of skeletal malocclusions include individuals with normal gene polymorphisms for signaling molecules and growth factors that attenuate the capacity of tissues and cells to reliably respond to orthopedic treatment.[208]

The efficacy of craniofacial growth modification has been a controversial subject for more than a century. At the onset of the 20th century, there was universal confidence by the orthodontic profession that forces applied through the dentition to the growing face could effectively treat craniofacial skeletal discrepancies. After the 1920s, there was a decline in this conviction by North American orthodontists. With the invention of the cephalostat, more precise skeletal assessment of treatment outcomes became possible during the 1950s. This resulted in renewed faith in facial growth modification, with the demonstration of skeletal changes from the use of extraoral force applied with a cervical headgear.

In Europe, there was less controversy regarding craniofacial growth modification efficacy throughout the first half of the 20th century. European orthodontists relied primarily on removable "functional" appliances, designed to provide forces from facial muscles and soft tissue function, for facial orthopedic treatment. The separate philosophic paths taken by European and American orthodontists united in the 1960s, resulting in a more global acceptance of either extraoral or intraoral appliances or a combination of both to facilitate craniofacial orthopedic treatment. This acceptance gained support and enthusiasm from results of basic research conducted during the 1970s using animal models. Although this enthusiasm reached its peak in the 1980s, it was considerably moderated in the 1990s from clinical experiences and the results of prospective clinical studies. There remains little argument that some craniofacial growth modification is feasible with specific skeletal discrepancies, but there continues to be controversy over the nature and extent of the skeletal change possible in individual patients as well as the optimal treatment timing and appliance type. In addition, a reliable and accurate method of predicting the direction, timing, and magnitude of craniofacial growth for an individual has not been devised.

The aim of craniofacial growth modification is to alter the growth pattern by changing the relationships of the jaws. If the skeletal unit is too large, the aim of the orthopedic treatment is to attenuate or redirect its growth to improve its relationship relative to the opposing smaller jaw. If the jaw is too small, the growth modification treatment is aimed at enhancing or redirecting its growth relative to the larger skeletal unit. Virtually all of the craniofacial growth modification appliances until the 1990s have been "toothborne" to some extent, so that the orthopedic forces applied to the skeletal units also create stress to the teeth that results in some dental movement. Although the goal of craniofacial growth modification is to limit the changes to the skeletal units while minimizing movement of the teeth, the reality is that most treatment is predominantly dentoalveolar with a possible minor skeletal component.

There is growing evidence that the long-term success of many forms of growth modification requires that the treatment be continued until facial growth is nearly complete, making early treatment a less efficient way to treat many jaw discrepancies. The following discussion summarizes the facial orthopedic options we have for clinical application of our present understanding of craniofacial growth in the three planes of space.

Transverse Orthopedic Treatment

Because transverse growth reaches completion earlier than anteroposterior or vertical craniofacial growth, it follows that transverse skeletal problems should be addressed early. The most common transverse skeletal problem is maxillary constriction, which can be treated in the preadolescent child even as early as during the primary dentition. The most recent federal epidemiologic study, the Third National Health and Nutrition Examination Survey (NHANES-III) conducted from 1989 through 1994, indicates the prevalence of posterior crossbite is about 5% of the U.S. population.[209] Significant facial or mandibular asymmetry represents approximately 0.1% of the total population.[210] Although maxillary orthopedic expansion devices have been used since 1860, they fell out of favor for a few decades prior to the 1940s due to unsubstantiated concerns regarding their safety and effectiveness.[211] Orthopedic expansion of the maxilla can be achieved with a variety of toothborne appliances (Figure 53-21). These appliances apply moderate to high forces to the teeth that are transmitted as stresses to the maxilla, primarily distracting the midpalatal sutures but also producing less pronounced stresses to the sphenoid and zygomatic bones and other adjacent structures.[212] The midpalatal sutural expansion outcome is wider anteriorly due to the buttressing effect of more posterior maxillary structures. This anteroposterior differential in opening becomes more exaggerated when treating older children due to the greater posterior resistance with age. Within days after initial expansion, new bone forms, eventually depositing both perpendicular and parallel to the edges of the expanded sutures.[213] Although a large amount of the skeletal expansion relapses during retention, overall stability is good if the extent of sutural patency and magnitude of expansion are great enough. A potential additional benefit to improvement in interarch transverse

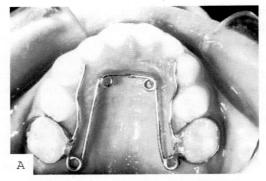

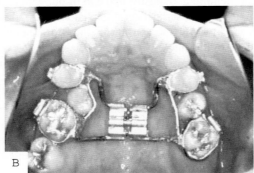

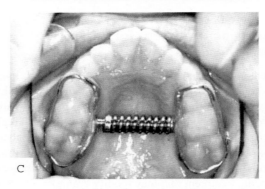

FIGURE 53-21.   Types of maxillary orthopedic expansion appliances. **A,** Quad-helix: An effective skeletal expansion appliance in the primary dentition. **B,** Banded hyrax: This traditional jackscrew also can be used as an activation component for an appliance bonded to the maxillary posterior teeth. **C,** Bonded Minne expander: This spring-loaded component also can be used as an activation component for an appliance banded to the maxillary posterior teeth.

compatibility is an increase in dental arch perimeter made possible by the maxillary orthopedic expansion.[214]

Although complete fusion of the midpalatal suture usually does not occur until the third postnatal decade, the process leading to fusion is a gradual one, characterized by progressive sutural interdigitation and ossification.[215] For this reason, more effective and parallel sutural separation, requiring less force and concomitant undesirable dental expansion, is possible in the younger child, especially before puberty, during a "phase 1" treatment in the mixed or early permanent dentition. Treatment before the peak pubertal growth velocity may result in greater long-term skeletal craniofacial transverse width.[216] Treatment may even be indicated as early as the

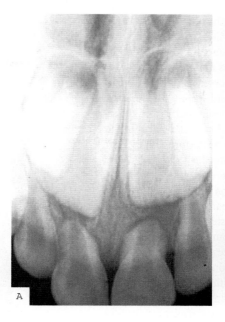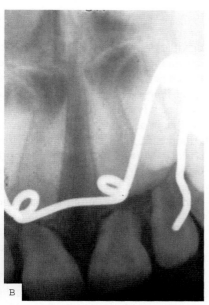

FIGURE 53-22.   Occlusal radiographs demonstrate maxillary skeletal expansion with a Quad-helix in the primary dentition. Note distraction of the midpalatal suture. Before **(A)** and after **(B)** initial palatal expansion.

primary dentition in the presence of a large transverse functional shift. This compensatory functional problem can result in asymmetrical condylar positioning that may lead to asymmetrical mandibular growth and uneven remodeling of the glenoid fossae, possibly resulting in permanent facial asymmetry, even if the constricted maxillary arch is corrected at a later date.[217–219] Maxillary constriction without a transverse functional shift does not carry the same urgency and is conveniently treated closer to the onset of puberty during the early permanent dentition.[220]

Maxillary orthopedic expansion in late adolescent or postadolescent patients should be attempted with caution. Even if skeletal expansion is possible in these older patients, the extent of circum-maxillary and midpalatal sutural patency is limited enough to compromise stability of the treatment outcome. It is appropriate to confirm intermaxillary expansion with an occlusal radiograph in these patients, because the development of a midline diastema may only indicate bending of maxillary bones. If the expansion is limited to lateral tipping of maxillary posterior teeth, buccal alveolar bone height reduction and gingival recession may occur. It usually is more prudent to consider surgically assisted palatal expansion (SARPE) for late adolescent or postadolescent patients to avoid periodontal compromises and instability. One should keep in mind that SARPE expansion will create much greater skeletal expansion across the canines as opposed to the more posterior expansion achieved by a conventional osteotomy.

The expansion appliance can be banded or bonded to the maxillary posterior teeth with a spring-loaded or non–spring-loaded palatal jackscrew that usually is activated by the patient 0.5 mm/day, delivering from 2 to more than 10 pounds of force (this may increase to cumulative loads of 20 pounds or more with multiple activations in the absence of adequate sutural separation). The conventional description for the expansion induced with this appliance is "rapid

palatal expansion." However, it is possible to affect slower expansion with less frequent activations (≤1 mm/wk), requiring more active treatment time but less retention time to ensure stability.[221] It is feasible to achieve skeletal expansion with simpler appliances such as a W-arch or Quad-helix that deliver only a few hundred grams of force, provided that the patient is in the primary or very early mixed dentition when the maxillary sutures are more patent or when a cleft of the hard palate is present (Figure 53-22).

Because all of these expansion appliances are toothborne, unwanted dentoalveolar expansion is an inevitable consequence.[222,223] An additional undesirable outcome is the long-term loss of about 30% of the skeletal expansion achieved during active treatment due to the rebound of stretched palatal tissues.[224] To compensate for these effects, maxillary expansion should be continued until adequate overexpansion is achieved, usually to the extent that the lingual cusps of the maxillary molars are opposing the buccal cusps of the mandibular molars (Figure 53-23). Once adequate expansion has

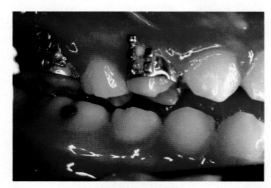

FIGURE 53-23.   Maxillary overexpansion to compensate for dentoalveolar expansion and skeletal relapse. Note the lingual cusps of maxillary posterior teeth are occluding with buccal cusps of the mandibular posterior teeth.

been accomplished, at least 3 to 6 months of retention is necessary to permit new bone to fill in the spaces created by maxillary separation and to permit time for dissipation of reaction forces stored in the facial bones that promote relapse. It is important to recognize that transverse maxillary skeletal expansion is notoriously unstable and prone to relapse, whether it is achieved orthopedically or surgically.[225,226] Overexpansion accounts for some of the relapse and permits the orthodontist to transversely upright the posterior teeth in their alveolar housing without compromising the final transverse occlusal correction after retention. More recently developed osseointegrated attachments or temporary skeletal anchorage devices hold some promise for a means of expanding the maxilla without buccally tipping posterior teeth and may improve the stability of the skeletal change (Figure 53-24).[227] However, there is preliminary evidence that skeletal anchorage for maxillary orthopedic expansion does not offer significant benefits over conventional toothborne appliances.[228]

A less common transverse skeletal problem than maxillary constriction is asymmetrical mandibular deficiency, usually caused from a previous trauma associated with unilateral mandibular condylar fracture or hemifacial microsomia, a congenital facial asymmetry. In both of these conditions, the affected side exhibits growth deficiency relative to the unaffected or normal side, resulting in a mandibular deviation toward the affected side. If left untreated in a growing individual, the alveolar processes compensate with limited eruption of the maxillary posterior teeth on the affected side and excessive eruption of the maxillary posterior teeth on the unaffected side, resulting in an occlusal cant that is higher on the affected side. It is best to start orthopedic treatment with these individuals before pubertal growth, as early as patient compliance will permit. The goal is to maximize the growth expression on the deficient side and minimize dentoalveolar compensation. The orthopedic appliance of choice is an asymmetrical "hybrid" functional appliance that is constructed to posture the mandible forward on the affected side, bringing the chin to the midline.[229] Posterior dental eruption is attenuated on the unaffected side with a bite block, and erup-

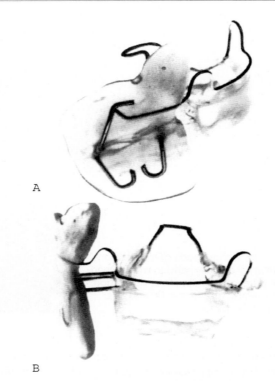

FIGURE 53-25. Asymmetrical "hybrid" functional appliance. **A,** Right lateral view. **B,** Frontal view. On the left, unaffected side, posterior dental eruption is restricted with an interocclusal acrylic block. On the right, affected side, the mandible is postured forward and posterior dental eruption is encouraged with a buccal shield and absence of an interocclusal acrylic block. (**A** and **B,** Reproduced with permission from Proffit WR, Fields HW. Contemporary orthodontics. 3rd ed. St. Louis (MO): Mosby; 2000. p. 370.)

tion is facilitated on the affected side with a buccal shield and the absence of interocclusal acrylic (Figure 53-25). Because untreated mandibular asymmetries of this nature invariably worsen with growth, orthopedic treatment is considered successful if the asymmetry remains stable or improves. Treatment should not continue if progressive asymmetry is apparent in spite of reliable appliance use by the patient.

Anteroposterior Orthopedic Treatment: Class II

A class II skeletal relationship can be the result of a retrusive and/or a deficient mandible, a protrusive or vertically excessive maxilla, or a combination of these skeletal problems. The prevalence of this type of malocclusion is approximately 15% to 20% of the U.S. population, with approximately 2% severe enough to be considered as handicapping.[209] Prospective clinical studies have supported that early growth modification during the mixed dentition may lead to an improvement in the skeletal class II malocclusion.[230–232] It should be kept in mind that regardless of whether orthopedic treatment is attempted during active facial growth, approximately 10% of patients ultimately require orthognathic surgery to fully correct the class II malocclusion.[232]

The headgear has been used as a means of class II orthopedic treatment in North America since the late 19th century

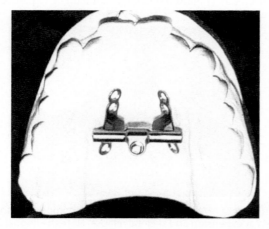

FIGURE 53-24. Bone-anchored palatal distraction appliance. Reproduced with permission from J Orofac Orthop 2003; 64:444.

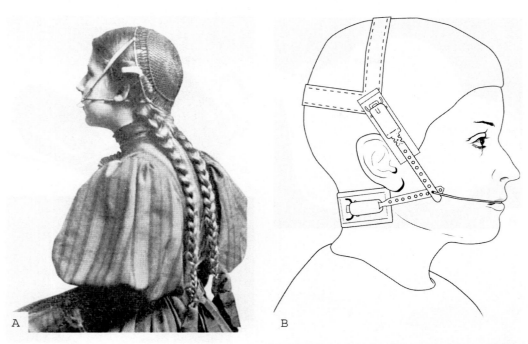

FIGURE 53-26. Headgear, past and present. An orthopedic force is directed posteriorly and superiorly to the maxilla, attenuating circum-maxillary sutural growth. **A,** Headgear from the late 19th century. **B,** Contemporary headgear appliance fabricated with more durable materials and with additional calibration and safety features, although the overall design has changed little in over a century. (**A,** Reproduced with permission from Angle EH. Treatment of malocclusion of the teeth. Philadelphia (PA): S.S. White Dental Manufacturing Co; 1907. p. 234; **B** adapted from McNamara JA, Brudon WL. Orthodontics and dentofacial orthopedics. Ann Arbor (MI): Needham Press, Inc.; 2001. p. 365.)

(Figure 53-26). An orthopedic force ranging from 16 to more than 32 ounces is delivered using elastic traction from the headgear to a cervical or cranial attachment for 12 to 14 hr/day, usually for 9 to 12 months. A safety release for the retractive mechanism and parent/patient education are essential to prevent potential traumatic injuries. Theoretically, the force is transmitted in a posterior and superior direction via the teeth through the maxilla to compress the circum-maxillary sutures, limiting or redirecting maxillary growth. Since the introduction of standardized cephalometric radiographs, many clinical studies have demonstrated that maxillary growth can be altered with the use of the headgear.[233–235] These clinical data have been supported by primate studies demonstrating that extraoral orthopedic force directed against the maxilla attenuates forward growth and alters bone apposition at the maxillary sutures.[236–239] Some retrospective studies suggest that mandibular growth may be enhanced as well. Because the headgear is a toothborne appliance, some maxillary dental retraction accompanies the skeletal change. Another dentoalveolar effect is the attenuation of maxillary molar eruption, resulting in anterior and superior mandibular rotation. There is some support for this being the only clinically relevant skeletal effect.[240] A significant treatment effect usually requires that a headgear be worn 12 to 14 hr/day. Human GH and other endocrine factors that promote growth and dental eruption are primarily released during the evening and night.[241–243] It is fortuitous that this is the only time of day that one can reliably expect an adolescent to wear a headgear.

Because it is a removable appliance, few adolescents after the peak of pubertal growth will reliably wear the appliance.

The alternative orthopedic method for treating a class II skeletal relationship is the class II functional appliance, which has been used since the early 20th century in Europe and since the 1960s in North America. These appliances include the removable toothborne activator, bionator, and twin block, the removable and primarily tissueborne Fränkel (functional regulator) appliance, or the fixed toothborne Herbst appliance (Figure 53-27). All of these appliances position the mandibular condyles downward and forward away from the glenoid fossae. Theoretically, the distracted condylar positions reduce the normal compressive joint pressure on the growing condylar cartilage and the forward mandibular posturing alters muscle tension on the condyles, stimulating or accelerating the endochondral condylar growth more than would normally occur. There is some support from animal studies that a histologic increase in condylar growth can be achieved.[244–246] Retrospective clinical studies have both supported[247–251] and refuted[252–255] that clinically significant lengthening of the mandible can be achieved with functional appliances. However, prospective, randomized clinical studies have more definitively confirmed that there is no greater absolute growth reflected by the long-term treatment outcome.[256] Much of the skeletal change demonstrated with a functional appliance may result from forces against the maxilla, similar to those applied with a headgear, that are created from the stretched facial muscles and soft tissues

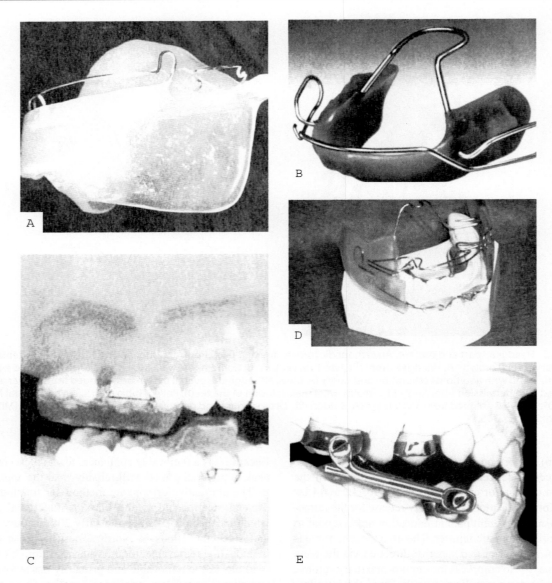

FIGURE 53-27. Class II functional appliances. All of these appliances position the mandible downward and forward, distracting the condyles from the glenoid fossae. This simultaneously creates posterior and superior forces on the maxilla from the facial muscles and soft tissues attempting to return the mandible to its normal position. **A,** Activator. **B,** Bionator. **C,** Twin block. **D,** Fränkel. **E,** Fixed Herbst. An alternative is to utilize occlusal acrylic and bond the maxillary portion of the appliance with a removable acrylic splint for the mandibular arch. (**A–E,** Reproduced with permission. A, C, and D from Bishara SE. Textbook of orthodontics. Philadelphia (PA): W.B. Saunders; 2001. p. 345. B from Graber TM, Vanarsdall RL. Orthodontics: current principles and techniques, 3rd ed. St. Louis (MO): Mosby; 2000. p. 488. E from McNamara JA, Brudon WL. Orthodontics and dentofacial orthopedics. Ann Arbor (MI): Needham Press, Inc.; 2001. p. 287.)

attempting to return the postured mandible back to its posterior and superior position.[257,258] Because of the toothborne nature of this appliance, dentoalveolar changes accompany the skeletal changes, including maxillary dental retraction and mandibular dental protrusion.

Retrospective clinical studies have demonstrated few differences in treatment outcome when comparing the skeletal response between headgear and functional appliance treatment.[251,259,260] In the last decade of the 20th century, three prospective, randomized class II clinical trials conducted in the United States. and Great Britain have all demonstrated that orthopedic treatment with either a headgear or a functional appliance in the mixed dentition results in an average improved short-term skeletal outcome. There is some evidence that there is more of a maxillary effect with headgears[232,260] and more of a mandibular effect with functional appliances.[231,232,260,261] Most functional appliances need to be worn for the same daily duration as the headgear (exceptions are the Fränkel and Herbst appliances, which are worn full time) for a significant treatment effect. Much like the headgear, dependable wear is more realistic during the evening and at night when the most active facial growth and dental eruption usually occur. However, like the headgear, its removable nature prevents it from being reliably worn by most adolescents after the peak of their pubertal growth.

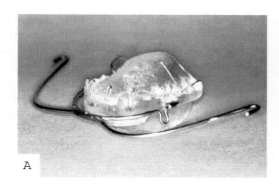

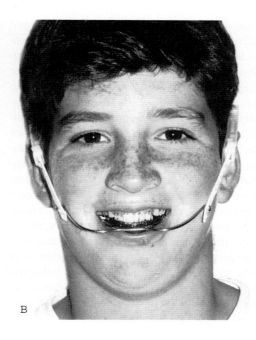

FIGURE 53-28. Combination headgear and removable functional appliance. The interocclusal acrylic permits orthopedic forces to be transmitted further anteriorly and superiorly through the center of the maxilla. **A,** Intraoral part of the appliance with headgear tubes embedded in the interocclusal acrylic. **B,** Extraoral application of the appliance. (**A** and **B,** Reproduced with permission from Bishara SE. Textbook of orthodontics. Philadelphia (PA): W.B. Saunders; 2001. p. 341.)

In the late 1960s, when European and American facial orthopedic philosophies were becoming more fully integrated, a method was introduced in Europe using a headgear in combination with a functional appliance (Figure 53-28).[262] This approach was intended to provide greater cumulative skeletal growth effects than use of either appliance alone, but this has yet to be demonstrated by clinical studies.

Although there is greater general acceptance that treatment with a headgear or functional appliance may achieve an improved long-term treatment outcome, there continues to be controversy over the optimum treatment time in the growing child. It has already been demonstrated that orthopedic class II treatment in the very young child, in the primary or early mixed dentition, results in substantial relapse and recurrence of the original facial skeletal pattern by late adolescence.[263] However, there is great debate regarding the long-term efficacy of orthopedic treatment during later mixed dentition as the first phase of a two-phase treatment versus delaying orthopedic treatment until definitive orthodontic treatment during puberty, after the eruption of the permanent dentition. Many orthodontists historically have preferred the earlier first phase because there is substantial potential growth remaining, compliance in wearing the orthopedic appliance often is greater, and the arch space for the remaining erupting dentition may be improved. The advocates for a delayed one-phase treatment have contended that comparable skeletal treatment effects can be achieved during definitive orthodontic treatment without putting the patient through an unnecessary initial phase.[264,265] The three prospective, randomized class II clinical trials mentioned earlier have supported this position, demonstrating that early skeletal improvement achieved from these appliances seems to represent accelerated growth and can be used just as effectively later during pubertal growth.[266–268] They also showed that there was substantial individual growth variability with no reliable predictors for a favorable growth response identified and early

treatment did not reduce the need for dental extraction or orthognathic surgery during the definitive phase. These studies indicate that there is no adequate additional benefit in treatment outcome to justify the greater burden to the patient, their parents, and the orthodontist, as represented by an early phase that precedes the definitive phase of orthodontic treatment.[256]

It can be concluded from past retrospective and more recent prospective clinical trials that headgear treatment tends to have more of a maxillary-restrictive effect whereas functional appliances have more of a mandibular-enhancing effect. Either approach can be satisfactory and should be selected on the basis of patient acceptance of the appliance and dentoalveolar side effects (there is more maxillary dental retrusion with headgear and more mandibular protrusion with a functional appliance). The American and British prospective, randomized trials have clearly demonstrated that class II orthopedic treatment during the mixed dentition is justified only in selected cases in which there is short face height with impinging anterior overbite, predisposed to root resorption or trauma risk coupled with excessive overjet, sufficient aesthetic/psychosocial concern by the patient, or a precocious adolescent growth that substantially precedes dental development.[269,270] Treatment at an earlier age has been further justified by the argument that there is lack of reliable means of predicting mandibular growth and that improved cooperation with a removable appliance usually is present with the younger patient.[271]

In summary, the most ideal patient for class II orthopedic treatment would be pubertal with facially inclined and spaced maxillary incisors, lingually inclined mandibular incisors, a mild skeletal discrepancy, and a short or normal anterior face height. Although improvement in skeletal discrepancy is expected, the class II correction usually is due to a combined response of both the dentoalveolar and the skeletal components. Both headgear and class II functional appliance use can be effective in limiting downward and forward eruption of the maxillary molars. However, the functional appliance tends to promote upward and forward eruption of mandibular molars, which may complement the correction in deep overbite cases but is counterproductive in patients with a long face. Because class II orthopedic appliances are toothborne, there may be some unwanted dentoalveolar change, including retraction of maxillary anterior teeth and protraction of mandibular anterior teeth. This compensatory change may be undesirable if the skeletal discrepancy ultimately requires orthognathic surgery for correction. With the advent of osseointegrated attachments or temporary skeletal anchorage devices, there may be the future possibility of preventing unwanted dentoalveolar change by attaching a force system directly to these attachments rather than using toothborne attachments. Orthodontic retention after class II orthopedic treatment as a part of definitive orthodontic treatment may require the use of a class II functional appliance at night for up to 24 months, particularly if they have significant adolescent growth remaining.

Anteroposterior Orthopedic Treatment: Class III

A class III skeletal relationship can be the result of a retrusive and/or deficient maxilla, a large and/or prognathic mandible, or most often, a combination of these skeletal problems. The prevalence of this type of malocclusion is approximately 3% to 5% of the U.S. population, with approximately 0.3% severe enough to be considered as handicapping.[209] Since the late 19th century, when headgear was being used for class II skeletal problems, the chin cup was the appliance used for orthopedic treatment of skeletal class III problems (Figure 53-29). Theoretically, an orthopedic force is transmitted to the mandibular condyles, compressing the condylar cartilage and limiting endochondral growth in order to decrease the ultimate length of the mandible.[272] Primate studies suggest that mandibular growth can be impeded with heavy full-time

forces directed against the mandibular condyles.(Janzen & Bluher, 1965) Full-time wear with such excessive forces is unrealistic with humans. Most clinical studies, using tolerable forces (12–16 oz/side) and realistic daily wear (12–14 hr), have demonstrated that mandibular growth is not restrained, but rather vertically redirected from chin cup wear, rotating the mandible down and back, resulting in decreased chin prominence while increasing face height.[273–276] Clinical studies also have suggested that the long-term stability of these changes is poor.[277,278] The stability is dependent on favorable facial growth after active treatment, which is unpredictable but usually results in a resumption of the original facial growth pattern and relapse of the skeletal discrepency during or after adolescent growth. An additional side effect from chin cup wear is more lingual inclination of lower incisors due to the force of the chin cup to the lower lip and base of the mandibular anterior alveolar process.[274] Although this effect may help in the dentoalveolar compensation for the skeletal discrepancy, it usually does so at the expense of lower incisor crowding and increased relative chin prominence. Treatment with a chin cup may be an acceptable option for an individual with mild mandibular excess associated with decreased facial height (only one third of the prognathic white population) but is contraindicated when there is a normal or excessive facial height, because the treatment outcome simply would be trading one deformity for another. East Asian populations may benefit more often from this treatment because they tend to have shorter face heights than whites. However, chin cup treatment for mandibular prognathism has very limited utility, with its benefits usually negated from subsequent growth and ultimately resulting in unnecessary additional treatment burden to the patient.

Class III functional appliances also have been developed, limiting eruption of mandibular posterior teeth and promoting eruption of maxillary posterior teeth and resulting in downward and backward mandibular rotation with increased facial

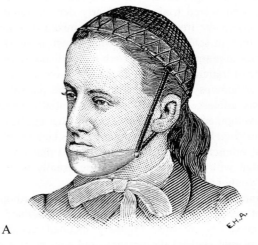

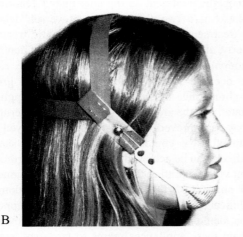

A

B

FIGURE 53-29. Class III chin cup appliance. A retractive orthopedic force is directed against the chin posteriorly and superiorly toward the condylar heads. **A,** Chin cup from the late 19th century. **B,** Contemporary chin cup, with minimal change in design, but fabricated with more comfortable and durable materials. (**A** and **B,** Reproduced with permission.) A from Angle EH. Treatment of malocclusion of the teeth. Philadelphia (PA): S.S. White Dental Manufacturing Co; 1907. p. 194. B from Proffit WR, Fields HW, Sarver DM. Contemporary orthodontics. 4th ed. St. Louis (MO): Mosby; 2007. p. 301.

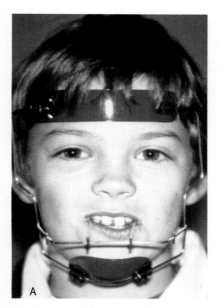

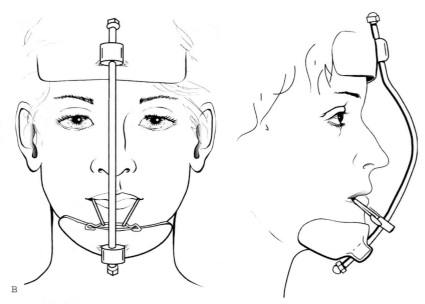

FIGURE 53-30. Class III maxillary protraction headgear, or facemask. A protractive orthopedic force is directed on the maxilla in a downward and forward direction, with the force being dissipated on the forehead and chin, distracting the circummaxillary sutures to augment AP maxillary growth. **A,** Delaire design. **B,** Petit design (frontal and lateral views). (**A,** Reproduced with permission from Proffit WR, White RP, Sarver DM. Contemporary treatment of dentofacial deformity. St Louis (MO): Mosby, 2003. p. 516. **B** adapted from McNamara JA, Brudon WL. Orthodontics and dentofacial orthopedics. Ann Arbor (MI): Needham Press, Inc.; 2001. p. 378.)

height. These functional appliances have few advocates owing to their effectiveness, similar to chin cup treatment, being limited to dentoalveolar changes and their inability to promote forward maxillary growth or attenuate mandibular growth.[279,280] Jean Delaire, a French dentist, was responsible for developing the protraction headgear or facemask, the most effective orthopedic appliance for skeletal class III problems since its introduction in the early 1970s (Figure 53-30).[281] Delaire recognized that the offending jaw in many of the skeletal class III problems was the maxilla, so he departed from the historic focus on the mandible and directed treatment at the retrusive or deficient maxilla. The appliance creates tension in the circum-maxillary sutures with elastics from the maxillary dental arch to a frame that uses the forehead and chin to dissipate the force anteriorly. Primate studies have demonstrated adaptive responses of the sutures to the stress from the distraction forces produced by this appliance.[213]

Depending on the developmental stage and size of the patient, a protractive force ranging from 2 to 4 pounds is applied to the facemask in an anterior and slightly inferior direction relative to the occlusal plane for 12 to 16 hr/day, usually for 6 to 9 months. Clinical studies have demonstrated clinically relevant maxillary skeletal protraction downward and forward on average with this appliance, with some concomitant protraction of the maxillary teeth due to the tooth-borne nature of the intraoral part of the appliance.[282–285] However, as with other forms of craniofacial orthopedic treatment, there is substantial variability and an unpredictable patient response to the appliance, ranging from no appreciable skeletal change to about 5 mm anterior maxillary movement.[286] It is important to achieve overcorrection of the anterior crossbite and anterior overbite because there is

some relapse after discontinuation of treatment.[287] Additional effects of maxillary orthopedic protraction often include rotation of the maxilla downward in the posterior and upward in the anterior, downward and backward rotation of the mandible, and retraction of the mandibular incisors due to the reactive posterior force dissipated on the chin. These additional orthopedic and dentoalveolar changes that accompany maxillary skeletal protraction would be contraindicated for a class III pattern with excessive vertical development (long anterior face height and obtuse gonial angle) or where mandibular excess is the underlying cause of the problem.[288] In summary, the most ideal patient for maxillary orthopedic protraction would be younger than 8 years old and would have a mild skeletal discrepancy without mandibular prognathism, a short anterior face height, and retrusive maxillary incisors.

Although some clinicians have promoted the orthopedic distraction of the midpalatal suture to enhance subsequent anterior protraction with the facemask,[289] this has not demonstrated improved treatment efficacy.[290] The timing of facemask therapy often is recommended for patients in the primary to early mixed dentition (i.e., ages 4–8) owing to the increased patency of the maxillary sutures and compliance with appliance wear at this age.[291,292] As the patient ages, there is more interdigitation and ossification of the circummaxillary sutures, resulting in less skeletal and more dental response to the protraction forces. However, the earliest practical time for starting treatment is after eruption of first permanent molars owing to the poor anchorage provided by the primary dentition alone for the intraoral portion of the appliance. Although some clinical studies have found few differences between early and late treatment up until puberty,[292–295] more controlled studies have shown that skeletal change diminishes after age 8 after which mostly tooth movement and backward mandibular rotation can be expected.[291] The limited skeletal change after this age is undoubtedly due to increased resistance from more mature sutures posterior and superior to the maxilla.

The stability of maxillary orthopedic protraction with a facemask is variable and dependent on whether mandibular growth ultimately overwhelms the skeletal improvement after active treatment. It should be expected that the original facial growth pattern will continue after treatment, often resulting in relapse of the skeletal discrepency. Approximately 30% of patients end up in anterior crossbite in late adolescence, most of whom will ultimately require orthognathic surgery to fully correct the class III malocclusion.[296,297] It should be kept in mind that long-term efficacy of facemask treatment has not been fully studied.

Toothborne class III orthopedic appliances, as with class II devices, result in dentoalveolar movements that accompany the skeletal changes. Treatment with the face-mask causes protraction of maxillary anterior teeth and retraction of mandibular anterior teeth. The development of osseointegrated attachments or temporary skeletal anchorage devices may make it possible to transmit the orthopedic protraction force to intraoral skeletal attachments that prevent undesirable dentoalveolar changes.[298,299] Orthodontic retention for class III orthopedic treatment may require the use of a class III functional appliance at night for up to 24 months after definitive orthodontic treatment, particularly if they have post-treatment adolescent growth remaining. However, it is wise to wait before initiating the definitive treatment as close as possible to the completion of adolescent growth to minimize overcompensation for a skeletal discrepancy that ultimately requires orthognathic surgery. A particularly challenging aspect of treating skeletal class III problems (as well as vertical skeletal excess problems) is that short-term successful treatment, whether it occurs during or at the completion of adolescent growth, may relapse due to the continued class III growth pattern during adulthood.[300]

A recently developed novel method of class III orthopedic treatment, termed "bone-anchored maxillary protraction" (BAMP), has used maxillary posterior and mandibular anterior miniplates as skeletal anchorage in children 10 to 12 years of age (Figure 53-31).[301] Relatively light (150–250 g/side) full-time use of class III maxillomandibular intraoral elastic traction used with this method has produced remarkable maxillary skeletal protraction within about 12 months without the concomitant maxillary dentoalveolar protraction seen in more conventional facemask treatment (Figure 53-32). Preliminary data indicate that this treatment often results in anterior movement of the zygoma and maxilla and corresponding soft tissue with variable effects on the mandible in different individuals.[302,303] There is evidence that treatment using this new method results in much larger maxillary advancement with better controlled vertical changes

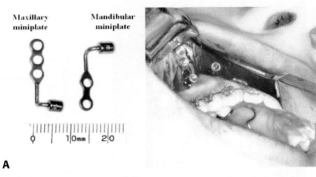

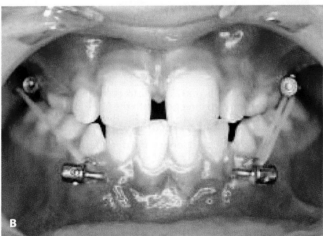

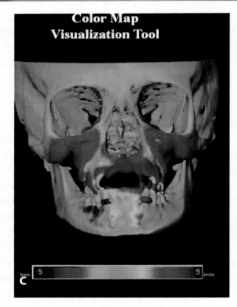

FIGURE 53-31. **A,** Modified titanium miniplates used as TADs for bone-anchored maxillary protraction (BAMP). **B,** Intermaxillary Class III elastics to customized attachment hooks on miniplates. **C,** Three-dimensional superimposition with color map tool used on individual patient. Areas on the red end of the spectrum represent outward movement during active treatment. Areas on the blue end of the spectrum represent inward movement during treatment. (**A-C,** Reproduced with permission from Am J Orthod Dentofacial Orthop 2010;137. pp. 276, 277).

Vertical Orthopedic Treatment

Excessive vertical face height is characterized by a posterior maxilla that is inferiorly positioned, resulting in downward and backward rotation of the mandible, resulting in an increased mandibular plane angle and incompetent lips. Although most individuals with excess vertical face height exhibit anterior open bite, a minority will have excessive eruption of maxillary anterior teeth preventing open bite but worsening the excess vertical display of the maxillary gingiva and anterior teeth. The prevalence of excess vertical facial problems is less than 5% of the U.S. population with approximately 0.3% considered as handicapping.[209,210]

The orthodontist has not historically had very effective nonsurgical options to manage vertical skeletal problems. Orthopedic treatment strategy has historically been directed at restraining vertical maxillary growth and posterior dental eruption in order to promote anterior and superior mandibular rotation because it is usually associated with a class II skeletal discrepancy. A high-pull headgear is used to apply a superior intrusive force of 2 to 4 pounds to inhibit eruption of maxillary posterior teeth and compress circum-maxillary sutures to limit the downward development of the maxilla. An alternative to the use of high-pull headgear is a removable orthopedic appliance that incorporates interocclusal acrylic bite blocks in order to stretch the facial musculature and soft tissue beyond the normal resting vertical dimension, creating a reactive intrusive force against the mandibular as well as the maxillary teeth.[304,305] Neither of these methods has been very effective, perhaps owing to the extensive duration of wear required by the patient daily and throughout adolescent growth. Repelling magnets have been embedded in the opposing acrylic bite blocks to accentuate the intrusive force with no significant treatment benefit.[306-309]

High-pull headgear and interocclusal acrylic have been combined into one appliance with the hope that this approach may provide greater cumulative skeletal growth effects than use of either appliance alone.[262] Unfortunately, this combined treatment demonstrates no appreciable additional benefit in controlling excess vertical growth.[310]

In summary, neither the high-pull headgear or interocclusal acrylic alone or in combination offer appreciable effective treatment for vertical skeletal excess. A final challenge in the use of either or both of these orthopedic appliances to treat vertical maxillary excess is the inability to direct the orthopedic force in a straight vertical manner. Both methods include some posteriorly directed force to the maxilla that is not appropriate unless the maxilla is protrusive as well as inferiorly positioned. It also is counterproductive in a patient with maxillary vertical excess combined with a class III skeletal relationship. Just as the protraction headgear should not be used with this individual to address the anteroposterior skeletal problem, the high-pull headgear and/or interocclusal bite block are contraindicated in this same clinical situation to address the vertical excess.

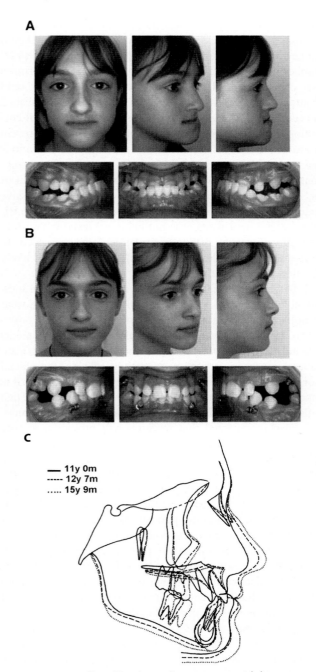

FIGURE 53-32.   Class III orthopedic treatment with bone-anchored maxillary protraction (BAMP). A reciprocal force of 300 to 500 g is produced by maxillomandibular elastics, resulting in a maxillary force directed downward and forward and a mandibular force directed upward and backward. **A,** Before treatment. **B,** After treatment. **C,** Superimposed cephalometric tracings show the beginning of treatment, end of treatment, and follow-up. (**A–C,** Reproduced with permission from J Oral Maxillofac Surg 2009;67. pp. 2126, 2128.)

than the conventional orthopedic treatment with facemask. There may be a short window of treatment opportunity with this technique because mandibular miniplates cannot be placed before canine eruption and circum-maxillary sutural patency is more limited at older ages.

— 11y 0m
----- 12y 7m
..... 15y 9m

The clinical introduction of temporary anchorage devices in the form of miniplates[311] or miniscrews[312,313] offers a new and potentially more successful way of orthopedically controlling mild to moderate vertical skeletal excess. Miniplates or miniscrews permit skeletal anchorage to intrude posterior teeth as a means of dentoalveolar compensation for the skeletal discrepancy. The posterior dental intrusion has shown short-term success in rotating the mandible upward and forward, closing mild to moderate anterior open bites. The extent to which posterior teeth can be orthodontically intruded by this means has not yet been determined. In addition, no substantial post-treatment data are yet available to confirm the long-term stability of this treatment approach. If this treatment takes place before the end of adolescent growth, it is likely that the continued vertical skeletal growth pattern will cause relapse. Even if this short-term successful treatment occurs after adolescent growth is complete, the continued vertical growth pattern during adulthood may lead to some return of the malocclusion. No studies to date have been able to demonstrate long-term stability with any nonsurgical orthopedic methods for correcting vertical maxillary excess, with or without an anterior open bite.[314] Achieving stability is particularly difficult owing to the extended duration of vertical facial growth continuing well beyond adolescence.[78] The long duration of active orthopedic treatment as well as duration of vertical growth makes the excessive vertical plane of space the most difficult to successfully manage by the orthodontist attempting facial growth modification.

Deficient vertical face height usually is a result of more posterior than anterior mandibular vertical growth with deficient vertical eruption of posterior teeth and anterior mandibular rotation, resulting in deep anterior overbite with lingual inclination of incisors. It is common for deficient face height to be associated with a mandibular or maxillary anteroposterior deficiency resulting in a class II or class III malocclusion. Orthodontic treatment directed at encouraging posterior eruption or extruding posterior teeth to improve facial height may include a functional appliance or a cervical headgear, in combination with an anterior bite plane, to disocclude posterior teeth. This may be successful with a class II malocclusion if upper molar eruption is limited, lower molar eruption is encouraged, and there is adequate mandibular growth to compensate for the resulting downward and backward mandibular rotation. It also may be successful with a class III malocclusion if upper molar eruption is encouraged, lower molar eruption is limited, and there is minimal mandibular growth after active orthodontic treatment. In contrast to the treatment stability of excess face height, long-term stability of treated deficient vertical face height is quite good.[315]

Conclusion

Facial orthopedic treatment may be effective in resolving mild to moderate skeletal discrepancies in some patients. The indications for craniofacial skeletal growth modification before adolescence is a maxillary deficiency in any plane of space or a progressive deformity, usually causing facial asymmetry. No growth modification can be justified for mandibular excess. Class II skeletal problems should not be addressed before adolescent growth except for a small number of selected cases involving trauma, root resorption risk, or psychosocial concerns. An orthopedic phase should be attempted with a specific treatment time frame established in order to assess treatment progress toward successful correction. This time frame must be honored in order to prevent protracted treatment with excessive dental compensations that need to be reversed for surgical correction. The orthodontist attempting growth modification must be mindful of the duration and extent of treatment to prevent excessive length and morbidity of the orthodontic treatment. If significant skeletal improvement is not being achieved within 6 to 8 months of starting orthopedic treatment, the case needs to be reevaluated and the growth modification treatment likely abandoned as a treatment choice.

It has become clear that there is great variability in individual treatment response, even when factoring out wear compliance and duration of treatment. It has not been possible to identify the variables to explain why some patients respond well and some do not demonstrate any significant skeletal improvement with treatment regardless of their facial morphology or the severity of their skeletal discrepancy. It is anticipated that future research will reveal the variables that will enable the clinician to better predict treatment response.

It also is expected that research will provide a greater understanding of the nature and extent of facial growth modification possible in individual patients as well as the type of appliance and timing of treatment to achieve the best outcome. The development of intraoral skeletal anchorage attachments holds promise for a future means of dissipating orthopedic forces to prevent unwanted dentoalveolar changes that at present occur with our toothborne appliances. Analogous attachments are at present undergoing clinical testing for surgically assisted orthopedic movements associated with distraction osteogenesis.[316,317] Recent and future advances in developmental biology and genomics hold great promise in increasing our understanding of the molecular and genetic mediators of craniofacial growth. This understanding will be crucial for us to make constructive modifications of our treatment methods to target these mediators in order to prevent or correct a craniofacial anomaly or developmental deformity.

Orthodontic Camouflage: Orthopedic Consequence versus Surgical Preparation

Orthodontic camouflage, rather than orthognathic surgery, may indeed be an appropriate treatment choice for some mild and moderate skeletal malocclusions in patients who are beyond pubertal growth. Successful camouflage is predicated on a favorable dental occlusion that will not be overly unfavorable to the patient's facial aesthetic appearance. Because aesthetic appearance is subjective in nature, it is essential to have the patient's and parent's perceptions dictate whether camouflage is a reasonable option. Camouflage can be considered when there are normal vertical facial proportions and minimal crowding of teeth so that extractions can be used for retraction of anterior teeth rather than to simply alleviate crowding.

Most mild and some moderate skeletal class II malocclusions can be effectively camouflaged with extraction of two maxillary premolars and retraction of maxillary anterior teeth, leaving the posterior teeth in a class II occlusion. However, these cases should mainly be limited to those that present without significant dental crowding, some protrusion of the maxillary incisors, and where there is not significant maxillary gingival display on smiling. If the maxillary incisors are normally or palatally inclined before treatment, orthodontic retraction of these teeth may result in an even poorer aesthetic result than the original problem even if the occlusion is acceptable. The unaesthetic appearance includes not just the incisor inclination but often an unattractive retrusive upper lip and increased maxillary gingival exposure during smiling as well. This is why the recent introduction of palatal implants, miniplates, and miniscrews as skeletal orthodontic anchorage, which provide the opportunity for the orthodontist to retract maxillary incisors even further than was previously possible, is a mixed blessing.

It is more challenging to camouflage class III than class II skeletal malocclusions because considerable natural dentoalveolar camouflage (proclined maxillary incisors, lingually inclined mandibular incisors) is often already present before treatment. Unlike camouflage class II treatment, successful class III camouflage treatment is only limited to mild skeletal discrepancies. Additional maxillary incisor proclination may be unaesthetic, and further lingual inclination of mandibular incisors usually accentuates an already prominent chin. For this reason, extraction of mandibular premolars to permit more retraction of mandibular incisors to obtain positive overjet often compromises the aesthetic outcome. If interarch tooth size compatibility can be maintained, extraction of one mandibular incisor rather than two premolars may provide an acceptable compromise. It is crucial not to begin class III camouflage as a definitive treatment until completion of adolescent growth to minimize post-treatment relapse. Camouflage of an anterior open bite that is due to maxillary vertical excess has been notoriously unsuccessful in the past. It remains to be seen whether the newly introduced skeletal anchorage devices for posterior orthodontic intrusion offer stable long-term treatment of mild to moderate skeletal anterior open bite problems. An orthodontic technique for stably extruding anterior teeth has been introduced.[318] Unfortunately, this only exacerbates the excessive vertical display of maxillary gingiva and anterior teeth.

SUMMARY

The surgeon's understanding of craniofacial growth has an important impact on clinical treatment decisions to alter craniofacial morphology. This understanding is relevant to the appreciation of the role of orthopedic treatment in the prepubertal and pubertal patient to limit or preclude the need for corrective surgery at a later age. Clinically relevant modification of craniofacial growth is possible, but substantial advances will be necessary to elucidate how growth modification can be accomplished in a controlled and predictable manner to achieve an efficacious outcome. Optimal timing and stability of craniofacial surgery are dependent on a thorough appreciation of the sequence, timing, magnitude, and differential expression of craniofacial growth. The recent dramatic advances in developmental genetics and molecular biology, highlighted by complete mapping of the human genome, familial genetic studies, and gene targeting in mice and humans, promises an explosive increase to our understanding of the complex interactions of the genetic, epigenetic, and environmental influences that determine human craniofacial morphogenesis, prenatal development, and postnatal growth. A more thorough understanding of these influences and their interactions will be necessary to determine the best timing and method of clinical intervention to achieve the optimum treatment outcome.

References

1. Trainor P, Nieto MA. Jawsfest: new perspectives on neural crest lineages and morphogenesis. Development 2003;130:5059–5063.
2. Kontges G, Lumsden A. Rhombencephalic neural crest segmentation is preserved throughout craniofacial ontogeny. Development 1996;122:3229–3242.
3. Bronner-Fraser M. Neural crest cell migration in the developing embryo. Trends Cell Biol 1993;3:392–397.
4. Noden DM. The role of the neural crest in patterning of avian cranial skeletal, connective, and muscle tissues. Dev Biol 1983;96:144–165.
5. LaBonne C, Bronner-Fraser M. Molecular mechanisms of neural crest formation. Annu Rev Cell Dev Biol 1999;15:81–112.
6. Le Douarin NM, Ziller C, Couly GF. Patterning of neural crest derivatives in the avian embryo: in vivo and in vitro studies. Dev Biol 1993;159:24–49.
7. Shah NM, Anderson DJ. Integration of multiple instructive cues by neural crest stem cells reveals cell-intrinsic biases in relative growth factor responsiveness. Proc Natl Acad Sci U S A 1997;94:11369–11374.
8. Selleck MA, Scherson TY, Bronner-Fraser M. Origins of neural crest cell diversity. Dev Biol 1993;159:1–11.
9. Serbedzija GN, Bronner-Fraser M, Fraser SE. Vital dye analysis of cranial neural crest cell migration in the mouse embryo. Development 1992; 116:297–307.
10. Graham A, Lumsden A. The role of segmentation in the development of the branchial region of higher vertebrate embryos. Birth Defects Orig Artic Ser 1993;29:103–112.
11. Imai H, Osumi-Yamashita N, Ninomiya Y, Eto K. Contribution of early-emigrating midbrain crest cells to the dental mesenchyme of mandibular molar teeth in rat embryos. Dev Biol 1996;176:151–165.
12. Trainor PA, Krumlauf R. Patterning the cranial neural crest: hindbrain segmentation and Hox gene plasticity. Nat Rev Neurosci 2000;1:116–124.

13. Baker CV, Bronner-Fraser M. Vertebrate cranial placodes I. Embryonic induction. Dev Biol 2001;232:1–61.

14. Couly G, Creuzet S, Bennaceur S, et al. Interactions between Hox-negative cephalic neural crest cells and the foregut endoderm in patterning the facial skeleton in the vertebrate head. Development 2002;129:1061–1073.

15. Trainor PA, Ariza-McNaughton L, Krumlauf R. Role of the isthmus and FGFs in resolving the paradox of neural crest plasticity and prepatterning. Science 2002;295:1288–1291.

16. Chai Y, Maxson RE Jr. Recent advances in craniofacial morphogenesis. Dev Dyn 2006;235:2353–2375.

17. Tucker GC, Aoyama H, Lipinski M, et al. Identical reactivity of monoclonal antibodies HNK-1 and NC-1: conservation in vertebrates on cells derived from the neural primordium and on some leukocytes. Cell Differ 1984;14:223–230.

18. Poelmann RE, Gittenberger-de Groot AC. A subpopulation of apoptosis-prone cardiac neural crest cells targets to the venous pole: multiple functions in heart development? Dev Biol 1999;207:271–286.

19. Chai Y, et al. Fate of the mammalian cranial neural crest during tooth and mandibular morphogenesis. Development 2000; 127:1671–1679.

20. Ito Y, et al. Receptor-regulated and inhibitory Smads are critical in regulating transforming growth factor beta–mediated Meckel's cartilage development. Dev Dyn 2002;224: 69–78.

21. Jiang X, Iseki S, Maxson RE, et al. Tissue origins and interactions in the mammalian skull vault. Dev Biol 2002;241: 106–116.

22. Soriano P. Generalized lacZ expression with the ROSA26 Cre reporter strain. Nat Genet 1999;21:70–71.

23. Brault V, et al. Inactivation of the beta-catenin gene by Wnt1-Cre–mediated deletion results in dramatic brain malformation and failure of craniofacial development. Development 2001; 128:1253–1264.

24. Francis-West PH, Robson L, Evans DJ. Craniofacial development: the tissue and molecular interactions that control development of the head. Adv Anat Embryol Cell Biol 2003;169: III–VI, 1–138.

25. Mallo M, Brandlin I. Segmental identity can change independently in the hindbrain and rhombencephalic neural crest. Dev Dyn 1997;210:146–156.

26. Schneider RA, Helms JA. The cellular and molecular origins of beak morphology. Science 2003;299:565–568.

27. Richman JM, Lee SH. About face: signals and genes controlling jaw patterning and identity in vertebrates. Bioessays 2003; 25:554–568.

28. Irving C, Mason I. Signalling by FGF8 from the isthmus patterns anterior hindbrain and establishes the anterior limit of Hox gene expression. Development 2000;127:177–186.

29. Trainor PA, Tam PP. Cranial paraxial mesoderm and neural crest cells of the mouse embryo: co-distribution in the craniofacial mesenchyme but distinct segregation in branchial arches. Development 1995; 121:2569–2582.

30. Young DL, Schneider RA, Hu D, Helms JA. Genetic and teratogenic approaches to craniofacial development. Crit Rev Oral Biol Med 2000;11:304–317.

31. McGonnell IM, Clarke JD, Tickle C. Fate map of the developing chick face: analysis of expansion of facial primordia and establishment of the primary palate. Dev Dyn 1998;212:102–118.

32. Johnston MC, Bronsky PT. Prenatal craniofacial development: new insights on normal and abnormal mechanisms. Crit Rev Oral Biol Med 1995;6:25–79.

33. Hu D, Helms JA. The role of sonic hedgehog in normal and abnormal craniofacial morphogenesis. Development 1999;126: 4873–4884.

34. Fujino M, et al. Disappearance of epidermal growth factor receptor is essential in the fusion of the nasal epithelium. Anat Sci Int 2003;78:25–35.

35. Wilkie AO, Morriss-Kay GM. Genetics of craniofacial development and malformation. Nat Rev 2001;2:458–468.

36. Helms JA, Cordero D, Tapadia MD. New insights into craniofacial morphogenesis. Development 2005;132:851–861.

37. Kjaer I. Human prenatal craniofacial development related to brain development under normal and pathologic conditions. Acta Odontol Scand 1995;53:135–143.

38. Brunet CL, Sharpe PM, Ferguson MW. Inhibition of TGF-beta 3 (but not TGF-beta 1 or TGF-beta 2) activity prevents normal mouse embryonic palate fusion. Int J Dev Biol 1995;39: 345–355.

39. Cameron N, editor. Human Growth and Development. London's Academic Press, Elsevier Science; 2002; pp. 6–7, 85.

40. Houpt MI. Growth of the craniofacial complex of the human fetus. Am J Orthod 1970;58:373–383.

41. Opperman LA, Passarelli RW, Morgan EP, et al. Cranial sutures require tissue interactions with dura mater to resist osseous obliteration in vitro. J Bone Miner Res 1995;10:1978–1987.

42. Kim HJ, Rice DP, Kettunen PJ, Thesleff I. FGF-, BMP- and Shh-mediated signalling pathways in the regulation of cranial suture morphogenesis and calvarial bone development. Development 1998; 125:1241–1251.

43. Roth DA, et al. Immunolocalization of transforming growth factor beta 1, beta 2, and beta 3 and insulin-like growth factor I in premature cranial suture fusion. Plast Reconstr Surg 1997; 99:300–309.

44. Nah H. Suture biology: Lessons from molecular genetics of craniosynostosis syndromes. Clin Orthod Res 2000;3:37–45.

45. Stottmann RW, Anderson RM, Klingensmith, J. The BMP antagonists Chordin and Noggin have essential but redundant roles in mouse mandibular outgrowth. Dev Biol 2001;240: 457–473.

46. Merida Velasco JR, et al. Development of the mandibular condylar cartilage in human specimens of 10-15 weeks' gestation. J Anat 2009;214:56–64.

47. Plavcan JM, German RZ. Quantitative evaluation of craniofacial growth in the third trimester human. Cleft Palate Craniofac J 1995;32:394–404.

48. Ronning O. Basicranial synchondroses and the mandibular condyle in craniofacial growth. Acta Odontol Scand 1995;53: 162–166.

49. Bareggi R, et al. Mandibular growth rates in human fetal development. Arch Oral Biol 1995;40:119–125.

50. Bentley RP, Sgouros S, Natarajan K, et al. Normal changes in orbital volume during childhood. J Neurosurg 2002;96: 742–746.

51. Hunter WS, Baumrind S, Moyers RE. An inventory of United States and Canadian growth record sets: preliminary report. Am J Orthod Dentofacial Orthop 1993;103:545–555.

52. Bellus GA, et al. Identical mutations in three different fibroblast growth factor receptor genes in autosomal dominant craniosynostosis syndromes. Nat Genet 1996;14:174–176.

53. Copray JC, Jansen HW, Duterloo HS. Growth and growth pressure of mandibular condylar and some primary cartilages of the rat in vitro. Am J Orthod Dentofacial Orthop 1986;90:19–28.

54. Peltomaki T, et al. Tissue-separating capacity of growth cartilages. Eur J Orthod 1997;19:473–481.

55. Wang X, Mao JJ. Chondrocyte proliferation of the cranial base cartilage upon in vivo mechanical stresses. J Dent Res 2002; 81:701–705.

56. Kiliaridis S. Masticatory muscle influence on craniofacial growth. Acta Odontol Scand 1995;53:196–202.

57. Bjork A, Skieller V. Contrasting mandibular growth and facial development in long face syndrome, juvenile rheumatoid polyarthritis, and mandibulofacial dysostosis. J Craniofac Genet Dev Biol Suppl 1985;1:127–138.

58. Sarnat BG. Normal and abnormal craniofacial growth. Some experimental and clinical considerations. Angle Orthod 1983; 53:263–289.

59. Rabie AB, Hagg U. Factors regulating mandibular condylar growth. Am J Orthod Dentofacial Orthop 2002;122:401–409.

60. Houston WJ. Mandibular growth rotations—their mechanisms and importance. Eur J Orthod 1988;10:369–373.

61. Liu YP, Behrents RG, Buschang PH. Mandibular growth, remodeling, and maturation during infancy and early childhood. Angle Orthod 2010;80:97–105.

62. Anderson DL, Thompson GW, Popovich F. Adolescent variation in weight, height, and mandibular length in 11 females. Hum Biol 1975;47:309–319.

63. Bjork A, Skieller V. Normal and abnormal growth of the mandible. A synthesis of longitudinal cephalometric implant studies over a period of 25 years. Eur J Orthod 1983;5:1–46.

64. Mamandras AH. Linear changes of the maxillary and mandibular lips. Am J Orthod Dentofacial Orthop 1988;94: 405–410.

65. Nanda RS, Meng H, Kapila S, Goorhuis J. Growth changes in the soft tissue facial profile. Angle Orthod 1990;60:177–190.

66. Vig PS, Cohen AM. Vertical growth of the lips: a serial cephalometric study. Am J Orthod 1979;75:405–415.

67. Subtelny JD. Intelligibility and associated physiological factors of cleft palate speakers. J Speech Hear Res 1959;2:353–360.

68. Chaconas SJ. A statistical evaluation of nasal growth. Am J Orthod 1969;56:403–414.

69. Scott JH. The growth of the human face. Proc R Soc Med 1954;47:91–100.

70. Edwards CB, et al. Longitudinal study of facial skeletal growth completion in 3 dimensions. Am J Orthod Dentofacial Orthop 2007;132:762–768.

71. Buschang PH, Baume RM, Nass GG. A craniofacial growth maturity gradient for males and females between 4 and 16 years of age. Am J Phys Anthropol 1983;61:373–381.

72. Ferrario VF, Sforza C, Poggio CE, Schmitz JH. Craniofacial growth: a three-dimensional soft-tissue study from 6 years to adulthood. J Craniofac Genet Dev Biol 1998;18:138–149.

73. Hrdlicka. Growth during adult life. Proc Am Phil Soc 1936; 76:847–897.

74. Hooton, Dupertuis. Age changes and selective survival in Irish males. Stud Phys Anthropol 1951;2:1–130.

75. Israel H. Recent knowledge concerning craniofacial aging. Angle Orthod 1973;43:176–184.

76. Lewis AB, Roche AF. Late growth changes in the craniofacial skeleton. Angle Orthod 1988;58:127–135.

77. Akgul AA, Toygar TU. Natural craniofacial changes in the third decade of life: a longitudinal study. Am J Orthod Dentofacial Orthop 2002;122:512–522.

78. Behrents RG. Growth in the aging craniofacial skeleton. Craniofacial growth monograph series Monograph 17. Ann Arbor: Center for Human Growth and Development, University of Michigan; 1985.

79. Bishara SE, Treder JE, Jakobsen JR. Facial and dental changes in adulthood. Am J Orthod Dentofacial Orthop 1994;106: 175–186.

80. Formby WA, Nanda RS, Currier GF. Longitudinal changes in the adult facial profile. Am J Orthod Dentofacial Orthop 1994;105:464–476.

81. West KS, McNamara JA Jr. Changes in the craniofacial complex from adolescence to midadulthood: a cephalometric study. Am J Orthod Dentofacial Orthop 1999;115:521–532.

82. Forsberg CM. Facial morphology and ageing: a longitudinal cephalometric investigation of young adults. Eur J Orthod 1979;1:15–23.

83. Fudalej P. Long-term changes of the upper lip position relative to the incisal edge. Am J Orthod Dentofacial Orthop 2008; 133:204–209; quiz 328, e201.

84. Pecora NG, Baccetti T, McNamara JA Jr. The aging craniofacial complex: a longitudinal cephalometric study from late adolescence to late adulthood. Am J Orthod Dentofacial Orthop 2008;134:496–505.

85. Dager MM, McNamara JA, Baccetti T, Franchi L. Aging in the craniofacial complex. Angle Orthod 2008;78:440–444.

86. Vig RG, Brundo GC. The kinetics of anterior tooth display. J Prosthet Dent 1978;39:502–504.

87. McKinney P, Cook JQ. Liposuction and the treatment of nasolabial folds. Aesthetic Plast Surg 1989;13:167–171.

88. Ellenbogen R, Karlin JV. Visual criteria for success in restoring the youthful neck. Plast Reconstr Surg 1980;66:826–837.

89. Spranger J, et al. Errors of morphogenesis: concepts and terms. Recommendations of an international working group. J Pediatr 1982;100:160–165.

90. Wilson GN. Genomics of human dysmorphogenesis. Am J Med Genet 1992;42:187–196.

91. Jabs EW, et al. A mutation in the homeodomain of the human MSX2 gene in a family affected with autosomal dominant craniosynostosis. Cell 1993;75:443–450.

92. Mooney MP, Siegel MI. Understanding craniofacial anomalies: the etiopathogenesis of craniosynostoses and facial clefting. New York (NY): Wiley-Liss, Inc.; 2002.

93. Johnston MC, Bronsky PT. Prenatal craniofacial development: new insights on normal and abnormal mechanisms. Crit Rev Oral Biol Med 1995;6:368–422.

94. Krusinskiene V, Alvesalo L, Sidlauskas A. The craniofacial complex in 47, XXX females. Eur J Orthod 2005;27:396–401.

95. Jones KL. Smith's recognizable patterns of human malformation. Philadelphia (PA): W.B. Saunders; 1988.

96. Proffit WR, Turvey TA, Phillips C. The hierarchy of stability and predictability in orthognathic surgery with rigid fixation: an update and extension. Head Face Med 2007;3:21.

97. Mikkelsen TS. Initial sequence of the chimpanzee genome and comparison with the human genome. Nature 2005;437:69–87.

98. Church DM, et al. Lineage-specific biology revealed by a finished genome assembly of the mouse. PLoS Biol 2009; 7:e1000112.

99. Shepard TH. Catalog of teratogenic agents. Baltimore (MD): John Hopkins University Press; 1995.

SECTION 7

100. Naidoo S, Norval G, Swanevelder S, Lombard C. Foetal alcohol syndrome: a dental and skeletal age analysis of patients and controls. Eur J Orthod 2006;28:247–253.

101. Gorlin RJ, Cohen MM, Levin LS. Syndromes of the head and neck. New York (NY): Oxford University Press; 1990.

102. Edwards LE, Alton IR, Barrada MI, Hakanson EY. Pregnancy in the underweight woman. Course, outcome, and growth patterns of the infant. Am J Obstet Gynecol 1979;135:297–302.

103. Abel EL. Consumption of alcohol during pregnancy: a review of effects on growth and development of offspring. Hum Biol 1982;54:421–453.

104. Haste FM, Anderson HR, Brooke OG, et al. The effects of smoking and drinking on the anthropometric measurements of neonates. Paediatr Perinat Epidemiol 1991;5:83–92.

105. Zuckerman B, et al. Effects of maternal marijuana and cocaine use on fetal growth. N Engl J Med 1989;320:762–768.

106. Misra DP, Nguyen RH. Environmental tobacco smoke and low birth weight: a hazard in the workplace? Environ Health Perspect 1999;107(Suppl 6):897–904.

107. Ando, Hattori. Statistical studies on the effects of intense noise during human fetal life. J Sound Vibr 1973;27:101–110.

108. Lejarraga H, Peckham CS. Birthweight and subsequent growth of children exposed to rubella infection in utero. Arch Dis Child 1974;49:50–54.

109. Higginbottom MC, Jones KL, James HE. Intrauterine constraint and craniosynostosis. Neurosurgery 1980;6:39–44.

110. Gluckman. Fetal hypothalamic-pituitary relationships: a review with particular reference to experimental studies of the somatotropic axis. Dev Endocrinol 1990;67.

111. Abdul-Karim RW, Marshall LD. Influence of maternal oophorectomy on the collagen and calcium contents of fetal bone. Obstet Gynecol 1969;34:837–840.

112. Abdul-Karim RW, Nesbitt RE Jr, Drucker MH, Rizk PT. The regulatory effect of estrogens on fetal growth. I. Placental and fetal body weights. Am J Obstet Gynecol 1971;109:656–661.

113. de Zegher F, et al. The prenatal role of thyroid hormone evidenced by fetomaternal Pit-1 deficiency. J Clin Endocrinol Metab 1995;80:3127–3130.

114. Warshaw. Intrauterine growth restriction revisited. Growth Genet Horm 1992;8:5–8.

115. D'Ercole AJ, Applewhite GT, Underwood LE. Evidence that somatomedin is synthesized by multiple tissues in the fetus. Dev Biol 1980;75:315–328.

116. Evain-Brion D. Hormonal regulation of fetal growth. Horm Res 1994;42:207–214.

117. Rotwein P. Peptide growth factors other than insulin-like growth factors or cytokines. In: Degroot LJ, Jameson JL, editors. Endocrinology. 4th edition. Philadelphia (PA): W.B. Saunders, 2001; 461–476.

118. Siler-Khodr TM. Endocrine and paracrine function of the human placenta. In: Polin RA, Fox WW, editors. Fetal and neonatal physiology. 2nd edition. Philadelphia (PA): W.B. Saunders, 1998;89–102.

119. Hall K, et al. Somatomedin levels in pregnancy: longitudinal study in healthy subjects and patients with growth hormone deficiency. J Clin Endocrinol Metab 1984;59:587–594.

120. Li Y, Behringer RR. Esx1 is an X-chromosome-imprinted regulator of placental development and fetal growth. Nat Genet 1998;20:309–311.

121. Towne B, Demerath EW, Czerwinski SA. The genetic epidemiology of growth and development. In: Cameron N, editor. Human growth and development. London: Academic Press, Elsevier Science, 2002;103–137.

122. Pirinen S. Genetic craniofacial aberrations. Acta Odontol Scand 1998;56:356–359.

123. Hughes T, Thomas C, Richards L, Townsend G. A study of occlusal variation in the primary dentition of Australian twins and singletons. Arch Oral Biol 2001;46:857–864.

124. King L, Harris EF, Tolley EA. Heritability of cephalometric and occlusal variables as assessed from siblings with overt malocclusions. Am J Orthod Dentofacial Orthop 1993;104:121–131.

125. Corruccini RS. An epidemiologic transition in dental occlusion in world populations. Am J Orthod 1984;86:419–426.

126. Evensen JP, Ogaard B. Are malocclusions more prevalent and severe now? A comparative study of medieval skulls from Norway. Am J Orthod Dentofacial Orthop 2007;131:710–716.

127. Chung CS, Niswander JD, Runck DW, et al. Genetic and epidemiologic studies of oral characteristics in Hawaii's schoolchildren. II. Malocclusion. Am J Hum Genet 1971;23:471–495.

128. Proffit WR, Fields HW Jr, Moray LJ. Prevalence of malocclusion and orthodontic treatment need in the United States: estimates from the NHANES III survey. Int J Adult Orthod Orthognath Surg 1998;13:97–106.

129. Lauweryns I, Carels C, Vlietinck R. The use of twins in dentofacial genetic research. Am J Orthod Dentofacial Orthop 1993;103:33–38.

130. Savoye I, Loos R, Carels C, et al. A genetic study of anteroposterior and vertical facial proportions using model-fitting. Angle Orthod 1998;68:467–470.

131. El-Gheriani AA, et al. Segregation analysis of mandibular prognathism in Libya. J Dent Res 2003;82:523–527.

132. Litton SF, Ackermann LV, Isaacson RJ, Shapiro BL. A genetic study of Class 3 malocclusion. Am J Orthod 1970;58:565–577.

133. Bui C, King T, Proffit W, Frazier-Bowers S. Phenotypic characterization of Class III patients. Angle Orthod 2006;76:564–569.

134. Frazier-Bowers S, Rincon-Rodriguez R, Zhou J, et al. Evidence of linkage in a Hispanic cohort with a Class III dentofacial phenotype. J Dent Res 2009;88:56–60.

135. Tomoyasu Y, et al. Further evidence for an association between mandibular height and the growth hormone receptor gene in a Japanese population. Am J Orthod Dentofacial Orthop 2009;136:536–541.

136. Johannsdottir B, Thorarinsson F, Thordarson A, Magnusson TE. Heritability of craniofacial characteristics between parents and offspring estimated from lateral cephalograms. Am J Orthod Dentofacial Orthop 2005;127:200–207; quiz 260–261.

137. Suzuki A, Takahama Y. Parental data used to predict growth of craniofacial form. Am J Orthod Dentofacial Orthop 1991;99:107–121.

138. Rabie AB, She TT, Harley VR. Forward mandibular positioning up-regulates SOX9 and type II collagen expression in the glenoid fossa. J Dent Res 2003;82:725–730.

139. Tang GH, Rabie AB. Runx2 regulates endochondral ossification in condyle during mandibular advancement. J Dent Res 2005;84:166–171.

140. Proffit WR. Equilibrium theory revisited: factors influencing position of the teeth. Angle Orthod 1978;48:175–186.

141. Buchman SR, Bartlett SP, Wornom IL 3rd, Whitaker LA. The role of pressure on regulation of craniofacial bone growth. J Craniofac Surg 1994;5:2–10.

142. Kean MR, Houghton P. The role of function in the development of human craniofacial form—a perspective. Anat Rec 1987;218:107–110.

143. Schumacher GH. Factors influencing craniofacial growth. Prog Clin Biol Res 1985;187:3–22.

144. Poikela A, Kantomaa T, Pirttiniemi P. Craniofacial growth after a period of unilateral masticatory function in young rabbits. Eur J Oral Sci 1997;105:331–337.

145. Bouvier M, Hylander WL. The effect of dietary consistency on gross and histologic morphology in the craniofacial region of young rats. Am J Anat 1984;170:117–126.

146. Luca L, Roberto D, Francesca SM, Francesca P. Consistency of diet and its effects on mandibular morphogenesis in the young rat. Progr Orthod 2003;4:3–7.

147. Gionhaku N, Lowe AA. Relationship between jaw muscle volume and craniofacial form. J Dent Res 1989;68:805–809.

148. Ingervall B, Thilander B. Relation between facial morphology and activity of the masticatory muscles. J Oral Rehabil 1974;1:131–147.

149. van Spronsen PH, Weijs WA, Valk J, et al. A comparison of jaw muscle cross-sections of long-face and normal adults. J Dent Res 1992;71:1279–1285.

150. Weijs WA, Hillen B. Relationships between masticatory muscle cross-section and skull shape. J Dent Res 1984;63:1154–1157.

151. Gardner DE, Luschei ES, Joondeph DR. Alterations in the facial skeleton of the guinea pig following a lesion of the trigeminal motor nucleus. Am J Orthod 1980;78:66–80.

152. Wolf G, Koskinen-Moffett L, Kokich V. Migration of craniofacial periosteum in guinea-pigs with unilateral masticatory muscle paralysis. J Anat 1985;140:259–268.

153. Hirabayashi S, Harii K, Sakurai A, et al. An experimental study of craniofacial growth in a heterotopic rat head transplant. Plast Reconstr Surg 1988;82:236–243.

154. Sakurai A, Hirabayashi S, Harii K, Fukuda O. Experimental studies on complete global brain ischemia using the isohistogenic infantile head transplant model in Lewis rats. J Reconstr Microsurg 1989;5:145–150.

155. Proffit WR, Fields HW. Occlusal forces in normal- and long-face children. J Dent Res 1983;62:571–574.

156. Vig KW. Nasal obstruction and facial growth: the strength of evidence for clinical assumptions. Am J Orthod Dentofacial Orthop 1998;113:603–611.

157. Tourne LP, Schweiger J. Immediate postural responses to total nasal obstruction. Am J Orthod Dentofacial Orthop 1996;110:606–611.

158. Fields HW, Warren DW, Black K, Phillips CL. Relationship between vertical dentofacial morphology and respiration in adolescents. Am J Orthod Dentofacial Orthop 1991;99:147–154.

159. Hermann NV, et al. Early craniofacial morphology and growth in children with bilateral complete cleft lip and palate. Cleft Palate Craniofac J 2004;41:424–438.

160. Will LA. Growth and development in patients with untreated clefts. Cleft Palate Craniofac J 2000;37:523–526.

161. Conrad AL, Richman L, Nopoulos P, Dailey S. Neuropsychological functioning in children with non-syndromic cleft of the lip and/or palate. Child Neuropsychol Epub ahead of print 2009;February 2;1–14.

162. Weinberg SM, Andreasen NC, Nopoulos P. Three-dimensional morphometric analysis of brain shape in nonsyndromic orofacial clefting. J Anat 2009;214:926–936.

163. Moyers RA, McNamara JA. In: McNamara JA, editor. Factors affecting growth of the midface. Craniofacial growth monograph series. Ann Arbor (MI): Center for Human Growth and Development, University of Michigan, 1976; 43–59, 169–204, 239–249.

164. Katsaros J, David DJ, Griffin PA, Moore MH. Facial dysmorphology in the neglected paediatric head and neck burn. Br J Plast Surg 1990;43:232–235.

165. Laurenzo JF, Canady JW, Zimmerman MB, Smith RJ. Craniofacial growth in rabbits. Effects of midfacial surgical trauma and rigid plate fixation. Arch Otolaryngol Head Neck Surg 1995;121:556–561.

166. Proffit WR, Vig KW, Turvey TA. Early fracture of the mandibular condyles: frequently an unsuspected cause of growth disturbances. Am J Orthod 1980;78:1–24.

167. Sahm G, Bartsch A, Witt E. Micro-electronic monitoring of functional appliance wear. Eur J Orthod 1990;12:297–301.

168. Proffit WR, White RP, Sarver DM. Contemporary treatment of dentofacial deformity. St. Louis (MO): Mosby, 2003; 43–51, 587–596.

169. Fujita T, et al. Influence of sex hormone disturbances on the internal structure of the mandible in newborn mice. Eur J Orthod 2006;28:190–194.

170. Ohlsson C, Isaksson O, Lindahl A. Clonal analysis of rat tibia growth plate chondrocytes in suspension culture—differential effects of growth hormone and insulin-like growth factor I. Growth Regul 1994;4:1–7.

171. Ramirez-Yanez GO, Smid JR, et al. Influence of growth hormone on the craniofacial complex of transgenic mice. Eur J Orthod 2005;27:494–500.

172. Berg MA, et al. Diverse growth hormone receptor gene mutations in Laron syndrome. Am J Hum Genet 1993;52:998–1005.

173. Schaefer GB, et al. Facial morphometry of Ecuadorian patients with growth hormone receptor deficiency/Laron syndrome. J Med Genet 1994;31:635–639.

174. Funatsu M, Sato K, Mitani H. Effects of growth hormone on craniofacial growth. Angle Orthod 2006;76:970–977.

175. Pirinen S. Endocrine regulation of craniofacial growth. Acta Odontol Scand 1995;53:179–185.

176. Barrett RL, Harris EF. Anabolic steroids and craniofacial growth in the rat. Angle Orthod 1993;63:289–298.

177. Petrovic A, Stutzmann J, Gasson N. [Is the final shape of the mandible, as such, genetically predetermined?] (French). Orthod Fr 1979;50:751–767.

178. Riesenfeld A. Endocrine and biomechanical control of craniofacial growth: an experimental study. Hum Biol 1974;46:531–572.

179. Rivkees SA, Danon M, Herrin J. Prednisone dose limitation of growth hormone treatment of steroid-induced growth failure. J Pediatr 1994;125:322–325.

180. Maor G, Silbermann M. Studies on hormonal regulation of the growth of the craniofacial skeleton: IV. Specific binding sites for glucocorticoids in condylar cartilage and their involvement in the biological effects of glucocorticoids on cartilage cell growth. J Craniofac Genet Dev Biol 1986;6:189–202.

181. Teng CM, Sobkowski FJ, Johnston LE Jr. The effect of cortisone on the eruption rate of root-resected incisors in the rat. Am J Orthod Dentofacial Orthop 1989;95:67–71.

182. Graham GG, Adrianzen B, Rabold J, Mellits ED. Later growth of malnourished infants and children. Comparison with "healthy" siblings and parents. Am J Dis Child 1982;136:348–352.

183. Soliman AT, et al. Serum insulin-like growth factors I and II concentrations and growth hormone and insulin responses to arginine infusion in children with protein-energy malnutrition before and after nutritional rehabilitation. Pediatr Res 1986;20:1122–1130.

184. Pucciarelli HM. The effects of race, sex, and nutrition on craniofacial differeniation in rats. A multivariate analysis. Am J Phys Anthropol 1980;53:359–368.

185. Pucciarelli HM. Growth of the functional components of the rat skull and its alteration by nutritional effects. A multivariate analysis. Am J Phys Anthropol 1981;56:33–41.

186. Engstrom C, Linde A, Thilander B. Craniofacial morphology and growth in the rat. Cephalometric analysis of the effects of a low calcium and vitamin D–deficient diet. J Anat 1982;134:299–314.

187. Baume LJ, Franquin JC, Korner WW. The prenatal effects of maternal vitamin A deficiency on the cranial and dental development of the progeny. Am J Orthod 1972;62:447–460.

188. Howe AM, Webster WS. Vitamin K—its essential role in craniofacial development. A review of the literature regarding vitamin K and craniofacial development. Aust Dent J 1994;39:88–92.

189. Li KW, Petro TM, Spalding PM. The effect of dietary protein deficiency and realimentation on serum growth hormone and insulin-like growth factor-I in growing mice. Nutrition Res. 1996;16:1211–1223.

190. Miller JP, German RZ. Protein malnutrition affects the growth trajectories of the craniofacial skeleton in rats. J Nutr 1999;129:2061–2069.

191. Russell GF. Premenarchal anorexia nervosa and its sequelae. J Psychiatr Res 1985;19:363–369.

192. Sadeghianrizi A, Forsberg CM, Marcus C, Dahllof G. Craniofacial development in obese adolescents. Eur J Orthod 2005;27:550–555.

193. Jantz RL. Cranial change in Americans: 1850–1975. J Forensic Sci 2001;46:784–787.

194. Salzer HR, Haschke F, Wimmer M, et al. Growth and nutritional intake of infants with congenital heart disease. Pediatr Cardiol 1989;10:17–23.

195. Berkowitz RJ, et al. Developmental orofacial deficits associated with multimodal cancer therapy: case report. Pediatr Dent 1989;11:227–231.

196. Cohen SR, Bartlett SP, Whitaker LA. Reconstruction of late craniofacial deformities after irradiation of the head and face during childhood. Plast Reconstr Surg 1990;86:229–237.

197. Yu JC, Fearon J, Havlik RJ, et al. Distraction osteogenesis of the craniofacial skeleton. Plast Reconstr Surg 2004;114:1E–20E.

198. Powell GF, Brasel JA, Blizzard RM. Emotional deprivation and growth retardation simulating idiopathic hypopituitarism. I. Clinical evaluation of the syndrome. N Engl J Med 1967;276:1271–1278.

199. Schell LM, Knutsen KL. Environmental effects on growth. In: Cameron N, editor. Human growth and development. London: Academic Press, Elsevier Science, 2002;165–195.

200. Schell LM, Norelli RJ. Airport noise exposure and the postnatal growth of children. Am J Phys Anthropol 1983;61:473–482.

201. Baccetti T, Reyes BC, McNamara JA Jr. Gender differences in Class III malocclusion. Angle Orthod 2005;75:510–520.

202. Gandini P, Mancini M, Andreani F. A comparison of hand-wrist bone and cervical vertebral analyses in measuring skeletal maturation. Angle Orthod 2006;76:984–989.

203. Chatzigianni A, Halazonetis DJ. Geometric morphometric evaluation of cervical vertebrae shape and its relationship to skeletal maturation. Am J Orthod Dentofacial Orthop 2009;136:481e1–9; discussion 481–483.

204. Fudalej P, Bollen AM. Effectiveness of the cervical vertebral maturation method to predict postpeak circumpubertal growth of craniofacial structures. Am J Orthod Dentofacial Orthop 2010;137:59–65.

205. Gabriel DB, et al. Cervical vertebrae maturation method: poor reproducibility. Am J Orthod Dentofacial Orthop 2009;136:478,e1–7; discussion 478–480.

206. Masoud MI, et al. Relationship between blood-spot insulin-like growth factor 1 levels and hand-wrist assessment of skeletal maturity. Am J Orthod Dentofacial Orthop 2009;136:59–64.

207. Mao JJ, Wang X, Kopher RA. Biomechanics of craniofacial sutures: orthopedic implications. Angle Orthod 2003;73:128–135.

208. Carlson DS. Biological rationale for early treatment of dentofacial deformities. Am J Orthod Dentofacial Orthop 2002;121:554–558.

209. Brunelle JA, Bhat M, Lipton JA. Prevalence and distribution of selected occlusal characteristics in the US population, 1988–1991. J Dent Res 1996;75(Spec No):706–713.

210. Proffit WR, White RP, Sarver DM. Contemporary treatment of dentofacial deformity. St Louis (MO): Mosby, 2003;23–24.

211. Haas AJ. Rapid expansion of the maxillary dental arch and nasal cavity by opening the mid-palatal suture. Angle Orthod 1961;31:73–90.

212. Jafari A, Shetty KS, Kumar M. Study of stress distribution and displacement of various craniofacial structures following application of transverse orthopedic forces—a three-dimensional FEM study. Angle Orthod 2003;73:12–20.

213. Wagemans PA, van de Velde JP, Kuijpers-Jagtman AM. Sutures and forces: a review. Am J Orthod Dentofacial Orthop 1988;94:129–141.

214. McNamara JA Jr. Early intervention in the transverse dimension: is it worth the effort? Am J Orthod Dentofacial Orthop 2002;121:572–574.

215. Melsen B, Melsen F. The postnatal development of the palatomaxillary region studied on human autopsy material. Am J Orthod 1982;82:329–342.

216. Baccetti T, Franchi L, Cameron CG, McNamara JA Jr. Treatment timing for rapid maxillary expansion. Angle Orthod 2001;71:343–350.

217. Hesse KL, Artun J, Joondeph DR, Kennedy DB. Changes in condylar postition and occlusion associated with maxillary expansion for correction of functional unilateral posterior crossbite. Am J Orthod Dentofacial Orthop 1997;111:410–418.

218. Liu C, Kaneko S, Soma K. Effects of a mandibular lateral shift on the condyle and mandibular bone in growing rats. Angle Orthod 2007;77:787–793.

219. Pirttiniemi P, Kantomaa T, Lahtela P. Relationship between craniofacial and condyle path asymmetry in unilateral crossbite patients. Eur J Orthod 1990;12:408–413.

220. Revelo B, Fishman LS. Maturational evaluation of ossification of the midpalatal suture. Am J Orthod Dentofacial Orthop 1994;105:288–292.

221. Hicks EP. Slow maxillary expansion. A clinical study of the skeletal versus dental response to low-magnitude force. Am J Orthod 1978;73:121–141.

222. Krebs AA. Expansion of mid palatal suture studied by means of metallic implants. Acta Odontol Scand 1959;17:491–501.

223. Wertz RA. Skeletal and dental changes accompanying rapid midpalatal suture opening. Am J Orthod 1970;58:41–66.

224. Krebs AA. Rapid expansion of mid palatal suture studied by fixed appliance. An implant study over a 7 year period. Trans Eur Orthod Soc 1964;141–142.

225. Lagravere MO, Major PW, Flores-Mir C. Long-term dental arch changes after rapid maxillary expansion treatment: a systematic review. Angle Orthod 2005;75:155–161.

226. Lagravere MO, Major PW, Flores-Mir C. Long-term skeletal changes with rapid maxillary expansion: a systematic review. Angle Orthod 2005;75:1046–1052.

227. Mommaerts MY. Transpalatal distraction as a method of maxillary expansion. Br J Oral Maxillofac Surg 1999;37:268–272.

228. Lagravère MO, Carey J, Heo G, et al. Transverse, vertical, and anteroposterior changes from bone-anchored maxillary expansion vs traditional rapid maxillary expansion: a randomized clinical trial. Am J Orthod Dentofacial Orthop 2010;137:304.e1–12; discussion 304–305.

229. Vig PS, Vig KW. Hybrid appliances: a component approach to dentofacial orthopedics. Am J Orthod Dentofacial Orthop 1986;90:273–285.

230. Ghafari J, Shofer FS, Jacobsson-Hunt U, et al. Headgear versus function regulator in the early treatment of Class II, Division 1 malocclusion: a randomized clinical trial. Am J Orthod Dentofacial Orthop 1998;113:51–61.

231. Keeling SD, et al. Anteroposterior skeletal and dental changes after early Class II treatment with bionators and headgear. Am J Orthod Dentofacial Orthop 1998;113:40–50.

232. Tulloch JF, Phillips C, Proffit WR. Benefit of early Class II treatment: progress report of a two-phase randomized clinical trial. Am J Orthod Dentofacial Orthop 1998;113:62–72, quiz 73–64.

233. Baumrind S, Molthen R, West EE, Miller DM. Distal displacement of the maxilla and the upper first molar. Am J Orthod 1979;75:630–640.

234. Howard RD. Skeletal changes with extra oral traction. Eur J Orthod 1982;4:197–202.

235. Melsen B. Effects of cervical anchorage during and after treatment: an implant study. Am J Orthod 1978;73:526–540.

236. Brandt HC, Shapiro PA, Kokich VG. Experimental and postexperimental effects of posteriorly directed extraoral traction in adult *Macaca fascicularis*. Am J Orthod 1979;75:301–317.

237. Droschl H. The effect of heavy orthopedic forces on the maxilla in the growing Saimiri sciureus (squirrel monkey). Am J Orthod 1973;63:449–461.

238. Elder JR, Tuenge RH. Cephalometric and histologic changes produced by extra-oral high pull traction to the maxilla of *Macaca mulatta*. Am J Orthod 1974;66:599–617.

239. Thompson RW. Extraoral high-pull forces with rapid palatal expansion in the *Macaca mulatta*. Am J Orthod 1974;66:302–317.

240. Dermaut LR, Aelbers CM. Orthopedics in orthodontics: fiction or reality. A review of the literature–Part II. Am J Orthod Dentofacial Orthop 1996;110:667–671.

241. Born J, Muth S, Fehm HL. The significance of sleep onset and slow wave sleep for nocturnal release of growth hormone (GH) and cortisol. Psychoneuroendocrinology 1988;13:233–243.

242. Risinger RK, Proffit WR. Continuous overnight observation of human premolar eruption. Arch Oral Biol 1996;41:779–789.

243. Stevenson S, Hunziker EB, Herrmann W, Schenk RK. Is longitudinal bone growth influenced by diurnal variation in the mitotic activity of chondrocytes of the growth plate? J Orthop Res 1990;8:132–135.

244. McNamara JA Jr, Bryan FA. Long-term mandibular adaptations to protrusive function: an experimental study in *Macaca mulatta*. Am J Orthod Dentofacial Orthop 1987;92:98–108.

245. Petrovic AG. Experimental and cybernetic approaches to the mechanism of action of functional appliances on mandibular growth. In: McNamara JA, Ribbons KA, editors. Malocclusion and the periodontium. Craniofacial growth monograph series. Ann Arbor (MI): Center for Human Growth and Development, University of Michigan, 1984;213–268.

246. Rabie AB, She TT, Hagg U. Functional appliance therapy accelerates and enhances condylar growth. Am J Orthod Dentofacial Orthop 2003;123:40–48.

247. Jakobsson SO, Paulin G. The influence of activator treatment on skeletal growth in Angle Class II: 1 cases. A roentgenocephalometric study. Eur J Orthod 1990; 12:174–184.

248. McNamara JA Jr, Bookstein FL, Shaughnessy TG. Skeletal and dental changes following functional regulator therapy on Class II patients. Am J Orthod 1985;88:91–110.

249. Pancherz H. The effect of continuous bite jumping on the dentofacial complex: a follow-up study after Herbst appliance treatment of Class II malocclusions. Eur J Orthod 1981;3:49–60.

250. Remmer KR, Mamandras AH, Hunter WS, Way DC. Cephalometric changes associated with treatment using the activator, the Frankel appliance, and the fixed appliance. Am J Orthod 1985;88:363–372.

251. Righellis EG. Treatment effects of Frankel, activator and extraoral traction appliances. Angle Orthod 1983;53:107–121.

252. Bjork A. The principle of the Andresen method of orthodontic treatment: a discussion based on cephalometric x-ray analysis of treated cases. Am J Orthod 1951;37:437–458.

253. Gianelly AA, Brosnan P, Martignoni M, Bernstein L. Mandibular growth, condyle position and Frankel appliance therapy. Angle Orthod 1983;53:131–142.

254. Nelson C, Harkness M. Herbison P. Mandibular changes during functional appliance treatment. Am J Orthod Dentofacial Orthop 1993;104:153–161.

255. Wieslander L, Lagerstrom L. The effect of activator treatment on Class II malocclusions. Am J Orthod 1979;75:20–26.

256. Harrison JE, O'Brien KD, Worthington HV. Orthodontic treatment for prominent upper front teeth in children. Cochrane Database Syst Rev 2007;3:CD003452.

257. Ahlgren J, Laurin C. Late results of activator-treatment: a cephalometric study. Br J Orthod 1976;3:181–187.

258. Freunthaller P. Cephalometric observation in Class II, Division I malocclusions treated with the activator. Angle Orthod 1967;37:18–25.

259. Baumrind S, Korn EL, Isaacson RJ, et al. Quantitative analysis of the orthodontic and orthopedic effects of maxillary traction. Am J Orthod 1983;84:384–398.

260. Baumrind S, Korn EL, Molthen R, West EE. Changes in facial dimensions associated with the use of forces to retract the maxilla. Am J Orthod 1981;80:17–30.

261. Baccetti T, Franchi L, Stahl F. Comparison of 2 comprehensive Class II treatment protocols including the bonded Herbst and headgear appliances: a double-blind study of consecutively treated patients at puberty. Am J Orthod Dentofacial Orthop 2009;135:698.e1–10; discussion 698–699.

262. Teuscher U. A growth-related concept for skeletal Class II treatment. Am J Orthod 1978;74:258–275.

263. Wieslander L. Long-term effect of treatment with the head-gear-Herbst appliance in the early mixed dentition. Stability or relapse? Am J Orthod Dentofacial Orthop 1993;104:319–329.

264. Pancherz H. The effects, limitations, and long-term dentofacial adaptations to treatment with the Herbst appliance. Semin Orthod 1997;3:232–243.

265. von Bremen J, Pancherz H. Efficiency of early and late Class II division 1 treatment. Am J Orthod Dentofacial Orthop 2002;121:31–37.

266. Dolce C, McGorray SP, Brazeau L, et al. Timing of Class II treatment: skeletal changes comparing 1-phase and 2-phase treatment. Am J Orthod Dentofacial Orthop 2007;132:481–489.

267. O'Brien K, et al. Prospective, multi-center study of the effectiveness of orthodontic/orthognathic surgery care in the United Kingdom. Am J Orthod Dentofacial Orthop 2009;135:709–714.

268. Tulloch JF, Proffit WR, Phillips C. Outcomes in a 2-phase randomized clinical trial of early Class II treatment. Am J Orthod Dentofacial Orthop 2004;125:657–667.

269. Brin I, Tulloch JF, Koroluk L, Philips C. External apical root resorption in Class II malocclusion: a retrospective review of 1- versus 2-phase treatment. Am J Orthod Dentofacial Orthop 2003;124:151–156.

270. Proffit WR, Tulloch JF. Preadolescent Class II problems: treat now or wait? Am J Orthod Dentofacial Orthop 2002;121:560–562.

271. Bishara SE. Facial and dental changes in adolescents and their clinical implications. Angle Orthod 2000;70:471–483.

272. Yamada S, et al. Diurnal variation in the response of the mandible to orthopedic force. J Dent Res 2002;81:711–715.

273. Allen RA, Connolly IH, Richardson A. Early treatment of Class III incisor relationship using the chincap appliance. Eur J Orthod 1993;15:371–376.

274. Sugawara J, Mitani H. Facial growth of skeletal Class III malocclusion and the effects, limitations, and long-term dentofacial adaptations to chincap therapy. Semin Orthod 1997;3:244–254.

275. Thilander B. Chin-cap treatment for Angle Class 3 malocclusion. Rep Congr Eur Orthod Soc 1965;41:311–327.

276. Vego L. Early orthopedic treatment for Class III skeletal patterns. Am J Orthod 1976;70:59–69.

277. Sakamoto T, Iwase I, Uka A, Nakamura S. A roentgenocephalometric study of skeletal changes during and after chin cup treatment. Am J Orthod 1984;85:341–350.

278. Sugawara J, Asano T, Endo N, Mitani H. Long-term effects of chincap therapy on skeletal profile in mandibular prognathism. Am J Orthod Dentofacial Orthop 1990;98:127–133.

279. Levin AS, McNamara JA Jr, Franchi L, et al. Short-term and long-term treatment outcomes with the FR-3 appliance of Frankel. Am J Orthod Dentofacial Orthop 2008;134:513–524.

280. Ulgen M, Firatli S. The effects of the Frankel's function regulator on the Class III malocclusion. Am J Orthod Dentofacial Orthop 1994;105:561–567.

281. Delaire J. [Considerations on facial growth (particularly of the maxilla). Therapeutic deductions] (French). Rev Stomatol Chir Maxillofac 71971;2:57–76.

282. Jackson GW, Kokich VG, Shapiro PA. Experimental and postexperimental response to anteriorly directed extraoral force in young *Macaca nemestrina*. Am J Orthod 1979;75:318–333.

283. Nartallo-Turley PE, Turley PK. Cephalometric effects of combined palatal expansion and facemask therapy on Class III malocclusion. Angle Orthod 1998;68:217–224.

284. Ngan P, Hagg U, Yiu C, et al. Treatment response to maxillary expansion and protraction. Eur J Orthod 1996;18:151–168.

285. Takada K, Petdachai S, Sakuda M. Changes in dentofacial morphology in skeletal Class III children treated by a modified maxillary protraction headgear and a chin cup: a longitudinal cephalometric appraisal. Eur J Orthod 1993;15:211–221.

286. Ngan PW, Hagg U, Yiu C, Wei SH. Treatment response and long-term dentofacial adaptations to maxillary expansion and protraction. Semin Orthod 1997;3:255–264.

287. Williams MD, Sarver DM, Sadowsky PL, Bradley E. Combined rapid maxillary expansion and protraction facemask in the treatment of Class III malocclusions in growing children: a prospective long-term study. Semin Orthod 1997;3:265–274.

288. da Silva Filho OG, Magro AC, Capelozza Filho L. Early treatment of the Class III malocclusion with rapid maxillary expansion and maxillary protraction. Am J Orthod Dentofacial Orthop 1998;113:196–203.

289. Gautam P, Valiathan A, Adhikari R. Skeletal response to maxillary protraction with and without maxillary expansion: a finite element study. Am J Orthod Dentofacial Orthop 2009;135:723–728.

290. Vaughn GA, Mason B, Moon HB, Turley PK. The effects of maxillary protraction therapy with or without rapid palatal expansion: a prospective, randomized clinical trial. Am J Orthod Dentofacial Orthop 2005;128:299–309.

291. Baccetti T, McGill JS, Franchi L, et al. Skeletal effects of early treatment of Class III malocclusion with maxillary expansion and face-mask therapy. Am J Orthod Dentofacial Orthop 1998;113:333–343.

292. Kapust AJ, Sinclair PM, Turley PK. Cephalometric effects of face mask/expansion therapy in Class III children: a comparison of three age groups. Am J Orthod Dentofacial Orthop 1998;113:204–212.

293. Baik HS. Clinical results of the maxillary protraction in Korean children. Am J Orthod Dentofacial Orthop 1995; 108:583–592.

294. Gallagher RW, Miranda F, Buschang PH. Maxillary protraction: treatment and posttreatment effects. Am J Orthod Dentofacial Orthop 1998;113:612–619.

295. Merwin D, Ngan P, Hagg U, et al. Timing for effective application of anteriorly directed orthopedic force to the maxilla. Am J Orthod Dentofacial Orthop 1997;112:292–299.

296. Baccetti T, Franchi L, McNamara JA Jr. Cephalometric variables predicting the long-term success or failure of combined rapid maxillary expansion and facial mask therapy. Am J Orthod Dentofacial Orthop 2004;126:16–22.

297. Hagg U, Tse A, Bendeus M, Rabie AB. Long-term follow-up of early treatment with reverse headgear. Eur J Orthod 2003; 25:95–102.

298. Kircelli BH, Pektas ZO. Midfacial protraction with skeletally anchored face mask therapy: a novel approach and preliminary results. Am J Orthod Dentofacial Orthop 2008;133:440–449.

299. Smalley WM, Shapiro PA, Hohl TH, et al. Osseointegrated titanium implants for maxillofacial protraction in monkeys. Am J Orthod Dentofacial Orthop 1988;94:285–295.

300. Baccetti T, Reyes BC, McNamara JA Jr. Craniofacial changes in Class III malocclusion as related to skeletal and dental maturation. Am J Orthod Dentofacial Orthop 2007;132:171.e1–171.e12.

301. De Clerck HJ, Cornelis MA, Cevidanes LH, et al. Orthopedic traction of the maxilla with miniplates: a new perspective for treatment of midface deficiency. J Oral Maxillofac Surg 2009;67:2123–2129.

302. Heymann GC, Cevidanes L, Cornelis M, et al. Three-dimensional analysis of maxillary protraction with intermaxillary elastics to miniplates. Am J Orthod Dentofacial Orthop 2010;137:274–284.

303. Cevidanes L, Baccette T, Franchi L, McNamara JA, De Clerck H. Comparison of two protocols for maxillary protraction: bone anchors versus face mask with rapid maxillary expansion. Angle Orthod 2010;80:799-806.

304. Lundstrom A, Woodside DG. Longitudinal changes in facial type in cases with vertical and horizontal mandibular growth directions. Eur J Orthod 1983;5:259–268.

305. Woodside DG, Altuna G, Harvold E, et al. Primate experiments in malocclusion and bone induction. Am J Orthod 1983; 83:460–468.

306. Barbre RE, Sinclair PM. A cephalometric evaluation of anterior openbite correction with the magnetic active vertical corrector. Angle Orthod 1991;61:93–102.

307. Iscan HN, Sarisoy L. Comparison of the effects of passive posterior bite-blocks with different construction bites on the craniofacial and dentoalveolar structures. Am J Orthod Dentofacial Orthop 1997;112:171–178.

308. Kalra V, Burstone CJ, Nanda R. Effects of a fixed magnetic appliance on the dentofacial complex. Am J Orthod Dentofacial Orthop 1989;95:467–478.

309. Kuster R, Ingervall B. The effect of treatment of skeletal open bite with two types of bite-blocks. Eur J Orthod 1992;14:489–499.

310. Freeman CS, McNamara JA Jr, Baccetti T, et al. Treatment effects of the bionator and high-pull facebow combination followed by fixed appliances in patients with increased vertical dimensions. Am J Orthod Dentofacial Orthop 2007;131:184–195.

311. Umemori M, Sugawara J, Mitani H, et al. Skeletal anchorage system for open-bite correction. Am J Orthod Dentofacial Orthop 1998;115:166–174.

312. Kuroda S, Sakai Y, Tamamura N, et al. Treatment of severe anterior open bite with skeletal anchorage in adults: comparison with orthognathic surgery outcomes. Am J Orthod Dentofacial Orthop 2007;132:599–605.

313. Park HS, Kwon TG, Kwon OW. Treatment of open bite with microscrew implant anchorage. Am J Orthod Dentofacial Orthop 2004;126:627–636.

314. Shapiro PA. Stability of open bite treatment. Am J Orthod Dentofacial Orthop 2002;121:566–568.

315. Schutz-Fransson U, Bjerklin K, Lindsten R. Long-term follow-up of orthodontically treated deep bite patients. Eur J Orthod 2006;28:503–512.

316. Cohen SR. Craniofacial distraction with a modular internal distraction system: evolution of design and surgical techniques. Plast Reconstr Surg 1999;103:1592–1607.

317. Sawaki Y, Ohkubo H, Hibi H, Ueda M. Mandibular lengthening by distraction osteogenesis using osseointegrated implants and an intraoral device: a preliminary report. J Oral Maxillofac Surg 1996;54:594–600.

318. Kim YH, Han UK, Lim DD, Serraon ML. Stability of anterior openbite correction with multiloop edgewise archwire therapy: A cephalometric follow-up study. Am J Orthod Dentofacial Orthop 2000;118:43–54.

Orthognathic Database Acquisition

Marc B. Ackerman, DMD, and David M. Sarver, DMD, MS

INTRODUCTION

Traditional methods of database acquisition remain the primary means of beginning the diagnostic and treatment planning phases of orthognathic surgery, although recent advances in imaging and improvements in accuracy have contributed to some improvements in this process. Prior to the new millennium, treatment planning in orthognathic surgery was based primarily on a system of clinical observations, a static set of records (dental models, two-dimensional radiographs), with the major goals of treatment directed toward satisfying lateral cephalometric goals (STOs [surgical treatment objectives]). These goals include the correction of specific measurements (sella-nasion–A point and A point–nasion–B point differences) or analytical norms (Steiner, Ricketts), or even comparison of lateral cephalometric film tracings of patients with craniofacial skeletal dysplasia[1-3] to templates having average skeletal proportions derived from longitudinal growth studies.[4] The most significant shortcoming of reliance on the lateral cephalometric film as the primary determinant of treatment goals is that it did not take into account the resting and dynamic hard-soft tissue relationships, which are the most critical aspects in treatment planning for both orthodontics and orthognathic surgery. Furthermore, cephalometric analysis quantifies dentoskeletal relationships in angular and linear measures, which are not entirely representative of the three-dimensioanl multidimensional interrelationship of craniofacial structures. In other words, the integumental soft tissue drape may, on occasion, be inconsistent with the underlying skeletal framework in an individual patient. Whereas the skeletal framework may be reasonably stable after adolescence, the soft tissues become more susceptible to maturational and age-related changes. The cephalometric approach to treatment planning is now considered "procrustean," after the story based on Greek mythology, in which Procrustes was an innkeeper with only one bed, and if a traveler was too tall for the bed, Procrustes would cut off the traveler's feet so that he or she would fit the bed. A traveler who was too short would be stretched on a rack to likewise fit the bed in length. This charming story relates to this chapter in that the inappropriate application of the same hard tissue lateral cephalometric analysis to all patients would result in all of our patients being crammed into the same bed, with the goal of creating patients with similar, or "normal," cephalometric measurements, but with poor final functional and aesthetic results.

The contemporary approach to the surgical-orthodontic treatment of dentofacial deformities illustrates the importance of the use of dentofacial proportionality instead of applying absolute linear or angular norms to individual patients. Individualized patient-specific treatment planning is the focus of this chapter.

CONTEMPORARY ORTHOGNATHIC TREATMENT PLANNING

The emphasis on orthognathic diagnosis and treatment planning will lead the clincan into a new era and methodology of patient analysis and establishment of treatment goals. In modern orthognathic surgery, treatment goals are determined through systematic clinical examination and quantification of the individual patient's dentofacial characteristics. Therefore, the purpose of this chapter is to introduce a method of systematic three-dimensional dentofacial analysis with emphasis on both static and dynamic relationships as well as both functional and aesthetic treatment objectives.

Problem-oriented treatment planning has served the orthodontist and oral and maxillofacial surgeon well in the past several decades by focusing on the problems in need of correction, including the identification of solutions for each problem. The natural progression of problem-oriented treatment planning should include both the identification of favorable attributes as well as the abnormal features and problems in facial proportions. The reason for this is the realization that focusing solely on the problems and their solutions may result

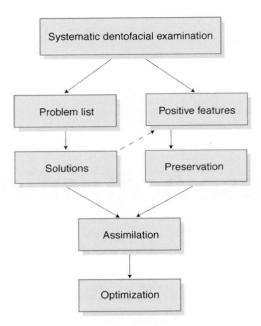

FIGURE 54-1. Contemporary treatment planning flow chart. After the clinical examination and databasing of the quantitative measurements, both problems and positive attributes are identified. Solutions for the problems are identified and the *dotted arrow* indicates that each potential solution can negatively affect a positive feature. Therefore, the advantage of measuring both problems and positive features permits the clinician to recognize the potential negative impact that any given solution has on the positive attributes. This "decision tree" leads to correction of the problems but also preservation of the positive attributes. The clinician then assimilates all of this information for optimization of treatment.

in a treatment plan that potentially has a negative effect on the positive attributes already present in a patient. A classic orthodontic example is one in which the extraction of maxillary premolars in the correction of a skeletal class II malocclusion, although satisfying functional and occlusal issues, may result in profile flattening and a negative effect on facial appearance. In orthognathic surgery, a good example is widening of the alar base secondary to maxillary advancement and/or impaction. The goal of orthognathic treatment is the correction or optimization of negative attributes, while at the same time preserving those attributes that are deemed favorable (Figure 54-1).

This systematic approach to clinical examination of the patient is essential for the development of an optimization-oriented database. All clinically detectable deviations from the optimal range fall into the two broad categories, function and aesthetics.

Oral Function and Dentofacial Deformity

Patients with severe discrepancies in the size and position of their jaws and teeth often have difficulty with oral function. Certain foods may be difficult to incise and chew, and speech may also be negatively affected by a jaw deformity. If the

patient cannot bring the tongue and lips into the proper position, it may not be possible to produce a specific sound properly. Other than a careful clinical examination of the patient, it is doubtful that diagnostic tests of oral function could be performed adequately in the dental or surgical office. The relationship of temporomandibular joint (TMJ) problems to severe malocclusions and dentofacial deformities is complex, but important. Although there is some evidence that patients with specific types of malocclusion are more susceptible to TMJ problems (e.g., prevalence of internal derangement in class II deformities), the increased risk is relatively small.[5] In general terms, patients with dentofacial deformity are similar to patients with normal facial proportions with regards to the prevalence of TMJ problems.[6] In addition, speech and mastication are commonly affected negatively by dentoskeletal deformities that may affect tongue position and lip competence, and much research has focused on the effects of correction of the skeletal deformity on speech and bite forces, with mixed results.

Facial Aesthetics and Dentofacial Deformity

Appearance and dentofacial aesthetics can be divided into three subcategories: macroaesthetics, miniaesthetics, and microaesthetics (Figure 54-2). The specific aesthetic concerns of the patient can be elucidated through open-ended doctor-patient communication and then integrated into the diagnostic decision-making tree. The surgeon and orthodontist should be sensitive to the patient's aesthetic desires, balancing them against cultural and familial standards and norms. The physical burden of orthodotnic and surgical treatment is borne by the patient and must be considered when determining the extent of treatment intervention. For example, when deciding whether treatment should involve orthodontics alone, orthodontics and orthognathic surgery, or acceptable orthodontic camouflage, the patient should understand the risk-benefit ratio of any given treatment sequence.

DATABASE COLLECTION

Primary database collection begins with the clinical examination and is supplemented with static and dynamic recordings of the patient in three spatial dimensions. Record-taking should replicate the functional and aesthetic facial presentation of the patient. Findings from the clinical examination should be either confirmed or challenged by data obtained from the records. The analysis of the clinical database will generate a diagnostic summary and optimized problem list. An emerging soft tissue paradigm in surgical orthodontic treatment planning has refocused analysis on facial proportionality and balance versus reliance on normative data derived from cephalometrics.[7] The art of surgical orthodontics rests in the ability to envisage the patient's desired three-dimensional soft tissue outcome and then retroengineer the dental and skeletal hard tissues to produce such a change. The concept of retroengineering is explained later in this

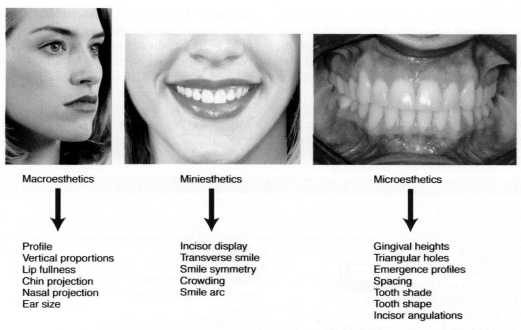

Macroesthetics	Miniesthetics	Microesthetics
Profile	Incisor display	Gingival heights
Vertical proportions	Transverse smile	Triangular holes
Lip fullness	Smile symmetry	Emergence profiles
Chin projection	Crowding	Spacing
Nasal projection	Smile arc	Tooth shade
Ear size		Tooth shape
		Incisor angulations

FIGURE 54-2. Recommended subcategories of appearance and aesthetics.

chapter under technologic applications to orthognathic treatment planning.

In today's clinical environment there are three methods of data collection. The first and most commonly used method includes still facial photography, dental study models, and lateral and posteroanterior cephalometric radiographs. The second is the use of databasing programs to document direct clinical measurement of the patient's resting and dynamic, or functional, relationships. The third involves the use of digital video to record the dynamics of facial movement. This methodology as it currently exists does not dynamically quantify movement, but emerging technologies should lead to research into the clinical application of quantification of dynamic facial movements.

Conventional Diagnostic Records

Standard orthodontic records have not changed significantly in many years, but contemporary records in surgical orthodontic treatment are changing rapidly. Surgical orthodontics demands three-dimensional treatment planning of all patients. In clinical practice, standard diagnostic records include digital photographs, two-dimensional radiographs, and dental study models (plaster, mounted or unmounted, or digitally scanned dental models [e.g., OrthoCAD]). The facial images, which are considered universally standard records, include a frontal view at rest, frontal smile, and profile at rest images. Whereas these orientations do provide an adequate amount of diagnostic information, they do not contain all of the information needed for three-dimensional visualization and quantification. Orthognathic surgery requires expansion of the database compared with conventional orthodontic treatment.

The suggested records can be divided into two groups: static and dynamic. The accepted facial photographic recordings should include frontal smile close-up, oblique (or three-quarter view) facial smile, oblique smile close-up, and profile smile, as well as bird's-eye and worm's-eye views, when indicated for facial syndromic or nonsyndromic asymmetries.[8]

Direct Measurement as a Biometric Tool

The goal of the clinical examination is to quantitatively assess soft and hard tissue attributes of the dentofacial complex and record what elements are satisfactory and which are in need of correction or optimization. Whereas clinical examination procedures vary greatly among practitioners, measurements should be thorough, systematic, and consistent, in an attempt to minimize the chance that something of importance will be overlooked. It is critical to avoid a situation in which the clinician performs a cursory examination, recording only brief notes regarding abnormalities observed, without recording any other descriptive data. This practice is often justified by the assumption that most diagnostic decisions can be made from the records after the patient leaves. This is a poor assumption for several reasons. First, static records cannot reflect the dynamic relationships that are important in the overall functional assessment of the patient. For example, the simple idea of the relationship of the upper incisor at rest and on smile is not reflected on radiographs or models and is poorly evaluated in photographs. Second, information that may have not looked important enough to document during a cursory examination may be important later and, therefore, would be unavailable because it was not recorded. Third, a thorough and comprehensive examination record that includes normal observations provides an accurate medicolegal document. It is difficult for an unhappy patient to prove negligence when it is clear that comprehensive clinical information was obtained and utilized in the treatment planning phases. The more thorough and well documented the record is, the more valuable it is if problems arise after treatment.

Contemporary clinical examination uses a computer-databasing program to facilitate data entry, and these data are then merged into reports and treatment planning screens or forms.[9] Each clinical characteristic in the examination has a pop-up menu containing all of the possible descriptions for that particular trait (Figure 54-3). By using a computer interface, the surgeon or orthodontist saves valuable time in both the clinical examination and the diagnostic and treatment planning workup. The information is then stored for recall and analysis and can even have predefined parameters that identify problematic measurements automatically.

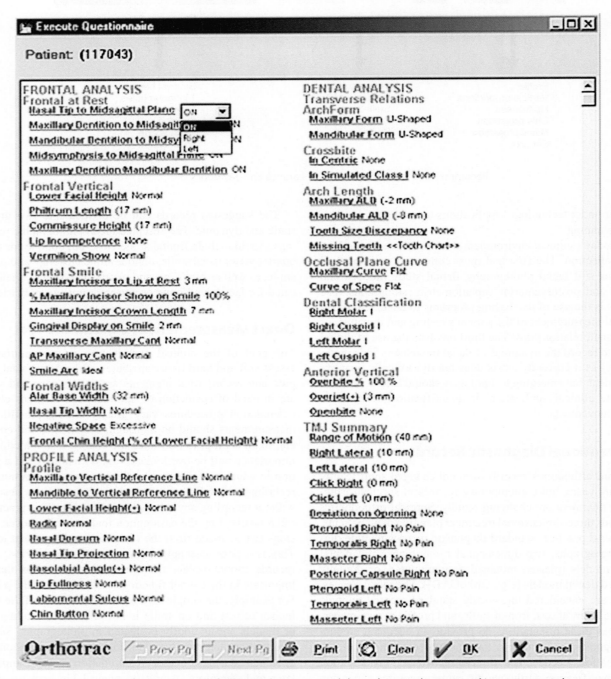

FIGURE 54-3. A computer databasing program facilitates data entry, and these data are then merged into reports and treatment planning screens or forms. Each clinical characteristic in the examination has a pop-up menu containing all of the possible descriptions for that particular trait.

As an example of how this interface facilitates the examination of dynamic hard-soft tissue relationships, the following frontal measurements may be performed systematically in evaluation of anterior dental display, both at rest and at smile:

■ Philtrum height: The philtrum height is measured in millimeters from subnasale (the base of the nose at the midline) to the most inferior portion of the upper lip on the vermilion tip beneath the philtral columns. The absolute linear measurement is not particularly important, but what is significant is its relationship to the upper incisor and the commissures of the mouth. In the adolescent, it is common to find the philtrum height to be shorter than the commissure height, and the difference can be explained in the differential in lip growth with maturation.

■ Commissure height: The commissure height is measured from a line constructed from the alar bases through subspinale, then from the commissures perpendicular to this line.

■ Interlabial gap: The interlabial gap is the distance in millimeters between the upper and the lower lips, when lip incompetence is present.

■ Amount of incisor show at rest: The amount of upper incisor display at rest is a critical aesthetic parameter because one of the inevitable characteristics of an aging tooth-lip relationship is diminished upper incisor show at rest and on smile. For example, an adult patient who displays 3 mm of gingival display on smile and 3 mm of upper incisor at rest should carefully consider only maxillary incisor intrusion or maxillary impaction to reduce gingival display, because reduction in gingival display also results in diminished incisor show at rest and during conversation (a characteristic of the aging face).

■ Amount of incisor display on smile: On smile, patients will show either their entire upper incisor or only a percentage of the incisor. Measurement of the percentage of incisor display, when combined with the crown height measured next, leads the clinician to decide how much tooth movement is required to attain the appropriate smile for that patient.

■ Crown height: The vertical height of the maxillary central incisors in the adult is measured in millimeters and is normally between 9 and 12 mm, with an average of 10.6 mm in males and 9.6 mm in females. The age of the patient is a factor in crown height because of the rate of apical migration in the adolescent.

■ Gingival display: There is variability in what is aesthetically acceptable for the amount of gingival display on smile, but it is important to always remember the relationship between gingival display and the amount of incisor shown at rest. In broad terms, it is better for a patient to be treated less aggressively in reducing smile gumminess when considering that the aging process will result in a natural diminishment of this characteristic. A gummy smile is often more aesthetic than a smile with diminished tooth display.

■ Smile arc: The smile arc should be defined as the relationship of the curvature of the incisal edges of the maxillary incisors and canines to the curvature of the lower lip in the posed social smile.[10,11] The ideal smile arc has the maxillary incisal edge curvature parallel to the curvature of the lower lip upon smile, and the term *consonant* is used to describe this parallel relationship. A *nonconsonant,* or flat, smile arc is characterized by the maxillary incisal curvature being flatter than the curvature of the lower lip on smile. The smile arc relationship is not as quantitatively measurable as the other attributes, so the qualitative observation of consonant, flat, or reverse smile arcs is generally cited.

It critically important to measure the previously described characteristics in orthognathic cases for a variety of reasons. The following case illustrates the significance of resting and dynamic soft tissue measurements, and how surgical or orthodontic treatment planning is determined by direct measurement as much as it is by indirect cephalometric radiographic analysis. The role of cephalometrics is discussed later in this chapter, and the emphasis is less on static comparisons to norms and more on its coordination with the soft tissue overlay of the individual face and the use of predictive algorithms to arrive at final macrotreatment decisions.

The patient in Figure 54-4 was a 16-year-old male who presented with a chief complaint of excessive gingival display on smile, or a "gummy smile" (see Figure 54–4A). He had finished orthodontic treatment 1 year ago, and the orthodontist believed that the only way to improve smile aesthetics further was to consider maxillary superior repositioning via a Le Fort I osteotomy. The oral and maxillofacial surgeon wanted to wait until growth completion, but the patient's mother pursued further investigation.

The examination revealed an excellent occlusion, and the macrorelations were also normal in terms of profile and facial proportions. The anterior tooth-lip relationships were as follows:

■ Resting relationships (see Figure 54-4B)
   ▪ Philtrum height: 25 mm
   ▪ Commissure height: 25 mm
   ▪ Maxillary incisor at rest: 2 mm
■ Dynamic relationships (see Figure 54-4C)
   ▪ Percentage of maxillary incisor display on smile: 100%
   ▪ Maxillary incisor crown height: 8 mm
   ▪ Gingival display on smile: 4 mm
   ▪ Smile arc: consonant

It is useful to outline the various etiologies of excessive gingival display on smile and characteristics seen with each in order to demonstrate the decision-making process in problem-oriented treatment planning with optimization:

■ Vertical maxillary excess: VME is characterized by a disproportionately long lower facial height, lip incompetence, excessive incisor display at rest, and excessive gingival display on smile.

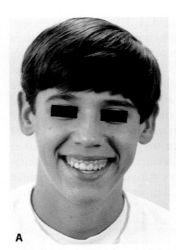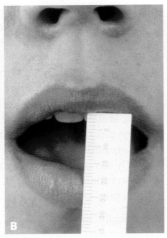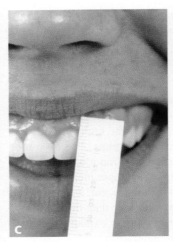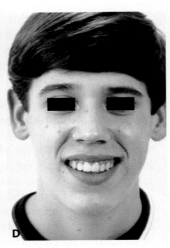

FIGURE 54-4. **A–D,** Case illustration of direct measurement of lip-tooth-gingival relationships.

■ Short philtrum: The philtrum height is shorter than the commissure, with excessive incisor display at rest, and a reverse resting upper lip line.
■ Excessive smile curtain: Excessive animation of the upper lip on smile is seen, displaying more tooth and gingiva than desired.
■ Short crown height: If the anterior incisor height is short, excessive gingival display may result.

In this case, VME was ruled out because facial proportionality was normal, no lip incompetence was present, and only 2 mm of upper incisor showed at rest. The second possibility, a short philtrum, was ruled out because the philtrum and commissure heights were the same and no reverse upper lip resting characteristics were noted. The third possibility, excessive curtain, was eliminated because the vermilion was adequate on smile and the margins of the commissure and philtrum even on posed smile. The fourth possibility, short crown height, was significant because the maxillary incisors measured to be only 8 mm in height.

Treatment options to decrease gingival display included maxillary impaction, orthodontic intrusion of maxillary incisors, or periodontal crown lengthening.

■ Maxillary impaction: A 4-mm superior repositioning of the maxilla would decrease the gumminess of the smile, but would result in a –2-mm upper incisor show at rest, greatly hastening the aging characteristics of the face and smile.
■ Orthodontic intrusion of the maxillary anterior teeth: This would likewise result in reduction of incisor display at rest but would also flatten the already consonant smile arc.
■ Periodontal crown lengthening: The increase in anterior crown height decreases the gumminess of the smile (appropriate because the teeth are short) and optimizes treatment by *not* decreasing incisor display at rest and by maintaining the consonant smile arc.

After discussing all these options with the family, the family decided to proceed with the third and recommended option

of crown lengthening, with an excellent aesthetic outcome (see Figure 54-4D).

In summary, this case demonstrates the new direction in dentofacial treatment planning, even though the final result was not an orthognathic treatment plan. This case was selected to make the point that through careful observation and measurement, the appropriate treatment plan was performed.

Digital Videography

Dynamic recording of patient's facial motion is accomplished with the use of digital videography.[12] This technology may be used to document and evaluate such characteristics as range of mandibular motion on opening and laterotrusive movements, deviations on opening, smile, and speech. Digital video and computer technology have primarily been used to record anterior tooth display during speech and smiling. Digital videos can be recorded in a standardized fashion with the camera at a fixed distance from the subject. It is recommended that these images be taken in a standard format with emphasis on natural head position, so that future analysis and research possibilities may be maximized. It is also recommended that video be taken in the frontal, oblique, and lateral dimensions. Clinically, an example of where this technology is most relevant is the patient with an asymmetrical smile. The question that arises is whether or not the patient has a dental asymmetry, skeletal asymmetry, or asymmetrical movement of the lip curtain during animation. The single smile photograph cannot corroborate the clinical impression gained during the data collection process. The video clip may be reviewed and evaluated during all planning phases of treatment as well as for comparison of the orthognathic treatment effects (Figure 54-5).

SYSTEMATIC CLINICAL EXAMINATION OF DENTOFACIAL DEFORMITIES

The importance of clinical observation and direct measurement of the interaction of hard and soft tissues in planning

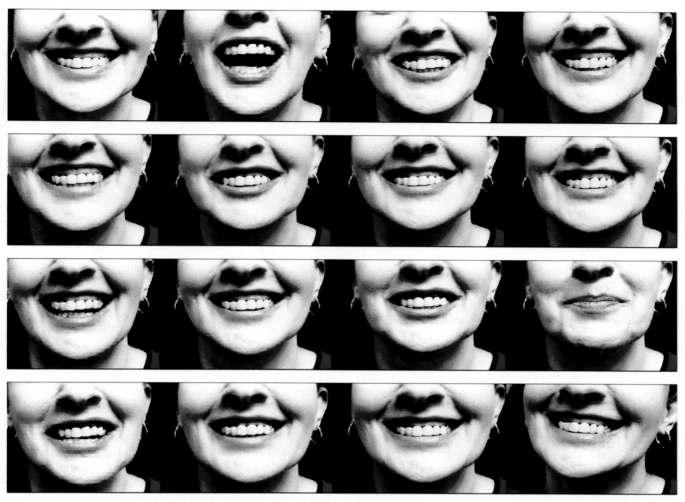

FIGURE 54-5. The video clip may be reviewed and evaluated during all planning phases of treatment as well as for comparison of the orthognathic treatment effects.

appropriate combined orthodontic and orthognathic treatments of dentofacial deformity has been discussed, and in this section, the components of the examination from the macro-, mini-, and microperspectives are described.

Macroaesthetic Examination: Frontal View

The facial areas for macroaesthetic examination, as investigated from the frontal view, can be summarized as follows:

- Vertical proportions
  - Facial heights:
  - Lower facial third
- Transverse proportions
  - Rule of fifths
  - Middle fifth
    - Inner canthi
    - Alar base
  - Medial two fifths
    - Outer canthi
    - Gonial angles of mandible
- Outer two fifths
  - Ear deformity
  - Ear projection
- Nasal anatomy
- Alar base
- Columella
- Nasal tip
- Dorsum
- Transverse symmetry
  - Nasal tip to midsagittal plane
  - Maxillary dental midline to midsagittal plane
  - Mandibular dental midline to symphysis
  - Mandibular asymmetry with or without functional shift
  - Maxillomandibular asymmetry
  - Chin asymmetry

The starting point for the macroaesthetic examination is the frontal perspective. Transverse and vertical relationships make up the major components of the frontal examination and analysis. As emphasized in the introduction, the *proportional* relationship of height and width is far more important

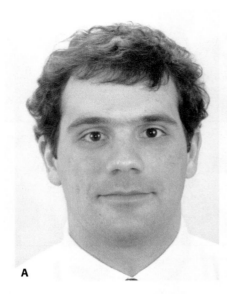
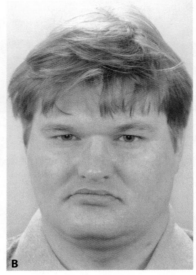
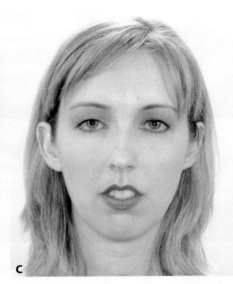

FIGURE 54-6.   **A,** The mesocephalic facial type is characterized by equal vertical facial thirds. **B,** The brachycephalic facial type appears square with a diminished lower third. **C,** The dolichocephalic facial type appears ovoid with an increased lower third.

than absolute values in establishing overall facial type. Faces can be broadly categorized as either mesocephalic, brachycephalic, or dolichocephalic (Figure 54-6).[13] The differentiation between these facial types has to do with the general proportionality of facial breadth to facial height, with brachycephalic faces being broader and shorter in comparison with the longer and more narrow dolichocephalic faces. Generally, the most attractive faces tend to have common proportions and relationships that generally differ from normative values.[14]

Vertical Facial Proportions

The ideal face is vertically divided into equal thirds by horizontal lines adjacent to the hairline, the nasal base, and the menton (Figure 54-7A). Surgical orthodontic treatment is in a large part limited to the lower facial third. Measurement of the upper face is often hindered by the variability in identification of broad landmarks such as the location of the hairline and radix.

The clinical examination begins with the evaluation of lower facial height. In the ideal lower third of the face, the upper lip makes up the upper third, and the lower lip and chin compose the lower two thirds (see Figure 54-7B). Disproportion of the vertical facial thirds may be a result of many dental and skeletal factors, and these proportional relationships may help us define the contributing factors related to vertical dentofacial deformities.

In the following sections, case illustrations of orthognathic changes in vertical proportionality are presented.

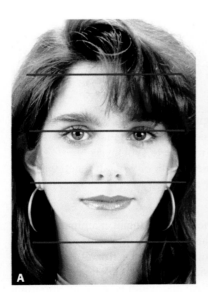
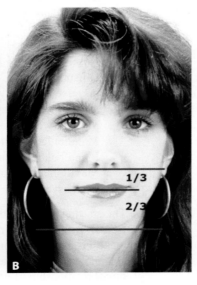

FIGURE 54-7.   **A,** The ideal face is vertically divided into equal thirds by horizontal lines adjacent to the hairline, the nasal base, and menton. **B,** In the ideal lower third of the face, the upper lip makes up the upper third, and the lower lip and chin compose the lower two thirds.

Short Vertical Proportions

The patient in Figure 54-8 presented for correction of her class II deep bite secondary to her mandibular deficiency. Her anterior vertical relationships were characterized by a short lower facial third relative to her upper thirds (see Figure 54-8A and B). In addition, the lower third was comprised of a 45:55 vertical relation of the upper lip to lower lip and chin height. Recalling that the ideal proportions of the lower face are one-third upper lip and two-thirds lower lip and chin, the treatment plan was clearly a result of the direct clinical examination rather than any cephalometric standard. Other important clinical measurements entered into the decision process. Differential diagnosis for a short lower facial height included the following:

- Vertical maxillary deficiencies, which are then characterized by the following features:
  - Short lower facial third
  - Diminished maxillary incisor display at rest
  - Diminished incisor display on smile
- Diminished chin height, ascertained through the proportionality in the lower face rather than a linear cephalometric value
- Posterior dental collapse secondary to the loss of posterior dental support

The functional goal of mandibular advancement to correct the class II dentoskeletal relationship was obvious, but an aesthetic adjunctive consideration was a vertical genioplasty to optimize the macroaesthetics of her vertical facial thirds. The final diagnosis depended not only on the vertical facial proportionality but on the measurement of the resting tooth-lip relationships as well in order to more clearly define the etiology of the lower facial height. In this case, our patient displayed 3 mm of maxillary incisor at rest and all of her maxillary incisor on smile (see Figure 54-8C), which was inconsistent with vertical

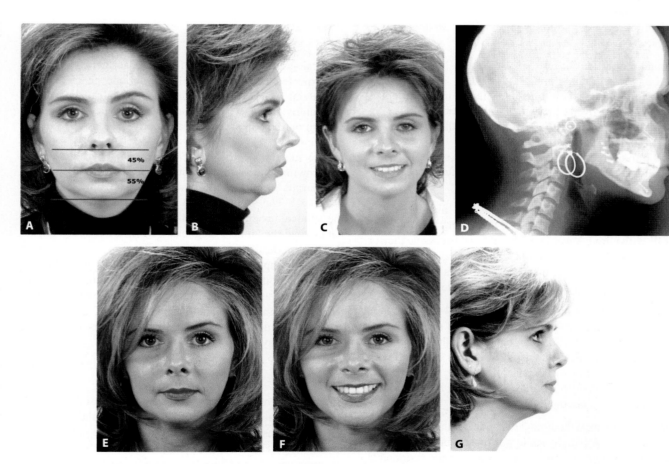

FIGURE 54-8. **A,** This patient was referred for correction of her class II deep bite secondary to her mandibular deficiency. **B,** Evaluation of her anterior vertical relationships was characterized by a short lower facial third relative to her upper thirds. The lower third was comprised of a 45:55 vertical relationship of the upper lip to lower lip and chin height. The ideal proportions of the lower face are one-third upper lip and two-thirds lower lip and chin; thus the treatment plan was derived from the direct clinical examination of this patient rather than any cephalometric standard. **C,** Our patient displayed 3 mm of maxillary incisor at rest, and all of her maxillary incisors on smile, inconsistent with vertical maxillary deficiency. **D,** The treatment plan was orthodontic preparation for mandibular advancement and vertical genioplasty. **E,** The post-treatment frontal view demonstrates balance of the vertical facial thirds. **F,** The vertical incisor position at smile was maintained, while the lower facial third was vertically augmented. **G,** The profile view shows improved mandibular projection relative to the upper face, improved chin-neck angle, and improved chin-neck length.

maxillary deficiency. Because the chin height was short, the final diagnosis was mandibular deficiency with short chin height. Therefore, the recommended treatment plan was orthodontic preparation for mandibular advancement and vertical genioplasty (see Figure 54-8D) to increase the lower facial height (see Figure 54-8E-G).

Long Vertical Proportions

Long lower facial height is due to one of two possibilities: (1) VME or (2) excessive chin height. The clinical keys that may be associated with VME are gummy smile, open bite, lip incompetence, and steep mandibular plane as evidenced by gonial angle form. Excessive chin height is measured from the lower vermilion to the soft tissue menton. The clinical keys that may be associated with excessive chin height are lower facial third disproportionate from the one-third upper lip to two-thirds low lip and chin ratio and the absence of VME characteristics.

The patient in Figure 54-9A was referred for correction of an anterior open bite and a gummy smile. Our systematic examination revealed the following problem list and characteristics:

■ Frontal proportions at rest
1. Long lower facial third
2. Disproportion of chin height with the upper lip occupying 25% of the lower facial third and the lower lip and chin occupying 75% of the lower third of the face
3. Lip incompetence of 5 mm
4. 8 mm of maxillary incisor display at rest
5. Midsymphysis to right 3 mm with no functional shift
6. Lip strain on closure (Figure 54-9B)

Clinical assessment of the frontal resting macroaesthetic evaluation: This patient had most of the macrocharacteristics of VME with a long lower facial height and excessive incisor display at rest. Excessive chin height was also a contributor to the lower facial height disproportion, as is evidenced by the upper lip and chin height clinical proportions.

■ Frontal proportions on smile (see Figure 54-9C)
1. 100% of maxillary incisor displayed on smile
2. Excessive gingival display on smile with 3 mm gingival display at the right cuspid and 5 mm at the left with a transverse cant to the palatal plane
3. Transverse cant to the maxilla with the left side down 2 mm more than the left

Clinical assessment of the frontal dynamic (smiling) macroaesthetic evaluation: A gummy smile was present but with normal incisor crown height. This would exclude cosmetic periodontal crown lengthening as the primary therapeutic choice for improvement of the gummy smile. The asymmetry of the maxilla is in compensation for the mandibular asymmetry and results in a canted frontal occlusal plane and smile line.

■ Oblique at-rest facial observation (see Figure 54-9D)
1. Excessive lower facial height
2. Lip strain and excessive chin height

3. Flat labiomental sulcus
4. Nasal form judged to be quite adequate

Clinical assessment of the oblique macroaesthetic evaluation: The flattened labiomental sulcus was secondary to the excessive lower facial height, lip incompetence, and chin deficiency.

■ Oblique smiling facial observation (see Figure 54-9E)
1. No noticeable anteroposterior cant to the maxillary occlusal plane
2. The smile arc was consonant
3. The excessive gingival display was also evident on the oblique smile

Clinical assessment from the oblique smiling macroaesthetic evaluation: Because the smile arc was consonant, alteration of the palatal plane would not have been indicated through either surgery or orthodontic incisor repositioning.

■ Profile evaluation (Figure 54-9F)
1. Long lower facial third
2. Long chin height
3. Flat labiomental sulcus
4. Lip strain on closure

Clinical assessment of the profile macroaesthetic evaluation: As expected from the frontal and oblique characteristics, the lateral profile reflected the overall skeletal and dental characteristics of VME, but the chin deficiency that became evident on the oblique view was clearly demonstrated on the profile view.

The functional problem of the anterior open bite in this nongrowing patient necessitated superior repositioning of the maxilla to correct the functional complaint (see Figure 54-9G-K). The exact surgical movements were directed by the clinical examination and measurements. Because the patient had the clinical diagnosis of VME, maxillary impaction was indicated, but some discretionary decisions were needed for appropriate position of the maxilla from the aesthetic standpoint. From the frontal dimension, the left side of the maxilla was impacted 2 mm more than the right in order to level the smile line. The differential degree of impaction reflected the degree of the maxillary compensation for the mandibular asymmetry.

Transverse Facial Proportions

The assessment of the transverse components of facial width is best described by the rule of fifths.[9] This method describes the ideal transverse relationships of the face. The face is divided sagittally into five equal parts from helix to helix of the outer ears (Figure 54-10). Each of the segments should be one eye distance in width. Each transverse fifth should be individually examined and then assessed as a complete group.

The middle fifth of the face is delineated by the inner canthus of the eyes. A vertical line from the inner canthus should be coincident with the alar base of the nose. Variation in this facial fifth could be due to transverse deficiencies or excesses in either the inner canthi or the alar base. For example,

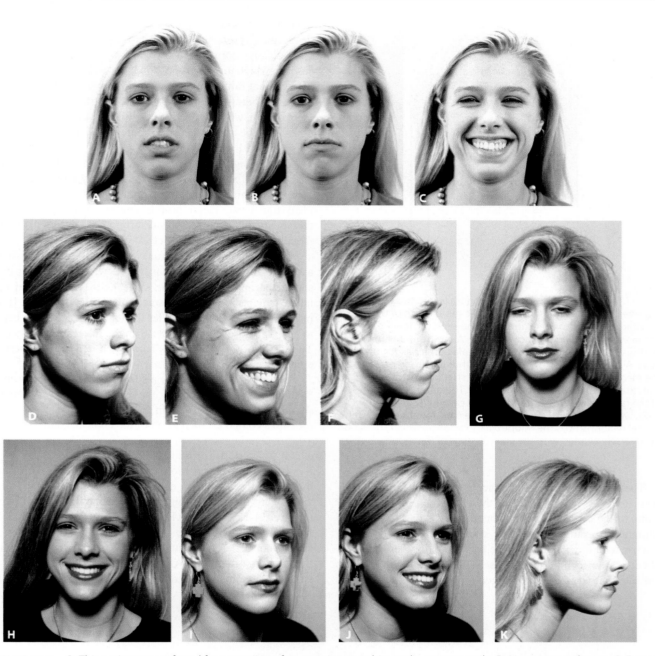

FIGURE 54-9.   **A,** This patient was referred for correction of an anterior open bite and a gummy smile. **B,** Lip strain on closure. **C,** Frontal proportions on smile with 100% of maxillary incisor displayed. There was excessive gingival display on smile with 3-mm gingival display at the right cuspid and 5 mm at the left with a transverse cant to the palatal plane. Transverse cant to the maxilla with the left side down 2 mm more than the left. **D,** Oblique at-rest facial observation with excessive lower facial height, lip strain and excessive chin height, and a flat labiomental sulcus. The nasal form was judged to be quite adequate. **E,** Oblique smiling facial observation with no noticeable anteroposterior cant to the maxillary occlusal plane. The smile arc was consonant. The excessive gingival display was also evident on the oblique smile. **F,** Profile evaluation with emphasis on a long lower facial third, long chin height, a flat labiomental sulcus, and lip strain on closure. **G–K,** The functional problem of the anterior open bite in this nongrowing patient necessitated superior repositioning of the maxilla to correct the functional complaint. The exact surgical movements were obtained from the clinical examination and measurements (see text).

hypertelorism in craniofacial syndromes can create disproportionate transverse facial aesthetics.

A vertical line from the outer canthus of the eyes frames the medial three fifths of the face, which should be coinci-

dent with the gonial angles of the mandible. Although disproportion may be very subtle, it is worth noting because our treatments can positively change the shape or relative proportion of the gonial angles.

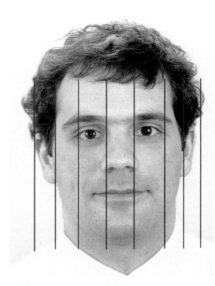

FIGURE 54-10.   The face is divided sagittally into five equal parts from helix to helix of the outer ears. The middle fifth of the face is delineated by the inner canthus of the eyes, the inner corner of the eye containing the lacrimal duct. A line from the inner canthus should be coincident with the ala of the base of the nose. A vertical line from the outer canthus of the eyes frames the medial two fifths of the face, which should be coincident with the gonial angles of the mandible. The outer two fifths of the face is measured from the lateral canthus to the lateral helix, which represents the width of the ears. Another significant frontal relationship is the midpupillary distance, which should be transversely aligned with the commissures of the mouth.

The outer two fifths of the face is measured from the lateral canthus to lateral helix of the ear, which represents the width of the ears. Unless this abnormality is part of the chief complaint, prominent ears are often a difficult feature to discuss with the patient because laypeople only recognize its effect on the face in severe cases. However, studies clearly indicate that large ears are judged by laypeople to be one of the most unaesthetic features, particularly in males. Otoplastic surgical procedures are relatively atraumatic and can dramatically improve facial appearance. In orthognathic cases in which this disproportion is noted by the clinician, we believel that failure to mention this feature violates informed consent. Therefore, otoplasty should be presented as a treatment option, whether received positively or not. These procedures can be performed on adolescents and adults as is illustrated in Figure 54-11.

Another significant frontal relationship is the midpupillary distance, which should be transversely aligned with the commissures of the mouth.[15] Although this is considered the ideal transverse facial proportionality, little can be done therapeutically to correct this disproportion, except in craniofacial synostosis such as Apert's syndrome.

Nasal anatomy in the transverse plane should also be assessed through proportionality. The width of the alar base should be approximately the same as the intercanthal distance, which should be the same as the width of an eye. If the intercanthal distance is smaller than an eye width, it is better to keep the nose slightly wider than the intercanthal distance. The width of the alar base is heavily influenced by inherited ethnic characteristics.

Asymmetry of the face is a somewhat natural occurrence. Systematic examination of the patient's facial symmetry should be directly measured in the frontal plane. The following measures compose this portion of the clinical examination.

Nasal Tip to Midsagittal Plane

Evaluation of the position of the nasal tip is performed by asking the patient to elevate the head slightly and then visualizing the nasal tip in relation to the midsagittal plane (Figure 54-12). Any deviation of the nasal tip should be noted in relation to the maxillary midline. The clinician should not make the mistake of treating the maxillary midline to a distorted nose. An attempt to obtain the etiology of nasal tip asymmetry is recommended. The patient should be

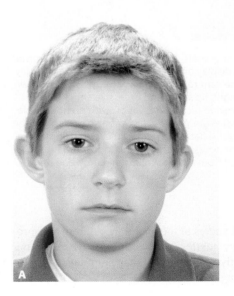

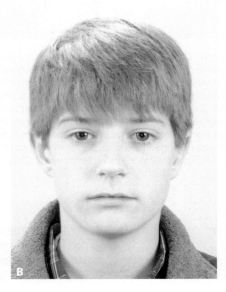

FIGURE 54-11.   **A,** An otoplastic surgical procedure was recommended for this patient's prominent ears. **B,** The facial transverse fifths were improved, resulting in a dramatic facial improvement.

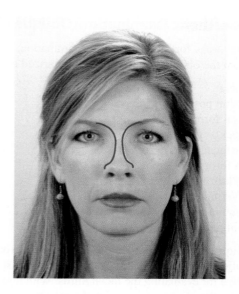

FIGURE 54-12.   The "gull in flight" contour of the base of the nose.

questioned as to any previous history of nasal trauma or nasal surgery for a deviated septum. Patients may then be advised appropriately as to whether this deviation is severe enough to consider correction.

Maxillary Dental Midline to Midsagittal Plane

The maxillary dental midline should be recorded relative to the midsagittal plane. A discrepancy could be due to either dental factors or skeletal maxillary rotation. Maxillary rotation is a rarely occurring clinical finding and is usually accompanied by posterior dental crossbite. The dental features of maxillary midline discrepancies are discussed in both the miniaesthetic and microaesthetic perspectives.

Mandibular Dental Midline to Midsymphysis

The mandibular dental midline to midsymphysis relationship is best visualized by standing behind the patient and then viewing the lower arch from above (Figure 54-13). The patient should open her or his mouth in order for the clinician to view the lower arch and its relationship to the body of the

mandible and symphysis. Lower dental midline discrepancies are usually due to tooth-related issues such as dental crowding with shifted incisors, premature exfoliation of primary teeth and subsequent space closure in preadolescents, congenitally missing teeth, or an extracted unilateral tooth. If the lower dental midline is not coincident with the midsymphysis, it usually indicates a dental shift. However, chin asymmetry should also be considered.

Mandibular Asymmetry with or without Functional Shift

Mandibular asymmetry is suspected when the midsymphysis is not coincident with the midsagittal plane. An important diagnostic factor is whether a lateral functional shift is present secondary to a functional shift of the mandible due to crossbite. When the patient is manipulated into centric relation, a bilateral, end-to-end crossbite usually is present, and as the patient moves the teeth into full occlusion, the patient must choose a side to move his or her mandible into maximum intercuspation. This lateral shift is indicative not of true mandibular asymmetry but of transverse maxillary deficiency and a resultant functional shift of the mandible.

True mandibular asymmetry is suspected when, in closure into centric relation, no lateral functional shift occurs. The truly asymmetrical mandible may be due to an inherited asymmetrical facial growth pattern or a result of localized or systemic factors. A thorough history of traumatic injuries and a review of systems of the patient will help ascertain potential etiologies of true mandibular asymmetry.

Chin Asymmetry

Facial asymmetry in some cases may be limited to the chin only. If the systematic evaluation of facial symmetry has dental and skeletal midlines and vertical relationships of the maxilla is normal and lower facial asymmetry is noted, the asymmetry may be isolated to the chin. Measurement of the midsymphysis to the midsagittal plane is a logical indicator of chin asymmetry, but the parasymphyseal heights should also be measured when chin asymmetry is suspected (Figure 54-14). The frontal view is recommended, but a view from the superior facial aspect (much like the evaluation of

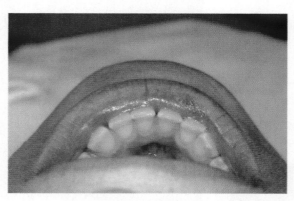

FIGURE 54-13.   If the lower dental midline is not coincident with the midsymphysis, it usually indicates a dental shift. However, chin asymmetry should also be considered.

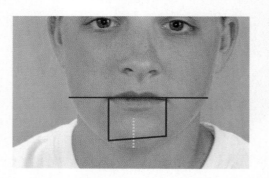

FIGURE 54-14.   Measurement of the midsymphysis to the midsagittal plane is a logical indicator of chin asymmetry, but the parasymphyseal heights should also be measured when chin asymmetry is suspected.

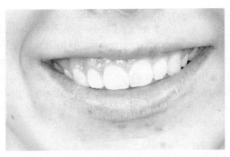

FIGURE 54-15. Transverse tilting of the maxilla may be detectable cephalometrically but is most evident during the macroaesthetic examination.

the mandibular dental midline) with the mouth closed also affords the clinician excellent visualization of the chin to the body of the mandible and the midsymphysis.

Maxillomandibular Asymmetry

Mandibular asymmetry is often accompanied by maxillary compensation, which is reflected clinically by a transverse cant of the maxilla. This means that evaluation of mandibular deformity should now include the possibility of maxillomandibular deformity. Transverse tilting of the maxilla may be detectable cephalometrically but is most evident during the macroaesthetic examination (Figure 54-15). Clinically, one notes this, for example, as *right maxilla 4 mm more superior than left.* The transverse cant of the maxilla is often determined by the relative difference in gingival show present at the level of the canine moving posterior at smile. Differentiation between the macro- and miniaesthetic factors that are related to the transverse cant of the maxilla are discussed later.

Macroaesthetic Examination: Oblique View

The facial areas for macroaesthetic examination, as investigated from the oblique view, can be summarized as follows:

- Midfacial
  - Orbital position
  - Nasal form
  - Cheek/zygomatic form
- Lower facial
  - Lip form
    - Philtrum
    - Vermilion
  - Mandibular form
  - Chin projection

The oblique view (Figure 54-16A) in the macroaesthetic examination affords the surgeon and orthodontist another perspective for evaluating the facial thirds. With regard to the upper face, the clinician may view the relative projection of the orbital rim and malar eminence. Orbital and malar retrusion is often seen in craniofacial syndromes. Cheek projection is evaluated in the area of the zygomaticus and malar scaffold. Skin laxity and atrophy of the malar fat pad in this area may actually be a characteristic of aging and, therefore, seen in the older orthognathic population.[16] This area can be described as "deficient," "balanced," or "prominent." Nasal anatomy, which was described in the frontal examination, may also be characterized in this dimension.

Lip anatomy is also examined in the oblique and lateral views. The philtral area and vermilion of the maxillary lip should be clearly demarcated. The height of the philtrum should be noted as "short," "balanced," or "excessive." Vermilion display should be termed as "excessive," "balanced," or "thin."

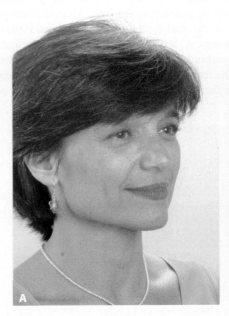
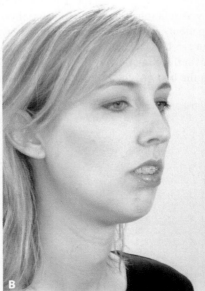
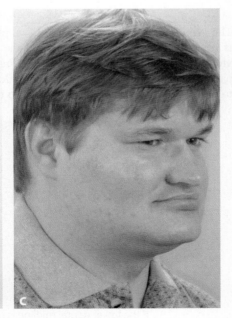

FIGURE 54-16. **A,** Desirable definition of the chin-neck anatomy. **B,** A dolichofacial skeletal pattern with a steeper mandibular plane, not as aesthetic as in **A. C,** A brachyfacial pattern with an obtuse cervicomental angle secondary to submental fat deposition.

The relative projection of the maxilla and mandible can be assessed in the oblique view. Midface deficiency can result in increased nasolabial folding, relaxed upper lip support, and altered columella and nasal tip support.

One of the greatest values of the oblique view is visualization of the body and gonial angle of the mandible as well as the cervicomental area. The patient in Figure 54-16A illustrates a desirable definition of the chin-neck anatomy. The patient in Figure 54-16B has a dolichofacial skeletal pattern with a steeper mandibular plane, not as aesthetically pleasing as the previous illustration. The patient in Figure 54-16C demonstrates a brachyfacial pattern with an obtuse cervicomental angle secondary to submental fat deposition. Mandibular deficiency with associated dental compensation may produce lower lip eversion, excessive vermilion display, and a pronounced labiomental sulcus.

A characterization of mandibular form is also very important. The oblique view also demonstrates the effects of animation on the appearance of lip and chin projection. The patient in Figure 54-17 shows a moderate anterior divergence and facial concavity at rest, but during the smile, animation reveals an increased chin projection with excessive concavity.

Macroaesthetic Examination: Profile View

The facial areas for macroaesthetic examination, as investigated from the profile view, can be summarized as follows:

- Lower facial
  - Maxillomandibular projection or facial divergence
  - Lip form
    - Size
    - Projection
    - Labiomental sulcus
    - Chin projection

The last view in the macroaesthetic examination is the profile perspective. Natural head position is essential for accurate evaluation of profile characteristics. The patient should be instructed to look straight ahead and, if possible, into her or his own image in an appropriately placed mirror. The visual axis is what determines "natural head position." This axis very often, but not always, approximates the Frankfort horizontal plane. The classic vertical facial thirds should also be applied in profile view. An assessment of lower facial deficiency or excess should be noted.

The *nasolabial angle* describes the inclination of the columella in relation to the upper lip. The nasolabial angle should be in the range of 90 to 120 degrees (Figure 54-18A).[17] The nasolabial angle is determined by several factors: (1) the anteroposterior position of the maxilla to some degree; (2) the anteroposterior position of the maxillary incisors; (3) vertical position or rotation of the nasal tip, which can result in a more obtuse or acute nasolabial angle; and (4) soft tissue thickness of the maxillary lip that contributes the nasolabial angle, in which a thin upper lip favors a flatter angle and a thicker lip favors an acute angle.

The characterization of the lower face in profile (see Figure 54-18B) is measured by the relative degree of lip projection, the labiomental sulcus, the chin-neck length, and the chin-neck angle. Maxillary and mandibular sagittal position can be described by means of facial divergence. The lower third of the face is evaluated in reference to the anterior soft tissue point at the glabella. Based on the position of the maxilla and mandible relative to this point, a patient's profile will be described as "straight," "convex," or "concave" and either anteriorly or posteriorly divergent.

Lip projection is a function of maxillomandibular protrusion or retrusion, dental protrusion or retrusion, and/or lip thickness. The description of lip projection should include pertinent information from any of the previous sources. For example, a patient with lower lip protrusion may be maxillary (midface) deficient with dentoalveolar compensation including flared incisors and a thin maxillary vermilion display or simply may have a thick lower lip that appears protrusive.

The *labiomental sulcus* is defined as the fold of soft tissue between the lower lip and the chin and may vary greatly in

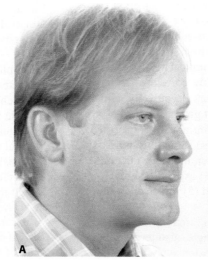 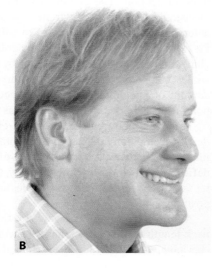

FIGURE 54-17.   **A,** The amount of facial concavity and chin projection at rest is within acceptable limits. **B,** When this patient animates, an excessive amount of chin projection and facial concavity is revealed.

A   B

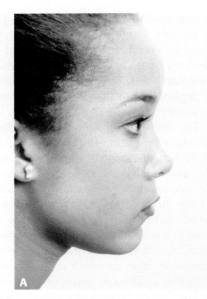 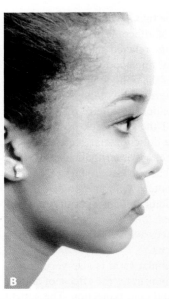

FIGURE 54-18. **A,** The facial profile view. Superiorly, the radix of the nose is characterized by an unbroken curve that begins in the superior orbital ridge and continues along the lateral nasal wall. The nasal dorsum is made up of both bony and cartilaginous tissues. The nasal tip is described as the most anterior point of the nose, and the supratip is just cephalic to the tip. The columella is the portion of the nose between the base of the nose (subspinale) and the nasal tip. **B,** The characterization of the lower face in profile is measured by the relative degree of lip projection, the labiomental sulcus, the chin-neck length, and the chin-neck angle.

form and depth. The clinical variables that can affect the labiomental sulcus include (1) lower incisor position, in which upright lower incisors tend to result in a shallow labiomental sulcus because of lack of lower lip projection, whereas excessive lower incisor proclination deepens the labiomental sulcus, and (2) vertical height of the lower facial third, which has a direct bearing on chin position and the labiomental sulcus. Diminished lower facial height will usually result in a deeper labiomental sulcus (just as in the overclosed full-denture patient), whereas a patient with a long lower facial third has a tendency toward a flat labiomental sulcus.

Chin projection is determined by the amount of anteroposterior bony projection of the anterior, inferior border of the mandible, and the amount of soft tissue that overlays that bony projection. The amount of profile chin projection is measured by the distance from pogonion (or Pg, the most anterior point on the bony chin) to soft tissue pogonion' (or Pg', the most anterior point on the soft tissue profile of the chin) and is not particularly alterable by surgical means. In the adolescent, the amount of chin is directly correlated to the amount of mandibular growth that occurs because the chin point itself is borne on the mandible as it grows anteriorly.

The angle between the lower lip, chin, and R point (the deepest point along the chin-neck contour) should be approximately 90 degrees. An obtuse angle often indicates (1) chin deficiency, (2) lower lip procumbency, (3) excessive submental fat, (4), retropositioned mandible, and (5) low hyoid bone position.

Another important measure in this area is the chin-neck length and chin-neck angle. The angle, also termed the *cervicomental angle,* has been studied extensively in plastic

surgery and orthognathic literature.[18] Studies report that a wide range of normal neck morphology exists, and that the cervicomental angle may vary between 105 and 120 degrees, with gender being a major consideration. Age of the patient must be considered with regard to this area. Soft tissue "sag" due to the loss of skin elasticity during aging is a major cause of change in the cervicomental region. Weight gain is another important factor in the morphology of this area.

Miniaesthetic Examination: Frontal View

The facial areas for miniaesthetic examination, as investigated from the frontal view, can be summarized as follows:

- Vertical characteristics of the smile
  - Lip-tooth-gingival relationships
  - Gingival display on smile
  - Excessive gingival display on smile
  - VME
  - Short philtrum height
  - Excessive curtain
  - Short clinical crown height
  - Upright maxillary incisors
  - Inadequate gingival display on smile
  - Vertical maxillary deficiency
  - Diminished curtain
  - Short clinical crown height
  - Flared maxillary incisors
- Transverse characteristics of the smile
  - Arch form
  - Buccal corridor
  - Cant of the transverse occlusal plane

Vertical Characteristics

Lip-Tooth-Gingival Relationships

A key feature of vertical facial aesthetic characteristics is the relationship between the incisal edges of the maxillary incisors relative to the lower lip as well as the relationship between the gingival margins of the maxillary incisors relative to the upper lip. The gingival margins of the cuspids should be coincident with the upper lip, and the lateral incisors positioned slightly inferior to the adjacent teeth. It is generally accepted that the gingival margins should be coincident with the upper lip in the social smile. However, this is very much a function of the age of the patient, because children show more teeth at rest and gingival display on smile than do adults.[19]

Excessive Gingival Display on Smile

The vertical characteristics of facial miniaesthetics affect the relative amount of gingival display at rest and during animation. Gingival display is the amount of "gumminess" of the smile. Measuring the amount of gingival display on smile easily quantitates a "gummy" smile. The decision as to whether the amount of gingival display is an aesthetic problem in which treatment is desirable is a personal choice. Orthodontists and oral and maxillofacial surgeons tend to see the "gummy" smile as an unaesthetic characteristic, whereas laypersons attach importance only in the more extreme cases. The use of computerized graphic simulation of the frontal view of the smile is useful in counseling a patient and showing potential treatment changes. The individual is then able to guide the clinician and express opinions about what should and should not be corrected. Computer imaging not only provides the patient with a visual template for treatment but also provides the clinician with a testing ground for treatment options. The patient in Figure 54-19A exhibits excessive gingival display on smile, secondary to VME. The diagnosis of VME is confirmed by the facial characteristics of a long lower facial third, lip incompetence, excessive incisor display at rest, and excessive gingival display on smile. Superior repositioning of the maxilla was performed with excellent facial proportions and smile aesthetics (see Figure 54-19B).

The patient in Figure 54-20A also exhibited excessive gingival display but has normal vertical facial proportions. Her incisor crown height, however, is only 8 mm. The etiology of her "gummy" smile is not an orthognathic problem or an orthodontic problem but a cosmetic or periodontal problem. This diagnosis was confirmed and further visualized through computerized image modification (see Figure 54-20B and C), simulating the crown-lengthening procedure. Orthodontic intrusion of maxillary incisors would have reduced gingival display but would also have adversely affected the smile arc with concomitant flattening. This case example emphasizes differential diagnosis of gingival display issues and also emphasizes the optimization of unaesthetic facial traits while preserving those positive facial aesthetic attributes.

Transverse Characteristics

The three transverse characteristics of facial aesthetics in the frontal dimension are (1) arch form, (2) buccal corridor, and (3) transverse cant of the maxillary occlusal plane.

Arch form plays a pivotal role in the transverse dimension. Recently, much attention has been focused on using broad square arch forms in orthodontic treatment and orthognathic surgical treatment. In cases in which the arch forms are narrow or collapsed, the smile may also appear narrow and, therefore, present inadequate transverse smile characteristics. An important consideration in widening a narrow arch form, particularly in the adult, is the axial inclination of the buccal segments. Cases in which the posterior teeth are already flared laterally are not good candidates for dental expansion. Upright premolars and molars allow for a more bodily transverse expansion of the buccal segments in both adolescent and adult patients but are particularly important in the adult in whom sutural expansion is less likely. Orthodontic expansion

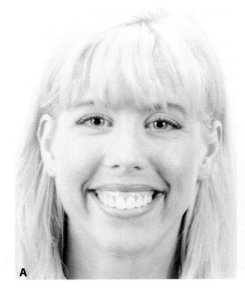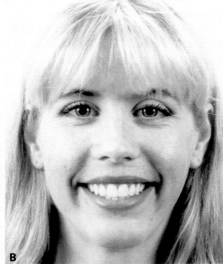

FIGURE 54-19.   **A,** This patient exhibits excessive gingival display on smile, secondary to vertical maxillary excess. **B,** The actual post-treatment outcome.

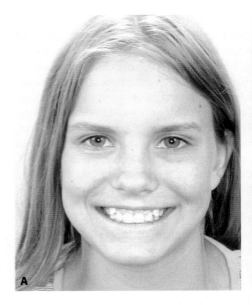

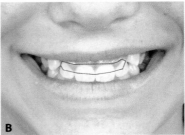

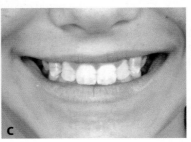

FIGURE 54-20. **A,** This patient exhibits excessive gingival display but has normal vertical facial proportions. Her incisor crown height, however, is only 8 mm. The etiology of her "gummy" smile is not an orthognathic problem or an orthodontic problem but a cosmetic or periodontal problem. **B** and **C,** This diagnosis was confirmed and further visualized through computerized image modification, simulating the crown-lengthening procedure.

and widening of a collapsed arch form can dramatically improve the appearance of facial aesthetics and smile by decreasing the size of the buccal corridors and improving the *transverse smile dimension* (Figure 54-21). The transverse smile dimension (and the buccal corridor) is related to the lateral projection of the premolars and the molars into the buccal corridors. The wider the arch form is in the premolar area, the greater would be the portion of the buccal corridor filled.

As alluded to in the previous cases, arch expansion can have undesirable effects. Expansion of the arch form may fill out the transverse dimension of the smile, but two undesirable side effects may result and careful observation should be made to avoid these side effects wherever possible. First, the buccal corridor can be obliterated and create a "denture"-like smile. Second, when the anterior sweep of the maxillary arch is broadened, the smile arc may be flattened. Although it may not be possible to avoid these undesirable aspects of expansion, the clinician must make a judgment in concert with the patient as to what "trade-offs" are acceptable in the pursuit of the ideal facial aesthetic outcome.

The last transverse characteristic of facial aesthetics is the transverse cant of the maxillary occlusal plane. Transverse cant of the maxilla can be due to differential eruption and placement of the anterior teeth and skeletal asymmetry of the skull base and/or mandible resulting in a compensatory cant to the maxilla. Intraoral images or even mounted dental casts do not adequately reflect the relationship of the maxilla to the smile. Only frontal smile visualization permits the orthodontist to visualize any tooth-related asymmetry transversely.

Smile asymmetry may also be due to soft tissue considerations such as an asymmetrical smile curtain. In the asymmetrical smile curtain, there is a differential elevation of the upper lip during smile, which gives the illusion of transverse cant to the maxilla. This smile characteristic emphasizes the importance of direct clinical examination in treatment planning the smile, because this soft tissue animation is not visible in a frontal radiograph or reflected in study models. It is not well documented in static photographic images and is documented best in digital video clips.

Miniaesthetic Examination: Oblique View

Miniaesthetic examination from the oblique view involves two main areas:

- Orientation of the palatal and occlusal planes
- Smile arc

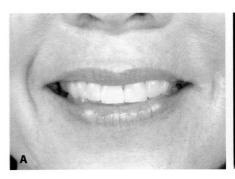

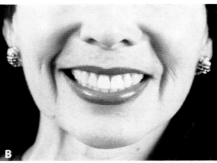

FIGURE 54-21. **A,** The transverse smile dimension in this patient was characterized by narrow arch form and excessive buccal corridor. In this adult, the axial inclinations of the molars and premolars were favorable for orthodontic expansion. **B,** The transverse smile dimension after orthodontic treatment.

The oblique view of the smile reveals characteristics of the smile that are not obtainable on the frontal view and certainly not obtainable through any cephalometric analysis. The palatal plane may be canted anteroposteriorly in a number of orientations. In the most desirable orientation, the occlusal plane is consonant with the curvature of the lower lip on smile (see discussion of *smile arc,* in the next paragraph). Deviations from this orientation include a downward cant of the posterior maxilla, upward cant of the anterior maxilla, or variations of both.[20] In the initial examination and diagnostic phase of treatment, it is important to visualize the occlusal plane in its relationship to the lower lip.

The *smile arc* should be defined as the relationship of the curvature of the incisal edges of the maxillary incisors, canines, premolars, and molars to the curvature of the lower lip in the posed social smile. The ideal smile arc has the maxillary incisal edge curvature parallel to the curvature of the lower lip upon smile, and the term *consonant* is used to describe this parallel relationship. A *nonconsonant,* or flat, smile arc is characterized by the maxillary incisal curvature being flatter than the curvature of the lower lip on smile. Early definitions of the smile arc were limited to the curvature of the canines and the incisors to the lower lip on smile because smile evaluation was made on direct frontal view. The visualization of the complete smile arc afforded by the oblique view expands the definition of the smile arc to include the molars and the premolars (Figure 54-22).

Miniaesthetic Examination: Profile View

The facial areas for miniaesthetic examination, as investigated from the profile view, can be summarized as follows:

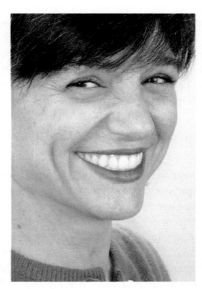

FIGURE 54-22.   The smile arc is best visualized in the oblique view and should be defined as the relationship of the curvature of the incisal edges of the maxillary incisors, canines, premolars, and molars to the curvature of the lower lip in the posed social smile. The 45-degree view permits visualization of vermilion display, lip fullness, and turgor not readily seen in another view.

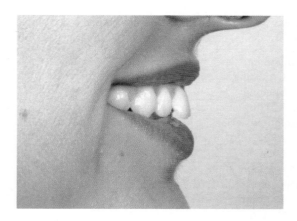

FIGURE 54-23.   The two miniaesthetic characteristics visualized in the sagittal dimension are overjet and incisor angulation.

- Overjet
- Incisor angulation
  - Upright maxillary incisors
  - Flared maxillary incisors
  - Retroclined mandibular incisors

The two miniaesthetic characteristics visualized in the sagittal dimension are overjet and incisor angulation (Figure 54-23). Excessively positive overjet is one of the most recognizable dental traits to the layperson. Adolescents tend to label unflattering names such as "Andy Gump" and "Bucky Beaver" onto children unfortunate enough to have inherited this dentoskeletal pattern. How overjet is orthodontically corrected involves macroelements such as jaw patterns and soft tissue elements such as nasal projection. Excessive positive overjet is not as readily perceived in the frontal dimension as it is in the sagittal dimension. Many class II patterns have very aesthetic smiles frontally but not when the patient's smile is observed from the side. In class III patterns, the same phenomenon may be true, in that the smile looks aesthetic on frontal smile, but on the oblique or sagittal view, the overall appearance reflects the underlying skeletal pattern and dental compensation. The patient and parents have to decide with the clinician whether this is an acceptable outcome.

The amount of anterior maxillary projection also has great influence on the transverse smile dimension in the frontal view. When the maxilla is retrusive, the wider portion of the dental arch is positioned more posteriorly relative to the anterior oral commissure. This creates the illusion of greater buccal corridor in the frontal dimension. Overall, the sagittal cant of the maxillary occlusal plane in natural head position can influence the smile arc in the frontal dimension, affecting vertical characteristics. A negative cant of this plane will diminish the apposition of the incisal edges of the maxillary anterior teeth to the superior vermilion border of the lower lip at smile.

Dental Examination

The dental component of the clinical examination is the evaluation of any standing periodontal or cariogenic disease process and the assessment of the patient's occlusion. The areas for dental examination can be summarized as follows:

- Alignment
  - Crowding
  - Spacing
  - Missing or supernumerary teeth
- Anteroposterior
  - Angle classification
  - Overjet
  - Compensation
- Bite depth
  - Anterior
  - Posterior
  - Compensation
- Transverse
  - Compensation
- Functional occlusal issues
  - Missing teeth and sequelae
  - Occlusal interferences and parafunction

Intra-arch and interarch relationships are described in the categories of dental alignment, anteroposterior occlusion, and bite depth. Clinically, the patient's occlusion should be examined in both a static and a dynamic sense.

The maxillary and mandibular dental arches are described as either "well aligned," "crowded," or "spaced." The extent of crowding or spacing is usually noted in millimeters. Individual teeth are described by virtue of their spatial position and degree of rotation. Therefore, an incisor could be described as "severely rotated" and "in linguoversion." Any congenitally missing, lost, or supernumerary teeth are noted. A description of teeth that have been severely worn or damaged due to trauma should be included.

In terms of the static occlusion, Angle's classification of the patient should be recorded. The Angle class I relationship is such that the mesiobuccal cusp of the maxillary first molar should rest in the buccal groove of the mandibular first molar. The Angle class II relationship exhibits a more anterior position of the mesiobuccal cusp of the maxillary first molar, The Angle class III relationship exhibits a more posterior position of the mesiobuccal cusp of the maxillary first molar. The degree of incisor overjet that accompanies an anteroposterior discrepancy should also be noted.

Concepts of Incisor Compensation

Incisor compensation in the sagittal view is very important in planning the presurgical orthodontics, yet not fully recognized by both orthodontists and surgeons alike. In most cases of skeletal dysplasia, whether in the range of surgical or nonsurgical treatment, dental compensation is a common feature. The forms and expression of this compensation are as complex as the myriad of dentoskeletal problems that exist, but common patterns are frequently encountered. In the diagnosis and proper treatment of these cases, the primary responsibility of the orthodontist is to recognize these compensations

and eliminate or *decompensate* them. The range of which compensations are problematic is not concrete, so the surgeon and the orthodontist must decide how much compensation is acceptable and what is to be done for decompensation. Although we tend to think of these compensations as an anteroposterior consideration (incisor angulation problems), dental compensation can occur in all planes of space.

Class II and Class III Problems

The classic pattern of compensation in class II skeletal patterns is the proclination of the mandibular incisors and retroclination of the maxillary incisors. Conversely, class III skeletal dysplasias often feature retroclination of the mandibular incisors and proclination of the maxillary incisors. The orthodontist must recognize these compensations and decide what degree of compensation is acceptable and what requires substantive treatment. For example, if lower incisor flare in the class II patient is only moderate, what is the value of removing two mandibular premolars to upright the incisors? These decompensation decisions affect the treatment outcome in three basic ways: (1) inadequate incisor positioning can compromise buccal interdigitation; (2) incisor positioning can substantially affect the aesthetic outcome; and (3) in certain types of functional problems such as obstructive sleep apnea syndrome, aesthetic considerations have a lower priority compared with correction of the functional problem.

The effect of incisor angulation on buccal occlusal relationships was advanced and best expressed by Andrews.[21] In presurgical preparation for mandibular advancement, maxillary incisors that are not properly flared or mandibular incisors that are left overly flared may result in (1) insufficient overjet to provide for adequate advancement of the mandible from the aesthetic standpoint and (2) the inability to achieve desired class I buccal segments because the advanced nature of the lower incisor edge does not permit interdigitation of the buccal segments (Figure 54-24). The appropriate amount of incisor angulation can be determined either through cephalometric investigation or by simply holding study models in a simulated class I molar relationship.

Vertical Characteristics and Compensations

Bite Depth

The vertical component of the dental examination describes *bite depth*. A patient's anterior bite depth is the amount of maxillary incisor overbite relative to the mandibular incisors. Therefore, a patient can be described as having "an anterior open bite," "a satisfactory bite (25–50% overbite), or "an anterior deep bite." The posterior bite depth is usually characterized as being "open," "satisfactory," or "collapsed." The latter is seen when the patient is missing unilateral or bilateral posterior dental units.

Curve of Spee

Dental compensation in the vertical plane has to do with aberrations in the curve of Spee. The curve of Spee is measured

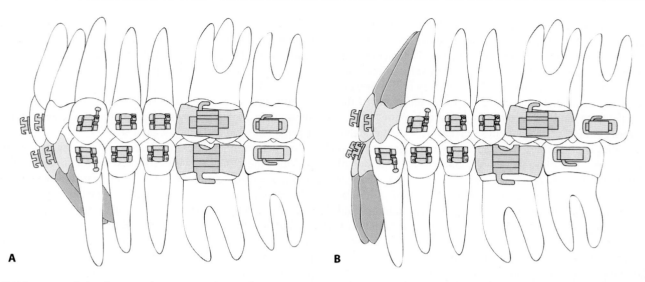

FIGURE 54-24. **A,** Inadequate decompensation in class II correction makes class I buccal segments not attainable because the flared lower incisors do not permit interdigitation of the posterior segments. **B,** Inadequate decompensation in class III correction makes class I buccal segments not attainable because the upright lower incisors or flared maxillary incisors do not permit interdigitation of the posterior segments.

by the arc extending from the cusp tips of the incisors posteriorly to the cusp tips of the molars in a sagittal view. Clinically, the study model can be placed on a flat surface and the cusp tips relative to that flat plane will give a rough estimate of the maxillary and mandibular curve of Spee. This is an important diagnostic feature of model analysis in recognizing potential pitfalls that may be encountered during orthodontic preparation for orthognathic surgery. For example, in a patient in whom the anterior segment is significantly superior (>2 mm) to the posterior segment, failure to recognize this occlusal plane differential may result in orthodontic flattening before surgery and postsurgical relapse, resulting in anterior open bite.[22]

Transverse Compensations

The class II patient often has narrowing of the maxilla in response to the narrower portion of the mandible being placed in the broader portion of the maxillary arch. In the class III patient, the maxillary posterior segments are often flared buccally in compensation for the wider portion of the mandible being placed into the narrower aspect of the maxilla. By holding the study models in a simulated class I relationship, these compensations can be easily recognized (Figure 54-25).

Functional Occlusal Issues

The last portion of the dental examination relates to dynamics of occlusal function. The clinician should ascertain whether the patient exhibits a discrepancy between maximum intercuspal position and retruded contact position in the anteroposterior dimension. In general, small differences exist in the vast majority of patients. Only large slides should be

recorded. If the patient's dentition is mutilated, the clinician should note the resultant occlusal compensations. Any supererupted teeth will create lateral and anteroposterior interferences. A history of bruxism or other parafunctional habits will affect orthodontic appliances and will affect the type of retention used post-treatment.

Microaesthetic Examination

The microaesthetic portion of the clinical examination focuses on the morphology of tooth-to-tooth contacts and the surrounding intraoral tissues, summarized as follows:

- Dentogingival relationships
- Tooth form/tooth contact/gingival architecture

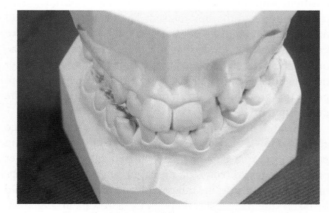

FIGURE 54-25. Transverse problems are first diagnosed by holding the study models together in a simulated class I relationship. The most commonly found transverse problem is that the maxilla is narrower than the mandible in cases similar to that of this patient who was being evaluated for class II correction by mandibular advancement.

As a structural unit, the dentogingival complex is defined by the relationship of the teeth to the alveolar bone and surrounding gingival and masticatory mucosa. The factors that influence the appearance of the dentogingival complex are the patient's periodontal status and past history of disease, the proximal and occlusal contacts of the teeth, the shape of the individual teeth, and the type of gingival architecture.

An assessment of the patient's current periodontal status is exceedingly important from an orthodontic and surgical point of view. The clinician should take an accurate dental history in order to ascertain whether the patient has had any periodontal disease and related treatment. Clinically, the teeth should be examined for plaque accumulation and any supragingival calculus. Patients who cannot maintain a satisfactory level of oral hygiene are at risk for gingival inflammation, attachment loss, and caries during presurgical orthodontic treatment. Periapical radiographs combined with a panoramic radiograph will reveal alveolar architecture and any evidence of horizontal or vertical bone loss. Suspected periodontal defects should be probed and the depths recorded. The extent of attachment loss and degree of tooth mobility will influence tooth movement.

Surgical treatment planning of the segmental Le Fort I osteotomy should consider gingival architecture in relation to maxillary segmentation. If the incisions are made mesial to the maxillary canines, the patient may lose the interdental papilla in between this tooth and the maxillary lateral incisor. By positioning the incisions distal to the maxillary canines, an obliterated papilla can be more easily camouflaged owing to the convexity of the canine.

COMPUTERIZED CEPHALOMETRIC PREDICTION

For computer image prediction, a digital model of the cephalometric tracing must be entered into computer memory. It is important that the radiograph be obtained in natural head position, with the teeth lightly together and in retruded contact position and the lips relaxed. The details of the digital model vary among the several currently available software programs but the similarities are more impressive than the differences. The more points in the digital model, the greater the anatomic fidelity of that model. Conversely, the more points that are digitized, the more time it takes to perform the digitization process.

A lateral image of the patient's profile, matching the cephalograms as closely as possible in head position and lip posture, must be captured and entered into the computer program (either directly via digital photography or by scanning a slide). Ideally, the radiograph and profile image would be taken simultaneously, although the hardware arrangement to do this does not yet exist.

The patient in Figure 54-26A presented for correction of a severe class II dentofacial deformity. After clinical examination and diagnostic records, digital image integration and algorithmic projections are used for consultation with the patient.

After the records are gathered, the next step in the treatment planning is to superimpose the profile image and radiograph, with the hard and soft tissues matched to each other as closely as possible. Most programs use the profile as the major method of image coordination. Once the images are coordinated, any cephalometric analysis can be displayed, although in contemporary surgical planning, the goal of treatment is not what the analysis indicates.

At that point, a "treatment screen" (see Figure 54-26B) provides the clinician with "handles" (the *blue squares*) by which selected sections of hard tissue can be moved (e.g., the mandible, the maxilla, or maxillary incisor segment); the procedures are similar to the use of templates and manual prediction. In this case illustration, surgical mandibular advancement is being contemplated. Dental compensation is present in the form of flared mandibular incisors, and decompensation is recommended to decompensate the dentition in order to increase the overjet, thus maximizing the magnitude of mandibular advancement. Simulation of lower first premolar extraction and lower incisor retraction is made on the treatment screen; the software applies its embedded algorithms for profile prediction and creates a new line drawing of the profile (see Figure 54-26C) reflecting the expected profile change after incisor decompensation. The algorithms may be ratios based on regressive equations and multiple correlations. They are not the same in all programs: the quality of the algorithms is the major determinant of how well or poorly the predicted profile matches the actual change produced by the treatment. The quantitative table on the right of Figure 54-26C provides to the clinician the measurements of the movements made on screen calibrated to actual movements required clinically to achieve the projected change.

After decompensation movements are simulated, the mandible is advanced on the treatment screen to ideal overjet, and the software then "warps" the original profile image to fit the prediction line drawing, producing an image that conveys much more visual information to the clinician and patient than the line drawing (see Figure 54-26D). As treatment is being planned, the amount of change is suggested until, within the limits of possible surgical change, it looks best. It is advantageous to include the patient in this process of adjusting the amount of change to provide an optimal outcome. In this case, a comparison image is generated so the patient may visualize the profile outcome expected with mandibular advancement (see Figure 54-26E). The profile was judged to be improved but was still clearly chin deficient. Simulation of chin advancement is then performed (see Figure 54-26F), not by using any cephalometric norm or predetermined value, but by simply using the facial outline as a guide. In other words, the chin is moved horizontally and vertically until it meets the approval of the patient. The projected final profile image is depicted in Figure 54-26G. The quantitative table reflects the exact movements in millimeters so that the surgeon and orthodontist have a precise plan for the amount of change needed to produce the desired result seen in Figure 54-26H. Presurgical planning using this

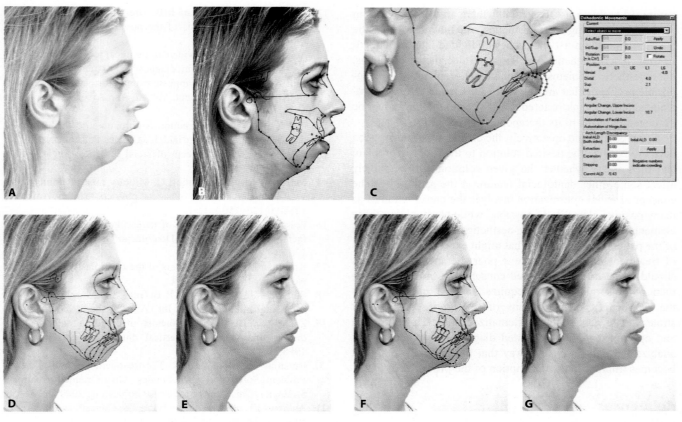

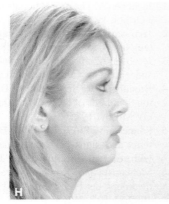

FIGURE 54-26.   **A,** This patient presented for correction of a severe class II dentofacial deformity. **B,** A "treatment screen" provides the clinician with "handles" (the *blue squares*) by which selected sections of hard tissue can be moved (e.g., the mandible, the maxilla, or the maxillary incisor segment); the procedures are similar to the use of templates and manual prediction. **C,** Simulation of lower first premolar extraction and lower incisor retraction is made on the treatment screen. The software applies its embedded algorithms for profile prediction and creates a new line drawing of the profile reflecting the expected profile change after incisor decompensation. **D,** After decompensation movements are simulated, the mandible is advanced on the treatment screen to ideal overjet, and the software then "warps" the original profile image to fit the prediction line drawing, producing an image that conveys much more visual information to the clinician and patient than the line drawing. **E,** In this case, a comparison image is generated so that the patient may visualize the profile outcome expected with mandibular advancement. **F,** Simulation of chin advancement is then performed, not by using any cephalometric norms or predetermined value, but by simply using the facial outline as a guide. **G,** The projected final profile image. **H,** The actual treatment result.

methodology should eliminate "on-the-table" estimates of whether or not the patient needs "a bit more chin." It is ludicrous to make aesthetic treatment decisions with the patient under general anesthesia, horizontal, fully draped, paralyzed, and with a nasal tube in place.

An important consideration is the accuracy of the computer prediction process. Although it is far from perfect (some computer programs are more accurate than others), it is good enough to be clinically useful.[23–27] Chin predictions are usually quite accurate and those of the upper lip are reasonably good, whereas predictions of the lower lip can be problematic. As the data on which algorithms are based become more extensive, as different algorithms are applied when vertical and anterior changes occur, and as multiple regression equa-

tions replace simple ratios, accuracy can be expected to improve.[28]

It could be said that in this era of informed consent and bioethical decision making, the patient should be actively involved in the process of computer prediction and treatment planning. Cultural and familial traits may be important to the patient. Surgeons and orthodontists tend to want to "optimize" all patients to the prevailing aesthetic norm, which diminishes any ethnic variation in dentofacial appearance.

SYNTHESIS OF AN OPTIMIZED PROBLEM LIST

The data derived from the systematic clinical examination and analysis of patient records are synthesized into a diagnostic optimized problem list. Essentially, there are two branches in the problem-solving tree: aesthetics and function. Thus, the diagnostic problem list should be subdivided into the categories of macroaesthetic problems, miniaesthetic problems, microaesthetic problems, and functional problems. All recognizable problems that are relevant to the patient's chief complaint should be rank-ordered. Lastly, each problem should be evaluated in terms of its therapeutic modifiability

Conceptually and operatively, the orthodontist and surgeon have to visualize the desired solution to the specific problem and then assess whether the given solution will negatively affect some other dentofacial feature at the same time. The concept of facial optimization involves the preservation of as many positive elements as possible, while harmonizing those elements that fall short of the aesthetic and functional needs of the patient. The problems that might exceed the limitations of treatment or perhaps have a poor therapeutic prognosis should be described. Informed consent and bioethical treatment of the surgical patient requires that the clinician explain the risk-benefit considerations of the proposed treatment strategy. The goal of the systematized clinical examination and optimized problem-oriented diagnosis is to record and analyze the data in such a way that the required treatment becomes implicit in the description of the problem.

References

1. Jacobson A. The proportionate template as a diagnostic aid. Am J Orthod 1979;75:156–172.
2. Jacobson A. Orthognathic diagnosis using the proportionate template. Oral Surg 1980;238:820.
3. Jacobson A, editor. Radiographic Cephalometry: From Basics to Videoimaging. Carol Stream, IL: Quintessence Publishing; 1995.
4. Broadbent BH Sr, Broadbent BH Jr, Golden WH, editors. Bolton Standards of Dentofacial Developmental Growth. St. Louis: CV Mosby; 1975.
5. Sonnesen L, Bakke M, Solow B. Malocclusion traits and symptoms and signs of temporomandibular disorders in children with severe malocclusion. Eur J Orthod 1998;10:543–559.
6. McNamara JA. Orthodontic treatment and temporomandibular disorders. Oral Surg Oral Med Oral Pathol Oral Radiol Endod 1997;83:107–117.
7. Sarver DM, Ackerman JL. About face—the reemerging soft tissue paradigm. Am J Orthod Dentofacial Orthop 2000;117:575–576.
8. Sarver DM, Ackerman MB. Dynamic smile visualization and quantification: part 1. Evolution of the concept and dynamic records for smile capture. Am J Orthod Dentofacial Orthop 2003:124:4–12.
9. Sarver DM, editor. Esthetic Orthodontics and Orthognathic Surgery. St. Louis: CV Mosby; 1997.
10. Sarver DM. The smile arc—the importance of incisor position in the dynamic smile. Am J Orthod Dentofacial Orthop 2001;120:98–111.
11. Ackerman JL, Ackerman MB, Brensinger CM, Landis JR. A morphometric analysis of the posed smile. Clin Orth Res 1998;1:1–11.
12. Ackerman MB. Digital video as a clinical tool in orthodontics: dynamic smile design in diagnosis and treatment planning. 29th Annual Moyers Symposium on Information Technology and Orthodontic Treatment. Vol 40. Ann Arbor: University of Michigan Press; 2003.
13. Farkas LG, Munro JR, editor. Anthropometric facial proportions in medicine. Springfield, IL: Charles C. Thomas; 1987.
14. Peck H, Peck S. A concept of facial esthetics. Angle Orthod 1970;40:284–317.
15. Mazur A, Mazur J, Keating C. Military rank attainment of a West Point class: effects of cadets' physical features. Am J Soc 1984;90:125–150.
16. Pessa JA. The potential role of stereolithography in the study of facial aging. Am J Orthod Dentofacial Orthop 2001;119:117–120.
17. Krugman ME. Photo analysis of the rhinoplasty patient. J Ear Nose Throat 1981;60:56–59.
18. Sommerville JM, Sperry TP, BeGole EA. Morphology of the submental and neck region. Int J Adult Orthod 1988;3:97–106.
19. Zachrisson BU. Esthetic factors involved in anterior tooth display and the smile: vertical dimension. J Clin Orthod 1998;32:432–445.
20. Burstone CJ, Marcotte MR. The treatment occlusal plane. In Problem Solving in Orthodontics: Goal-Oriented Treatment Strategies. Chicago: Quintessence Publishing; 2000; pp. 31–50.
21. Andrews LF, editor. Straight Wire: The Concept and the Appliance. San Diego, CA): LA Wells; 1989.
22. Lo FM, Shapiro PA. Effect of presurgical incisor extension on stability of anterior open bite malocclusion treated with orthognathic surgery. Int J Adult Orthod Orthognath Surg 1998;13:23–34.
23. Sinclair PM, Kilpelainen P, Phillips C, et al. The accuracy of video imaging in orthognathic surgery. Am J Orthod Dentofacial Orthop 1995;107:177–185.
24. Upton PM, Sadowsky PL, Sarver DM, Heaven TJ. Evaluation of video imaging prediction in combined maxillary and mandibular orthognathic surgery. Am J Orthod Dentofacial Orthop 1997;112:656–665.
25. Syliangco ST, Sameshima GT, Kaminishi RM, Sinclair PM. Predicting soft tissue changes in mandibular advancement surgery: a comparison of two video imaging systems. Angle Orthod 1997;67:337–346.
26. Sameshima GT, Kawakami RK, Kaminishi RM, Sinclair PM. Predicting soft tissue changes in maxillary impaction surgery: a comparison of two video imaging systems. Angle Orthod 1997;67:346–354.
27. Kazandjian S, Sameshima GT, Champlin T, Sinclair PM. Accuracy of video imaging for predicting the soft tissue profile after mandibular set-back surgery. Am J Orthod Dentofacial Orthop 1999;115:382–389.
28. Peters DG. Lower lip changes in surgical correction of Class I malocclusion [Master's dissertation]. Chapel Hill: University of North Carolina; 2001.

Orthodontics for Orthognathic Surgery

Larry M. Wolford, DMD, Eber L. L. Stevao, DDS, PhD, C. Moody Alexander, DDS, MS,
Joao Roberto Goncalves, DDS, PhD, and Daniel B. Rodrigues, DDS

An understanding of the role of the orthodontist, as well as specifics of orthodontic therapy as it relates to orthognathic surgery, is essential for the oral and maxillofacial (OMF) surgeon. Moderate to severe occlusal discrepancies and dentofacial deformities in adolescents and adults usually require combined orthodontic treatment and orthognathic surgery to obtain optimal, stable, functional, and aesthetic results. The basic goals of orthodontics and orthognathic surgery are to (1) satisfy the patients' concerns, (2) establish optimal functional outcomes, and (3) provide good aesthetic results. To accomplish this, the orthodontist and the OMF surgeon must be able to correctly diagnose existing dental and skeletal deformities, establish an appropriate treatment plan, and properly execute the recommended treatment. The orthodontist is limited, to a great extent, by growth, and although the orthodontist can move teeth and, to some degree, the alveolar bone, she or he does not have any appreciable effect on the basal bone of the jaws. The orthodontist's role is to align the teeth relative to the maxillary and mandibular jaws, whereas the OMF surgeon is responsible for surgically repositioning the jaw(s) and associated structures.

It is very important to listen to, and understand, the patient's concerns. Empathetic listening from the first appointment and throughout the treatment will build trust, improve communication, and help provide a quality end result for all parties involved. Comprehensive analysis of the patient and the complete orthodontic records (cephalograms, panoramic films, computed tomography, photographs, dental models, occlusal registration, and face-bow transfer) is important for diagnosis and development of the presurgical orthodontic goals. Although detailed analysis of the patient's facial and jaw structures from a clinical and radiographic perspective is vitally important, the focus of this chapter is

the teeth and orthodontic considerations in preparation for orthognathic surgery and postsurgical orthodontic management. Other important factors in diagnosis, treatment planning, and outcomes, such as patient concerns, psychosocial factors, masticatory dysfunction, airway problems, speech difficulties, temporomandibular joint (TMJ) pathologies, and comprehensive orthognathic surgery workup are not discussed in this chapter. Note that the normal values provided in this chapter are not absolutes for every patient because of individual size, morphologic variances, and racial and ethnic differences. They are provided as a guide to help the clinician evaluate each individual patient. Establishing an all-inclusive diagnosis is paramount to developing a comprehensive prioritized treatment plan. The orthodontist must determine the orthodontic goals based on the pretreatment findings and on the projected treatment outcome. This chapter first presents orthodontic diagnostic information, then orthodontic treatment considerations, followed by postsurgical orthodontic management.

CLINICAL EXAMINATION AND DENTAL MODEL ANALYSIS

From an orthodontic standpoint, in evaluating the occlusion and other dental factors, the clinical and dental model analyses, when correlated with the cephalometric analysis, provide the most information for proper diagnosis and treatment planning. There are 13 basic clinical and dental model evaluations that are helpful for making these determinations:

1. **Arch length:** This measurement correlates the mesiodistal widths of the teeth relative to the amount of alveolar bone available and aids in identifying the presence of crowding

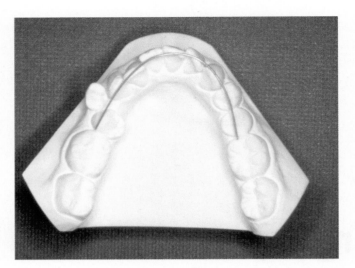

FIGURE 55-1. Arch length analysis measures mesiodistal widths of the teeth relative to the amount of alveolar bone available to identify the presence of crowding or spacing. The curved wire shows ideal cuspid and incisor tip position relative to the basal bone.

or spacing. This helps determine whether teeth need to be extracted or whether spaces need to be either created or closed (Figure 55-1). Clinical and dental model assessment, when correlated to the cephalometric analysis, will aid in determining arch length requirements. Generally, class II patients will tend to have more crowding in the mandibular arch and less in the maxillary arch, whereas class III patients may have spacing in the mandibular arch but a tendency for crowding in the maxillary arch.

2. **Tooth size analysis:** This assessment relates the mesiodistal width of the maxillary teeth compared with the mandibular teeth. A tooth size discrepancy (TSD) causes an incompatibility of dental alignment and may occur in the anterior teeth, premolars, and molar regions. Approximately 40% of patients with dentofacial deformities will have an anterior TSD affecting the anterior six teeth of the

maxillary and mandibular arches (the mandibular arch is commonly too large compared with the maxillary arch), usually owing to small maxillary lateral incisors. In such cases, proper tooth alignment, with all spaces closed, often precludes the establishment of a good class I cuspid-molar relationship with treatment, and instead, a class II end-on cuspid-molar occlusal relationship may result. Occasionally, the maxillary anterior six teeth may be too large for the mandibular anterior teeth, creating an excessive anterior overjet when in a class I cuspid relationship. Determination of a TSD pretreatment will provide the best opportunity to correct the TSD during the presurgical orthodontic phase of treatment. Explaining to the patient before treatment that small maxillary lateral incisors may need restorative crown enlargement to maximize the quality aesthetic and functional outcome is important, so that the patient is aware from the onset of the time and financial commitment necessary for treatment. The normal mesiodistal widths of each of the permanent teeth are recorded in Tables 55-1 and 55-2. Variations from the norm may create difficulties in tooth alignment and occlusal interdigitation.

Bolton's analysis is a method used to correlate the widths of the maxillary and mandibular anterior six teeth. Needle-point calipers can be used to measure each individual tooth at its widest dimension and successive holes punched into a tablet for each of the anterior six teeth for each arch. Then, a measurement from the first to the last holes will give the summation of mesiodistal widths of the anterior six teeth for each arch (Figures 55-2 and 55-3). The summation of the mesiodistal widths of the maxillary anterior six teeth, divided into the combined width of the mandibular anterior six teeth, yields a value called the *intermaxillary (Bolton's) index.* The average index (percentage) is 77.5 ± 3.5.[1] A simple conversion of this factor would be to measure the width of the mandibular anterior six teeth and then multiply that sum by 1.3. This results in a calculated ideal maxillary arch width. The difference between the calculated and the actual maxillary arch

TABLE 55-1. **Maxillary Mesiodistal Teeth Diameters***

	Central Incisor	Lateral Incisor	Cuspid	First Bicuspid	Second Bicuspid	First Molar	Second Molar
Males	8.9 (0.59)	6.9 (0.64)	8.0 (0.42)	6.8 (0.47)	6.7 (0.37)	10.6 (0.56)	9.5 (0.71)
Females	8.7 (0.57)	6.8 (0.64)	7.5 (0.36)	6.6 (0.46)	6.5 (0.46)	10.2 (0.58)	8.8 (0.73)

*Measurements in millimeters (standard deviation [SD]).
Adapted from Moyers RE, van der Linden FPGM, Riolo ML, McNamara JA, editors. Standards of Human Occlusal Development. Ann Arbor: The University of Michigan. The Center for Human Growth and Development; 1976; pp. 53–94.

TABLE 55-2. **Mandibular Mesiodistal Teeth Diameters***

	Central Incisor	Lateral Incisor	Cuspid	First Bicuspid	Second Bicuspid	First Molar	Second Molar
Males	5.5 (0.32)	6.0 (0.37)	7.0 (0.40)	6.9 (0.63)	7.2 (0.47)	10.7 (0.60)	10.0 (0.67)
Females	5.5 (0.34)	5.9 (0.34)	6.6 (0.34)	6.8 (0.70)	7.1 (0.46)	10.3 (0.74)	9.5 (0.59)

*Measurements in millimeters (standard deviation [SD]).
Adapted from Moyers RE, van der Linden FPGM, Riolo ML, McNamara JA, editors. Standards of Human Occlusal Development. Ann Arbor, MI: The University of Michigan. The Center for Human Growth and Development; 1976; pp. 53–94.

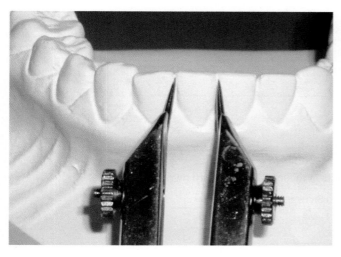

FIGURE 55-2. Bolton's analysis. Needle-point calipers are used to measure each tooth at the contact-point level to aid in tooth-size analysis.

width values determines the TSD (see Figure 55-3). This evaluation is very helpful in determining presurgical orthodontic and surgical goals. TSDs can also occur in the premolar and molar areas (normally the same maxillary and mandibular teeth are similar in size) in which the mandibular teeth may be significantly larger than the maxillary teeth.

Bolton's analysis is not perfect and functions only as a guide in assessing the tooth size compatibility of the anterior teeth because it does not take into consideration the labiolingual thickness of the incisors, the axial inclination

of the teeth, or the thickness and prominence of the marginal ridges. A thin labiolingual dimension of the maxillary incisors may compensate for small TSDs, but thicker than normal dimensions or prominent marginal ridges may preclude a class I cuspid relationship even though Bolton's index is normal. An accurate dental model orthodontic wax setup or computer rendering may achieve a more accurate assessment.

3. **Incisor inclination:** This refers to the inclination of the maxillary and mandibular incisors relative to their respective basal bones. The dental models are correlated to the cephalometric analysis and the ideal axial inclination of the incisors determined (Figure 55-4). The incisor inclination analysis contributes to the determination of whether extractions are necessary, spaces need to be created or eliminated, and what mechanics are required to align and level the arches or segments of the arches. The key is to remove any anterior dental compensations by repositioning the incisors in their proper position and inclination over basal bone.

4. **Arch width analysis:** This refers to the evaluation of the intra-arch transverse widths between the maxillary and

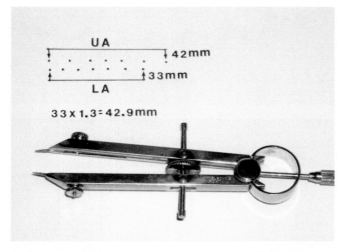

FIGURE 55-3. Bolton's analysis. Seven successive holes are punched into a tablet for the contact points of each of the anterior six teeth for each arch. The distance from the first hole to the last hole is the summation of mesiodistal widths of the anterior six teeth in each arch. Multiplying the summation of the mandibular anterior six teeth (LA) by 1.3 yields the calculated arch width for the maxillary anterior six teeth (UA). Subtracting the actual maxillary anterior arch width from the calculated width yields the tooth-size discrepancy (0.9 mm, in this example).

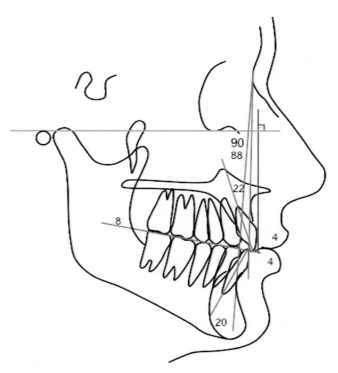

FIGURE 55-4. Cephalometric analysis. Normal maxillary depth angle is 90 degrees ± 3 degrees and mandibular depth is 88 degrees ± 3 degrees. Normal occlusal plane angulation is 8 degrees ± 4 degrees. Normal maxillary incisor inclination to the nasion point A (NA) line is 22 degrees ± 2 degrees with the labial surface of the incisor being 4 mm ± 2 mm anterior to the NA line. The angle between Frankfort horizontal plane and a line drawn tangent to the facial aspect of the maxillary central incisor crown should be at 90 degrees ± 2 degrees. Normal mandibular incisor inclination to the nasion point B (NB) line is 20 degrees ± 2 degrees with the labial surface of the incisor being 4 mm ± 2 mm anterior to the NB line.

TABLE 55-3. **Maxillary Arch Width* Measurements in millimeters (standard deviation [SD])**

	Cuspid	First Bicuspid	Second Bicuspid	First Molar	Second Molar
Males	32.3 (1.7)	36.7 (2.0)	41.5 (2.5)	47.1 (2.8)	52.3 (3.4)
Females	31.2 (2.45)	34.6 (3.2)	39.3 (2.2)	44.3 (2.3)	49.3 (2.8)

*All measurements at centroid.

Adapted from Moyers RE, van der Linden FPGM, Riolo ML, McNamara JA, editors. Standards of Human Occlusal Development. Ann Arbor, MI: The University of Michigan. The Center for Human Growth and Development; 1976; pp. 53–94.

TABLE 55-4. **Mandibular Arch Width* Measurements in millimeters (standard deviation [SD])**

	Cuspid	First Bicuspid	Second Bicuspid	First Molar	Second Molar
Males	24.8 (1.3)	32.8 (1.5)	37.6 (2.3)	43.0 (2.7)	49.0 (2.3)
Females	23.1(2.0)	31.8 (1.4)	36.8 (1.3)	41.7 (2.3)	47.2 (2.1)

*All measurements at centroid.

Adapted from Moyers RE, van der Linden FPGM, Riolo ML, McNamara JA, editors. Standards of Human Occlusal Development. Ann Arbor, MI: The University of Michigan. The Center for Human Growth and Development; 1976; pp. 53–94.

the mandibular arches. The average maxillary and mandibular arch widths for adults are listed in Tables 55-3 and 55-4.[2] These averages are only guidelines and do not account for patient size or racial or ethnic differences. However, from a practical standpoint, a good way to analyze the arch width is to relate the models to the occlusal position that is to be achieved with the surgical correction and then assess the transverse relationship. For example, if a patient has a class II occlusion, position the models in a class I cuspid-molar relation and evaluate the transverse width relationship. Similarly, a patient with a class III occlusion is evaluated by positioning the models into a class I cuspid-molar relationship. When a class II relationship is shifted to a class I relationship, the maxilla may be narrow and require expansion. In some cases, it may be indicated to evaluate the transverse relationship by placing the models into a class II molar position to determine whether a class I cuspid and class II molar relationship (this would require maxillary bicuspid extractions) would be best for that particular patient; this may be beneficial when there is significant crowding in the maxillary arch and no crowding in the mandibular arch. Transverse discrepancies will influence the presurgical orthodontics and dictate the surgical procedures required.

5. **Curve of Spee:** This evaluates the vertical position of the anterior teeth compared with the posterior teeth. This assessment can be determined by placing the occlusion of the maxillary dental model on a flat plane; the incisors should be about 1 mm above the flat plane (Figure 55-5A). Placing the occlusion of the mandibular dental model on a flat plane should see the mandibular incisors elevated 1 mm above the midbuccal teeth. A significant accentuated curve of Spee in the maxilla is usually associated with an anterior open bite and a reverse curve associated with an anterior deep bite. An accentuated curve of Spee in the mandible (see Figure 55-5B) is commonly

associated with an anterior deep bite and a reverse curve associated with an open bite. Accentuated or reverse curves of Spee will influence whether the curve in each arch requires correction, and if so, whether the correction will be achieved by orthodontics, with or without extractions, opening spaces, or surgical intervention.

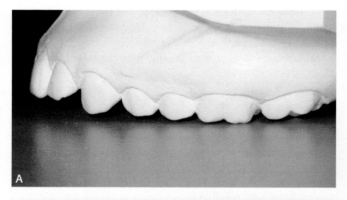

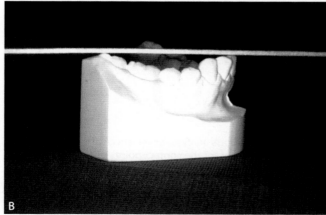

FIGURE 55-5. Increased curve of Spee in the maxillary arch **(A)** and in the mandibular arch **(B).**

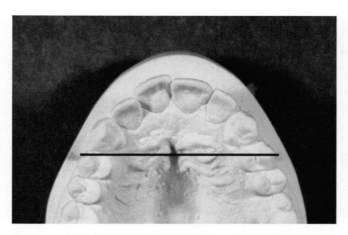

FIGURE 55-6.   Tooth arch symmetry. The left cuspid is significantly more anteriorly positioned in the arch compared with the right cuspid.

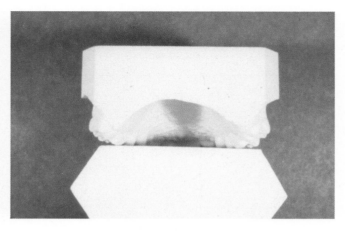

FIGURE 55-7.   Curve of Wilson. This assesses the mediolateral position of the occlusal surfaces of the maxillary and mandibular posterior teeth.

6. **Cuspid-molar position:** This identifies the Angle classification and dental interrelationships. It is usually preferable to have a class I cuspid-molar relationship as an optimal outcome result; however, a class II molar relationship is acceptable. A class III molar relationship is less desirable because the mandibular first molar functions against the maxillary second bicuspid, although this may be indicated in select cases.

7. **Tooth arch symmetry:** This compares the left with the right side symmetry within each arch. There may be a significant asymmetry within the arch, such as a cuspid on one side being more anteriorly positioned in the arch than the cuspid on the opposite side (Figure 55-6). This problem often occurs with a unilateral missing tooth. Also, vertical asymmetries can occur with individual teeth, sections of the dentoalveolus, or the entire dental arches, creating a cant in the transverse occlusal plane. Correcting these types of asymmetrical conditions may require special orthodontic mechanics, unilateral or asymmetrical extractions or creation of arch space, and/or segmental surgical procedures.

8. **Curve of Wilson** (degree of buccal tooth tipping): This evaluates the mediolateral position of the occlusal surfaces of the maxillary (Figure 55-7) and mandibular posterior teeth. If the occlusal surfaces of the maxillary or mandibular posterior teeth are tipped too far buccally, it may be difficult to achieve a proper occlusal interdigitation relationship. In the presence of a transverse maxillary deficiency with preexisting increased curve of Wilson and posterior cross-bites, it is very difficult, if not impossible, to correct the problem orthodontically, orthopedically, or even with surgically assisted rapid palatal expansion (SARPE). The curve of Wilson will usually get much worse with these mechanics. In these types of cases, surgical expansion by multiple maxillary osteotomies may be indicated to decrease the curve of Wilson.

When the mandibular posterior teeth are tipped buccally, it is often related to macroglossia or habitual tongue posturing. Orthodontic lingual tipping of the posterior teeth is very difficult when macroglossia is present and will likely be unstable. A reduction glossectomy may be indicated before orthodontics in order to permit a more stable final orthodontic result.

9. **Dental problems,** including missing teeth, severe caries, extensive dental restorations, or root resorption: These must be identified because they may influence treatment design. If a tooth is nonrestorable and requires extraction, it must be determined whether the extraction space requires orthodontic closure or the space maintained for later dental prosthetic reconstruction. In some cases, it may be helpful to maintain the condemned tooth to improve stability during surgical alignment of the jaws or segments thereof, with extraction after surgery. Crowns on previously restored teeth may need to be refabricated after orthodontics and orthognathic surgery, because the crown anatomy may need to be changed for proper occlusion with the new dental relationships. Evaluation for the presence of developmentally short roots or root resorption is necessary because this will have an effect on orthodontics and specific design of the surgical procedures. Determination of salvageable teeth and restorative requirements is an integral component in the planning and treatment of patients.

10. **Tooth ankylosis:** If undiagnosed, ankylosed teeth can have devastating effects on presurgical orthodontics. Tooth ankylosis, the fusion of alveolar bone and cementum, results from damage to the periodontal ligament (PDL). An ankylosed tooth may be identified by failure to move with orthodontic forces (Figure 55-8), failure of a tooth to erupt, submerged or incomplete tooth eruption (Figure 55-9), or lack of eruption of a tooth compared with adjacent teeth and alveolar bone growth. The most sensitive diagnostic test is percussion, performed by tapping the crown with the end of a mouth mirror, in which the ankylosed tooth has a high, clear, solid metallic sound. A normal tooth has a dull sound, being protected

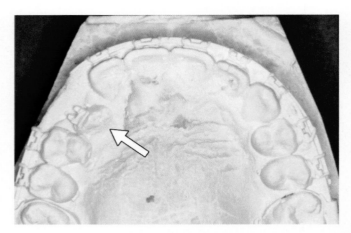

FIGURE 55-8. Dental cast shows a palatally displaced cuspid, unresponsive to orthodontic mechanics, indicating probable ankylosis.

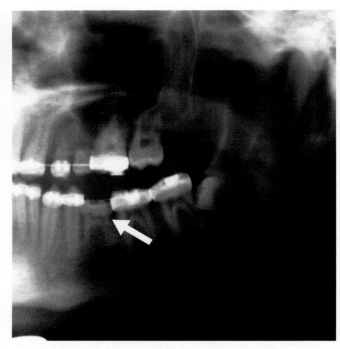

FIGURE 55-9. Panorex shows incomplete eruption of primary tooth without a permanent successor, indicating ankylosis.

by the PDL. However, an erupted tooth with an impacted tooth directly against it may also have a solid sound to percussion. Normal multirooted teeth present a more solid sound than single-rooted teeth. Therefore, percussion testing should be compared with similar teeth (i.e., test bicuspids vs. bicuspids, molars vs. molars, using both sides of the arch). An ankylosed tooth lacks any mobility. Over 90% of ankylosed teeth are deciduous, most often, the second molar followed by the first molar.[3] Ankylosed primary teeth are not susceptible to resorption by the follicle of the underlying permanent tooth and may result in impaction of the permanent tooth.[3]

Ankylosed teeth can cause significant problems with jaw growth and development. Early ankylosis results in noneruption or partial eruption, resulting in incomplete development of the alveolar process.[4] Permanent teeth may be displaced from normal eruption pathways with resulting loss of alveolar bone height. The failure of an ankylosed tooth to erupt may allow adjacent teeth to drift and permit supereruption of the tooth in the opposing arch. Ankylosed teeth do not respond to orthodontic

forces and can create significant orthodontic problems when malaligned and tied into the orthodontic arch wire (Figure 55-10).[5] The ankylosed tooth functions as an anchor and, in active uncontrolled orthodontics, will move adjacent teeth to align with its position, with subsequent development of an occlusal, alveolar, and possibly, a visible facial deformity.

11. **Periodontal status:** This is very important, because preexisting periodontal pathologies could be exacerbated during orthodontic and orthognathic surgical treatments.[6] Factors that can adversely affect the health and outcome of the periodontal tissues as well as the orthodontics and orthognathic surgery include smoking, excessive consumption of alcohol or caffeine, habitual patterns such as bruxism and clenching, preexisting con-

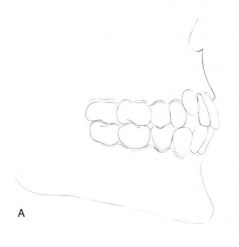

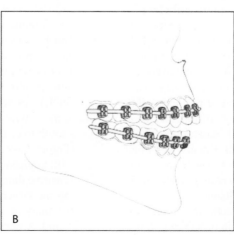

FIGURE 55-10. **A,** This illustration depicts a partially submerged ankylosed maxillary cuspid. **B,** If tied into an active straight arch wire, the adjacent teeth will be orthodontically moved toward the ankylosed tooth, resulting in the development of a significant malocclusion (in this case, an open bite due to incisor intrusion).

A

B

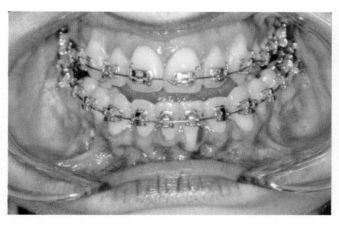

FIGURE 55-11.   Periodontal concerns. A lack of attached gingiva in the lower incisor region before initiation of orthodontics if left untreated will cause severe gingival retraction and loss of supporting bone. Gingival grafting should be considered before initiation of orthodontics.

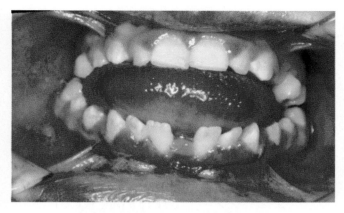

FIGURE 55-12.   Macroglossia may cause anterior open bite, diastema between the teeth, accentuated maxillary curve of Spee, and reverse mandibular curve of Spee.

nective tissue/autoimmune diseases, diabetes, malnutrition, and other diseases that could affect the local tissue blood supply perfusion and wound healing. Any pretreatment of acute or chronic periodontal disease should be addressed before the orthodontics and surgery. The lack of attached gingiva around the teeth (most commonly seen in the mandibular anterior arch) can cause gingival retraction, loss of bone, and loosening of teeth if orthodontics is initiated and the mandibular incisors are tipped forward (Figure 55-11). Gingival grafting may be indicated before orthodontics to provide attached gingiva so as to prevent these problems. Good communication between the periodontist, the orthodontist, and the OMF surgeon is of utmost importance.

Orthodontics can help prepare interdental osteotomy sites by tipping the roots of the adjacent teeth away from each other to increase the interosseous space between the roots. A number of studies have demonstrated that interdental osteotomies have a minimal effect on the periodontium when they are properly performed.[7-11] Having healthy stable dental tissues to work with during the orthodontics and surgery will maximize the periodontal outcome as well as the overall outcome. The failure to recognize preexisting periodontal pathology, identify risk factors, poor performance of surgery, and/or lack of attention to detail could result in significant periodontal problems as well as other problems that could compromise the final result.

12. **Tongue assessment:** An enlarged tongue (macroglossia) can cause dentoskeletal deformities and instability of orthodontic and orthognathic surgical treatments and create masticatory, speech, and airway management problems. There are a number of congenital and acquired causes of true macroglossia, including muscular hypertrophy, glandular hyperplasia, hemangioma, lymphangioma,

Down syndrome, and Beckwith-Wiedemann syndrome. Acquired factors include acromegaly, myxedema, amyloidosis, tertiary syphilis, cysts or tumors, and neurologic injury.[12] Specific clinical and cephalometric features may help the clinician identify the presence or absence of macroglossia, although not all of these features are always present. Specific clinical features of macroglossia include the following (Figure 55-12):

■ Grossly enlarged, wide, broad, flat tongue
■ Open bite (anterior or posterior)
■ Mandibular prognathism
■ Class III malocclusion with or without anterior or posterior cross-bite
■ Chronic posturing of the tongue between the teeth at rest (rule out habitual posturing of normal-sized tongue)
■ Increased curve of Wilson of the maxillary posterior teeth
■ Reverse curve of Wilson of the mandibular posterior teeth
■ Accentuated curve of Spee in the maxillary arch
■ Reverse curve of Spee in the mandibular arch
■ Increased transverse width of the maxillary and mandibular arches
■ Diastema, with increased incisor inclination, in the mandible and/or maxilla
■ Crenations (scalloping) of the tongue
■ Glossitis (due to excessive mouth breathing)
■ Speech articulation disorders
■ Asymmetry in the maxilla or mandible associated with an asymmetrical tongue
■ Difficulty with mastication and swallowing (severe cases)
■ Instability in "stable" orthodontic mechanics or orthognathic surgeries
■ Airway difficulties (obstructive sleep apnea) due to oropharyngeal obstruction
■ Chronic drooling

SECTION 7

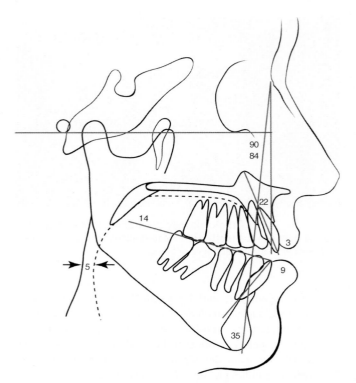

FIGURE 55-13. Macroglossia. Cephalometric analysis shows mandibular dentoalveolar protrusion and proclination of the mandibular anterior teeth. The tongue fills the oral cavity (dotted line) and the oropharyngeal airway is decreased (normal distance from posterior aspect of tongue to posterior pharyngeal wall is 11 mm; in this case, 5 mm).

Cephalometric radiographic features commonly seen with macroglossia (Figure 55-13) include the following:

- Tongue filling the oral cavity and extrudes through anterior open bite
- Mandibular or bimaxillary dentoalveolar protrusion
- Increased inclination of the maxillary and mandibular anterior teeth
- Disproportionately excessive mandibular growth
- Decreased oropharyngeal airway
- Increased gonial angle
- Increased mandibular plane angle
- Increased mandibular occlusal plane angle

Most open bite cases are not related to macroglossia. In fact, it has been established that closing open bites with orthognathic surgery will allow a normal tongue (which is a very adaptable organ) to readjust to the altered volume of the oral cavity, with little tendency toward relapse.[13,14] Most anterior open bite deformities that develop in the teenage years or later are commonly related to TMJ pathology.[15] However, if true macroglossia is present with the open bite, then instability of the orthodontics and orthognathic surgery will likely occur, with a tendency for the open bite to return. Pseudomacroglossia is a condition in which the tongue may be normal in size, but it appears large relative to its anatomic interrelationships. This can be created by (1) habitual posturing of the tongue; (2) hypertrophied tonsils and adenoid tissue displacing the tongue forward; (3) low palatal vault, decreasing the oral cavity volume; (4) transverse, vertical, or anteroposterior deficiency of the maxillary and/or mandibular arches decreasing oral cavity volume; and (5) tumors that displace the tongue. Pseudomacroglossia must be distinguished from true macroglossia because the methods of management are different.

13. **TMJ assessment.** Jaw deformities requiring orthognathic surgery often coexist with TMJ pathology. Unrecognized or untreated TMJ pathologies are one of the primary factors leading to postsurgical complications, resulting in poor quality and unpredictable outcomes. TMJ surgery may be required in these coexisting situations to obtain the highest quality results for patients. However, the TMJ surgery should be done before the orthognathic surgery in separate operations or perform the TMJ surgery followed by the orthognathic surgery at the same operation.[1,2] It is important that TMJ problems be identified and properly managed in the orthognathic surgery patient.

DIAGNOSTIC PROBLEM LIST AND PRIORITIZED TREATMENT PLAN

Before an orthodontic and surgical treatment plan can be properly developed, a diagnostic list of the existing problems is established based on patient concerns; a clinical, radiographic, dental model analyses; and other indicated evaluations. This will include all findings relative to musculoskeletal and dental imbalances, occlusal problems, aesthetic concerns, TMJ pathology, myofascial pain problems, missing teeth, crowns, bridges, endodontically treated teeth (occasionally ankylosed), periodontal problems, other functional disorders as well as any other medical factors that may affect treatment outcomes. The prioritized treatment plan is formulated from the diagnostic problem list and may include one or more ideal treatment plans and several other treatment options that may have one or more compromises, but may be appropriate based upon each individual patient situation. All potential treatment options should be presented to the patient; the final determination is made by the patient and the orthodontist and OMF surgeon.

PRESURGICAL ORTHODONTIC GOALS

The basic presurgical orthodontic goals are

- Align and position the teeth over the basal bone.
- Avoid excessive intrusion or extrusion of the teeth.
- Decompensate teeth.
- Avoid unstable expansion of the arches.
- Avoid class II and class III mechanics (unless required for dental decompensation).
- Perform stable and predictable orthodontics.
- Avoid orthodontic movements that can be performed more predictably with surgery.

Relative to the position of the maxillary and mandibular incisors, the ideal presurgical orthodontic goals are

1. Position the long axis of the maxillary central incisors approximately 22 degrees ± 2 degrees to the nasion-point A (NA) line, with the labial surface of the incisors 4 mm anterior to the NA line relative to a normally positioned maxilla and normal occlusal plane angle (see Figure 55-4).
2. The aesthetic crown angle is a line drawn tangent to the facial aspect of the maxillary central incisor crown extending through Frankfort horizontal plane. The angle created should be at 90 degrees ± 2 degrees. This places the crown into the best aesthetic position (see Figure 55-4).
3. Position the long axis of the mandibular central incisors 20 degrees ± 2 degrees to the nasion-point B (NB) line with the labial surface of the incisors 4 mm anterior to that line relative to a normally positioned mandible and normal occlusal plane angle (see Figure 55-4).
4. Satisfy arch length requirements (with regards to crowding or spacing).

Assessment of the ideal position of the maxillary and mandibular incisors to the NA and NB lines, respectively (see Figure 55-4), is the most convenient and practical method to establish the presurgical orthodontic goals for the incisors. However, these presurgical orthodontic goals may be different if the occlusal plane angle is to be altered surgically. Removal of dental compensations is helpful before surgery so that maximum skeletal correction can be achieved. An exact orthodontic treatment plan, including the specific mechanics and anchorage requirements necessary to position the teeth to satisfy the presurgical orthodontic goals, must be developed and executed.

INITIAL SURGICAL TREATMENT OBJECTIVE

The *surgical treatment objective (STO)*, also known as a *cephalometric prediction tracing,* is a two-dimensional visual projection of the changes in osseous, dental, and soft tissues as a result of orthodontics and orthognathic surgical correction of the dentofacial and occlusal deformity. The purpose of the STO is threefold: (1) establish presurgical orthodontic goals, (2) develop an accurate surgical objective that will achieve the best functional and aesthetic result, and (3) create a facial profile objective that can be used as a visual aid in consultation with the patient and family members. A prediction tracing of the anticipated presurgical orthodontic dental movements is created by placing an acetate sheet over the original cephalometric tracing and retracing the teeth into the position they will be placed with the presurgical orthodontics, based on the goals and available mechanics (Figure 55-14A). The initial STO is then constructed with the teeth in their presurgical orthodontic final position.

The STO has significant importance in two phases of treatment planning: (1) the initial STO is prepared before treatment to determine the orthodontic and surgical goals and (2) the final STO is prepared after the presurgical orthodontics are completed but before surgery to determine the exact vertical and anteroposterior skeletal and soft tissue

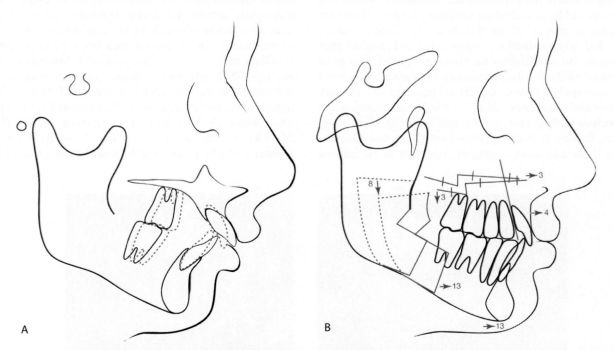

FIGURE 55-14.   **A,** Presurgical orthodontics. The predicted orthodontic tooth movements are traced on acetate paper overlying the original lateral cephalometric tracing. The *solid lines* show the original position of the teeth. The *dashed lines* shoe the new position of the teeth after simulated extraction of four first bicuspids and orthodontic closure of the spaces. **B,** Surgical treatment objective (STO). This is an example of a completed final STO showing the predicted outcome of the presurgical orthodontics and the anticipated surgical treatment. The *arrows* and *numbers* indicate the direction and millimeters of movement.

movements to be achieved (see Figure 55-14B). These determinations can also be done through computer software programs, but these techniques may be less accurate than a manual STO because these programs have only the central incisor and first molar present to represent the entire dentition. However, the software programs are adequate for single-jaw and double-jaw planning when the maxilla is repositioned as a single unit. The STO is invaluable to the orthodontist and surgeon in establishing treatment objectives and projected results, acting as the blueprint for the entire treatment plan.

DEFINITIVE INTERDISCIPLINARY TREATMENT PLAN

The definitive treatment plan is formulated after consideration of all possible treatment options, and it is finalized based upon the patient's concerns, clinical evaluation, radiographic analysis, dental model evaluation, TMJ assessment, initial STO, and other relevant evaluations. Although the specific treatment plan may vary throughout the course of treatment, the general sequencing of the treatment that may be involved in a typical patient is described in the following sections.

Dental and Periodontal Treatment

Any indicated periodontal or general dental care related to maintaining teeth or improving dental health should be performed before orthodontics and surgical intervention. The objective is to maintain as many teeth as possible and maximize the health of the periodontium. Temporary crowns and bridges should be placed where necessary for the orthodontic and surgical phases of the treatment. Permanent crowns, inlays, and bridges should be constructed and inserted after the surgery and orthodontics have been completed. This gives the restorative dentist the opportunity to provide escapement grooves, cuspid protection, and incisal guidance for optimum function and aesthetics. Initial periodontal management may include scaling, root planing, and curettage, eliminating pockets, as well as grafting procedures to provide adequate alveolar bone and attached gingiva, especially in the anterior

mandible. Occasionally, in patients with several missing teeth, osseointegrated implant placement before orthodontics and orthognathic surgery may provide anchorage for orthodontics and additional dental units to help in repositioning the jaw structures at surgery.

Presurgical Orthodontics

The orthodontist is responsible for positioning the teeth to the most desirable position over basal bone in preparation for surgery. The development of prescription brackets and straight wire orthodontic techniques has helped simplify orthodontics. Most prescription bracket systems are designed to tip the cuspid roots distally, creating space between the roots of the lateral incisors and the cuspids. In cases requiring segmentalization of the maxilla, this interdental space may be adequate through which to perform interdental osteotomies; but if inadequate, additional room can be created by tipping the lateral incisor roots mesially and the cuspids more distally. Bonded brackets are clean and eliminate interdental spacing problems created by circumferential bands. Bonded brackets with the currently available resins are quite adequate for orthognathic surgery procedures. However, inaccurate placement of the brackets on the teeth can result in undesired rotations, vertical discrepancies between teeth, malalignment of marginal ridges and labial surfaces of adjacent teeth, and unfavorable root positions. Careful placement of brackets is paramount in helping to achieve high-quality results.

Nickel-titanium or similarly shaped memory arch wires can be advantageous for many orthognathic cases to aid in presurgical orthodontic dental alignment goals. However, there are cases in which shape memory wires could be detrimental, such as in an anterior open bite with an accentuated maxillary curve of Spee. The use of nickel-titanium wires or any type of straight wire in these cases can create unstable orthodontic movements such as extrusion of teeth and buccal tipping of the molars as a result of reciprocal forces. Stainless steel wires (SSWs) with compensating bends (Figure 55-15A), or sectional wires (see Figure 55-15B), may provide a better controlled mechanical force in these types of cases.

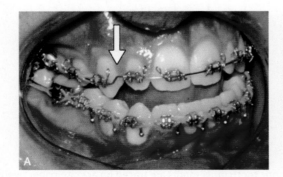
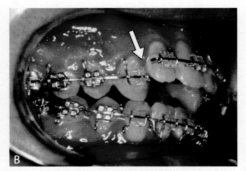

FIGURE 55-15. **A,** Compensating steps *(arrow)* in the orthodontic arch wire to align the anterior teeth at an elevated level compared with the posterior teeth to eliminate extrusion or intrusion of teeth that may result in unstable orthodontic movements. **B,** Sectioning the arch wire *(arrow)* is another approach to align teeth at independent levels to avoid extrusion or intrusion of teeth. However, sectional wires may decrease positional control of teeth adjacent to the ends of the cut wire.

The type of arch wire, and how long each is left in place, is critical and must be carefully monitored by the orthodontist.

Lingual orthodontic appliance are sometimes requested by patients for aesthetic reasons. Lingual appliances can work satisfactorily for single-piece maxillary osteotomies and mandibular osteotomies but will require the placement of brackets or buttons on the lateral aspect of the teeth at surgery to facilitate intraoperative intermaxillary fixation for application of rigid skeletal fixation to stabilize the osteotomies and to use postsurgical elastics, if necessary. When segmentation of the maxilla is required, lingual appliances present a greater challenge. Construction of palatal or occlusal covering surgical splints is much more difficult because of distortion of the lingual appliance on the surgical models that interfere with the fit of the splint at surgery. In addition, postsurgical changing of the arch wire is more difficult, uncomfortable, and painful for the patient. It may be several months after surgery before the lingual arch wire can be changed. It is much more difficult to finalize the occlusion and may require labial appliances to finalize the occlusal results.

To follow are basic presurgical orthodontic factors that commonly must be addressed in preparing patients for orthognathic surgery. It is important to avoid interarch class II mechanics (i.e., class II elastics, growth appliances, TMJ "disk recapturing" splints, Herbst appliances) unless they are specifically required during the presurgical orthodontics (e.g., to correct arch asymmetry to decompensate mandibular arch with lingually inclined mandibular incisors). Long-term class II mechanics positions the mandibular condyle downward and forward in the fossa and may allow hypertrophy (thickening) of the TMJ bilaminar tissues (Figure 55-16). This same condition can occur in patients with a "Sunday" bite. In these

situations, after surgical mandibular advancement, the bilaminar tissue will slowly thin out over time, causing a slow relapse of the mandible toward a class II relationship. In addition, posturing the mandible forward for an extended time could result in foreshortening of the anterior articular disk attachments, increasing the risk of TMJ articular disk displacement postsurgery.

If a patient has been treated with long-term class II mechanics or has a "Sunday" bite, it may be an advantage to use light class III mechanics for a few months presurgery to eliminate the hypertrophied bilaminar tissue and to decompensate for any unstable orthodontics that may have been created. If the TMJ articular disk does become displaced, it would be better to have that occur before surgery because the articular disk can be surgically repositioned and stabilized with high predictability at the same time as the orthognathic surgery.[16–19] Attempts to recapture a TMJ displaced disk with splint therapy before surgery could be detrimental to the patient relative to outcome stability and pain. In most cases, nonsurgical disk "recapturing" procedures have proved clinically unsuccessful.

TREATMENT OPTIONS FOR SPECIFIC ORTHODONTIC PROBLEMS

This section presents specific dental malrelationships and the orthodontic and surgical treatment options for consideration. Comprehensive assessment of the patient and developing treatment objectives will aid in selecting the appropriate treatment.

Adjustment for TSD

Usually, TSDs occur because of small maxillary lateral incisors, making the combined mesiodistal width of the maxillary anterior six teeth too small to fit properly around the mandibular anterior six teeth, so that when the teeth are properly aligned, an end-on class II cuspid relationship will result (Figure 55-17). If Bolton's analysis indicates a significant

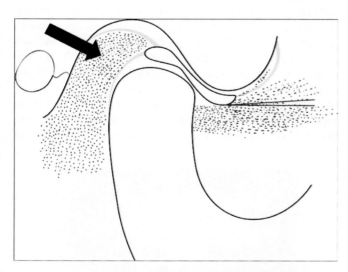

FIGURE 55-16. Temporomandibular joint (TMJ) effects of long-term class II mechanics, anterior repositioning splints, growth devices, or "Sunday" bite relationships can cause hypertrophy of the posterior bilaminar tissue (arrow), positioning the condyle downward and forward in the fossa. After mandibular advancement, this tissue will slowly thin out, and the condyles will move posteriorly in the fossa, causing a shift of the mandible and occlusion toward a class II relapse position.

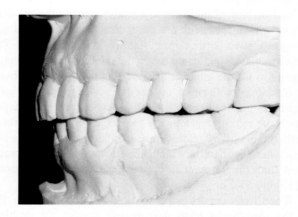

FIGURE 55-17. Tooth size discrepancy (TSD). These casts show well-aligned and leveled teeth in each arch, but because the maxillary laterals are small creating a TSD, even with the best possible occlusal fit, there is an end-on class II occlusion due to the TSD.

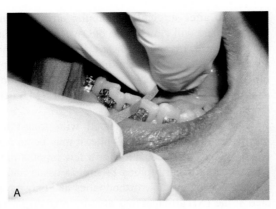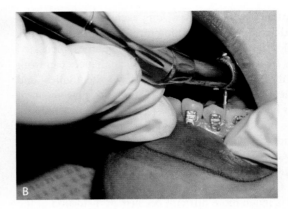

FIGURE 55-18. Interproximal reduction. Mesiodistal tooth width can be reduced with a diamond strip **(A)** or a thin cylindrical diamond bur **(B)**, and the space created can be closed orthodontically.

TSD, presurgical orthodontic adjustments can usually correct the discrepancy and aid in providing a solid class I cuspid relationship at surgery and in the final outcome. TSDs can also occur in the bicuspids and molars, with the maxillary teeth usually being too small compared with the mandibular teeth. The following are treatment options that can be used to correct TSDs.

Interproximal Tooth Size Reduction

Interproximal tooth size reduction (IPR) reduces the mesiodistal dimension of the involved teeth. Because most TSDs involve larger mandibular anterior teeth compared with the maxillary anterior teeth, slenderizing the mandibular anterior teeth can address the issue (Figure 55-18). Approximately 10% to 12% of the mesiodistal width can be safely removed from each tooth with 50% of the interproximal enamel remaining. Up to 3 mm of IPR can usually be safely achieved in the mandibular anterior six teeth. Slenderizing the mandibular anterior teeth is an advantageous procedure, in which the maximum width of the incisors is toward the incisor edge, particularly in the presence of crowding and/or increased inclination of the mandibular incisors. It may not be advantageous if the mandibular anterior teeth are in a normal or lingual inclination, because closing the resultant spaces will further decrease the incisor inclination and may adversely affect orthodontic stability and aesthetics. This technique is not indicated when the contact points are positioned toward the gingiva, because this could result in tissue strangulation with loss of papilla and interdental bone, creating significant periodontal issues. In the rare case in which the maxillary teeth are too large for the mandibular teeth, the maxillary teeth can be slenderized, but this is best used when the maxillary teeth are crowded and/or overangulated and the individual crowns are wider than normal (see Table 55-1).

When TSDs occurs in the bicuspid and/or molar area, IPR of the mandibular teeth will usually correct the problem, unless the IPR will cause excessive retraction of the mandibular anterior teeth. If this appears to be a potential outcome, careful closure of the spacing by loosing (slipping)

posterior anchorage (using mechanics that will move the posterior teeth forward instead of the anterior teeth backward) may solve the problem. This approach may include class II mechanics to provide forward forces on the posterior teeth or moving one tooth at a time on each side. Dental implants or temporary anchoring devices (TADs) placed in the posterior or anterior dentoalveolus could provide stable anchorage to aid in applying mechanics necessary to push the posterior teeth forward.

Creation of Arch Space

Additional arch space can enlarge the circumference of each involved arch. Because TSDs are often related to small maxillary lateral incisors, creating space around the maxillary lateral incisors may be a logical approach. A simple technique involves placement of coil springs between the cuspids and the lateral incisors and, if needed, between the lateral incisors and the central incisors to open spaces (Figure 55-19). At the end of treatment, the lateral incisors can be built up by bonding, veneers, or crowns. This technique can also be used in the mandibular arch when the mandibular anterior teeth are too small compared with the maxillary anterior teeth. In either arch, this technique is most applicable when the teeth are decreased in inclination, because opening space will increase the axial inclination of

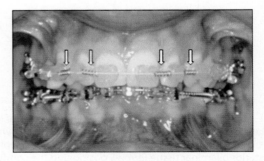

FIGURE 55-19. Orthodontic coil springs between teeth can create spaces around the lateral incisors to correct tooth size discrepancies. Post-treatment, the lateral incisors can be built up by bonding, veneers, or crowns.

the incisors. It may not be indicated when the maxillary or mandibular incisors are increased in inclination or crowded, because the resultant increased inclination may be unstable and cause untoward periodontal changes. However, if there is significant crowding or increased inclination of the incisors requiring extraction of bicuspids, during closure of the bicuspid spacing by retraction of the anterior teeth, space could be created around the lateral incisors.

When maxillary incisors are already increased in inclination, it is not feasible to open spaces during the presurgical orthodontics. In this situation, performing interdental osteotomies between the maxillary cuspids and the lateral incisors will permit opening space at surgery and the incisors can also be uprighted to decrease their axial inclination. A maximum 3 mm of spacing (1.5 mm on each side) can usually be acquired with this approach.

When the TSD occurs in the bicuspid or molar area, space can be opened around the maxillary bicuspids and/or molars to compensate for the tooth mass deficiency. Bonding, veneers, or crowns can then be placed to eliminate the created space.

Altering Axial Inclination of Incisors

This technique can affect the labial circumference of the anterior teeth. Increased axial inclination slightly increases the arch length, and decreased axial inclination slightly decreases it. Application of this technique would result in increasing the maxillary incisors' inclination above normal and decreasing the mandibular incisors' inclination below normal. This technique can accommodate small TSD differences but may place the teeth in a compromised position relative to stability and aesthetics.

Surgery can alter the axial inclination of the anterior teeth. In the maxillary arch, interdental osteotomies between the lateral incisors and the cuspids, and in the mandibular arch anterior subapical osteotomies, will provide a means to alter and control axial inclination of the incisors.

Altering Mesiodistal Angulation of Maxillary Incisors

Tipping the roots of the maxillary central incisors distally away from each other alters the position of the contact points, making the intercontact distance on each tooth slightly wider.

This can be used only for small differences. However, it then usually requires recontouring of the distal aspect of the incisor edges and could cause a soft tissue void between the mesial contact points and the gingival tissues ("the black triangle"), creating an aesthetic concern for the patient. This technique is rarely recommended.

Extraction of Mandibular Incisors

This technique should be used only for large TSDs (5 mm) and only if there is significant crowding and/or significant increased inclination of the mandibular incisors. Removing a mandibular incisor usually creates a significant space (the width of the tooth), and closure of that space may significantly decrease the axial inclination of the mandibular incisors. In addition, it may cause a decreased transverse width between the cuspids, resulting in relative narrowing of both maxillary and mandibular arches, affecting the dental aesthetics. Extraction of a mandibular incisor may produce an increased overjet. If the patient has a good maxillary arch but mandibular crowding and increased incisor inclination, large TSD, and an end-on or slight class III anterior occlusion, the single mandibular incisor extraction may be the treatment of choice. An alternative in cases with large TSDs would be to slenderize the mandibular anterior teeth and create spacing around the maxillary lateral incisors.

A surgical alternative for a large TSD, when the teeth are not crowded and have good axial inclination, would be to extract the mandibular incisor and perform a vertical ostectomy through the mandible at the extraction site and rotate the segments together to eliminate the extraction space (Figure 55-20). This would prevent further decreased inclination of the incisors with subsequent orthodontics but will narrow the transverse dimension of the anterior mandibular dental arch.

Correction of Maxillary Anterior Crowding or Increased Inclination

Increased inclination and/or crowding of maxillary anterior teeth are most commonly seen in patients with maxillary deficiency (hypoplasia). The following treatment methods can be used to correct this type of situation:

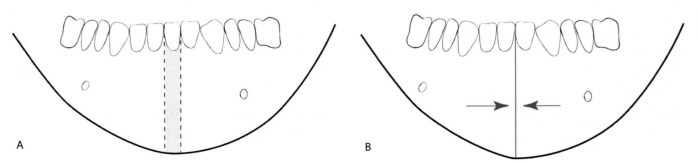

A   B

FIGURE 55-20.   With a TSD of 5 mm or greater, in the presence of well-aligned teeth in proper inclination, the TSD can be managed by removing a mandibular central incisor and performing a vertical midline ostectomy **(A)** with space closure **(B)** and stabilization with a bone plate and screws.

IPR and Incisor Retraction

This technique involves removal of tooth structure at the contact points and is applicable when there is a rare reverse TSD with the maxillary anterior teeth too large for the mandibular anterior teeth. Usually, up to 3 mm of tooth structure can be safely removed from the contact area of the maxillary anterior six teeth with a margin of 50% of enamel remaining at the contact areas. However, this could make the maxillary incisors slightly smaller in size unless they are significantly oversized in the first place.

Extraction and Incisor Retraction

First or second bicuspids can be extracted depending on the amount of crowding, the anchorage requirements, and the amount of retraction of the incisors necessary. Every 1 mm of incisor retraction will require 1 mm of space on each side of the arch. Therefore, if the orthodontic goal is to retract the maxillary incisors by 3 mm, 6 mm of maxillary arch space will be required to accomplish this. Extracting first bicuspids will result in greater incisor retraction, because six multi-rooted posterior dental units (compared with six single-rooted anterior dental units) provide greater posterior anchorage. Extracting second bicuspids will result in less incisor retraction, because four posterior dental units (compared with eight anterior units) provide less posterior anchorage so that the posterior teeth will move forward a greater amount compared with first bicuspid extractions. The occlusal plane angle will also affect the posterior anchorage. Low–occlusal plane angle cases will have greater posterior anchorage stability, even with second bicuspid extraction, than will high–occlusal plane angle cases. High–occlusal plane angle cases will have less posterior anchorage stability, even with first bicuspid extraction, than low–occlusal plane angle cases. These factors are probably related to bite force influences. The amount of crowding may also influence which teeth to extract.

Distalization of Posterior Teeth

This objective can be accomplished using pendulum-type appliances, headgear, class II mechanics, osseointegrated dental implants, or TADs (i.e., implants posterior to molars, zygomatic implants, palatal implants, or buccal or lingual cortex implants). Distalizing maxillary posterior teeth can be augmented with class II mechanics but should be used only short term and discontinued several months before surgery to minimize postsurgical skeletal relapse potential that can occur with the use of long-term class II mechanics and the subsequent adverse effects on the TMJs. Another option is to distalize one tooth at a time on each side of the arch, beginning with the second molars (2 teeth moved against 12 anchor teeth). Another feasible approach is to use osseointegrated dental implants or TADs to distalize the maxillary arch, with implants either placed in the zygoma buttress, posterior to the second molars, or attached to the buccal cortex.

Anterior Maxillary Segmental Osteotomies

This technique permits uprighting of the anterior teeth but will cause the apical base of the segment to shift forward

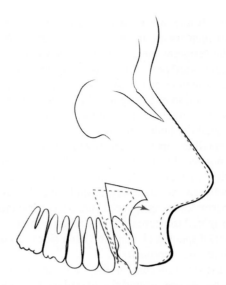

FIGURE 55-21.   An anterior maxillary segmental osteotomy can be used to upright maxillary incisors, but the dentoalveolar base will rotate anteriorly if no teeth are extracted. Because this will affect the position of the nose and upper lip, careful evaluation of facial aesthetics is necessary to determine whether this approach is appropriate. *Dashed line* represents the original position of the anterior maxilla, and the *solid line* represents the uprighted segment and associated soft tissue changes.

relative to the incisor edges unless teeth are extracted to reposition the incisal edges of the anterior teeth posteriorly. Careful assessment of the profile aesthetics is necessary to determine whether the patient can aesthetically benefit from this change. The interdental osteotomies should be done between the lateral incisors and the cuspids because this offers the best control in uprighting the segments (Figure 55-21), vertically leveling the segments, and correcting arch asymmetry and also allows opening of space between the lateral incisors and the cuspids (≤3 mm with 1.5 mm/side) that can be used for correction of crowding or TSD.

Maxillary Expansion by Orthodontics, Orthopedic Palatal Expansion, and SARPE

These techniques will increase arch length and may allow retraction of the anterior teeth. However, they will also increase the curve of Wilson because the transverse width of the maxillary arch increases because the crowns of the posterior teeth will expand three times as much as the palate expands (Figure 55-22). In addition, with SARPE, the palate moves inferiorly The expanded arches may not be as orthodontically stable, requiring long-term or permanent retention.

Correction of Mandibular Anterior Crowding or Increased Inclination

Increased inclination and/or crowding of mandibular teeth occurs most often with mandibular deficiency (hypoplasia). The following treatment options can be used to correct these types of conditions.

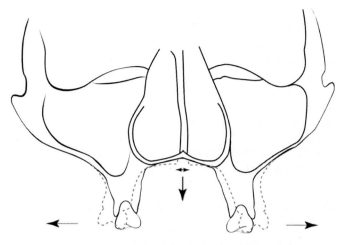

FIGURE 55-22. Maxillary expansion by orthodontics, orthopedics, or surgically assisted rapid palatal expansion (SARPE) will cause an increase of the curve of Wilson. Even with SARPE, the occlusal surface will expand three times as much as the palate expands, thus increasing the curve of Wilson. The palate also moves inferiorly.

IPR and Incisor Retraction

This technique involves removal of tooth structure at the contact points and is most applicable when there is a TSD with the mandibular anterior teeth being too large for the maxillary anterior teeth. Up to 3 mm of tooth structure can be safely removed from the contact areas of the mandibular anterior six teeth with a margin of 50% of enamel remaining at the contact areas. Subsequent retraction will decrease the axial inclination of the incisors providing that no major crowding is present.

Extraction and Retraction

First or second bicuspids can be extracted depending on the degree of incisor inclination, the amount of crowding, the anchorage requirements, and the amount of retraction of the incisors necessary. Every 1 mm of incisor retraction will require 1 mm of space on each side of the arch. Therefore, if the orthodontic goal is to retract the mandibular incisors by 3 mm, 6 mm of mandibular arch space will be required to accomplish this. Extracting first bicuspids will result in greater incisor retraction, because six multirooted posterior dental units (compared with six single-rooted anterior dental units) provide greater posterior anchorage. Extracting the second bicuspids will result in less incisor retraction, because four posterior dental units (compared with eight anterior units) provide less posterior anchorage, so that the posterior teeth will move forward a greater amount compared with first bicuspid extractions. The occlusal plane angle will also affect the posterior anchorage. Low–occlusal plane angle cases will have greater posterior anchorage stability, even with second bicuspid extraction, than will high–occlusal plane angle cases. High–occlusal plane angle cases will have less posterior anchorage stability even with first bicuspid extraction than low-angle cases. These factors are probably

related to bite force influences. The amount of crowding may also influence which teeth to extract. If there is a large TSD (>5 mm), extraction of a mandibular incisor could be considered.

Distalization of Posterior Teeth

The mechanics to accomplish this include intra-arch, inter-arch, extraoral, or implant mechanics. Class III mechanics (i.e., elastics, headgear) can be used to distalize the mandibular teeth but may increase loading on the TMJs and could initiate TMJ problems. Another option is to distalize one tooth at a time on each side of the arch, beginning with the second molars (2 teeth moved against 12 anchor teeth). However, this technique takes a lot of time. The placement of dental implants or TADs posterior to the molar teeth or in the posterior buccal cortex could facilitate retraction without appreciably increasing the load to the TMJs.

Anterior Mandibular Subapical Osteotomies

This technique permits uprighting of the anterior teeth but will cause the apical base of the segment to shift forward relative to the chin (Figure 55-23), unless teeth are extracted at the time of surgery to reposition the incisal edges of the anterior teeth posteriorly.

Bilateral Mandibular Body Osteotomies

This technique will permit uprighting of the anterior teeth and forward rotation of the chin (Figure 55-24), unless teeth are extracted. Without extraction, bilateral body bone grafting will be required to provide bony continuity between the segments and facilitate healing. This technique would be indicated only if the chin is anteroposteriorly deficient before surgery.

Mandibular Symphyseal Distraction Osteogenesis

This technique, usually performed with a midline vertical osteotomy, will allow expansion of the dentoalveolus and

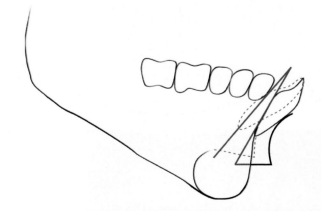

FIGURE 55-23. The anterior mandibular subapical osteotomy can be used to upright the mandibular anterior teeth, causing the apical base of the segment to shift forward relative to the chin, if teeth (bicuspids) are not extracted at the time of surgery. This may or may not be desirable. A chin augmentation may be required to achieve optimal aesthetics.

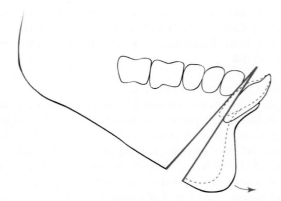

FIGURE 55-24. Bilateral body osteotomies can be used to upright mandibular anterior teeth, but the chin will rotate forward unless teeth are extracted. A gap created in the mandibular body area will require bone grafting unless teeth are extracted (first bicuspids) to allow the mandibular anterior teeth to move posteriorly, thus decreasing the forward movement of the chin.

widening of the mandibular arch, providing room to retract and/or align the teeth. This is an excellent treatment method to gain space for major arch length discrepancies. However, it is done as a prerequisite surgery to achieve the orthodontic goals before the major orthognathic surgery. Orthodontic preparation may be necessary before performing the midline vertical osteotomy. The roots of the central incisors (or the adjacent teeth, wherever the osteotomy is to be performed) must be tipped away from each other to make room for the interdental osteotomy. This can be accomplished by placing the mesial aspect of the bracket higher than the distal aspect on each of the central incisors. Placing a short segment straight arch wire will then tip the roots distally, creating

space to safely perform the vertical interdental osteotomy (Figure 55-25). If a toothborne distraction device is used, orthodontic treatment on any other teeth should *not* be initiated until adequate healing of the distraction area has occurred (~4 mo from initiation of the distraction). Otherwise, it may result in developing dental mobility and orthodontic instability, with the teeth expanding more than the basal bone. This can result in transverse dental relapse postdistraction with less expansion of the dental arch than desired. Bone-borne devices are not affected by predistraction orthodontics.

Correct Decreased Inclination of Maxillary Incisors

Decreased inclination of maxillary incisors is most commonly seen in class II division 2 malocclusions or with missing teeth in the arch. The following approaches can be used to correct this type of condition.

Correct Crowding
Crowding of the maxillary anterior teeth can accompany vertically inclined teeth. Therefore, correcting the crowding will increase the incisor inclination.

Open Space
In class I and class II patients, decreased inclination of the incisors may be present because of previous extractions (i.e., bicuspids), congenitally missing teeth, previous trauma resulting in loss of teeth, or small maxillary anterior teeth (i.e., small maxillary lateral incisors). Opening space in the bicuspid areas, if the problem exists because of previous extractions, can correct this problem and provide additional

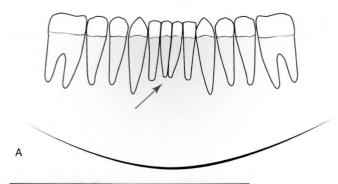

A

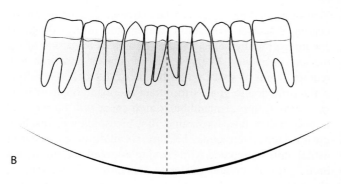

B

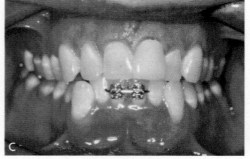

C

FIGURE 55-25. Mandibular symphysis distraction osteogenesis. **A,** Often, the incisor roots are very close together. **B,** Space must be created between the roots of teeth adjacent to the intended midline vertical osteotomy. **C,** Placing brackets on only the central incisors with the mesial aspect of the brackets higher than the distal aspect on each tooth and placing a short straight wire segment will tip the roots distally away from each other, creating space to perform the vertical interdental osteotomy.

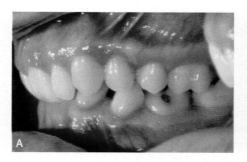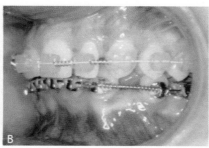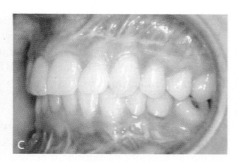

FIGURE 55-26. Coil springs to create arch space. Retroclined incisors may result from a division 2 malocclusion, crowding, missing dental units, or small teeth. Space can be created using coil springs that tip the incisors forward. **A,** Small maxillary laterals and missing mandibular bicuspids. **B,** Coiled springs create interdental spaces around the maxillary laterals (to correct an anterior TSD) and in the mandibular first bicuspid area (to replace a missing tooth and increase inclination of anterior teeth). **C,** The spaces around the maxillary lateral can be eliminated by bonding, veneer, or crown. In the mandibular arch, the space can be eliminated by surgical ostectomy, or replacement of the missing tooth with a bridge or dental implant.

dental units for a more complete occlusal result. The use of coil springs usually works well for this situation. If the problem is in the lateral incisor area, opening space can help correct the TSD as well as increase the incisor inclination (Figure 55-26).

Interarch Mechanics

The use of class III mechanics (i.e., elastics) can increase maxillary incisor inclination. However, the class III mechanics can be detrimental by overloading the TMJs.

Interdental Osteotomies

An anterior maxillary subapical osteotomy or segmentalized Le Fort I osteotomy will permit rotation of the anterior teeth to increase their inclination. However, significant room must be created between the roots of the adjacent teeth (lateral incisors and cuspids) at the osteotomy areas. Because bone removal between the teeth may be required, there is an increased risk of damage to the adjacent teeth. If the maxilla requires surgical expansion, segmentalization between the lateral incisors and the cuspids will allow the anterior segment to rotate posteriorly between the expanded posterior segments with fewer requirements for bone removal, if required at all.

Correct Decreased Inclination of Mandibular Incisors

Decreased inclination of mandibular incisors is more commonly seen in patients with a prognathic mandible or with missing teeth. The following treatment methods can be used to correct this condition.

Correction of Crowding

Crowding of the mandibular anterior teeth often accompanies vertically inclined teeth. Therefore, correcting the crowding will increase the incisor inclination.

Creation of Arch Space

In class I and class II patients, decreased inclination of mandibular incisors may be present because of previous extrac-

tions, congenitally missing teeth, previous trauma resulting in loss of teeth, or small mandibular teeth. In class III patients, decreased inclination of incisors may be present owing to an excessive amount of alveolar bone compared with the size of the teeth. If bicuspids are missing, opening space in the bicuspid areas can correct this problem and provide additional dental units for a more complete occlusal result. The use of coil springs usually works well for this situation (see Figure 55-26).

Occasionally, a mandibular incisor may be missing for various reasons. Viable options include opening appropriate space around the remaining three incisors and building up the crowns by bonding, veneers, or crowns. This technique works best if there is a TSD that is less than the width of the missing tooth. However, the maxillary dental midline will be in the center of a mandibular incisor. Another option would be to open space in the area of the missing tooth and replace it with a dental implant or bridge. This technique may work best when there is no TSD with a full-size dental replacement.

Interarch Mechanics

The use of class II mechanics (i.e., elastics, Herbst appliance) can increase mandibular incisor inclination. However, long-term class II mechanics can be detrimental to outcome stability and results, because of the potential untoward effects on the TMJs.

Interdental Osteotomies

An anterior subapical osteotomy or bilateral anterior body osteotomies will permit rotation of the anterior teeth to increase their inclination. However, significant room must be created between the roots of the teeth adjacent to the osteotomy areas. Because bone removal between the teeth may be required, there is an increased risk of damage to the adjacent teeth.

Correction of Excessive Curve of Spee: Maxillary Arch

This condition is most often seen with anterior open bite situations and high–occlusal plane facial types. Careful assessment of the curve of Spee is important because using only orthodontic mechanics to correct this condition may not be very stable. An increased curve of Spee usually makes it difficult to get the occlusion to fit together. The condition can be addressed by the following treatment options.

Anterior Tooth Extrusion

Conventional orthodontics with straight wire techniques will tend to extrude the anterior teeth and, as a byproduct, will tip the molars buccally, increasing the curve of Wilson. These dental changes may be unstable and fraught with relapse potential.

Midbuccal Tooth Intrusion

This is a very difficult technique, unless high-pull headgear or osseointegrated implants or TADs are used to provide intrusive forces. Placing TADs palatally and bucally would provide the best force vector for the intrusion of these teeth.

Extraction and Retraction

Extraction of maxillary first or second bicuspids with retraction will usually decrease the curve of Spee, providing the incisors are increased in inclination in the first place.

Orthodontic, Orthopedic Palatal Expansion, or SARPE with Retraction

Expansion of the maxillary arch by any of these techniques will increase the arch length and allow some retraction of the anterior teeth. In late adolescence or adulthood, SARPE may provide better stability than the other two techniques. However, note that the curve of Wilson will increase because the expansion at the occlusal level compared with the palate will be a 3:1 ratio.[20]

Orthognathic Surgical Correction

The maxilla can be orthodontically aligned in segments by aligning the four incisors at a different level, compared with the posterior teeth, to avoid extrusion, intrusion, and buccal tipping of teeth. Placing compensating vertical steps between the lateral incisors and the cuspids (see Figure 55-15A) will accomplish alignment at different levels. For some cases, the vertical positional difference may occur between the cuspids and the bicuspids or could occur asymmetrically on one side of the arch compared with the other side. The step in the arch would then be made between the appropriate teeth. Another technique involves cutting the arch wire into two or more segments and aligning groups of teeth in individual units (see Figure 55-15B). However, it may be more difficult to control rotations and root position, particularly of the teeth adjacent to the ends of the segmented wires, compared with using a continuous wire with compensating vertical steps. The arch can then be leveled surgically with a three-piece maxilla performing osteotomies between the lateral incisors and the cuspids. If a segmental arch wire has been used, the cuspid crowns tend to tip palatally presurgery and may require surgical expansion of the cuspids to a greater extent than using a continuous arch wire with a vertical step. The three-piece Le Fort I osteotomy, with interdental osteotomies performed between the lateral incisors and the cuspids, will permit repositioning of the anterior segment independent of the posterior segments (Figure 55-27). The anterior segment can be reoriented vertically and anteroposteriorly, and the axial inclination of the incisors can be changed to correct the curve of Spee and achieve the best interdigitation of the segments.

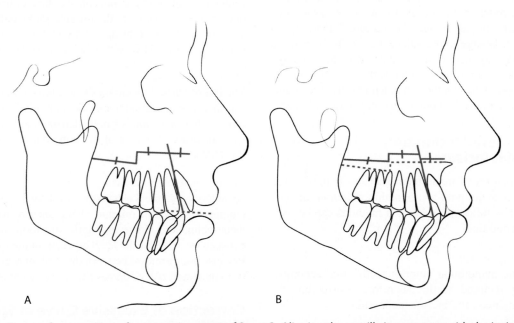

A   B

FIGURE 55-27.   Surgery for correction of an excessive curve of Spee. **A,** Aligning the maxilla in segments with the incisors at an elevated level compared with the posterior teeth will permit interdental osteotomies to be performed. **B,** Surgical leveling of the occlusal plane *(dotted line)* from a predictability and stability standpoint is superior to orthodontic means alone, particularly when no extractions are performed.

Correction of Excessive Curve of Spee: Mandibular Arch

An accentuated curve of Spee in the mandibular arch most often occurs in anterior deep-bite relationships. The condition can be addressed by the following treatment options.

Mandibular Anterior Tooth Intrusion

Intrusion mechanics can predictably inferiorly position mandibular anterior teeth approximately 2 mm. Beyond 2 mm, the vertical relapse approaches 60%. With accentuated curves of Spee, the contact area of the teeth will be at a different level in which the teeth are more narrow, below the normal contact level. Therefore, for every 1 mm of leveling of the mandibular arch, the mandibular incisor edges will move forward 0.6 mm to 1 mm as the contact points align. Any crowding of the arch will further contribute to flaring of the incisors. Intruding teeth will decrease the anterior mandibular vertical height and must also be taken into consideration so that the anterior mandibular height is not excessively shortened.

Midbuccal Tooth Extrusion

Extrusion of midbuccal teeth may be more stable than intrusion of anterior teeth. However, this technique is difficult to perform without special considerations. If the patient's malocclusion has the bicuspids and first molars in occlusion, extrusion will be virtually impossible. However, constructing a splint or using turbos that will open the bite and engage only the mandibular anterior teeth and second molars, with the bicuspids and first molars out of contact, will permit extrusion of the midbuccal teeth. Another alternative would be to correct the accentuated curve of Spee after the mandible and occlusion are surgically repositioned, placing the incisors and molars into proper contact, and then extrude the midbuccal teeth postsurgery. With this approach, the molars may tip distally and the arch may widen.

Interdental Osteotomies

An anterior subapical osteotomy (Figure 55-28) or bilateral anterior body osteotomies (Figure 55-29) will permit downward repositioning of the anterior teeth, with very stable

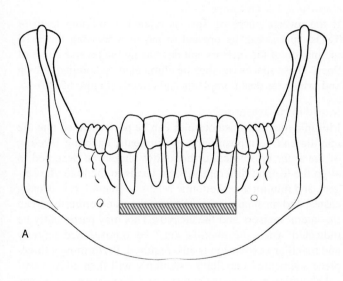

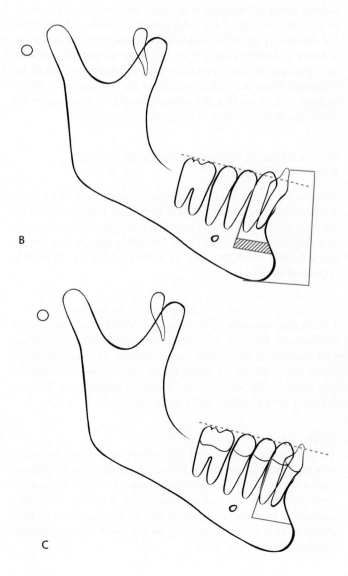

FIGURE 55-28. Subapical osteotomy correcting an accentuated mandibular curve of Spee. **A,** A subapical osteotomy, composed of two interdental osteotomies, with a subapical ostectomy to set the anterior teeth inferiorly. **B** and **C,** This is indicated when the anterior mandibular height is increased, because this will decrease anterior mandibular height. This technique, with grafting, can be used to elevate the anterior mandibular segment to correct a reverse curve of Spee.

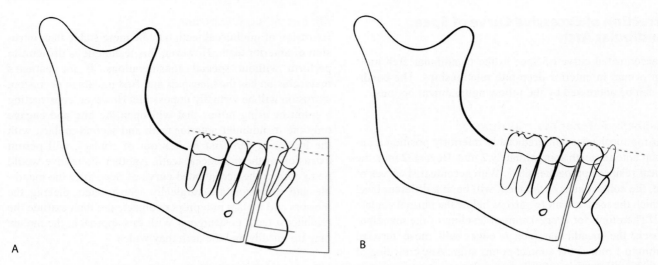

FIGURE 55-29. **A** and **B,** Bilateral mandibular body osteotomies will permit leveling of an excessive curve of Spee without shortening the vertical height of the mandible and are indicated when the mandibular anterior dental height is normal or slightly decreased vertically. This can also be used to correct a reverse curve of Spee by elevating the anterior segment.

results when the surgery is properly performed. If the anterior vertical height of the mandible is excessive, the subapical osteotomy would be indicated because it will shorten the anterior mandibular height by the amount that the incisors are lowered. Bilateral anterior body osteotomies would be indicated when the vertical height of the anterior mandible is normal or less, so that the anterior height remains unaltered while the curve of Spee is corrected (Figure 55-29).

Correction of Reverse Curve of Spee: Maxillary Arch

Reverse curves of Spee are more commonly seen in division 2 malocclusions and in vertical maxillary deficiencies with an anterior deep bite. The maxillary incisors are commonly in a decreased axial inclination. Crowding may or may not be present. The condition can be addressed by the following treatment options.

Correction of Crowding or Division 2 Relations
Eliminating crowding and division 2 dental positions will tip the incisors forward, increasing the incisor axial inclination and decreasing the reverse curve of Spee. These movements will usually fill out the upper lip but may decrease the maxillary tooth–to–lip relationship. Maxillary incisors may become intruded with a straight wire technique.

Midbuccal Tooth Extrusion
This technique is difficult if the midbuccal teeth are in occlusion with mandibular teeth. However, the bite can be opened with a splint or turbos that affords contact on only the maxillary second molars and anterior teeth, with the maxillary midbuccal teeth out of contact. The midbuccal teeth (bicuspids and first molars) can then be extruded into position to improve the curve of Spee.

Creation of Arch Space
If the reverse curve of Spee is related to missing teeth or TSDs, spaces can be opened to aid in increasing the axial inclination of the incisors and decreasing the reverse curve of Spee. These spaces can then be eliminated by bonding, crown and bridge, or dental implants and crowns (Figure 55-26).

Interdental Osteotomies
Multiple maxillary osteotomies can be performed so that the maxilla can be repositioned in segments, enabling leveling of the arch. Presurgical orthodontics should be designed to align the teeth at different vertical levels to facilitate the surgery and minimize orthodontic relapse potential. It is usually easiest and most applicable to make the osteotomies between the lateral incisors and the cuspids. This may particularly be indicated when the maxilla must be repositioned anyway and maxillary expansion is also required. Performing a three-piece segmented maxillary osteotomy will then allow vertical alteration between the anterior and the posterior segments to level the curve of Spee.

Correction of Reverse Curve of Spee: Mandibular Arch

This condition is most commonly seen in patients with macroglossia, habitual tongue posturing, or tongue thrust, with an associated anterior open bite. The following techniques can be used to correct this type of condition.

Anterior Tooth Extrusion
Extrusion of anterior teeth may not be very stable long term and, without permanent retention, could result in re-intrusion and redevelopment of an anterior open bite.

Midbuccal Tooth Intrusion
This technique may be accomplished with osseointegrated implants or TADs placed as anchors in the buccal and lingual

cortical bone of the dentoalveolus. However, no studies support the stability long term.

Extraction and Retraction

If the mandibular incisors are significantly increased in inclination, with or without crowding, bicuspid extractions can be performed and the incisors retracted, which will decrease the reverse curve of Spee.

Bonding the Mandibular Anterior Teeth

This technique can be used to level the arch by building up the incisors, increasing the crown height. However, care must be taken not to exceed a safe crown-root ratio and/or create an aesthetic compromise.

Interdental Osteotomies

Anterior subapical (see Figure 55-28) or anterior bilateral mandibular body osteotomies (see Figure 55-29) can be used to elevate the anterior teeth. If the anterior mandibular height is short, the subapical osteotomy can also be used to increase the anterior height of the mandible. If the anterior mandibular height is normal, the bilateral anterior body osteotomies will permit elevation of the anterior teeth while maintaining the anterior height of the mandible.

Anteroposterior Arch Asymmetry (Maxilla or Mandible)

Anteroposterior arch asymmetry, when the cuspid on one side of the arch is anterior to the cuspid on the opposite side of the arch, is fairly common in patients with dentofacial deformities. Arch asymmetries can be related to developmental abnormalities, missing teeth, or ankylosed teeth. Dental midlines may not align with the facial midline. The condition can be addressed by the following treatment options.

Unilateral Extractions

In some cases, unilateral extraction and retraction will correct the problem. The decision must be made as to which tooth to extract. Extraction of a first bicuspid will allow greater anterior retraction compared with extracting a second bicuspid. This extraction would be indicated only if there were significant increased inclination of the incisors, crowding, and/or significant midline dental shift.

Unilateral Creation of Arch Space

This technique would be indicated if a tooth is missing, there is significant decreased inclination of the incisors, and/or the midline is significantly deviated to one side.

Interarch Mechanics

This technique can be effectively used by incorporating class II mechanics on one side and class III mechanics on the opposite side. Anterior cross-arch elastics can also be helpful. If only one arch is involved, maximizing anchorage in the other arch is very important so that an asymmetry does not develop in the normal arch. Osseointegrated implants or TADs can be used as anchors to correct asymmetry in an arch without having to use interarch mechanics.

Segmental Osteotomies

Osteotomies can be used in the maxillary arch by segmentalization of the maxilla and advancing one side more than the other side. Osteotomies in the mandibular arch to correct arch asymmetry can become somewhat complex. Anterior subapical osteotomies with removal of a unilateral tooth can correct some large discrepancies (6–9 mm). However, the subapical osteotomy may need to be combined with ramus sagittal split osteotomies and a unilateral or bilateral body osteotomy, with or without extraction, to shift the occlusion into a symmetrical position. These types of movements require a high degree of surgical skill, but can provide high-quality outcomes.

Divergence of Roots Adjacent to Interdental Osteotomy Sites

When interdental osteotomies are planned, it may be necessary for the orthodontist to tip the adjacent tooth roots away from the area of the planned osteotomy to prevent damage to the teeth (Figure 55-30). If the roots are too close together, postsurgical periodontal problems may develop with possible loss of interdental bone and teeth. Creating interdental space between the roots significantly improves the margin of safety. This can be easily achieved by selective bracket placement. For the tooth mesial to the osteotomy, the bracket is slightly rotated so that the mesial aspect of the bracket is positioned slightly more gingivally than the distal aspect of the bracket (Figure 55-31). Conversely, the distal tooth bracket is positioned so that the distal aspect of the bracket is placed slightly more gingivally than the mesial aspect of the bracket. With a straight wire technique, the roots will diverge.

Postsurgically, periapical radiography may be necessary for the orthodontist to check for rebonding the adjacent teeth brackets to ensure proper root angulation at completion of treatment.

Extraction versus Nonextraction Orthodontic and Surgical Treatment

The decision to extract or not to extract can sometimes be difficult. A number of factors may contribute to this determination:

Increased Inclination Anterior Teeth

Increased inclination anterior teeth may require extraction to set the teeth over basal bone. However, if the arch is to be expanded or teeth slenderized with IPR for treatment of a TSD, for example, extraction may not be necessary.

Crowding

This is a common indicator, particularly with major crowding or increased inclination of the incisor teeth. However, if

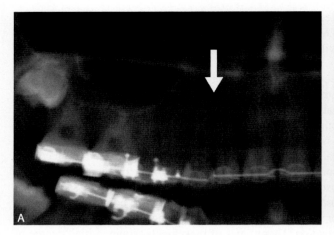
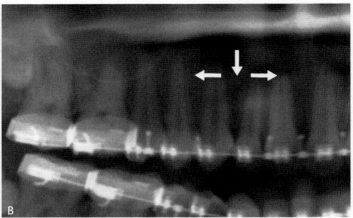

FIGURE 55-30. Interdental osteotomies. **A,** Panorex demonstrates inadequate room between the roots of the lateral incisors and the cuspids, and performing osteotomies with roots in this position may cause periodontal problems and loss of teeth. **B,** Adequate spaces for interdental osteotomies can be created by selective bracket placement on adjacent teeth.

crowding is mild to moderate, widening of the arch or teeth slenderizing for TSD may eliminate the need for extraction.

Tooth-Size Discrepancy

TSDs of significant magnitude may indicate the need for extraction, particularly if the TSD of the anterior mandibular teeth is 5 mm or greater and the mandibular incisors are increased in inclination and/or crowded, in which case a mandibular incisor extraction could be considered.

Curve of Spee

Accentuated curves of Spee in the maxillary arch usually have overangulated maxillary incisors, and reverse curves of Spee in the mandibular arch usually have increased inclination of mandibular incisors. Extraction of bilateral first or second bicuspids and retraction will result in leveling of the

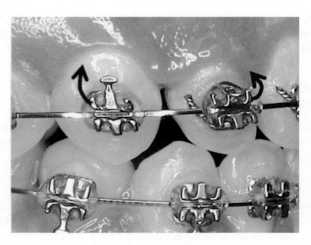

FIGURE 55-31. Selective bracket placement can create adequate interdental space for osteotomies. On the tooth mesial to the osteotomy, the mesial aspect of the bracket is rotated slightly gingival, and on the distal tooth, the distal aspect of the bracket is rotated slightly gingival, and a straight wire will then cause root divergence.

arches. However, arch expansion, when indicated, may create enough room so that extractions are not necessary.

Arch Asymmetries

With significant anteroposterior arch asymmetries, unilateral or bilateral asymmetrical extractions (i.e., first bicuspid on one side and a second bicuspid on the opposite side) may be indicated when there is coexisting crowding, increased inclination of incisors, or midline shift.

Arch Width Coordination of Maxilla and Mandible

In some cases. transverse arch width discrepancies can be corrected with stable and predictable orthodontic movements, but in other cases. orthodontic correction may be very unstable and fraught with relapse. It must be determined whether to correct width problems by orthodontics, orthopedics, SARPE, or surgical expansion. Even with SARPE using a fixed device, the palate expands only approximately one-third the amount of the expansion that occurs at the occlusal level, thus increasing the curve of Wilson.[20] For example, if the maxilla is expanded with SARPE and the expansion at the occlusal level is 6 mm, the expansion at the palatal level will only be 2 mm (see Figure 55-22). Patients with reverse curves of Wilson in the maxillary arch may benefit more from these techniques, but those with a pretreatment accentuated curve of Wilson may have unfavorable results, with subsequent difficulty getting the buccal cusps to interdigitate. The following predictable changes will occur with maxillary arch expansion by orthodontic, orthopedic, or SARPE procedures.

1. The bite may open anteriorly, particularly if the maxillary incisors have significant initial vertical inclination. If the maxillary incisors are overangulated, the bite may deepen anteriorly as the spacing is closed.

2. Buccal tipping of the maxillary posterior teeth will increase the curve of Wilson, because the lingual cusps will move downward relative to the buccal cusps. This may make it very difficult to properly interdigitate the buccal cusps orthodontically. Therefore, these techniques are not recommended, especially when there is a preexisting accentuated curve of Wilson.

3. Long-term or perhaps permanent retention may be necessary to counterbalance the orthodontic relapse potential seen in a high percentage of these patients.

4. In late adolescent and adult patients, SARPE will likely be necessary to expand the maxilla orthopedically because the midpalatal suture is usually closed.

Surgical expansion of the maxilla at the time of the Le Fort I procedure using multiple segmentation of the maxilla, stabilization with bone plates and palatal or occlusal splints, and autogenous bone or hydroxyapatite synthetic bone grafting along the lateral maxillary walls can provide a good outcome. This technique when properly performed is very stable and eliminates the orthodontic relapse potential inherent with the other techniques.

Missing Teeth

Teeth can be missing from the arches for a number of reasons such as congenital absence, uneruption, previous orthodontic extractions, extractions for periodontal or dental pathology, and trauma. In some cases (i.e., congenital absence of maxillary lateral incisors, previous inappropriate bicuspid extraction), opening space to accommodate replacement teeth may be indicated. This is most applicable when the incisors are decreased in inclination without appreciable crowding. If the incisors are already increased in inclination and/or crowding is present, opening space orthodontically may be detrimental to stability and periodontal health. In this situation with missing maxillary lateral incisors, the cuspids can be used as lateral incisors but may require considerable recontouring to aesthetically and functionally conform to lateral incisor morphology. Although this cuspid substitution can work well for missing lateral incisors, it is done less frequently now that dental implants are so predictable and successful, thereby allowing the canine to be placed in its normal and more functional position.

When conditions permit, opening space for replacement teeth can be accomplished by appropriate mechanics to achieve the required space. Surgery can also be used to create spacing in some areas. In the mandibular arch, distraction osteogenesis can be used to create space. The missing teeth can then be replaced with dental implants, bridges, or partial dentures, for example.

Correction of Tooth Rotations

Bracket placement and arch wire adaptation are the primary keys to correcting rotated teeth, and it is usually best to achieve these corrections presurgery. However, if the malrotations do not interfere with the establishment of the desired dentoskeletal relationship, the rotations can be corrected postsurgery. Severe rotations may require supracrestal fiberotomy to prevent relapse and improve permanent retention. This can often be done at the time of orthognathic surgery.

Management of Short Roots

The two most common causes of short roots are developmental or root resorption. There are a numbers of reasons for root resorption including (1) orthodontic tooth movement with high forces; (2) presence of multinucleated odontoclasts possibly stimulated by transforming growth factor-Beta, cytokins, and interleukins; (3) systemic factors such as nutritional abnormalities, metabolic bone disease, age, and use of drugs; (4) systemic or innate predisposition including genetics; (5) impairment of alveolar bone resorption; (6) endocrine disturbances such as hyperphosphotemia, Papillon-Lefreve syndrome, Paget's disease, hyperparathyroidism, hypophosphatasia, Gaucher's disease, Turner's syndrome, or anachoresis; (7) inflammation of collagen in the periodontal ligaments; and (8) idiopathic root resorption. When these conditions are present pretreatment, orthodontic mechanics must be designed to place minimal forces on the teeth and minimize tooth movement with no extrusion, intrusion, or bodily repositioning because these forces may increase root resorption. Surgical management may require segmentation of the maxilla and/or mandible so that sections of the maxillary and mandibular alveolar bone and teeth can be moved independently to achieve a good dental interrelationship, minimizing pre- and postsurgical orthodontic forces. The interdental osteotomies, when performed properly, should have no adverse affect on root resorption.

Management of Ankylosed Teeth

Treatment of ankylosed teeth depends on (1) whether the tooth is primary or permanent, (2) the surrounding dentition, (3) the eruption status, (4) tooth position and orientation, (5) the time of onset and diagnosis, (6) the age of the patient, and (7) the treatment goals. Some of the considerations are discussed in the following sections.

Ankylosed Primary Tooth

This can impede the development and eruption of the permanent successor. If a primary tooth has a permanent successor, treatment is immediate extraction followed by space maintenance until the permanent tooth erupts. If no permanent successor is present and the primary tooth ankylosis occurs at an early stage in jaw growth and development with submergence of the tooth eminent, treatment includes extraction and space maintenance.[21] If the ankylosis occurs late with no permanent successor, the occlusal and proximal contacts can be reestablished with restorative dentistry to provide aesthetics and function with perhaps many years of service.[22]

It is important to diagnose and treat the ankylosed tooth before the adolescent growth phase. Retaining an ankylosed tooth during jaw growth leads to arrested development of the alveolar ridge. The severity of alveolar growth loss depends on the amount of facial growth left at the time that the ankylosis occurs. Timing the removal of an ankylosed tooth just at the start of the pubertal phase of adolescent growth may achieve the treatment objective of maintaining alveolar ridge height while allowing the tooth to remain long enough to act as a space maintainer and aesthetic temporary.[23]

Ankylosed Permanent Tooth

An unrecognized ankylosed permanent tooth tied into the arch wire can result in a significant malocclusion (Figure 55-32). There are several ways of treating the permanent ankylosed tooth. If ankylosis of the permanent tooth has an early onset during eruption, the tooth should be luxated, allowing for further eruption.[2] If repeated luxation proves ineffective, the tooth should be extracted to prevent submergence. If the onset of ankylosis occurs late in the normal eruption pattern, the tooth should be luxated. If the attempt is unsuccessful and the tooth does not submerge, it may be vertically restored on growth maturity. A composite buildup or crown can be added to a partially erupted ankylosed tooth to level and align the arch.[22] A deeply unerupted ankylosed tooth, primary or permanent, may be left undisturbed unless it is infected, alters the alveolar bone growth potential, constitutes an immediate threat to the occlusion or adjacent teeth, or would impede the placement of an osseointegrated implant.[3]

Other treatment options include extraction followed by reimplantation, osseointegrated implant, or prosthetic replacement.[24] The patient's developmental age is very important in considering replacing an ankylosed tooth with an osseointegrated implant. The implant will have the same effect on growth of the alveolar ridge as the ankylosed tooth and, therefore, should be considered for placement after alveolar growth is essentially complete.[25]

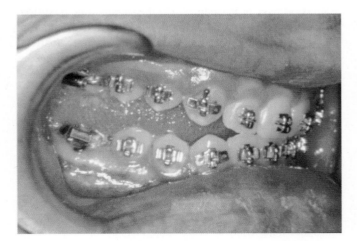

FIGURE 55-32. An ankylosed first molar tied into the arch wire has prevented alveolar development and created a posterior open bite.

Proffit[21] suggests surgical luxation of the tooth with extraction forceps disrupting the cementum-bone fusion followed by immediate orthodontic traction to move the tooth into position. Luxation involves breaking the bony bridge of ankylosis without damaging the apical nutrient vessels. This procedure forms fibrous inflammation tissue in the reparative process. This tissue forms a false periodontal membrane, and tooth eruption may resume. Orthodontic movement should begin immediately. Complications include possible crown, root, and alveolar fractures, loss of viability and vitality, as well as reankylosis. When an ankylosed tooth is impacted, a similar technique can bring an impacted tooth (usually canines) into the arch. Exposure involves surgical uncovering, application of orthodontic bonding, and tension forces applied to direct the tooth into occlusion. However, if the tooth becomes reankylosed, the orthodontic forces will intrude adjacent teeth.

Orthodontics for Surgical Management of Ankylosed Teeth

Presurgical orthodontics may be indicated to create adequate space (minimum of 2–3 mm) between the roots of the adjacent teeth to safely accommodate interdental osteotomies around the ankylosed tooth. Spacing is best assessed with cone beam or periapical radiographs. The ankylosed tooth is left out of the arch wire, and all other teeth are properly aligned. If orthognathic surgery is required to correct a dentofacial deformity, the orthodontics are performed in the traditional manner, but the ankylosed tooth must remain out of the arch wire, unless it aligns well with one of the dental segments. After surgery, orthodontic mechanics can be initiated immediately to help get the mobilized dental segment with the ankylosed tooth into the best possible position.

Segmental Osteotomies

Performing single-tooth osteotomies or sectional arch osteotomies with mobilization of the segment will permit immediate repositioning of the ankylosed tooth (Figure 55-33), or facilitate repositioning by distraction osteogenesis (DO).

In select cases in which an ankylosed primary molar is present, without a successor, a treatment option is to remove the ankylosed tooth and eliminate the extraction space by performing a vertical body ostectomy in conjunction with a mandibular ramus osteotomy and advance the posterior teeth and mandibular body forward (Figure 55-34). This eliminates the need for osseointegrated implants and extensive dental reconstruction.

Final Presurgical Orthodontic Preparation

As presurgical orthodontic treatment progresses, new diagnostic records (lateral cephalograms, pantomograms, dental models) are taken to determine the feasibility and timing of surgical procedures. This will also aid the orthodontist in identifying specific areas that may need to be addressed in completing the presurgical orthodontic goals (i.e., sectional leveling of the arch segments, marginal ridge alignment,

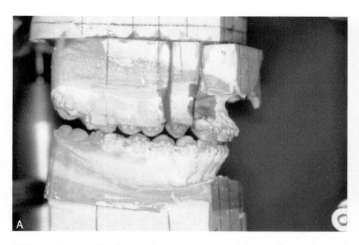
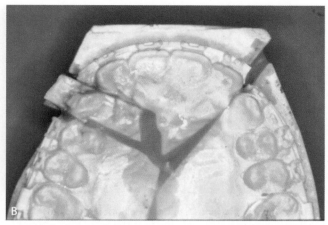

FIGURE 55-33. Single-tooth osteotomies can be performed as isolated cases or in combination with multiple maxillary osteotomies to allow individual movement of the dental osseous segments or application of immediate distraction osteogenesis (DO). **A** and **B,** This case had an ankylosed maxillary right cuspid (Figure 55-8) treated with segmental maxillary osteotomies including a single tooth segment containing the right cuspid.

vertical dental alignment, buccal surface alignment, additional TSD correction).

During surgery, the jaws are usually wired together once or twice, as each jaw is independently mobilized and stabilized with rigid fixation. To facilitate wiring the jaws together as well as provide a means of using postsurgical elastics if required, fixtures attached to the brackets or arch wires are usually necessary. Fixtures attached to the brackets are dependent on the manufacturer but may include ball hooks built onto the brackets, T pins, and K (Kobayashi) hooks (Figure 55-35). Fixtures attached to the arch wire include crimped-on hooks and soldered pins (Figure 55-36). Hooks built onto the brackets are preferred, followed by the other hooks placed on the brackets (T pins, K hooks). The least

preferred are the hooks on the arch wire. The reason is that if postsurgery elastics are required for an extended time, the elastics and hooks on the arch wire will activate the arch wire, possibly creating unwanted orthodontic forces and movements (i.e., tipping the crowns lingually and the roots buccally). This undesirable torquing occurs to a much lesser degree when the hooks are directly on the brackets.

When the maxilla or mandible are to be segmentalized, it may be better for the orthodontist to section the arch wire (see Figure 55-15B) and bend the ends inward at the predetermined osteotomy areas immediately before surgery, or the surgeon can cut the wire at surgery.

The best type of arch wire to place before surgery is a rectangular SSW that fills the bracket slot. For example, with

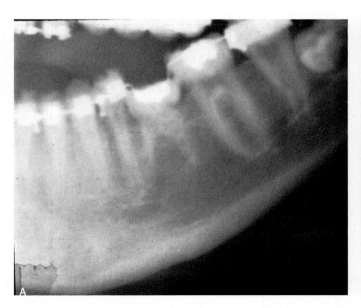
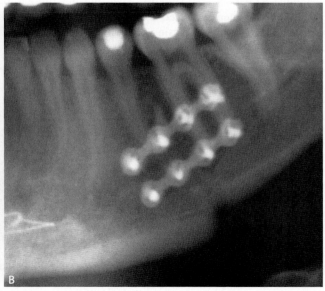

FIGURE 55-34. **A** and **B,** An ankylosed submerged primary tooth without a permanent successor can be treated with extraction of the primary tooth as well as a vertical body ostectomy with a mandibular ramus sagittal split osteotomy to advance the posterior teeth forward to eliminate the ankylosed tooth and space. This eliminates the need for an osseointegrated implant or a fixed prosthesis.

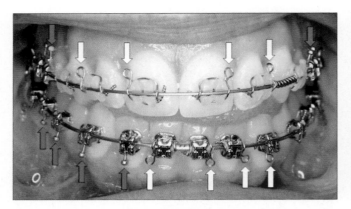

FIGURE 55-35. Orthodontic hooks. Ball hooks built onto the brackets *(blue arrows)* provide the best stability. Other options include T pins and K (Kobayashi) hooks *(white arrows)* or other methods to provide attachments directly on the brackets.

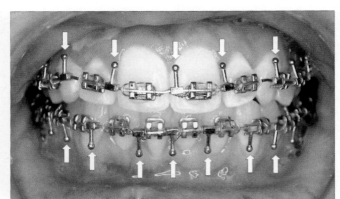

FIGURE 55-36. Soldered pins or crimped hooks *(white arrows)* onto the arch wire can also be used but are not preferred because the use of postsurgical elastics will activate the arch wire, possibly creating unwanted orthodontic movements.

an 18 slot, a 17 × 25-gauge wire is recommended, and for a 22 slot, a 21 × 25-gauge wire is indicated. This will help stabilize the individual dental units together as a whole arch or in segments when segmental surgery is required. The final wire should be placed 2 to 3 months before surgery.

POSTSURGICAL ORTHODONTIC TREATMENT

At the completion of surgery, a surgical stabilizing splint may be present and wired to the upper teeth and light elastics (3½ oz) are usually placed between the upper and the lower arches in the cuspid and molar areas and/or elsewhere, if indicated. If the occlusion is good, elastics may not be necessary if appropriate rigid fixation was used at surgery. Surgical stabilizing splints are indicated to provide the following: (1) stability in multiple segmental surgery of the maxilla or mandible, (2) transverse stability when the maxilla and/or mandible have been expanded or narrowed, (3) occlusal support when key teeth are missing (i.e., first, second, and third

molars are missing in a quadrant), and (4) a means to interdigitate the occlusion if teeth are severely worn or missing. There are two basic types of maxillary splints for orthognathic surgery; the *palatal splint* (Figure 55-37) and the *occlusal coverage splint* (Figure 55-38). If the maxilla and mandible are single pieces and the teeth can be appropriately interdigitated, a final splint is usually not necessary in single- or double-jaw surgery.

Palatal Splint

This horseshoe-shaped splint (see Figure 55-37) is preferred because (1) it provides excellent stability, (2) the occlusal interrelationship can be maximized and observed (the teeth and occlusal relationships are not covered and hidden by the splint), (3) it is easier to keep the teeth and splint clean, (4) orthodontic treatment can be performed with the splint in place, including arch wire changes (see Figure 55-37B), (5) it can be left in place for extended time (2–3 mo or longer

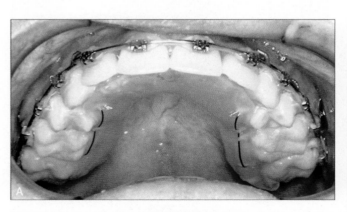

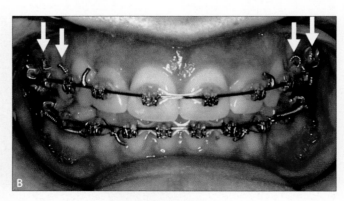

FIGURE 55-37. The horseshoe-shaped palatal splint is constructed to help stabilize the maxillary segments to enhance healing. **A,** The splint design does not cover the occlusal surfaces but fits snugly around the palatal aspect of the tooth crowns. The splint is stabilized to the maxilla with 28-gauge stainless steel wire (SSW) placed through the splint and circumferentially around the first molars and first bicuspids, or as in this case, the second bicuspids, because the first bicuspids are missing. **B,** The wires are twisted on the labial side of the teeth *(white arrows).* The splint design allows for maximal interocclusal fit at surgery as well as transverse and intersegmental stabilization. Orthodontic mechanics can be performed with the splint in position.

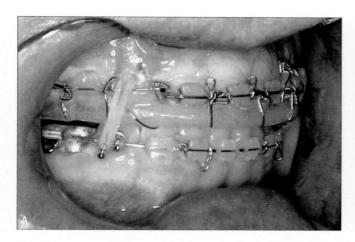
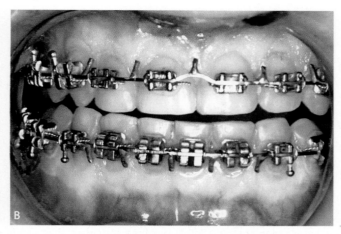

FIGURE 55-38.   **A,** The occlusal coverage splint fits between the occlusal surfaces of the maxillary and the mandibular teeth. It is usually stabilized to the maxillary arch with wires placed through the buccal flange of the splint and around the adjacent orthodontic brackets on the teeth. **B,** Upon removal of the splint, a malocclusion can occur (as in this case) as a result of a defect in the occlusal surfaces of the models, teeth not set fully into the splint, occlusal interferences, or a warped splint. This may require considerable orthodontic efforts to optimize the occlusion.

if necessary), and (6) after removal, the splint can be modified to function as a retention splint by adding clasps. When making the splint, the palatal tissues beneath the splint must have wax relief of approximately 1 to 2 mm on the dental model so the splint does not impinge on the soft tissues. If the splint is constructed to sit against the soft tissues, a major risk of vascular compromise to the maxilla could occur resulting in a potential disastrous outcome. The splint is stabilized to the maxilla with light, 28-gauge SSW placed through the splint and circumferentially around the first molars and first bicuspids (second bicuspids if the first bicuspids are missing) and wires twisted on the labial side of the teeth (see Figure 55-37). The anterior teeth are not tied into the splint because the anterior segment could become displaced because of the cingulum morphology that will displace the segment superiorly and posteriorly. At surgery, the anterior segment is stabilized with bone plates.[26]

Occlusal Coverage Splint

The occlusal coverage splint is the most common type of maxillary splint used and has the following advantages: (1) it is easy to construct, (2) it provides transverse stability, and (3) it can "lock-in" the occlusion perhaps better than the palatal splint (see Figure 55-38A). However, the occlusal coverage splint presents the following possible complicating factors: (1) the clinician cannot see the occlusal interrelationship of the teeth with the splint in place, (2) an occlusal interference caused by the splint could result in a malocclusion (see Figure 55-38B), (3) postsurgical orthodontics can be much more difficult, (4) the arch wire cannot be changed with the splint in place, (5) orthodontics cannot be performed with the splint in place, 6) oral hygiene is more difficult to maintain, and (7) it can cause discoloration, decalcification, and caries of the teeth where covered by the splint. The splint

is usually stabilized to the maxillary arch with wires placed through the buccal flange of the splint and around the adjacent orthodontic brackets on the teeth.

Mandibular Splint

Mandibular splints may be indicated for the following reasons: (1) they assist in stabilizing the mandible and segments after body osteotomies, subapical osteotomies, symphysis and sagittal split osteotomies, and other procedures, (2) they provide transverse stability if the mandible is expanded or narrowed by osteotomies or distraction osteogenesis, and (3) they temporarily replace missing teeth (Figure 55-39). Splints for providing transverse stability can be constructed to fit around the lingual aspect of the mandibular crowns, similar to the maxillary palatal splint. Therefore, these splints can be maintained in position for an extended time (2–3 mo or longer) if required. The splints can be secured to the mandibular arch by placing retention wires through the splint and circumferentially around the first molars and first bicuspids (second bicuspids if the first bicuspids are absent) (see Figure 55-39). Using this splint design, orthodontic arch wire changes and mechanics can progress with the splint remaining in place. Clasps can be placed on the splint after removal of the surgical retention wires so that the splint can be used as a removable retainer.

Splint Removal

This process requires cutting and removing the retention wires and then removing the splint. For most cases, the palatal or occlusal coverage splints can be removed at 1 month postsurgery. An exception is in maxillary expansions (>3–4 mm), in which the palatal splint can remain in position for 2 to 3 months or longer if required. After removal of the splint,

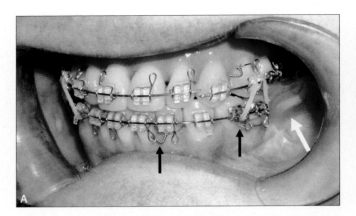
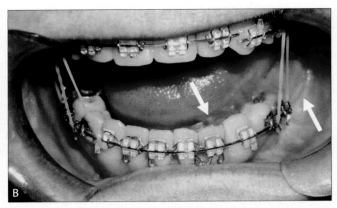

FIGURE 55-39. **A,** A mandibular splint *(white arrows)* can be constructed similar to the palatal splint design. It may be indicated to stabilize a segmented mandible, provide transverse stability, and temporarily replace missing teeth (as in this case). **B,** The splint can be stabilized to the mandibular teeth with wires placed through the splint and circumferentially around the adjacent teeth and twisted on the labial side *(black arrows).*

a transpalatal arch bar, removable palatal splint, or heavy labial arch wire followed by postorthodontic retainers can be used to maintain the maxillary expansions for an extended time period. The palatal splint can be modified to function as a removable splint by adding retention clasps. Maxillary or mandibular arches that have been expanded orthodontically, orthopedically, surgically assisted, or by osteotomies will require long-term transverse stabilization post-treatment to ensure a predictable outcome.[26]

Postsurgical Follow-up

The surgeon and/or orthodontist should see the patient on a weekly basis, or more often if indicated, for the first 1 to 2 months postsurgery to check the occlusion and patient progress and make any indicated changes in the elastic or orthodontic mechanics to maximize the occlusal interrelationship. If the occlusion fits properly, elastics may not be necessary. Then, as long as the occlusion remains stable, the time span between appointments can be increased. The surgeon and orthodontist must coordinate this postoperative patient management.

Patient Positioning at Follow-up

Patient position is important when evaluating postorthognathic surgery occlusal relationships. Patients should be in an upright or slightly reclined position; not in a horizontal position as used for routine orthodontic treatment. The mandibular condyles may set more inferior and posterior than usual, particularly shortly after surgery. Conversely, if the surgeon was somewhat rough with the surgery or TMJ surgery was done simultaneously, there may be intercapsular edema that could cause the mandible to be postured slightly forward. If there was preexisting TMJ pathology that was not corrected, patients may "splint" by holding the mandible forward to decrease pressure on the TMJs, altering the centric relation occlusion. Of particular concern is when TMJ surgery has

also been performed at the same operation as the orthognathic surgery. The capsular ligaments have been cut and with the patient in a reclined position, the condyles can slide posterior and inferior to the centric relation position, yielding a false class II end-on occlusal relationship. Setting the patient in an upright or only slightly reclined position and pushing gently upward at the angles of the mandible should seat the condyles into a centric relationship to more accurately evaluate the occlusal interrelationship.[26]

Aggressive Postsurgical Orthodontics

If the occlusion is not "perfect" initially postsurgery, the surgeon and/or orthodontist must aggressively apply the appropriate elastic mechanics. Relatively light strength elastics ($3\frac{1}{2}$ oz) will usually be adequate to correct the situation. However, occasionally, heavier elastics may be necessary. This can be accomplished by doubling-up the $3\frac{1}{2}$-oz elastics or using a stronger elastic. Delays in addressing postsurgical occlusal imbalances will result in much greater difficulties in correcting the problem at a later time. If the occlusion was good at the completion of surgery, but a shift has occurred or open bite developed, this is often due to minor posterior occlusal changes that have caused interference. If light elastics do not reapproximate the occlusion, placing heavy elastics in the appropriate direction for 30 minutes to an hour may settle the occlusion into position so that light elastics can then be used again. Although heavy-strength elastics are occasionally necessary, it is unusual to require them when the surgery has been properly and accurately performed. Occasionally, equilibration of the teeth may be necessary to settle the occlusion into position. If there is a major postsurgical malocclusion, assessment of postsurgical lateral cephalograms and TMJ tomograms may help determine whether it is a correctable problem orthodontically or whether additional surgical intervention is required. If required, the sooner the surgical intervention is performed, usually the better situation for the patient and surgeon.

Postsurgical Elastic Traction

Postsurgical interarch elastics are indicated for the following reasons: (1) to maximize the occlusal fit; (2) to provide orthodontic forces to correct postsurgical occlusal discrepancies; (3) to take stress off the muscles of mastication to improve patient comfort immediately postsurgery; (4) to finalize the occlusion; and (5) to minimize edema in the bilaminar tissues if simultaneous TMJ surgery was performed. Controlling the occlusion postsurgery can generally be accomplished using elastics with one or more of the following vectors depending of the situation; that is, class II, class III, vertical, box, triangle, trapezoidal, rhomboidal, cross-arch, anterior tangential, or others. Usually, only light-force elastics of $3^{1}/_{2}$ ounces with sizes of $^{1}/_{8}$", $^{3}/_{16}$", $^{1}/_{4}$", and $^{5}/_{16}$" are needed because teeth and bone segments (maxilla particularly) can move faster postsurgery. If the occlusion fits together very well, elastics may not be necessary, unless the patient requires elastics for improved comfort by providing vertical support for relieving tension on the muscles of mastication. As soon as possible postsurgery, patients should be instructed on the placement and removal of their elastics to facilitate their dietary intake, oral hygiene, and jaw exercises. When TMJ surgery is simultaneously done with the orthognathic surgery, using light class III directional elastics for a few days postsurgery will minimize TMJ edema. If postsurgical TMJ edema develops, the occlusion can shift toward a class III end-on relationship. Class III elastics will then be necessary to reapproximate the occlusion into a class I relationship. It is usually easier to minimize the TMJ edema immediately after surgery with class III elastics than to recapture the occlusion later.[26]

Vertical Elastics

The use of anterior vertical elastics must be closely monitored. Although often necessary initially postsurgery to provide vertical support to the jaws to decrease masticatory muscle tension and to maximize the occlusal fit, these elastics can also create unwanted dentoalveolar changes (Figure 55-40). Patients that may be predisposed to these unwanted changes include (1) patients with nasal airway obstruction that was not corrected at surgery and who continue to be mouth breathers; (2) patients who habitually hold their jaws apart or in their work or play activities talk a lot requiring the jaws to be held open; and (3) patients with short roots. Holding the jaws apart for extended periods of time with anterior vertical elastics will extrude the anterior teeth and, over time, increase the alveolar bone height. Also, a degree of DO may occur in the maxilla. These changes may result in the development of posterior open bites, premature contact of the incisors, increased upper tooth-to-lip relationship, and increased mandibular and maxillary anterior vertical height. Avoiding these factors may include one or more of the following: (1) perform stable presurgical orthodontics and accurate surgery to decrease requirements for vertical elastics; (2) discontinue vertical elastics as soon as possible; (3) decrease daily time requirements for wearing elastics, particularly during activities in which the jaws will function

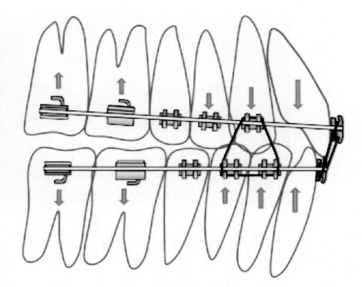

FIGURE 55-40. The use of anterior vertical elastics must be closely monitored. These elastics can create undesirable dentoalveolar effects including development of posterior open bites, premature contact of the incisors, increased tooth-to-lip relationship, and increased mandibular and maxillary anterior vertical height.

in an open position; (4) use very light vertical therapeutic clenching to minimize adverse vertical forces; (5) correct nasal airway obstruction and sleep apnea issues by performing the appropriate surgical procedures so the patients can breathe through their noses instead of requiring mouth breathing.

Power Chains

Avoid the use of power chains (Figure 55-41A) in the upper arch postsurgery. The use of power chains is a relatively common technique in the orthodontic finishing phase of treatment. However, power chain forces can create increased torque on the incisors, tipping the incisor edges posteriorly and tipping the root tips anteriorly (see Figure 55-41 B and C). This can cause premature contact of the incisors with subsequent end-on incisor relationship and development of posterior open bites. This can be a major problem, particularly in patients in whom spacing was created in the anterior arch around the lateral incisors to compensate for the TSD. When this problem develops, the power chain should be removed immediately and mechanics reversed to tip the incisor edges forward and the root tips posteriorly. This may involve reopening space between the lateral incisors and the cuspids that may have been inadvertently closed. This spacing can be eliminated postorthodontically with bonding, veneers, or crowns on the lateral incisors.

Changing Arch Wires

Segmental osteotomies in the maxilla or mandible commonly require the arch wire to be cut into sections. Crimping the wire ends, placing a bead of acrylic over the ends, or using

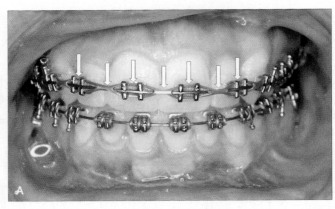

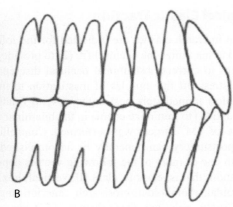

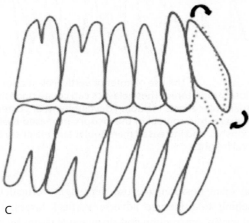

FIGURE 55-41. **A,** Power chains create increased torque on the incisors, tipping the incisors edges posteriorly and tipping the root apices anteriorly. **B** and **C,** This can cause premature contact of the incisors with subsequent end-on incisor relationship and development of posterior open bites.

wax postsurgery to cover the cut ends of the wire are techniques to protect the lips and cheeks from trauma caused by the cut wire ends. Generally, the arch wires can be changed at about 4 to 6 weeks postsurgery, at about the same time that the splint is ordinarily removed. It is usually too uncomfortable for patients to tolerate the arch wire change before that time. If a palatal splint is in place, it can remain in place because it should not interfere with the arch wire change and the splint can continue to help with maxillary transverse stability. Occlusal coverage splints usually require removal before the arch wire can be changed.

Dental Arch Spacing

The correction of significant anterior TSDs may require the creation of space in the upper arch between the lateral incisors and the cuspids and/or the lateral incisors and the central incisors to ensure a good class I occlusal fit with proper overjet/over bite relationship (see Figure 55-26B). It is very important in the postsurgical patient management phase that the space is maintained for subsequent bonding, veneers, or crowns (see Figure 55-26C). DO NOT CLOSE THE SPACE! because this can result in malocclusion. A common postsurgery orthodontic practice is to close interdental spaces. This can create major occlusal problems by downward and backward retraction of the maxillary incisors resulting in an end-on incisor relationship, posterior open bites, downward and

backward rotation of the mandible, increased stress on the TMJs, and pain. If this situation occurs where the spaces have been closed, the spaces need to be opened again with forward rotation of the incisors to improve the occlusal fit with subsequent restorative dentistry to eliminate the spaces with bonding, veneers, or crowns.

Tooth Movement

Teeth move more rapidly for approximately the first 6 months postsurgery as compared with presurgery. Relative to tooth movement, the orthodontist can usually accomplish in 1 to 2 weeks postsurgery what took 4 to 6 weeks presurgery. This is because the bone metabolism and bone "turnover" increase substantially after surgery, allowing more rapid bone resorption and apposition in response to orthodontic forces, so the teeth move more quickly. In addition, with segmental maxillary surgery, the individual bone segments can also move some, providing increased flexibility of the teeth and bone segments.

Finishing Orthodontics

It is important for the patient to keep the orthodontic appliances on for a minimum of 4 to 6 months postorthognathic surgery, when appropriate rigid fixation techniques are used, to allow for initial bone healing as well as finish aligning, leveling, and stabilizing the occlusion. It usually takes 4 months to complete the initial postsurgical bone healing phase to where the maxilla and mandible should be skeletally stable.[27] If inadequate rigid fixation was used or the maxillary bone was exceptionally thin, or uncontrolled clenching/bruxism is present, orthodontic appliances may be required for a significantly extended time. The greater and more complex required surgical movements and presurgical orthodontic treatment mechanics, generally the longer the time requirements for the postsurgical orthodontic management. The orthodontist will determine when the occlusion is maximized and stabilized and the patient is ready for debanding and retainers.

Orthodontic Retainers

For patients who have undergone orthognathic surgery, rigid retainers (Hawley or wraparound types) without occlusal coverage (Figure 55-42A) are recommended to provide trans-verse support to the width of the maxillary and mandibular dental arches, maintain the dental alignment, and allow for maximal interdigitation of the occlusion (see Figure 55-42B). Occlusal coverage retainers (see Figure 55-42C) should not be used because of vertical separation of the occlusion as this can create a malocclusion, usually with open bite situations anteriorly or posteriorly, unilaterally or bilaterally. In addition, occlusal coverage retainers are often flexible (see Figure 55-42D) and do not provide any transverse stability, resulting in transverse relapse in cases of surgical or orthodontic expansion or narrowing of the dental arches that can result in anterior open bite and posterior cross-bite relationships.[26]

Relapse

Orthodontic or surgical instability and relapse can also cause changes and is particularly related to transverse or vertical relapse of the orthodontically expanded maxilla or unstable

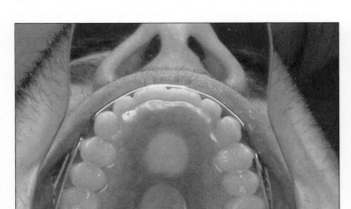
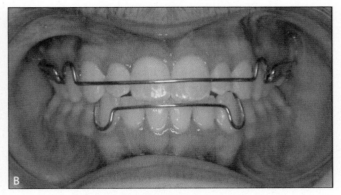
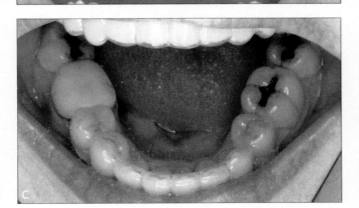
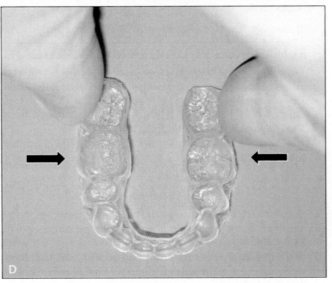

FIGURE 55-42. **A,** For patients who have undergone orthognathic surgery, rigid retainers (Hawley-type) without occlusal coverage, are recommended to provide transverse support to the width of the maxillary dental arch as well as maintain the dental alignment. **B,** These retainers should allow maximal interdigitation of the occlusion. **C,** Occlusal coverage retainers should not be used because of vertical separation of the occlusion as this can create a malocclusion. **D,** Occlusal coverage retainers are usually flexible and do not provide any transverse stability resulting in transverse relapse in cases of surgical or orthodontic expansion or narrowing of the dental arches that can result in anterior open bite and posterior cross-bite relationships.

dental extrusions or intrusions. Transverse collapse of the maxillary dentition will usually cause posterior cross-bites and dental interferences as well as an anterior open bite. Transverse stability is paramount to provide predictable treatment outcomes. Also, inappropriate orthodontic closure of spaces created for correcting TSDs is another orthodontic factor contributing to unwanted postsurgical occlusal changes. Performing careful stable orthodontics, providing good surgical results, no indiscriminate closing of spaces, and appropriate retention, should prevent these types of problems, providing that the TMJs are healthy and stable.

Postsurgical orthodontic patient management is a very important aspect of the treatment for providing optimal patient outcomes. Immediate postsurgical orthodontics should be approached aggressively to maximize high-quality occlusal results in the shortest time frame. However, orthodontic appliances should remain for a minimum of 4 to 6 months postsurgery to get through the primary bone healing phase. This will help minimize orthodontic and surgical relapse potential. Splints play an important role in providing stability for the segmentalized maxilla at surgery and postsurgery. Splints can usually be maintained in position for 1 month or longer for large arch expansions.

The TMJs are a vital component of orthognathic surgery but are often ignored. Failure to diagnose and properly treat TMJ conditions can result in orthodontic and orthognathic surgery relapse, unsatisfactory results relative to functional and aesthetic outcomes, as well as pain and headaches. Proper management of TMJ pathology can provide highly predictable treatment outcomes with usual significant reduction in pain and improved jaw function.

References

1. Bolton WA. The clinical application of a toothsize analysis. Am J Orthod 1962;48:504–529.
2. Moyers RE, van der Linden FPGM, Riolo ML, McNamara JA, editors. Standards of Human Occlusal Development. Ann Arbor: The University of Michigan. The Center for Human Growth and Development; 1976; pp. 53–94.
3. Alling CC III, Helfrick JF, Alling RD, editors. Impacted Teeth. Philadelphia: WB Saunders; 1993; p. 4.
4. Biederman W. The problem of the ankylosed tooth. In Spengeman WG, editor. Dental Clinics of North America. Philadelphia: WB Saunders; 1968; pp. 409–424.
5. Jacobs SG. Ankylosis of permanent teeth: a case report and literature review. Aust Orthod J 1989;11:38–44.
6. Schultes G, Gaggl A, Karcher H. Periodontal disease associated with interdental osteotomies after orthognathic surgery. J Oral Maxillofac Surg 1998;56:414–417.
7. Wolford LM. Periodontal disease associated with interdental osteotomies after orthognathic surgery. J Oral Maxillofac Surg. 1998;56:417–419.
8. Dorfman HS, Turvey TA. Alterations in osseous crestal height following interdental osteotomies. Oral Surg Oral Med Oral Pathol 1979;48:120–125.
9. Shepherd JP. Long-term effects of segmental alveolar osteotomy. Int J Oral Surg 1979;8:327–332.
10. Kwon H, Philstrom B, Waite DE. Effects on the periodontium of vertical bone cutting for segmental osteotomy. J Oral Maxillofac Surg 1985;43:953–955.
11. Fox ME, Stephens WF, Wolford LM, el Deeb M. Effects of interdental osteotomies on the periodontal and osseous supporting tissues. Int J Adult Orthod Orthogn Surg 1991;6:39–46.
12. Wolford LM, Cottrell DA. Diagnosis of macroglossia and indications for reduction glossectomy. Am J Orthod Dentofacial Orthop 1996;110:170–177.
13. Turvey TA, Journot V, Epker BN. Correction of anterior open bite deformity: a study of tongue function, speech changes, and stability. J Maxillofac Surg 1976;4:93–101.
14. Wickwire NA, White RP Jr, Proffit WR. The effect of mandibular osteotomy on tongue position. J Oral Surg 1972;30:184–190.
15. Wolford LM, Cassano DS, Goncalves JR. Common TMJ disorders: orthodontic and surgical management. In McNamara JA, Kapila SD, editors. Temporomandibular Disorders and Orofacial Pain: Separating Controversy from Consensus. Monograph 46, Craniofacial Growth Series, Department of Orthodontics and Pediatric Dentistry and Center for Human Growth and Development. Ann Arbor, MI: The University of Michigan; 2009; pp. 159–198.
16. Wolford LM, Karras S, Mehra P. Concomitant temporomandibular joint and orthognathic surgery: a preliminary report. J Oral Maxillofac Surg 2002;60:356–362.
17. Wolford LM, Mehra P, Reiche-Fischel O, et al. Efficacy of high condylectomy for management of condylar hyperplasia. Am J Orthod Dentofacial Orthop 2002;121:136–151.
18. Mehra P, Wolford LM. The Mitek mini anchor for TMJ disc repositioning: surgical technique and results. Int J Oral Maxillofac Surg 2001;30:497–503.
19. Wolford LM, Cardenas L. Idiopathic condylar resorption: diagnosis, treatment protocol, and outcomes. Am J Orthod Dentofacial Orthop 1999;116:667–676.
20. Schwarz GM, Thrash WJ, Byrd DL, Jacobs JD. Tomographic assessment of nasal septal changes following surgical-orthodontic rapid maxillary expansion. Am J Orthod 1985;87:39–45.
21. Proffit WR. Contemporary Orthodontics. St. Louis: CV Mosby; 1986; pp. 191–192, 352.
22. Williams HS, Zwemer, JD, Hoyt DJ. Treating ankylosed primary teeth in adult patients: a case report. Quintessence Int 1995;26:161–166.
23. Steiner DR. Timing of extraction of ankylosed teeth to maximize ridge development. J Endod 1997;23:242–245.
24. Geiger AM, Bronsky MJ. Orthodontic management of ankylosed permanent posterior teeth: a clinical report of three cases. Am J Orthod Dentofacial Orthop 1994;106:543–548.
25. Oesterle LJ. Implant consideration in the growing child. In Higuchi KW, editor. Orthodontic Applications of Osseointegrated Implants. Chicago: Quintessence Publishing 2000; pp. 133–159.
26. Wolford LM. Postsurgical patient management. In Fonseca R, Marciani R, Turvey T, editors. Oral and Maxillofacial Surgery. 2nd ed. Vol III. St. Louis. Saunders Elsevier. 2008; pp. 396–418.
27. Ayers RA, Simske SJ, Nunes CR, et al. Long-term bone ingrowth and residual mocrohardness of porous block hydroxyapatite implants in humans. J Oral Maxillofac Surg 1998;56:1297–1301.

56
CHAPTER

Model Surgery and Virtual Planning for Orthognathics

Martin B. Steed, DDS, Vincent J. Perciaccante, DDS, and Robert A. Bays, DDS

INTRODUCTION

Traditional model surgery is one of the first examples of preoperative surgical simulation and template fabrication widely used to guide orthognathic surgical movements. The complex three-dimensional movements of the maxilla, mandible, and chin achieved with orthognathic surgery necessitate the significant precision that can be obtained through this process, if care is taken when performing each sequential step. Models are used throughout the course of the patient's treatment, beginning with the pretreatment planning stage, proceeding to an immediate preoperative analytical model surgery, and ultimately resulting in splint construction that is transferred intraoperatively to the orthognathic procedure. The diagnostic information gained from the pretreatment clinical facial and dental measurements, radiographic assessment, and model analysis is integrated to establish a treatment plan. The articulated anatomically mounted models can be utilized in this pretreatment planning stage. These help in the determination of the type of surgery needed and can direct the presurgical orthodontic movements and decompensations.

Presurgical records that provide the ability to surgically simulate surgery include dental impressions, a bite registration with the patient in centric relation (CR), a facebow transfer, and facial measurements made from a standardized clinical examination. Standardized clinical photos and a standardized cephalometric film are also obtained, but their analysis and use are addressed elsewhere in the text. The dental models are placed on a semiadjustable articulator using the CR bite registration and facebow transfer. The treatment plan is expressed in the model surgery that simulates the proposed surgical changes. These models are used to fabricate the occlusal wafers (splints) that facilitate jaw positioning during the actual surgery.

Advances in technology have begun to revolutionize the preparation and performance of orthognathic surgery. Imaging and software innovations have brought fully compu-terized three-dimensional treatment planning, virtual dental models, virtual simulated surgery, and computer-assisted manufacturing of surgical splints or custom onlay implants. A virtual three-dimensional model of the patient can be created and interactive software can be used to provide preoperative evaluation and treatment planning as well as simulated surgery and splint fabrication Virtual surgical planning and splint manufacturing is not always indicated for straightforward routine orthognathic cases, but these advances currently lend themselves well to the correction of complex facial asymmetry cases.[1] Outcome studies on the accuracy of virtual surgical simulation in orthognathic surgery and its cost-benefit analyses continue to be explored.

TRADITIONAL IMMEDIATE PREOPERATIVE ANALYTICAL MODEL SURGERY

Presurgical Clinical Database

The clinical examination of the patient is the first, and most important, step in the orthognathic surgical workup. A comprehensive variety of measurements are obtained that can characterize the patient's skeletal deformity. These measurements reflect not only the position of the maxilla and mandible but also help identify the symmetry of other facial structures. The clinical measurements used to identify the three planes of space—transverse, vertical, and anteroposterior (AP)—can be categorized into those measured at facial frontal view, facial lateral view, and oral examination (Figure 56-1). A small millimeter ruler is used to make most linear measurements and an angle ruler can be utilized for angle measurements.

The transverse measurements include the evaluation of the midlines—relating the facial midline to the maxillary dental midline, the maxillary midline to the mandibular

Orthognathic Physical Examination Database			
Transverse	Date:	Date:	Date:
Maxilla to face			
Mandible to maxilla			
Chin to maxilla			
Occlusal plane			
Mandibular angles			
Arch width			
Vertical			
Crown length			
Upper lip length			
Upper lip—resting			
Upper lip—speech			
Upper lip—smiling			
Open bite/overbite			
Anteroposterior			
Overjet			
Nasolabial angle			
Nasal contour			
Labiomental fold			
Chin			

FIGURE 56-1.   Clinical orthognathic physical examination database.

midline, as well as the chin point to the maxilla. In patients with a notable deviation of their nasal structure or in those with hemifacial asymmetries, there will be added complexity in evaluating midlines. In these instances, utilizing a glabellar mark with a skin marker and holding a perpendicular plumb line from this point will help to measure facial and dental midlines. Occlusal cant is measured at both the maxillary canines and the first maxillary molars. It is quantified by measuring from each orbital rim or medial canthus to the tip of the maxillary canine on the same side. The difference between the two sides defines the cant (e.g., 1.5 mm down at the left maxillary canine). Whereas occlusal cant is often found in the maxilla with mandibular adaptation, there may be an isolated mandibular cant in rare instances. Another measurement of the asymmetry in the transverse plane is assessment of the symmetry of the left and right mandibular angles as measured from the most lateral aspect of the infraorbital rims.

The measurement of maxillary and mandibular arch widths is accomplished through the oral examination and on study models. In areas in which a tooth cross-bite exists within the mouth, hand articulating the study models will reveal whether this represents a true arch width discrepancy or is merely a reflection of the relative skeletal discrepancy manifested by the position of the mandible or maxilla. When a unilateral cross-bite is observed clinically, more often than not the cross-bite is actually bilateral, but the mandible slides to one side upon closure to achieve better interdigitation of the teeth. The examiner should carefully manipulate the mandible to a seated condylar position and then close the teeth together to determine where the first point of contact occurs.

This can be crucial in determining whether the mandible is truly asymmetrical or has deviated from a bilateral end-to-end occlusion to a unilateral full cross-bite in "centric occlusion." This assessment can also be made on carefully mounted models.

The maxillary central incisors are key to treatment planning in orthognathic surgery. Their preoperative position must be assessed when the patient is smiling, speaking, and most important, in repose. In addition, any additional gingival show must be noted and quantified. Open bite in the area of the central incisors must be measured preoperatively as well as the length of the upper lip. Overbite, positive or negative, should be noted pretreatment and after orthodontic decompensations. The importance of this evaluation is to detect any orthodontic closure of a pretreatment open bite that may relapse after completion of all treatment. In addition, the nasolabial angle and the labiomental fold often help assess the soft tissue contour that accompanies the jaw relation discrepancies. One must also be mindful of the nasal contour while treatment planning upper jaw procedures. Typically, maxillary advancements or impactions widen the alar base and elevate the nasal tip. Concomitant procedures can be performed to correct significant nasal functional and aesthetic concerns such as osseous recontouring, alar cinch, turbinate reduction, and septoplasty.

The position and structure of the chin play a major role in the final aesthetic perspective of most patients. Although model surgery may or may not reveal the final position of the chin, it will predict the final position of "B" point, which can then be used with the cephalometric analysis and prediction tracing to predict final chin position. Thus, a preoperative assessment of the chin position at baseline is important to assess the need for change.

Presurgical Records

Dental Impressions

Dental impressions are obtained with alginate at the final presurgical records appointment. They must be obtained after all preoperative orthodontic tooth movement is complete and the surgical stabilizing arch wires have been in place for several weeks and are passive. Recently placed surgical arch wires cause tooth movement, which may continue to take place after the impressions are obtained. Any tooth movement that occurs after the impressions are made will lead to inaccuracies in how well the splint fits intraoperatively. The dental impressions must include the occlusal surfaces of each of the teeth and be without voids or alginate tears. The impressions are poured up using dental die stone and a dental vibrating platform for a hard and precise model. Indentations may be placed within the base of the cast in order to allow for future separation and re-indexing of the cast from its plaster mounting.

Facebow Transfer

The transfer of the maxillary cast to the articulator by using a facebow (Figure 56-2) gives a reliable estimation of the distance between the dentition and the intercondylar hinge

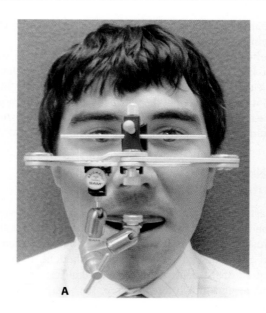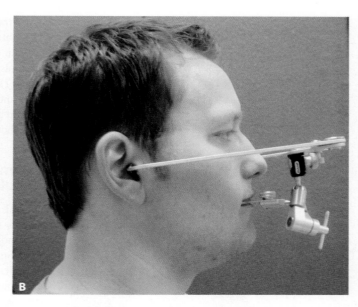

FIGURE 56-2.   **A,** The Student Articulator of Munich (SAM) facebow is used to relate the maxillary occlusal plane to the axis-orbital plane (AOP). **B,** The AOP is formed by the intercondylar axis of the mandible and the lowest point of the inferior orbital rim known as the *orbitale*. This plane is approximately 7 degrees different from true Frankfurt horizontal (FH). This often results in cases in which the maxillary occlusal plane is too steep when mounted.

axis. This is important when vertical movements of the maxilla and/or mandible are planned, because autorotation changes the position of the jaws in both vertical and horizontal dimensions. The more accurately the maxillary model is mounted with respect to the true hinge axis, the more accurate will be the information provided about the horizontal and vertical movements of the jaws during model surgery. Traditionally, a facebow device is used to register the three-dimensional relationship of the maxillary dental arch to the Frankfort horizontal plane (FHP) using either the patient's external auditory meatus or the condylar heads (depending on the requirements of the facebow) as the posterior reference.

It is universally accepted that the upper arm of the articulator represents Frankfort horizontal (FH). However, this assumption can introduce error. The semiadjustable articulator used for model surgery was originally created for use in prosthetic dentistry. Its facebow was designed to transfer the relationship of the maxilla to the terminal hinge axis of the mandible. To accomplish this, the posterior end of the facebow was aligned to the terminal hinge axis (middle of the condyle), and the anterior end was aligned to orbitale. These points defined a plane called the *axis-orbital plane (AOP),* which is 7 degrees off from FH. Modifications have been made for surgical cases to minimize this error. Facebows equipped with an adjustable nasal rest and an infraorbital pointer provide an additional point of reference. The pointer arbitrarily lowers the anterior part of the facebow below orbitale by 6.8 mm, thereby reducing the inclination of the occlusal plane. This facebow registration is transferred to the articulator to position and mount the maxillary dental model.

There are other reasons for the inaccuracy in the traditional facebow mounting of dental models[2]: (1) the position of the patient's external auditory meatus or mandibular condyles (depending on the reference for the facebow) may be asymmetrical from side to side compared with the fixed symmetrical position of the facebow mounting rods on the articulator; (2) owing to anatomic variances, the patient's FHP as determined by the facebow may be significantly different than the fixed FHP of the articulator; (3) the facebow may be improperly positioned on the patient, or facebow components could shift when tightening the bolts, nuts, and/ or screws during the registration procedure; (4) cranial base and jaw aberrations may be present that are not reproducible on the articulator; (5) anatomic structures may be absent (i.e., hemifacial microsomia), rendering the facebow mounting totally arbitrary; and (6) shifting of the facebow components can occur during the mounting of the maxillary model. Despite these limitations, a carefully obtained and clinically correlated arbitrary facebow is essential to mount the models correctly without compromising the patient's surgical results.

CR Bite Registration

The mandibular dental model is then mounted with a CR bite registration. This registration is usually obtained with either wax or polyvinylsiloxane (PVS; Figure 56-3). An accurate registration of the relationship between the maxilla and the mandible *independent of the occlusion* must be obtained for proper mounting and model surgery to be carried out. This has historically been termed *centric relation (CR)* and a record of CR can be obtained in a number of manners. The definition of CR, however, is controversial and frequently misstated. The definition of CR underwent a change in terminology in 1987 from a mandibular position in which the condyles are seated in the most "posterior

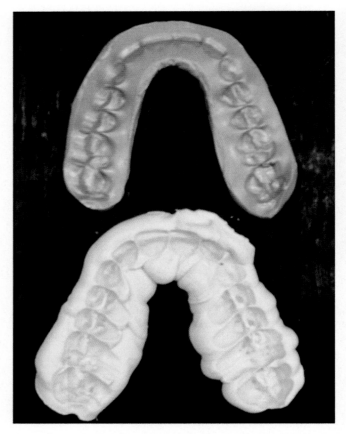

FIGURE 56-3. Centric relation (CR) bite registration in wax and in polyvinylsiloxane (PVS).

superior" position to one in which they are placed in the most "superior anterior" position in the glenoid fossa. The most recent Academy of Denture Prosthetics' "Glossary of Prosthodontic Terms" (GPT) from 2005 defines CR as a maxillomandibular relation in which the condyles articulate with the thinnest avascular portion of their respective disks with the complex in the anterosuperior position against the slopes of the articular eminences.[3] It is essential to locate a mandibular position that is reproducible (without the assistance of the patient) and that can be reliably accomplished both preoperatively and intraoperatively. This position must also be transferable to the articulator in order for model surgery planning to be accomplished accurately. If an inaccurate bite registration is obtained from the patient preoperatively, this will be transferred to the articulated models, leading to inaccurate model surgery and resulting in intraoperative error. Obtaining an accurate and reproducible bite registration in CR is essential if the surgeon is to avoid this error.

The clinical methods to obtain a correct CR registration vary.[4] The "chin point guidance" procedure involves the patient opening wide while the interocclusal record material is applied over the occlusal surfaces of the mandibular teeth. The surgeon then gently manipulates the chin and guides the mandible closure until the mandibular incisors have encoun-

tered the material and the patient is held in this position until the material has set.

The effects of the material used to record CR (i.e., wax) have also been considered as a potential source of introducing error. The error introduced is directly proportional to its thickness and it is suggested that the wax between the distal molars should be as thin as possible. The wax should not be punctured and should retain its rigidity to avoid distorting contacts.

Mounting Dental Models for Simulated Surgery

Dental articulators allow the surgeon to measure surgical moves and carry out multidimensional surgical simulation. Semiadjustable hinge axis articulators commonly used by oral and maxillofacial surgeons and orthodontists permit visualization of the dentoalveolar units, their relationship to one another, and to a limited degree, the position of these structures relative to other parts of the craniofacial skeleton. Typically, the upper member of a semiadjustable or fully adjustable articulator is said to represent one of the cephalometric planes (i.e., FH), and the intercondylar distance is set to approximate that measurement in the average adult. The diagnostic utility of the articulator is enhanced when predictive mock surgery is carried out on mounted dental casts.

In order to ensure that the articulator is calibrated correctly, it is appropriate to periodically calibrate the instrument with a split cast check. To perform the split cast check:

1. Set the horizontal condylar inclination at 30 degrees and the Bennett side shift at 5 degrees (average setting) on each side.
2. The incisal pin should be at the zero mark or less.
3. Attach the metal portion of the split cast to the lower member and attach the plaster portion of the split cast to the upper member (Figure 56-4).
4. The two portions of the split cast should fit together without any discrepancy (Figure 56-5).
5. If these two parts do not fit together, make sure the incisal pin is out of contact with the incisal table and check the articulator for wax or plaster debris under the split cast or in the condylar housing area.

Mounting the maxillary cast using facebow transfer (Figure 56-6) requires that the angle between the occlusal plane of the maxillary model and the upper member of the articulator are the same as the occlusal plane angle. If the maxillary model is mounted at a different angle, the intermediate splint utilized in combined maxillary and mandibular cases will convey an aberrant position during surgery. Comparison of the maxillary plane angle (once the facebow is attached to the articulator) to patient's cephalogram may be required in the laboratory when mounting the maxillary cast. Accurate mounting of the mandibular cast using a CR interocclusal registration is mandatory.

The base of the mounting and the cast are best prepared for separation by application of a layer of separating media

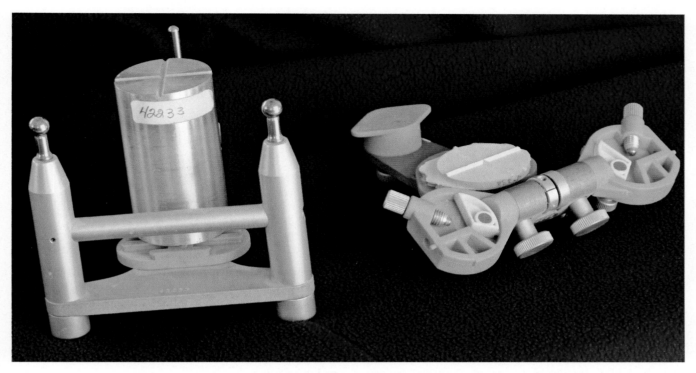

FIGURE 56-4. Calibration of a SAM articulator with a split cast. The metal portion of the split cast has been attached to the lower member and the plaster portion has been attached to the upper member.

at the time of mounting. They also may be made in two separate colored stone products. For instance, the model may be poured in green stone and the mounting in white dental plaster. The base must be smooth and parallel to the base of the cast so that measuring marks can be made easily and smoothly. Trimming of maxillary cast should be parallel to the AOP. The incisal guide pin setting is recorded after mounting.

Marking and Measuring Final Models and Surgical Simulation

Mandibular Surgery

ISOLATED MANDIBULAR SURGERY (SAGITTAL SPLIT OSTEOTOMY OR VERTICAL RAMUS OSTEOTOMY ONLY)

Once the models have been correctly mounted, they are marked with points for measuring. When mandibular

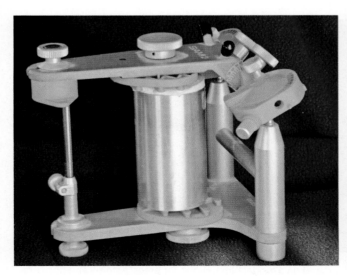

FIGURE 56-5. The two portions of the split cast should fit together without any discrepancy.

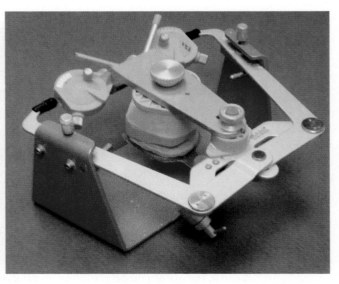

FIGURE 56-6. Mounting the maxillary model on a SAM articulator using a facebow transfer.

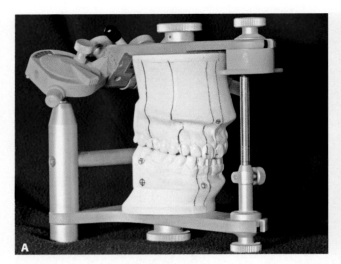
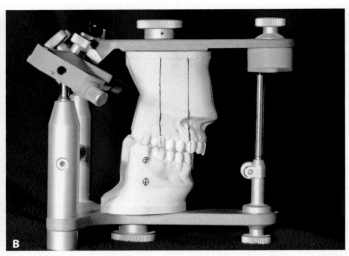

FIGURE 56-7. **A** and **B,** Mandibular models marked for surgery with representative points made on the mandibular cast at the region of the vertical corticotomy or Dal Pont and at the mandibular incisors and genial region.

surgery alone is planned, the mandibular anterior, posterior, or rotational movements are dictated by the maxillary dentition. Because of this, many surgeons use a simple hinge (nonadjustable) articulator to mount the final models. Although the maxillary position will remain constant throughout surgery, there are several benefits to using a semiadjustable articulator and facebow mounting even in straightforward cases. This provides the surgeon with information regarding the distance of the surgical move at the osteotomy site and possible proximal segment positioning challenges, especially when correcting large mandibular asymmetries.

In cases of isolated mandibular surgery, representative points are made on the mandibular cast at the region of the vertical corticotomy or Dal Pont and at the mandibular incisors and genial region (Figure 56-7). These points in the Dal

Pont should be spaced as widely as possible in order to glean the most information about the move. Vertical lines are made at the posterior of the cast descending from the retromolar pad inferiorly.

There are two options to obtain the preoperative measurements now that the models are marked. One way utilizes an Erickson model platform (Great Lakes Orthodontic Products, Ltd., Tonawanda, NY), which is an orientation block with an attached caliper that allows for marking and measuring models to an accuracy of 0.01 mm. With the model secured on a model block, the platform and caliper allow for preosteotomy and postosteotomy measurements in an AP dimension and a vertical dimension (Figure 56-8). This technique eliminates the parallax error that may be introduced by use of the second measuring option, the freehand ruler technique measuring AP to the articulator's pin (Figure 56-9).

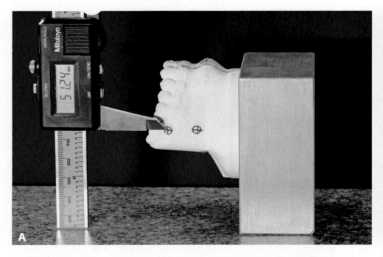
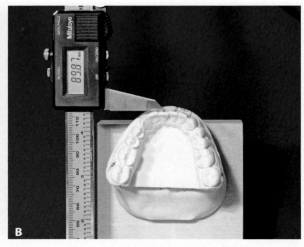

FIGURE 56-8. **A** and **B,** The use of a model platform with the model secured on a model block allows for preosteotomy and postosteotomy measurements in an anteroposterior dimension. Precise thin cross-hatch marks are made on the mandibular cast at the region of the site of the mandibular osteotomy, central incisors, and genial region.

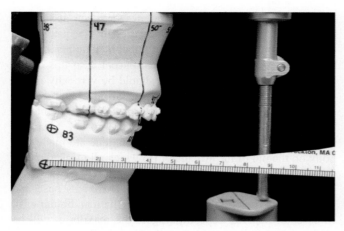

FIGURE 56-9. Utilizing the freehand technique to measure anteroposterior distance at the inferior border of the anticipated right Dal Pont osteotomy. Parallax error is introduced when viewing the same object (in this case the markings on a ruler) from different places.

Parallax error results when viewing the same object (in this case, the markings on a ruler) from different places. Attempts to minimize this error include placing a straight black line on the pin platform (Figure 56-9) and measuring consistently to the anterior portion of the pin while viewing from a position at which the black line becomes a point (perpendicular to the ruler). The measurements obtained are recorded onto a laboratory data sheet (orthognathic roadmap) that can be taken to the operating room for reference (Figure 56-10).

The mandibular model can then be separated from its original cast and repositioned to the planned occlusion. Setting of bite should take into consideration the surgery that will be done (bilateral sagittal split osteotomy [BSSO] or intraoral vertical subcondylar ramus osteotomy [IVRO]) and should involve close communication with the patient's orthodontist. The mandibular model is secured to the maxillary with hot glue or sticky wax. The model is then remounted with plaster and a final acrylic surgical splint is fabricated. Postoperative measurements can then be obtained that will inform the surgeon of the distance the mandible is being advanced or set back on each side (the surgical move). In patients in whom an asymmetry is being corrected, a view of the models from a posterior vantage point will help identify regions in which proximal and distal segment interferences can be anticipated (Figure 56-11).

Maxillary Surgery

ISOLATED MAXILLARY SURGERY
Pretreatment model surgery is essential when contemplating maxillary surgery alone and very useful when planning two-jaw surgery. Pretreatment model surgery permits the evaluation of the maxilla and the mandible whether the mandible is autorotated without surgery or also osteotomized. If the goals of the surgery can be accomplished with a single-jaw surgery, the orthodontic preparation and patient's expectations can be influenced appropriately.

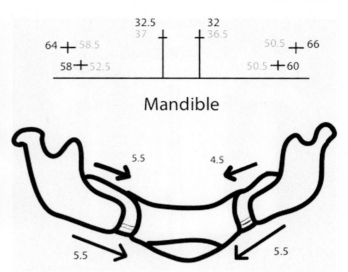

FIGURE 56-10. Mandibular roadmap for an isolated mandibular bilateral sagittal split osteotomy (BSSO) planned for 5.5-mm advancement on each side. The *numbers denoted in black* are made before the surgical move and the *numbers in gray* are made after remounting the mandible in its prescribed final occlusion. The differences between the two numbers reflect the surgical move at that point.

In this scenario, the mandible will serve as a template for final position of the maxilla. A clinical example would be a single-piece Le Fort I maxillary osteotomy for correction of posterior maxillary excess resulting in a skeletal class I open bite malocclusion. The models are mounted as previously discussed. A semiadjustable articulator is strongly recommended for these cases. The advantage of using such an articulator lies in its simulation of the appropriate arc of autorotation of the mandible when properly mounted. When performing isolated maxillary impaction, the incisal pin will be shortened.

Marking the midline is the first step in marking models. This can be done by making lines parallel to the articulating

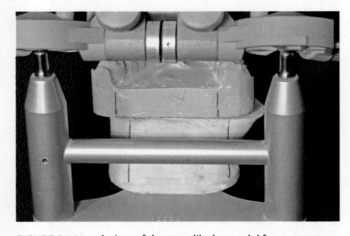

FIGURE 56-11. A view of the mandibular model from a posterior vantage point after surgical move will help identify regions in which proximal and distal segment interferences can be anticipated.

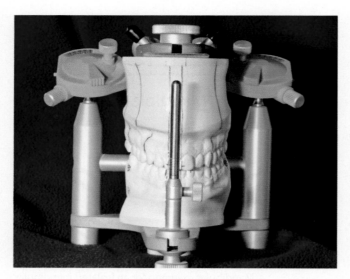

FIGURE 56-12. Red vertical lines are drawn on each side of the midline, using the articulating pin as a guide. The position of these lines is entirely dependent on a correct facebow transfer and the maxillary midline should correlate to the clinical examination.

pin on either side of it from a frontal view, avoiding paralleling errors (Figure 56-12). This step is done on both the maxilla and the mandible mounted together in the presurgical occlusion. A mounted maxillary model requires measurements in the AP, vertical, and transverse planes. This can be accomplished with the maxilla removed from the articulator or while on it. Where the models are measured will depend upon which of the two options is used to measure these distances: the model block or a freehand technique (Figure 56-13). When measuring vertical distances on the model block, it is necessary to "zero" the electronic caliper at the level of the mounting base before obtaining a measurement. The freehand

technique uses a caliper for vertical measurements and a ruler for AP measurements. Vertical measures of the maxilla are made at both the central incisors at premarked points, both of the canine cusp tips, and the mesial-buccal cusp tips of the first molars. In addition, the cast should be vertically measured at both tuberosities. AP measurements are then recorded at the central incisors and a point representing the anterior nasal spine on the base of the cast (Figure 56-14). Measurements obtained with the "freehand" technique are made to a point on the pin of the articulator (to which all measurements should be consistently made).

The maxillary cast is now separated from its base and positioned in the proper occlusion with the mandibular cast. In cases of superior repositioning of the maxilla, it will be necessary to remove additional plaster from the mounting to provide clearance for the superior repositioning of the maxilla. A layer of wax or hot glue is added to the gap between the base and the model. Any AP changes are usually limited by the mandibular position. The incisal guide pin is adjusted as needed to provide the proper vertical measurement at the maxillary incisor. Shortening of the incisal guide pin height in maxillary impaction cases will allow the proper arc of autorotation of the mandible to this newly positioned maxilla. The final measurements are recorded (Figure 56-15) and the roadmap is prepared (Figure 56-16). A final splint is made to this occlusion.

VERTICAL MEASUREMENTS IN MAXILLARY SURGERY

Despite meticulous presurgical planning and model surgery, vertical positioning in maxillary surgery will depend entirely upon intraoperative measurements and will not be ensured from only model surgery or surgical splints. How best to control the positional change of the maxilla has been debated. The unfortunate use of the terms "internal" and "external" reference marks has led to confusion because "internal" has been used to describe an antiquated technique of scribing

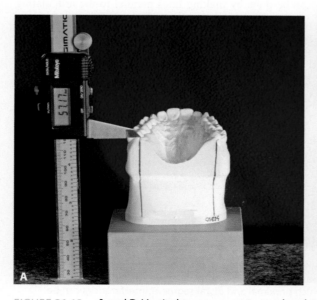

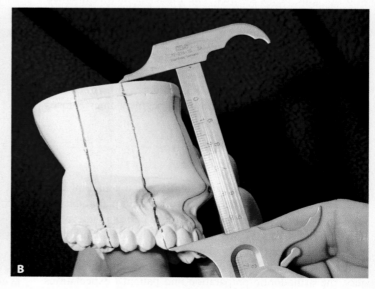

FIGURE 56-13. **A** and **B**, Vertical measurements may be obtained with either a model block (**A**) or a handheld caliper (**B**).

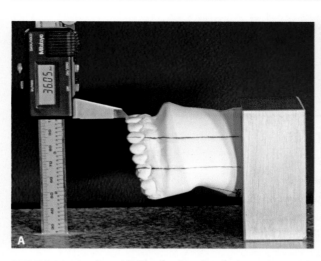
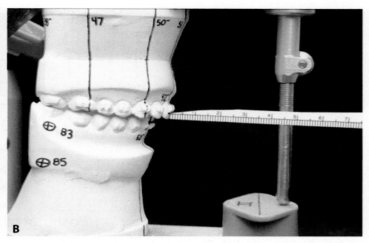

FIGURE 56-14.   **A** and **B,** The freehand technique measures anteroposterior distance from a point marked on the maxillary right central incisor to the anterior of the mounting pin.

lines above and below the osteotomy in an attempt to measure the vertical position of the maxilla intraoperatively. The term "external" has come to mean placing a referencing device somewhere outside of the wound above the osteotomy and measuring to the mobilized maxilla, usually the central incisor brackets. But the issue is not whether the reference marks are inside or outside of the mouth or the wound, but rather that they are superior to the osteotomy and are in stable bone. The use of superior bony reference marks (SBRMs), inside or outside of the wound, has proved to be more accurate than scribing lines along the osteotomy. This makes outside of the wound reference marks unnecessary if SBRMs are placed as described later. The technique presented here provides four SBRMs in two bilateral locations. Measurement is made from the SBRM to the gingival crest rather than orthodontic brackets, which can be loosened resulting in the loss of that measuring point.

Method 1: Utilizing four SBRMs for point-to-point intraoperative measurements This method simultaneously employs two different manners of measuring. Preoperatively, the Erickson model block is used for pure horizontal or vertical measurements whereas bilateral "point-to-point" measurements are made with a Boley gauge or calipers that correlate to intraoperative measurements. Premovement measurements at the canine and molar areas bilaterally are repeated postmovement, in a point-to-point fashion, using a Boley gauge to measure vertical change.

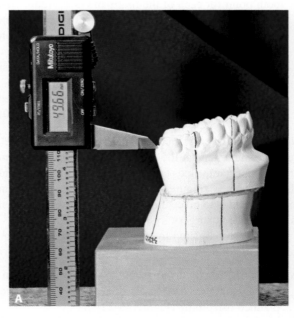
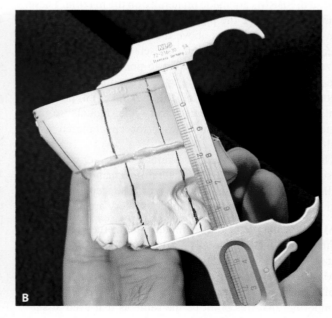

FIGURE 56-15.   **A** and **B,** Final measurements are made at the left and right maxillary incisor, canine, and first molar teeth, as well as at the tuberosity and anterior nasal spine region. These new measurements reflect the change in vertical positioning.

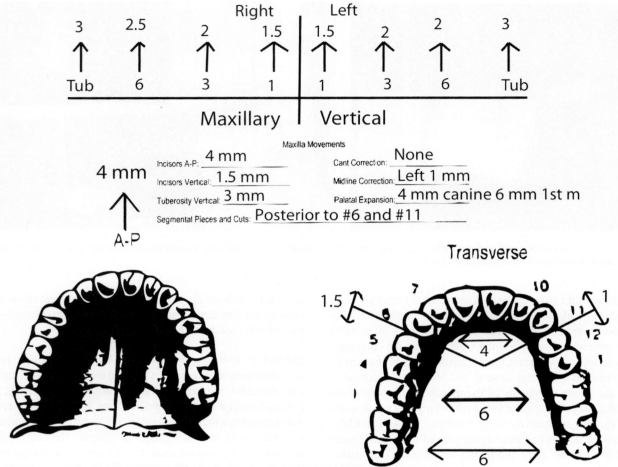

FIGURE 56-16. Maxillary orthognathic roadmap denotes planned maxillary movements.

Intraoperatively, the model surgery measurements are replicated. SBRMs are made bilaterally on the maxilla. These are made well above the planned osteotomy line in the piriform and buttress regions above the canine and molar. The difference in the two measurements sets from the models is utilized intraoperatively, in a point-to-point fashion, with a caliper, obtaining the same difference in the preoperative and postoperative measurements on the maxilla. This point-to-point measurement transferred from the models to the surgical measurements eliminates error encountered as a result of AP movement.

This method does not require a reference marker outside of the surgical wound and gives bilateral information regarding the three-dimensional maxillary moves. The steps necessary for this technique at the time of model surgery are as follows:

1. Mark a stable point on the models above the canine and first molar teeth bilaterally—a total of four stable points (see Figure 56-17, points *A* and *P*).
2. Mark a corresponding point on the canine and molar teeth bilaterally. The incisal edge is usually used. It is not important that this point be the same as that used at surgery so long as it is stable from before model surgical positioning until after (see Figure 56-17, points *B* and *C*).

3. Measure and record the distances from stable point to the tooth point for each of the four pairs (see Figure 56-17).
4. Measure the anterior maxilla from FH to the upper incisor using either the model block or the freehand technique (Figure 56-18).
5. Perform model surgery to the desired three-dimensional position (Figure 56-19).
6. Remeasure all five distances and record the difference between pre- and postmodel surgeries (Figure 56-20).

Note: The *differences* between the pre- and postmodel surgery measurements at the piriform rims and the first molars are the important values to have at the time of surgery, not the absolute values (Figure 56-21). The FH to upper incisor measurement is to place the model at the desired vertical and is not needed at surgery.

The steps completed for this technique at the time of surgery are as follows:

A. Place SBRMs by drilling small holes in the piriform rims and zygomatic buttresses bilaterally well above the planned osteotomy (Figure 56-22A).
B. Measure and record the distance from these holes (SBRMs) to the gingival crest of the canines and first

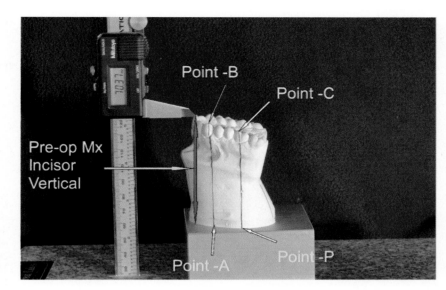

FIGURE 56-17. Measurement of preoperative maxillary vertical at right canine and mesial buccal cusp tip of right first molar with a model block.

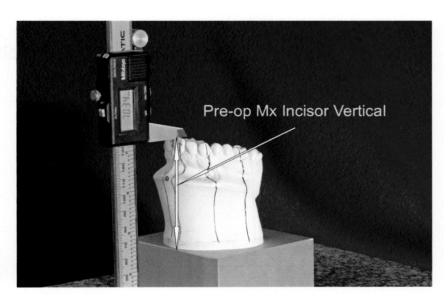

FIGURE 56-18. Measurement of preoperative maxillary vertical at the right central incisor with a model block.

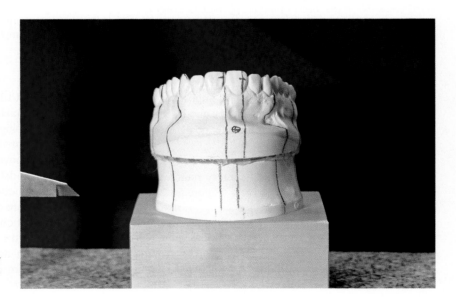

FIGURE 56-19. Cut and repositioned maxillary model placed onto the model block for postoperative measurement.

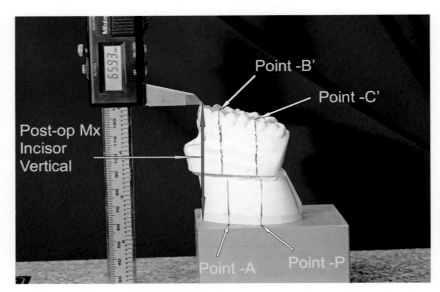

FIGURE 56-20. Postoperative vertical measurements are obtained in the same fashion as was done before cutting and repositioning the maxilla. Here, the new vertical measurements are obtained at the right canine and mesial buccal cusp tip of right first molar with a model block. The differences between the pre- and postoperative numbers should reflect the treatment plan.

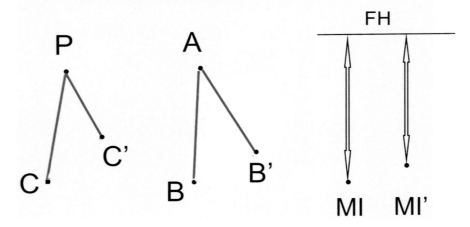

Maxillary impaction with clockwise rotation

If PC minus PC' = planned impaction @ M1 bilaterally &
If AB minus AB' = planned impaction @ Ca bilaterally
then MI minus MI' will be planned amount of impaction @ Ce Incisor

FIGURE 56-21. The differences between the pre- and the postmodel surgery measurements are the important values to have at the time of surgery.

molars bilaterally. Again, it is *not* important that this point on the teeth is the same as the model surgery so long as it is a stable, reproducible point (see Figure 56-22B).

C. After mobilization, position the maxilla so that the four *differences* measured at model surgery match those differences measured intraoperatively (Figure 56-23).

If the maxilla is positioned according to this method, the anterior maxillary vertical will be as planned. No SBRM outside of the wound is needed and the canine and molar vertical positions will also be as planned (see Figure 56-21).

Method 2: Utilizing one midline superior bony external reference mark This external reference point method provides a single measurement to assess proper vertical positioning of the maxilla and the anterior maxillary teeth. All other movements (AP and transverse) are provided from the model surgery and prefabricated surgical splints. After anesthetic induction and patient positioning and preparation are completed, the face is widely draped to allow for visualization of the nose. A 0.062 Kirschner pin (K wire) is placed in the nasal bones at the nasion of approximately 8 to 12 mm depth, and a measurement is obtained from the fixed wire to the maxillary central incisor orthodontic bracket before maxillary mobilization with a Boley gauge

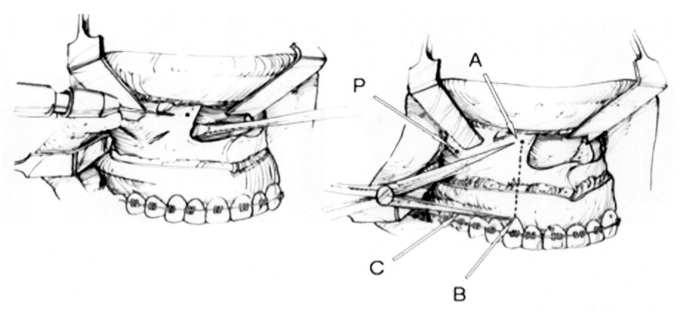

FIGURE 56-22.   Intraoperative placement of superior bony reference marks (SBRMs) by drilling small holes in the piriform rims and zygomatic buttresses bilaterally well above the planned osteotomy with a 703 straight fissure bur.

or Perkins device. Measurements are then repeated after the osteotomy and positioning of the maxilla until the planned change in vertical is achieved. The use of external reference points is also an accurate and predictable technique to measure and confirm vertical maxillary position.

SEGMENTAL MAXILLARY SURGERY

When performing model surgery for a segmental maxillary procedure, differences in the workup begin with the obtaining dental casts. It may be desirable to have more than one maxillary cast to test the planned segmentalization to

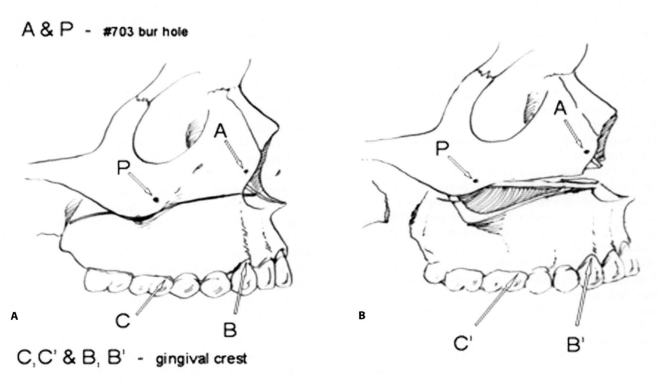

FIGURE 56-23.   **A** and **B,** After mobilization, the maxilla is positioned so that the four *differences* measured at model surgery match those differences measured intraoperatively.

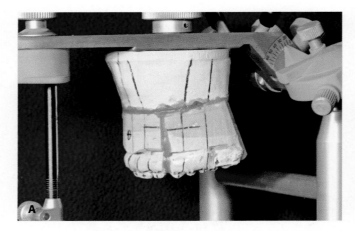 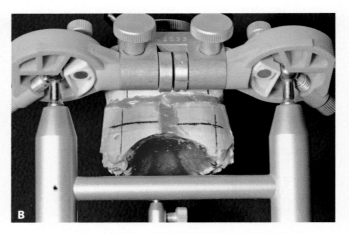

FIGURE 56-24. **A** and **B.** Additional markings placed on the maxillary cast for segmental surgery. Vertical lines should be drawn on both sides of the planned interdental osteotomy. Because segmentalization is often done on either side of the canine, some of these lines will already be present, but a line at the tooth on the opposite side of the interdental osteotomy must also be placed. In addition, horizontal lines should be placed across the posterior of the cast between the vertical tuberosity lines and also between the vertical lines at the interdental cuts. These lines are used for points of measurement and also to aid in appreciation of any tipping of the model of vertical changes in these areas.

determine whether the surgical cast should, in fact, be sectioned in a particular manner. Periapical radiographs should be made of the interdental osteotomy sites.

Marking and measuring of the surgical cast also has some variation (Figure 56-24). The casts are marked and measured as any other maxillary cast plus some additional markings and measurements. Vertical lines should be drawn on both sides of the planned interdental osteotomy. Because segmentalization is often done on either side of the canine, some of these lines will already be present, but a line at the tooth on the opposite side of the interdental osteotomy must also be placed. In addition, horizontal lines should be placed across the posterior of the cast between the vertical tuberosity lines and also between the vertical lines at the interdental cuts. These lines are used for points of measurement and also to aid in appreciation of any tipping of the models or vertical changes in these areas.

Transverse measurements are made with a Boley gauge at the intersection of the vertical and horizontal lines at the backside of the model, at the mesiobuccal cusps of the first molar, and at the canine. If there is an interdental cut behind the canine, this measurement should be made at the premolar. Additional measurements are made at the cusps of the teeth on either side of the interdental osteotomy and at the roots (the intersection of the vertical and horizontal lines at the interdental cut). Knowing the measurement at the cusp and root of the teeth is important to ensure that the planned surgery will not impinge upon the tooth roots. Even with separation at the cusps, the roots could converge with certain tipping movements.

After all marking and measuring is complete, the maxillary cast is sectioned in the areas of the interdental osteotomy. This is done with the thinnest diamond disk available and, in the area closest to the teeth, is best done by just scoring the cast with a #15 blade and breaking this last bit of the

cast along the score (after sectioning the remainder of the cast). This will prevent any removal of stone in areas of the teeth and creating an unrealistic simulation of the surgery. Once the cast is sectioned, the next step is establishment of the maxillary arch form

The proper maxillary arch form is the set on the mandible. Feasibility of the planned movements is determined by comparing the postmovement measurements to the pre sectioning measurements described previously. Once the maxillary arch form is set, the remainder of maxillary moves can be done is the same fashion as for a nonsegmental surgery.

In a single-jaw case, the final interocclusal splint with a transpalatal strap (which is sufficiently relieved so as not to impinge on the palatal mucosa and blood supply) is fabricated (Figure 56-25). Alternatively, a palatal style splint can be fabricated, without occlusal coverage, and a separate interocclusal splint can be fabricated to position the remainder of the maxillary movements. In a two-jaw orthognathic case, which involves segmental maxillary surgery, the final splint must be made first in this manner. It must be trimmed and polished to completion. Because this splint will be wired into place on the maxilla and left, postsurgically, for a period of time, the intermediate splint is made as a "piggy-back" splint or a "splint within a splint." That is, the upper surface will articulate with the final splint in the final maxillary position, and the lower surface will articulate to the uncut maxilla. The highly polished final maxillary splint must be adequately lubricated to prevent curing to the intermediate splint.

COMBINED MAXILLARY AND MANDIBULAR SURGERY
Examination and orthognathic workup of a patient will often reveal a skeletal deformity in both the maxilla and the mandible. If the maxilla is the first jaw to be mobilized in combined surgery, the following steps are carried out in the model surgery.

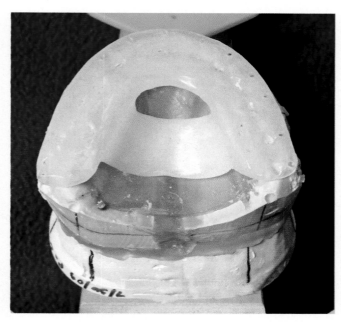

FIGURE 56-25.   Final interocclusal splint with a transpalatal strap, fabricated over a layer of wax to provide relief and not impinge on the palatal mucosa and blood supply once inserted and secured. Holes are made in the flange to allow for the splint to be secured to the orthodontic brackets.

The models are articulated as per the previously described standard mounting technique utilizing a facebow transfer and CR registration. The articulator's pin is not changed at all during the case. The previously described vertical and horizontal measurements are made on the casts and recorded on the models and plaster as well as on the laboratory data sheet (orthognathic roadmap).

The maxillary cast is then separated from the base. The base of the cast is trimmed sufficiently to accommodate impaction, advancement, cant correction, or rotation. The new position of the maxilla must be considered in all three planes of space. The movement is correlated to the clinical database and photos to place the maxillary midline in concordance with the facial midline. Any cant correction is achieved by correcting vertical measurements that may be unequal at first. For instance, if on clinical examination, the maxillary left canine is 2 mm lower than the right canine, this is leveled in the final position of the cast. Relating the clinical database and cephalometric prediction tracing, the maxilla is then moved in an AP dimension to the prescribed position. The vertical position of the maxilla is also prescribed by the clinical orthognathic database.

A number of methods can be used to hold the maxillary cast in this new position while making the movements and verifying through measurements. Three small balls of white dental wax can be used during the "move and measure" phase followed by placing yellow sticky wax in between the model and the base to secure the maxilla to the base more securely in that position once the correct position is obtained. Some clinicians use dental plaster whereas others utilize a glue gun for the same purpose.

Caution must be exercised while making multidimensional movements to constantly reevaluate the measurements in all planes and also ensure that the heels of the cast are not kicked off in one direction that would be difficult to replicate during surgery. This is especially possible while attempting to correct the midline. As the anterior part of the cast moves to one side or another, it is easy for the heels to move in the opposite direction (sometimes in a manner that will be difficult to accommodate at the time of surgery). This can be avoided by placing the fulcrum of rotation as anterior as possible.

With the maxilla secured in its desired position, it will provide the surgeon its orientation to the unoperated mandible. Following the placement of maxilla in its new prescribed position; the mandibular cast is separated from its base, placed into the planned occlusion, and a new base is created for it, preferably in a stone of a different color as opposed to the original mounting. This will be the final position of the mandible. Ideally, occlusal adjustments that are needed are performed before impressions are obtained; however, if this was unanticipated, these adjustments are now accomplished on the casts and marked with red pencil in order to facilitate replication at the beginning of surgery.

A final splint is fabricated first in this position. Once that splint is complete, the mandibular model can be repositioned onto the initial base and the intermediate splint is constructed. Postsurgical measurements are then obtained and recorded on the roadmap for surgery.

Sequence of bimaxillary orthognathic surgery The model surgery for bimaxillary surgery will depend upon which sequence the surgeon will perform the osteotomies in the operation. The model surgery will be performed in the same sequence to allow for correct intermediate splints to be fabricated. The majority of surgeons prefer to operate on the maxilla first, fixate it against the unoperated mandible using an intermediate splint, and then move the mandible to occlude with this new maxillary position for the final maxilla-mandible relation. Specific situations in which this sequence may be altered and the mandible operated on first include cases in which there will be counterclockwise rotation of the maxillomandibular complex and a large (temporary intraoperative) anterior open bite created if the maxilla is moved first.[5] Other times, the mandible may be operated first purely as a matter of surgeon preference.

Splint Fabrication

Most surgical splints are made with cold cure acrylic material. An ideal splint must be thin, yet strong, and devoid of interferences, air bubbles, and imperfections (Figure 56-26). Most clinicians prefer coverage of the splint to include at least the first molar tooth. However, this may allow extrusion of the second molars before splint removal; therefore, coverage of all teeth in the arch is recommended.

The steps involved in splint fabrication begin with application of separating media on the casts. A self-cure acrylic

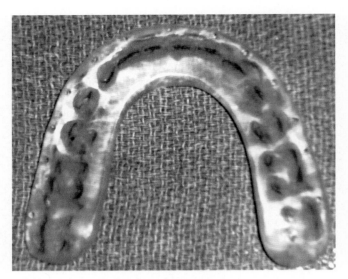

FIGURE 56-26. A final occlusal splint for an orthognathic surgical procedure that does not require a segmentalized maxilla. The regions that will accommodate the incisal tips of the teeth are marked with pencil to facilitate trimming. Holes are placed between the teeth within the flange of the splint for wires to be passed.

form is created and pressed between articulated casts. It is then cured in a pressure cooker and trimmed. Marks may be made with a pencil at the regions of the cusp tip indentations to prevent excessive trimming. Once the splint has been trimmed to be sufficiently thin, it is polished and small holes are made in the flange to allow for passing wires for assisting in intraoperative maxilla-mandible fixation.

While performing bimaxillary procedures that involve a segmental maxilla, the intermediate splint is a composite splint. This splint is constructed to fit over the final splint that remains attached to the maxilla (Figure 56-27). In segmental maxillary surgery, the final splint is often created with an additional palatal strap to prevent collapse of segments in the immediate postoperative phase. This splint is often left in place for several weeks to allow support for the

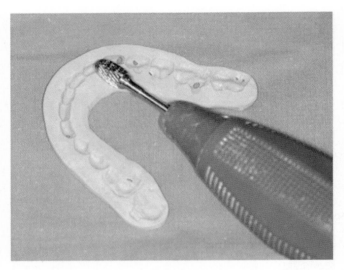

FIGURE 56-27. PVS intermediate splint trimmed, final occlusal splint surface.

segments. In cases that do not involve segmentalization, a splint fabricated from PVS may be used for both the intermediate and he final splint (Figure 56-28). When segmental maxillary surgery is performed, the final splint must be a rigid acrylic or composite splint, but the intermediate "piggy-back" splint may still be PVS. A PVS splint requires much less time and material to create and offers similar results (Figure 56-29).

Three-Dimensional Virtual Model Surgical Simulation

Introduction

Traditional model surgical planning has provided oral and maxillofacial surgeons with the ability to meticulously plan and perform orthognathic surgical procedures. Limitations and opportunities for the introduction of error through traditional model planning remain, however. The stone models are three-dimensional representations of the dentoalveolar

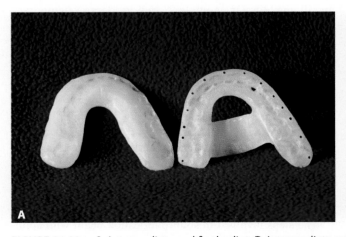

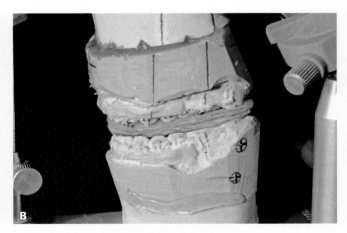

FIGURE 56-28. **A,** Intermediate and final splint. **B,** Intermediate splint *(red)* and final splint *(blue)* interdigitation on mounted casts.

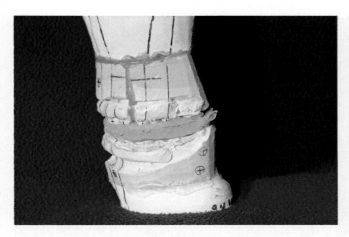

FIGURE 56-29. Intermediate splint fabricated with PVS and interdigitation to the acrylic final splint for this segmental bimaxillary case.

structure but cannot reflect the maxillofacial bony anatomy. Error can be introduced through an inaccurate facebow transfer, bite registration, mounting, or in obtaining model measurements. The entire process, even in experienced surgeons, is time- and labor-intensive. It also involves assimilating multiple unrelated data sets (such as the cephalometric film and clinical photos), which are two-dimensional representations. The use of a cephalometric radiograph analysis and cephalometric prediction tracings provides some level of simulation and prediction but is extremely limited because they are two-dimensional representations.

Advances in three-dimensional medical imaging and virtual surgical simulation software for orthognathic surgery have enabled a major breakthrough and allowed unprecedented virtual diagnosis, treatment planning, and evaluation of treatment outcomes of maxillofacial deformities. Virtual simulation allows for inclusion of the bony anatomy into the treatment plan, not relying solely on the position of the teeth and allows the surgeon to be able to

- Analyze three-dimensional anatomic discrepancies in pitch, roll, and yaw.
- Analyze how occlusal movements affect surrounding bony anatomy.
- Utilize simulated postoperative soft tissue and bony predictions for patient education and surgical resident teaching purposes.
- Investigate multiple surgical approaches for the same patient.
- Digitally create intermediate and final orthognathic splints using computer-aided design and computer-aided modeling (CAD/CAM) technology.
- Reduce surgeon planning time, especially for complex cases.

History

Xia and coworkers are the first group who used computer-aided surgical simulation (CASS) for treatment planning of complex craniomaxillofacial deformities.[6] The first step of the CASS process is to create a composite skull model. This

is accomplished with a bite jig that is used to relate the upper and lower dental casts to each other and to support a set of fiducial markers. Fiducial markers are selected points on an image that are used as a frame of reference in locating objects or in positioning (registering) images containing the same markers. After the bite jig is created, a computed tomography (CT) scan of the patient's craniofacial skeleton is obtained with the patient biting on the same bite jig. Scanning the stone dental models with a laser surface scanner then creates digital dental models. The markers are then used to register (superimpose) the digital dental models on to the three-dimensional CT skull model. The result is a computerized composite skull model with an accurate rendition of the bone and the teeth.

The second step of the CASS is to quantify the deformity with cephalometric analyses and virtual anthropometric measurements. The third step in the process is to simulate the surgery on the computer by moving the bony segments to the desired position. Using this software, the maxilla and mandible can be repositioned in all three planes of space. Hence, deformities of yaw, pitch, and roll can be accurately corrected in a virtual environment. The final step is to transfer the virtual plan to the operating room through surgical splints and templates that are created using a specialized CAD/CAM technique.

Whereas a number of CAD/CAM programs are currently commercially available for applications in craniofacial surgery and orthognathic surgery, CASS with the use of Simplant OMS (Materialise Dental, Ann Arbor, MI) software and the Medical Modeling Corporation (Golden, CO) are discussed and used as an example to illustrate a case sequence here.

Sequence of Virtual Simulated Surgery for an Orthognathic Surgical Procedure

1. The patient is clinically physically examined in the same fashion as one would for carrying out a traditional analytic model surgery and the same orthognathic database measurements are obtained and analyzed.
2. Digital photos of the patient in repose from the frontal, left, right, and while smiling, are obtained with the patient in a natural head position (NHP).
3. High-quality alginate impressions are obtained of the maxillary and mandibular dentition and stone casts are poured.
4. A final desired postoperative occlusion registration splint is fabricated from the models. This has the maxillary and mandibular teeth placed in their postoperative relationship. A cut and repositioned maxillary stone model is required if a segmental maxilla is planned.
5. A patient-specific bite jig is then created with the patient in CR. The jig will be used for the purpose of aligning a laser scan of the stone models and allows for detailed reorientation of the CT scan to the patient's NHP.
6. The jig is attached to a facebow and the patient's NHP is identified. Three Euler angle (pitch, roll, and yaw) readings (in degrees) are recorded with a gyroscope. The NHP may be established by asking the patient to look at a wall

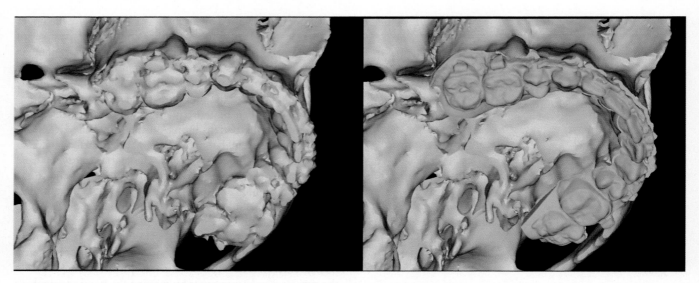

FIGURE 56-30. For an accurate occlusal surface, high-resolution laser scans of stone models are taken and integrated into the computed tomography/cone beam computed tomography (CT/CBCT) scan using fiducial marker registration.

without looking at a specific point or by the patient looking into his or her own eyes in a mirror with a plumb line hanging down the center of the mirror. If the patient has a tendency to orient his or her head forcefully (seen predominantly in asymmetry cases), the surgeon should intervene as necessary.

7. Following the appropriate CT scan protocol, a standard CT or cone beam computed tomography (CBCT) scan is obtained. This scan is obtained with the patient occluding on the bite jig, in CR, attached to the facebow.

Image Acquisition for Three-Dimensional Virtual Orthognathic Surgery

The surgeon must consider three important concepts in preparing data for successful digital orthognathic planning:

1. CT technology currently lacks the ability to capture the teeth and their occlusal surfaces with high accuracy. To produce accurate CAD/CAM splints, it is necessary to replace inaccurate occlusal surfaces from CT or CBCT scans with either a high-resolution laser scan or CT scan of the stone models (Figure 56-30).
2. Reorientation of the patient's CT/CBCT scan is needed to reflect their NHP for more accurate planning. This is accomplished utilizing the preoperative gyroscope Euler angle readings (Figure 56-31).
3. The quality of the CT scan is the most important aspect of creating a patient-specific anatomic model. The patient must wear the bite jig and attached fiducial facebow throughout the entire scan. For a standard CT, scans should be acquired at a high spatial resolution with thin (0.75–1.25 mm) image slices, a field of view of 20.0 to 25.0 cm, 0-degree gantry tilt with the patient's occlusal plane parallel to the gantry, and no motion artifact. The scans should be archived in DICOM (digital imaging and communications in medicine) format on a CD-R.

The digital clinical photos, upper and lower stone casts, clinical orthognathic database measurements, the acrylic bite jig, final occlusion registration, CT datasets, and the gyroscopic natural head position readings are then shipped to a software engineer for computer rendering.

Virtual Treatment Planning of Orthognathic Surgery

The software engineer then creates digital dental models by scanning the stone casts with a laser surface scanner. The digital dental casts are integrated into the digital CT skull using a best-fit model (Figure 56-32). This software offers the possibility of planning surgical procedures in multiplanar and three-dimensional views. Therefore, segmentation, measurement, repositioning, and importing tools are incorporated. All planning steps are based on virtual segmentation procedures, which are necessary for performing repositioning. By using predefined Le Fort I and sagittal (or vertical ramus) osteotomy lines, the upper (Figure 56-33) and lower jaws (Figure 56-34) can be segmented and virtually moved in all three planes of space.

A surgical plan is outlined and executed during a web conference with a software engineer. The maxillary and mandibular osteotomies are performed and movements are made with the patient's composite CT scan in the previously defined NHP. Deformities of yaw, pitch, and roll can be virtually corrected and accurately assessed using precise angular and linear digital measurements. Any inaccuracies in the virtual plan can then be corrected based on the virtual image analysis.

TRANSFERRING VIRTUAL TREATMENT PLANNING TO THE OPERATING ROOM
After the surgical plan has been finalized, it is necessary to transfer the plan to the patient at surgery. Similar to traditional model surgery, dental splints are created for this purpose, but in this case, the intermediate (see Figure 56-33) and final (see Figure 56-34) digital surgical splints are fabricated by CAD/

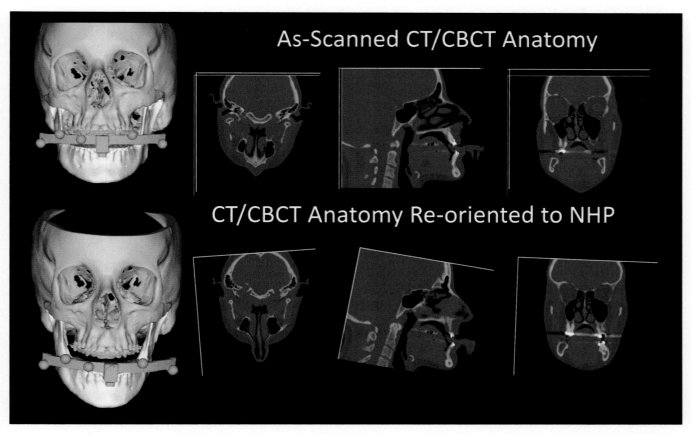

FIGURE 56-31.   The patient is CT/CBCT scanned in centric relation wearing a facebow device and neutral head posture (NHP) is clinically recorded by the surgeon using a gyroscope device. These orientation measurements are applied to the CT/CBCT scan to reorient the patient's digital data into the proper NHP.

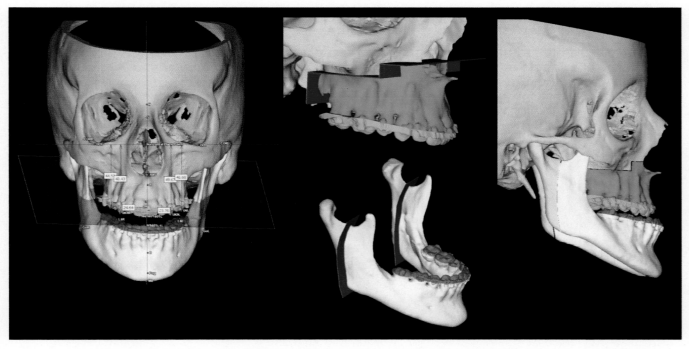

FIGURE 56-32.   The patient's asymmetry is quantified using digital bony landmarks and measurements to orthogonal reference planes. Digital osteotomies are performed on both the upper and the lower jaws.

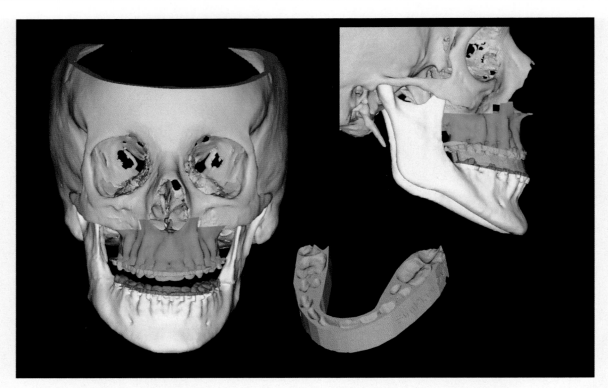

FIGURE 56-33. The maxilla is moved to its final position, and a computer-aided design and computer-aided modeling (CAD/CAM) intermediate splint is designed from the digital plan.

CAM technique. In procedures that require bone grafts to achieve symmetry, the computerized mirror-imaging technique can be used to provide a mirror image of the geometry from the healthy side to the affected side. The difference between the two sides can then be computed, resulting in a digital template that is used at surgery to harvest the graft and sculpt it or the implant. Vertical measurement is accomplished in either of the two methods mentioned earlier.

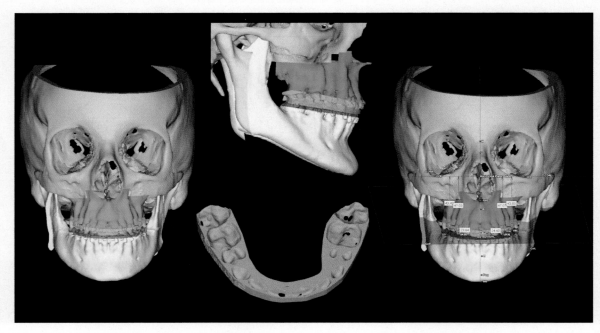

FIGURE 56-34. The mandible is moved into final occlusion and a final position CAD/CAM splint is designed from the digital plan. The simulated final position of the bony anatomy can be assessed using digital cephalometric analyses.

Much can be gained planning these cases in a virtual manner, similar to virtual planning of implant cases. The stumbling blocks at this time are need for the CT scan and the overall cost of the process.

REFERENCES

1. Bell RB. Computer planning and intraoperative navigation in craniomaxillofacial surgery. Oral Maxillofacial Surg Clin North Am 2010; 22:135–156.
2. Ellis E, Tharanon W, Gambrell K. A study on the accuracy of facebow transfer: effect of surgical prediction and postsurgical result. J Oral Maxillofac Surg 1992; 50:562–567.
3. The glossary of prosthodontic terms. J of Prosthet Dent 2005; 94: 10–92.
4. Posnick JC, Ricalde P, Ng P. A modified approach to "model planning" in orthognathic surgery for patients without a reliable centric relation. J Oral Maxillofac Surg 2006; 64:347–356.
5. Cottrell DA, Wolford LM. Altered orthognathic surgical sequencing and a modified approach to model surgery. J Oral Maxillofac Surg 1994; 52:1010–1020.
6. Xia JJ, Samman N, Wang D. Computer assisted three dimensional surgical planning and simulation: 3D virtual osteotomy. Int J Oral Maxillofac Surg 2000;29: 1–17.

Suggested Readings

Traditional Analytical Model Surgery

Anwar M, Harris M. Model surgery for orthognathic planning. Br J Oral Maxillofac Surg 1990;28:393.

Bamber MA, Firouzai R, Harris M, Linney AD. A comparative study of two arbitrary face bow transfer systems for orthognathic surgery planning. Int J Oral Maxillofac Surg 1996;25:339–343.

Bamber MA, Harris M. The role of occlusal wafers in orthognathic surgery: a comparison of thick and thin intermediate osteotomy wafers. J Craniomaxillofac Surg 1995;23:396–400.

Campos AA, Nathanson D, Rose L. Reproducibility and condylar position of a physiologic maxillomandibular centric relation in upright and supine body position. J Prosth Dent 1996;76:282.

Ellis E. Accuracy of model surgery: evaluation of old technique and introduction of a new one. J Oral Maxillofac Surg 1990;48:1161.

Ellis E. Bimaxillary surgery using an intermediate splint to reposition the maxilla. J Oral Maxillofac Surg 1999;57:53.

Ellis E, Johnson DG, Hayward JR. Use of the orthognathic simulating instrument in the presurgical evaluation of facial asymmetry. J Oral Maxillofac Surg 1984;42:805–811.

Erickson KL, Bell WH, Goldsmith DH. Analytical model surgery. In Bell WH, editor Modern Practice in Orthognathic and Reconstructive Surgery. Vol I. Philadelphia: WB Saunders; 1992; pp. 154–216.

Miles BA, Hansen BJ, Stella JP. Polyvinylsiloxane as an alternative material for the intermediate orthognathic occlusal splint. J Oral Maxillofac Surg 2006;64:1318.

O'Malley MA, Milosevic A. Comparison of three face bow/semi adjustable articulator systems for planning orthognathic surgery. Br J Oral Maxillofac Surg 2000;38:185–190.

Ong TK, Banks RJ, Hildreth AJ. Surgical accuracy in Lefort I maxillary osteotomies. Br J Oral Maxillofac Surg 2001;39: 96–102.

Polido WD, Ellis E, Sinn DP. An assessment of the predictability of maxillary repositioning. Int J Oral Maxillofac Surg 1991;20:349.

Renzi G, Carboni A, Gasparini G, et al. Intraoperative measurement of maxillary repositioning in a series of 30 patients with maxillomandibular asymmetries. Int J Adult Orthod Orthognath Surg 2002;17:111–115.

Rinchuse DJ, Kandasamy S. Centric relation: a historical and contemporary orthodontic perspective J Am Dent Assoc 2006;137:494.

Truitt J, Strauss RA, Best A. Centric relation: a survey study to determine whether a consensus exists between oral and maxillofacial surgeons and orthodontists. J Oral Maxillofac Surg 2009;67:1058.

Virtual Simulated Orthognathic Surgery

Gateno J, Teichgraeber JF, Xia JJ. Three-dimensional surgical planning for maxillary and midface distraction osteogenesis. J Craniofac Surg 2003;14:833.

Gateno J, Xia JJ, Teichgraeber JF, et al. Clinical feasibility of computer aided surgical simulation (CASS) in the treatment of complex craniomaxillofacial deformities. J Oral Maxillofac Surg 2007;65:728–734.

Gateno J, Xia J, Teichgraeber JF, et al. A new technique for the creation of a computerized composite skull model. J Oral Maxillofac Surg 2003;61:222.

Metzger MC, Hohlwe-Majert B, Schwarz U, et al. Manufacturing splints of orthognathic surgery using a three dimensional printer. Oral Surg Oral Med Oral Pathol Oral Radiol Endod 2008;105:e1–e7.

Noguchi N, Tsuji M, Shigematsu M, et al. An orthognathic simulation system integrating teeth, jaw and face data using 3D cephalometry. Int J Oral Maxillofac Surg 2007;36:640–645.

Olszewski R, Villamil MB, Trevisan DG, et al. Towards an integrated system for planning and assisting maxillofacial orthognathic surgery. Comput Methods Programs Biomed 2008;91: 13–21.

Papadopoulos MA, Christou PK, Athanasiou AE, et al. Three-dimensional craniofacial reconstruction imaging. Oral Surg Oral Med Oral Pathol Oral Radiol Endod 2002;93:382.

Santler G. 3D COSMOS: a new 3D model based computerized operation simulation and navigation system. J Maxillofac Surg 2000;28:287.

Santler G. The Graz hemisphere splint: a new precise, non-invasive method of replacing the dental arch of 3D models by plaster models. J Craniomaxillofac Surg 1998;26:169.

Swennen GRJ, Mollemans W, Schutyser F. Three-dimensional treatment planning for orthognathic surgery in the era of virtual imaging. J Oral Maxillofac Surg 2009;67:2080.

Swennen GR, Mommaerts MY, Abeloos J, et al. The use of a wax bite wafer and a double computed tomography scan procedure to obtain a three dimensional model. J Craniofac Surg 2007;18:533–539.

Troulis MJ, Everett P, Seldin EB, et al. Development of a three-dimensional treatment planning system based on computed tomographic data. Int J Oral Maxillofac Surg 2002;31:349.

Xia JJ, Gateno J, Teichgraeber JF. New clinical protocol to evaluate craniomaxillofacial deformity and plan surgical correction. J Oral Maxillofac Surg 2009;67:2093–2106.

Xia JJ, Gateno J, Teichgraeber JF. Three-dimensional computer-aided surgical simulation for maxillofacial surgery. Atlas Oral Maxillofac Surg Clin North Am 2005;13:25–72.

Mandibular Orthognathic Surgery

Dale S. Bloomquist, DDS, MS, and Jessica J. Lee, DDS

The development of mandibular osteotomies for correction of dentofacial deformities closely parallels the advancement of oral and maxillofacial surgery as a specialty more than any other group of surgical techniques. From Hullihen in 1849, who was the first to describe a mandibular osteotomy, to Obwegeser in 1955, who developed the sagittal osteotomy of the vertical ramus, there has been dramatic progress in the techniques of mandibular osteotomies. After Obwegeser's original paper in German, and especially since his description of techniques in the English literature, orthognathic surgery has seen dramatic changes in use as well as refinement of the osteotomies. Although the development of osteotomy techniques is ongoing, the purpose of this chapter is to describe the most commonly used surgical procedures for the mandible and also to emphasize the refinements in technique that have been the result of the most recent clinical as well as basic science research.

HISTORY

Hullihen[1] corrected a burn patient with an anterior open bite and mandibular dentoalveolar protrusion with an intraoral osteotomy, similar to an anterior subapical osteotomy (Figure 57-1). His efforts did not stimulate much interest, because it was almost 50 years later when Angle[2] described a body osteotomy done by V. P. Blair[3] (Figure 57-2A) for a patient with mandibular horizontal excess. This technique, with minor modifications, was advocated until the 1970s. Since then, the only major modifications in the body osteotomy that have occurred are a greater emphasis on preserving the inferior alveolar nerve (IAN) and a change to an intraoral approach.

The horizontal osteotomy of the vertical ramus popularized by Blair[4] (see Figure 57-2B) was performed through an extraoral approach. As with many of the early mandibular procedures, a horizontal bone cut was made above the lingula and was described for correction of both mandibular horizontal deficiency and horizontal excess. An intraoral technique was not suggested until Ernst[5] discussed his procedure approximately 25 years later. This method of correcting mandibular deformities was used for almost 60 years, but because of its lack of postoperative stability, it has fallen into disuse.

The subcondylar osteotomy (see Figure 57-2C), a description of which was first reported by Limberg[6] as an extraoral technique, has undergone relatively minor refinements to the intraoral vertical subcondylar osteotomy (VSO) that is used today. There has, however, been a substantial number of osteotomy designs involving the vertical ramus that begin in the sigmoid notch, which has led to some confusion in the nomenclature of what is a fairly closely related group of ramus osteotomies. The names that have been developed have generally been based upon the length and direction of the cuts made in the posterior portion of the vertical ramus. The subcondylar osteotomy was used to describe the condylar neck osteotomies of Kostecka[7] and Moose.[8] Generally, longer cuts that extended to the posterior border above the angle, such as described by Limberg, Thoma, and Robinson, were referred to as "oblique osteotomies."[5–10] Shira, however, coined the term "oblique sliding osteotomy" for this particular surgical procedure.[11] Finally, Caldwell and Letterman[12] described a vertical osteotomy of the mandibular ramus that included a cut from the sigmoid notch to the inferior border, in front of the angle of the mandible. The cut was posterior to the mandibular foramen, and a portion of the lateral cortex

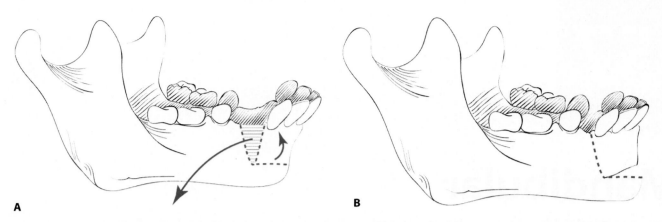

A   **B**

FIGURE 57-1.   Hullihen's mandibular subapical osteotomy. (Adapted from Bloomquist DS. Principles of mandibular orthognathic surgery. In Peterson LJ, Indresano AT, Marciani RD, Roser SM, editors. Principles of Oral and Maxillofacial Surgery. Vol 3. Philadelphia: JB Lippincott; 1992; p. 1416.)

of the distal fragment was decorticated to allow a larger area of bony contact. In general, these latter two groups of osteotomies are now called "vertical osteotomies," but some semantic differences still persist. Specifically, the terms *vertical subcondylar osteotomy (VSO)* and *vertical ramus osteotomy (VRO)* are still used interchangeably in the literature. Primarily, this type of osteotomy was designed for correction of mandibular horizontal excess, or mandibular asymmetries, although Robinson[10] described its use with a bone graft for advancement in horizontal deficiencies of the mandible.

The intraoral approach to the subcondylar osteotomy was first described by Moose in 1964.[13] He approached the condylar neck medially with a straight bur. Winstanley[14] suggested a lateral approach in 1968, but it was not until Hebert and colleagues[15] described the use of a special oscillating saw that this approach became popular.

A variation of the VSO was suggested by Wassmund in 1927[16] (Figure 57-3A), which is similar to what is now called the *inverted-L osteotomy*. Pichler and Trauner[17] later suggested inserting bone grafts into the defect created by advancement of the mandible. Caldwell and coworkers[18] further modified the inverted-L by adding a horizontal cut just above the inferior border of the mandible to create what is now called the *C osteotomy* (see Figure 57-3B). The stated advantage of the C osteotomy was that the bone cut design made the use of a bone graft unnecessary. This advantage

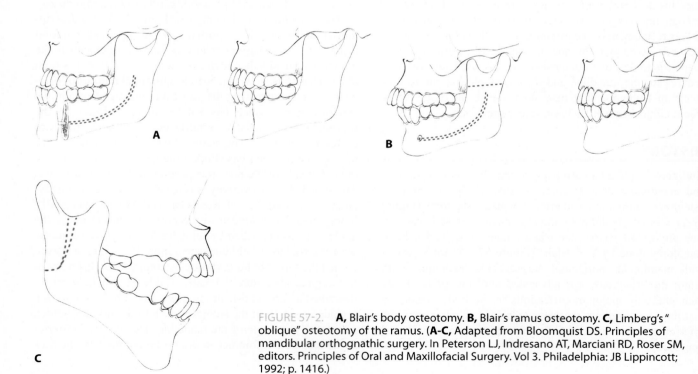

A

B

C

FIGURE 57-2.   **A,** Blair's body osteotomy. **B,** Blair's ramus osteotomy. **C,** Limberg's "oblique" osteotomy of the ramus. (**A-C,** Adapted from Bloomquist DS. Principles of mandibular orthognathic surgery. In Peterson LJ, Indresano AT, Marciani RD, Roser SM, editors. Principles of Oral and Maxillofacial Surgery. Vol 3. Philadelphia: JB Lippincott; 1992; p. 1416.)

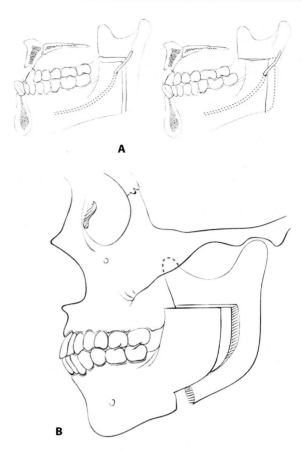

FIGURE 57-3.   **A,** L osteotomy. **B,** C osteotomy. (**A** and **B,** Adapted from Bloomquist DS. Principles of mandibular orthognathic surgery. In Peterson LJ, Indresano AT, Marciani RD, Roser SM, editors. Principles of Oral and Maxillofacial Surgery. Vol 3. Philadelphia: JB Lippincott; 1992; p. 1417.)

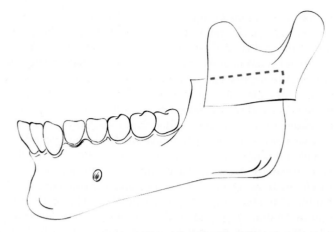

FIGURE 57-4.   Lane's osteotomy. (Adapted from Bloomquist DS. Principles of mandibular orthognathic surgery. In Peterson LJ, Indresano AT, Marciani RD, Roser SM, editors. Principles of Oral and Maxillofacial Surgery. Vol 3. Philadelphia: JB Lippincott; 1992; p. 1417.)

vertical cut through the lateral cortex as well as the suggestion that the medial horizontal cut be extended only to a point above the lingula and not to the posterior border (Figure 57-5). This latter technique shortens the split posteriorly, to the area of the retrolingular fossa and not to the posterior border, and as was further discussed by Hunsuck,[25] decreases the trauma to the overlying soft tissues. Many clinicians have

was further enhanced by the modification suggested by Hayes,[19] with the splitting of the inferior limb sagittally so that more bone contact could be achieved. A further interesting approach to this group of VROs used for horizontal mandibular deficiency is the modified-L osteotomy described by Fox and Tilson.[20] They eliminated the superior horizontal cut of the C osteotomy and, instead, extended the vertical cut to the sigmoid notch. Then the coronoid process was removed and added as a free graft into the defect resulting from the mandibular advancement.

The greatest development in osteotomies of the vertical ramus is the sagittal osteotomy, credited to Obwegeser and Trauner, but generally now used in a fashion modified from the original technique described in 1955.[21] Lane has been referred to as the developer of a form of the sagittal osteotomy, with parallel horizontal bone cuts made through the medial and lateral cortices of the vertical ramus (Figure 57-4).[22] The medial cut was made just above the lingula, with the lateral cut made just below it. This idea was expanded by Schuchardt[23] before being refined and popularized by Obwegeser and Trauner.[21] The major modifications in the osteotomy design were first made by DalPont[24] with his

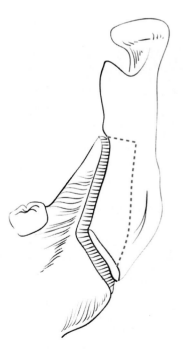

FIGURE 57-5.   DalPont's modification of the sagittal osteotomy. (Adapted from Bloomquist DS. Principles of mandibular orthognathic surgery. In Peterson LJ, Indresano AT, Marciani RD, Roser SM, editors. Principles of Oral and Maxillofacial Surgery. Vol 3. Philadelphia: JB Lippincott; 1992; p. 1418.)

offered suggestions for improving the sagittal osteotomy, but the only other major innovation to this technique has been the use of internal rigid fixation. Spiessl[26] suggested the use of screws for fixation of the fragments in the sagittal osteotomy. Although wire osseous fixation is still used by some surgeons, rigid internal fixation in some form (bicortical screws or monocortical plates and screws) has become the standard technique for the bilateral sagittal split osteotomy (BSSO).

Osteotomies of the mandibular body do not generally receive the same degree of attention as osteotomies of the vertical ramus, but they have undergone refinements and variations from the original anterior alveolar osteotomies of Hullihen[1] and the body osteotomies of Blair.[3] The first variation of Hullihen's procedure did not appear until 90 years after the original description, when Hofer[27] described an anterior mandibular alveolar osteotomy to advance anterior teeth in correction of mandibular dentoalveolar retrusion (Figure 57-6A). Kole[28] modified this procedure by suggesting the use of bone grafts from the mental region to the defect caused by the rotation of the anterior dentoalveolar segment (see Figure 57-6B). Clinicians now employing Hofer's osteotomy generally use some form of bone graft in the alveolar defect if significant movement of the fragment is planned. Mandibular alveolar osteotomies have expanded

primarily in two ways from Hofer's original procedure. Kent and Hinds[29] initially presented the use of the single-tooth osteotomies of the mandible in 1971, and MacIntosh[30] closely followed with his description of the total mandibular alveolar osteotomy in 1974. The latter procedure continues to be popular, with minor variations recommended by other clinicians.

Osteotomies of the body of the mandible have been described in almost every conceivable form, with the most durable advancements being the step osteotomy, initially described by Von Eiselberg in 1906[31] (Figure 57-7A), and the horizontal osteotomy of the symphysis described by Hofer in 1942[32] (see Figure 57-7B). The step osteotomy was originally described for treatment of mandibular horizontal deficiency,

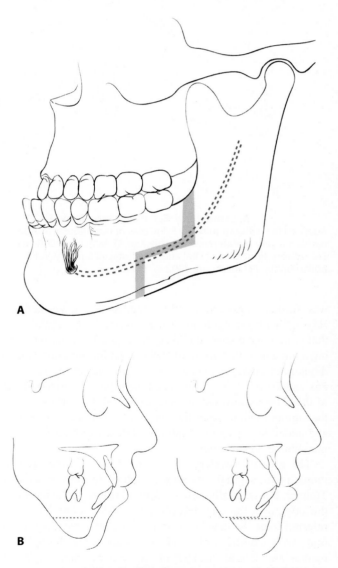

FIGURE 57-7. **A,** Von Eiselberg's step osteotomy. **B,** Hofer's horizontal osteotomy. (**A** and **B,** Adapted from Bloomquist DS. Principles of mandibular orthognathic surgery. In Peterson LJ, Indresano AT, Marciani RD, Roser SM, editors. Principles of Oral and Maxillofacial Surgery. Vol 3. Philadelphia: JB Lippincott; 1992; p. 1419.)

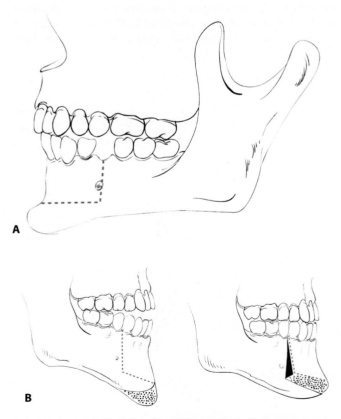

FIGURE 57-6. **A,** Hofer's subapical osteotomy. **B,** Kole's subapical osteotomy. (**A** and **B,** Adapted from Bloomquist DS. Principles of mandibular orthognathic surgery. In Peterson LJ, Indresano AT, Marciani RD, Roser SM, editors. Principles of Oral and Maxillofacial Surgery. Vol 3. Philadelphia: JB Lippincott; 1992; p. 1418.)

but it has been used in various forms for mandibular horizontal excess as well as asymmetry. The horizontal osteotomy of the symphysis has also developed a large degree of versatility, with its use in various forms being suggested for almost any skeletal deformity of the bony chin.

ANATOMIC AND PHYSIOLOGIC CONSIDERATIONS OF MANDIBULAR SURGERIES

Vascular Supply

A major concern with surgery of the facial skeleton is the vascular supply to the bony segments. This was demonstrated dramatically by the explosion of orthognathic surgery in the United States, after Bell and Levy's studies of vascular effects of the osteotomies.[33] Although all of the techniques they evaluated had been previously used in patients, there had not been any experimental evaluations of the physiologic basis for many of the procedures. Bell and Levy's work demonstrated that blood flow through the mandibular periosteum could easily maintain a sufficient blood supply to the teeth of a mobile segment, even when the labial periosteum was degloved. Blood flow from the periosteum was considered to be centripetal, to distinguish it from the blood flowing from endosteal vessels outward (centrifugal) that was associated with long bones. Previously, clinicians believed that the inferior alveolar artery had a primary role in nourishing the mandible, but Bell and Levy[33] demonstrated that there is also a sufficient blood supply from the surrounding soft tissues, even if the inferior alveolar artery was compromised. More recent work in animals suggests that the blood supply to the body of the mandible under normal conditions comes almost entirely from the inferior alveolar artery.[34] However, when this source is obstructed, the peripheral blood vessels quickly take over for the anterior mandible. The posterior mandibular dentoalveolus, however, does not benefit from this kind of collateral blood supply, which calls into question the safety of posterior mandibular segmental alveolar osteotomies. Zisser and Gattinger[35] showed pulpal necrosis in the molars of horizontal osteotomies done above the IAN in the body of the mandible of dogs.

The safety of combined mandibular osteotomies, such as ramal procedures and body osteotomies, has been a concern because of the predominant role of the inferior alveolar artery.[36] The fragility of the vascular supply to the mandibular alveolus engenders some concern over the common use of subapical osteotomies. Although their relative safety has been demonstrated by both animal studies and substantial clinical experience, subapical osteotomies need to be carefully planned to ensure as large a vascular pedicle as possible.[33,37] Complications, such as pulpal necrosis, soft tissue defects, and loss of teeth and bone, have demonstrated the delicate nature of the blood supply, especially when attempts to move small dentoalveolar fragments are made. The effect of aging on the vascular supply to the mandibular body is an area about which very little information is known, particu-

larly whether aging causes a switch from the centrifugal to the centripetal blood supply. Bradley[38] has demonstrated an apparent decreasing capacity of the inferior alveolar vessels that occurs with aging, but the impact of this effect on mandibular osteotomies is unknown. Subapical osteotomies are not routinely performed today.

Osteotomy designs of the vertical ramus have profited from studies of the effects of surgery on vascular supply. The proximal segment of the vertical subsigmoid osteotomy maintains its blood supply through the temporomandibular joint (TMJ) capsule and the attachment of the lateral pterygoid muscle. However, the inferior tip of this fragment may undergo vascular necrosis based upon prior experimental studies.[39] This observation led to the suggestion that fewer problems may occur if the cut is made above the angle of the mandible.[39]

The importance of the periosteal blood supply as well as the endosteal supply in the vertical ramus has been explored by animal research.[40–43] When the medial pterygoid and masseter muscles are stripped, both blood flow and blood supply studies have demonstrated the possibility of avascular necrosis in the proximal segment. Comparisons of extensive muscle stripping of the vertical ramus versus preservation of the masseter attachment have demonstrated a significant difference in the vascularity of the inferior portion of the proximal fragment. These studies of blood supply of the vertical ramus may be of value in predicting the vascular effects of the C or L osteotomies. However, resorption of the proximal fragment has not been reported in these particular bone cuts, possibly because of the rarity of their use. However, given the available research, it is prudent to minimize the periosteal and muscle attachment stripping on the medial surface of the proximal fragment with either the C or the L osteotomy, or any of their variations.

The last unanswered question concerning vascular supply in mandibular orthognathic surgery is the determination of a safe distance away from the apex of the teeth to make horizontal bone cuts. Much of the data addressing this question are based upon research about the maxilla.[44] From these early animal studies, the pulpal blood supply of a tooth should not be affected if a cut is made at least 5 mm away from the apex of the tooth root. Zisser and Gattinger,[35] however, saw pulpal changes in dogs with some horizontal cuts that were made 10 mm away from the apex. Whether these distances have any relevance to humans is unknown. Clinically, the incidence of tooth devitalization from horizontal subapical osteotomies is extremely low and it can be assumed that, for the most part, 5 mm is an adequate guideline. A cut made 10 mm from the apices, although allowing a greater safety margin, is often impractical because of other anatomic limitations. The greater distance from the apices of the teeth not only minimizes direct pulpal injury but also increases the vascular pedicle to the mobilized segment.

Nerves

The surgeon working around the face must be constantly aware of the nerve network that exists in this area.

Fortunately, in considering the mandible, these concerns can be narrowed down to essentially two major nerves: the marginal mandibular branch of the seventh cranial nerve and the third division of the trigeminal nerve, and most frequently, one of its branches, the IAN. The marginal mandibular branch is usually at risk only during extraoral procedures. Although trauma to this nerve has been reported to occur during an intraoral approach, it is rare and, for the most part, appears to be preventable. Avoiding damage to this nerve during extraoral approaches to the mandible is a major surgical goal; in most cases of orthognathic surgery, it is achieved because soft tissue anatomy in patients undergoing the surgery has not been disturbed by disease or trauma. The techniques of these approaches, as well as the methods for minimizing the risks of damage to the marginal mandibular branch, are covered elsewhere in this text. Damage to the third division of the trigeminal nerve is, however, a much-discussed issue in mandibular surgery. The course of the IAN into the vertical ramus and then through the body of the mandible makes it extremely susceptible to damage from almost every mandibular surgical procedure. In most cases, the surgeon's main goal relative to this nerve is to minimize the trauma, because its avoidance is almost impossible. In the past, surgeons stressed the importance of looking for and sometimes freeing up the nerve as it either entered or left the mandible before making osteotomies in the areas of the foramina. However, there is a trend toward avoiding this step, unless it is absolutely necessary to make the osteotomy as close to the nerve as possible. The simple act of exposing the nerve seems to increase the chance for postoperative sensory deficiency.

Often, the debates regarding whether one mandibular osteotomy is preferable to another are primarily based on the potential of damaging the IAN. This has resulted in many clinicians trivializing the damage found after certain technique. Well-defined standards for both long- and short-term follow-up of nerve damage during mandibular procedures have been discussed[45]; however, in most papers, these have not been used to evaluate sensory deficits. In addition, very few controlled studies have been published comparing procedures, so, as a result, not much can be concluded regarding any of the various attempts to minimize nerve damage.

Studies evaluating the loss of tooth sensibility from horizontal osteotomies below the dental apices, however, have been quite consistent. Most authors found a relatively high loss of response to pulp testing immediately after osteotomies, especially when teeth are close to a vertical osteotomy.[46-48] However, this loss may not correlate with actual loss of tooth vitality and, thus, either tooth loss secondary to an osteotomy or the need for endodontic therapy is very low.

Muscles

Orthognathic surgery affects muscles in primarily in one of two ways: it may change the length of a muscle or it may change the direction of muscle function. Effects of these changes are still not understood, although various authors have emphasized the importance of recognizing and controlling muscular alterations of orthognathic surgery. The muscles commonly discussed in orthognathic surgery of the mandible have been the muscles of mastication and the suprahyoid group of muscles. Recent interest on the soft tissue effects of facial skeletal surgery has expanded interest to the other facial mimetic muscles. This latter group, however, has generally not been discussed relative to mandibular osteotomies, with the possible exception of the effect of anterior mandibular osteotomies on the attachment of the mentalis muscle. The muscles of mastication, however, have received considerable attention, dating back to the early vertical ramus procedures. Research interest on the effects of altering these muscles concentrated either on their effect on skeletal changes, especially relapse after mandibular osteotomies, or on the changes in function of these muscles.

Distraction of the superior segment of a horizontal osteotomy of the vertical ramus owing to the temporalis muscle influence after surgery was noted early by surgeons who used this technique.[49] Evaluation of this procedure after correction of prognathism found a superior movement of the mandible in the gonial region as well as a downward and backward movement at the symphysis. This change, which was attributed to the forces of the pterygomasseteric sling, has received considerable attention, not only in mandibular setbacks done with osteotomies through the vertical ramus but also in mandibular advancements.[50-55] The apparent shortening of the vertical ramus has been noted in a number of studies, and in some, a correlation has been demonstrated between this change and the posterior movement of the symphysis. The exact reason for the change in the gonion has not been clearly demonstrated. Kohn[54] demonstrated the movement of this point inferoanteriorly in mandibular advancements by way of a measurement he termed the "gonial arc" (Figure 57-8). Most investigators believe this represents distraction of the condyle from the fossa, and this hypothesis was further supported by the migration of the gonion back during the postoperative period.[54,55] The long-term postoperative decrease in gonial arc was generally believed to be due to remodeling, especially resorption that occurred at the mandibular angle.[40,43] Especially in early studies, resorption could have accounted for this change because of the accepted technique of completely stripping muscle attachments from the proximal segment. However, in more recent studies in which minimal muscle stripping was done, a similar result has been noted.[56,57] Will and associates[58] noted condylar distraction followed by an "overshoot" in the resettling of the condyle in the fossa. This change in condylar position may be due to either displacement of the disk within the TMJ or compression of the soft tissues of the joint by increased pressures secondary to the muscles of the pterygomasseteric sling.

The rotational change in the proximal segment of a mandibular osteotomy has been implicated in relapse by multiple clinicians who believe that the muscles of the pterygomasseteric sling reassert themselves after the surgery.[59,60]

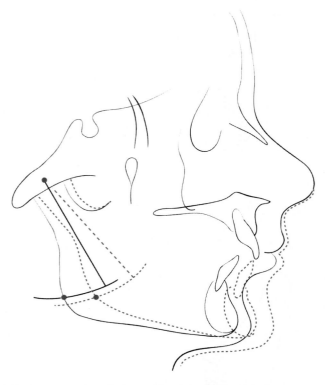

FIGURE 57-8.   Gonial arc used for showing condylar position change with a mandibular osteotomy. (Adapted from Bloomquist DS. Principles of mandibular orthognathic surgery. In Peterson LJ, Indresano AT, Marciani RD, Roser SM, editors. Principles of Oral and Maxillofacial Surgery. Vol 3. Philadelphia: JB Lippincott; 1992; p. 1422.)

Therefore, there has been an emphasis on carefully repositioning the proximal segment as close as possible to its preoperative position, which is a difficult task because there are many variable influences acting on condylar position that are different when records are obtained in an upright and awake position as opposed to supine under general anesthesia. Unfortunately, a correlation between mandibular ramus positioning and relapse in the case of mandibular advancements has never been demonstrated. A few studies have shown a relation between relapse of mandibular setback surgeries and the position of the vertical ramus.[61] It has been noted in these surgeries that the degree of clockwise rotation of the proximal fragment in a sagittal osteotomy seems to relate to the amount of forward relapse of the distal segment. Franco and colleagues[61] theorized that both a stretching of the medial pterygoid muscle as well as the elongation of the anterior fibers of the masseter and temporalis muscles from the clockwise rotation of the proximal segment can contribute to relapse in lengthening the muscles of the pterygomasseteric sling. This can result in a change in mandibular position as has been documented by Yellich and coworkers.[62] The degree to which this is active in orthognathic surgery remains unclear.

The contribution of the suprahyoid muscles to relapse in mandibular advancement surgery is equivocal, with many clinicians supporting an existence of this relationship. Ellis and Carlson[63] demonstrated in monkeys that relieving the suprahyoid muscles from the symphysis of the mandible decreased the amount of relapse when the mandibles were advanced. Clinical studies, however, have failed to show a relation between suprahyoid myotomies and relapse.[64,65] Animal studies have also demonstrated that adaptive changes occur in the connective tissues at the muscle-tendon and tendon-bone interfaces but only with large advancements.[66]

The belief, however unsubstantiated, that muscle pull in some way does affect the stability of mandibular osteotomies has led to a variety of recommendations. Historically, the most common method advocated is the attempt at minimizing the change in muscle position and length. The cutting of muscle attachments, such as has been recommended for the suprahyoid group, has the potential for increasing morbidity. Without significant evidence that this is of much value, this additional surgery cannot be justified. However, there has been recognition that muscles and their attachments seem to adapt fairly quickly if the bone is held rigidly for a long enough time.[66,67] It is important to recognize that intermaxillary fixation (IMF) does not provide a completely stable method of bone fixation, especially if the teeth have been under active orthodontic movement. In addition, the greatest amount of relapse of mandibular osteotomies seems to occur in the first 3 to 6 weeks after surgery. Whatever the causes of the instability during this time, several techniques have designed to provide increased stability for this initial period, to improve the stability of mandibular osteotomies. Primarily two techniques have been attempted: external supporting mechanisms and internal rigid fixation. The only external technique that has been of much value has been the wiring technique termed *skeletal fixation*. With this procedure, the bony skeletons are tied to one another, circumventing the periodontal ligaments of the teeth. This has been used with IMF, maintaining mandibular immobilization for 6 to 8 weeks (Figure 57-9).[58,67,68] The alternative procedures of internal rigid fixation techniques using plates or screws are discussed in the next section.

MANDIBULAR OSTEOTOMY TECHNIQUES

Mandibular Ramus Osteotomies

Osteotomies in the vertical ramus have been the preferred technique for correcting developmental deformities of the mandible. This preference has increased with closer cooperation between orthodontists and surgeons inztreating dentofacial deformities. Most of the time, the dental arch discrepancies can be corrected orthodontically, leaving to the surgeon the responsibility for moving the coordinated dental arch into its appropriate position, as dictated by functional and aesthetic demands. Operations in the vertical ramus, therefore, are considered primarily when the dental arch as a unit has to be moved. As previously noted, there are

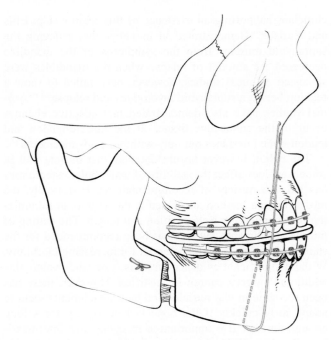

FIGURE 57-9.   Skeletal fixation used with maxillomandibular fixation or mandibular advancement. (Adapted from Bloomquist DS. Principles of mandibular orthognathic surgery. In Peterson LJ, Indresano AT, Marciani RD, Roser SM, editors. Principles of Oral and Maxillofacial Surgery. Vol 3. Philadelphia: JB Lippincott; 1992; p. 1423.)

numerous techniques for osteotomies of the ramus, but essentially three different procedures, with minor variations, are currently accepted techniques.

Vertical Ramus Osteotomy

Osteotomies extending from the sigmoid notch vertically behind the IAN foramen to the inferior border or angle have had several different names, but generally, the VRO seems to describe the procedure best (Figure 57-10). This osteotomy was initially done through an extraoral approach, but with the development of small offset oscillating blades with a long shaft, and adequate retraction, the intraoral route has become preferred.

Indications

The VRO has been limited to deformities requiring the mandible to be set back for mandibular horizontal excess or to be rotated for mandibular asymmetry. Robinson and Lytle[69] stated that this osteotomy can be used for mandibular advancement, but generally this recommendation was not accepted owing to questionable stability. Hall and Mc-Kenna[70] later revived this indication for minor (2–3 mm) advancements.

Technique

When preparing for an intraoral VRO, one needs to closely evaluate the panoramic and lateral head films for the position

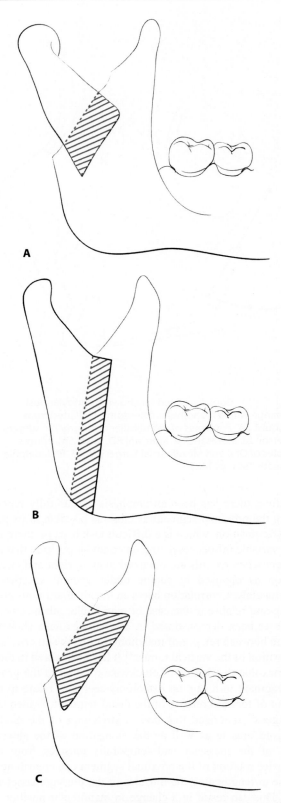

A

B

C

FIGURE 57-10.   Different lengths of the osteotomy in the vertical subcondylar osteotomies (VSOs). (Adapted from Bloomquist DS. Principles of mandibular orthognathic surgery. In Peterson LJ, Indresano AT, Marciani RD, Roser SM, editors. Principles of Oral and Maxillofacial Surgery. Vol 3. Philadelphia: JB Lippincott; 1992; p. 1423.)

of the inferior alveolar foramen relative to the posterior border of the mandible. The incision is made in the mucosa from midway up the anterior border of the ramus to the first molar area. The periosteum is reflected laterally to expose the entire ramus, with the exception of the condyle neck and coronoid tip. The posterior and inferior borders can be cleared of periosteum; but muscle attachments at the angle are generally difficult to elevate and should be left to ensure blood supply to this area. A special retractor, Merrill-Levaseur, fits around the posterior border and retracts tissue laterally, so that an oscillating saw can be used (Figure 57-11A). Also, Bauer retractors, left and right, can be used superiorly in the sigmoid notch and inferiorly in the antegonial notch for additional retraction and visualization.

The saw chosen should have a rounded blade that is set at an obtuse angle to the long shaft of the drill to facilitate the osteotomy. The blade should be used first to score the proposed osteotomy line on the lateral cortex. This line is then closely checked for its position relative to the sigmoid notch, posterior border, and angle. The use of the so-called antilingula has been proposed as the landmark for the mandibular foramen, but has generally fallen into disfavor, because of

both the difficulties with its identification and its lack of predictable relation to the foramen.[12,71,72] The cut should be made no more than 5 to 7 mm anterior to the posterior border at the anticipated level of the foramen, using the retractor as a guide to the posterior border.[73] The cut is carried through the medial cortex, starting in the middle of the ramus. It is carried superiorly to the sigmoid notch and then finished at the inferior border (see Figure 57-11B). In considering the three locations of the osteotomy cut, the vascular hazards should be recognized, including the maxillary artery superiorly, the inferior alveolar artery in the middle, and the facial artery inferiorly. Therefore, the surgical ability to control a bleed from one of these three sources should factor into the decision regarding where to begin and where to end the osteotomy. As the cut is completed, anterolateral tension is maintained on the Merril-Levaseur retractor so that the proximal fragment will be brought out laterally and prevent medial displacement. A straight clamp can be used to rotate the segment laterally after the cut is made and then to stabilize it while periosteum and muscle are stripped from the medial cortex down to the angle (see Figure 57-11C). Again, a small attachment is left at the angle to ensure a blood supply. This

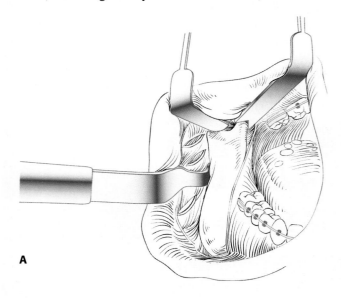

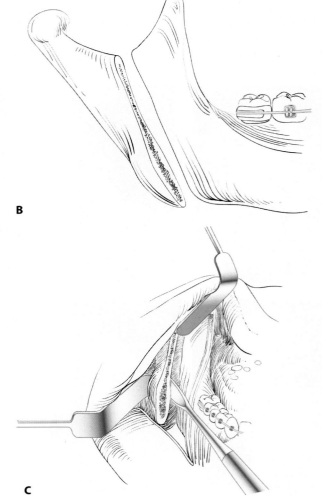

FIGURE 57-11.   The intraoral VSO. **A,** Exposure. **B,** Vertical ramus osteotomy. **C,** Proximal fragment displaced laterally. (**A-C,** Adapted from Bloomquist DS. Principles of mandibular orthognathic surgery. In Peterson LJ, Indresano AT, Marciani RD, Roser SM, editors. Principles of Oral and Maxillofacial Surgery. Vol 3. Philadelphia: JB Lippincott; 1992; p. 1424.)

proximal fragment can be held forward and laterally by a small gauze pack while the opposite side is being completed. If the proximal fragment is lost medially, it usually can be brought into the field with the help of a small periosteal elevator that is inserted posteromedially at the level of the sigmoid notch while the distal fragment is being pulled forward. The mandibular dentition is brought into its new position after the completion of both osteotomies, as established by a preformed occlusal splint and stabilized with maxillomandibular fixation.

Attention is directed back into the wound and toward placement, or reduction, and stabilization of the proximal fragment. Wire osseous fixation is generally not needed, although advocated by some surgeons. Most important is achieving as broad a bone contact area as possible, without displacing or rotating the condyle. Adjustment of the lateral cortex of the distal fragment may be performed with a straight fissure bur or small acrylic bur to permit the proximal fragment to lie as flat as possible against the vertical ramus. Care should be taken to ensure that the long axis of the proximal fragment does not differ considerably from its preoperative position. After a thorough irrigation of the wound, the mucosa is closed with a running stitch, using a resorbable suture. No drains or external dressings are placed, and IMF is used for 4 to 6 weeks, depending upon patient age and other factors. Postsurgical radiographs should be taken as soon as possible to confirm that the condyles have not been displaced or dislocated. A small amount of forward and

downward position of the condyle is common, and this generally resolves during the period of IMF (Figure 57-12).

Preoperative submentovertex radiographs have been recommended to identify divergence of the posterior border. It has been suggested that an angle smaller than 130 degrees produces such a significant surgical problem that in this type of patient, a VRO procedure should be avoided and another technique used. The use of this radiograph as a criterion for choosing this technique has been questioned, but some still believe that it can be used to identify the more difficult cases.[73,74]

A large number of variations of the VRO technique have come in the osteotomy design. Oblique versions, with the cut ending above the angle, have been described by many clinicians, with the only apparent benefit being the relative ease in performing the technique. Theoretically, there should also be less chance of damaging the IAN, but there has been no study to confirm this benefit. Interestingly, the one potential drawback, that of decreased skeletal stability, also appears to be difficult to demonstrate.[75] In contrast with this shorter cut, surgeons have recommended that a larger portion of the inferior border be left with the proximal fragment, especially in the larger mandibular setbacks.[70] This permits a good attachment of the medial pterygoid muscle to be maintained at the mandibular angle, which has been claimed to help seat the condyle in the fossa as the patient wakens from anesthesia. This variation, including the use of 8 weeks of IMF, is claimed to decrease one of the problems of the intraoral VRO, specifically that of condylar sag and the resulting open

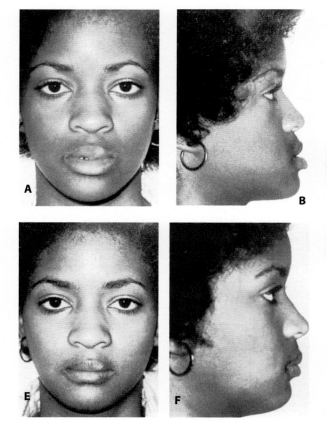

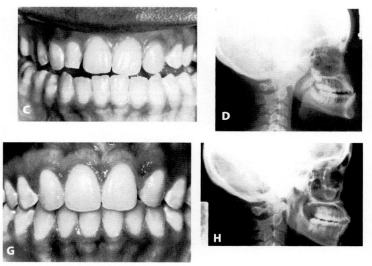

FIGURE 57-12. Patient who was treated with an intraoral VSO for mandibular horizontal excess. **A-D,** Preoperative photographs and radiograph. **E-H,** Postoperative photographs and radiograph. (**A-H,** Reproduced with permission from Bloomquist DS. Principles of mandibular orthognathic surgery. In Peterson LJ, Indresano AT, Marciani RD, Roser SM, editors. Principles of Oral and Maxillofacial Surgery. Vol 3. Philadelphia: JB Lippincott; 1992; p. 1426.)

bite that can occur on the release of fixation. Unfortunately, no clinical data have been reported that support this claim. The use of osseous wire fixation has been advocated to ensure the seating of the condyle. Again, no study comparing wire osseous fixation with no fixation has shown any advantage for the use of the wire.[76–78] This may be explained in the intraoral procedures by the technical difficulties of wire placement. However, Ritzau and associates[77] showed in an excellent prospective study that even from an extraoral approach, the position of the condyle in the fossa is not improved with the use of wire osseous fixation.

The effect of the temporalis pull on relapse has led to other recommendations that include either stripping the temporalis attachment completely off of the coronoid process or coronoidotomy. The use of coronoidotomy has been recommended by some clinicians for large setbacks, with a few using this modification routinely. The advantage of the coronoidotomy relative to prevention of relapse has not been studied, but the stability of the intraoral vertical subcondylar ramus osteotomy (IVRO) with coronoidotomy, compared with the sagittal split osteotomy (SSO) of the vertical ramus in mandibular setbacks, has been investigated and the IVRO seemed to be more stable.[79]

The use of the inverted-L osteotomy is another method used to neutralize the temporalis influence. This modification of the IVRO requires stripping of the medial periosteum to identify the lingula so that a horizontal cut can be made without increasing the risk of damaging the IAN. A further modification of the inverted-L osteotomy has been the use of

rigid internal fixation. Although technically a difficult surgery, it permits the early release from IMF. Unfortunately, there are no long-term studies that evaluate stability of any of the inverted-L techniques.

Alternative Techniques

The major variation of the described VRO technique is the use of an extraoral approach. The soft tissue incision is similar to that commonly used for an external approach to a fracture of the mandibular angle, with an approximately 4-cm incision made 2 cm below the angle and the inferior border of the mandible (Figure 57-13A). A combination of sharp and blunt dissection is used to access the inferior border of the mandible. Care is taken to avoid damaging the marginal mandibular branch of the facial nerve. After incising through the periosteum, the bone cuts are similar to those that have been described (see Figure 57-13B).

The external approach has been advocated for large mandibular setbacks of greater than 10 mm, difficult asymmetries, or large vertical moves in patients with unusual facial structure. Except for the risk of the scar, the risks of this technique have been reported as being comparable with the intraoral technique.[50,80]

Complications

STABILITY

Postoperative change in skeletal and dental position after the use of VRO in the treatment of mandibular horizontal excess

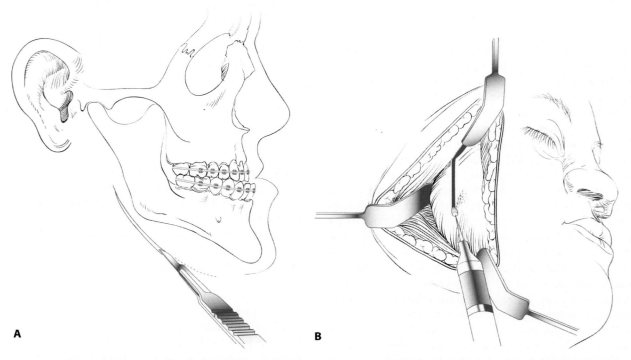

A and **B,** The extraoral VSO. (**A** and **B,** Adapted from Bloomquist DS. Principles of mandibular orthognathic surgery. In Peterson LJ, Indresano AT, Marciani RD, Roser SM, editors. Principles of Oral and Maxillofacial Surgery. Vol 3. Philadelphia: JB Lippincott; 1992; p. 1428.)

FIGURE 57-13.

A   **B**

SECTION 7

has received much attention. Goldstein[81] was the first to use serial cephalograms to evaluate the postoperative change of the mandible after surgical correction of the mandibular prognathism. He noted the anterior relapse that has now been well documented. Poulton and colleagues[82] recommended overcorrecting the mandibular setback by 2 mm to provide for the relapse that they noted. This amount of average relapse has, surprisingly, remained fairly consistent throughout the history of this technique, even though technical changes in procedures have been made.[80,83] Stella and coworkers[84] noted that the variation in the amount of relapse in mandibular setbacks was large and attempts at identifying controllable variables should be made. They suggested that the proximal fragment rotation affects the short-term pogonion changes, although they did not present any corroborative research. The finding that the pogonion tends to move posteroinferiorly during IMF has been well documented.[52] This movement, later followed by the anterosuperior "relapse" that occurs after skeletal fixation wires, does seem to stabilize the initial movement but does not affect the long-term relapse.[50,51,56]

Vertical instability of the VRO develops soon after the release of IMF in many patients. This problem was initially attributed to the "condylar sag" seen on x-ray films taken soon after surgery.[73] Although condylar sag may be one cause of relapse, a major contributor seems to be insufficient time of IMF. The VRO is generally not considered an appropriate surgery for correction of anterior open bite. In Scandinavian countries, however, this surgical procedure has been successfully used for patients with mandibular horizontal excess and anterior open bite.[85]

Nerve Damage

The chance of damaging the marginal mandibular branch of the facial nerve is one of the reasons given by several surgeons for avoiding the extraoral approach to the VRO. This concern, however, seems to be unsubstantiated, in that almost all of the clinicians reporting on the results of this approach have noted very little, if any, motor nerve damage. Damage to the IAN, however, is a concern in using a VRO. The incidence of trauma to the IAN at the time of surgery has been reported to vary from being "rare" to occurring 36% of the time.[70] Long-term sensory defects have also been reported to vary from none to 35%.[45,86] These apparent discrepancies can be explained by the differences in the sensitivity of the measurement techniques; in addition, there is a wide variation in the time after surgery during which the patients were tested. Other variables, such as whether the osteotomy was approached intraorally or extraorally as well as variations in the length of the cut, theoretically could affect the incidence of sensory problems, but comparison studies have not been done. From studies that have been done, the incidence of damage to the IAN is low with the VRO compared with the SSO.[86,87] The patient, however, should be warned that short-term sensory loss is a definite risk and permanent paresthesia is possible.

TMJ Dysfunction

Interesting literature has been published on changes in TMJ function after a VRO. These have included a number of radiographic studies documenting positional change of the condyle relative to the fossa. Radiographically, there is an initial downward and forward movement of the condyle, with a subsequent tendency to return to its preoperative position.[77,78,82] Sometimes, a double contour of the condyle appears approximately 6 months postoperatively, which has been attributed to condylar remodeling after the surgery.[88] Remodeling of the glenoid fossa has also been documented.[78]

In one early review of 100 cases, 6 patients were reported to have TMJ problems at 1 year after surgery.[89] A form of the VRO has been used to treat patients with TMJ pain and dysfunction. It appears that the VRO does not put the TMJ at any significant risk, and it may in fact be salutary for patients with preexisting TMJ dysfunction.[90–92]

Other Complications

Among the other reported complications of the VRO, vascular necrosis of the proximal segment seems to be the most potentially devastating. The maintenance of some muscle attachment to the angles makes this possibility unlikely.

Inverted-L and C Ramus Osteotomies

Osteotomy designs in the vertical ramus that include both the condyle and the coronoid in the same segment have varied from Blair's simple horizontal osteotomy to the modified C osteotomy of Hayes. The horizontal osteotomy of the vertical ramus has generally fallen into disuse because of the substantial relapse potential, but many of the remaining suggested variations continue to have treatment value. The two procedures that seem to be the most popular are the inverted-L and the C osteotomites. Both are generally approached extraorally, although intraoral variants are possible.[93] Clinical studies of either technique are rare, but those that exist seem to demonstrate reasonable success in correcting skeletal deformities with minimal complications.

Indications

The C osteotomy is generally reserved for treatment of horizontal mandibular deficiency, with some authors suggesting that it can be used to close an anterior open bite. The inverted-L, however, has been used for the correction of most types of mandibular horizontal discrepancies, including an anterior open bite. Generally, advancements of the distal segment with either technique require bone grafting to ensure adequate bone union.

Techniques

The basic techniques for an extraoral approach to perform a C and an inverted-L are the same, with the only modification being the inferior horizontal cut in the C osteotomy. For that reason, the inverted-L is described first, with various modifications of the C discussed later. The patient is prepared and draped, such that access to both the mouth and the submandibular incision area can occur without contamination of the skin wound by oral organisms. This can be accomplished in a variety of ways, but most surgeons use a plastic drape with adhesive on one edge to separate the two areas. The external drapes should be arranged so that they allow turning of the head for access to the submandibular wounds as well as access to the mouth.

The submandibular incision is made 2 cm below the angle and inferior border of the mandible. The posterior portion is curved superiorly to follow the cervical skin line as well as to improve the access to the entire vertical ramus. Generally, the incision is approximately 6 cm in length. Sharp dissection is used down through the platysma, and then blunt dissection is begun to minimize risk to the marginal mandibular branch of the facial nerve. The incision through the pterygomandibular sling and periosteum is made along the inferior border and is carried around the angle and up the posterior border about 2 cm. Periosteum and attachments for the masseter are completely stripped off the lateral cortex of the vertical ramus up to the level of the sigmoid notch. Very little periosteum is stripped off the medial side, especially at the angle, to retain as much blood supply as possible to the proximal fragment. The posterior vertical osteotomy is made at least 7 mm in front of the posterior border and extends to a point of the inferior border just in front of the angle. The horizontal cut is made above the anticipated position of the inferior alveolar foramen (Figure 57-14A). As mentioned previously with the VRO, it is wise to have a good radiographic view of the ramus so that the position of this foramen can be more accurately located. It is helpful to review the study by Reitzik and associates[72] of the position of the foramen relative to the lateral landmarks to lessen trauma to the neurovascular bundle.

Once the cuts are made, the medial periosteum may have to be elevated from some of the distal fragment to allow its advancement. Moist gauze is placed in the wound, and a similar procedure is done on the opposite side. After completion of the contralateral side, drapes are pulled back and shifted such that the oral cavity can be entered to place the mandibular teeth into the new occlusal position and secured with IMF. The surgeons who are involved in the intraoral fixation should change gloves and surgical gowns before the drapes are replaced so that the skin incisions can again be approached. The next step varies depending on the type of mandibular movement that occurred; however, the importance of maintaining the proximal fragment close to its preoperative position remains. If the distal segment is set back, the proximal segment has to be overlapped laterally (see Figure 57-14B). As described with the VRO, some adjustments of the lateral cortex of the distal segment may be necessary to permit passive position of the proximal fragment as well as to provide a good area of bone contact. The use of some form of fixation is generally recommended, although the use of no interosseous fixation has been suggested.[93] The type of osseous fixation varies widely; however, rigid internal

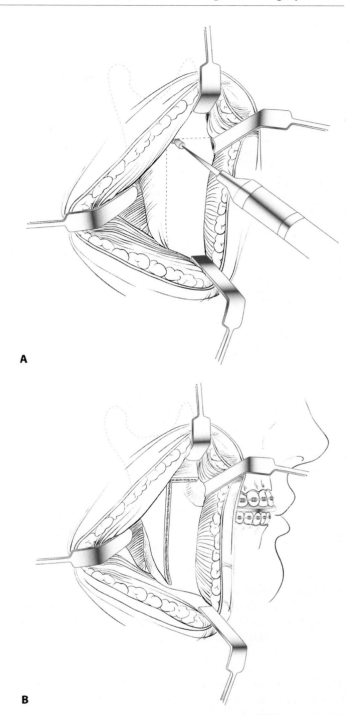

A

B

FIGURE 57-14.   A and **B,** The extraoral inverted L osteotomy. (**A** and **B,** Adapted from Bloomquist DS. Principles of mandibular orthognathic surgery. In Peterson LJ, Indresano AT, Marciani RD, Roser SM, editors. Principles of Oral and Maxillofacial Surgery. Vol 3. Philadelphia: JB Lippincott; 1992; p. 1430.)

fixation with metal plates or mesh secured with screws has become more popular.[93] After irrigation, the wound is closed in layers by whatever suturing method and material the surgeon prefers. Care should be taken to ensure hemostasis as the wound is closed. If there is any concern about hematoma

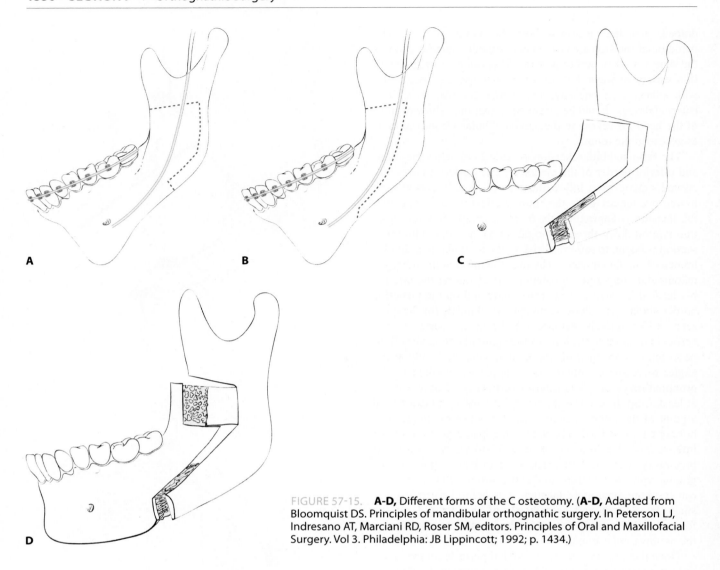

FIGURE 57-15. **A-D,** Different forms of the C osteotomy. (**A-D,** Adapted from Bloomquist DS. Principles of mandibular orthognathic surgery. In Peterson LJ, Indresano AT, Marciani RD, Roser SM, editors. Principles of Oral and Maxillofacial Surgery. Vol 3. Philadelphia: JB Lippincott; 1992; p. 1434.)

formation, a small drain should be placed. External pressure dressings are maintained for 24 to 48 hours. When the bone has been stabilized with wire fixation, IMF is used for at least 6 weeks and preferably 8 weeks.

Alternative Techniques

The most commonly used variation of the previously mentioned technique is the C osteotomy. This technique was first described jointly by Caldwell and coworkers[18] in an article reviewing their experiences with what they called a *vertical-L osteotomy.* They described a variation of their basic vertical-L with the addition of a horizontal cut that extended forward from the vertical cut below the inferior alveolar canal (Figure 57-15A). This permitted a larger amount of bone contact when the mandible was advanced. They also realized the problems caused by advancing the coronoid process and recommended either cutting the coronoid loose (coronoidotomy) or including it with the proximal segment (C osteotomy). Arcing the inferior cut was suggested to permit increased bone contact as the distal segment was advanced (see Figure

57-15B).[94] Unfortunately, the proposed arc cannot always be made because the position of the neurovascular bundle may interfere. Sagittal splitting of the inferior limb of the C osteotomy was proposed both to increase the bone contact area when the mandible was advanced and to decrease the problem of "notching" of the inferior border (see Figure 57-15C).[19] This latter problem, which is noticeable in some patients, is caused by the defect along the inferior border resulting from the advanced distal segment of the mandible. A further variation used to improve bone healing includes a bone graft taken from the lateral cortex of the distal segment and transferred back into the gap of the midramus area (see Figure 57-15D). The coronoid process has also been recommended as a free graft in to this defect.[20]

A further major modification of the described techniques is the use of rigid internal fixation.[95–97] The use of vitalium mesh with two screws in each fragment has been demonstrated as being effective, but any rigid plate with screws can be used to permit the early release of maxillomandibular dental fixation.

Complications

The skeletal stability of the inverted-L and its modifications, unlike the VRO, seems to be technique-sensitive to the type of fixation used. Like stability studies for almost all aspects of orthognathic surgery, controlled clinical studies are nonexistent, and the comparison of techniques by a single institution, if reported, lacks sufficient numbers of patients to make valid conclusions. Farrell and Kent[93] evaluated inverted-L and C osteotomies and reported skeletal relapse similar to what had been reported for the BSSO. However, because there were different criteria for the use of these two types of osteotomies, comparisons between them are questionable. Greebe and Tuinzing[98] compared the stability of mandibular advancement by way of an inverted-L or a BSSO. With only a few patients, they did not show any difference between the groups, but they did claim that skeletal relapse was dependent on the ratio of posterior facial height to anterior facial height. The largest studies of the stability of the inverted L included the use of rigid internal fixation in patients who had the mandible advanced. These seem to demonstrate that the use of rigid fixation for this type of procedure is more stable than simple IMF.[96,97] However, statements relative to stability of mandibular setbacks or the closure of open bites cannot be made, although a few authors seem to advocate these skeletal deformities as indications for the use of the inverted-L osteotomy.[96,99]

The incidence of facial nerve damage has not been mentioned in any review of these techniques, although it can be inferred to be quite low, given the reports for the external approach to the VRO. The incidence of damage to the IAN should be higher than the extraoral VRO because of the horizontal portions of the osteotomy, but Reitzik and colleagues[96] reported only a 6% incidence of permanent anesthesia with inverted-L osteotomies. The incidence of unsightly scars, which many clinicians claim deters them from using this approach, is unknown with this group of osteotomies.

Bilateral Sagittal Split Osteotomy

The BSSO of the vertical ramus has in a relatively short time become the predominant orthognathic procedure of the man-dible. Schuchardt[23] is credited for the use of an intraoral approach to what was called the "step" osteotomy of the vertical ramus. Specifically, he described parallel horizontal cuts through the cortex of the vertical ramus, the medial cut located above the lingual, and the lateral cut made about 1 cm below that level. A split was then made between these two cortices, and the distal segment could then be advanced or set back. Lane evidently described a very similar procedure earlier, but it probably was done extraorally (see Figure 57-4).[22] The singular credit for improving on this osteotomy, as well as being its strongest advocate, belongs to Obwegeser, who together with Trauner in 1955, described a sagittal split of the vertical ramus.[21] This intraoral technique included the medial horizontal cut above the lingula, but the lateral horizontal cut was lower than that of Schuchardt and extended to a point just above the angle, at least 25 mm below the lingual cortical cut (Figure 57-16A). A wide-splitting osteotome was then used to obtain a split between the cortices, with care taken to preserve the IAN and vascular bundle. This procedure was later slightly modified by Obwegeser by angling the lateral cut more toward the inferior border of the mandible (see Figure 57-16B). The major modifications still in use today were suggested by Dal-Pont.[24] The change commonly attributed to DalPont is the forward extension of the vertical cut through the lateral cortex just behind the second molar. But he also suggested the use of a medial cut that extends just past the lingula so that the posterior split would occur in the mylohyoid groove instead at the inferior border. Multiple other modifications have been suggested, but surprisingly, the present-day osteotomy remains very similar to that initially described by Obwegeser and Dal-Pont. Also in use today is the description by Hunsuck[25] to terminate the medial horizontal cut in the retrolingular fossa, and not attempt to cut through the posterior border; this would ensure that the induced fracture would occur posterior to lingula, in the thin bone, rather than in the thick cortical bone of the posterior border of the ramus.

Indications

The BSSO has been advocated for all types of mandibular deformities and for each possible mandibular movement that includes the entire horizontal ramus of the mandible.

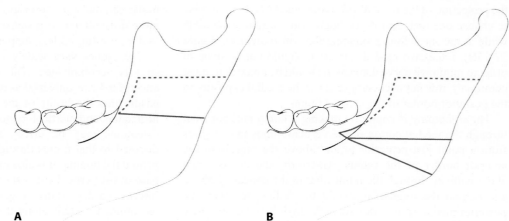

FIGURE 57-16.   Obwegeser's osteotomies of the ramus. **A,** Original cortical cuts. **B,** Later lateral cortex cuts. (**A** and **B,** Adapted from Bloomquist DS. Principles of mandibular orthognathic surgery. In Peterson LJ, Indresano AT, Marciani RD, Roser SM, editors. Principles of Oral and Maxillofacial Surgery. Vol 3. Philadelphia: JB Lippincott; 1992; p. 1435.)   **A**   **B**

Technique

This osteotomy has had multiple variations described, as would be expected for such a popular procedure, but many of them are based upon one surgeon's individual preferences, and the effect of these alterations of the osteotomy on the outcome of the procedure is questionable. Therefore, only the basic procedures are outlined, as well as the significant modifications that have been shown to affect the outcome or seem to have a solid theoretical foundation.

The incision is made on the anterior portion of the vertical ramus, midway between the occlusal planes. It is carried downward through the middle of the retromolar fossa to a point about 5 mm behind the second molar. Then the incisions wind laterally and forward to a point distal just to the first molar (Figure 57-17A). The incision should be kept lateral enough to allow easy closure of the wound later in the procedure when the teeth are in IMF. The periosteum is reflected to expose the lateral cortex of the mandible down to the inferior border for the vertical cut only. The exposure should be limited posteriorly to maximize the blood supply to the proximal fragment; this usually means the exposure ends at about the antegonial notch, and the masseter muscle is reflected minimally. A lateral channel retractor, or Minnesota retractor, can be placed at this time to assist in retraction as the periosteum is elevated from the retromolar area up the anterior border of the vertical ramus. Periosteal elevators are used during this portion of the surgery. The attachment of the temporalis muscle can be tenacious, but it may be reflected off of the coronoid process to the level of the sigmoid notch to ensure adequate access for the medial horizontal cut. Most times, this means stripping approximately 1 cm of the temporalis attachment off the anterior border of the coronoid process. The periosteum is then elevated from the medial surface of the vertical ramus, starting at about the level of the sigmoid notch and extending back to the medial flare at the start of the condylar neck. Inferiorly, the medial cortex is exposed to the lingula, with care being taken to minimize trauma to the IAN just below this area. The periosteal elevation can be extended inferoanteriorly along the internal oblique line to the distal of the second molar to allow better exposure of the osteotomy site, with care taken to protect the lingual nerve. A variety of retractors are available for the protection of the medial soft tissues and IAN, but it is wise to choose one that permits as much visualization as possible while at the same time protecting the soft tissue (see Figure 57-17B). Excessive medial retraction should not be done in order to minimize nerve damage. It should be noted that, most commonly, it is not necessary to carry the medial exposure to the posterior border of the vertical ramus.

The osteotomy is begun by making a horizontal bone cut through the medial cortex of the vertical ramus that extends from a point just posterior to and above the lingula to the anterior border of the ramus. Anteriorly, the cut is made about halfway through the ramus, but in the concavity above and behind the lingula, it should be shallow to allow the posterior medial split to initiate in the mylohyoid groove (see

Figure 57-17C). Sometimes, it is helpful to use a large round or acrylic bur to remove bone from the internal oblique ridge so that the depth of this concavity can be visualized. Occasionally, at the level of this horizontal cut, there is no significant cancellous bone to delineate the cortices. Here, the use of a half thickness of the ramus is the most practical guideline for judging the appropriate depth of this cut.

The vertical cut through the buccal cortex is generally made just distal to the second molar and extends from the inferior border superiorly to the external oblique ridge. Sometimes, the mandible is thin and the external oblique ridge ends at the distobuccal aspect of the second molar. In this case, the superior aspect of the vertical cut should be posterolateral enough so that the roots of the second molar are not placed at risk. The cut should be as close to perpendicular to the inferior border as possible and extended just into cancellous bone. Caution must be used such that the cut is not made any deeper because the IAN may be just medial to the buccal cortex in this region.

The vertical and horizontal cortical cuts are connected, starting superiorly at the anterior border of vertical ramus and continuing down just inside the external oblique ridge to the vertical cut (see Figure 57-17D). Again, the cut is made into cancellous bone, when at all possible, with the superior part of this connection being as deep as possible, especially if no cancellous bone is present. This will minimize the chance of an inadvertent fracture of the medial cortex. Some surgeons recommend that the corners between the horizontal and the connecting cuts, as well as the vertical and the connecting cuts, be rounded again to minimize a fracture. Difficulty is encountered often and can occur if a third molar is present and has been planned to be removed at the time of surgery. It is generally prudent to plan for the mandibular third molars to be removed well in advance of the SSO because they can make the surgery more difficult. Preferably, these third molars should be removed at least 9 to 12 months in advance of the SSO. Even experienced surgeons who remove third molars at the same time as the osteotomy may have difficulty in obtaining a successful split, but in general, the presence of third molars is a significant risk factor for bad splits, such as inadvertent buccal or lingual cortical plate fractures. Also, the bone defect left by removal of the third molar can make the use rigid fixation with bicortical screws more difficult and also weaken the bone distal to the second molar, resulting in less support.

Techniques vary widely regarding how the actual bone split is accomplished. The method described here is an attempt to be as universal as possible. First, steps are taken to ensure that the limits of the split occur as defined by the horizontal and vertical bone cuts. A narrow (4-mm) thin osteotome may be driven along the horizontal cut and directed so that it cuts through the medial cortex above and behind the lingula. It is also used to ensure that the split at the base of the vertical cut is started through the midpoint of the inferior border. Many surgeons also use this type of thin osteotome to "step" along the connecting cut to help ensure

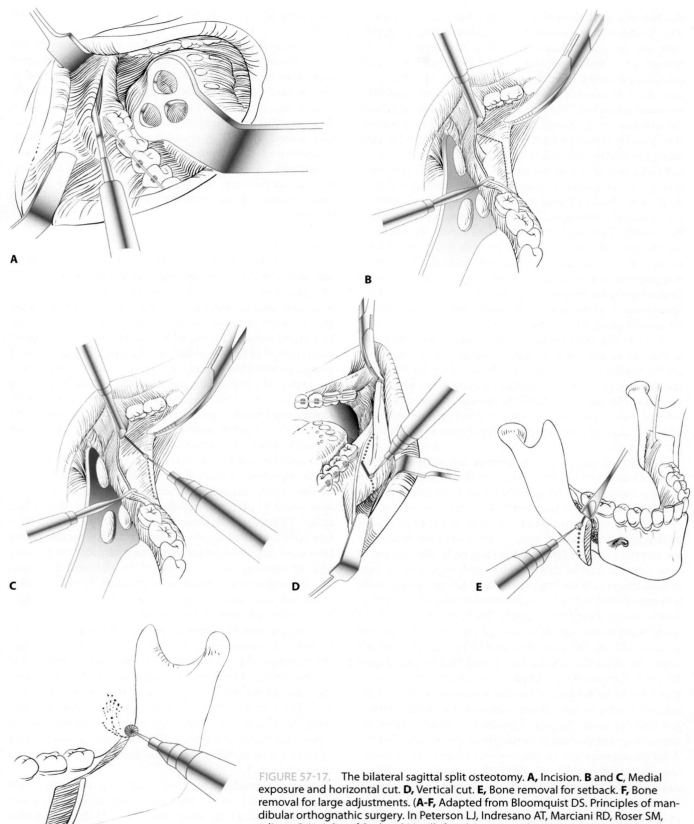

FIGURE 57-17. The bilateral sagittal split osteotomy. **A,** Incision. **B** and **C,** Medial exposure and horizontal cut. **D,** Vertical cut. **E,** Bone removal for setback. **F,** Bone removal for large adjustments. (**A-F,** Adapted from Bloomquist DS. Principles of mandibular orthognathic surgery. In Peterson LJ, Indresano AT, Marciani RD, Roser SM, editors. Principles of Oral and Maxillofacial Surgery. Vol 3. Philadelphia: JB Lippincott; 1992; pp. 1436–1437.)

that the split stays close to the lateral bone cortex. Traditionally, wide-wedging osteotomes have been used to slowly complete the split. More often today, a special spreading instrument, a Smith spreader, is used along with a smaller osteotome to allow more control of the split. Generally, the movement is initiated along the vertical cut and carefully extended posteriorly. The fine osteotome can be used to keep the split close to the lateral cortex. If the IAN is encountered, it is carefully separated from the proximal fragment. The split along the inferior border can be difficult to control, and the judicious use of a thin osteotome will assist in this area. Finally, as the posterior split through the medial cortex is made, care should be used to prevent the split from continuing behind the mylohyoid fossa and starting up the neck of the condyle. The speed of the split often varies, depending on the elasticity of the bone. In older patients, in whom the bone is not as elastic, the split can occur very suddenly. Preventing inappropriate fractures is dependent on the care used not only in making the cortical bone cuts but also in ensuring that the splits occur as planned at the posterior aspect of the horizontal cut and along the inferior border.

The two key areas necessary to ensure that an appropriate osteotomy occurs and to minimize the chance of a bad split are the medial horizontal cut into the retrolingular fossa and the cut through the inferior border on to the lingual aspect of the mandible. Attention should be directed to the area of the inferior border osteotomy to assist if a bad split is noted, and control in this area could prevent propagation of an inadvertent osteotomy.

The medial pterygoid attachments are stripped off the proximal fragment to permit freedom of movement between the two fragments. If the mandibular teeth are planned to be retropositioned, either unilaterally to correct an asymmetry or bilaterally for correction of horizontal mandibular excess, an appropriate amount of bone is removed at this time from the anterior portion of the proximal fragment. The amount of bone removal may be based upon model surgery or the prediction tracings. With large setbacks or advancements, bone will need to be removed from the anterior edge of the vertical ramus. When setting the mandible back, this needs to leave space between the vertical ramus and the mandibular second molar to prevent this area from interfering with the patient's ability to clean the mandibular second molars (see Figure 57-17E). Conversely, in large advancements, bone sometimes has to be removed from the remaining portion of the anterior border of the vertical ramus of the distal segment just anterior to the lingula to prevent encroachment of the segment against the maxillary tuberosity (see Figure 57-17F). After the opposite side is split, the mandible is moved into its new position and stabilized with IMF. It may be preferable to use an interocclusal splint to ensure accurate positioning of the mandible relative to the maxilla, based on the presurgical model surgery. It is unusual for teeth to interdigitate accurately enough to obviate the use of a splint, although, if there is a full dentition and the occlusion is deemed stable, it is acceptable to apply IMF without the use of an interocclusal splint.

The placement of osseous fixation is performed at this point. Because multiple techniques are possible, different options are described in the following section on "Alternative Techniques." For the SSO, rigid fixation techniques generally include bicortical screws or monocortical plate and screw fixation. After placement of osseous fixation, if rigid fixation is used, the IMF is released, allowing the occlusion to be evaluated. The wounds are thoroughly irrigated and closed with the use of a resorbable running suture. No drains or external dressings are generally necessary, and guiding elastic intermaxillary traction may be used postoperatively (Figure 57-18).

Alternative Techniques

There are many variations to the technique described here, and in this section only the major variations are discussed. The design of the osteotomy itself has received much attention, with each variation representing an attempt to decrease the incidence of complications, although there is very little supportive research for any of the modifications. Obwegeser was responsible for two variations, the first being his original design, in which the buccal cut was horizontal and parallel to the lingual cut through the cortex of the vertical ramus (see Figure 57-16A). This original technique was modified by making the lateral cortical cut at an angle to the medial cut so that the posterior portion of the osteotomy ended just above the angle (see Figure 57-16B).[100]

A popular modification of DalPont's vertical osteotomy is the continuation of this cut completely through the inferior border, which, according to surgeon advocates, made the split easier to perform, and decreased the chance of a bad split.[59] This technique, however, makes the use of rigid fixation with bicortical screws difficult.[101] A few modifications have been suggested for the connecting cut, with the primary goal of allowing better control of the proximal fragment. These modifications appear to be primarily personal preferences because there is no evidence that these changes improve the outcome of the procedure.

A major area of variation for the SSO is in the use, or nonuse, of osseous fixation.[21,25,102,103] The original Obwegeser technique[104] used wire through the superior lateral and medial cortices. This technique, with minor variation, became the standard for the SSO until rigid fixation became popular.[59] The use of circumandibular wires and inferior border wires have also been suggested as improved methods to control the proximal fragment.[105] No evidence exists that any of these wiring techniques have an advantage for minimizing complications.[26]

Spiessl[26] introduced the concept of using screws for "rigid internal fixation" of the SSO. Following its introduction in 1974, there was a slow acceptance of this method of osseous fixation. Currently, there is little debate on the advantages of using rigid internal fixation; however, a wide variety of

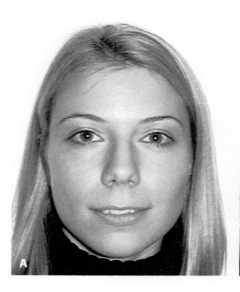

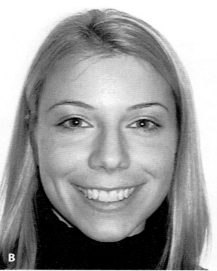

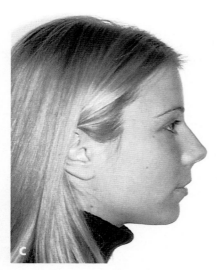

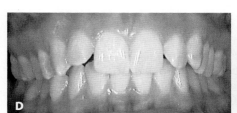

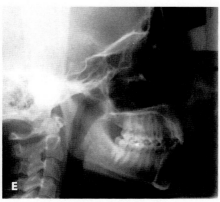

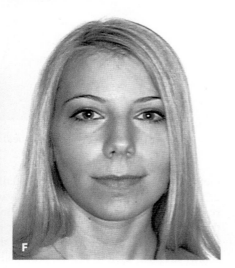

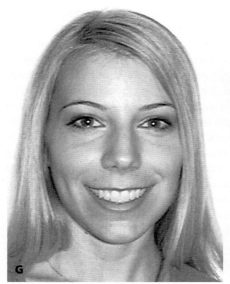

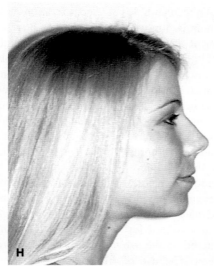

FIGURE 57-18. Patient who was treated with bilateral sagittal split osteotomies (for mandibular horizontal deficiency). **A-E,** Preoperative photographs and head radiograph. **F,** Presurgery head radiograph. **G-L,** Postoperative photographs and radiographs. (**A-L,** Courtesy of Dr. S. Lake.) *(Continued)*

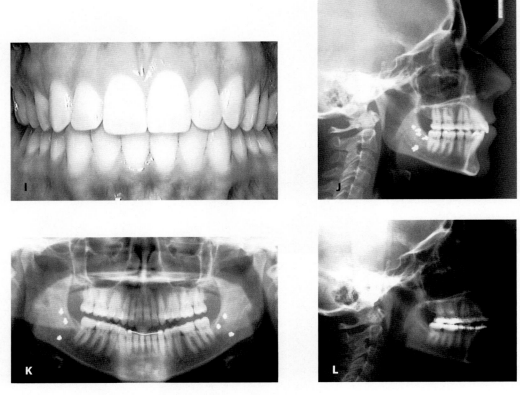

FIGURE 57-18. *(Continued)*

methods and materials are used. Initially, the use of three 2.7-mm "lag" screws on each side was advocated. A lag screw is placed by drilling a "guiding" hole with a larger drill through the lateral cortex, followed by a smaller hole through the medial cortex that is threaded with the use of a tap. Lag screws are then used to fix the proximal fragment tightly to the distal fragment. Compression across the osteotomy site was believed to be important to speed the healing of the osteotomy as well as to ensure the stability of the mandible. Concern developed among surgeons that compression may cause increased IAN damage and displacement of the condyles, with subsequent TMJ dysfunction.[106,107] An alternative technique, the positional screw, or bicortical screw, in which both cortices are drilled of equal diameter, has been advocated for stabilizing the osteotomy segments.[100] This technique permits maintenance of the gaps that may occur between the proximal and the distal fragments due to minor bony interferences, with no effort being made to compress the two segments together that may torque the condyle or compress the IAN. Standardization of techniques does not exist in rigid fixation of the SSO because there are many differences in screw sizes, number of screws, materials used, and whether plates are used across the osteotomy sites. Most of the research in the United States has centered on the use of three screws that are 2.0 mm in diameter. The use of monocortical screws and plates has become more widely used and a large multicenter study has provided clinical evidence to support this as routine practice. Direct comparisons of the various rigid fixation techniques in the literature are scarce and do not demonstrate that any one technique has any advantages.[109-110] One exception was noted by Fujioka and coworkers,[111] who found that there was more rotation through the osteotomy sites in patients with monocortical plate and screw fixation, perhaps justifying the need to consider additional fixation with counterclockwise rotation movements.

The use of resorbable screws has been a recent addition to fixation schemes. First attempted in Finland, the screws are made from polyglycolic acid using different manufacturing techniques and formulas. Development of these self-reinforced polylactic acid/polyglycolic acid copolymers that have reliable strength to withstand forces of mastication has made their use applicable in orthognathic surgery. The obvious advantage of resorbable fixation is to obviate future hardware removal, which is rarely necessary in the United States, but it has become an issue with patient concerns of risks of any permanent implant. The key features that are crucial in its application in orthognathic surgery are the rigidity and strength of the material, with the ability to resorb in a timely fashion. A few small studies have shown apparent stability of these resorbable implants comparable to metallic fixation; however, some inherent problems with material handling and early fixation failures have been reported.[112–114]

Suuronen and associates[112] reported the use of poly-L-lactic acid (PLLA) screws for fixation in SSO, with no apparent malocclusion or skeletal relapse. Harada and Enomoto[113] and, later, Ferretti and Reyneke[114] compared titanium and resorbable screws and noted no difference in healing between two groups, and no statistically significant difference in skeletal relapse. However, Harada and Enomoto's patients used IMF for a period ranging from 9 to 14 days after surgery.[113] Kallela and colleagues[115] used self-reinforced poly-L-lactic acid (SR-PLLA) screws for mandibular osteotomies and no IMF postoperatively. The mean advancement was 4.57 mm at B point, and the mean relapse was 17%. In their 2-year follow-up study in 1999, the authors reported osteolytic changes seen around the resorbable screws in 27% of cases, and the screw canals remained as radiolucent shadows without complete bony fill.[115] Turvey and coworkers[116] reported experience with resorbable fixation for 194 osteotomies of the maxilla and/or mandible. Forty-three of the patients had SSOs with 2-mm resorbable screws placed on each side for fixation. They reported only 1 infection at the SSO site and 1 patient who exhibited excessive masticatory forces that resulted in loosening of the fixation. More recently, the use of resorbable plates with monocortical screws has been advocated. A large group of 272 patients were evaluated for complications other than neurosensory changes. Titanium plates were used in 152 patients and resorbable plates, a copolymer of L-lactic acid and D-lactic acid, were used in 120 patients. The authors conclude that complications, including relapse, which was 18.3% for resorbable plates and 8.6% for titanium plates, must be questioned owing to the large number of variables in the study. However, the apparent successful treatment of that number of patients is impressive.[117]

Acceptance of the routine use of resorbable fixation with the SSO will require long-term evaluation with well-designed studies comparing these materials with the metal hardware. The major potential risk of permanent metal fixation is the possibility of bone remodeling, causing the hardware to become noticeable and possibly irritating to the patient. Although rarely reported in the literature, oral and maxillofacial surgeons have had experience with patients returning to have plates and screws removed simply because these implants have become noticeable or palpable. This problem must be weighed against the still unknown side effects of the resorbable materials. A prime example of these unknowns is the precise time required for total resorption and degradation of poly-L-lactic acid (PLLA) and poly-D,L-lactic acid (PDLLA) in human tissues, which is reported to range anywhere from 90 days to 5 years. Surgeons must closely follow the literature to determine the practicality of these new materials.

An interesting suggested modification in the SSO technique is the purposeful changing of the rotational position of the proximal fragment to control the direction of mandibular growth. It has generally been recommended that the proximal segment be maintained as close as possible to its preoperative position. O'Ryan and Epker[118] have further suggested that rotating the proximal fragment in a growing patient can change the vector of condylar growth and, thereby, influence the final mandibular position. Studies have failed to support this contention.[119] There is also concern with an SSO in growing children, especially those requiring significant advancement. Huang and Ross[120] demonstrated what they believed to be a cessation of mandibular growth and condylar resorption in growing patients in whom SSO procedures were performed. Whether this was a problem with the techniques used or a problem with performing surgery in such a young group of patients is unknown, but this effect has not been noted in any further literature.

A final modification of the SSO is the concomitant use of a midsymphyseal osteotomy to allow for correction of width discrepancies in the dental arch. For example, this could be used to narrow the mandibular arch form in lieu of a two-piece maxillary osteotomy, and this may be a more stable procedure. Although this procedure may be used with any of the ramal osteotomies, it has only been described with the SSO. First mentioned by Bell,[121] it has become more practical with the use of rigid internal fixation. A single four-hole plate across the bone cut between the mandibular central incisors, along with an intact orthodontic arch wire, provides sufficient postoperative stability.[122] Concerns regarding adverse effects on the TMJ and periodontium have been shown to be insignificant.[123]

Complications

STABILITY

The stability of the SSO of the vertical ramus is arguably the most studied complication in orthognathic surgery. Because the relapse patterns differ between mandibular advancements and setbacks, their particular etiologies most likely differ as well; however, many of the important principles for preventing relapse in each scenario may be the same. Whereas much of the research on mandibular advancement has been done in the United States, mandibular prognathism has generally received the greatest interest in the Scandinavian countries and the Far East. This highlights one of the major problems for surgeons attempting to decide on which techniques to use to minimize undesirable postoperative skeletal change. There are large variations in research techniques as well as surgical approaches that exist not only between surgical centers in different countries but also within the same country. Fortunately, there is enough corroboration in the literature that some general statements and conclusions can be made.

One of the most important findings made regarding the stability of mandibular osteotomies was that IMF does not prevent postoperative skeletal change. Intermaxillary elastics may have a minor influence on bony remodeling at the osteotomy sites, but the rigid fixation used may be difficult to overcome with elastic traction. More likely, the elastics provide some dental changes (extrusive movements), and possibly some condylar remodeling, that may serve to correct minor postoperative malocclusions. Although the influence of postoperative elastic traction on occlusion applies to any type of maxillary or mandibular osteotomy, it was first recognized in the evaluation of mandibular SSO. It is generally believed that paramandibular connective tissue pressures and muscle vectors are the major factors influencing relapse, especially in cases of mandibular advancement.[52,53,123] However, early attempts at minimizing these effects, such as suprahyoid myotomies and external supportive devices, have not been shown to be effective.[64] Internal support techniques, however, have been shown to be effective. Prior to rigid fixation screws and plates, a type of internal support called *skeletal fixation* was shown to be effective in decreasing the downward and backward relapse pattern of mandibular advancements.[64] This fixation was used in addition to IMF and consists of wires placed from the piriform rim to circumandibular wires placed in the cuspid or molar regions (see Figure 57-9). Interestingly, Van Sickels[124] noted a decrease in relapse in patients with large advancements when skeletal fixation was combined with rigid internal screw fixation.

Other possible causes of relapse include patient age, preoperative mandibular plane angle, rotational position of the proximal fragment, amount of distal segment advancement, and displacement of condyle within the fossa. The effect of mandibular plane angle is controversial because of conflicting reported in the literature, most of which evaluated patients who had wire osseous fixation with IMF. Mobarak and associates[125] clearly found decreased stability in patients with steep mandibular plane angles when rigid internal fixation was used. Of the remaining variables evaluated, only the last two appear to be definitively supported by clinical studies. In their multicenter study, Schendel and Epker[64] found that displacement/dislocation of the condyle from the glenoid fossa was a significant predictor of relapse. This was further confirmed by Lake and coworkers,[55] who showed a correlation between the amount of advancement and the amount of relapse.

The final area that must considered in relapse in both mandibular advancement and setback is the rigidity of the fixation across the osteotomy site. Early investigators thought that fixation across the osteotomy site may hinder the natural repositioning of the condyle in the fossa that occurs during IMF.[103] Later studies showed that wire osteosynthesis was superior to no osseous fixation in fragment positioning, and the incidence of relapse was decreased.[102] However, the search for an improved osseous wiring technique that would decrease relapse was not successful, with most studies on osseous wiring techniques consistently reporting a mean relapse of approximately 30%. The large range of individual relapses that does exist has led many surgeons to believe multiple factors influence relapse.

The use of rigid internal fixation techniques has become the preferred method for minimizing skeletal relapse in the SSO. Schmoker and colleagues[126] discussed the advantages of lag screws in SSO. Their initial study of skeletal stability evaluated mandibular setbacks, comparing the use of three 2.7-mm screws versus wire fixation and one or two screws. It was not until 1985 that Van Sickels and Flanary[127] showed

evidence that a similar rigid fixation technique provided increased stability in mandibular advancements. Furthermore, larger and longer studies have clearly shown the stability of using three bicortical screws for fixation of the SSO.[128–131] These studies have reported a mean relapse rate between 0.0% and 8.0%. The majority of studies comparing rigid internal fixation techniques versus the use of wire osseous fixation have also confirmed a significant difference in stability between the techniques.[132–136] Interestingly, the only clinical study that evaluated the stability of osseous wire fixation versus rigid screw fixation on patients treated at the same center seemed to show a comparable long-term stability.[137] This study, however, reported an unusually high stability of the wire osseous fixation group and did nothing to dispute the stability of the screw fixation. Dolce and associates[136] found, in their long-term follow-up of the multicenter study in which the patients were randomly assigned between internal rigid fixation with screws and wire osseous fixation, that at 5 years, the rigidly fixed mandibles were skeletally more stable, and there was no significant difference between the two groups in anterior overbite and overjet. This particular effect is difficult to explain except for some instability in the orthodontics. The number of screws may very well influence the stability, although only Spiessl's original study[26] demonstrated a difference. Knaup and associates[131] tried to demonstrate some difference in stability on large advancements in evaluating three versus four bicortical screws per side. They found no difference in horizontal changes but did show more stability with four screws when there was counterclockwise rotation of the distal fragment. This finding then led to an early attempt to reevaluate the possibility that anterior open bites can be successfully closed with BSSO stabilized with rigid screw fixation. Recently, the possibility of closing open bites with mandibular osteotomies in a stable fashion has been supported by other studies.[138]

Finally, several biomechanical studies have shown that the placement of three bicortical positional screws to fixate an SSO is more stable in an L configuration (two near the superior border, one near the inferior border) than in a linear configuration (three placed near the superior border), although there is concern that the inferior screw may iatrogenically injure the IAN or not engage the lingual aspect of the distal segment, resulting in less stability.

Another common method for rigid internal fixation of the SSO is the use of miniplates with monocortical screw fixation. Generally, 2.0-mm systems are used with two monocortical screws placed on either side of the osteotomy to secure one four-hole plate.[139–142] Questions remain over the minimum number of screws necessary to prevent relapse and whether more or larger screws, or plates, will improve stability in longer advancements. It has been shown that a single 2.0-mm screw does not seem to increase mandibular stability over wire osseous fixation, and therefore, it could be argued, in light of the previously reviewed research, that an increase in number or size of screws, and/or plates, may result in more osseous stability.[131,143]

With the exception of Schmoker and colleagues' original studies[126] on the stability of using rigid internal fixation in the correction of mandibular prognathism, a majority of the clinical research on the use of these fixation techniques has focused on mandibular advancements using SSOs. Proffit and associates[79] evaluated stability of using rigid internal fixation with screws in patients with mandibular setbacks. They compared these patients with patients who were treated VRO as well as patients who had wire IMF with SSO. Interestingly, they found that the rigid internal fixation seemed to be the less stable, with almost 50% of patients having more than 4.0 mm of skeletal relapse. In one of the largest retrospective studies of mandibular setbacks, Chou found a large skeletal relapse of 21% at 1 year after surgery.[144] This relatively large amount of skeletal relapse with rigid internal fixation has been verified by a comparison of bicortical positional screws with plate and monocortical screw fixation by Chung,[145] as well as an excellent systematic review by Joss and Vassalli.[146] It is clear from the literature that mandibular setback using rigid internal fixation is relatively unstable and that, unlike mandibular advancement, consideration for overcorrection is warranted.

Nerve Damage

The possibility of damage to the IAN during SSO has been well known since the technique was first described, but surprisingly, the issue was minimized early on. Kole[147] first mentioned a high incidence of neurosensory problems immediately after surgery for patients with SSOs, but most clinicians claimed a very low incidence of long-term neurosensory problems.[148] In contrast, Walter and Gregg,[45] in an objective study of sensory problems, noted a large incidence of long-term problems. Since this first definitive study, there has continued to be a variety of reported instances of both immediate postsurgical as well as chronic sensory disturbances.

Westermark and coworkers[149] evaluated 496 SSOs for possible correlations between neurosensory dysfunction and other variables, such as age of the patient, mandibular movement, type of split technique and fixation, degree of intraoperative nerve encounter, and surgeon skill. Nerve dysfunction developed in 40% of cases. Age had a significant influence on the recovery of the neurosensory function as well as the severity of neurosensory disturbance. Intraoperative nerve encounter and nerve manipulation as well as surgical experience were also reported to have an effect on nerve dysfunction. Other variables had no significant effects on the incidence of neurosensory dysfunction. Ylikontiola and colleagues[150] also found a statistically significant positive correlation between subjective neurosensory loss and patient age and, in addition, magnitude of mandibular movement and degree of manipulation of the IAN intraoperatively.

Other clinical research has noted a significant relation between patient age and nerve recovery. This finding was noted early on by MacIntosh,[151] who emphasized that this osteotomy should not be used for patients older than 40 years. Another interesting correlation was made by Van

Sickels and associates[152] who reported that patients with a concurrent genioplasty had a greater loss of IAN sensation initially. Unfortunately, the wide variation in neurosensory testing protocols makes comparisons of these various reports difficult and makes the evaluation of techniques that have been suggested to decrease the incidence of nerve damage difficult as well.

White and colleagues[153] indicated that damage to the IAN most likely occurs either during the medial retraction of the soft tissues for the horizontal osteotomy in the vicinity of the IAN as it enters the mandibular foramen or during the vertical bone cut anteriorly where the nerve may be close to the buccal cortex. Guernsey and DeChamplain[154] believed that IAN damage occurred during the actual splitting of the mandible and reported that segments of the neurovascular bundle may remain in the proximal fragment after the split. This has led some surgeons to recommend the use of a small flat (spatula) osteotome during the split, instead of the wide-splitting osteotome, although this remains controversial.[155] The fine osteotome is malleted carefully along the lateral cortex and cancellous bone junction but may also place the nerve at risk for iatrogenic injury because its actual position in three dimensions is unknown in each patient. It has been reported that the nerve is exposed less often during the split by this technique, and consequently, it has been assumed that this results in less sensory disturbances.[156,157] Unfortunately, this technique has not been directly compared with any other, and the comparison of the occurrence of sensory disturbance between reports is not possible. Yoshida and coworkers[157] and, later, Yamamoto and associates[158] found that nerves that were close to the lateral cortex, as determined by radiographs, were more likely to have severe sensory alteration after surgery. The deficits were also more likely to be present 1 year after surgery when the marrow space between the mandibular canal and the external cortical bone was 0.8 mm or less. Some authors believe that by making the vertical cut in the lateral cortex more posterior, a lower incidence of sensory problems occurs.[157,159] This has not been substantiated in comparison studies, and in fact, the IAN may be closer to the buccal cortex in the third molar region than further anteriorly.

Another possible cause of sensory loss to the IAN may be due to sharp medullary bone irregularities of the proximal or distal fragments or to compression of the IAN when the proximal fragment is positioned and fixated, especially if there is a "lag screw" component to the fixation.[160,161] A round or acrylic bur can be used cautiously to remove any bone spicules as well as to widen and deepen the canal in the proximal fragment to prevent this nerve compression effect. Care must be taken when working around the nerve so that instruments used during the osteotomy do not themselves cause direct iatrogenic nerve damage. This concern has been heightened with the use of screw fixation. Paulis and Steinhauser[162] noted slightly higher incidences of long-term sensory loss in patients with rigid screw fixation compared with simple osseous fixation, but statistics were not used and the significance of their numbers is questionable. Nishioka and colleagues[163] performed a comprehensive study involving sensory loss after the use of screw fixation and found the incidence of IAN sensory loss to be high but within the range of sensory loss reported by other well-designed objective studies. Subsequently, the effect of type of fixation on neurosensory functional outcome was extensively studied by a number of authors using different methods of clinical neurosensory testing.[164-167] Brushstroke directional discrimination was diminished to a greater extent in the rigid fixation group compared with the wire fixation group from 8 weeks through 2 years postoperatively; however, monofilament contact detectional discrimination did not show significant difference between types of fixation throughout the 2-year follow-up.[164] Despite a high number of studies on neurosensory disturbance after orthognathic surgery, the severity of IAN injury is difficult to compare across different studies because there is lack of standardization regarding which neurosensory tests were used, methods in which the tests were performed, and how the results were interpreted. Certain neurosensory tests are more sensitive in detecting sensory nerve deficit than others. Tests that evaluate patients' abilities to discriminate direction have been shown to be more sensitive indicators of trigeminal neurosensory impairment than other tests such as light touch detection. Westermark and coworkers[165] used a visual analogue scale (VAS), light touch perception, and temperature testing and concluded that there is a positive correlation with nerve dysfunction. Alternatively, Chen and associates[166] compared three methods of assessing neurosensory disturbance after SSO: two-point discrimination, pressure-pain thresholds, and perceived sensation changes in specific facial regions. The two-point discrimination test was consistent with patients' self-ratings of neurosensory problems using facial maps, but the pressure-pain test was the least sensitive to neurosensory changes. The frequency of IAN disturbance ranged from 10.0% to 94.0% depending upon the testing method and the testing site used. In a well-controlled study by Nakagawa and colleagues,[167] the occurrence of a long-lasting postoperative trigeminal sensory hypoesthesia was found to be dependent on the nerve involvement at the bone split interface, the manner of fixation, or the intraoperative handling of the tissue surrounding the nerve. Essick demonstrated improved return of sensation and less patient concerns following the SSO with the use of biofeedback sensory retraining exercises.[168] The biofeedback sessions, which occurred 1 week and 1 and 3 months after surgery, resulted in significantly less pain, "unusual feeling," and numbness than the control group. This training seems to be the only postoperative variable, other than time from surgery, that can influence spontaneous neurosensory recovery.

Although the neurosensory function of the IAN after SSO has received a great deal of attention, few studies have documented the incidence of lingual nerve dysfunction, mostly related to bicortical screw overpenetration of the lingual cortex. Jacks and associates[169] retrospectively reviewed the patient-reported incidence, duration, and perceived deficit associated with lingual nerve function. In the SSO patients,

19% reported lingual nerve sensory changes, of whom 69% reported a resolution of symptoms within 1 year and 88% reported altered activities of daily living. When compared with the IAN, lingual nerve sensory changes occurred much less frequently and resolved more frequently and sooner, but they were associated with greater perceived deficits in patients' daily activities. Zuniga and colleagues[170] were the first to report on studies performed to assess the effect of lingual nerve injury and repair on human taste perception. Gent and coworkers[171] examined perceived taste intensity and taste quality identification on localized regions of the tongue after orthognathic surgery. Lingual nerve function in taste perception was diminished at 1 to 2 months after surgery, likely due to impaired chorda tympani nerve function, but it improved by 6 to 9 months after surgery.

TMJ Dysfunction

The incidence of TMJ dysfunction is considered in two ways: first, the incidence of TMJ symptoms that are present after surgery compared with preoperative findings; and second, the change in mandibular range of motion. The latter may obviously not be related to TMJ dysfunction; conversely, it must be considered when evaluating the effects of the surgery on the TMJ. Unfortunately, few authors related these two areas when they reported on the effect of the SSO. Another factor that must be taken into account in evaluating the effects on the TMJ from orthognathic surgery is the possible contribution from presurgical orthodontics. There is certainly debate regarding the influence of orthodontics on TMJ dysfunction, in both the short and the long term.

Similar to neurosensory loss, the potential of the SSO to cause TMJ dysfunction was recognized early.[24] Reporting on the incidence of TMJ problems, however, has been highly variable, with most authors recording only the postoperative complaint without any reference to the preoperative condition. Some of the first reviews that did look at pre- and postoperative TMJ symptoms seemed to imply an increase in joint noise, but not in pain, after the SSO.[56,172,173] The use of rigid screw fixation was believed by some to cause an increase in TMJ problems by fixating the condyle into a position that may not be natural or adaptable after surgery.[174] This concern was highlighted by radiographic findings of condylar changes that occurred with rigid screw fixation. Kundert and Hadjianghelou[106] demonstrated that this tendency occurred with both wires and screws but was greater with rigid fixation than with a wire osseous fixation technique. In neither study was there a discussion of whether these changes had any clinical consequences. Hackney and associates[175] found that with bicortical screw fixation for SSO used for mandibular advancement, little change in condylar position occurred and there was no significant effect of the surgery on TMJ symptoms. Paulis and Steinhauser[162] compared preoperative and postoperative TMJ symptoms in two large groups who had either rigid screw fixation or wire osseous fixation of SSO. They found no difference in postoperative incidence of TMD between the two groups and, in fact, found a notable decrease in TMJ pain in both groups. The possibility that the SSO may benefit patients with TMJ symptoms was suggested by Martis[176] and Karabouta and Martis.[177] They reported that only 11% of the patients who had TMJ symptoms before surgery had any symptoms after surgery, whereas about 4% of the asymptomatic patients had TMJ problems after surgery. These results were better than, but consistent with, a study of all types of orthognathic surgery patients, which showed an improvement in a large percentage of patients, with relatively small risk for the asymptomatic patient.[178]

There is, surprisingly, a body of evidence in the literature that suggests that the SSO may have a beneficial effect on preexisting TMJ dysfunction. It is generally believed that TMJ dysfunction (internal derangement, anterior disk displacement) is found at a higher incidence in class II patients compared with patients with classes I and III malocclusions. The use of the SSO as an alternative to the mandibular condylotomy to treat patients with painful TMJ dysfunction has been proposed by some authors.[179] They suggest repositioning the proximal segment and increasing the joint space, both of which are thought to have an unloading effect on the highly innervated neurovascular retrodiskal tissues. However, this is controversial and there has not been adequate research to confirm this impression. Other studies have indicated the trend that class II patients who undergo SSO advancement may have improvement in TMJ symptoms, whereas class III patients who undergo SSO mandibular setback are less likely to improve or more likely to develop worsening TMJ symptomatology. Each patient must be treated individually based upon their age, dentoskeletal deformity, and preexisting TMJ symptoms.

Debate on rigid versus wire fixation relative to the effect on the TMJ has led to a number of studies that have shown no significant difference in the incidence of TMJ symptoms between patients who received rigid fixation versus wire osteosynthesis during SSO.[180] Feinerman and Piecuch[181] compared the TMJ outcomes of the miniplate with monocortical screw group versus the superior border wire fixation with IMF group. They found no demonstrable long-term differences between the two groups with respect to mandibular vertical opening, crepitus, and TMJ pain. In fact, masticatory muscle pain and TMJ clicking improved with rigid fixation and worsened with nonrigid wire fixation. One of the reported findings of a large prospective study comparing rigid screw fixation with wire IMF was that, although large mandibular advancements along with counterclockwise rotation of the distal segment resulted in more muscle as well as TMJ symptoms soon after surgery, at 2 years, there was significant decrease in both myofascial and TMJ symptoms.

The only negative report on the effects of SSO on the TMJ was by Wolford and colleagues,[182] who evaluated changes in TMJ dysfunction in patients with presurgical TMJ internal derangement as well as the long-term stability of orthognathic surgery. Unlike other clinicians, they noted the development of new TMJ symptoms, or an aggravation of existing

TMJ symptoms, in a group of patients at 14 months postsurgery. Therefore, the authors recommended that surgical correction of preexisting TMJ pathology with formal TMJ surgery be considered, either preceding or concurrently with the orthognathic procedure. In summary, it appears that there is a low risk of worsening TMJ symptoms in patients who have preexisting TMJ dysfunction with the SSO procedure. In addition, conversely, the SSO may result in improved TMJ symptoms in a greater number of symptomatic patients owing to changes in the orientation of the TMJ apparatus and subsequent TMJ adaptation. Unfortunately, standardized methods of predicting TMJ outcome in individual patients after SSOs have not been developed.

Mechanical displacement of the condyle out of its correct position has been implicated as a significant factor in postsurgical skeletal relapse after SSO. For this reason, as well as in an attempt to minimize TMJ problems, a great deal of interest has been focused by early investigators on the issues of condylar position after SSO.[183] There have been a myriad of technical notes on how to maintain the preoperative condylar position and use of different condylar repositioning devices, based on anecdotal reports of individual surgeon experiences. Harris and coworkers[184] examined factors influencing condylar position after SSO fixated with rigid fixation. The amount of advancement did not correlate with condylar displacement. Condyle angulation and superoinferior movement did correlate somewhat with the amount of advancement. In addition, Van Sickels and associates[185] found that the condylar position was slightly different with rigid fixation versus wire osteosynthesis beyond 8 weeks postoperatively, but the ultimate position of the condyle was not significantly different. They found, as have many others, that the final condylar position was posterior and superior to its preoperative location after mandibular advancement. Renzi and colleagues[186] specifically examined class III patients without preoperative TMJ dysfunction; half of the patient population was treated with a condylar positioning device and the other half was treated with manual intraoperative control of condylar position. The condylar repositioning device did not prevent the changes in condyle positions in all cases. Neither group had any skeletal or occlusal relapse or postsurgical TMJ dysfunction. The value of using condylar positioning devices was reviewed by Costa[187], who concluded that there was no scientific evidence until 2008 to support the routine use of these devices. However, some surgeons continue to use some form of positioning devices and to attempt to demonstrate benefit in the extra time required for these methods. magnetic resonance imaging (MRI) was used by Saka for evaluation of not only condylar position but also position of the disk in this prospective study comparing a condylar repositioning device versus regular manual positioning.[188] Postoperatively, they found a significant difference between these two groups, with anterior disk displacement significantly more common without the repositioning device. The condylar position after surgery, however, was found to be similar. Unfortunately, there was no mention of postoperative TMJ symptoms, although there was an assumption that problems would occur in those patients with a displaced disk. However, it is important to understand that the incidence of new-onset TMJ dysfunction in healthy individuals after orthognathic surgery is known to be low as previously mentioned. The assumption of many surgeons that changes found with TMJ imaging have clinical consequences may be unfounded, and this study included only patients without preoperative TMJ symptoms. Therefore, it is not surprising that the patients did not develop any postsurgical TMJ dysfunction. Also, the clinical implication of condylar and disk position in the healthy versus preexisting TMJ dysfunction groups may be different; therefore, the true clinical significance of condylar and disk position in exacerbation of TMJ symptoms remains unknown.

Computed tomography (CT) has enabled clinicians to assess and quantify condylar position changes in three planes of space. Alder and colleagues[189] reported that changes in condylar position occurred in all planes of space, but the most common postoperative condylar position was more lateral with increased condylar angle, a higher coronoid process, and a condyle located more superior and posterior in the fossa. Rebellato and coworkers[190] found an increased superior postsurgical movement of the condyle with increasing magnitudes of surgical advancement of the mandible.

MRI has revolutionized the examination of the TMJ, in that it not only allows the evaluation of condylar position but also provides information on disk position and morphology. Gaggl and associates[191] reported clinical and MRI findings of the TMJ in class II patients, preoperatively and 3 months postoperatively. Clinically, patients had improvements in joint pain and abnormal joint sounds such as clicking. The MRI showed displacement of the disk in 38 of the 50 joints preoperatively and in 28 postoperatively. No correlation was made between the change in disk position and improvement in TMJ symptoms, which is consistent with other MRI studies. Ueki and colleagues[192] made interesting comparisons of the condylar and disk positions after SSO and IVRO and correlated these findings with TMJ symptoms postoperatively. Fewer or no TMJ symptoms were reported by 88% of patients who underwent IVRO and by 66% of patients who underwent SSO. MRI studies showed no change in anterior disk displacement after BSSO; however, improvement was seen in 44% of patients who underwent IVRO, at least in the early postsurgical period.

The effect of SSO on mandibular range of motion has been studied extensively. Whereas Stacy[193] found that patients who underwent mandibular setbacks with IMF generally returned to presurgical function within 9 months after surgery without any physical therapy, other authors have found very different results. Storum and Bell[194] found that without active physical therapy after the release of IMF, there was a decrease in the patient's ability to achieve preoperative opening when compared with patients who had an active rehabilitation program. This latter study is consistent with most clinicians' experience, and some form of active physical

therapy is recommended after release from IMF. However, there is some research and intuitive evidence that rigid internal fixation that permits mandibular movement soon after surgery may result in a more rapid return to preoperative mandibular movement without active physiotherapy.[195] However, the literature remains inconclusive.[195,196] Nishimura and coworkers[196] found that final postoperative mouth opening was not significantly influenced by the type of fixation. Hatch[197] also found in a large prospective study of wire versus rigid internal fixation that at 5 years, that there was no significant difference between the two groups. Interestingly, they also noted that neither group returned to completely normal preoperative mouth opening levels.

Another poorly understood TMJ complication is idiopathic condylar resorption, or spontaneous resorption of the condyles, after SSO.[198] This process is different from standard orthognathic relapse with the abnormal resorption being seen primarily in a specific group of patient; specifically young female patients who have had a history of TMJ dysfunction before surgery, with a steep mandibular plane angle, and who have undergone a large mandibular advancement. Some remodeling of the condyles is expected to occur after SSO, but fortunately, only rarely does this condylar resorption result in significant clinical changes with pain and apertognathia. Cutbirth and colleagues[199] evaluated long-term condylar resorption after mandibular advancement stabilized with bicortical screws. Large advancements and preoperative TMJ symptoms significantly correlated with long-term postoperative condylar resorption at the mean follow-up of 3 years. The amount of vertical resorption did not directly correlate with the amount of relapse seen between 6 to 8 weeks or in the long term. Surprisingly, there was an improvement in TMJ symptoms for the group as a whole and even among the group who developed condylar resorption. It should be noted, however, that it is often difficult to distinguish between normal condylar remodeling and significant condylar resorption. In the Cutbirth and colleagues study,[190] the authors arbitrarily established a parameter of less than 10% loss of condylar height to be considered as "normal remodeling." Attempts to delineate the normal versus pathologic processes are difficult and may lead to an underestimation of the actual number of clinically significant condylar resorption cases that may occur.

Hoppenreijs and coworkers[200] evaluated the long-term treatment results of 26 patients (23 women and 3 men) who developed progressive condylar resorption after orthognathic surgery. The preoperative condylar configuration was noted in patients with deep bites to have more resorption on the superior aspect of the condyle, whereas patients with anterior open bites had resorption on the superior and anterior surfaces of the condyle. Thirteen patients were managed without surgery after the diagnosis of condylar resorption, and only 3 patients had class I occlusion at the end of treatment. Thirteen patients underwent a second surgical correction, with 7 patients having satisfactory occlusal results. Four of the patients had relapse with a stable occlusion not requiring further treatment, and 2 patients had complete relapse requiring a third surgical procedure. It was suggested that without surgical intervention after condylar resorption, further resorption ceased after approximately 2 years. The authors speculated that either the mechanical loading during or after SSO and/or the impediment of blood flow to the condylar segment and the TMJ capsule may play a role in condylar resorption. However, the etiology of this process is still unclear, but it does seem to be self-limiting and the resulting dental skeletal deformity can usually be successfully treated with further mandibular surgery.

Miscellaneous Complications

A wide variety of other complications have been reported after SSO. Early reviews of complications from this procedure noted excessive blood loss, postoperative airway compromise, aseptic necrosis of bone segments, and facial nerve damage. Better experience and improved instrumentation seem to have dramatically decreased the incidence of these problems. Bleeding is generally easily managed by direct or indirect pressure over the bleeding soft tissue and vessels. Lanigan and associates,[201] reporting on a questionnaire sent to a large number of oral and maxillofacial surgeons, found only 21 cases of significant bleeding after mandibular osteotomies. Suspected sources of bleeding included the inferior alveolar artery, facial artery, maxillary artery, and retromandibular vein. Management primarily included direct pressure packing or ligation of the vessel at the point of severance through the open wound. Extraoral approaches to gain access to the facial or external carotid artery can be ineffective owing to the collateral circulation. Angiography with embolization is considered appropriate in cases of acute persistent postoperative arterial bleeding of more than 0.5 mL/min.

A group of problems that seems to persist is the inadvertent fracture in the anterior buccal aspect of the proximal segment or the posterior lingual aspect of the distal segment. Good surgical technique with extension of the osteotomies into the marrow space minimizes these problems, and care used during the split is worth the effort because correcting a "bad" split can be difficult. Fortunately, the use of screws and plates does improve the chance of obtaining a satisfactory result, in light of an unexpected fracture, with minimum further morbidity to the patient.[202] It has been believed that one of the major risk factors predisposing to buccal cortex fracture is the presence of impacted third molars. Precious and colleagues[203] retrospectively reviewed two groups of patients: one group with retained impacted third molars removed during BSSO and the other group with third molars having been removed at least 6 months before BSSO. There was a 1.9% incidence of unfavorable fractures, and the majority of fractures occurred with the group who had the third molars removed at least 6 months before the BSSO. Mehra and coworkers[204] reported 2.2% unfavorable fractures in 500 procedures. They noted a larger percentage of unfavorable fractures in the patients with retained third molars (3.2% vs. 1.2%).

This finding is consistent with that of Reyneke and associates[205] who found that the presence of unerupted third molars increased the degree of difficulty of SSO, and in all 4 out of 139 patients, unfavorable fractures occurred in patients with unerupted third molars present at the time of surgery. Ideally, third molars should be extracted at least 9 to 12 months or more before the SSO, both to minimize unfavorable fractures and to allow optimal bony healing, especially when planning on the use of internal rigid fixation.

Airway patency and induction of iatrogenic obstructive sleep apnea (OSA) has become an area of concern to some clinicians, especially in the cases in which the mandible is retropositioned. Riley and colleagues[206] reported two patients who were surgically treated for prognathism and later developed OSA. Kawamata and coworkers[207] studied patients with mandibular prognathism who were treated with either SSO or VRO for mandibular setback. Using three-dimensional CT imaging, they quantified the posterior airway space after surgery and found that the lateral and frontal widths of the pharyngeal airway had decreased by 23% and 11%, respectively, and this reduction in airway dimension did not resolve at 1 year after surgery. However, in the longer postoperative period, a visible recovery of pharyngeal width was seen in some cases. The finding of decreased airway dimension secondary to mandibular setback has been confirmed by other studies. Therefore, one should be cognizant of any physiologic and medical etiologic factors, including preexisting OSA, that may have contributed to the emergence of OSA symptoms, rather than simply using the measurement of the posterior airway space after mandibular osteotomy as the sole means of predicting the development of new-onset OSA.

In general, the risk of infection seems to be low with the SSO owing to the vascularity in the head and neck region. In their clinical review of 700 consecutive cases of mandibular osteotomies, Bouwman and associates[208] reported that screw removal owing to infection was performed in 2.8% of cases. Screw loosening occurred in the first postoperative week, which resulted in an occlusal discrepancy in 4 patients. Fifteen sides required one or more screws to be removed as a result of infection. In a large study of complications in orthognathic surgery, Acebal-Bianco and colleagues[209] reported 36 infections out of 802 mandibular osteotomies (0.05%), but only 5 patients had hardware removed owing to infections.

Horizontal Ramus Osteotomies

Since Blair's first description of his osteotomy of the horizontal ramus,[3] a variety of osteotomy designs have been documented. Initially, the surgeons used extraoral, or a combination of extraoral and intraoral techniques, but since the early 1950s, the advocated approaches have primarily been intraoral. It is difficult to choose a representative technique for the body osteotomies because of the wide variations described as well as the relative infrequency of these techniques. Of the described procedures, the step osteotomy is reviewed because of its versatility and its apparent common use in some centers.

Indications

The greatest limitations of body osteotomies are that the osteotomy must be made through the dental alveolus so edentulous spaces are usually required and the IAN is at risk for injury during these procedures. Because these osteotomies are made anterior to the pterygomasseteric sling, some surgeons believe that the results are more stable and, therefore, prefer body osteotomies in the treatment of prognathism when there are edentulous spaces. Other unusual mandibular abnormalities, such as asymmetries, may also be treated more appropriately with one of these forms of osteotomy as opposed to an osteotomy of the vertical ramus.

With the step osteotomy, the surgeon must be concerned about the horizontal component of the "step," which often has to be performed between the IAN and the apices of the tooth roots. Sufficient room should, therefore, be available for this cut, unless the surgeon plans to externalize part of the IAN so that the cut can be made at the level of or below the inferior alveolar canal.

Technique

An incision is made 4 to 5 mm below the level of the attached gingiva (enough tissue is left superiorly to permit later suturing) and is carried forward at this level to the cuspid, where it can be dropped down 5 mm and extended forward to the midline (Figure 57-19A). The periosteum is elevated inferiorly until the mental foramen is located and then the remainder of the periosteum is stripped to expose the area of the osteotomy. The attached gingiva is also carefully elevated in the area of the dental alveolar cut so that it can be protected during the osteotomy.

The vertical cut through the alveolus is made with either a saw or a bur. A finger should be kept on the lingual aspect of the mandible to prevent the power instrument from penetrating the mucosa. Because the lingual mucosa is very thin, some surgeons may find it helpful to place a fine ribbon retractor between the bone and the mucosa. This is done by making a horizontal incision a few millimeters lingual to the teeth and the edentulous area and then carefully elevating the mucosa down below the floor of the mouth. The retractor is then placed and supported with the surgeon's finger to ensure it is not displaced while making the cuts. When the surgical plan includes a mandibular setback, a block of bone must be removed to permit posterior positioning of the mandible. The distance between the parallel cuts necessary to remove the bone should be as close as possible to the planned setback, as determined by the model surgery. The vertical cuts are carried inferiorly to the level of the planned horizontal cut, which would be at least 5 mm below the dental apices. The inferior vertical cuts are then made, again using parallel cuts as necessary for a setback of the distal fragment. Finally, the horizontal cut is made, preferably by a saw, to minimize bone

removal and endangering of the apices or the IAN (see Figure 57-19B).

The distal segment is related to the proximal segment with an occlusal splint and fixed with IMF. If the mandible is set back any significant distance, a wedge of attached tissue over

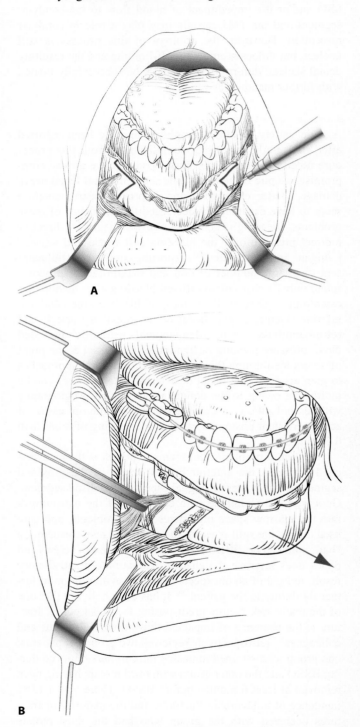

FIGURE 57-19. **A** and **B,** The step osteotomy. (**A** and **B,** Adapted from Bloomquist DS. Principles of mandibular orthognathic surgery. In Peterson LJ, Indresano AT, Marciani RD, Roser SM, editors. Principles of Oral and Maxillofacial Surgery. Vol 3. Philadelphia: JB Lippincott; 1992; p. 1444.)

the alveolar vertical osteotomy must be removed to permit the setback. This wedge should be narrower than the planned movement to allow tight mucosal contact. This eliminates the need for suturing in this area, which is often difficult. Osseous wire fixation can be placed at the inferior border, or if a rigid fixation technique is preferable, straight four-holed plates with monocortical screws can be placed above and below the nerve. With a rigid fixation technique, the IMF wires can be cut and the segment stability and position checked before closure of the wound. The surgical sites are thoroughly irrigated and the mucosa is then closed with a resorbable suture. IMF, if used, is maintained for 6 to 8 weeks (Figure 57-20).

Alternative Techniques

There are multiple variations of mandibular body osteotomies. Generally, the mucosal approaches are similar, although some surgeons prefer to make a cervical incision posterior to the mental foramen and then carry it below the attached tissue in the anterior symphyseal region. This approach unfortunately presents some difficulty with wound closure, especially if IMF is used.

One of the most difficult variations in the surgical approach occurs when there is a need for visualization or exteriorization of the IAN, if an osteotomy is planned through the inferior alveolar canal. The easiest method for this is similar to that described by Epker.[210]

After the lateral surface of the mandible is exposed in the area of the planned osteotomies, parallel horizontal cortical cuts are made on either side of the anticipated route of the IAN. These cuts are extended beyond either side of the planned osteotomy, sufficient to permit adequate approach to the nerve as well as to permit enough freedom of the nerve during stretching or compression that will occur with the planned segment movements. Perpendicular cuts are made just through the cortex at approximately 1-cm intervals (Figure 57-21). Starting with the forward cuts, a thin sharp 4-mm osteotome is used to carefully start a cleavage line through the cancellous bone, preferably just below the cortex. As each individual section is broken away, the medial aspect of the fragment must be checked to ensure that a nerve is not still attached to it. After all the small lateral cortical segments have been removed, often the nerve has been exposed and judicious use of a small surgical curette is all that is needed to remove any bone spicules over the nerve as well as to carefully lift the nerve out of its canal. If cancellous bone is still covering the nerve, a medium-sized round bur can be used to carefully remove the overlying bone. A small periosteal elevator or a surgical curette can be positioned in the lateral aspect of the canal when the nerve is exposed and the thin bur used to remove the remaining overlying bone. Following the visualization or exteriorization of the IAN, the osteotomies can proceed as planned.

Although primarily used for distal fragment setback, the step osteotomy can be used for advancement. To accomplish this, a horizontal incision must be made on the lingual side of the alveolus, posterior to the vertical alveolar bone cut. The mucoperiosteum below this cut can then be elevated to allow it to be stretched with the advancement. The lateral incision is designed to permit the labial tissue to be pulled lingually, without tension, so that soft tissue closure can be done. Bone grafts are generally used in the gaps created by the advancements, especially in the alveolar area, where prostheses may later be placed.

Sagittal osteotomies of the horizontal ramus have been described with either an extraoral or an intraoral approach possible.[211,212] With the intraoral approach, the lingual exposure has to be increased to make the vertical cortical cut. This generally requires that the incision on the lingual side of the teeth be brought forward, close to the midline, so that retraction may occur without endangering the surrounding soft tissue. The advantage of this type of osteotomy is that it allows the use of rigid internal fixation with bicortical screws, and generally, a bone graft is not needed if the distal segment is advanced.

Complications

Reports of body osteotomies in the literature include mostly case reports; therefore, there are few series reporting incidence of complications. The wide variety of techniques makes it impossible to make any definitive statements about body osteotomies. Therefore, this section is primarily limited to the listing of the reported complications, many of which can be anticipated simply from the knowledge of the anatomy of the area.

RELAPSE

One of the primary reasons given by surgeons for using a body osteotomy procedure is the stability of the technique. Sandor and coworkers[213] assessed relapse of the step osteotomy and found it to be very stable. Most other authors have not strictly analyzed the results but claim a good long-term stability with their particular technique.[214,215]

NEURAL COMPLICATIONS

Those studies that include reports of the incidence or duration of neurosensory damage report a high spontaneous recovery rate.[214,215] Unfortunately, these studies are of questionable value because of the inadequate testing methods used. It can be expected, however, that immediate postoperative sensory loss will be present after any of the body osteotomies, especially those that require visualization or exteriorization of the IAN. The incidence of devitalization of teeth on either side of the osteotomy or of those teeth above the horizontal cut of the step osteotomy is unknown, although it is probably similar to those reported with mandibular subapical osteotomies.

The increased potential of nonunion in body osteotomies has been discussed, but the incidence is unknown. The possibility of this occurring is very low if, as has been suggested, care is used in osteotomy design to ensure sufficient bone contact as well as in the provision of adequate fixation.

The possibility of periodontal defects does exist for osteotomies made close to the teeth where the surrounding soft

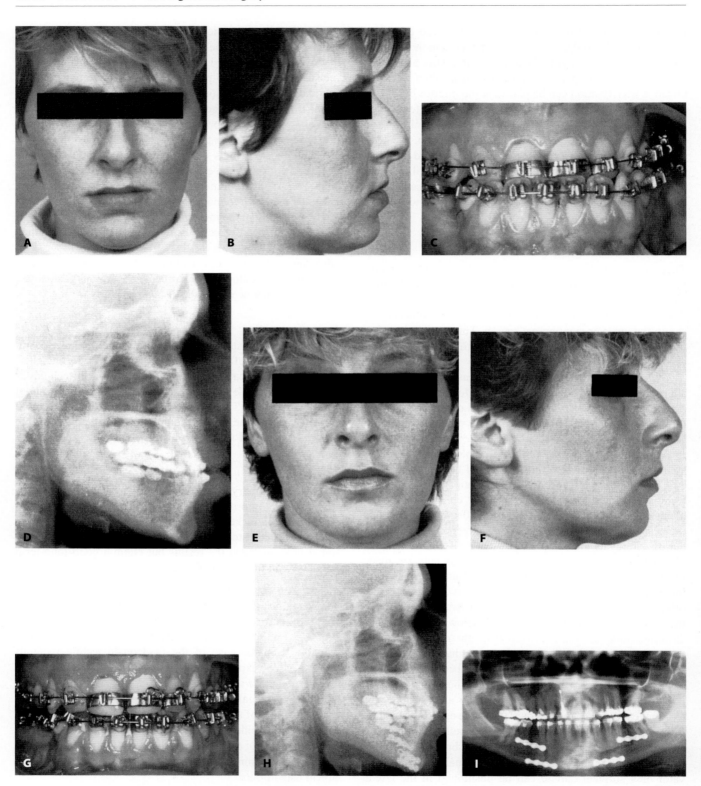

FIGURE 57-20. Patient who was treated with a step osteotomy for mandibular horizontal excess. **A-D,** Preoperative photographs and radiograph. **E-I,** Postoperative photographs and radiographs. (**A-I,** Reproduced with permission from Bloomquist DS. Principles of mandibular orthognathic surgery. In Peterson LJ, Indresano AT, Marciani RD, Roser SM, editors. Principles of Oral and Maxillofacial Surgery. Vol 3. Philadelphia: JB Lippincott; 1992; pp. 1446–1447.)

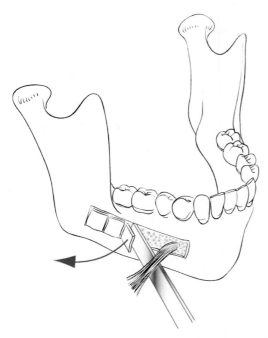

FIGURE 57-21. Decortication for exposure of the inferior alveolar nerve and vessels. (Adapted from Bloomquist DS. Principles of mandibular orthognathic surgery. In Peterson LJ, Indresano AT, Marciani RD, Roser SM, editors. Principles of Oral and Maxillofacial Surgery. Vol 3. Philadelphia: JB Lippincott; 1992; p. 1448.)

tissue pedicle may be injured. As has been noted earlier, the possibility of this occurring in midline osteotomies is low, but whether this can be related to other parts of the dental alveolus is doubtful.[216]

Subapical Osteotomies

There are essentially three types of mandibular subapical osteotomies: the anterior subapical, the posterior subapical, and the total alveolar osteotomy. Whereas these techniques have fallen out of favor as primary treatment options, each has a small place in orthognathic surgery; therefore, the indications and techniques of each are described individually, and because the complications are similar, these are discussed together as well.

Anterior Subapical Osteotomy

INDICATIONS

The subapical osteotomy has historically been popular because of its versatility to move the anterior mandibular teeth and alveolus in almost every possible direction, although it is not commonly performed today. The greatest concern in this procedure is the potential for damaging teeth, and therefore, space must be present or created to permit safe vertical cuts in the dental alveolus.

PROCEDURE

If necessary, teeth are removed to permit osteotomies or to provide space for the planned alveolar movement. The inci-

sion begins about 1 cm behind the planned vertical osteotomy and is carried forward about 4 to 5 mm below the attached tissue until reaching the cuspid, at which time, it can be positioned inferiorly and carried to the midline to connect with a contralateral incision. The periosteum is elevated, exposing the lateral cortex of the mandible, with care around the mental foramen as well as attention paid to leaving soft tissue attachments at the inferior border to ensure stability of the soft tissue–chin morphology. The attached tissue at the planned vertical osteotomy site must be elevated, and if posterior movement of the segment is anticipated, some of this tissue may have to be removed. As mentioned with the step osteotomy, the width of the tissue removed should be less than the planned posterior movement to ensure adequate soft tissue contact and coverage.

The vertical osteotomies are made using parallel cuts when the posterior movement of the segment is planned. Adequate preoperative radiologic evaluation and planning will minimize the chance of damage to the IAN. Most anterior subapical osteotomies are designed to include the cuspids and the incisors, which generally place the vertical cuts anterior to the mental foramen. Difficulties arise if the planned osteotomy includes extraction of the first bicuspid or if the cut is planned behind this area. The importance of being able to make the horizontal cut at least 5 mm below the tooth apices cannot be overemphasized. Not only is the vitality of the teeth potentially compromised, but the entire dentoosseous segment may be affected by the level of the horizontal cut. If parallel horizontal cuts are planned to move the anterior segment apically, the superior cut is made first. The inferior cut is then made, and the segment of bone is removed without overmanipulation of the dental alveolar segment that might increase the likelihood of injuring the soft tissue pedicle (Figure 57-22A). Beveling the cut from anterior to posteroinferior will minimize the amount of bone to be removed and increase the size of the lingual soft tissue pedicle. Usually, when attempting to reposition the mobile dentoalveolar segment to the rest of the mandible, further bony interferences are encountered. These exist primarily on the lingual cortex of the vertical cuts, and care must be used in the rotation of the mobile segment to access this cortex. As mentioned earlier for the step osteotomy, when possible, a retractor should be placed between the bone and the thin lingual mucosa to minimize iatrogenic soft tissue trauma.

After ensuring an adequate seating of the teeth into the surgical splint, the segment is stabilized by either wiring the splint to the teeth individually (see Figure 57-22B) or placing circumferential mandibular wires that can be combined with IMF. Osseous wires or plates with monocortical screws are rarely needed for stability, but can be used if desired. Plates and monocortical screws can be used with the splint but, generally, do not provide sufficient stability by themselves. Bone gaps caused by movement of the segment, especially by vertical movement necessary for the closure of an anterior open bite, should be grafted. The use of cortical bone from the symphysis, as advocated by Kole,[28] has been popular

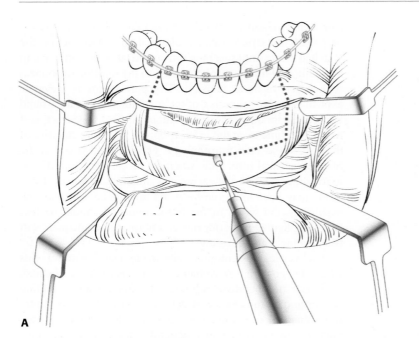

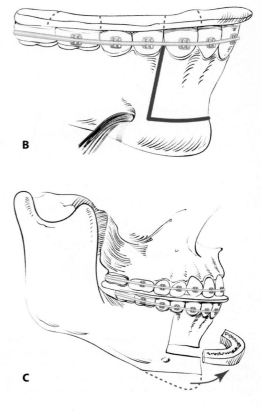

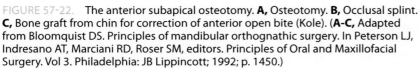

FIGURE 57-22. The anterior subapical osteotomy. **A,** Osteotomy. **B,** Occlusal splint. **C,** Bone graft from chin for correction of anterior open bite (Kole). (**A-C,** Adapted from Bloomquist DS. Principles of mandibular orthognathic surgery. In Peterson LJ, Indresano AT, Marciani RD, Roser SM, editors. Principles of Oral and Maxillofacial Surgery. Vol 3. Philadelphia: JB Lippincott; 1992; p. 1450.)

because many patients with an anterior open bite have the long anterior face, which can be improved by removal of a segment of the genial bone (see Figure 57-22C). The surgical site is then irrigated thoroughly and closed with resorbable sutures.

Posterior Subapical Osteotomy

INDICATIONS

The posterior subapical osteotomy has few indications, especially if orthodontics are an option. Primarily, it can be used as an aid in the correction of supereruption of posterior mandibular teeth or ankylosis of one or more posterior teeth. Abnormal buccal or lingual positioning of these teeth can also be improved upon with this technique, when orthodontics is not available or feasible.[217]

TECHNIQUE

The technique of Peterson, who first described this osteotomy,[208] can be done with local anesthesia and sedation or with general anesthesia. An incision begins 3 to 4 mm lateral to the attached gingiva, beginning at the anterior border of the vertical ramus. This incision is made down to bone and carried forward to the cuspid region. The periosteum is stripped superiorly and inferiorly sufficiently to expose the lateral cortex for the planned osteotomies (Figure 57-23). The osteotomy is outlined with a bur, based on the preoperative radiographic analysis of the length of the roots and the position of the inferior alveolar canal. The vertical cuts

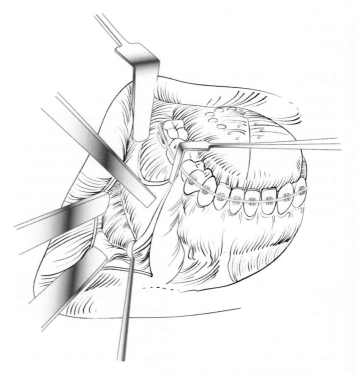

FIGURE 57-23. The posterior subapical osteotomy. (Adapted from Bloomquist DS. Principles of mandibular orthognathic surgery. In Peterson LJ, Indresano AT, Marciani RD, Roser SM, editors. Principles of Oral and Maxillofacial Surgery. Vol 3. Philadelphia: JB Lippincott Company; 1992; p. 1451.)

are made first through both cortices with a fine osteotome or thin saws. The horizontal cut is carried only through the buccal cortex, and a thick splitting osteotome is used to complete the osteotomy. Care is taken to ensure that the IAN is not caught in the mobile segment and that appropriate bony adjustments are made to permit the planned movement. The segment is positioned and stabilized with an acrylic splint and wire. Grafting is used if a bone gap is significant, and the mucosa is closed with a running resorbable suture.

ALTERNATIVE TECHNIQUES

Major modification of this technique would be appropriate if insufficient distance exists between the dental apices and the inferior alveolar canal. In such a situation, the IAN may be externalized, as described previously, and a horizontal cut made through the inferior alveolar canal. Periapical radiographs taken intraoperatively after the buccal horizontal cut will ensure that the osteotomies are made at a safe distance from the teeth and canal. This latter technique has been found to be useful because adequate visualization is difficult with the presence of posterior teeth. Also, with either of these techniques, the horizontal cut can be made safely through the lingual cortex, which eliminates the lack of predictability of the induced lingual cortical fracture.

Total Mandibular Subapical Alveolar Osteotomy

Indications

The total mandibular subapical alveolar osteotomy, first described by MacIntosh and Carlotti,[218] has limited applica-

tion today, but can prove valuable in isolated mandibular dentoalveolar protrusion or retrusion. It has also been advocated for closure of an anterior open bite when used with a bone graft.

Technique

An incision begins on the external oblique ridge of the base of the vertical ramus. The incision is carried down to bone and extends forward 4 to 5 mm below the attached gingiva. The incision can be positioned inferiorly in the region of the canine and forward where it meets the contralateral incision at the midline. The periosteum is elevated to expose the lateral cortex, with care taken around the mental nerve, as well as leaving some attachment at the inferior border of the symphysis for the soft tissue chin. The vertical cut posterior to the terminal molar is made first and carried down to the level of the planned horizontal osteotomy. As with the step osteotomies, the horizontal cut needs to be placed appropriately, based upon preoperative periapical radiographs. If this cut cannot be made safely between the dental apices and the inferior alveolar canal, the IAN needs to be exteriorized or the cut placed below the canal (Figure 57-24A). The horizontal cut can then be placed low enough to be at a safe distance from the dental root apices, as well as maintaining an adequate vascular pedicle to the dental alveolus. The angle of the horizontal cut should be made to facilitate segment movement; for instance, a flat cut paralleling the maxillary occlusal plane permits the straight advancement of the segment without significantly changing mandibular vertical height while at the same time maintaining a large area of bone contact.

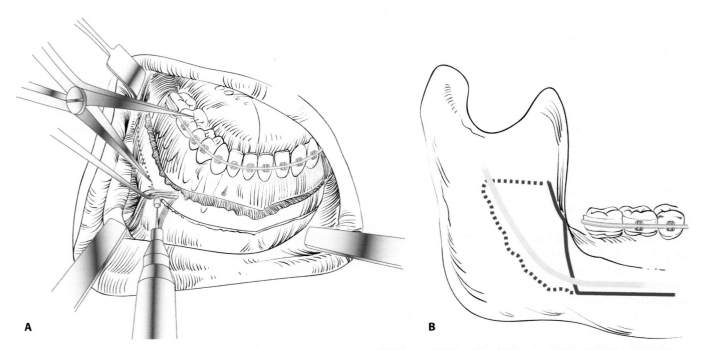

A   **B**

FIGURE 57-24.   **A** and **B,** Variations of the total mandibular alveolar osteotomy. (**A** and **B,** Adapted from Bloomquist DS. Principles of mandibular orthognathic surgery. In Peterson LJ, Indresano AT, Marciani RD, Roser SM, editors. Principles of Oral and Maxillofacial Surgery. Vol 3. Philadelphia: JB Lippincott; 1992; p. 1451.)

SECTION 7

The mobile segment is related to the maxilla with an acrylic interocclusal splint and IMF. Osseous fixation can be achieved either with the lateral cortical wires placed in the first bicuspid area along with maintaining IMF or by rigid internal fixation with monocortical plates and screws. As with correction of an anterior open bite, any significant bone gaps created may be filled with graft material. The wound is thoroughly irrigated and closed with resorbable suture.

Technique Variations

Booth and associates[219] suggested a variation of the total mandibular subapical osteotomy that combines the SSO of the vertical ramus with the total mandibular alveolar osteotomy (see Figure 57-24B). This modification has a number of advantages over the original technique. First, the osteotomy is made below the inferior alveolar canal, thereby decreasing the risk of damaging the IAN and tooth roots, at the same time preserving the vascular supply to the mobilized segment. Also, the sagittal part of the osteotomy allows a larger bone contact area to assist in bony healing.

The total mandibular alveolar osteotomy can also be divided into interdental segments to correct axial inclination of teeth or close edentulous sites. These modifications are not easily performed with Booth's osteotomy, but can be valuable as a variation of the original procedure.

Complications

The complications of all mandibular subapical alveolar osteotomies are considered together owing to their similarities. Stability is often mentioned as one of the advantages of the alveolar osteotomies because of the minimal soft tissue forces acting on these areas. Unfortunately, there have been very few studies to document this claim, and the technique has limited use. Available studies question the stability of these segmental osteotomies. Theisen and Guernsey[220] evaluated six patients who had anterior subapical osteotomies. At 1 year after surgery, an average of 1.0 mm of movement of the incisors was noted on lateral cephalograms. In contrast, Kloosterman[48] evaluated a much larger group and found a 30% recurrence of an open bite after anterior maxillary osteotomies. Pangrazio-Kulbersh and MacIntosh[221] compared the hard and soft tissue changes in a retrospective study comparing total subapical osteotomies with BSSOs for treatment of mandibular retrognathia. They found no significant difference in skeletal changes at 1 year. Interestingly, the major difference between the two groups was at soft tissue "B" point, with the subapical osteotomy resulting in a significant decrease in the labiomental angle.

Unlike segment stability, neurologic and vascular complications of segmental osteotomies have received a great deal of attention. Much of the research has focused on pulpal changes and not on peripheral IAN sensory loss or avascular necrosis with bone loss. Both of these latter problems are recognized complications of mandibular subapical osteotomies, but there are no clinical studies noting their exact incidence.[28,36] Many authors report some incidence of sensory change of the lower lip and chin but claim that there have been no permanent problems with the return of normal sensation in about 3 months.[218,229,221]

Clinical and animal studies on the effect of mandibular osteotomies on pulpal blood flow are numerous.[35,37,39,40] An early animal study did not note many vascular changes when a lingual vascular pedicle was maintained.[33] However, all subsequent studies have noted a significant decrease in blood flow, especially to the dental pulp.[222] Histologic studies of dental pulp after subapical osteotomies reveal some pulpal necrosis in most teeth.[35,223] Whether this is of clinical importance is questionable, because there were relatively few teeth in clinical series that required endodontics or extraction.[47,48] It is likely that some pulpal necrosis occurs in greater numbers of teeth than are clinically evident.[224] The only way that pulpal changes have been assessed clinically is with "vitality testing" and laser Doppler flow studies. A change in pulpal nerve sensation does not necessarily correlate with a decrease in pulpal vascularity. However, the rate of recovery of sensory loss seems to give some measure of the iatrogenic trauma to the teeth. Early clinical studies seem to show that teeth in mandibular alveolar osteotomies fare better than their maxillary counterparts.[225] More recent and larger studies, however, have demonstrated the reverse.[47,48] One report found that approximately 40% of the teeth in the repositioned mandibular segment remain unreactive to vitality testing at 1 year.[47] This high incidence of pulpal trauma was attributed to technical errors during surgeries. The incidence of teeth requiring endodontics range from 1.5% to 10%. The teeth at greatest risk for damage are those in the mobile segment directly adjacent to the vertical osteotomies. The teeth immediately posterior to the vertical cut are approximately equal in risk to the teeth in the center of the mobile segment.

Periodontal problems have been mentioned by authors reviewing mandibular alveolar osteotomies.[48,220] The incidence and quantitative evaluations of soft and hard tissue loss have not been done, although individual cases of significant interdental bone loss have been noted. Periodontal problems are seen less frequently when the vertical cuts are made in extraction sites than when the cuts are attempted between teeth without extraction.[48]

Horizontal Osteotomy of the Symphysis (Genioplasty)

The horizontal osteotomy of the symphysis, or genioplasty procedure, differs very little from that originally described by Hofer,[32] except that the procedure is routinely performed intraorally. The versatility of this procedure for correction of skeletal deformities of the chin is impressive, and the results are superior to those of synthetic implant placement in most cases.

Indications

This osteotomy of the anterior inferior border of the mandible, with minor variations, can be used to improve almost every conceivable skeletal abnormality of the chin. The technique is primarily used only for aesthetic reasons, and therefore, its use depends upon the patient's concern about appearance of this area of the face, more commonly in syndromic cases. Often, the surgeon has to bring the genioplasty to the patient's attention when other facial osteotomies are planned because of the impact that these osteotomies will have on chin prominence and aesthetics. The indications, therefore, are often made apparent by comprehensive presurgical treatment planning.

Technique

The horizontal osteotomy of the symphysis is often done in conjunction with other major osteotomies and, thus, is frequently accomplished under general anesthesia. However, it can be performed as a separate procedure on an outpatient basis with sedation and local anesthesia.

The mucosal incision is made on the labial side of the vestibule at approximately 1 cm above its depth and extends posteriorly to the first bicuspid region. This incision is carried just below the mucosa to the depth of the vestibule and then angled directly to the labial cortex through the mentalis muscle (Figure 57-25A) in an "apron" fashion with the posterior limbs closer to the attached gingiva to avoid the terminal branches of the mental nerve exiting from the mental foramen. The periosteum is elevated inferiorly to a point just below the intended level of the osteotomy. Laterally, the periosteum is elevated to the mental foramen and then extended posteroinferiorly to the mandibular inferior border below the mental foramen bilaterally. The extent of the posterior cortical exposure is generally determined by the position of the mental foramen and the vertical height of the mandible in this area. In most cases, the exposure terminates in about the first molar area. Caution must be taken if the genioplasty is performed at the same time as a BSSO procedure, because not only with the incisions closely approximate one another but also the osteotomies nearly overlap. In general, no attempt is made to expose the mental nerve by releasing the soft tissue around it, primarily because the nerve can be small and friable, making inadvertent severing a possibility. Therefore, "skeletonization" of the mental nerve should be avoided in all cases. The periosteal elevation posterior to the mental foramen is minimized to only what is necessary for placement of a narrow channel retractor and the reciprocating saw blade or bur.

It is helpful at this point to inscribe a vertical mark (or two or three marks) into the bone across the planned osteotomy site in the anterior mandible so that the transverse position of the inferior fragment can be more easily reoriented after completion of the osteotomy. The osteotomy cut is then made with a reciprocating saw, preferably because this technique minimizes soft tissue trauma on the lingual aspect of the mandible (see Figure 57-25B). The length and angle of the horizontal cut may have profound effects on positioning of the mobilized segment as well as the final postsurgical results. Further osteotomies or osteoplasties of the chin are made after mobilization of the inferior segment. The stabili-

zation of the segment in its new position can be done with cortical wires, circumandibular wires, or plates and screws; prebent chin plates are available with varying degrees of advancement in millimeters, and these may be used in a reverse fashion for setback procedures of the chin. For vertical augmentation or reduction, standard four-hole plates with screws may be used, possibly using a bone graft, if necessary. The wound is irrigated and closed in two layers, mentalis muscle and mucosa, with resorbable suture. Care should be taken to reapproximate the mentalis muscle formally in order to prevent chin ptosis ("witch's chin") postoperatively. Elastoplast tape, or similar tape, should be placed across the lip and chin to support and maintain mentalis position, and it is continued for 2 to 5 days to minimize hematoma formation and to support the suture repair. Patients should be instructed

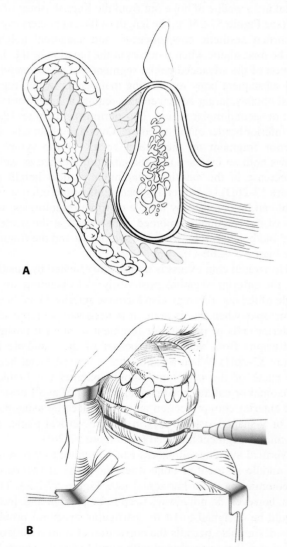

FIGURE 57-25.   The surgical approach for the horizontal osteotomy. **A,** Soft tissue approach. **B,** Osteotomy. (**A** and **B,** Adapted from Bloomquist DS. Principles of mandibular orthognathic surgery. In Peterson LJ, Indresano AT, Marciani RD, Roser SM, editors. Principles of Oral and Maxillofacial Surgery. Vol 3. Philadelphia: JB Lippincott; 1992; p. 1453.)

not to pull on their lip in order to minimize the possibility of wound dehiscence.

Alternative Techniques

The primary technical alterations in the horizontal osteotomy are based upon variations in the osteotomy design; and these design differences depend upon the preexisting symphyseal deformity that is being corrected with genioplasty. Obwegeser[100] concentrated on correction of horizontal deficiency of the chin when he described the basic procedure (Figure 57-26A). He suggested that a midsagittal osteotomy of the inferior fragment may be helpful in preventing the prominence of the posterior ends of the fragment, relative to the body of the mandible, as the fragment is advanced (see Figure 57-26B). A narrower chin point can also be obtained by taking a wedge of bone out from the lingual aspect of this cut (see Figure 57-26C). The length of the cut posteriorly has important aesthetic consequences, and anegonial notching can be unaesthetic when it occurs at the junction of the distal portion of the advanced genial segment and native mandible and subsequent bony remodeling that occurs in that region. Most notably, larger advancements require a larger cut to the first or second molar region. This permits a smoother line to the inferior border of the mandible. Overlapping an advanced inferior fragment on the lateral cortex of the symphysis allows both an increase in horizontal prominence as well as a decrease in the anterior mandibular vertical height (see Figure 57-26D).[226] Larger advancements of the inferior fragment can be obtained by double or triple osteotomies, rotation of the fragment combined with a graft at the posterior gap, and bone graft between the symphysis and the fragment (see Figure 57-26E-G).[227,228]

Horizontal chin excess is traditionally treated by positioning the inferior segment posteriorly.[229] Depending on the angle of the cut, this may also increase anterior facial height. Sometimes when this is done, it is necessary to remove the posterior ends of the inferior fragment to prevent unsightly protrusions from the inferior border of the mandible (see Figure 57-26H). When a patient has a normal facial height, the plane of the osteotomy should parallel the Frankfort horizontal or natural head position (NHP), if at all possible. The anterior chin projection may be reduced by using parallel, or V-shaped, osteotomies in a more vertical plane, with the middle segment removed (see Figure 57-26I).

Vertical symphyseal excess can be reduced by removing the middle segment of bone when the plane of two parallel osteotomies is more horizontal (see Figure 57-26J). These cuts, however, do not always need to be parallel and, in fact, should be designed to fit the particular structural problem. This design also permits the correction of a mild horizontal deficiency that is combined with a mild vertical excess (see Figure 57-26K). This skeletal problem can also be corrected with a single osteotomy placed more vertically and by repositioning the segment anteriorly (see Figure 57-26L). Vertical symphyseal deficiency can be addressed only with an interpositional graft, with either bone or other implant material

(see Figure 57-26M). The use of plates and screws alone to hold the segment in an inferior position has been suggested as well (Figures 57-27 and 57-28).

The use of wires, pins, screws, or plate and screws for the fixation of the inferior segment is common. Precious and associates[230] evaluated the changes that occur as the bone remodels after a horizontal osteotomy. They recommended that the fixation take into account these changes, especially the positioning of rigid fixation devices. Plates placed along the superior border of the inferior fragment may become noticeable to the patient as the bone remodels.

Finally, a horizontal osteotomy can be used in combination with a midline osteotomy and BSSO to allow narrowing of the mandibular arch form and at the same time advancing or setting back the chin. In this situation, the inferior segment acts as a plate and with two screws placed on either side of the vertical cut in order to stabilize the segments (Figure 57-29).

Complications

The incidence of postoperative problems after a horizontal osteotomy of the symphysis is rarely mentioned. This may be because genioplasties are frequently done in conjunction with other osteotomies, which makes the designation of various complications to one particular portion of the surgery difficult. Van Sickels evaluated sensory loss from SSOs and the effect of other factors, including genioplasty.[152] He found that there was greater initial sensory loss with genioplasty in all age groups, but prolonged neurosensory dysfunction persisted only in older patients. It is intuitive that a BSSO combined with a genioplasty would have a higher incidence of IAN dysfunction than either procedure performed alone, and the literature confirms this suspicion. The possibility of sensory loss from genioplasty alone has not been adequately evaluated, although in one study, it was noted that postsurgical sensory loss was found in all patients, but it was temporary, with normal sensation returning within 12 months.[231] Another study reported a 3.5% long-term incidence of sensory deficits after genioplasties.

Most of the literature concerning genioplasties concentrates on the soft tissue response to the skeletal movement. Reports of relapse after genioplasty are few and conflicting. Some clinicians report that there is essentially no relapse after a genioplasty, noting only a spontaneous remodeling of the sharp corners of the advanced segment occurring with time.[232–235] These studies, however, follow patients for only up to 1 year. Two other studies with follow-up of at least 1 year do seem to show some instability of the skeletal chin advancement.[236,237] The mean relapse with a genial advancement varies widely (from 2.6% to 30%), and the one consistent finding is that most of the skeletal relapse occurs within the first year. As with stability studies of other osteotomies, there exists a large variation in individual relapse, and no attempt has been made to identify the specific etiologies. However, there are probably many factors involved, including patient age and the magnitude of advancement. There have been no studies on the stability of this surgery in correction

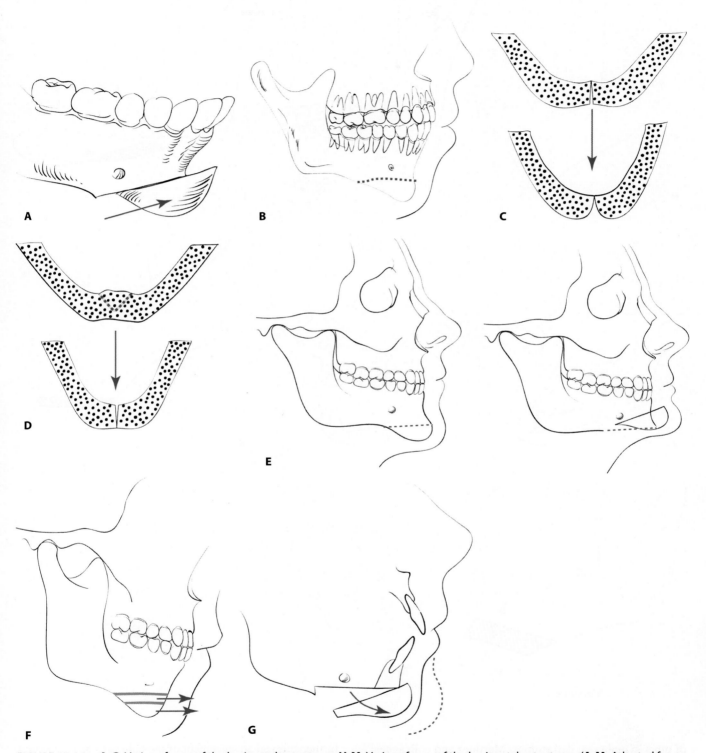

FIGURE 57-26. **A-G,** Various forms of the horizontal osteotomy. **H-M,** Various forms of the horizontal osteotomy. (**A-M,** Adapted from Bloomquist DS. Principles of mandibular orthognathic surgery. In Peterson LJ, Indresano AT, Marciani RD, Roser SM, editors. Principles of Oral and Maxillofacial Surgery. Vol 3. Philadelphia: JB Lippincott; 1992; pp. 1454–1455.) *(Continued)*

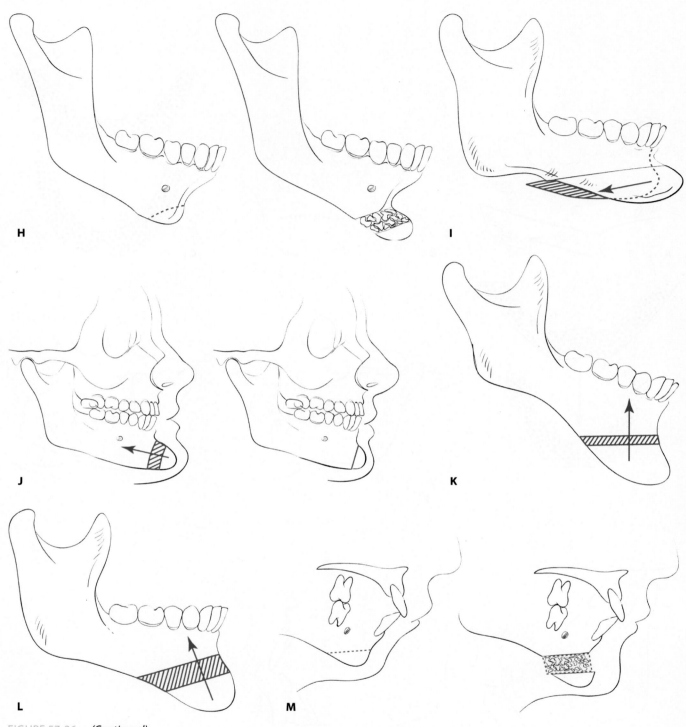

FIGURE 57-26. *(Continued)*

of other symphyseal deformities. Martinez and colleagues[234] found that regeneration of the cortical thickness of the symphysis was significantly better in patients younger than 15 years of age. They suggested that this may be beneficial if further surgical advancement of the chin is to be considered. Other complications, such as bone loss and infection, have been reported, but small samples preclude any definitive conclusions regarding precise incidence.[238]

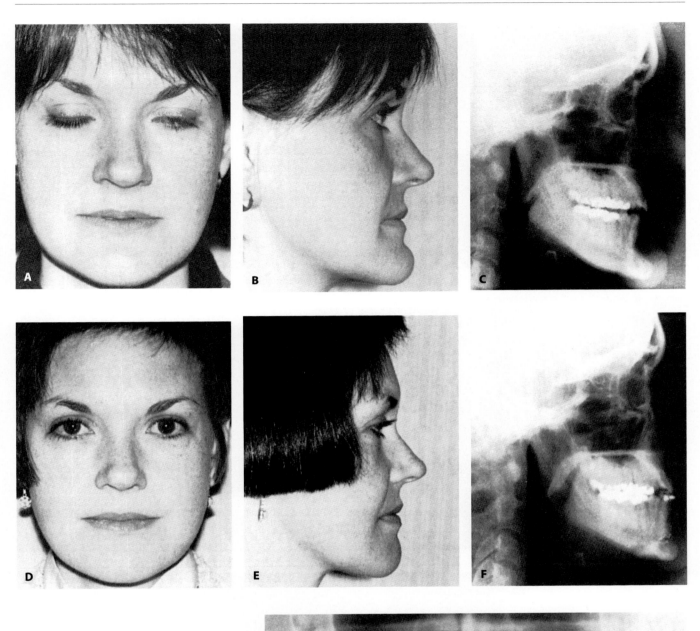

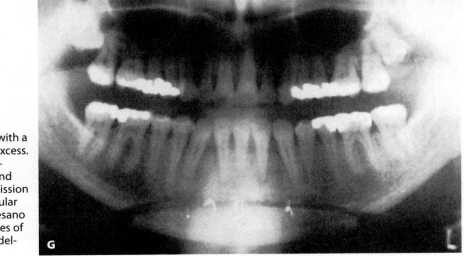

FIGURE 57-27.　Patient who was treated with a horizontal osteotomy for horizontal chin excess. **A–C,** Preoperative photographs and radiograph. **D–G,** Postoperative photographs and radiographs. (**A-G,** Reproduced with permission from Bloomquist DS. Principles of mandibular orthognathic surgery. In Peterson LJ, Indresano AT, Marciani RD, Roser SM, editors. Principles of Oral and Maxillofacial Surgery. Vol 3. Philadelphia: JB Lippincott; 1992; p. 1456.)

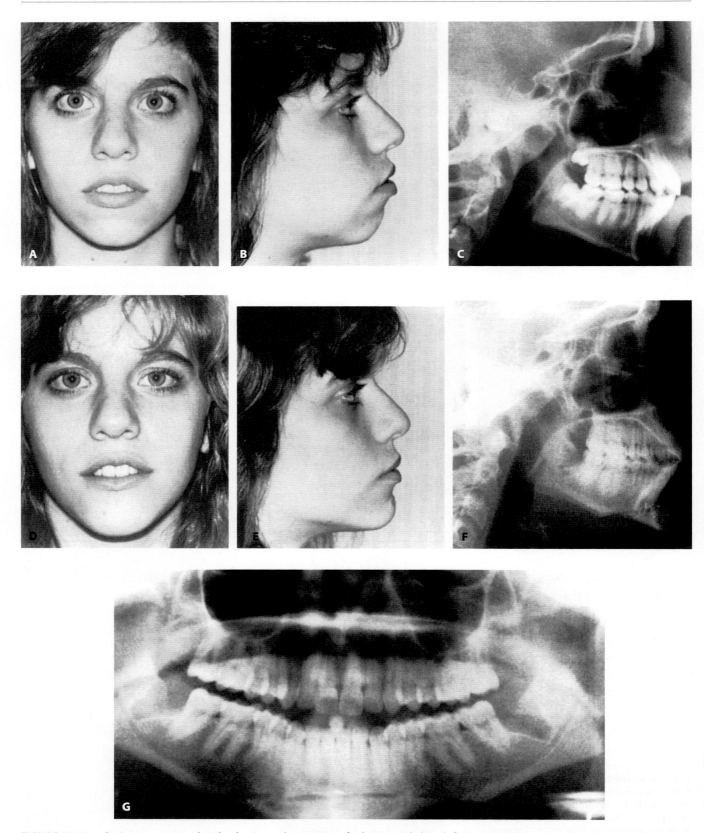

FIGURE 57-28. Patient was treated with a horizontal osteotomy for horizontal chin deficiency. **A–C,** Preoperative photographs and radiograph. **D–G,** Postoperative photographs and radiographs. (**A-G,** Reproduced with permission from Bloomquist DS. Principles of mandibular orthognathic surgery. In Peterson LJ, Indresano AT, Marciani RD, Roser SM, editors. Principles of Oral and Maxillofacial Surgery. Vol 3. Philadelphia: JB Lippincott; 1992; p. 1457.)

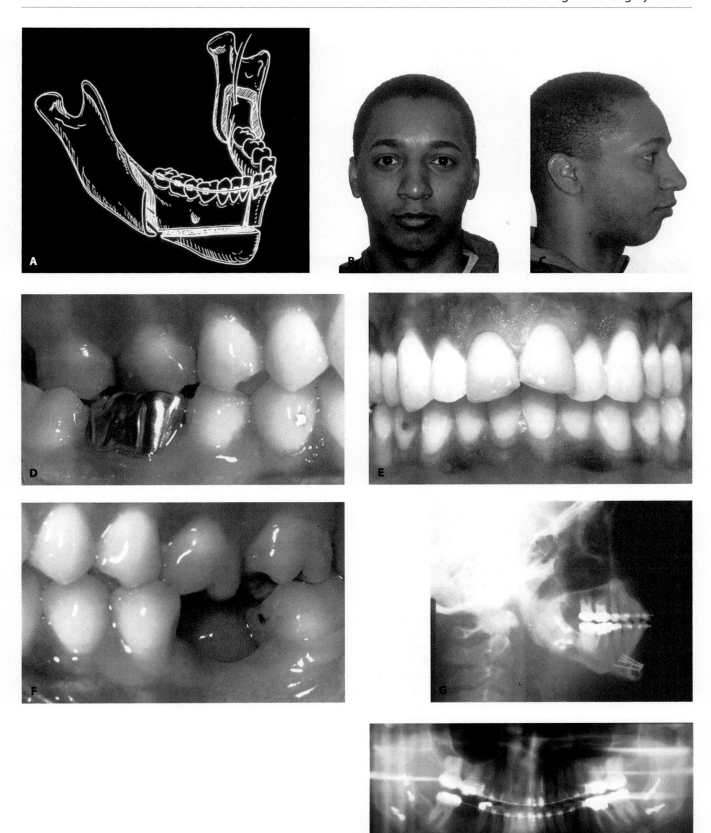

FIGURE 57-29. BSSO combined with midline mandibular osteotomy for mandibular narrowing, and genioplasty. **A,** Osteotomy designs. **B-F,** Pretreatment records. **G-M,** Postoperative records. *(Continued)*

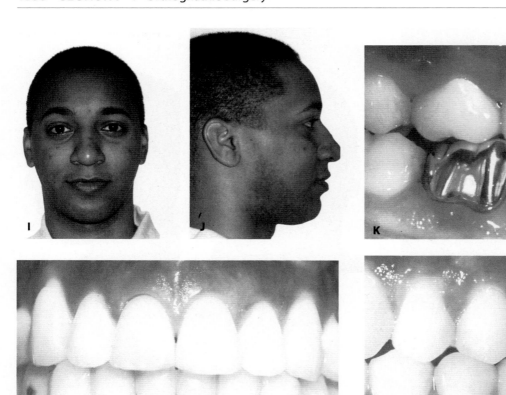

FIGURE 57-29. *(Continued)*

References

1. Hullihen SP. Case of elongation of the under jaw and distortion of the face and neck, caused by a burn, successfully treated. Am J Dent Sci 1849;9:157.
2. Angle EH. Double resection of the lower maxilla. Dent Cosmos 1889;40:635.
3. Blair VP. Report of a case of double resection for the correction of protrusion of the mandible. Dent Cosmos 1906;48:817.
4. Blair VP. Operations on the jaw bone and face. Surg Gynecol Obstet 1907;4:67.
5. Ernst F. Progenie. In Kirshhner M, Nordmann O, editors. Die Chirurgie. IV. Berlin: Urban & Schwarzenberg; 1927; p. 802.
6. Limberg A. Treatment of open-bite by means of plastic oblique osteotomy of the ascending rami of the mandible. Dent Cosmos 1925;67:1191.
7. Kostecka P. A contribution to the surgical treatment of open-bite. Int J Orthod 1934;28:1082.
8. Moose SM. Surgical correction of mandibular prognathism by intra-oral subcondylar osteotomy. Br J Oral Surg 1964;39:172.
9. Thoma KH. Oblique osteotomy of mandibular ramus-speical technique for correction of various types of facial defects and malocclusion. Oral Surg 1961;14(Suppl 1):23.
10. Robinson M. Prognathism corrected by open vertical subcondylotomy. J Oral Surg 1958;16:215.
11. Shira RB. Surgical correction of open bite deformities by oblique sliding osteotomy. J Oral Surg 1961;19:275.
12. Caldwell JB, Letterman GS. Vertical osteotomy in the mandibular rami for correction of prognathism. J Oral Surg 1954;12:185.
13. Moose SM. Surgical correction of mandibular prognathism by intraoral subcondylar osteotomy. J Oral Surg Anesth Hosp D Serv 1964;22:197.
14. Winstanley RP. Subcondylar osteotomy of the mandible and the intraoral approach. Br J Oral Surg 1968;6:134.
15. Hebert JM, Kent JN, Hinds EC. Correction of prognathism by an intraoral vertical subcondylar osteotomy. J Oral Surg 1970;28:651.
16. Wassmund M. Frakturen und luxationen des gesichtesschadels. 1927.
17. Pichler H, Trauner R. Lehrbuch der mundund kieferchirurgie. Wien: 1948.
18. Caldwell JB, Hayward JR, Lister RL. Correction of mandibular retrognathia by vertical L osteotomy: a new technique. J Oral Surg 1968;26:259.
19. Hayes PA. Correction of retrognathia by modified "C" osteotomy of the ramus and sagittal osteotomy of the mandibular body. Oral Surg 1973;31:682.

20. Fox GL, Tilson HB. Mandibular retrognathia: a review of the literature and selected cases. J Oral Surg 1976;34:53.

21. Obwegeser H, Trauner R. Zur operationstechnik bei der progenie und anderen unterkieferanomalien. Dtsch Zahn Mund Kieferheilkd 1955;23:H1–H2.

22. Lane WA. Cleft Palate and Hare Lip. The Medical Publishing Co, London, 2906.

23. Schuchardt K. Ein beitrag zur chirurgischen kieferorthopadie unter berucksichtigung ihrer bedeutung fur die behandlung ang-eborener und erworbener kieferdeformitaten Uei soldaten. Dtsch Zahn Mund Kieferhielkd 1942;9:73.

24. DalPont G. Retromolar osteotomy for the correction of prognathism. J Oral Surg Anesth Hosp D Serv 1961;19:42.

25. Hunsuck EE. Modified intraoral sagittal splitting technique for correction of mandibular prognathism. J Oral Surg 1968; 26:250.

26. Spiessl B. Ostoesynthese abei sagittaler osteotomie nach Obwegeser/dal Pont. Fortschr Kiefer Gesichtschir 1974;18:145.

27. Hofer O. Die vertikale osteotomie zur verlangerung des einseitig verkurzten aufsteigenden unterkieferastes. Atschr Stomatol 1936;34:826.

28. Kole H. Surgical operations on the alveolar ridge to correct occlusal abnormalities. Oral Surg Oral Med Oral Pathol 1959; 12:277.

29. Kent JN, Hinds EC. Management of dental facial deformities by anterior alveolar surgery. J Oral Surg 1971;29:13.

30. MacIntosh RB. Total mandibular alveolar osteotomy: encouraging experiences with an infrequently indicated procedure. J Maxillofac Surg 1974;2:210.

31. Von Eiselberg A. Uber plastik bei ektropium des unterkeifers (progenie). Klin Wochenschr 1906;19:1505.

32. Hofer O. Operation der prognathie und mikrogenie. Dtsch Zahn Mund Kieferheilkd 1942;9:121.

33. Bell WH, Levy BM. Revascularization and bone healing after anterior mandibular osteotomy. J Oral Surg 1970;28:196.

34. Hellem S, Ostrup LT. Normal and retrograde blood supply to the body of the mandible in the dog. Int J Oral Surg 1981; 10:31.

35. Zisser G, Gattinger B. Histologic investigation of pulpal changes following maxillary and mandibular alveolar osteotomies in the dog. J Oral Surg 1982;40:322.

36. Epker BN. Vascular considerations in orthognathic surgery. Oral Surg 1984;57:467.

37. Boc T, Peterson L. Revascularization after posterior mandibular alveolar osteotomy. J Oral Surg 1981;39:177.

38. Bradley JC. Age changes in the vascular supply of the mandible. Br Dent J 1972;132:142.

39. Bell WH, Kennedy JW III. Biological basis for vertical ramus osteotomies—a study of bone healing and revascularization in adult rhesus monkeys. J Oral Surg 1976;34:215.

40. Grammer FC, Meyer MW, Richter KJ. A radioisotope study of the vascular response to sagittal split osteotomy of the mandibular ramus. J Oral Surg 1974;32:578.

41. Bell WH, Schendel SA. Biologic basis for modification of the sagittal ramus split operation. J Oral Surg 1977;35:362.

42. Path MG, Nelson RL, Morgan PR, Meyer MW. Blood flow changes after sagittal split of the mandibular ramus. J Oral Surg 1977;35:98.

43. Grammer FC, Carpenter AM. A quantitative histologic study of tissue responses to ramal sagittal splitting procedures. J Oral Surg 1979;37:482.

44. Bell WH. Revascularization and bone healing after anterior maxillary osteotomy: a study using adult rhesus monkeys. J Oral Surg 1969;27:249.

45. Walter JM, Gregg JM. Analysis of postsurgical neurologic alteration in the trigeminal nerve. J Oral Surg 1979;37:410.

46. Hutchinson D, MacGregor AJ. Tooth survival following various methods of subapical osteotomy. Int J Oral Surg 1972;1:181.

47. Pepersack WJ. Tooth vitality after alveolar segmental osteotomy. J Maxillofac Surg 1973;1:85.

48. Kloosterman J. Kole's osteotomy: a follow-up study. J Maxillofac Surg 1985;13:59.

49. Ridell A, Soremark R, Lundberg M. Positional changes of the mandible after surgical correction of mandibular protrusion by horizontal osteotomy of the rami. Acta Odontol Scand 1971;29:123.

50. Tornes K, Wisth PJ. Stability after vertical subcondylar ramus osteotomy for correction of mandibular prognathism. Int J Oral Maxillofac Surg 1988;17:242.

51. Astrand P, Ridell A. Positional changes of the mandible and upper and lower anterior teeth after oblique sliding osteotomy of the mandibular rami. Scand J Plast Reconstr Surg 1973;7: 120.

52. Poulton DR, Ware WH. Surgical-orthodontic treatment of severe mandibular retrusion. Am J Orthod 1971;58:244.

53. Poulton DR, Ware WH. Surgical-orthodontic treatment of severe mandibular retrusion (part II). Am J Orthod 1973;63:237.

54. Kohn MW. Analysis of relapse after mandibular advancement surgery. J Oral Surg 1978;36:676.

55. Lake SL, McNeill RNA, Little RM, West RA. Surgical mandibular advancement: a cephalometric analysis of treatment response. Am J Orthod 1981;80:376.

56. Smith GC, Moloney FB, West RA. Mandibular advancement surgery: a study of the lower border wiring technique for osteosynthesis. Oral Surg 1985;60:461.

57. Komiri E, Aigase K, Sugisaki M, Tanabe H. Skeletal fixation versus skeletal relapse. Am J Orthod Dentofacial Orthop 1987;92:412.

58. Will LA, Joondeph DR, Hold TH, West RA. Condylar position following mandibular advancement: its relationship to relapse. J Oral Maxillofac Surg 1984;42:578.

59. Epker BN. Modifications in the sagittal osteotomy of the mandible. J Oral Surg 1977;35:157.

60. Komiri E, Aigase K, Sugisaki M. Cause of early skeletal relapse after mandibular setback. Am J Orthod Dentofacial Orthop 1989;95:29.

61. Franco JE, Van Sickels JE, Thrash WJ. Factors contributing to relapse in rigidly fixed mandibular setbacks. J Oral Maxillofac Surg 1989;47:451.

62. Yellich GM, McNamara JA, Ungerleider JC. Muscular and mandibular adaptation after lengthening, detachment, and reattachment of the masseter muscle. J Oral Surg 1981;39:656.

63. Ellis E III, Carlson DS. Stability two years after mandibular advancement with and without suprahyoid myotomy: an experimental study. J Oral Maxillofac Surg 1983;41:426.

64. Schendel SA, Epker BN. Results after mandibular advancement surgery: an analysis of 87 cases. J Oral Surg 1980;38:265.

65. Bhatia SN, Yant B, Behbehanit I, Harris M. Nature of relapse after surgical mandibular advancement. Br J Orthod 1985;12:58.

66. Reynolds ST, Ellis E III, Carlson DS. Adaptation of the suprahyoid muscle complex to large mandibular advancements. J Oral Maxillofac Surg 1988;46:1077.

67. Ellis E III, Reyolds S, Carlson DS. Stability of the mandible following advancement: a comparison of three postsurgical fixation techniques. Am J Orthod Dentofacial Orthop 1988; 94:38.

68. Ellis E III, Gallo JW. Relapse following mandibular advancement with dental plus skeletal maxillomandibular fixation. J Oral Maxillofac Surg 1986;44:509.

69. Robinson M, Lytle JJ. Micrognathism corrected by vertical osteotomies of the rami without bone grafts. Oral Surg Oral Med Oral Pathol 1962;15:641.

70. Hall HD, McKenna SJ. Further refinement and evaluation of intraoral vertical ramus osteotomy. J Oral Maxillofac Surg 1987;45:684.

71. Bereni B. Open subcondylar osteotomy in the treatment of mandibular deformities. Int J Oral Surg 1973;2:81.

72. Reitzik M, Griffiths RR, Mirels H. Surgical anatomy of the ascending ramus of the mandible. Br J Oral Surg 1976;14:150.

73. Hall HD, Chase DC, Payor LG. Evaluation and refinement of the intraoral vertical subcondylar osteotomy. J Oral Surg 1975;33:333.

74. Massey GB, Chase DC, Thomas PM, Kohn MW. Intraoral oblique osteotomy of the mandibular ramus. J Oral Surg 1974;32:755.

75. Tornes K. Osteotomy length and postoperative stability in vertical subcondylar ramus osteotomy. Acta Odontol Stand 1989;47:81.

76. Sund G, Eckerdal O, Astrand P. Changes in the temporomandibular joint after oblique osteotomy of the mandibular rami: a longitudinal radiological study. J Maxillofac Surg 1983; 11:81.

77. Ritzau M, Wenzel A, Williams S. Changes in condyle position after bilateral vertical ramus osteotomy with and without osteosynthesis. Am J Orthod Dentofacial Orthop 1989;96:507.

78. Sund G, Eckerdal O, Astrand P. Skeletal remodeling in the temporomandibular joint after oblique sliding osteotomy of the mandibular rami. Int J Oral Maxillofac Surg 1986;15:233.

79. Proffit WR, Phillips C, Denn C IV, Turvey TA. Stability after surgical-orthodontic correction of skeletal class III malocclusion. I: mandibular setback. Int J Adult Orthodont Orthognath Surg 1991;6:7.

80. Nystrom E, Rosenquist J, Astrand P, Nordin T. Intraoral or extraoral approach in oblique sliding osteotomy of the mandibular ramus. J Maxillofac Surg 1984;12:277.

81. Goldstein A. Appraisal of results of surgical correction of class III malocclusions. Angle Orthod 1974;17(3–4):59.

82. Poulton DR, Taylor RC, Ware WH. Cephalometric x-ray evaluation of the vertical osteotomy correction of mandibular prognathism. Oral Surg Oral Med Oral Pathol 1963;16:807.

83. Morrill LR, Baumrind S, Miller D. Surgical correction of mandibular prognathism. Am J Orthod 1974;65:503.

84. Stella JP, Astrand P, Epker BN. Patterns and etiology of relapse after correction of class III open bite via subcondylar ramus osteotomy. Int J Adult Orthod Orthogn Surg 1986;1:191.

85. Kahnberg KE, Widmark G. Surgical treatment of the open bite deformity: surgical correction of combined mandibular prognathism and open bite by oblique sliding osteotomy of the mandibular rami. Int J Oral Maxillofac Surg 1988;17:45.

86. Zaytoun HS, Phillips C, Terry BC. Long-term neurosensory deficits following transoral vertical ramus and sagittal split osteotomies for mandibular prognathism. J Oral Maxillofac Surg 1986;44:193.

87. Wang JH, Waite DE. Vertical osteotomy vs sagittal split osteotomy of the mandibular ramus: comparison of operative and postoperative factors. J Oral Surg 1975;33:596.

88. Hollender L, Ridell A. Radiography of the temporomandibular joint after oblique sliding osteotomy of the mandibular rami. Scand J Dent Res 1974;82:466.

89. Egyedi P, Houwing M, Juten E. The oblique subcondylar osteotomy: report of results of 100 cases. J Oral Surg 1981;39:871.

90. Bell WH, Yamaguchi Y, Poor MR. Treatment of temporomandibular joint dysfunction by intraoral vertical ramus osteotomy. Int J Adult Orthod Orthogn Surg 1990;5:9.

91. Upton LG, Sullivan SM. Modified condylotomies for management of mandibular prognathism and temporomandibular joint internal derangement. Clin Orthod 1990;24:697.

92. Hu J, Wang D, Zou S. Effects of mandibular setback on the temporomandibular joint: a comparison of oblique and sagittal split ramus osteotomy. J Oral Maxillofac Surg 2000;58:375.

93. Farrell CD, Kent JN. Evaluation of the surgical stability of 20 cases of inverted-L and C osteotomies. J Oral Surg 1977; 3:239.

94. Hawkinson RT. Retrognathia correction by means of an arcing osteotomy in the ascending ramus. J Prosthet Dent 1968; 20:77.

95. Reitzik M. Mandibular advancement surgery: stability following a modified fixation technique. J Oral Surg 1980;38:893.

96. Reitzik M, Barer PC, Wainwright WM, Lim B. The surgical treatment of skeletal anterior open-bite deformities with rigid internal fixation in the mandible. Am J Orthod Dentofacial Orthop 1990;97:52.

97. Barer PC, Wallen TR, McNeill RW, Reitzik M. Stability of mandibular advancement osteotomy using rigid internal fixation. Am J Orthod Dentofacial Orthop 1987;92:403.

98. Greebe RB, Tuinzing DR. Mandibular advancement procedures: predictable stability and relapse. Oral Surg 1984;57:13.

99. Dattilo DJ, Braun TW, Sotereanos GC. The inverted L osteotomy for treatment of skeletal open-bite deformities. J Oral Maxillofac Surg 1985;43:440.

100. Obwegeser H. The surgical correction of mandibular prognathism and retrognathia with consideration of genioplasty. Oral Surg 1957;10:681.

101. Jeter TS, Van Sickels JE, Dolwick MR. Modified techniques for internal fixation of sagittal ramus osteotomies. J Oral Maxillofac Surg 1984;42:270.

102. Sandor GKB, Stoelinga PJW, Tideman H, Leenen RJ. The role of the intraosseous osteosynthesis wire in sagittal split osteotomies for mandibular advancement. J Oral Maxillofac Surg 1984;42:231.

103. Isaacson RJ, Kopytov OS, Bevis RR, Waite DE. Movement of the proximal and distal segments after mandibular ramus osteotomies. J Oral Surg 1978;36:263.

104. Obwegeser H. The indications for surgical correction of mandibular deformity by the sagittal splitting technique. Br J Oral Surg 1962;1:157.

105. Booth DF. Control of the proximal segment by lower border wiring in the sagittal split osteotomy. J Maxillofac Surg 1981;9:126.

106. Kundert M, Hadjianghelou O. Condylar displacement after sagittal splitting of the mandibular rami: a short-term radiographic study. J Maxillofac Surg 1980;8:278.

107. Spitzer W, Rettinger C, Sitzman F. Computerized tomography examination for the detection of positional changes in the

temporomandibular joint after ramus osteotomies with screw fixation. J Maxillofac Surg 1984;12:139.

108. Watzke IM, Tucker MR, Turvey TA. Lag screw versus position screw techniques for rigid internal fixation of sagittal osteotomies: a comparison of stability. Int J Adult Orthod Orthogn Surg 1991;6:19.

109. Bloomqvist JE, Isaksson S. Skeletal stability after mandibular advancement: a comparison of two rigid internal fixation techniques. J Oral Maxillofac Surg 1994;52:1133.

110. Bloomqvist JE, Ahlborg G, Isaksson S, Svartz K. A comparison of skeletal stability after mandibular advancement and use of two rigid internal fixation techniques. J Oral Maxillofac Surg 1997;55:568.

111. Fujioka M, Fujii T, Hirano A. Comparative study of mandibular stability after sagittal split osteotomies: bicortical versus monocortical osteosynthesis. Cleft Palate Craniofac J 2000;37:551.

112. Suuronen R, Laine P, Pohjonen T, Lindqvist C. Sagittal ramus osteotomies fixed with biodegradable screws: a preliminary report. J Oral Maxillofac Surg 1994;52:715.

113. Harada K, Enomoto S. Stability after surgical correction of mandibular prognathism using the sagittal split ramus osteotomy and fixation with poly-L-lactic acid (PLLA) screws. J Oral Maxillofac Surg 1997;55:464.

114. Ferretti C, Reyneke JP. Mandibular sagittal split osteotomies fixed with biodegradable or titanium screws: a prospective, comparative study of postoperative stability. Oral Surg Oral Med Oral Pathol Oral Radiol Endod 2002;93:534.

115. Kallela I, Laine P, Suuronen R, et al. Skeletal stability following mandibular advancement and rigid fixation with polylactide biodegradable screws. Int J Oral Maxillofac Surg 1998;27:3.

116. Turvey TA, Bell RB, Tejera TJ, Proffit WR. The use of self-reinforced biodegradable bone plates and screws in orthognathic surgery. J Oral Maxillofac Surg 2002;60:59.

117. Ahn YS, Kim SG, Baik SM, et al. Comparative Study Between Resorbable & Nonresorbable Plates in Orthognathic Surgery. J Oral Maxillofac Surg 2010;117.

118. O'Ryan F, Epker BN. Deliberate surgical control of mandibulargrowth: 1. A biomechanical theory. Oral Surg 1982;53:2.

119. Killiany DM, Johnston LE Jr. Surgical control of mandibular growth: test of a recent biomechanical hypothesis. Oral Surg 1986;62:500.

120. Huang CS, Ross RB. Surgical advancement of the retrognathic mandible in growing children. Am J Orthod 1982;82:89.

121. Bell WH. Augmentation of the nasomaxillary and nasolabial regions. Oral Surg Oral Med Oral Pathol 1976;41:691.

122. Alexander C, Bloomquist D, Wallen T. Stability of mandibular constriction with a symphyseal osteotomy. Am J Orthod Dentofacial Orthop 1993;103:15.

123. McNeill RW, Hooley JR, Sundberg RJ. Skeletal relapse during intermaxillary fixation. J Oral Surg 1973;31:212.

124. Van Sickels JE. A comparative study of bicortical screws and suspension wires versus bicortical screws in large mandibular advancements. J Oral Maxillofac Surg. 1991;49:1293.

125. Mobarak KA, Espeland L, Rogstad O, Lyberg T. Mandibular advancement surgery in high-angle and low-angle class II patients: different long-term skeletal responses. Am J Orthod Dentofacial Orthop 2001;119:368.

126. Schmoker R, Speissl B, Gensheimer T. Functionally stable osteosynthesis and simulography in sagittal osteotomy of

the ascending ramus: a comparative clinical study. Schweiz Monatsschr Zahnheilkd 1976;86:582.

127. Van Sickels JE, Flanary CM. Stability associated with mandibular advancement treated by rigid osseous fixation. J Oral Maxillofac Surg 1985;43:338.

128. Van Sickels JE, Larsen AJ, Thrash WJ. Relapse after rigid fixation of mandibular advancement. J Oral Maxillofac Surg 1986;44:698.

129. Van Sickels JE, Larsen AJ, Thrash WJ. A retrospective study of relapse in rigidly fixated sagittal split osteotomies: contributing factors. Am J Orthod Dentofacial Orthop 1988;93:413.

130. Caskey RT, Turpin DL, Bloomquist DS. Stability of mandibular lengthening using bicortical screw fixation. Am J Orthod Dentofacial Orthop 1989;96:320.

131. Knaup CA, Wallen TW, Bloomquist DS. Linear and rotational changes in large mandibular advancements using three or four fixation screws. Int J Adult Orthod Orthogn Surg 1993; 8:245.

132. Douma E, Kuftinec MM, Moshiri F. A comparative study of stability after mandibular advancement surgery. Am J Orthod Dentofacial Orthop 1991;100:141.

133. Mommaerts MY. Lag screw versus wire osteosynthesis in mandibular advancement. Int J Adult Orthod Orthogn Surg 1991;6:153.

134. Moenning JE, Bussard DA, Lapp TH, Garrison BT A comparison of relapse in bilateral sagittal split osteotomies for mandibular advancement: rigid internal fixation (screws) versus inferior border wiring with anterior skeletal fixation. Int J Adult Orthod Orthogn Surg 1990;5:175.

135. Berger JL, Pangrazio-Kulbersh V, Bacchus SN, Kasczynski R. Stability of bilateral sagittal split ramus osteotomy: rigid fixation versus transosseous wiring. Am J Orthod Dentofacial Orthop 2000;118:397.

136. Dolce C, Hatch JP, Van Sickels JE, Rugh JD. Rigid versus wire fixation for mandibular advancement: skeletal and dental changes after 5 years. Am J Orthod Dentofacial Orthop 2002;121:610.

137. Watzke IM, Turvey TA, Phillips C, Proffit WR. Stability of mandibular advancement after sagittal osteotomy with screw or wire fixation: a comparative study. J Oral Maxillofac Surg 1990;48:101.

138. Stansbury CD, Evans CA, Miloro M, et al. Stability of open bite correction with sagittal split osteotomy and closing rotation of the mandible. J Oral Maxillofac Surg 2010;68:149.

139. Rubens BC, Stoelinga PJW, Blijdorp PA, et al. Skeletal stability following sagittal split osteotomy using monocortical miniplate internal fixation. Int J Oral Maxillofac Surg 1985;17:371.

140. Lee J, Piecuch JF. The sagittal ramus osteotomy. Stability of fixation with internal miniplates. Int J Oral Maxillofac Surg 1992;21:326.

141. Abeloos J, Le Clercq C, Neyt L. Skeletal stability following miniplate fixation after bilateral sagittal split osteotomy for mandibular advancement. J Oral Maxillofac Surg 1993; 51:366.

142. Scheerlinck JP, Stoelinga PJ, Blijdorp PA, et al. Sagittal split advancement osteotomies stabilized with miniplate fixation. A 2-5 year follow-up. Int J Oral Maxillofac Surg 1994;23:127.

143. Bloomquist D. The use of a single lag screw in the mandibular sagittal osteotomy. Presentation at the AAO-ASOMFS Conference on Surgical Orthodontics. 1983; New Orleans.

SECTION 7

144. Chou J, Fong H, Kuang S, et al. A retrospective analysis of the stability and relapse of soft and hard tissue change after bilateral sagittal split osteotomy for mandibular setback of 64 Taiwanese patients. J Oral Maxillofac Surg 2005;63:355.

145. Chung IH, Yoo CK, Lee EK et al. Postoperative stability after sagittal split ramus osteotomies for a mandibular setback with monocortical plate fixation or bicortical screw fixation. J Oral Maxillofac Surg 2008;66:446.

146. Joss C, Vassalli I. Stability after bilateral sagittal split osteotomy setback surgery with rigid fixation: a systematic review. J Oral Maxillofac Surg 2008;66:1634.

147. Kole H. Results, experience, and problems in the operative treatment of anomalies with reverse overbite (mandibular protrusion). Oral Surg 1965;19:427.

148. Behrman SJ. Complications of sagittal osteotomy of the mandibular ramus. J Oral Surg 1972;30:554.

149. Westermark SA, Bystedt H, von Konow L. Inferior alveolar nerve function after sagittal split osteotomy of the mandible: correlation with degree of intraoperative nerve encounter and other variables in 496 operations. Br J Oral Maxillofac Surg 1998;36:429.

150. Ylikontiola L, Kinnunen J, Laukkanen P, Oikarinen K. Prediction of recovery from neurosensory deficit after bilateral sagittal split osteotomy. Oral Surg Oral Med Oral Pathol Oral Radiol Endod 2000;90:275.

151. MacIntosh RB. Experience with the sagittal osteotomy of the mandibular ramus: a 13-year review. J Maxillofac Surg 1981;8:151.

152. Van Sickels JE, Hatch JP, Dolce C, et al. Effects of age, amount of advancement, and genioplasty on neurosensory disturbance after a bilateral sagittal split osteotomy. J Oral Maxillofac Surg 2002;60:1012.

153. White RP, Peters PB, Costich ER, Page HL Jr. Evaluation of sagittal split-ramus osteotomy in 17 patients. J Oral Surg 1969;27:851.

154. Guernsey LH, DeChamplain RW. Sequelae and complications of the intraoral sagittal osteotomy in the mandibular rami. Oral Surg 1971;32:176.

155. Fiamminghi L, Aversa C. Lesions of the inferior alveolar nerve in sagittal osteotomy of the ramus: experimental study. J Maxillofac Surg 1979;7:125.

156. Brusati R, Fiamminghi L, Sesenna E, Gazzotti A. Functional disturbance of the inferior alveolar nerve after sagittal osteotomy of the mandibular ramus: operating technique for prevention. J Maxillofac Surg 1981;9:123.

157. Yoshida T, Nagamine T, Kobayashi T, et al. Impairment of the inferior alveolar nerve after sagittal split osteotomy. J Craniomaxillofac Surg 1989;17:271.

158. Yamamoto R, Nakamura A, Ohno K, Michi KI. Relationship of the mandibular canal to the lateral cortex of the mandibular ramus as a factor in the development of neurosensory disturbance after bilateral sagittal split osteotomy. J Oral Maxillofac Surg 2002;60:490.

159. Freihofer HP Jr. Probleme der behandlung der progenie durch sagittler spaltung der auf-steigenden unterkieferaste. Schweiz Monatsschr Zahnheilkd 1976;86:679.

160. Wolford LM, Bennett MA, Rafferty CG. Modification of the mandibular ramus sagittal split osteotomy. Oral Surg Oral Med Oral Pathol 1987;64:146.

161. Converse JM. Surgical treatment of facial injuries. In Kazanjian VH, Converse JM, editors. Surgical Treatment of Facial Injuries. Baltimore: Williams & Wilkins; 1974.

162. Paulis GW, Steinhauser EW. A comparative study of wire osteosynthesis versus bone screws in the treatment of mandibular prognathism. Oral Surg 1982;54:2.

163. Nishioka GJ, Zysset ME, Van Sickels JE. Neurosensory disturbance with rigid fixation of the bilateral sagittal split osteotomy. J Oral Maxillofac Surg 1987;45:20.

164. Lemke RR, Rugh JD, Van Sickels J, et al. Neurosensory differences after wire and rigid fixation in patients with mandibular advancement. J Oral Maxillofac Surg 2000;58:1354.

165. Westermark A, Englesson L, Bongenhielm U. Neurosensory function after sagittal split osteotomy of the mandible: a comparison between subjective evaluation and objective assessment. Int J Adult Orthod Orthogn Surg 1999;14:268.

166. Chen N, Neal CE, Lingenbrink P, et al. Neurosensory changes following orthognathic surgery. Int J Adult Orthod Orthogn Surg 1999;14:259.

167. Nakagawa K, Ueki K, Takasuka S, et al. Somatosensory-evoked potential to evaluate the trigeminal nerve after sagittal split osteotomy. Oral Surg Oral Med Oral Pathol Oral Radiol Endod 2001;91:146.

168. Essick G, Phillips, Turvey T, Tucker M. Facial altered sensation and sensory impairment after orthognathic surgery. Int J Oral Maxillofac Surg 2007;36:577.

169. Jacks SC, Zuniga JR, Turvey TA, Schalit C. A retrospective analysis of lingual nerve sensory changes after mandibular bilateral sagittal split osteotomy. J Oral Maxillofac Surg 1998; 56:700.

170. Zuniga Jr, Chen N, Phillips CL. Chemosensory and somatosensory regeneration after lingual nerve repair in humans. J Oral Maxillofac Surg 1997;55:2.

171. Gent JF, Shafer DM, Frank ME. The effect of orthognathic surgery on taste function on the palate and tongue. J Oral Maxillofac Surg 2003;61:766.

172. Freihofer HPM Jr, Petresevic D. Late results after advancing the mandible by sagittal splitting of the rami. J Maxillofac Surg 1975;3:250.

173. O'Ryan F, Epker BN. Surgical orthodontics and the temporomandibular joint II: mandibular advancement via modified sagittal split ramus osteotomies. Am J Orthod 1983;83: 418.

174. Buckley MJ, Tulloch JFC, White RP, Tucker MR. Complications of orthognathic surgery: a comparison between wire fixation and rigid internal fixation. Int J Adult Orthod Orthogn Surg 1989;4:69.

175. Hackney FL, Van Sickels JE, Nummikoski PV. Condylar displacement and temporomandibular joint dysfunction following bilateral sagittal split osteotomy and rigid fixation. J Oral Maxillofac Surg 1989;47:223.

176. Martis CS. Complications after mandibular sagittal split osteotomy. J Oral Maxillofac Surg 1984;42:101.

177. Karabouta I, Martis C. The TMJ dysfunction syndrome before and after sagittal split osteotomy of the rami. J Maxillofac Surg 1985;13:185.

178. Kerstens HCJ, Tuinzing DB, van der Kwast WAM. Temporomandibular joint symptoms in orthognathic surgery. J Craniomaxillofac Surg 1989;17:215.

179. Pruitt JW, Moenning JE, Lapp TH, Bussard DA. Treatment of painful temporomandibular joint dysfunction with the sagittal split ramus osteotomy. J Oral Maxillofac Surg 2002;60: 996.

180. Flynn B, Brown DT, Lapp TH, et al. A comparative study of temporomandibular symptoms following mandibular advancement

by bilateral sagittal split osteotomies: rigid versus nonrigid fixation. Oral Surg Oral Med Oral Pathol 1990;70:372.

181. Feinerman DM, Piecuch JF. Long-term effects of orthognathic surgery on the temporomandibular joint: comparison of rigid and nonrigid fixation methods. Int J Oral Maxillofac Surg 1995;24:268.

182. Wolford LM, Reiche-Fischel U, Mehra P. Changes in temporomandibular joint dysfunction after orthognathic surgery. J Oral Maxillofac Surg 2003;61:655.

183. Luhr HG. The significance of condylar position using rigid fixation in orthognathic surgery. Clin Plast Surg 1989;16:147.

184. Harris MD, Van Sickels JE, Alder M. Factors influencing condylar position after the bilateral sagittal split osteotomy fixed with bicortical screws. J Oral Maxillofac Surg 1999; 57:650.

185. Van Sickels JE, Tiner BD, Keeling SD, et al. Condylar position with rigid fixation versus wire osteosynthesis of a sagittal split advancement. J Oral Maxillofac Surg 1999;57:31.

186. Renzi G, Becelli R, Di Paolo C, Iannetti G. Indications to the use of condylar repositioning devices in the surgical treatment of dental-skeletal class III. J Oral Maxillofac Surg 2003;61:304.

187. Costa F, Robiony M, Toro C, et al.Condylar positioning devices for orthognathic surgery: a literature review. Oral Surg Oral Med Oral Pathol Oral Radiol Endod 2008;106:179.

188. Saka B, Petsch I, Hingst V, Hartel J. The influence of pre- and intraoperative positioning of the condyle in the centre of the articular fossa on the position of the disc in orthognathic surgery. A magnetic resonance study. Brit J Oral Maxillofac Surg 2004;42:120.

189. Alder ME, Deahl ST, Matteson SR, et al. Short-term changes of condylar position after sagittal split osteotomy for mandibular advancement. Oral Surg Oral Med Oral Pathol Oral Radiol Endod 1999;87:159.

190. Rebellato J, Lindauer SJ, Sheats RD, Isaacson RJ. Condylar positional changes after mandibular advancement surgery with rigid internal fixation. Am J Orthod Dentofacial Orthop 1999;116:93.

191. Gaggl A, Schultes G, Santler G, et al. Clinical and magnetic resonance findings in the temporomandibular joints of patients before and after orthognathic surgery. Br J Oral Maxillofac Surg 1999;37:41.

192. Ueki K, Marukawa K, Nakagawa K, Yamamoto E. Condylar and temporomandibular joint disc positions after mandibular osteotomy for prognathism. J Oral Maxillofac Surg 2002;60:1424.

193. Stacy GC. Recovery of oral opening following sagittal ramus osteotomy for mandibular prognathism. J Oral Maxillofac Surg 1987;45:487.

194. Storum KA, Bell WH. The effect of physical rehabilitation on mandibular function after ramus osteotomies. J Oral Maxillofac Surg 1986;44:94.

195. Aragon SB, Van Sickels JE. Mandibular range of motion with rigid/nonrigid fixation. Oral Surg Oral Med Oral Pathol 1987;63:408.

196. Nishimura A, Sakurada S, Iwase M, Nagumo M. Positional changes in the mandibular condyle and amount of mouth opening after sagittal split ramus osteotomy with rigid or nonrigid osteosynthesis. J Oral Maxillofac Surg 1997;55:672.

197. Hatch JP, Van Sickels JE, Rugh JD, et al. Mandibular range of motion after bilateral sagittal split ramus osteotomy with wire osteosynthesis or rigid fixation. Oral Surg Oral Med Oral Pathol Oral Radiol Endod 2001;91:274.

198. Phillips RM, Bell WH. Atrophy of mandibular condyles after sagittal ramus split osteotomy: report of case. J Oral Surg 1978;36:45.

199. Cutbirth M, Van Sickels JE, Thrash WJ. Condylar resorption after bicortical screw fixation of mandibular advancement. J Oral Maxillofac Surg 1998;56:178.

200. Hoppenreijs TJ, Stoelinga PJ, Grace KL, Robben CM. Long-term evaluation of patients with progressive condylar resorption following orthognathic surgery. Int J Oral Maxillofac Surg 1999;28:411.

201. Lanigan DT, Hey J, West RA. Hemorrhage following mandibular osteotomies: a report of 21 cases. J Oral Maxillofac Surg 1991; 49:713.

202. Tucker MR, Ochs MW Use of rigid internal fixation for management of intraoperative complications of mandibular sagittal split osteotomy. Int J Adult Orthod Orthogn Surg 1988; 2:71.

203. Precious DS, Lung KE, Rynn BR, Goodday RH. Presence of impacted teeth as a determining factor of unfavorable splits in 1256 sagittal-split osteotomies. Oral Surg Oral Med Oral Pathol Oral Radiol Endod 1998;85:362.

204. Mehra P, Castro V, Freitas RZ, Wolford LM. Complications of the mandibular sagittal split ramus osteotomy associated with the presence or absence of third molars. J Oral Maxillofac Surg 2001;59:854.

205. Reyneke JP, Tsakiris P, Becker P. Age as a factor in the complication rate after removal of unerupted/impacted third molars at the time of mandibular sagittal split osteotomy. J Oral Maxillofac Surg 2002;60:654.

206. Riley RW, Powell NB, Guilleminault C, Ware W. Obstructive sleep apnea syndrome following surgery for mandibular prognathism. J Oral Maxillofac Surg 1987;45:450.

207. Kawamata A, Fujishita M, Ariji Y, Ariji E. Three-dimensional computed tomographic evaluation of morphologic airway changes after mandibular setback osteotomy for prognathism. Oral Surg Oral Med Oral Pathol Oral Radiol Endod 2000;89:278.

208. Bouwman JPB, Husak A, Putnam GD, et al. Screw fixation following bilateral sagittal ramus osteotomy for mandibular advancement: complications in 700 consecutive cases. Br J Oral Maxillofac Surg 1995;33:231.

209. Acebal-Bianco F, Vuylsteke PL, Mommaerts MY, De Clercq CA. Perioperative complications in corrective facial orthopedic surgery: a 5-year retrospective study. J Oral Maxillofac Surg 2000;58:754.

210. Epker BN. Dentofacial deformities. In Integrated Orthodontic and Surgical Correction. St. Louis: CV Mosby; 1986.

211. Beke AL, Yahner VB. Surgical correction of overbite and overjet with sagittal osteotomy of the mandibular horizontal ramus: report of case. J Oral Surg 1969;27:358.

212. Bloomquist DS. Mandibular body sagittal osteotomy in the correction of malunited edentulous mandibular fractures. J Maxillofac Surg 1982;10:18.

213. Sandor GK, Stoelinga PJ, Tideman H. Reappraisal of the mandibular step osteotomy. J Oral Maxillofac Surg 1982;40: 78.

214. Keller EE, Hill AJ Jr, Sather AH. Orthognathic surgery: review of mandibular body procedures. Mayo Clin Proc 1976;51: 117.

215. Nakajima T, Kajikawa Y, Ueda K, Hanada K. Sliding osteotomy in the mandibular body for correction of prognathism. J Oral Surg 1978;36:361.

216. Kavanaugh SH. Maxillary midline split surgery [dissertation]. University of Washington, Department of Orthodontics; 1985.

217. Peterson LJ. Posterior mandibular segmental alveolar osteotomy. J Oral Surg 1978;36:454.

218. MacIntosh RB, Carlotti AE. Total mandibular alveolar osteotomy in the management of skeletal (infantile) apertognathia. J Oral Surg 1975;33:921.

219. Booth DF, Dietz V, Gianelly AA. Correction of class III malocclusion by combined sagittal ramus and subapical body osteotomy. J Oral Surg 1976;34:630.

220. Theisen FC, Guernsey LH. Postoperative sequelae after anterior segmental osteotomies. Oral Surg Oral Med Oral Pathol 1976;41:139.

221. Pangrazio-Kulbersh V, MacIntosh RB. Total mandibular alveolar osteotomy: an alternate choice to other surgical procedures. Am J Orthod 1985;87:319.

222. Meyer MW, Cavanaugh GD. Blood flow changes after orthognathic surgery: maxillary and mandibular subapical osteotomy. J Oral Surg 1976;34:495.

223. Banks P. Pulp changes after anterior mandibular subapical osteotomy in a primate model. J Maxillofac Surg 1977;5:39.

224. Scheideman GB, Kawamura H, Finn RA, Bell WH. Wound healing after anterior and posterior subapical osteotomy. J Oral Maxillofac Surg 1985;43:408.

225. Johnson JV, Hinds EC. Evaluation of teeth vitality after subapical osteotomy. J Oral Surg 1969;27:256.

226. Converse JM, Wood-Smith D. Horizontal osteotomy of the mandible. Plast Reconstr Surg 1964;34:464.

227. Neuner O. Correction of mandibular deformities. Oral Surg Oral Med Oral Pathol 1973;36:779.

228. Fitzpatrick B. Reconstruction of the chin in cosmetic surgery (genioplasty). Oral Surg 1975;39:522.

229. Hinds EC, Kent JN. Genioplasty: the versatility of horizontal osteotomy. J Oral Surg 1969;27:690.

230. Precious DS, Armstrong JE, Morais D. Anatomic placement of fixation devices in genioplasty. Oral Surg Oral Med Oral Pathol 1992;73:2.

231. Hohl TH, Epker BN. Microgenia: a study of treatment results, with surgical recommendations. Oral Surg Oral Med Oral Pathol 1976;41:545.

232. Scheideman GB, Legan HL, Bell WH. Soft tissue changes with combined mandibular setback and advancement genioplasty. J Oral Surg 1981;39:505.

233. Gallagher DM, Bell WH, Storum KA. Soft tissue changes associated with advancement genioplasty performed concomitantly with superior repositioning of the maxilla. J Oral Maxillofac Surg 1984;42:238.

234. Martinez JT, Turvey TA, Proffitt WR. Osseous remodeling after inferior border osteotomy for chin augmentation: an indication for early surgery. J Oral Maxillofac Surg 1999;57:1175.

235. Talebzadeh N, Pogrel MA. Long-term hard and soft tissue relapse rate after genioplasty. Oral Surg Oral Med Oral Pathol Oral Radiol Endod 2001;91:153.

236. Fitzpatrick BN. Genioplasty with reference to resorption and the hinge sliding osteotomy. Int J Oral Surg 1974;3:247.

237. McDonnell JP, McNeill RW, West RA. Advancement genioplasty: a retrospective cephalometric analysis of osseous and soft tissue changes. J Oral Surg 1977;35:640.

238. Nishioka GJ, Mason M, Van Sickels JE. Neurosensory disturbance associated with the anterior mandibular horizontal osteotomy. J Oral Maxillofac Surg 1988;46:107.

Principles of Maxillary Orthognathic Surgery

Vincent J. Perciaccante, DDS, and Robert A. Bays, DDS

HISTORICAL PERSPECTIVES

Orthognathic surgery involving the maxilla was first described in 1859 by von Langenbeck[1] to provide surgical access for the removal of nasopharyngeal polyps. The first report of a maxillary osteotomy in the United States was by Cheever in 1867[2] for the treatment of complete nasal obstruction secondary to recurrent epistaxis for which a right hemimaxillary down-fracture was performed. Throughout the next century, numerous authors described various osteotomy designs and techniques that included mobilization of the entire maxilla, mostly for access and treatment of pathologic processes. In 1901, Rene Le Fort[3] published his classic and vivid descriptions of the natural planes of maxillary fracture by applying blunt forces to cadaver head specimens. In 1927, Wassmund[4] first described the Le Fort I osteotomy for the correction of midface deformities. However, complete mobilization of the maxilla with immediate repositioning was not performed until 1934 by Axhausen.[5] Separation of the pterygomaxillary junction was advocated by Schuchardt in 1942.[6] Moore and Ward in 1949[7] recommended that a horizontal transsection of the pterygoid plates is necessary for maxillary advancement. Willmar[8] reported on over 40 patients treated in this manner with a horizontal osteotomy through the pterygoid plates and described severe bleeding in most cases likely due to laceration of one of the pterygoid branches of the maxillary artery; this technique was abandoned in favor of a vertical separation of the maxilla from the pterygoid plates at the pterygomaxillary suture or junction. Most of the early technical descriptions simply mobilized the maxilla by releasing at least some bony attachments and then placing orthopedic forces with elastic traction on the maxilla to achieve the desired movement, in a sort of unintentional distraction osteogenesis procedure. As expected, owing to

soft tissue restriction, uncontrolled distraction forces, and the lack of wire or rigid fixation of the maxilla, these techniques were associated with a high degree of bony relapse. In 1965, Obwegeser[9] recommended complete mobilization of the maxilla so that repositioning could be accomplished without soft tissue or bony resistance, and this notion proved to be a major advancement in the concept of maxillary stability, as documented later by Hogeman and Willmar,[10] and Perko.[11]

Due to early concerns regarding vascular supply to the maxilla, and the belief that complete mobilization would result in complete loss of vascularity to the entire maxilla, anterior segmentalization of the maxilla was advocated in the early descriptions of maxillary surgery in order to preserve blood supply to the posterior segments, including reports by Cohn-Stock,[12] Wassmund,[4] and Spanier.[13] Because complete mobilization of the maxilla was not performed, instability and relapse occurred commonly. In addition, because surgical access was performed through palatal incisions, vascularity to the anterior maxillary segment was severely compromised. Cupar,[14,15] Kole,[16] and Wunderer[17] reported a more direct surgical access to the anterior maxilla via vestibular incisions with improved mobilization of the maxilla and maintenance of blood supply to the anterior maxillary segment. Posterior segmentalization of the maxilla was used by Schuchardt,[18] but owing to incomplete mobilization, it had limited stability with hard and soft tissue relapse. Kufner[19] improved on this posterior segmental osteotomy technique in attempt to decrease relapse by complete mobilization of the osteotomized segments before surgical repositioning. The next logical step in the evolution of maxillary surgery was to combine the techniques of anterior and posterior segmental osteotomies in order to accomplish a total maxillary alveolar osteotomy (TMAO) for segmental manipulation and surgical repositioning simultaneously.[20,21] Several forms of TMAOs were described by Converse and Shapiro,[22] Cupar,[14] and Kole.[23] Willmar[8] further established the stability achieved by performing a complete Le Fort I osteotomy, and Bell[24] documented the overall superiority of the total down-fracture Le Fort I osteotomy for segmental and one-piece maxillary osteotomies. In addition, in 1975, Bell[24] documented that the vascular supply to the down-fractured, completely mobilized maxilla is preserved via the buccal and palatal soft tissues and that the descending palatine vessels may be sacrificed without vascular compromise to the surgically repositioned maxilla.

In further consideration of maxillary stability before rigid fixation techniques, block bone grafting to improve stability was advocated by Gillies and Rowe,[25] Cupar,[14,15] and Obwegeser[26] who first advocated grafting in the pterygomaxillary fissure. Throughout the years, clinicians have advocated block grafting, using autogenous iliac crest blocks, allogeneic block grafts, or synthetic materials (e.g., block hydroxylapatite) in the bony gaps created by maxillary osteotomy but specifically placed in the pterygomaxillary buttress or piriform rims. The use of block grafting to improve stability remained a controversial procedure despite the promulgation of certain guidelines for grafting (i.e., >6 mm of maxillary advancement, or cleft lip and palate cases), and interestingly, Willmar[8] did not find a difference in stability with and without bone grafting in a series of noncleft maxillary osteotomies. Early descriptions of rigid fixation of maxillary osteotomies were published by Michelet in 1973,[27] Horster in 1980,[28] Drommer and Luhr in 1981,[29] and Luyk and Ward-Booth in 1985.[30] Since that time, a wide variety of methods have been advocated for rigid internal fixation of maxillary osteotomies, including stainless steel or titanium bone plates and screws, metallic mesh, pins, rigid adjustable pin (RAP) system and resorbable (polyglycolic acid [PGLA], poly-L-lactic acid [PLLA] polymers) fixation.[31–33] Despite these descriptions of various surgical techniques throughout the past century, there remains a lack of consensus among surgeons regarding the specifics of the surgical technique utilized for maxillary mobilization, the considerations for maxillary distraction osteogenesis versus one-stage Le Fort surgery, the need for adjunctive bone grafting, the specific "rigid fixation" devices used (e.g., number of plates needed, appropriate plate and screw thickness and diameter), and the use of postoperative intermaxillary fixation (IMF).

BASIC PRINCIPLES OF MAXILLARY SURGERY

Maxillary deformities may manifest in any of the three planes of space: sagittal, axial, and coronal. Patients display abnormal facial anatomy and exhibit elements of maxillary and mandibular deformities, and therefore, the clinician must be able to recognize and treat a variety of maxillary and midface deformities. Subjectively, patients with maxillary deformities often describe their dentofacial problem in terms of the relative mandibular appearance, such that maxillary hypoplasia may be attributed to mandibular hyperplasia ("pseudoprognathism"). Patient expectations clearly demonstrate the importance of the position of the mandible and the chin in patient aesthetic satisfaction.[34] This perceptual preoccupation with apparent mandibular excess or deficiency in the absence of a significant absolute mandibular abnormality may require additional patient education and guidance from the surgeon in order to assist the patient in recognizing the contribution of the midface and maxilla to her or his overall facial appearance. In a similar fashion, the patient may attribute a convex facial profile to an abnormal nasal prominence in describing the chief complaint, which may be due to maxillary anteroposterior (AP) excess and/or mandibular AP deficiency.

Therefore, the clinical data base should include a comprehensive history and physical examination, dental model analysis and model surgery, and cephalometric analysis with prediction tracings in order to determine the list of treatment options. These important diagnostic and treatment planning modalities are discussed extensively in Chapter 56; however, model surgery may be the most valuable tool in preparing for orthognathic surgical correction of skeletal facial deformities. Whereas model surgery is essential for immediate preoperative surgical simulation and splint construction, it may be even more important in the early phases of treatment planning. Before initiating orthodontic or surgical treatment, model surgery is the best method to determine the final postoperative position of the mandible as well as the maxilla. No cephalometric prediction (computer-generated or hand-drawn) or photographic image manipulation can detail all of the three-dimensional and occlusal information obtained from accurate model surgery. In the pretreatment stages, the teeth may not fit together perfectly during preliminary model surgery, but orthodontic tooth movement can be simulated to permit an accurate prediction of the specific movements required in the maxilla and mandible to achieve the desired final surgical result. The model surgery measurements made at the time of this pretreatment setup should be exactly the same as those used for the actual preoperative model surgery. Pretreatment model surgery is essential when contemplating maxillary surgery alone and is also very useful when planning two-jaw surgery. Pretreatment model surgery permits three-dimensional evaluation of the maxilla and the mandible, independent of whether autorotation or osteotomy of the mandible is part of the final surgical treatment plan. It should be mentioned that the entire process of presurgical assessment and treatment planning for orthognathic surgery is undergoing major advances with three-dimensional technology, which may improve efficiency and accuracy for severe, syndromic, and/or asymmetrical skeletal discrepancies.

MODEL SURGERY

Model surgery may be useful in mandibular surgery from an academic standpoint, although the final mandibular position is determined by the occlusion in all three planes of space, but it is particularly important in maxillary, and two-jaw, orthognathic surgical planning. The information obtained from precise model surgery permits accurate surgical planning, reveals the three-dimensional changes that are planned in the surgery, and facilitates the exact positioning of the jaws. Model surgery is critical for two-jaw surgery and fabrication of intermediate and final surgical splints, and when applied to isolated maxillary surgery, model analysis may reveal that, in fact, maxillary surgery alone is not sufficient to most appropriately treat the skeletal deformity. The principles of model surgery for orthognathic surgery, including both one- and two-jaw surgery, are covered in Chapter 56.

SURGICAL ANATOMY

Osseous Structures

The body of the maxilla contains the maxillary sinus in its entirety, except rarely when the apex of the sinus extends into the zygomatic bone.[35] The anterior, or facial, surface of the maxilla is composed of the anterolateral wall of the sinus. The infraorbital foramen is located at variable distances between the inferior orbital rim and the maxillary alveolus. The alveolar jugae, or root prominences, visible through the facial surface of the maxillary alveolar process are more prominent anteriorly, and the longest root in the maxilla of the canine tooth, form the canine fossa just lateral to the root juga. The anterior aspect of the alveolar process of each side of the maxilla surrounds the piriform aperture, or rim, and the maxillary suture in the anterior midline unites to form the anterior nasal spine (ANS). This bony prominence forms the most anterior and inferior, or caudal, support for the flexible anterior cartilaginous nasal septum. Proceeding posteriorly from the ANS, the nasal crest of the maxilla rises sharply to form a crest at the junction of the anterior and nasal surfaces of the maxilla, which forms the nasal floor and results in an inclination of this structure superiorly, or cranially, at the piriform aperture. The body of the maxilla and its frontal process form the superolateral boundary of the piriform aperture as a thin edge of bone. The piriform rim itself represents a vertical pillar of midfacial support (Figure 58-1).

In the midline between the nasal cavities, the nasal crest of the maxilla articulates with the septal, or quadrangular, cartilage, the vomer, and the perpendicular plate of the ethmoid bone.[36,37] The nasal septal cartilage rests in a central groove of the nasomaxillary crest, which extends posterior from the ANS to the posterior nasal spine (PNS). This bony-cartilagenous articulation is flexible, but it is stabilized by the perichondrial-periosteal continuity and interposed connective tissue. In the midline, at the junction of the premaxilla and the maxilla, or the primary and secondary palate, is the incisive foramen or fossa, which typically contains the openings of four canals through which the nasopalatine arteries and nerves pass.

The hard palate is formed by the midline fusion of the palatine processes of the two hemimaxillae and the horizontal lamina of the palatine bones.[38] The transverse suture

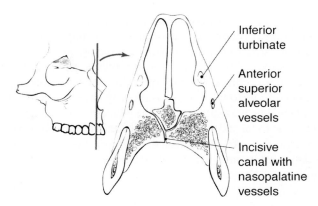

FIGURE 58-1.   Cross-sectional anatomy of the maxilla at the piriform rim.

between the maxilla and the palatine bones is located approximately 1 cm anterior to the posterior margin of the hard palate or the junction of the hard and soft palate. At its most lateral extension, this suture widens into the greater and lesser palatine foramina, which are located approximately 1 cm posteromedially to the second molar (Figure 58-2). The greater palatine canal superiorly, or cranially, is also formed by the perpendicular laminae of the palatine and maxillary bones, which continue cranially to form the inferior lateral nasal wall. The inferior nasal turbinate, an isolated bony structure, articulates with the maxillary and palatine components of the lateral nasal wall in this region, and the superior and middle turbinates are part of the ethmoid bone. Posterolaterally, the maxillary tuberosity is located behind the third molar tooth, when present. Superior to the tuberosity is the posterosuperior alveolar foramina through which the posterosuperior alveolar nerves and vessels emerge. The pyramidal processes of the palatine bones unite the medial and lateral pterygoid plates of the sphenoid bone with each other, as well as to the maxilla. The pterygomaxillary junction, formed by the palatine bone, ends superiorly in the pterygomaxillary fissure leading into the pterygopalatine

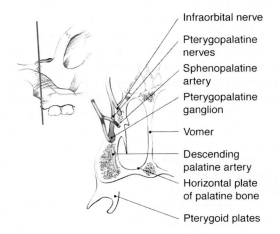

FIGURE 58-2.   Cross-sectional anatomy at the pterygomaxillary junction. Note the position of the greater palatine foramen and the perpendicular plate of the palatine bone.

fossa.[39,40] The foramen rotundum, containing the second division of the trigeminal nerve, opens into the posterior wall of the pterygopalatine fossa. In addition, the pterygoid (vidian) canal also communicates into the pterygopalatine fossa. From this point extending medially, the sphenopalatine foramen leads to the lateral nasal cavity beginning posterior to the middle nasal turbinate of the ethmoid bone. Anteriorly, the infraorbital and zygomatic nerves and infraorbital vessels traverse the infraorbital canal; inferiorly, the descending palatine artery and greater palatine nerves course within the greater palatine canal.

Vascular Structures

The vascular supply to the maxilla is extensive, and it originates from large and small vessels as well as soft tissue perfusion. The normal vascular supply is derived from the terminal branches of the maxillary artery, which traverses the pterygopalatine fossa approximately 20 mm superior to the pterygomaxillary suture. The pterygoid and pterygomaxillary divisions of the maxillary artery supply various portions of the maxilla via a complex network of tributary vessels and collateral circulation. Additional perfusion is supplied via the anastomosis of the greater palatine artery with the lesser palatine artery. The lesser palatine connects with the ascending pharyngeal artery off of the external carotid artery and the ascending palatine artery off of the facial artery. This three-way junction of the lesser, greater, and descending palatine arteries at the opening of the greater palatine foramen is a critical crossroads in the blood supply to the maxilla after down-fracture. The venous outflow tracts mimic the vascular anatomy with a confluence of veins located posteriorly as the pterygoid venous plexus.

Although numerous texts concerning head and neck anatomy describe the detailed vascular anatomy of the intact maxilla, several aspects of maxillary blood flow during and after maxillary osteotomy remain controversial or unknown. The Le Fort I osteotomy had been performed for over 100 years before Bell[41,42] first identified the exact nature of the blood supply in the osteotomized maxilla, which provided detailed information regarding the viability of the pedicled maxilla. It was obvious that even though the direct blood supply to the maxillary teeth and periodontal tissues was interrupted, collateral circulation existed to provide perfusion of the dental pulp and surrounding structures[43] (Figures 58-3 and 58-4). This same circulation is also responsible for the survival of the remainder of the maxilla; however, the exact nature of the various factors affecting maxillary perfusion is still not well documented or understood. During the classic down-fracture maxillary osteotomy, the entire blood supply to the maxilla is severed except for posterior remaining buccal pedicle and that heading for the greater palatine artery distal to the greater palatine foramen. If the greater palatine artery is disrupted anterior to this junction, severe ischemia will result unless an anterior pedicle has been retained. Bell[41,42] has shown that preservation or sacrifice of the

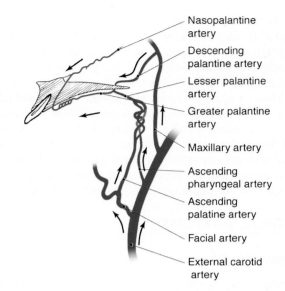

FIGURE 58-3. Pathway of the ascending palatine, ascending pharyngeal, and descending palatine arteries as they continue into the greater palatine arteries.

descending palatine artery is inconsequential and can be ligated, thereby shifting the perfusion of the greater palatine artery via the lesser palatine artery. However, the pressure head from the lesser palatine artery to the greater palatine artery will be possible only if the descending palatine artery has been ligated and not lacerated. Laceration of the descending palatine artery will not only increase uncontrolled hemorrhage but also reduce the perfusion distally through the greater palatine artery to the maxilla.

Bell[42] also verified the revascularization process after anterior maxillary osteotomy using the microangiographic technique. Brusati and Bottoli[44] performed revascularization studies similar to those of Bell and found quite different results in that the tunneling technique to access the anterior maxillary bone[16] was superior to the anterior maxillary labial pedicle technique in maintaining the blood supply, especially

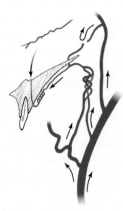

FIGURE 58-4. Soft palatal, ascending pharyngeal, and ascending palatal vessels anastomose with the greater palatine artery. Major vessels have been sectioned and tied. The *arrows* signify direction of blood flow.

Labels for Figure 58-3:
Nasopalantine artery
Descending palantine artery
Lesser palantine artery
Greater palantine artery
Maxillary artery
Ascending pharyngeal artery
Ascending palatine artery
Facial artery
External carotid artery

to the pulpal tissues.[17] One possible explanation for this discrepancy is that Bell used a monkey model whereas Brusati and Bottoli used the dog model, which they claimed possess a more similar maxillary vasculature to that of the human.[44] The clinical significance of these differences remains unclear, and in none of these studies were the maxillae moved to a new position, which may, in fact, represent the greatest insult to the blood supply at the time of actual maxillary osteotomy surgery. It should be remembered that revascularization does not necessarily represent the reestablishment of adequate blood flow, and therefore, Nelson and coworkers[45,46] used a radioactive microsphere technique to evaluate maxillary blood flow. Unfortunately, several variables were present in this study that make interpretation difficult, including the fact that severance of the descending palatine vessels was inadvertent, and no ligation was performed, which allowed bleeding to occur through the lacerated vessels and prevented a pressure head from developing that would serve to maintain distal blood flow to the anterior maxillary segment. In other studies involving anterior maxillary osteotomies, Nelson and coworkers[46] found no significant differences among three different techniques, including the labial pedicle, tunnel technique (as described by Brusati and Bottoli)[44], plus a third procedure using only a palatal pedicle. Although no statistical difference was seen, the palatal flap seemed to be slightly superior to the others, and owing to the presence of multiple confounding variables, clinical significance could not be determined.

The Soft Tissue Envelope of the Maxilla

The midfacial superficial fascia, or subcutaneous tissues, contain variable amounts of adipose tissue as well as the muscles of facial expression within the deep fascial layer. This fascia is tightly bound to bone in most locations in the midface, except directly adjacent to the buccal fat pad and in the lower eyelids. In *Anatomy for Surgeons: The Head and Neck,* Hollinshead[39] divides the mimetic or facial muscles into five chief groups: mouth, nose, orbit, ear, and scalp. The muscle groups of the mouth and nose, which are innervated at their posteroinferior aspect by the facial nerve, are of greatest concern with regards to maxillary orthognathic surgery. These muscle groups insert into the skin and mostly arise from periosteum surrounding the midfacial facial skeleton. The upper oral group of muscles radiate from their insertions near the corner of the labial commissure (modiolus region). From a horizontal to vertical, and inferior to superior, orientation the risorius, zygomaticus major and minor, and levators (levator labii superioris alaeque nasi) insert and blend with the skin and orbicularis oris muscle. The risorius does not arise from bone but originates from the superficial fascia over the parotid gland. The risorius, zygomaticus major, and zygomaticus minor elevate and retract the corner of the mouth and upper lip laterally. The superficial levator muscles and a third deeper muscle, the levator anguli oris, elevate the lateral portion of the upper lip. In addition, the levator labii superioris alaeque nasi muscle attaches to the

skin and greater alar cartilage of the nose, thus lifting the ala and widening the naris.

The orbicularis oris muscle is composed of many multidirectional fiber groups that blend with other surrounding facial muscles, encircle the mouth, originate from periosteum covering the roots of the canine teeth, insert laterally at the corner of the mouth, and pass at right angles to the encircling sphincter fillers connecting skin to labial mucosa. This diverse muscle draws the lips together, purses the lips, presses the lips against the teeth, and pulls the corners of the lips inward. The buccinator muscle arises from the mandible and maxilla and the pterygomandibular raphe, which separates it from the superior pharyngeal constrictor muscle. The fibers pass forward and slightly inferiorly to blend with the orbicularis oris and attach to the mucosa and skin of the labial region. The buccinator muscle acts to flatten the cheek against the teeth and alveolus.

Lightoller[47] and Nairn[48] place emphasis on the modiolus, which is the point at the lateral aspect and just superior to the corner of the mouth where muscles of the oral group of the mimetic muscles converge. The orbicularis oris and buccinator muscles join at the modiolus region to form a continuous muscular sheet on either side of the midline. The zygomaticus major, levator anguli oris, and depressor anguli oris (this group is referred to as the "modiolar stays") immobilize the modiolus in any position. In addition the marginal and peripheral parts of the orbicularis oris muscle are distinguishable by the fact that the peripheral aspect of the muscle lies parallel to the inner labial mucosal surface and the marginal part curls outward following the vermilion surface. As tension is expressed in the orbicularis oris, the marginal aspect of the muscle is thought to straighten and decrease vermilion exposure, thereby pulling the upper and lower lips toward each other and against the facial surfaces of the dentition.

When contemplating maxillary orthognathic surgery, consideration must be given to the nasal group of facial muscles that act to both dilate and compress the nares and whose length and function may be affected by Le Fort surgery. The nasalis muscle arises from the anterior aspect of the maxilla in a position lateral and inferior to the ala. The transverse portion of the nasalis muscle unites with the contralateral nasalis muscle over the dorsum of the nose. The alar portion of the nasalis muscle inserts into the greater alar cartilage. Thus, the two parts of the nasalis compress and dilate the nasal apertures, respectively. The depressor septi muscle lies beneath the orbicularis oris and attaches to the base of the columella and posterior ala; it functions to narrow the naris. The posterior and anterior dilator muscles are intrinsic muscles of the nose that course from the alar cartilages to the margin of the alar fat pads. The nasal mucoperiosteum is firmly fixated to the elevated piriform rim above the floor of the nose, to the lateral margin of the nasal aperture, and to the ANS. The premaxillary wings that flare laterally from the anterior midline nasal crest provide an irregular attachment of the mucoperiosteum along the inferoanterior nasal floor.

The hard palate is covered by mucosa firmly adherent to the periosteum and containing mucous minor salivary glands. The mucosa is thin in the midline region of the palate and thickens toward the alveolar process. The palatine crest is a transverse elevation at the posterior border of the horizontal plate of the palatine bone that gives attachment to the tensor veli palatini muscle. The larger, lateral pterygoid plate is the origin of the inferior head of the lateral pterygoid and the medial pterygoid muscles. A small part of the medial pterygoid muscle also arises from the maxillary tuberosity. The tensor veli palatini muscle that functions during speech and swallowing curves around the hamulus, which is the caudal, or inferior, termination of the medial pterygoid plate. From the hamulus, the tensor muscle of the palate enters the soft palatal tissues. The tensor aponeurosis is an adherent connective tissue sheath continuous with the periosteum, which covers the posterior hard palate attaching laterally to the submucosal layer of the pharynx and the tensor veli palatini tendon.

SURGICAL TECHNIQUES

Incisions, Dissection, and Exposure of the Maxilla

Exposure of the anterior, lateral, and pterygomaxillary regions of the maxilla is most commonly achieved via a circumvestibular incision horizontally through the mucoperiosteum above the attached gingival margin at the level of the maxillary teeth apices (Figure 58-5A). The circumvestibular incision typically extends from the first molar to the contralateral first molar region (see Figure 58-5B). Care is taken to avoid the parotid papilla of Stensen's duct at approximately the maxillary second molar region superior to the occlusal plane. The incision may be made with electrocautery or a scalpel, and there are no studies evaluating the two techniques, A full mucoperiosteal incision is made to the anterior wall of the maxillary sinus, and care should be taken in the anterior region to keep the incision below the ANS and avoid a superiorly placed incision that may perforate the nasal mucosa and enter the nasal cavity. The tissues above the incision are reflected superiorly in a subperiosteal plane first at

the area of the piriform rims, using a periosteal elevator (#9) (see Figure 58-5C). Further superior exposure lateral to the nasal aperture will lead to exposure of the infraorbital nerve exiting from the infraorbital foramen. This subperiosteal dissection also elevates the insertions of the muscles mentioned previously, including the upper lip muscles, nasal muscles, and zygomatic muscles. Further posterior subperiosteal tissue reflection from the infraorbital foramen will reveal the zygomaticomaxillary suture, the zygomatic buttress, and the most anterior aspect of the zygomatic arch. Continuing posteriorly and inferiorly with subperiosteal tunneling, the lateral aspect of the maxillary tuberosity and its junction with pterygoid plates of the sphenoid bone are exposed. Care should be taken to avoid vascular structures by directing the subperiosteal dissection posteroinferiorly, more toward the mucogingival junction, as dissection progresses toward the pterygomaxillary fissure. Meticulous maintenance of the subperiosteal plane of dissection may prevent troublesome exposure of buccal fat pad tissue, which impairs visualization and retraction of soft tissue during the subsequent osseous surgery. A reverse-angled Obwegeser retractor ("toe-out" or "up-turned") is placed in the pterygomaxillary junction to facilitate bony exposure. Close attention should be paid to the placement of this retractor because it can be responsible for iatrogenic laceration of the periosteum and/or exposure of the buccal fat pad. The attached and unattached mucogingival tissues inferior to the incision are elevated minimally, if at all. In areas of planned interdental osteotomies for segmentalization of the maxillary arch, the attached gingiva and periosteum are elevated conservatively using a Woodson elevator, while retraction can be provided, if necessary (Figure 58-6). Because the alveolar osteotomy will be accomplished with a thin osteotome, osseous exposure requirements at the alveolar crest level are minimal and minimal soft tissue dissection is usually required. Infrequently, the intersegment osteotomy may be larger, and more exposure may be necessary to prevent tearing of the gingival papilla. In addition, a wider exposure of alveolar bone is frequently needed when the osteotomy is planned in an edentulous site or in a simultaneous extraction space. In these rare situations, a vertical releasing mucosal incision at the line angle one tooth away from the ostectomy site will facilitate

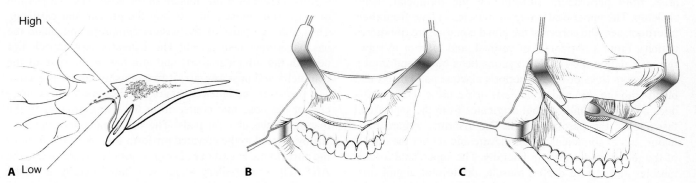

FIGURE 58-5. **A,** The soft tissue incision for maxillary surgery. **B,** The circumvestibular incision extends from the area of the first molar to the same location on the opposite side. **C,** The nasal mucosa is elevated beginning on the superolateral surface of the piriform rim.

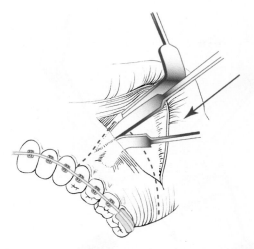

FIGURE 58-6.   If segmentalization is necessary, it is best to perform interdental osteotomies before horizontal osteotomies and down-fracture. Use minimal exposure technique for interdental osteotomies.

wider exposure for the osseous procedure. This ancillary vertical incision should be used only when an anterior labial pedicle can be maintained to maximize the existing vascular pedicle during multisegment osteotomy procedures (Figure 58-7). As mentioned, for one-, two-, and most routine three-piece maxillary osteotomies, a circumvestibular incision, with minimal interdental exposure, is preferred. For three-piece maxillary osteotomies involving wide expansion or other extreme changes, four-piece maxillary osteotomies, and osteotomies in cleft maxillas, soft tissue incisions can be isolated from second molar to first premolar to maintain a wide anterior labial soft tissue and vascular pedicle to the anterior maxillary segment(s) (see Figure 58-7). In some cases, a midline vertical incision is utilized to gain access to the anterior maxillary segments, if necessary.

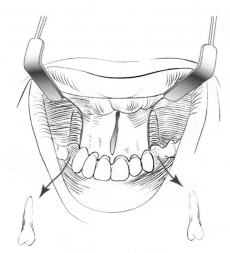

FIGURE 58-7.   Modified incision for cases in which anterior perfusion is questionable. Bilateral vestibular incisions are made from the first premolar to the second molar; shown with a midline vertical incision.

Once the labial incision(s) and soft tissue and muscle dissection are completed, the nasal mucoperiosteum is elevated to complete soft tissue exposure of the osseous surgical site (see Figure 58-5C). A meticulous initial subperiosteal plane of dissection is imperative for complete elevation of the nasal mucosa without disruption of mucoperiosteal integrity, leading to persistent nasal bleeding both intraoperatively and postoperatively. Because the nasal cavity is more voluminous inside the piriform rim than at the entrance to the piriform aperture, the periosteal elevator should be held at an oblique angle to the surrounding maxillary bone adjacent to the nasal aperture; alternatively a Woodson elevator may be used to initiate the dissection at the piriform rim. While maintaining the elevator tip against the bone within the nasal cavity, the mucoperiosteum is reflected from the nasal floor, lateral nasal wall, and nasal crest of the maxilla. The dissection should continue superiorly 1 cm along both lateral nasal walls and both sides of the nasal septum to prevent nasal mucosal tearing during the nasal septal osteotomy and the lateral nasal osteotomies or during the down-fracture of the maxilla. The AP depth of this nasal mucosal dissection is approximately 15 to 20 mm. The remaining posterior soft tissue of the nasal floor is reflected more precisely after the initial down-fracture of the maxilla. At this point, in preparation for osseous surgery, there should be two reverse-angle ("toe-out") Obwegeser retractors, one on each side posteriorly at the pterygomaxillary junction; two Obwegeser retractors ("toe-in") elevating the soft tissues, upper lip muscles, nasal muscles, and zygomatic muscles and protecting the infraorbital neurovascular bundles superiorly; and two periosteal elevators, one in the inferolateral aspect of the piriform rims bilaterally protecting the lateral nasal mucosa.

Osseous Surgery

Before osseous surgery, vertical reference points must be recorded, and these may be made either inside or outside of the wound. The internal reference points are small holes made with a #701 bur in the piriform rim and the zygomatic buttress, well above the osteotomy. Measurements are made from the reference points to the gingival crest corresponding to the point-to-point measurements made at the time of model surgery using a caliper as described in Chapter 56. External reference using a Kirshner wire or Steinmann pin may also be used. An external reference is created by using a wire or Steinmann pin placed in the nasal bones, and then using a measuring device (e.g.. Perkins device) to make reproducible vertical measurements to the central incisor bracket or other inferior reference that will not be obscured if an interocclusal splint is used later during surgery. In addition, a horizontal measurement can be made using the same Perkins device with a millimeter calibrated rod placed in the lower portion of the device. After making the initial vertical and horizontal measurements, the device can be set to the planned movements and used subsequently during osseous surgery to confirm that the planned movements have been

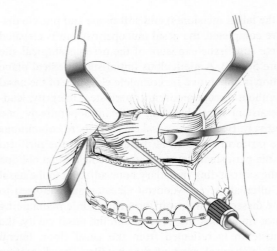

FIGURE 58-8. Lateral wall osteotomy is begun at greatest convexity of the buttress and brought forward to the piriform rim with a periosteal elevator protecting the nasal mucosa and the endotracheal tube.

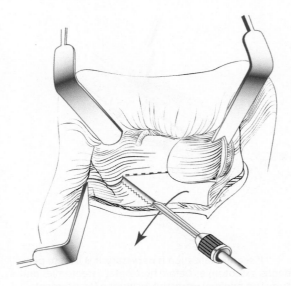

FIGURE 58-9. The saw is then turned inside out and the osteotomy from the buttress to the pterygomaxillary junction is made angling downward as it goes posteriorly.

achieved. Many studies have shown that external reference points are more predictable and reproducible than traditional scribed lines, and, similar to model surgery, the external technique (and the technique described in Chapter 56) utilize reference points that are located at a distance from the osteotomy site. This minimizes parallax error, especially with a significant maxillary advancement. It also prevents obliteration of landmarks inappropriately placed adjacent to the osteotomy, especially with a significant maxillary impaction procedure.

The design of the osteotomy will depend upon the maxillary movement desired. The initial lateral maxillary osteotomy (Figure 58-8) is generally begun at the greatest convexity of the zygomatic buttress because this area provides a convex surface for the reciprocating saw. The saw is advanced anteriorly through the lateral piriform rim below the inferior nasal turbinate while the nasal mucoperiosteum is protected with the periosteal elevator. For a standard maxillary osteotomy, the horizontal bony cut is made parallel to the maxillary arch wire and maxillary occlusal plane, in an attempt to simulate the cut performed previously during model surgery. Any modifications to the standard osteotomy are taken into consideration at this point and altered as necessary (e.g., a Z or a step osteotomy). After the anterior osteotomy is completed, the bony cut is continued posteriorly by tapering inferiorly toward the pterygomaxillary junction, using the reciprocating saw in an "inside-out" fashion (Figure 58-9).

After completion of the osteotomy of the anterior and lateral wall of the maxillary sinus, a bayonet or double-guarded nasal septal osteotome is directed slightly downward and posterior (Figure 58-10), beginning just above the ANS while the anterior nasal mucoperiosteum is retracted. Proceeding posteriorly, the osteotome is carefully maintained in the midline along the nasal crest of the maxilla. There is a tendency toward superior deviation of the osteotome while separating the cartilaginous and vomerine septum from the

nasal crest of the maxilla; this necessitates slight downward inclination of the nasal septal osteotome. A finger placed at the PNS region near the soft palate confirms that the osteotome has been carried sufficiently posterior. Next, the lateral nasal walls are osteotomized using a thin spatula or single guarded nasal osteotome directed posteriorly and inferiorly if necessary, while medial retraction of the nasal mucoperiosteum is accomplished with a periosteal elevator. The osteotome is gently malleted posteriorly for a distance of approximately 20 mm to avoid premature injury to the descending palatine neurovascular bundle that resides in the lateral posterior nasal wall. In many cases, the use of these osteotomes will initiate the down-fracture of the maxilla, and some surgeons may choose to perform this portion of the osteotomy after all other osteotomies have been completed, including the pterygoid plate osteotomy, in which the pterygoid plates are separated from the maxillary tuberosity (Figure 58-11) using a small, sharp, curved osteotome (pterygoid

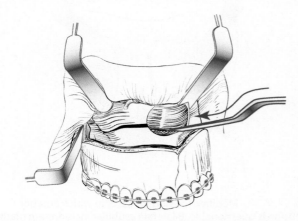

FIGURE 58-10. Separation of the nasal septum from the septal crest of the maxilla with a special osteotome.

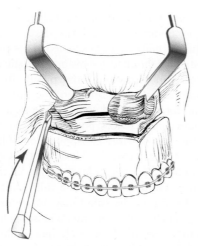

FIGURE 58-11.   Pterygomaxillary separation with a small, sharp, curved osteotome directed medially.

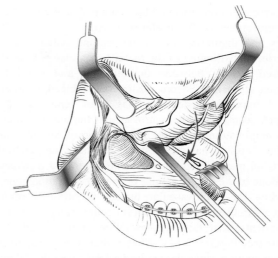

FIGURE 58-12.   Down-fracture is accomplished with a sharp-toothed Senn retractor, with simultaneous elevation of nasal mucoperiosteum.

osteotome). This instrument is preferred over the traditional large thick pterygomaxillary osteotome (swan-neck osteotome) because the thin cutting edge and more gentle curve limit the extent of fracture[49] and promotes precise division of this bony junction, although studies indicate that the pterygoid osteotomy may occur in a variety of erroneous locations, including the alveolus, through the plates horizontally, and close to the skull base, as well as other locations. The tip of the curved pterygoid osteotome is directed as anteriorly, inferiorly, and medially as the tunneled buccal soft tissue pedicle will allow. A finger placed on the palatal side of the maxilla and posterior to the maxillary tuberosity will help verify complete separation of the maxilla from the pterygoid plates while avoiding trauma to the palatal vascular pedicle. Because the maxillary artery has been shown to lie in the pterygomaxillary fossa approximately 20 to 25 mm above the pterygomaxillary fissure, the use of a 10-mm pterygoid chisel will allow a 10- to 15-mm margin of safety during performance of the osteotomy. At this point, all osteotomies have been completed, and downward pressure is placed on the anterior maxilla using digital manipulation or the sharp hooks of a Senn retractor to facilitate initial down-fracture of the maxilla (Figure 58-12). If moderate pressure does not result in mobilization of the maxilla, an evaluation and verification of all osteotomies should be performed, and typically, the pterygoid disjunction is found to be incomplete. The curved pterygoid osteotome is again placed into the pterygomaxillary junction, malleted gently, and then torqued to attempt to mobilize the maxilla. If no significant movement is achieved, the pterygoid osteotome may be carefully placed further superiorly in the pterygomaxillary fissure, directed anteriorly, and malleted again until the separation is complete. Another area of possible incomplete osteotomy is the lateral nasal wall, which can be checked with a guarded osteotome and completed if necessary.

When mobilization occurs, the nasal mucoperiosteum is elevated in a progressive fashion posteriorly until the posterior edge of the hard palate is encountered (see Figure

58-12). Any significant tears in the nasal mucosa should be repaired at this point with resorbable suture to prevent persistent nasal bleeding. Portions of the pterygoid plates or perpendicular process of the palatine bone that resist fracture may be completely separated from the maxilla using a carefully placed double-action rongeur under direct visualization (Figure 58-13). After initial mobilization of the maxilla, the descending palatine neurovascular bundle may be identified, isolated, and either protected or ligated with hemoclips and divided. If the descending palatine vessels are maintained, care must be taken to avoid inadvertent laceration or the presence of sharp bony edges that may contribute to intraoperative bleeding during maxillary repositioning or postoperative

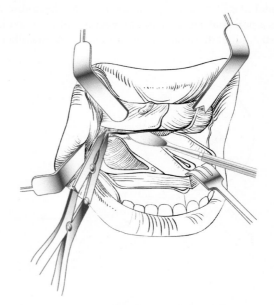

FIGURE 58-13.   Complete removal of bone around the perpendicular plate of palatine bone. The descending palatine artery is isolated, ligated, and divided.

hemorrhage, as documented by Lanigan and West.[50] Significant movement of the posterior maxilla can cause tensile forces and disruption of the descending palatine vessels. Superior repositioning of the maxilla may also compress the exposed vessels between the superior and the inferior osseous segments. Severe postoperative bleeding after Le Fort I maxillary osteotomy has been reported,[51–54] and attempts to preserve the neurovascular bundle may increase this complication. Ligation and division of the descending palatine vessels has been shown to have no deleterious effects on maxillary perfusion or neurosensory recovery.[55,56] The bone of the perpendicular plate of the palatine bone surrounding the neurovascular bundle is carefully removed using a Woodson elevator and a rongeur (preferable to rotary instruments) that facilitates isolation of the neurovascular bundle (see Figure 58-13). Other clinicians argue against the routine ligation of the descending palatine vessels if they can be protected adequately, especially during segmental maxillary procedures. After maxillary down-fracture, if additional mobilization of the maxilla is needed, a J stripper, typically used during mandibular sagittal osteotomies, may be placed over the posterior border of the midline of the nasal floor at the PNS region (Figure 58-14), and anterolateral pressure is exerted to progressively mobilize the maxilla. A Tessier retromaxillary lever or similar instrument may also be placed posterior to the tuberosity region with anterior pressure. Finally, with extreme caution, two Rowe disimpaction forceps may be used with the straight arm of the forceps placed on one side of the nasal floor and the curved arm placed on the palatal mucosa. With two of these forceps, significant torque may be placed on the maxilla to achieve mobility, but significant pressure on the palatal vascular pedicle may compromise blood flow to the anterior maxilla if used inappropriately or for an extended period of time, especially during segmental maxillary surgery and their use has been discouraged as a potential cause of aseptic necrosis of the maxilla.[57] The goal of all of these maneuvers is to move the maxilla into

the approximate final position with only gentle digital pressure and a minimum of soft and hard tissue restriction. After down-fracture, significant, unexpected sinus pathology may be débrided and submitted for histopathologic evaluation, if indicated. After mobilization of the maxilla from the cranial base is completed, a reassessment of the surgical movement should be performed. Based upon the planned movement all potential bony interferences posterior to the second molar should be eliminated before the application of IMF or maxillomandibular fixation (MMF). Next, MMF is applied, either with or without the interocclusal splint fabricated during model surgery. On occasion, with a full dentition and good interocclusal contacts, the splint may not be used. However, even in cases such as this, an interocclusal splint provides a more definitive seating of the teeth than tooth-to-tooth contact. If there is instability in the occlusion, a planned open bite posteriorly, or a tripod plan for the occlusion to be corrected orthodontically after surgery, the interocclusal splint should be used. Also, the splint may or may not be left in place, typically wired to the maxilla, after surgery.

Condylar positioning during rotation of the maxillomandibular complex and application of rigid fixation to the maxilla are paramount to success, and some surgeons prefer complete paralysis of the patient during this process. The physiologic position of the condyle is thought to be in a superoanterior orientation relative to the glenoid fossae against the posterior slopes of the articular eminences, with the disk interposed between the condyle and the fossa, and the surgeon should position the condyles appropriately before autorotation (Figure 58-15). The importance of this stage of the surgery cannot be overstated, and the most likely points of unrecognized bony interferences are in the areas of

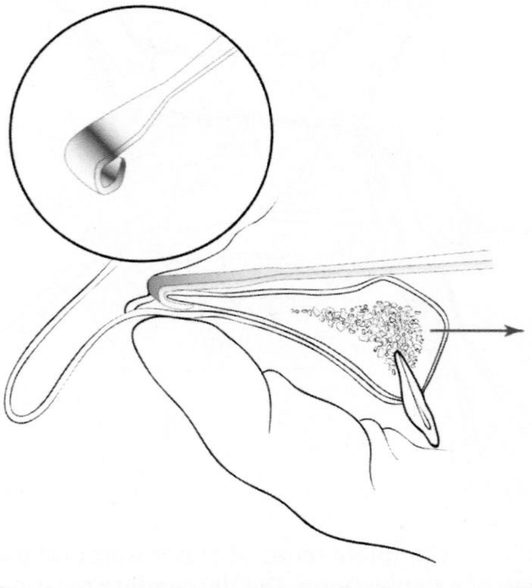

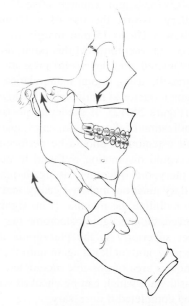

FIGURE 58-15. Manual positioning of the maxillomandibular complex with condyles seated. Note the posterior pivot point that must be removed.

FIGURE 58-14. Mobilization of the maxilla with a J stripper.

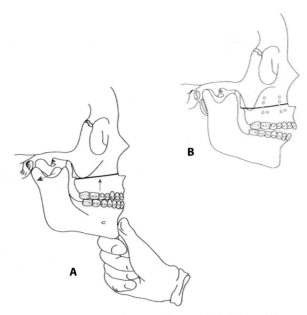

FIGURE 58-16.   Inappropriate positioning of the condyles around posterior pivot points **(A)** will result in open bite **(B)** after release from maxillomandibular fixation.

the pterygoid plates, the maxillary tuberosities, and the perpendicular plate of the palatine bone. It is possible to rotate the maxillomandibular complex while being unaware of a premature pivot point in these posterior bony areas (Figure 58-16A). This will result in immediate malpositioning and a class II open bite discrepancy upon release of MMF. If a significant period of MMF or training elastics is used postoperatively, this discrepancy may not become apparent for weeks or months (see Figure 58-16B). Once these posterior interferences have been removed, the surgeon continues to rotate the entire complex around the temporomandibular joints until the appropriate vertical relationship is achieved. The cartilaginous septum and vomer as well as the nasal crest

of the maxilla are reduced in height equal to the planned movement of the maxilla. This may require a submucous resection of the cartilaginous nasal septum to prevent buckling of the septum from pressure as the maxilla is repositioned. A groove can be fashioned in the midline of the nasal floor to accommodate the recontoured septum and prevent nasal septal deviation postoperatively. A portion of the inferior edge of the cartilaginous septum should also be removed, and the tendency is to not remove enough because there may be unequal areas of contact between septum and maxilla. Even if the maxilla is inferiorly repositioned, buckling of the septum may occur because the cartilaginous septum extends anterior and inferior to the ANS and, therefore, may be buckled as the maxilla moves forward even with some downward movement (Figure 58-17). This is the reason that the surgeon should err on overreduction, rather than underreduction, of the nasal septum and nasomaxillary crest. As mentioned, the maxillary movements have been predetermined by model surgery, and splint fabrication dictates the horizontal and transverse maxillary movements but not the vertical position. At the time of surgery, as the maxilla is rotated around the condyles, bony interferences are removed only at the points of contact, not as a full wedge reduction of bone planned upon the movement,[58] because "telescoping" of the bony edges may occur without the need for bony reduction (Figure 58-18). Selective bony reduction of interferences only results in improved bone-to-bone contact and avoids large gaps between bony segments. Once the desired vertical relationship has been achieved based on the measurements and reference points as described in Chapter 56, the maxilla should be fixated in position with internal rigid fixation, typically using four 2.0-mm plates with 16 self-drilling screws, placed at the piriform rim and zygomaticomaxillary buttress regions, because these represent the structural pillars of the midface. Next, MMF is removed and the mandible is rotated based upon the condylar position into the interocclusal splint while the splint is held against the maxillary dentition. This step is

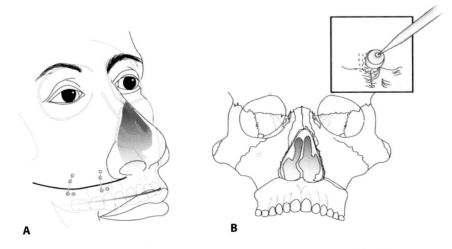

FIGURE 58-17.   **A,** Anterior aspect of the cartilaginous nasal septum extends anteroinferiorly to the anterior nasal spine. **B,** Pure horizontal advancement of the maxilla will buckle the septum unless adequate bony and cartilaginous relief is provided.

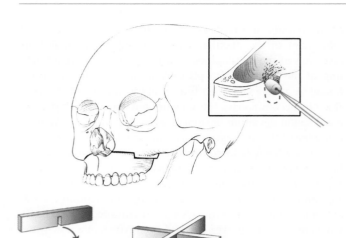

FIGURE 58-18. Removal of bony walls and slotting of the contact points.

critical to determine whether the condyles were adequately seated during fixation of the maxilla. An immediate anterior open bite or significant malocclusion at this point necessitates removal of rigid fixation and inspection and reduction of bony interferences to allow correct condylar positioning in order to achieve the appropriate maxillary movements. After release of MMF and verification of the correct, stable and repeatable occlusion, the surgical splint is usually removed unless the planned postoperative surgical occlusion is unstable, as mentioned previously. Variations in the previously discussed basic osteotomy design may enhance osseous contact, facilitate bone graft placement, or assist in the application of rigid fixation devices and result in improved stability of the repositioned maxilla. These variations are described later as they apply to specific maxillary movements. To prevent nasal septal deviation, despite adequate bone and cartilage removal, it is desirable to suture the nasal septum to the

ANS in the midline. This is done by drilling a hole through the ANS and passing a 2-0 resorbable or nonresorbable suture through the hole and then through the cartilaginous nasal septum (Figure 58-19). This will also contribute to prevention of postoperative displacement of the septum during nasal extubation. The use of alar base cinch sutures to control alar base widening using 2-0 nonresorbable suture and V-Y or double V-Y closure to preserve vermilion display using 4-0 chromic gut sutures are discussed in Chapter 60. Recontouring of the bony inferior piriform rim and reduction of the ANS are often useful in preventing widening of the alar base and preventing overrotation with elevation of the nasal tip. After copious irrigation, wound closure is performed by suturing the periosteum using a polyglycolic acid suture followed by mucosal closure with chromic gut. Alternatively, a single 3-0 chromic gut suture may be used to close the mucosa and periosteum from the superior tissue to the inferior alveolar unattached periosteum and mucosa.

Segmental Maxillary Procedures

A variety of surgical options exist when segmental maxillary surgery is required. Whereas there are regional variations and specific orthodontic preferences for preparing the dentition for surgery, the need for segmentation of the maxilla occurs in up to 30% of cases. Whereas two-piece maxillary surgery is frequently required for a surgically assisted maxillary expansion procedure, the three-piece maxillary osteotomy is perhaps performed most commonly when segmentation of the maxilla is required. Once again, the decision-making process regarding which of the options will be utilized in each case is determined by pretreatment and preoperative assessment and model surgery simulation. The need for dental extractions, most commonly of the premolar teeth with the segmental osteotomies performed through the extraction sites, is also determined at this stage of treatment planning. If no extractions are required, the interdental osteotomies

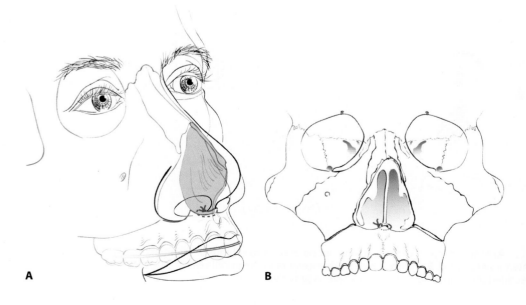

FIGURE 58-19. **A** and **B,** To avoid septal deviation, the cartilaginous septum should be sutured to the anterior nasal spine.

A   B

may be made reliably between the parallel or divergent roots of the canine and the lateral incisors or posteriorly between the canine and the premolar teeth. When possible, the osteotomy should be performed between the canine and the premolar teeth to preserve more hard and soft tissue with the associated vascular pedicle to the anterior maxillary segment. If the anterior six maxillary teeth interdigitate well with the lower anterior teeth, the interdental osteotomy is performed between the canine and the premolar teeth. This places a potential periodontal defect at the interdental osteotomy site more posterior in the oral cavity, removed from the aesthetic zone. If extractions are required based upon by the coordinated orthodontic and surgical treatment plans, the teeth may be removed early during presurgical orthodontic treatment or during the orthognathic surgical procedure. The indications and considerations that influence this decision are covered in Chapter 55. Regarding the specific surgical technique, the interdental osteotomy is created with gentle soft tissue retraction and the use of a thin cement spatula osteotome while palpating the palatal mucosa in the area of the osteotomy. As described, the standard circumvestibular incision can be performed, and a conservative tunneling technique can be created from the circumvestibular incision inferiorly to the alveolar crest on the facial aspect of the alveolus. The osteotome is malleted through the interdental alveolus until the tip is just palpable under the palatal mucosa (see Figure 58-6). With care, the osteotomy can be carried superiorly to the level of the planned horizontal maxillary osteotomy and medially to the horizontal surface of the hard palate. This should be performed before any of the other maxillary osteotomies are done because the maxilla must be stable at the time to withstand the forces of the mallet. If teeth are to be extracted at the time of the interdental osteotomy, an alternative flap design is recommended in order to maintain an anterior soft tissue pedicle for blood supply to the anterior segment (see Figure 58-7). It should be remembered that segmentalization with a standard, or modified, interdental osteotomy may be more difficult when alternative Le Fort osteotomy designs are used, such as high Le Fort I, II, or III designs, because access and ability to fully complete the segmental osteotomies may be compromised; for example, when Z osteotomies are used, interdental cuts between canines and premolars are more difficult than between canines and lateral incisors.

After complete maxillary down-fracture and full mobilization of the maxilla, the remainder of the segmental osteotomies can be completed. The palatal soft tissue is very thin in the midline and the bone is very thick, but the opposite is true in the area between 5 and 10 mm lateral to the midline. For that reason, two parasagittal osteotomies are frequently utilized along the floor of the nose using a bur with a rounded tip, such as a Steiger bur, or 1703 fissure bur (Figure 58-20). The use of two parasagittal, or paramedian, osteotomies creates a bony island in the midline to avoid perforation of the thin palatal mucosa in the midline region; this creates a separate "island" of bone in the midline of the palate. The

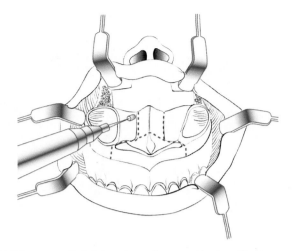

FIGURE 58-20.   Following down-fracture, the maxilla is segmentalized with a rounded-end cutting bur such as a Steiger bur by making two parasagittal cuts that join across the midline and connect with the interdental osteotomies.

parasagittal cuts are joined with the interdental cuts in order to perform the three-piece maxillary osteotomy and release the three dentoalveolar segments. If significant torquing of the anterior maxillary segment is planned, the two parasagittal cuts must be joined across the midline so that there are three dentoalveolar segments and one midpalatal bony fragment (i.e., a total of four bony segments). In two-piece maxillary osteotomy designs, the two parasagittal cuts are joined with one midline interdental cut between the central incisors at the incisive canal (i.e., three bony segments). It must be remembered that the orthodontic arch wire must be sectioned at the interdental osteotomy sites in order to ensure complete segment mobilization and allow any necessary recontouring in the osteotomy site. Finally, if large interdental bone removal is necessary to close an extraction space, surgical access may be needed from the palate, especially in the midline (Figure 58-21). In this case, it is recommended that an anterior labial mucoperiosteal pedicle is maintained with a small midline vertical incision in order to access the ANS region (see Figure 58-7). This technique allows for a midline palatal incision and the use of conservative circumdental incisions to access the palate for bone removal. The individual segments are then wired to the final surgical splint The splint should have some palatal coverage for segmental maxillary surgery, with relief so that pressure is not placed on the palatal vascular pedicle. If bone grafting is required on the palate, for example, with a significant transverse expansion, this must be done before the maxilla is repositioned and stabilized vertically. In contrast, any interdental and/or buttress bone grafting, if necessary, can be performed just before closure of the soft tissue wounds owing to access from the facial aspect of the maxilla. After splint fixation, the orthodontic arch wire can be luted together with rapid-curing acrylic or a new orthodontic arch wire can be placed. The length of time the splint is left in place depends upon the magnitude and direction of segment movement. Typically,

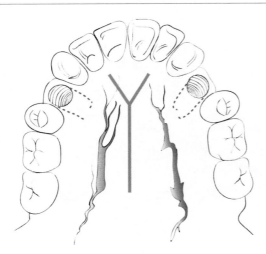

FIGURE 58-21. A midline palatal incision with a Y at the anterior aspect can be used with caution to access the palate for interdental bone removal in closing large extraction spaces.

splints are left in place for segmental cases for approximately 3 weeks for smaller movements and up to 8 weeks for greater degrees of expansive movements. After splint removal, the patient returns to the orthodontist for fabrication of the appropriate retention devices and completion of postsurgical orthodontic treatment.

Superior Maxillary Repositioning

When considering maxillary impaction surgery, historical descriptions suggested a lateral maxillary wedge ostectomy based upon the amount of the planned superior maxillary movement. However, this should be avoided because it often results in large gaps in the bony interfaces as the maxilla is moved superiorly because the contour of the maxilla is not consistent and has several bends and turns that may result in unpredictable superior movement of the maxilla, with some areas having premature contacts that require reduction and others exhibiting a "telescoping" effect of the bones with desirable overlap.[58] Furthermore, any shifting, tilting, or advancement of the maxilla may further reduce bone-to-bone contact, making premature bony removal unnecessary and potentially deleterious. Instead, sequential intermittent bony reduction of premature osseous contacts avoids unnecessary loss of bone and ensures a more predictable final contact between the maxilla and the cranial base (see Figure 58-18). Therefore, the standard horizontal osteotomy is performed, and no bone is removed until the splint is in place with IMF, and the maxillomandibular complex is rotated superiorly, with the condyles seated appropriately, to determine the specific location of bony interferences (see Figures 58-15 and 58-16). The areas of premature bone contact can now be determined as the maxilla is positioned superiorly, and bone is removed minimally at the contact points to permit the planned superior repositioning based upon the reference landmarks. In many cases, isolated interferences of the

anterior wall of the maxillary sinus may be managed with the creation of slots, or grooves, in the zygomatic buttress region or anywhere necessary along the lateral maxillary wall (see Figure 58-18). One must be careful that the grooves do not inhibit the free rotational movement of the maxillomandibular complex and cause displacement of the maxilla with condylar malpositioning. This technique is particularly valuable when the maxilla is shifted laterally or torqued in a transverse direction, which would make prediction of a predetermined ostectomy difficult. In most cases of maxillary superior movement, significant bony reduction is required on the superior aspect of the maxilla as well, especially in the posterior regions. This bony reduction can be performed using a rongeur initially followed by a large round, or pineapple-shaped, bur while protecting the nasal tissues and the descending palatine vessels. If these vessels were not sacrificed previously, they may require ligation at this point if significant bony interferences are present in these areas. Once the maxillary vertical position is ideal based upon the reference points, the maxilla is rigidly fixated, the MMF is released, and the occlusion is assessed for accuracy, stability, and repeatability.

Anterior Maxillary Repositioning

The traditional standard Le Fort I osteotomy is ideally horizontal in angulation parallel to the maxillary occlusal dentition. However, in an attempt to avoid the long maxillary canine root, there may be a tendency to incline the angle of the osteotomy in a superior direction from posterior to anterior into the piriform rim. Such an inclination in the osteotomy design may not coincide with the desired forward maxillary movement, and if the angulations of the left and right sides are not coincident, an asymmetry may be created with the maxillary movement.

For this reason, a variety of straight, stepped, and Z osteotomies have been described in the literature and may be individually designed to accommodate the planned maxillary movements[59-64] (Figures 58-22 to 58-25). If bone grafting

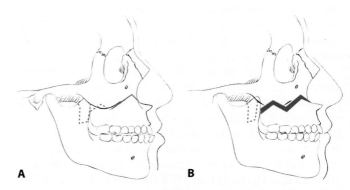

FIGURE 58-22. A Z-shaped osteotomy can be designed in the lateral walls of the pirifom rims and the buttresses **(A)** so that the maxilla may be moved downward and forward **(B)** without loss of all bony contact.

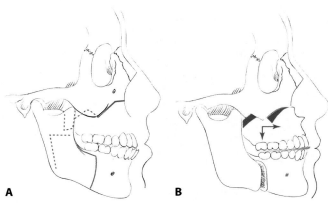

FIGURE 58-23.   A Z osteotomy with the posterior cut steeper than the anterior one to increase posterior facial height **(A)** and to rotate the maxilla downward and forward with adjustment to the occlusal plane **(B)**.

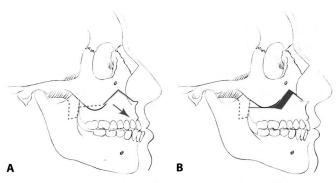

FIGURE 58-24.   A Z osteotomy with the posterior cut shallower than the anterior one to increase anterior facial height **(A)** and to rotate the maxilla down in the front and adjust the occlusal plane to a steeper angle **(B)**.

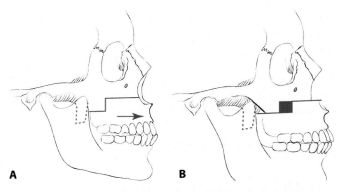

FIGURE 58-25.   An alternative method for advancement is to create a step **(A)** in the buttress and place a bone graft **(B)** in the step after repositioning.

(Figure 58-26) is planned for stability with a large maxillary advancement, the vertical steps in the osteotomy design, or Z osteotomies, can provide additional, and improved, sites for placement of the bone grafts. In many cases of AP maxillary deficiency, there is an additional component of

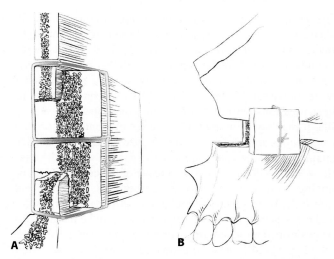

FIGURE 58-26.   **A,** A single hole is placed in the middle of the bone graft and a loop of 28-gauge stainless steel wire is placed through the hole from inside out. The two ends are divided, with one placed through the superior cranial base wall and the other through the inferior maxillary segment. Finally, one end is passed through the loop and twisted to the other, much like an Ivy loop. **B,** Bone graft shown in place.

midface, or malar, hypoplasia, and various osteotomy designs have been advocated to simultaneously attempt to advance the zygomatic bone and or infraorbital rim (e.g., high Le Fort I, or Le Fort II, or modified Le Fort III, zygoma osteotomies, zygomatic arch osteotomies, quadrangular osteotomies, or double-step osteotomies of the maxilla and infraorbital rim). Unfortunately, many of these techniques fail to improve the malar hypoplasia and result in a worsening of the facial profile, such that a "dish-face" deformity may result (Obwegeser). Perhaps the most predictable method by which to address malar hypoplasia is to consider prosthetic malar augmentation using stock or custom implants (e.g., high-molecular-weight porous polyethylene). This option may be used at the time of the Le Fort advancement surgery or in a delayed fashion to determine whether the maxillary surgery itself had a significant enough positive impact on the malar hypoplasia to result in the patient declining any future surgery for aesthetic reasons. These prosthetic implants may also be placed in the paranasal regions for augmentation in this area, if necessary. Finally, severe maxillary hypoplasia, due to a cleft lip and palate or other syndrome or etiology, may be managed with distraction osteogenesis, which is covered in Chapters 62 and 63.

Inferior Maxillary Repositioning

Inferior repositioning of the maxilla presents a unique challenge in orthognathic surgery owing to the increased relapse potential resulting from impingement of the maxilla on the pterygomandibular sling of the medial pterygoid and masseter muscles.[65–68] In the pre–rigid fixation era, various techniques were recommended for additional stabilization and fixation of the maxilla after inferior repositioning, including skeletal suspension wires (circumzygomatic, frontozygomatic suture, and piriform rim wiring), interosseous wires, Steinmann pins, Wessberg pins, and RAPs, until the introduction of rigid fixation plates and screws in the United States in the early 1980s.[32,60,63,69–71] Whereas bone grafting has been used for stabilization of the inferiorly repositioned maxilla, it may not be required if a series of slanted Z, or step, osteotomies are used[59,63,64,72] (see Figure 58-22). The specific angulations of these osteotomies are planned so that the maxilla will slide down the inclined plane of the cuts while maintaining bony contact as it is repositioned anteriorly and inferiorly. Based upon the inclination of the anterior portion and the posterior portion of the osteotomies, the maxilla may be positioned more anteriorly or more inferiorly (see Figures 58-22 to 58-24). Most surgeons use bone grafts and rigid fixation to stabilize the maxilla that has been inferiorly repositioned with a resultant lack of bone-to-bone contact. Bone grafts may be secured with bone screws or plates if sufficient bone is available, or with stainless steel wires (see Figure 58-26). Patients who are candidates for inferior maxillary repositioning often have paper-thin maxillary bone due to the vertical skeletal growth pattern or lack of occlusal forces. Although rigid internal fixation with plates and screws is the stabilization method of choice, occasionally insufficient bone is available adjacent to the osteotomy sites for plate placement, and in these cases, the RAP system can be a useful alternative.[63]

Posterior Maxillary Repositioning

Posteriorly repositioning, or setback, of the maxilla must be considered carefully because there will be a resultant loss of upper lip support as well as paranasal osseous support for the overlying soft tissues. At the pterygomaxillary disjunction of the Le Fort osteotomy, bone must be removed from either the pterygoid plates (with great caution) or the maxillary tuberosity, which extends into the alveolar process. An alternative technique is to intentionally direct the osteotomy through the maxillary tuberosity or alveolus just posterior to the second molar to ensure a predictable osteotomy and guide the position where bone will be removed.[73,74] Also, this technique will leave tuberosity bone attached to the pterygoid plates, which may then be more safely removed. A possible complication of this technique is damage to the greater palatine artery distal to its anastomosis with the lesser palatine vessel. Alternatively, maxillary horizontal excess may also be addressed with an anterior maxillary osteotomy, especially when extractions are planned, or if edentulous sites are present; this is discussed later in this chapter.

Rigid Internal Fixation for Maxillary Osteotomy

Rigid internal fixation with bone plates and screws is the current standard for maxillary stabilization after Le Fort surgery. Although this technique has eliminated many of the

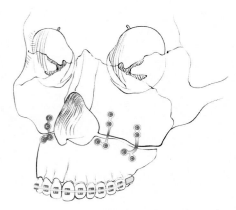

FIGURE 58-27. Bone plating encompasses a wide variety of plates and screws, ranging from very rigid to very malleable. Generally, 2.0-mm plates are used in the piriform rims and either 2.0- or 1.5-mm plates in the buttresses.

concerns with postoperative stability and relapse from wire fixation or no fixation, the technique is less forgiving than wire fixation and, therefore, precise intraoperative positioning is even more critical. A wide variety of plating systems and sizes are available, and there is no consensus on the number of plates and screws necessary or the thickness of the plates or diameter of the screws required for stable fixation. Typical midface plating sets have 1.5- and 2.0-mm plates and screws that work well for maxillary fixation, and most surgeons prefer to use four 2.0-mm plates in the pillar regions of the midface at the piriform rims and zygomaticomaxillary buttress regions (Figure 58-27). Preformed plates are available with specific bends for specific maxillary advancements, and computer planning may allow fabrication of customized fixation devices in the future. Whereas resorbable plates and screws are available for midface applications, most surgeons do not use these on a routine basis and reserve these for the pediatric age group, when indicated. The use of rigid internal fixation for maxillary surgery has also decreased the need for adjunctive bone grafting for large maxillary advancements and has essentially eliminated the need for skeletal suspension wiring techniques, because relapse is no longer a significant concern with the current fixation techniques.

SPECIFIC PROCEDURES

Anterior Maxillary Osteotomy

Numerous surgical techniques have been advocated to perform the anterior maxillary osteotomy, and the three main options involve the use of one of three vascular pedicles: labial (Figure 58-28), palatal (Figure 58-29), or a combination of these, with the use of vertical incisions in both (Figure 58-30). The anterior segmental maxillary osteotomy can be performed successfully and, when done properly with attention to detail and respect for the hard and soft tissues, generally has few complications. However, if there is compromise

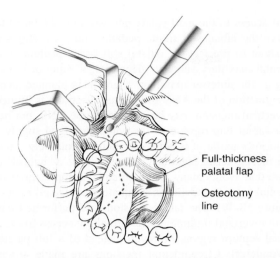

FIGURE 58-28.   Labial pedicle for anterior maxillary osteotomy; the palate is flapped open.

Full-thickness palatal flap

Osteotomy line

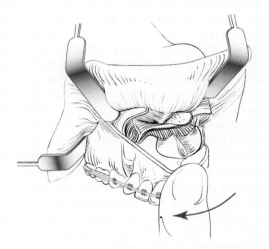

FIGURE 58-29.   Palatal pedicle for anterior maxillary osteotomy is created with a horizontal labial incision.

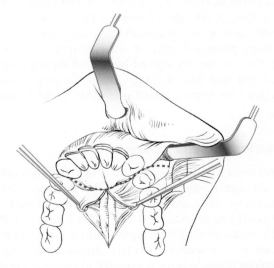

FIGURE 58-30.   A combination of labial and palatal pedicles can be used for an anterior maxillary osteotomy without extractions.

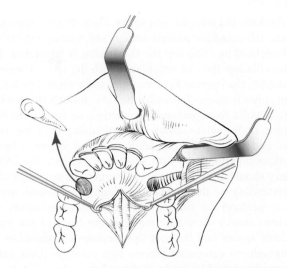

FIGURE 58-31.   A midline palatal incision can be used with caution to access the palate for interdental bone removal in closing large extraction spaces.

of the vascular pedicle to the anterior maxillary segment, the complications can range from minor periodontal defects, which can be devastating in the aesthetic zone, to loss of teeth, bone, or the entire anterior maxillary segment due to avascular necrosis. Anterior maxillary osteotomies are generally used to treat horizontal maxillary excess when the posterior occlusion is ideal or if the posterior occlusion can be corrected with mandibular surgery. Commonly, an anterior maxillary osteotomy, with simultaneous premolar extractions, is used for bimaxillary protrusion in which both the anterior maxilla and the anterior mandible require retraction (Figure 58-31). These procedures can also be used for correction of an anterior open bite occlusal relationship. On occasion, an anterior maxillary osteotomy may be combined with a mandibular advancement and anterior mandibular segmental osteotomy in cases planned for correction of a severe curve of Spee. The specific surgical sequence must be considered carefully when both jaws are involved because the surgical procedures must be done systematically so that the surgeon does not lose orientation. There are two possible scenarios: (1) the posterior occlusion will not change because the posterior maxillary and mandibular teeth will not be moved, or (2) mandibular surgery will be performed to correct the posterior occlusion. This a critical difference because, if the posterior occlusion is not going to be changed by surgery, the models must be mounted in centric occlusion, not centric relation, for model surgery. If the posterior occlusion will be altered by mandibular surgery, a new centric relation will be established by the surgery and model surgery can be done as usual. In the first scenario, the maxillary anterior model is cut and repositioned to the best relationship against the uncut mandible in centric occlusion and the remaining maxillary dentition, and then a splint is constructed. In the second scenario, if mandibular surgery is planned, two mandibular models are mounted, with one mandibular model cut, and the other left intact to preserve the intermediate phase

SECTION 7

and fabricate the intermediate splint. Then, the anterior maxilla and the mandible models are cut and repositioned to the final occlusal position and the final splint is fabricated. The cut maxilla can then be articulated with the uncut mandible to establish the intermediate position, and a second (intermediate) splint is made. Typically, the final splint will be wired to the maxilla for a postoperative period, so there must be a separate intermediate splint that articulates with the final splint and the mandibular teeth (a splint within a splint technique). Particularly with segmental surgery, the model surgery should simulate the actual surgery to provide a clear understanding of the three-dimensional movements necessary to perform the surgical procedure. Measurements and reference marks should be made at the level of the interproximal spaces and the root tips, perhaps correlated to the radiographs to determine precise root position. Also, reference marks should be made on the palate at the root tips and the maxillary midline. If maxillary widening is planned, transpalatal reference marks should also be used. The use of intermediate splints in segmental cases is different from total arch cases because the posterior maxilla is not mobilized and the anterior maxillary positioning is more difficult to determine precisely. For example, the anterior maxilla may fit into the splint and appear ideal until the mandible is rotated into occlusion, and if the mandible does not fit ideally, it is possible that the anterior maxilla can be rotated or tipped superiorly or inferiorly within the splint, and this must be adjusted before fixation. For this reason, the mandible should not be wired into MMF but left to freely rotate into the maxillary splint. Also, at surgery if the mandible is held into MMF during the fixation process for the anterior maxilla, it is possible for the condyles to be pulled out of the fossae resulting in an immediate postoperative malocclusion (anterior open bite). Therefore, the splint must be ligated to the posterior maxilla first, and then the anterior maxilla is brought into the splint and ligated. If the mandible rotates freely into the desired occlusion, the maxilla is in the correct position, and rigid fixation may be applied. Next, if mandibular surgery is planned, it may be initiated at this time.

In cases of segmental maxillary surgery, the choice of surgical technique depends upon surgical access to the areas that will be most difficult to visualize intraoperatively. For example, in the case of an anterior open bite in which no teeth are to be extracted, the anterior segment will be rotated clockwise and downward after the interdental osteotomies. Access to the interdental area, the midline of the palate, and the ANS is not as critical as it is with other surgical movements. This procedure can be done with a circumvestibular incision, or with bilateral horizontal incisions, in the canine-molar regions, and a vertical incision in the midline between the central incisors. Conversely, if first premolars have been extracted, or are planned to be extracted, and the anterior maxilla is planned for retraction, access to the midpalatal region is essential. The original description of the Wunderer technique, in which a transverse palatal incision allows the palatal soft tissues to be elevated posteriorly, provides excellent access to the hard palate but care must be taken to preserve the labial soft tissue pedicle, and most surgeons are hesitant to transect the palatal soft tissue pedicle with segmental maxillary surgery.[16] However, if superior repositioning of the anterior maxillary segment is planned, access to the junction of the ANS and the nasal septum is limited, and a vertical incision may be made over the ANS, but because this labial flap represents the complete blood supply to the anterior maxilla, it is not recommended routinely. An option for most anterior maxillary osteotomies is a "hybrid" procedure that avoids many of the potential complications of segmental surgery and allows adequate access to all regions (see Figure 58-30). The labial incisions are performed laterally, with a vertical midline incision to allow access to the ANS–nasal septum region, however, instead of a full palatal flap (Wunderer). Circumdental incisions are made around the necks of the teeth on either side of the interdental osteotomies with a midline incision over the midpalatal suture, with a small anterior Y incision, if necessary. This Y incision extension should be performed anterior to the interdental osteotomy cut and should be as conservative as possible.

Fixation techniques for anterior maxillary osteotomies are as varied as the surgical techniques themselves.[75] Orthodontic arch wires and cast splints represent the two extremes for fixation; however, orthodontic appliances are the simplest and easiest to use, at least as a part of the fixation scheme, and supplemental fixation may be required. An occlusal splint with a skeletal suspension wire from the ANS or piriform rim region is helpful in such cases, especially if there is any significant tension on the free maxillary segment. Interosseous wires or smaller profile plates and screws can be carefully used to fixate the segment, perhaps in the 1.0- to 1.5-mm range rather than 2.0-mm plates and screws used for standard Le Fort surgery. Although Erich arch bars have been used for additional fixation and in certain cases may be appropriate, a lower level of precision can be expected owing to torque of the maxillary segment from the circumdental wires. The most critical factor with segmental maxillary surgery is that, at the time of surgery, the anterior maxillary segment must be mobile enough that it does not require any significant pressure to place it in the desired final position. Then, fixation can be applied by one of the methods discussed that will hold the segment in the proper position throughout the healing period, and MMF is not commonly used.

Posterior Maxillary Osteotomy

The posterior maxillary osteotomy (PMO) and its modifications are rarely indicated today[17,20,76-81] because open bite correction or transverse maxillary expansion is performed more easily and predictably with Le Fort I surgery. PMO is usually indicated for preprosthetic reasons to correct hypereruption of a posterior maxillary dentoalveolar segment. Meticulous model surgery is essential to visualize the three-dimensional movements and anticipate osseous interferences

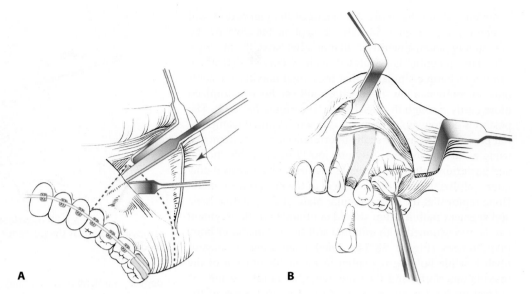

FIGURE 58-32. **A,** Posterior maxillary osteotomy. Horizontal vestibular incision with tunneling access to the interdental papilla. The *dashed line* marks horizontal and interdental osteotomies. **B,** An alternative soft tissue flap design can add a vertical releasing incision from the horizontal incision inferiorly through the gingiva at the mesial line angle of the canine tooth.

of the individual segments. Periapical radiographs are useful for evaluating interdental and subapical osteotomy sites. Once again, the dental models should be mounted on the articulator in the centric occlusion relationship, not centric relation, unless the mandible is also planned for surgery. In general, outpatient intravenous anesthesia with airway protection can be used for isolated posterior segmental procedures. A high palatal vault allows access to the palatal osteotomy via a transantral approach beneath the nasal floor. The soft tissue incision is made horizontally in the maxillary buccal vestibule from the anticipated anterior interdental osteotomy site to the second molar region (Figure 58-32A). A mucoperiosteal dissection beneath the superior aspect of the incision exposes the lateral maxilla, and the pterygomaxillary region is exposed via soft tissue retraction in a tunneling technique. At the anterior interdental osteotomy site, conservative tunneling of the periosteum exposes the full vertical extent of the dentoalveolar segments. After retraction

of the soft tissue with skin hooks and right-angle retractors, the facial interdental osteotomy may be outlined with a small fissure bur, or it can be completed directly with a thin cement-spatula osteotome. An alternative soft tissue flap design can add a vertical releasing incision from the horizontal incision inferiorly through the gingiva at the mesial line angle of the canine tooth (see Figure 58-32B). A horizontal osteotomy is performed approximately 5 mm above the roots of the teeth and joined with the anterior interdental osteotomy (see Figure 58-32A). The vertical interdental osteotomy should be completed first so that the segment is not mobile while using interdental osteotomes. The palatal osteotomy is accomplished with a small, sharp, curved osteotome directed at the junction of the vertical alveolus and the horizontal palatal shelf. The surgeon may place a finger on the palatal mucosa to detect complete osseous sectioning while minimizing palatal mucosal trauma (Figure 58-33A). In patients with a high palatal vault, the transantral osteotomy is

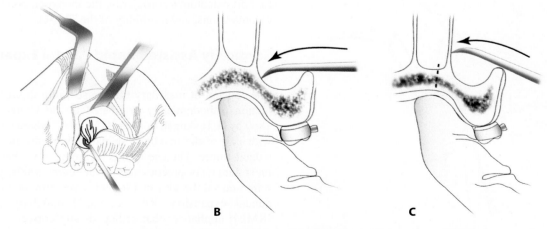

FIGURE 58-33. **A,** Transantral osteotomy is made at the junction of the horizontal palate and vertical alveolar process. **B,** Approach for deep vaulted palates. **C,** Approach for flat shallow palates.

completed along the entire AP extent of the planned palatal osteotomy (see Figure 58-33B), except in the area of the descending palatine neurovascular bundle. Next, the pterygomaxillary junction is separated with a curved osteotome using a technique similar to that for a total maxillary osteotomy. In contrast, a low, flat palatal vault can be osteotomized more easily through the nasal floor (see Figure 58-33C). The posterior dentoalveolar segment is down-fractured using digital pressure, and any osseous interferences may be removed using a bur or rongeurs. Any previously inaccessible medial and posterior walls of the mobile segment are addressed now after mobilization and displacement of the posterior segment. Bone removal at the perpendicular plate of the palatine bone and segment mobilization should continue until the segment can be repositioned with minimal soft tissue tension or bony interferences (Figure 58-34). Final contouring is accomplished while holding the splint in the stable portion of the maxilla anteriorly, and then the mandible is rotated into its correct occlusal position to ensure that no distortion of the splint has occurred. A splint modification should be considered that results is a slightly thicker splint with transpalatal acrylic or wire reinforcement that will add rigidity to prevent inadvertent distortion of the posterior extension of the splint and to support the osseous segments postsurgically. Once the segments are ligated to the splint, the repositioned posterior maxillary segment(s) may be fixated with interosseous wires, suspension wires, stable pin fixation, or bone plates and screws. Bone grafts are rarely required, and additional stability may be obtained by luting the orthodontic arch wire back together with quick-curing acrylic or by placing a new rectangular surgical arch wire across the interdental osteotomy site; MMF is usually not required. If the posterior segment is repositioned laterally or medially to a significant

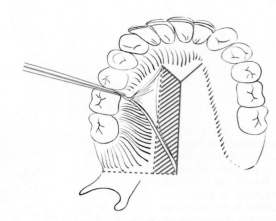

FIGURE 58-35. A midline palatal incision gives access for the removal of bone as the posterior maxillary segment is moved medially.

degree, additional access may be necessary; this can be performed via a midline palatal incision with palatal tissue reflection laterally (Figure 58-35). Meticulous surgical dissection can ensure maintenance of the integrity of the descending palatine vessels. This approach also provides access to the sinus and nasal cavity, especially if the palatal vault is high and the osteotomy is performed through the sinus as mentioned (see Figure 58-33B). If the alveolus is short and the palatal vault is flat or shallow, the osteotomy usually traverses the medial sinus wall and passes through the floor of the nose (see Figure 58-33C).

Total Maxillary Alveolar Osteotomy

The TMAO was designed to avoid some of the problems encountered with the Le Fort I down-fracture technique; however, the hypothesized advantages, including improved nasal airway, improved stability due to better bony contact, improved ability to widen the maxilla, and better maxillary perfusion, have not been realized clinically.[82–88] Throughout the past several decades, there has been very little need to consider this surgical option over the traditional standard Le Fort osteotomy, considering the increased potential risks, complications, and morbidity of the TMAO.

Surgically Assisted Rapid Palatal Expansion

History

The concept of maxillary transverse width discrepancy correction orthodontically originated in the United States in 1860 by G. H. Angell in *Dental Cosmos,*[89] where he described widening of the maxillary dental arch by opening the midpalatal suture. The use of this technique was abandoned by most American practitioners by the early 1900s, until Haas reintroduced the idea in 1961 with the introduction of rapid palatal expansion (RPE, or rapid maxillary expansion [RME]) appliances that orthopedically corrected maxillary arch width discrepancies.[90] In growing children, nonsurgical RPE resulted in fairly predictable opening of the midpalatal

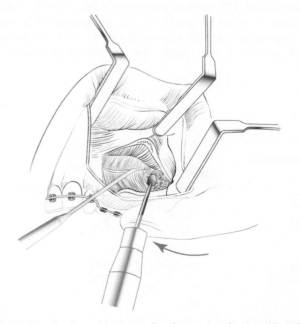

FIGURE 58-34. Bone is removed at the perpendicular plate of the palatine bone using a transantral approach.

suture with bony expansion, but in adults, the stability of RPE has been questioned and potentially results in dental tipping and periodontal defects rather than true bony expansion. Several authors including Timms and Moss[91] and Haas[90,92] have shown that orthodontic RPE results in alveolar bending, periodontal ligament compression, lateral tooth displacement, and tooth extrusion.[94] For these reasons, Haas advocated overexpansion to allow for some degree of relapse; however, even with 50% overexpansion, nonsurgical RPE has been associated with significant relapse and subsequent failure in the skeletally mature adult patient, although orthopedic RPE is relatively successful and stable in children and adolescents who have not yet experienced closure of the midpalatal suture. Although historically the midpalatal suture was thought to be the area of greatest resistance to expansion, Isaacson and Ingram[93] have shown that the major site of resistance to expansion is not the midpalatal suture, but all of the remaining maxillary articulations. Lines[94] and Bell and Epker[95] demonstrated that increased facial skeletal resistance to expansion was located at the zygomaticotemporal, zygomaticofrontal, and zygomaticomaxillary sutures, whereas Wertz[96] hypothesized that the resistance was attributable to the zygomatic arches. This controversy regarding the specific areas of resistance in the midfacial skeleton stimulated the development of a variety of maxillary osteotomy designs to expand the maxilla using orthodontic appliances. Lehman and coworkers[97] demonstrated that there was improved expansion with surgery and the use of an RPE orthopedic appliance. Kennedy and colleagues[98] reported a significant increase in the amount of lateral osseous movement possible in animals that underwent surgical osteotomies before orthodontic RPE. Whereas the results reported in the literature varied with the specific techniques used as well as the timing of orthopedic expansion device activation, the majority of studies show that surgically assisted rapid maxillary (or palatal) expansion (SARME or SARPE) is more stable than orthodontic expansion alone. SARPE is one of the earliest forms of distraction osteogenesis of the maxilla used to widen the maxilla in the transverse plane. The benefits of its use are gradual callous distraction that allows the soft tissues to accommodate to the bony movements thereby resulting in improved long-term stability. The role of surgery with RPE is to release the areas of resistance in the maxilla before orthopedic RPE. Whether transverse maxillary expansion will be performed alone or in conjunction with surgery will depend on the patient's age, the magnitude of expansion required (if > 5 mm is required, a SARPE may be indicated), and the condition of the midpalatal suture and will not be based solely upon the maxillomandibular relationship. Lines[95] found SARPE to be extremely valuable in young patients (growing children) exhibiting maxillary collapse, maxillary retrusion, and pseudo–class III malocclusions. When maxillary expansion and total maxillary osteotomy are required, two treatment regimens are possible: (1) SARPE followed by a one-piece maxillary osteotomy at a later date or (2) two-piece (or multiple-piece) maxillary osteotomy in

one procedure. Several factors must be considered when determining which method is preferable for each individual patient.

SARPE versus Multiple-Piece Maxillary Osteotomy

There is controversy regarding the relative risks and benefits of SARPE followed by Le Fort I in two procedures as opposed to a single-stage, multiple-piece maxillary osteotomy; of the many factors involved in each of these two approaches, only the issue of transverse stability has been studied extensively. The vast majority of the data supports the fact that the transverse stability of SARPE far exceeds multipiece osteotomy.[99–106] It should be mentioned that the poorest results reported for SARPE are nearly as unstable as those reported for multiple-piece maxillary surgery; however, the surgical technique is not described.[107] In general, a SARPE will increase total arch length, permitting extraction-free orthodontic leveling and aligning and allowing a greater degree of transverse expansion with lower morbidity than segmental maxillary surgery. It has been suggested that vertical and horizontal repositioning of the maxilla are better managed in a single-stage procedure with segmental maxillary surgery,[109] and although no data to substantiate or refute this suggestion have been offered, typically when SARPE is performed before orthodontic therapy, the maxillary arch can be leveled and aligned orthodontically, within the basal bone without extrusion of teeth, which is then followed by a one-piece maxillary osteotomy to correct any vertical and horizontal discrepancies. The main reasons for this preference is that segmental maxillary surgery has a much higher incidence of both minor and major complications than SARPE and one-piece maxillary surgery, and also segmental surgery often requires premolar extractions that add another surgical procedure and additional morbidity and potential complications.[52,110] In addition, surgical splints must be left in place postoperatively for several weeks after segmental maxillary surgery, thereby increasing postoperative discomfort and negatively affecting the performance of adequate oral hygiene. Finally, issues of cost, not only from a financial standpoint but also including time off from work or school as well as the psychological impact of surgery, must be taken into consideration.[109] Therefore, SARPE followed by Le Fort I single-piece osteotomy is used most often, and the use of multisegment maxillary surgery is reserved for two specific case scenarios. The first example involves cases in which there are different occlusal planes in the maxilla that are not amenable to correction solely with an SARPE and cannot be adequately addressed with orthodontic leveling and aligning within a reasonable time period. But, with SARPE, the creation of a large midline diastema between the maxillary central incisors and the two hemimaxillae allows considerable orthodontic leveling options without tooth extrusion so that these cases requiring segmental surgery to correct variable maxillary occlusal planes are not common. The second example requiring segmental surgery includes the patient who has undergone orthodontic therapy for months or years before referral for a surgical option and the dentition has reached a maximum limit of movement, possibly with root resorption, which would make a single-stage segmental maxillary procedure more desirable.

SARPE Technique

It should be mentioned that a variety of techniques exist for the SARPE procedure based upon where the surgeon and orthodontist believe that the major points of resistance to expansion exist. In addition, some limited osteotomy design SARPE surgeries may be performed in the outpatient setting using intravenous sedation, although if the SARPE is performed as a standard Le Fort I two-piece osteotomy without down-fracture, an operating room setting with endotracheal intubation may be preferred. A typical SARPE surgery begins with local anesthesia and bilateral mucoperiosteal incisions that extend from the piriform rim to zygomatic buttress region in the area of the maxillary first molar (Figure 58-36A). Bilateral osteotomies are then performed from the piriform rims to low in the pterygomaxillary junction (see Figure 58-36A). A simple linear AP osteotomy from the piriform rim to the pterygomaxillary junction is recommended for the SARPE.

More complicated designs[108,110,111] appear to offer advantages in theory and on paper but, in fact, are not clinically relevant when applied to the three-dimensional geometric structures such as the maxilla and the movements realized with the procedure. A sloped variation of the osteotomy of the lateral maxillary wall[110] is based upon the expectation that as the maxilla is expanded, it will "ride down" this slope laterally and inferiorly. This concept appears valid in a two-dimensional drawing; however, in three dimensions, if the osteotomy is flat from lateral to medial, as expansion occurs, the bone at the piriform region slides laterally over the flat surface lateral to it, and the bone in the buttress region slides laterally over the flat surface lateral to this area. Therefore, if the lateral maxillary wall cuts are straight and horizontal, perpendicular to the midsagittal plane, from lateral to medial, the angulation of the cut from anterior to posterior does not affect the vertical position of the segments as they are expanded. As a result, a standard horizontal osteotomy may be used for the SARPE procedure. Next, osteotomies are made in the anterior 1.5 cm of the lateral nasal walls, because this is the thickest portion of the anterior maxillary wall. Separation of the hemimaxillae is performed by driving a thin spatula osteotome between the central incisors in the

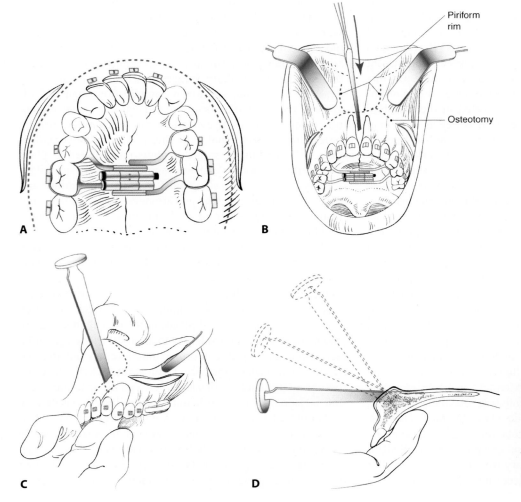

FIGURE 58-36. Surgically assisted rapid palatal expansion. **A,** Bilateral horizontal mucoperiosteal incisions are made, followed by bilateral osteotomies from the piriform rims to pterygomaxillary junctions. **B–D,** Division of the hemimaxillae is accomplished by inserting an osteotome in the midline.

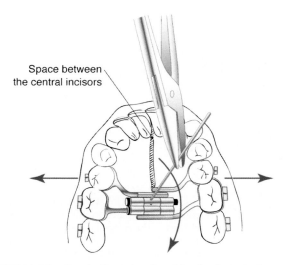

Space between the central incisors

FIGURE 58-37.   Surgically assisted rapid palatal expansion. Expansion device is turned to separate the hemimaxillae.

alveolus in the midline and parallel to the palate posteriorly for approximately 1 to 1.5 cm (see Figure 58-36B-D). The expansion device is turned three or four activations ($\frac{1}{4}$ mm each activation, although some devices are 0.2 mm/ activation) until separation is noted between the central incisor teeth (Figure 58-37). Both segments are mobilized until equal mobility is seen bilaterally in each hemimaxillary segment. Some authors recommend a subtotal Le Fort I osteotomy with a horizontal osteotomy, vertical midline osteotomy, and with pterygoid and nasal septal separation.[109,111] Shetty demonstrated with a photoelastic model that the midpalatal and pterygomaxillary articulations were the primary anatomic sites of resistance to expansion forces.[112] This study used only incomplete cuts of the lateral maxillary wall, from second bicuspid to second molar. It is unclear whether these findings would be as significant with complete cuts from the piriform to the pterygomaxillary fissure. Need for separation of the pterygomaxillary junction is, therefore, a subject of debate. Several studies have shown minimal relapse without pterygomaxillary disjunction and, therefore, do not advocate a pterygoid osteotomy for improved stability.[99,103] However, a reasonable argument for pterygomaxillary separation is that potential complications may be minimized because pterygoid separation will reduce forces transmitted to the skull base upon expansion.[111] Of course, additional sutural release will obviously contribute to improved segment mobility with an SARPE, and the potential morbidity, although significant, is typically uncommon. In addition, nasal septal separation from the nasal crest of the maxilla will avoid postoperative nasal septal deviation because the septum may remain attached to one of the two maxillary segments. Also, two sources of potential hemorrhage, via manipulation of the pterygomaxillary junction and separation of the nasal septum from the nasal crest of the maxilla, should be avoided if this procedure is performed as an office-based procedure or on an outpatient basis under intravenous sedation. Steroids are used routinely, but systemic antibiotics

are not necessary. As with distraction osteogenesis, a latency period after the SARPE procedure of approximately 5 days should be used to allow some soft tissue healing and the formation of a fibrovascular bridge to support future bone formation in the distraction gap. The activation period can begin after 5 days and the expansion appliance is activated, or turned with a special "key," according to specific instructions (usually a rate and rhythm of twice-daily activations of 0.25 mm each turn), until the desired expansion is achieved based upon the orthodontic requirements. After completion of the distraction phase, a consolidation period should be allowed for bony healing with the device locked in place to prevent counterclockwise rotation, using a stainless steel wire through the activation device or composite resin, or some other material, placed to prevent device deactivation. This is usually held in place for a period of 8 to 12 weeks after completion of bony movement. An alternative use of SARPE is unilateral SARPE that can be achieved by completing a vertical interdental osteotomy between the appropriate teeth and connecting that cut with a unilateral horizontal osteotomy extending posteriorly to the pterygomaxillary junction. If the entire hemimaxilla is planned to be mobilized, the surgical procedure is performed the same as described for a standard bilateral SARPE case, with the horizontal Le Fort osteotomy performed on one side only. If widening of an isolated portion of one posterior hemimaxilla is planned, the interdental osteotomy must be completed to the midline palatal suture (Figure 58-38). The posterior maxillary segment is mobilized (Figure 58-39A) and expanded in the same manner as for the bilateral SARPE procedure (see Figure 58-39B). The long-term effects on nasal airway resistance after the SARPE procedure are unknown, although some studies have shown increased nasal airflow whereas others have not shown changes in nasal airflow in long-term follow-up.[113,114]

Zygomatic Osteotomy and Modified Le Fort Osteotomies

As discussed in the section on anterior maxillary repositioning, patients with severe midface deficiency may benefit from enhancement of the prominence of the zygoma region. From an aesthetic standpoint, prominent malar prominences are desirable, and with a growing public awareness of surgical capabilities, there is an increased demand for cosmetic procedures designed to enhance this region of the face. Numerous methods have been developed to augment the malar eminences and the paranasal regions, mostly using bone grafts or synthetic implants. Autologous grafts, from the ramus, chin, or coronoid process, are disappointing because of resorption and the donor site morbidity. Allogeneic transplants such as lyophilized cartilage have been used with some success but are prone to migration, inflammation, and resorption. At the present time, the preferred method for malar augmentation is the use of alloplastic implants, most commonly with high-molecular-weight porous polyethylene

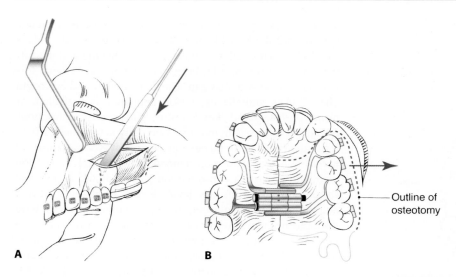

A   **B**

Outline of osteotomy

FIGURE 58-38.   Unilateral surgically assisted rapid palatal expansion. **A,** The osteotomy is driven to the midpalatal suture. **B,** The horizontal osteotomy is completed in the same manner as the bilateral osteotomy.

or silicone. If alloplasts are contraindicated or declined by the patient, the zygomatic osteotomy may be a useful alternative. The zygomatic osteotomy is approached through an intraoral incision, and a reciprocating saw is used to create a parasagittal osteotomy through the zygoma immediately adjacent to the root of the zygoma (Figure 58-40A and B). This is performed as close to the lateral orbital rim as possible, and the zygoma is out-fractured gently so that an inter-

positional material can be placed in the gap to hold the zygoma in a lateral position. The interpositional material (bone graft or synthetic implant) can be stabilized in a traditional fashion in this area. This technique provides lateral zygomatic projection, but it does not provide anterior projection, unless the interpositional material is fashioned in such a way as to project the zygoma in a forward position (see Figure 58-40C).

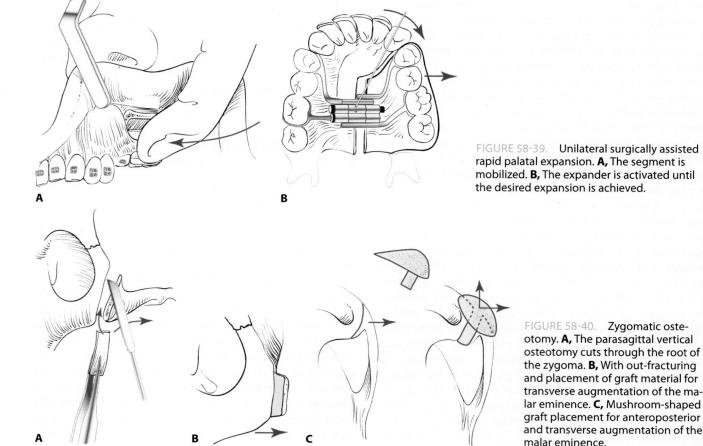

A   **B**

FIGURE 58-39.   Unilateral surgically assisted rapid palatal expansion. **A,** The segment is mobilized. **B,** The expander is activated until the desired expansion is achieved.

A   **B**   **C**

FIGURE 58-40.   Zygomatic osteotomy. **A,** The parasagittal vertical osteotomy cuts through the root of the zygoma. **B,** With out-fracturing and placement of graft material for transverse augmentation of the malar eminence. **C,** Mushroom-shaped graft placement for anteroposterior and transverse augmentation of the malar eminence.

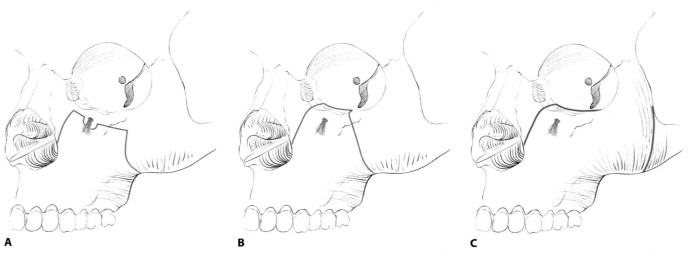

FIGURE 58-41. Modified Le Fort I osteotomy. **A,** High Le Fort I below the infraorbital rims. **B,** Quadrangular Le Fort I extending into the orbital floor. **C,** Quadrangular Le Fort I including the lateral orbital rim and zygoma.

The wide range and variety of maxillary osteotomies that represent modifications of the traditional Le Fort I procedure have been referred to by many terms including the *modified Le Fort I, II, III, high Le Fort I, pyramidal, middle, intermediary, quadrangular,* and *maxillary-malar-infraorbital osteotomies* (Figure 58-41). These techniques or modifications to these procedures have been described previously[115]; however, this group of maxillary osteotomies is limited clinically with regards to their use for maxillary expansion, rotation, and torque, or yaw, movements. Therefore, with the clinical successes of silicone and porous polyethylene and other synthetic implants to the malar, infraorbital, lateral orbital, and paranasal regions, these more invasive and potentially hazardous osteotomy designs are rarely used clinically (Figure 58-42).

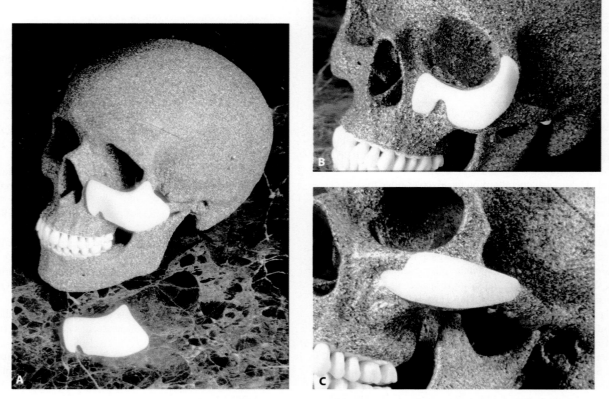

FIGURE 58-42. Porous polyethylene implants. **A,** Infraorbital augmentation with the zygoma. **B,** Infraorbital augmentation with the zygoma and lateral orbital rim. **C,** Zygoma augmentation.

References

1. Langenbeck B. Beitrange zur Osteoplastik—Die osteoplastiche Resektion des Oberkierers. Deutsche Klinik. G oschen A (Hrsg) A, editor. Berlin: Reimer; 1859.

2. Cheever D. Naso-pharyngeal polpus, attached to the basilar process of occipital and body of the sphenoid bone successfully removed by a section, displacement, and subsequent replacement and reunion of the superior maxillary bone. Boston Med Surg 1867;8:162.

3. Le Fort R. Fractures de la machoire superieure. Rev Chir 1901; 4:360.

4. Wassmund M. Frakturen und Lurationen des Gesichtsschadels. Leipzig Meusser Verlag: 1927.

5. Axhauser G. Zur Behandlung veralteter desloziert verheilter Oberkieferbrunche. Dtsch Zahn Mund Kieferheilkd 1934; I:334.

6. Schuchardt D. Ein Beitrag zur chirurgeschen Kieferorthopadie unter Berucksichtigung ihrer Bedertung fur die Behandlung angeborener und erworbener Kieferdeformitaten bei Soldaten. Dtsch Zahn Mund Kieferheilkd 1942;9:73.

7. Moore F, Ward F. Complications and sequelae of untreated fractures of the facial bones and their treatment. Plast Surg 1949;1:262.

8. Willmar K. On Le Fort I osteotomy: a follow-up study of 106 operated patients with maxillofacial deformity. Scand J Plast Reconstr Surg 1974;12(Suppl):1–68.

9. Obwegeser H. Eingriffe an Oberkiefer zur Korrektur des progenen. Zahnbheilk 1965;75:356.

10. Hogeman K, Willmar K. Die Vorverlagerung des Oberkiefers zur Korrektur von Gebisanomalien. Fortschr Kiefer Gesichtschir 1967;12:275–8

11. Perko M. Maxillary sinus and surgical movement of the maxilla. Int J Oral Surg 1972;1:177–184.

12. Cohn-Stock G. Die Chirugische-Immediatre-Julierung der Kiefer speziell die Chirurgische Behandlung der Prognathie. Vjischr Zahnheilk (Berlin) 1921;37:320.

13. Spanier F. Prognathie-Operationen Z zahnarytl. Orthop Munchen 1932;24:76.

14. Cupar I. Die Chirurgische Behandlung der Formund Stellungsveranderungen des Oberkiefers. Ost Z Stomat 1954;51:565.

15. Cupar I. Die Chirurgische Behandlung def Formund Stellungsveranderungen des Oberkiefers. Buss Sc Cons Acad RPF Yougosl 1955;2:60.

16. Kole H. Surgical operations on the alveolar ridge to correct occlusal abnormalities. Oral Surg 1959;12:277.

17. Wunderer S. Erfahrungen mit der operatiren Behandlung hochgradiger Prognathien. Dtsch Zahn Mund Kieferheilkd 1963;39:451.

18. Schuchardt K. Experiences with surgical treatment of some deformities of the jaws: Prognathia, micrognathia and open bite. In Wallace AG, editor. Transactions of Second Congress of International Society of Plastic Surgeons. Edinburgh. E & S Livingstone; 1961:73–78.

19. Kufner J. Experience with a modified procedure for correction of open bite. In Walker, RV, editor. Transactions of the Third Interantional Congerence on Oral Surgery. Vol. 18. London: E & S Livingstone; 1970:18–23.

20. West R, McNeill R. Maxillary alveolar hyperplasia, diagnosis and treatment planning. J Maxillofac Surg 1975;3:239–350.

21. Bell WH. Correction of skeletal type anterior open bite. J Oral Surg 1971;29:706–714.

22. Converse J, Shapiro H. Treatment of developmental malformation of the jaws. Plast Reconstr Surg 1952;10:473.

23. Kole H. Kieferorthopadie. In Reischenback K., Brueckel K, editors. Chir. Leipzig: Barth; 1965.

24. Bell WH, et al. Bone healing and revascularization after total maxillary osteotomy. J Oral Surg 1975;33:253–260.

25. Gillies J, Rowe N. L'osteotomie du maxillaire superieur envisagee essentiellement dans les cas de bec-de-lievre totale. Rev Stomat 1954;55:545.

26. Obwegeser H. Surgical correction of small or retrodisplaced maxillae. The "dish-face" deformity. Plast Reconstr Surg 1969;43:351–365.

27. Michelet FX, Deymes J, Dessus B. Osteosynthesis with miniaturized screwed plates in maxillofacial surgery. J Maxillofac Surg 1973;1:79–84.

28. Horster W. Experience with functionally stable plate osteosynthesis after forward displacement of the upper jaw. J Maxillofac Surg 1980;8:176–181.

29. Drommer R, Luhr HG. The stabilization of osteotomized maxillary segments with Luhr mini-plates in secondary cleft surgery. J Oral Maxillofac Surg 1981;9:166–169.

30. Luyk NH, Ward-Booth RP. The stability of Le Fort I advancement osteotomies using bone plates without bone grafts. J Maxillofac Surg 1985;13:250–253.

31. Edwards RC, Kiely KD. Resorbable fixation of Le Fort I osteotomies. J Craniofac Surg 1998;9:210–214.

32. Bays RA. Rigid stabilization system for maxillary osteotomies. Oral Maxillofac Surg 1985;43:60–63.

33. Stringer DE, Boyne PJ. Modification of the maxillary step osteotomy and stabilization with titanium mesh. J Oral Maxillofac Surg 1986;44:487–488.

34. Olson R, Laskin D. Expectations of patients from orthognathic surgery. J Oral Surg 1980;38:283–285.

35. Schaeffer J., The sinus maxillaires and its relations in the embryo, child and adult man. Anat 1910;10:313.

36. Klaff D. The surgical anatomy of the antero caudal portion of the nasal septum: a study of the area of the premaxilla. Laryngoscope 1956;66: 995.

37. Cottle M, et al. The maxilla-premaxilla approach to extensive nasal septum surgery. Arch Otolaryngol 1958;68:301.

38. Hollinshead WH. The Palate. In Anatomy for Surgeons. The Head and Neck. 3rd ed. Philadelphia: J.B. Lippincott; 1982; pp 331–345

39. Hollinshead WH. The Facial Muscles. In Anatomy for Surgeons. The Head and Neck. 3rd ed. Philadelphia: J.B. Lippincott; 1982; pp 292–300

40. Sewall E. Surgical removal of the sphenopalatine ganglien. Ann Otol Rhinol Laryngol 1937;46:79.

41. Bell WH. Le Forte I osteotomy for correction of maxillary deformities. J Oral Surg 1975;33:412–426.

42. Bell W. Revascularization and bone healing after anterior maxillary osteotomy: a study using adult rhesus monkeys. Oral Surg 1960;27:249.

43. Siebert JW, et al. Blood supply of the Le Fort I maxillary segment: an anatomic study. Plast Reconstr Surg 1997;100:843–851.

44. Brusati R, Bottoli V. Maxillary anterior segmental osteotomy, experimental research on vascular supply of osteotomized segments. Fortschr Kiefer Gesichts Chir 1974;18: 90–93.

45. Nelson R, et al. Quantitation of blood flow after Le Fort I osteotomy. J Oral Surg 1977;35:10–16.

46. Nelson R, et al. Quantitation of blood flow after anterior maxillary osteotmy: investigation of three surgical approaches. J Oral Surg 1978;36:106–111.
47. Lightoller G. Facial muscles. Anat (Lond) 1925;60:1.
48. Nairn R. The circumoral musculature: structure and function. Br Dent J 1975;138:49–56.
49. Robinson P, Hendy C. Pterygoid plate fracture caused by the Le Fort I osteotomy. Br J Oral Maxillofac Surg 1986;24:198–202.
50. Lanigan DT, West RA. Management of postoperative hemorrhage following Le Fort I maxillary osteotomy. J Oral Maxillofac Surg 1984;42:367–375.
51. Lanegan D, West R. Management of postoperative hemorrhage following Le Fort I maxillary osteotomy. Oral Maxillofac Surg 1984;42:367.
52. Hemmig S, Johnson R., Ferraro N. Mangement of a ruptured pseudoaneurysm of the sphenopalatine artery following a Le Fort I osteotomy. J Oral Maxillofac Surg 1987;45:533–536.
53. Solomons N, Blumgart R. Severe late-onset epistaxis following Le Fort I osteotmy: angiographic localization and embolization. Laryngol Otol 1988;102:260–263.
54. Newhouse R, et al. Life threatening hemorrhage from a Le Fort I osteotomy. J Oral Maxillofac Surg 1982;40:117–119.
55. Dodson TB, Bays RA, Neuenschwander MC. Maxillary perfusion during Le Fort I osteotomy after ligation of the descending palatine artery.[comment]. J Oral Maxillofac Surg 1997;55:51–55.
56. Bouloux GF, Bays RA. Neurosensory recovery after ligation of the descending palatine neurovascular bundle during Le Fort I osteotomy. J Oral Maxillofac Surg 2000;58:841–845; discussion 846.
57. Bell WH, Profitt WP. Maxillary excess. In Bell WH, Proffitt WP, White RP Jr, editors. Surgical Correction of Dentofacial Deformities. Philadelphia: WB Saunders; 1980; pp. 234–441.
58. Lanigan DT, Hey JH, West RA. Aseptic necrosis following maxillary osteotomies: report of 36 cases. J Oral Maxillofac Surg 1990;48:142–156.
59. Reyneke JP, Masureik C. Treatment of maxillary deficiency by a Le Fort I downsliding techniques. J Oral Maxillofac Surg 1985;43:914–916.
60. Bennett MA, Wolford LM. The maxillary step osteotomy and Steinmann pin stabilization. J Oral Maxillofac Surg 1985;43:307–311.
61. Kaminishi RM, et al. Improved maxillary stability with modified Le Fort I technique. J Oral Maxillofac Surg 1983;41:203–205.
62. Stringer DE, Boyne PJ. Modification of the maxillary step osteotomy and stabilization with titanium mesh. J Oral Maxillofac Surg 1986;44:487–488.
63. Bays RA. Maxillary osteotmies utilizing the rigid adjustable pin (RAP) system: a review of 31 clinical cases. Adult Orthod Orthogn Surg 1986;1:275–297.
64. Wagner S, Reyneke JP. The Le Fort I downsliding osteotomy: a study of long-term hard tissue stability. Int J Adult Orthod Orthogn Surg 2000;15:37–49.
65. Hedemark A, Freihofer HP Jr. The behaviour of the maxilla in vertical movements after Le Fort I osteotomy. J Maxillofac Surg 1978;6:244–249.
66. Epker BN, Fish LC, Paulus PJ. The surgical-orthodontic correction of maxillary deficiency. Oral Surg Oral Med Oral Pathol 1978;46:171–205.
67. Wolford L, Epker B. The surgical orthodontic correction of vertical dentofacial deformities. J Oral Surg 1981;39:883–897.
68. Freihofer HP Jr. Results of osteotomies of the facial skeleton in adolescence. J Maxillofac Surg 1977;5:267–297.
69. Bell WH, Jacobs J, Quejada J. Simultaneous repositioning of the maxilla, mandible, and chin. Treatment planning and analysis of soft tissues. Am J Orthod 1986;89:28–50.
70. Persson G, Hellem S, Nord P. Bone plates for stabilizing Le Fort I osteotomies. Maxillofac Surg 1986;14: 69.
71. Wessberg G, Epker BN. Intraoral skeletal fixation appliance. J Oral Maxillofac Surg 1982;40:827–829.
72. Junger TH, Krenkel C, Howaldt HP. Le Fort I sliding osteotomy— a procedure for stable inferior repositioning of the maxilla. J Craniomaxillofac Surg 2003;31:92–96.
73. Dupont C, Ciaburro T, Prevost Y. Simplifying the Le Fort I type of maxillary osteotomy. Plast Reconstr Surg 1974;54:142–147.
74. Trimble L, Tideman H, Stoelinga PJ. A modification of the pterygoid plate separation in low-level maxillary osteotomies. J Oral Maxillofac Surg 1983;41:544–546.
75. Bays RA, Fonseca RJ, Turvey TA. Single arch stabilization devices for segmental orthognathic surgery. Oral Surg 1978; 46:467–476.
76. West R, Epker BN. Posterior maxillary surgery: its place in treatment of dentofacial deformities. J Oral Surg 1972;30:562–563.
77. Sailer HF. [Routine methods in orthodontic surgery] (French). Rev Orthop Dento-Fac 1982;16:307–326.
78. Merville L, Princ G. Postero-lateral expansion osteotomy of maxilla. A case report. J Craniomaxillofac Surg 1987;15:20–23.
79. Bell WH, Turvey TA. Surgical correction of posterior crossbite. J Oral Surg 1974;32:811–812.
80. Perko M. [Late surgical correction of tooth malpositions and jaw abnormalities in patients with clefts] (German). Schweiz Monatsschr Zahnheilk 1969;79:179–213.
81. Moloney F, S toelinga. PJ, and Tedeman H, The posterior segmental maxillary osteotomy: recent applications. Oral Maxillofac Surg 1984;42:771.
82. Wolford L, Epker BN. The combined anterior and posterior maxillary ostectomy: a new technique. J Oral Surg 1975;33:842–851.
83. Hooley JR, West RA. Vertical repositioning of total maxillary alveolus to compensate for "short upper lip" [abstract]. Second Congress Europe an [European] Association for Maxillofacial Surgery. Zurich, Sept 16–24:1974.
84. Guenthner T, Sather AH, Kern E. The effect of Le Fort I maxillary impaction on nasal airway resistance. Am J Orthod 1984;85:308–315.
85. Turvey TA, Hall DJ, Warren DW. Alterations in nasal airway resistance following superior repositioning of the maxilla. Am J Orthod 1984;85:109–114.
86. Warren DW. A quanitative technique for assessing nasal airway impairment. Am J Orthod 1984;86:306–314.
87. Walker D, Turvey TA, Warren DW., Alterations in nasal respiration and nasal airway size following superior repositioning of the maxilla. J Oral Maxillofac Surg 1988;46:276–281.
88. Maloney F, West R, McNeil R. Surgical correction of the vertical maxillary excess: A re-evaluation. Maxillofac Surg 1982;10:84.
89. Angell E. Treatment of irregulariteis of the permanent adult tooth. Dent Cosmos 1860;1:540.
90. Haas A. Rapid expansion of the maxillary dental arch and nasal cavity by opening the mid palatal structure. Angle Orthod 1961;31:73.
91. Timms D, Moss JP. An histological investigation into the effects of rapid maxillary expansion on the teeth and their supporting tissues. Trans Eur Orthod Soc 1971:263–271.

92. Haas A. Long-term postreatment evaluation of rapid palate expansion. Angle Orthod 1980;50:189–217.

93. Isaacson R, Ingram A. Forces produced by rapid maxillary expansion: forces present during treatment. Angle Orthod 1964;34:256.

94. Lines P. Adult rapid maxillary expansion with corticotomy. Am J Orthod 1975;67:44–56.

95. Bell WH, Epker BN. Surgical-orthodontic expansion of the maxilla. Am J Orthod 1976;70:517–528.

96. Wertz R. Skeletal and dental changes accompanying rapid midpalatal suture opening. Am J Orthod 1970;58:41–66.

97. Lehman JA Jr, Haas AJ, Haas DG. Surgical correction of transverse maxillary deficiency: a simplified approach. Plast Reconstr Surg 1984;73:62–68.

98. Kennedy JW 3rd, et al. Ostectomy as an adjunct to rapid maxillary expansion. Am J Orthod 1976;70:123–137.

99. Bays RA, Greco JM. Surgically assisted rapid palatal expansion: an outpatient technique with long-term stability. J Oral Maxillofac Surg 1992;50:110–113; discussion 114–115.

100. Pogrel MA, et al. Surgically assisted rapid maxillary expansion in adults. Int J Adult Orthod Orthogn Surg 1992;7: 37–41.

101. Phillips C, et al. Stability of surgical maxillary expansion. Intl J Adult Orthod Orthogn Surg 1992;7:139–146.

102. Suri L, Taneja P. Surgically assisted rapid palatal expansion: a literature review. Am J Orthod Dentofacial Orthop 2008;133:290–302.

103. Marin C, Gil JN, Lima SM Jr. Surgically assisted palatine expansion in adult patients: evaluation of a conservative technique. J Oral Maxillofac Surg 2009;67:1274–1279.

104. Proffit WR, Turvey TA, Phillips C. Orthognathic surgery: a hierarchy of stability. Int J Adult Orthod Orthogn Surg 1996;11:191–204.

105. Stromberg C, Holm J. Surgically assisted, rapid maxillary expansion in adults. A retrospective long-term follow-up study. J Craniomaxillofac Surg 1995;23:222–227.

106. Lagravere MO, Major PW, Flores-Mir C. Dental and skeletal changes following surgically assisted rapid maxillary expansion. Int J Oral Maxillofac Surg 2006;35:481–487.

107. Chamberland S, Proffit WR. Closer look at the stability of surgically assisted rapid palatal expansion. J Oral Maxillofac Surg 2008;66:1895–1900.

108. Vandersea BA, Ruvo AT, Frost DE. Maxillary transverse deficiency—surgical alternatives to management. Oral Maxillofac Surg Clin North Am 2007;19:351–368, vi.

109. Betts NJ, et al. Diagnosis and treatment of transverse maxillary deficiency. Int J Adult Orthod Orthogn Surg 1995;10:75–96.

110. Turvey TA, Schardt-Sacco D. Lefort I Osteotomy. In Fonseca R, editor. Oral and Maxillofacial Surgery. Philadelphia: WB Saunders; 2000; pp. 232–238.

111. Lanigan DT, Mintz SM. Complications of surgically assisted rapid palatal expansion: review of the literature and report of a case. J Oral Maxillofac Surg 2002;60:104–110.

112. Shetty V, et al. Biomechanical rationale for surgical-orthodontic expansion of the adult maxilla. J Oral Maxillofac Surg 1994;52:742–749; discussion 750–751.

113. Babacan H, et al, Rapid maxillary expansion and surgically assisted rapid maxillary expansion effects on nasal volume. Angle Orthod 2006;76:66–71.

114. Berretin-Felix G, et al. Short- and long-term effect of surgically assisted maxillary expansion on nasal airway size. J Craniofac Surg 2006;17:1045–1049.

115. Bays RA, Timmis DP, Hegtvedt AK. Maxillary orthognathic surgery. In Peterson LJ, et al, editors. Principles of Oral and Maxillofacial Surgery. Philadelphia: JB Lippincott; 1992; pp. 1349–1414.

59

Facial Asymmetry

Peter D. Waite, MPH, DDS, MD, and Scott D. Urban, DMD, MD

Facial asymmetries comprise a heterogeneous group of craniofacial disorders charcterized by significant alterations in dental relationships as well as facial form that are readily apparent even to the untrained individual, and these present significant psychosocial issues for patients and families. During the 1960s, surgical treatment of orthognathic deformities developed when satisfactory results were not attainable with orthodontic therapy alone. On occasion, mild cases of jaw deformities and dental malocclusions may be camouflaged by dental treatment and growth modification.[1] In contrast, severe skeletal malocclusions are often beyond the envelope of discrepancy for orthodontic treatment and growth modification; therefore, a variety of surgical procedures of the maxilla and mandible have been developed. Some severe malocclusions are beyond the scope of orthodontic therapy alone, and some orthognathic deformities are beyond single-jaw surgery. Although a one-jaw osteotomy might improve function and aesthetics, bimaxillary, two-jaw, or double-jaw, surgery is often indicated for larger-magnitude anteroposterior (AP) discrepancies, most open bite deformities, and most cases of skeletal asymmetries.[2-5] With refinements in orthognathic surgery, it has become clear that some skeletal problems are beyond the envelope of one-jaw surgery, and although the novice might assume that one-jaw surgery is indicated owing to simplicity, the final functional and aesthetic outcome is often compromised and the bony movements are unstable. In general, two-jaw surgery allows a much greater degree of flexibility with regards to a three-dimensional approach to treatment of facial asymmetries.

In the 1960s and 1970s, surgeons attempted to limit orthognathic surgery to one jaw, usually the mandible, for fear of vascular compromise with maxillary osteotomies. Mandibular ramus osteotomies performed in conjunction with maxillary osteotomies were complex, technically difficult, time-consuming, and unstable procedures and were associated with higher patient morbidity.[6] It is difficult to correct a maxillary occlusal cant in the nongrowing patient without adjustment of the mandibular plane of occlusion. Similarly, midline discrepancies resulting from unilateral tooth loss are more rapidly corrected by mild asymmetrical rotational changes in the maxilla and/or mandible rather than with a prolonged course of orthodontics with possible gingival and periodontal problems.

This chapter focuses on the unique characteristics of asymmetrical orthognathic deformities as an indication for two-jaw surgery. The most important concept to understand about bimaxillary surgery is not the ability to perform simultaneous maxillary and mandibular procedures but to know the indications for surgery as well as the sequential treatment plan and also how to maintain a stable reference during complex asymmetrical bimaxllary surgery. Although little information is available on orthognathic asymmetry as an indication for bimaxillary surgery, it is well recognized that an inappropriate diagnosis, inaccurate treatment planning, and lack of intraoperative surgical reference points and planes are common errors in the approach to these patients. Skeletal asymmetries require three-dimensional bony and soft tissue changes with complex skeletal movements that result in aesthetic facial changes, and facial symmetry has a high degree of correlation with perceived facial attractiveness. Even mild facial asymmetries may be easily perceived by the untrained individual, and higher degrees of asymmetry are correlated with clinical depression, neurosis, feelings of inferiority, poor self-esteem, and general poor quality of life health-related problems.[7]

ETIOLOGY OF FACIAL ASYMMETRY

Although there are multiple potential causes of facial asymmetry, the differential diagnosis can be grouped into three general classes: congenital, developmental, and acquired deformities.[8,9] *Congenital* anomalies are conditions acquired during in utero development and can be further subdivided into malformations, deformities, and disruptions. Malformations are the result of an intrinsically abnormal developmental process during embryogenesis. For example, unilateral cleft lip is a type of malformation.[9] Deformities represent an abnormal form, or position, of a part of the body caused by a nondisruptive mechanical force applied during the fetal period.[9] Mandibular deformation may result from a prolonged, acute lateral flexion position of the head, with the shoulder pressed against the mandible, during late intrauterine growth. Lastly, disruptions are morphologic defects resulting from a breakdown of an otherwise normal developmental process.[9] Examples of disrution are facial clefting and limb amputation from in utero formation of amniotic banding.[9] *Developmental* anomalies are conditions arising during postuterine growth through adulthood, and *acquired* anomalies are clinicial conditions arising from either traumatic injuries or pathologic lesions. Finally, the etiology of facial asymmetry may be idiopathic without any identifiable cause.

CONGENITAL ANOMALIES

Hemifacial Microsomia

Hemifacial microsomia (HFM) is a craniofacial malformation resulting from defects in the first and second branchial arches that presents with asymmetrical unilateral, or bilateral, hypoplasia of the orbit(s), maxilla, mandible, ear, cranial nerves, and facial soft tissues (Figure 59-1).[10] Current

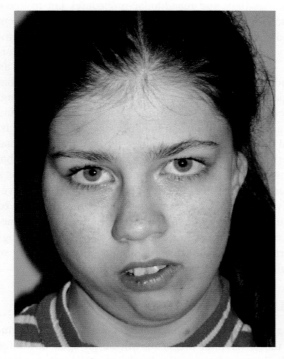

FIGURE 59-1. A 16-year-old with hemifacial microsomia (HFM) type I, with maxillary cant, dental midline deviation, and facial asymmetry.

evidence supports the theory that HFM results from a defect in the proliferation and migration of embryonic neural crest cells,[11,12] whereas another theory maintains that hemorrhage, or thrombosis, of the stapedial artery during fetal development leads to impaired unilateral facial growth.[13,14] In fact, the exact etiologic factors involved in the development of HFM still remain unknown.

Two important factors need to be considered in the treatment planning of the patient with HFM: (1) the facial growth potential and magnitude of growth restriction and the effect on surrounding hard and soft tissue structures and (2) the degree of hypoplasia of the glenoid fossa, mandibular condyle, and ramus unit.[15,16] Appropriate classification of the extent of the HFM deformity can provide useful information in order to determine an accurate diagnosis and ideal reconstruction options and a valid estimation of prognosis. The Pruzansky classification of HFM,[17] modified by Kaban and coworkers,[18] currently provides a clinically useful framework to help guide the treatment plan, based upon the presence or absence of critical structures of the condyle-fossa-ramus complex.[18,19] HFM type I deformity can be summarized as a generalized mild hypoplastic state involving the muscles of mastication, the glenoid fossa, and the mandibular condyle and ramus unit. The temporomandibular joint (TMJ) functions with normal rotation but restricted translation movements. Patients typically present with mild mandibular retrognathia and facial asymmetry. Because there is acceptable TMJ function and mild facial dysmorphology, surgical therapy is usually not indicated. HFM type IIA deformity involves a hypoplastic cone-shaped condylar head that is located medial and anterior to a hypoplastic glenoid fossa. TMJ function is often satisfactory so, again, surgical intervention is usually not indicated. HFM type IIB deformity involves a moderate to severe hypoplasia of the glenoid fossa, condyle, and mandibular ramus. Unlike the type IIA deformity, these patients have no functional articulation between the temporal bone and the condyle. However, manual jaw manipulation usually reveals a posterior stop of the condyle when placed in contact with posterior slope of the glenoid fossa.[20] HFM type III has a complete absence of the mandibular ramus and condyle. No manual condylar seating or posterior stop is achievable with jaw mamipulation. In contrast to types I and II, type III patients present with severe mandibular dysmorphology and often require surgical reconstruction of the fossa-condyle-ramus complex (Figure 59-2).[20]

The treatment protocols for HFM remain an area of controversy. The treatment philosophy of using interceptive orthodontic therapy, combined with early surgical treatment in growing children, is based upon the hypothesis that HFM is a progressive deformity and that early treatment can positively affect future facial growth.[15] Alternatively, a treatment protocol based upon the theory that HFM is not progressive in nature has been well described by Posnick,[16] and with this philosophy, treatment is considered primarily later in life during the adolescent period.

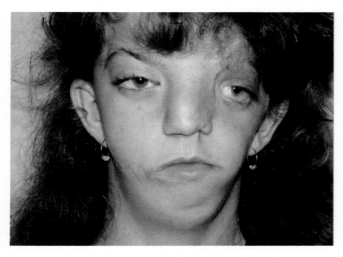

FIGURE 59-2.   A 14-year-old with HFM type III, associated with facial clefting and lack of a condyle.

Cleft Lip and Cleft Palate

Patients with cleft lip and palate often present with bilateral or unilateral midface deficiency resulting in an apparent increased AP projection of the paranasal, nasal, infraorbital, and zygomatic regions as well as at the occlusal level.[21] However, the degree and location of maxillofacial growth deficiency in children with cleft lip and palate are largely dependent upon the location and type of cleft lip and cleft palate repair performed and the patient age at the time of repair.[22–24] Most studies show that children with a repaired cleft lip and palate have a decreased vertical and horizontal maxillary growth pattern and a decreased vertical growth of the mandibular ramus with a steep mandibular plane angle.[25–27] Ross[28] has shown that approximately 25% of patients with a repaired cleft lip or cleft palate have a midface deficiency and class III malocclusion that require skeletal orthognathic surgery in adolescence.

Craniosynostosis: Plagiocephaly

The term *plagiocephaly* is derived from the Greek word *plagios,* which refers to the twisted shape of the skull when viewed from a craniocaudal perspective. The etiology of this type of craniosynostosis is often a unilateral premature fusion of the coronal or lambdoid sutures. Unilateral synostosis of the coronal suture results in an asymmetrical parallelogram-shaped forehead and brow. The affected side is usually flattened, and the contralateral side may show compensatory overgrowth with frontal bulging or frontal bossing. In addition, synostosis of the coronal suture often indirectly affects the lower facial morphology, with deviation of the root of the nose toward the affected side and chin deviation to the unaffected side, opposite to the flattened forehead. The mandible generally develops normally but may exhibit secondary dysmorphology as well.[29,30]

Congenital Hemifacial Hyperplasia

Congenital hemifacial hyperplasia is a rare unilateral enlargement of the craniofacial soft and/or hard tissues. Although the term "hemihypertrophy" has commonly been used, it is inappropriate because the condition is due to tissue hyperplasia (increased number of cells) and not tissue hypertrophy (enlargement of individual cells).[31] Pollock and colleagues[32] have hypothesized that the asymmetrical facial development results from abnormal neural crest cell migration. Yoshimoto and associates[33] found increased proliferative activity of osteoblasts in a patient with congenital hemifacial hyperplasia and hypothesized that fibroblast growth factor (FGF), and its receptor signal transduction axis in osteoblasts, may be selectively involved resulting in the progression of hemifacial overgrowth.

DEVELOPMENTAL FACIAL ASYMMETRIES

Primary Growth Deformities

Facial Hemiatrophy

Facial hemiatrophy (Parry-Romberg syndrome) is characterized by a progressive unilateral facial loss of skin, associated soft tissues, cartilage, and hard tissues (Figure 59-3). The left side is more often affected than the right side. Associated clinical findings include Jacksonian epilepsy, cutaneous dyspigmentations, and ipsilateral alopecia.[31] An internet survey of 205 facial hemiatrophy patients revealed a median age

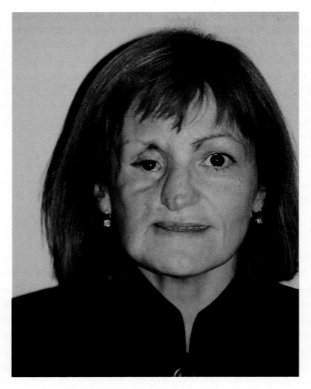

FIGURE 59-3.   Right facial hemiatrophy (Parry-Romberg syndrome), after skin and bone grafting.

SECTION 7

of onset of 10 years with a range of 1 to 50 years. In most patients (71%), the facial hemiatrophy began before age 15 years.[34-36] The etiology of facial hemiatrophy remains unknown, but there have been associations established with Lyme disease, ablation of the superior cervical sympathetic ganglia, localized scleroderma, Rasmussen's encephalitis, and systemic lupus erythematosus (SLE).[37-41] Alterations in the peripheral trophic sympathetic system is one of the more commonly accepted theories of the etiology of this disorder.[31] The various treatments for the soft tissue deficiencies of facial hemiatrophy, or hemifacial atrophy, have included silicone injections, alloplastic implants, microfat injections, and microvascular free tissue transfer.[42-44]

Hemimandibular Hyperplasia

Another developmental anomaly resulting in facial asymmetry is hemimandibular hyperplasia, which is characterized by a diffuse enlargement of the condyle, the condylar neck, and the mandibular ramus and body regions.[45] In 1986, Obwegeser and Makek[46] described the deformity as hemimandibular hyperplasia or hemimandibular elongation. In 1996, Chen and coworkers[47] proposed that all cases of hemimandibular hyperplasia actually represent a spectrum of variations in condylar overgrowth, and it was proposed that if condylar overgrowth is not arrested, it can progress into hemimandibular hyperplasia. In spite of the differences in nomenclature, no specific etiologic factor has been established. Condylar growth patterns can be evaluated by serial clinical comparisons, including serial cephalometric tracings, and bone scan techniques. However, no ideal method has been found to assess whether condylar overgrowth is active or inactive, or quiescent. Treatment for hemimandibular hyperplasia is guided by patient age and condylar growth activity; these range from orthopedic maxillary management to condylectomy. Although it is generally accepted that surgical treatment should be delayed until growth activity has ceased,[45] others believe that early surgery, performed while condylar growth is still active, may cause a surgical insult and postsurgical scarring that can beneficially halt the condylar growth. Also, in some severe cases, condylar resection during active growth of the condyle may be necessary for correction of a significantly asymmetrical, or socially unacceptable, facial appearance.

Secondary Growth Deformities

Sternocleidomastoid torticollis is a condition resulting from a birth trauma–induced hematoma of the sternocleidomastoid muscle that gradually undergoes fibrosis over time and leads to muscular contraction and torticollis. However, the precise etiologic factors of this entity are still unknown. If the condition is not corrected early enough with proper physical therapy, or surgery, for neck and sternocleidomastoid muscle mobility, malformed facial development will usually result ipsilateral to the side affected by the torticollis.[48,49] Duchenne's muscular dystrophy and cerebral palsy often result in areas of decreased muscle tone, which can affect the develop-

ment of facial form by limiting the amount of bone formation at sites of normal muscle attachment and function. Consequently, facial asymmetry and dysmorphology may be a clinical finding seen in patients with Duchenne's muscular dystrophy and cerebral palsy.[50]

ACQUIRED FACIAL ASYMMETRIES

Condylar Trauma

A common cause of facial asymmetry in the growing child is trauma to the mandibular condyle, although in many cases, neither the child nor the parent can recall the traumatic event (Figures 59-4 and 59-5).[51] Trauma-induced injury to the condyle can lead to a hemarthrosis that results in intra-articular scarring and restriction of condylar translation. Proffit and Turvey[52] described this clinical scenario as a functional ankylosis, or soft tissue extracapsular ankylosis, because, in most cases, condylar function is acceptable. In addition to limitation of jaw movement caused by fibro-osseous TMJ ankylosis and coronoid process elongation and temporalis tendon scarring, complete bony ankylosis of the condyle to the temporal bone and skull base may also occur after intracapsular hemarthrosis, resulting in no rotation or any condylar movement. Consequently, trauma-induced scarring or bony ankylosis of the TMJ can also result in relative degrees of restricted skeletal growth. In other words, the greater the degree of translational restriction, the greater the resultant facial deformity. A similar clinical scenario involves whether open reduction with internal fixation (ORIF) of a condylar fracture is required to stabilize the condylar cartilaginous growth center in skeletally immature patients. Studies in skelettaly immature primates and in children have revealed that the displaced condylar segment undergoes resorption and replacement with a new condylar head with regeneration

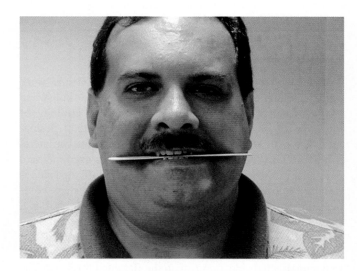

FIGURE 59-4. A 38-year-old who had a right condylar fracture during adolescence resulting in excessive growth of the right condyle and jaw deviation to the left.

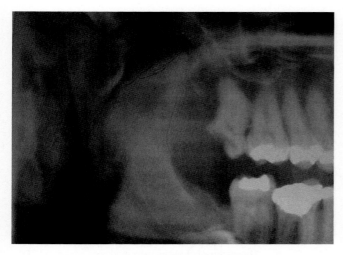

FIGURE 59-5. Panorex of the patient in Figure 59-4 shows right condylar overgrowth and asymmetry.

of the overlying cartilage based upon functional remodeling. Therefore, there is nothing intrinsically critical about the condylar head as a mandibular growth center, and because the condylar head in children is regenerated spontaneously, the necessity of ORIF of a displaced condylar segment is unnecessary. Moreover, the surgical procedure is not without potentially significant morbidity, and the resulting scar and possible soft and hard tissue restriction from the ORIF procedure may outweigh the benefits of surgical anatomic condylar reduction. Several studies have indicated that ORIF of condylar fractures in children should be avoided.[52–54]

Juvenile Idiopathic Arthritis

Facial asymmetry may be found in patients affected with juvenile idiopathic arthritis (JIA) of the TMJ.[55] JIA is a disease characterized by chronic inflammation of one or more joints, affecting children up to the age of 18 years. The TMJ is frequently involved and can lead to facial growth disturbances, including facial asymmetry.[55] TMJ involvement may be asymmetrical and very apparent or may be mild or asymptomatic and not be clinically detectable.[56,57] However, symptomatic TMJ involvement may not be associated with any evidence of facial growth disturbances; and conversely, facial growth disturbances may be present without any clinical TMJ symptoms.[56] Both polyarticular-onset and pauciarticular-onset JIA have been found to have a negative impact on the form, function, and aesthetics of the face. However, the effects are more pronounced with polyarticular JIA.[58,59] Characteristic facial features of patients with JIA include a small mandible, class II malocclusion, and anterior open bite occlusion. Patients with polyarticular JIA with TMJ involvement tend to have small, short faces with underdeveloped mandibles.[60] Currently, no effective therapeutic method is available to eliminate the progression of the disease and its effect on facial development, although methotrexate therapy has been shown to minimize TMJ destruction and craniofa-

cial dysmorphology in patients with polyarticular JIA.[61] Corticosteroids have been used in the treatment of JIA, but their therapeutic benefit is controversial.

Degenerative Joint Disease

Degenerative joint disease (DJD) is considered an end-stage result of progressive internal derangement and osteoarthritis of the TMJ. Usually, patients have bilateral involvement of the TMJ, but unilateral involvement is not uncommon. The wear and tear effects of DJD on the TMJ results in condylar-glenoid erosion and decreased condylar ramus height with asymmetry. Clinically, patients often present with preauricular noise or crepitus, limitation of mandibular motion, preauricular pain, and an anterior open bite occlusion.[62]

CLINICAL PATIENT ASSESSMENT

The usual comprehensive methods of patient evaluation includes the chief complaint, and with additional information gained from the history of the present illness, the answers to pertinent questions regarding a history of facial trauma, arthritis involving other joints, and genetic or congenital malformations may be identified. A physical examination of the head and neck region in the patient with a facial asymmetry should include[63]

1. Visual inspection of the entire face including facial subunits for symmetry in the vertical and horizontal planes.
2. Palpation of the face to differentiate between soft and hard tissue defects.
3. Comparison of dental and facial midlines with each other and with the central facial axis.
4. Inspection for gonial angle asymmetry or differences in the degree of antegonial notching.
5. Analysis of the relationship between the upper lip and the maxillary central incisors.
6. Inspection for malocclusion, occlusal cants, excessive inclination of anterior teeth, dental crowding, open bite occlusal relationships, the maximal interincisal opening, and the presence of mandibular deviation upon opening.
7. Comprehensive examination of TMJ function including protrusion and lateral excursion movements.

Following the data gathering including the chief complaint, history of present illness, past medical history, family history, social history, and physical examination, radiographic and laboratory studies may be indicated, and articulator-mounted diagnostic dental casts are evaluated, a prioritized problem list and corresponding treatment plan options may be developed and presented to the patient and family.

Radiographic Assessment

Panoramic Radiograph

The Panorex can provide information about the relative size and shape of the mandibular condyle as well as ramus height and antegonial notching. Degenerative changes of the TMJ or asymmetrical mandibular ramus morphology may be identified with a comparative vertical measurement of the condylar head apex (condylion) to the base of the sigmoid notch and the sigmoid notch to the mandibular angle (gonion) bilaterally.[63] Also, dental and sinus abnormalities as well as orbital and ear deformities may be detected if the field of view includes these structures.

Posteroanterior Cephalometric Radiograph

The posteroanterior (PA) cephalometric radiograph enables one to evaluate the magnitude of the facial skeletal deformity relative to the cranial base. Acetate overlay tracings soft and hard tissue features can be created and compared with true vertical and horizontal axes. These reference landmarks may not be easy to determine, especially in severe deformties or where the landmark may be missing (e.g., zygomatic bone or condylar hypoplasia or aplasia). Although the most appropriate midline reference is controversial and may include a midpoint between two lateral measurements (e.g., medial aspect of the frontozygomatic suture), a consistent midline reference is the crista galli of the ethmoid bone. In cases of ear abnormalities, the ear rod on the involved side should rest against the temporal bone in the area where the normal ear should be so that horizontal references can be compared without the need to account for an abnormal head posture. Also, owing to the overlap of several skeletal structures, there are limitations to the use of the PA cephalogram in the diagnosis of facial asymmetries, but in general, deviations of the dental and skeletal midlines, occlusal cants, orbital asymmetries, ear and external auditory canal (EAC) abnormalities, and vertical ramus discrepancies may be determined with this radiograph.[63]

Lateral Cephalometric Radiograph

A lateral cephalometric radiograph can provide an indication of vertical ramus height differences by the finding of two separate radiographic mandibular inferior border outlines. However, to determine the relative significance of the differences in dentofacial superimposition, one must know whether the EACs are level with the patient's natural head position, and as mentioned, only a single cephalometric ear rod should be used if the patient's EACs are abnormal or not located at the same level.[63]

Computed Tomography

Computed tomography (CT) can provide two-dimensional localized views of the facial skeleton, or it can be developed further into three-dimensional views that can provide excellent overall detail necessary for the proper diagnosis and treatment planning of a complex facial dysmorphology (Figure 59-6).

Stereolithographic Modeling

Three-dimensional CT scans can provide information to allow the fabrication of an actual three-dimensional skeletal

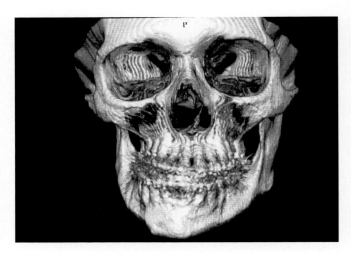

FIGURE 59-6.　Three-dimensional computed tomography (CT) scan of asymmetrical craniofacial skeleton (right HFM).

model via stereolithography (SLA) or computer-aided design/computer-aided manufacturing (CAD/CAM). These models can assist the surgeon with physical three-dimensional assessment and formulation of surgical predictions; however, owing to the high cost, these models are primarily used for planning of complex dentofacial and craniofacial deformities.[64]

Most recently, three-dimensional CT treatment planning has become a popular technique for planning three-dimensional orthognathic and skeletal jaw movements, especially in cases of severe asymmetries planned for complex rotation and transverse jaw movements, and fabrication of SLA intermediate and final occlusal splints during the treatment planning process.

Bone Scans

Radionuclide skeletal scintigraphy, including technetium 99m pertechnetate, gallium, and indium-labelling, as well as positron-emission tomography (PET) scans, have been shown to be sensitive diagnostic methods for identifying mandibular overgrowth in the patient with a facial asymmetry and to determine activity or quiescence of the increased growth. However, bone scan findings are nonspecific and may be the result of a variety of bone and soft tissue abnormalities, including soft and hard tissue carcinomas, sarcomas, metastatic disease, hematologic disease, infections, inflammatory processes, metabolic diseases, and trauma, including recent dental extractions.[65] In patients with asymmetrical mandibular overgrowth, nucleotide uptake is not imaged in a symmetrical fashion bilaterally, and in most cases, patients demonstrate an increased nucleotide uptake and activity on the affected side. However, caution must be exercised when evaluating an area of increased uptake in order not to confuse condylar overgrowth with other conditions (e.g., arthritis, TMJ disorders, trauma) that can mimic nucleotide uptake activity.[66] Additional diagnostic radiographic techniques of fusing PET-CT images to high-resolution structural CT images have been shown to provide improved resolution and delineation of the precise area of bone activity.[67]

SURGICAL TREATMENT

Some facial asymmetries may not always be apparent to the patient and family, and therefore, appropriate treatment can begin only when a proper diagnosis has been established. The face should be evaluated in all dimensions, with a careful analysis of the vertical and horizontal proportions and the corresponding facial subunits. Failure to recognize asymmetry until after surgery is complete is generally the reason for the poor final outcome. In general, treatment planning of facial asymmetry is similar to that of orthognathic surgery, except that, depending upon the specific skeletal abnormality, more emphasis is placed on the frontal, as opposed to the profile, view during the examination. As mentioned, cephalometric analysis may be grossly inaccurate owing to inappropriate ear rod positioning during lateral and PA cephalograms, and whereas these radiographs are simple screening tools, standard and three-dimensional CT scans are much more accurate. CT data can be converted by CAD/CAM imaging into an actual acrylic SLA model that can be used for predictive model surgery, customized facial implant fabrication, and design of custom distraction osteogenesis devices. Despite the available radiologic studies, the clinical examination is the most important diagnostic tool, and it should be remembered that body posture, mannerisms, and the presence of facial hair and various hairstyles may mask a facial asymmetry and may direct the treatment plan in an erroneous direction. In one study of 495 patients with facial asymmetry, the mandible was the facial bone most often affected.[68] Upper face and midface asymmetry was found only in 5% of patients, but mandibular asymmetry with chin point deviation was present in 75% of cases. Chin deviation, usually apparent on clinical examination, is most often to the left, indicating a tendency for increased right-sided mandibular growth.

Delayed Treatment

In many cases, a delayed treatment approach may be most appropriate because the management of facial asymmetry in preadolescent children is extremely complex and the results are not always predictable owing to continued facial growth. The interpretation of studies on growth modification using functional appliances have been difficult because of a variety of treatment designs with lack of standardization of treatment and control group populations and difficulties with randomization of the groups, as well as other confounding variables in the studies. Although noninvasive techniques, such as growth modification, will not cause irreversible harm to the patient, most asymmetrical craniofacial syndromes, condylar deformities, and traumatic injuries sustained at an early age do require surgery. Bite block therapy can be helpful in reorienting the plane of occlusion in children with occlusal cants, but it rarely obviates the need for surgery, and typically, bite block therapy is mainly used as an intervention for secondary growth deformities. The functional status of the TMJ is a critical component to consider in the overall treatment planning process for the patient with facial asymmetry, and mild asymmetries in the growing patient with functional TMJs should be considered for early interceptive orthodontics only, and growth completion should be permitted to occur before consideration for surgical intervention. It is well accepted that jaw movement is critical after condylar fractures to prevent limitation of mandibular motion and the development of ankylosis and that physical therapy and rehabilitation stimulate continued condylar and mandibular growth. Lack of function usually results in an asymmetrical mandible and secondary maxillary and midface asymmetries. After condylar trauma, mandibular hypoplasia with growth retardation is seen much more frequently than mandibular hyperplasia or overgrowth. In general, mandibular hyperplasia may be accelerated after an adolescent growth spurt, whereas delayed growth with mandibular hypoplasia is more often present in the preadolescent years and childhood. Regardless of the exact etiology of the mandibular asymmetry, it is important to establish a surgical treatment plan that will achieve the most functional, stable, and aesthetic outcomes. Orthognathic asymmetries should be treated after growth completion because this surgery will require a combination of maxillary and mandibular surgery with the application of rigid internal fixation.

Orthodontic Considerations

Human facial symmetry is directly associated with facial attractiveness. It is also well documented that true symmetry is not the norm, and comparison mirror-imaging of the right sides of a face compared with the left side reveals two completely different facial forms.[69,70] For the typical orthodontic patient, minor facial asymmetries become a concern only when they present with aesthetic complaints. Severe asymmetries often result in cross-bites, malocclusions, cheek biting, poor masticatory forces, condylar dysfunction, myositis, tendinitis, and chronic head and neck pain. From a diagnostic standpoint, patients with asymmetries differ from the typical orthodontic patient in several ways, and the clinical examination and data gathering process should generate sufficient information for accurate diagnosis and formulation of the most appropriate treatment plan. The data should include photographs from multiple views, lateral and PA cephalometric radiographs, and facebow-mounted dental models.[62–71] Facial structures may be evaluated with a reference grid formed by the midsagittal plane and several perpendicular reference lines, according to the area being evaluated (e.g., interpupillary, subnasal, stomion). A tongue blade, or Fox plane, can be used to determine whether an occlusal cant is present, because unilateral vertical maxillary excess and mandibular asymmetries are usually associated with an occlusal plane cant;[63] and this is the reason why most asymmetries cannot be effectively treated with single-jaw surgery. Typical orthodontic diagnostic records rely heavily on the profile view, because the lateral approach is derived from traditional diagnoses based upon cephalometric radiographs; however, patients are more aware of their aesthetic presentation from the frontal view. Additional diagnostic records may include a PA cephalometric radiograph, a submentovertex radiograph, and an accurate facebow transfer with casts mounted on a semiadjustable articulator.[65–73]

The orthodontic management of patients with asymmetries does not differ a great deal from the typical orthognathic surgical patient. Good communication and a team approach during all phases of treatment are essential. Once the diagnosis and treatment plan have been established, the presurgical orthodontic phase is initiated, and basic principles of presurgical orthodontics must be observed. All tooth movements that may compromise stability should be avoided, especially if the intended movement may be more easily accomplished with the surgical movements of bony segments (e.g., transverse maxillary expansion is more effectively managed with two-piece segmental maxillary surgery rather than orthodontic maxillary expansion, especially in the adult patient). Dentoalveolar decompensation in the maxillary arch must take into account the postsurgical position of the maxillary central incisor. Maxillary AP movements, as well as posterior impactions, have the greatest effect on the upper incisors with regards to AP positioning and dental torque, respectively. Dentoalveolar decompensations in the mandibular arch must observe the anatomic limits of the outlines of the bony symphysis. It must be remembered that the morphogenetic pattern in patients with maxillomandibular discrepancies results in variable abnormal bony architectural changes, and therefore, cephalometric norms cannot be applied to all asymmetries. In addition, there should not be any compromise in the presurgical orthodontic treatment plan that might severely limit the final orthodontic and surgical treatment outcomes. The need for extractions should be assessed and performed if indicated, and dental impressions and early model surgery can be helpful in confirming that the presurgical goals are appropriate and/or that the treatment objectives have been achieved.

Common orthodontic problems in the asymmetry patient include improper buccal root torque in the upper arch, improper arch coordination (especially when AP movements are planned), and a lack of sufficient incisor overjet that can limit placement of the jaws into an ideal class I canine and molar occlusal relationship. The decision to extract teeth is often difficult, and perhaps the first issue that must be addressed is whether there is significant dental crowding or a Bolton discrepancy. This determination is based primarily on the ideal planned final position of the upper and lower incisors in the basal bone of the maxilla and mandible. The relationships of the upper incisors to the sella-nasion (SN) (104 degrees), palatal plane (104 degrees), and nasion point A (NA) line (4 mm and 22 degrees) are excellent indicators of whether these teeth require decompensation. It must be

kept in mind that posterior impaction of the maxilla decreases the torque, or protrusion, of the upper incisors, so the orthodontic treatment must take this into consideration and not retrocline the incisors because they will be further uprighted by the surgical movement. In addition, large unilateral vertical changes, such as maxillary impaction or down-grafting, will rotate the midline of the maxillary incisors. However, when this is anticipated, the upper incisors should be maintained in a slightly proclined angulation. As a surgical treatment objective (STO), the position of the upper incisor, and a point relative to N-perpendicular, can be used as reasonable cephalometric references. Therefore, dental crowding as well as the ideal position of the upper incisors within basal bone of the maxilla will ultimately determine the need for extractions. Upper second bicuspid extractions are preferred when minimal incisor decompensation is required anteriorly; and maxillary first bicuspids are extracted when the upper incisors require greater degrees of decompensation, such as in class III cases. If mild crowding is present (≤4 mm) and no dentoalveolar decompensation is needed, a nonextraction approach is acceptable, and some interproximal reduction (IPR) may be required. If significant incisor decompensation is required, the cephalometric correction must be factored into the assessment of the degree of crowding. For every 3 degrees of change in the angulation between the lower incisor and the mandibular plane, it is necessary to add or subtract 2.5 mm to the measured clinical crowding. In patients with class II malocclusions, cephalometric correction most often adds to the clinical crowding assessment because the lower incisor typically requires a more upright repositioning, whereas with class III malocclusions, cephalometric correction usually alleviates this crowding. In other words, cephalometric correction takes into account the goals for the lower incisor into the crowding assessment; moreover, it helps to decide which teeth should be extracted. When the measured crowding in the lower arch is moderate (5–9 mm), mandibular second bicuspids should be extracted, which will result in alignment of lower incisor angulation and complete closure of the extraction spaces. When crowding is severe (>10 mm) after cephalometric correction, mandibular first bicuspids should be extracted to allow alignment and proper positioning of the lower incisor. The rationale is that when two bicuspids are extracted, an average of 14 mm of total arch space is created. If the total crowding is 10 mm including cephalometric correction, then 4 mm of space is left. These 4 mm are used by the forward movement of the posterior teeth as lost anchorage during the alignment and retraction of the lower incisors. Maximum decompensation is often required with minimal clinical crowding, therefore, requiring first bicuspid extractions. If crowding exceeds 14 mm, extractions alone are not sufficient to alleviate the crowding and achieve an ideal position of the lower incisors. IPR may help to create another 3 to 4 mm of total arch space to accomplish these goals simultaneously.

Patients with hyperdivergent facial forms who present with an asymmetry may require differential maxillary impaction; in such cases, there is a need to flatten the curve of Spee in both arches before surgery. The curve of Spee is often different from left to right, and flattening the curve allows for maximum intercuspation to be achieved between the anterior teeth and the bicuspid teeth, with the creation of minimum posterior open bites. If the posterior maxilla is intentionally overimpacted when relapse is expected, the result will be a posterior open bite, and no vertical elastics are placed distal to the bicuspids for the first 8 weeks after surgery. The goal should be to achieve maximal intercuspation, although in the patient with a facial asymmetry, the occlusion on one side may be more open than on the other; it is usually the hypoplastic side that remains slightly open, and generally teeth can be extruded with vertical elastics postsurgically. An open bite of 2 mm or less is acceptable, and occasionally desirable, because some settling and relapse occur after surgery; and in general, no orthodontic forces should be applied in the direction of the potential surgical relapse. Patients with hypodivergent asymmetrical faces typically require mandibular advancement with an increase in the lower anterior facial height. The original malocclusion is often characterized by an excessive overbite, overjet, and accentuated curve of Spee, which may be different from side to side. The maxillary curve of Spee should be flattened and the ideal position of the upper incisors achieved. No attempt should be made to level the lower curve of Spee because forward movement of the mandible to an ideal overbite and overjet will increase the lower anterior facial height and the curve of Spee is maintained. If the lower mandibular plane angle has been maintained during mandibular advancement, this may result in a posterior open bite in the bicuspid or molar region. The increased interocclusal space with this postsurgical tripod occlusion will allow leveling of the mandibular curve of Spee with minimal effort after surgery, using a flexible braided wire in the lower arch as vertical intercuspation elastics are applied to extrude the lower posterior teeth and close the posterior open bite. A class II or class III vector may be incorporated in the postsurgical period in order to achieve optimum occlusal intercuspation. The maxillary arch should be stabilized with a heavy rectangular arch wire. Postsurgical orthodontic procedures are usually completed within 6 to 8 months after surgery if all other phases of treatment have been successful. Vertical elastics may be directed by the orthodontist depending on the occlusion and the unique differences of the hyperplastic or hypoplastic side of the face. Severe orthognathic asymmetries are often difficult from an orthodontic standpoint owing to the presence of unilateral differences in a hyperplastic jaw, with a contralateral hypoplastic dental and skeletal compensation.

Surgical Options

In rare cases, facial asymmetries may be treated in a single jaw, although generally, asymmetrical growth results in compensation of the teeth, alveolus, and the other jaw and the rest of the facial skeleton and soft tissues. Furthermore, this com-

pensation may be significantly different from side to side and will require different orthodontic mechanics. Facial asymmetry may be improved from an aesthetic standpoint without standard orthognathic surgery, using a variety of techniques including an inferior border ostectomy or recontouring procedure, inferior border augmentation, and genioplasty procedures. The aesthetic impact of an asymmetry involves both the hard and the soft tissues, and commonly, the zygoma and periorbital and nasal structures may be involved, as well as the adjacent soft tissues, such as the salivary glands, muscles, and adipose tissue, with quantitative differences from side to side. The expectations of the patient as well as the surgical possibilities should be discussed at length, because asymmetrical deformities can rarely be corrected completely. Most patients notice horizontal or transverse facial discrepancies more often than vertical asymmetries (e.g., maxillary occlusal cants are difficult to detect clinically). Horizontal asymmetries resulting in maxillary dental midline, chin, and nasal deviations are typically very obvious clinically. Asymmetries in vertical facial height are less apparent clinically, and in severe cases, such as HFM or other syndromes, soft tissue augmentation and even free vascularized tissue may be necessary for correction.

The oral and maxillofacial surgeon should make a note of even minor anatomic asymmetries such as orbital, nasal, and upper lip position; maxillary dental midline position; smile arch; amount of gingival display on each side of the midline; cheek mass and malar prominence; the presence of dimples or clefts; mandibular dental midline position; mandibular deviations on opening or protrusion; TMJ articulation, rotation, and translation; gonial angle position; and cervical and neck anatomy. All of these should be documented. The surgical procedure should be selected based upon the etiology of the asymmetry with a healthy concern for stability and relapse in these patients. For example, when correcting a maxillary cant, vertical impaction is more stable than vertical down-grafting, and often the discrepancy may be corrected by a combination of both types of vertical maxillary movements. Severe asymmetries with a short mandibular ramus height may require an extraoral inverted-L osteotomy with bone grafting and rigid internal fixation. This technique releases the pterygomasseteric sling and provides excellent access to the hypoplastic ramus for bone grafting and application of rigid fixation. Vertical changes of less than 6 to 8 mm may be treated via an intraoral approach with a bilateral sagittal split osteotomy (SSO) and rigid fixation. Rotational movements of the mandible produce proximal segment flaring on the side that the mandible rotates away from and ramus collapse on the side that the mandible is rotating toward. Proximal segment flaring may require bony modification within the SSO site to allow a more appropriate relationship of the proximal and distal segments. Some surgeons prefer a unilateral vertical oblique ramus osteotomy (VRO) (on the side that the mandible rotates toward) combined with a unilateral SSO (on the side that the mandible rotates away from). This combination surgery usually requires intermaxillary fixation, which may be beneficial in asymmetrical cases. With current techniques, monocortical plate and screw fixation can be applied to a VRO, using intraoral right-angle instrumentation, a transbuccal trocar technique, or an extraoral, or endoscope-assisted, approach. Conversely, intermaxillary fixation is often necessary, and even beneficial, because alignment of the segments with rigid fixation is not always possible and the soft tissue tension will attempt to retract the mandible to the original asymmetrical position.

As mentioned previously, a treatment plan should be established with an accurate clinical examination, cephalometric analysis, and model surgery, and the surgical procedure should be executed efficiently and with minimal patient morbidity, and the issues of relapse, stability, and mode of fixation should be determined before surgery and discussed with the patient. The first, and perhaps most important, treatment plan decision the surgeon must make is the ideal position of the maxillary central incisor. This is a critical decision and will essentially determine the three-dimensional position of both the maxilla and the mandible. The surgeon must consider dental midline discrepancies, incisor proclination or retraction excesses, occlusal plane abnormalities, smile arch aesthetics, dental/gingival display at rest and upon smiling, and upper and lower lip support. An intermediate splint is useful in repositioning the maxilla, assuming that an accurate facebow transfer and model surgery have been performed. The intermediate splint is only one method used to align the maxilla and correct the asymmetry, although surgical experience and a thorough appreciation of aesthetics and facial symmetry are often more valuable tools for the surgeon. The maxilla must be placed in the proper and most symmetrical position, and then consideration should be given to the occlusion in relation to the uncut mandible; this position should be evaluated in relation to the overall treatment plan. The maxillary position can best be measured using a combination of an external landmark reference (nasal bone pin), Fox plane, upper lip position, as well as internal reference marks on the anterior maxillary wall. The intermediate splint helps to position and maintain the maxilla in the correct position during application of rigid fixation. The concept of an intermediate splint is based upon proper condylar position which is difficult to similate because functional condylar position in an awake, upright patient is not the same as it is in a supine, paralyzed patient. Furthermore, asymmetrical problems often originate from abnormal condylar (TMJ) disorders, and many patients with facial asymmetries do not have bilateral symmetrical condylar rotation and, therefore, exhibit a great deal of muscular compensation during jaw posturing. If an intermediate splint does not seem to position the maxilla properly in all three dimensions, the surgeon should consider other references to determine facial symmetry; however, no specific measurements can replace surgical experience. In bimaxillary surgery, the osteotomies are performed in the mandible first, without completion of the osteotomy until after maxillary surgery is complete and rigid internal fixation has been applied to the repositioned maxilla. This surgical

sequence prevents the creation of excessive forces on the new maxillary position via vibration of the drill or saw used for the mandible with a bite block in position and the forces transmitted to the maxilla. In addition, some surgeons believe that this sequence seems to expedite the overall surgery. An alternative surgical sequence completes the mandibular surgery with rigid fixation before the maxillary surgery, with the premise that it is more appropriate to reposition a mobile structure (the mandible) to a more stable structure (the maxilla and cranium), but this plan requires the precise predetermination of both the mandibular and the maxillary positions.

Mandibular ramus surgery is often difficult in cases of asymmetry because the ramus and body of the mandible are usually deformed and may be hypoplastic with a limited range of motion. Limited surgical access and a smaller soft tissue envelope create a difficult surgical challenge. If the mandible is cut first but not split, the osteotomies are made and a moist sponge is packed into the wound for hemostasis while the maxillary surgery is completed. The mandible is later split and moved to the proper position with the maxilla and held in the proper occlusion with an occlusal wafer, or final splint, with intermaxillary fixation wires. Rigid fixation of the mandible can be achieved with either bicortical positional screws or monocortical plates and screws, assuming that condylar position is appropriate. In large horizontal rotations of the mandible, bicortical screws cannot be placed as true compression screws (lag screws) without significant torque placed on the condyles. Modifications of the lingual cortical plate, and selective grinding of the bony interferences, can be helpful to increase the bony contacts. In most cases, monocortical plates and screws provide adequate stability, without compression of the inferior alveolar nerve, or torquing of the condyles; these can be placed transorally without the need for a transbuccal trocar used with bicortical screw fixation.

Adequate surgical mobilization of the maxilla and mandible is a key step that must be performed during bimaxillary surgery. The mandible and maxilla should be mobile enough to be positioned passively without tension on the soft tissues. This can be a significant concern because jaw repositioning can create tension and restriction in the pterygomasseteric sling, and and if the mandibular segments are stretched into position under tension, long-term stability may be compromised. A balance must be achieved between adequate reflection of periosteum and loss of vascularity and maintenance of an adequate connective tissue envelope. Therefore, in severely hypoplastic mandibles with only rudimentary condyles, considerations for condylar reconstruction should include extraoral procedures of the mandibular ramus with costochondral grafting, or in some situations, distraction osteogenesis may be more appropriate in order to achieve soft tissue expansion with the gradual bony movements. Adjunctive simultaneous soft tissue procedures may be considered after bony repositioning of the maxilla and mandible and occlusal correction orthognathic surgery and internal rigid fixation. Alignment of the chin, nose, and malar complex should be performed after the functional anatomy of the maxilla and mandible has been established. Although simultaneous hard and soft tissue surgery has multiple advantages, it may not always be feasible, and some surgeons choose to wait to see the unpredicatble soft tissues changes after bimaxillary surgery before addressing the soft tissue asymmetries.

Facial Asymmetry Case Examples

Case 1

This is a 20-year-old woman with facial asymmetry resulting from trauma who required bimaxillary surgery (Figure 59-7). She has a chief complaint of difficulty eating and chewing, with a history of chronic myofascial pain and masticatory dysfunction. She sustained a jaw fracture as a young child without treatment, and she has experienced the development of gradual facial asymmetry. She had an orthodontic consultation and it was determined that orthodontic treatment alone or single-jaw surgery would be insufficient to correct her asymmetry.

The physical examination revealed the obvious facial deformity, more pronounced from a basal view, which can often better demonstrate the deformity; also upon biting on a tongue blade, occlusal cant can be demonstrated (Figure 59-8). She was normocephalic and asymmetrical, with a short face and a jaw deviation to the right (Figure 59-9). The TMJ articulation, rotation, and tramslation function was normal without clicking or popping. The maximum incisal opening was 56 mm, with a deviation to the right. The mandibular midline was 7 mm to the right, the overjet was 5 mm, the overbite was 2 mm; there was excessive lower incisor dental display. She had a right buccal crossbite, an anterior cross-bite, maxillary hypoplasia, a canted maxilla, and a short mandibular condyle (Figure 59-10).

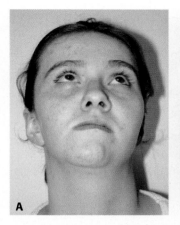
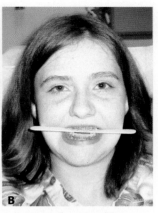

FIGURE 59-8.   **A,** Worm's-eye view shows asymmetry with chin deviation to the right. **B,** Tongue blade demonstrates the occlusal cant plane relative to the normal orbital level.

The presurgical workup included a three-dimensional CT scan, cephalometric and panoramic radiographs, and facebow mounting for fabrication of an accurate intermediate splint and predictive model surgery (Figures 59-11 to 59-13). The Erickson model block was used to measure the vertical changes in the maxilla and to fabricate an intermediate splint to assist in positioning the maxilla (Figures 59-14 and 59-15). The surgical plan included a Le Fort I advancement of 4 mm with a differential maxillary down-grafting of 4 mm on the right

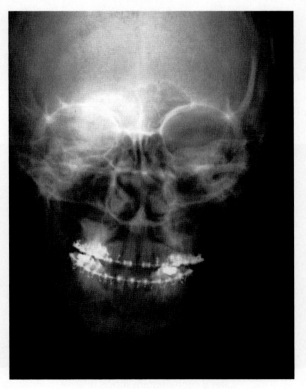

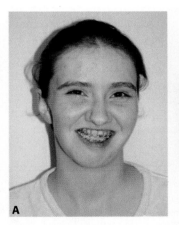
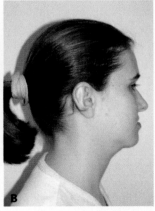

FIGURE 59-7.   **A,** A 20-year-old who had an untreated jaw fracture in childhood; note facial asymmetry. **B,** Profile view shows midface deficiency and relative mandibular prognathism.

FIGURE 59-9.   Posteroanterior (PA) cephalogram shows decreased right facial height and severe asymmetry.

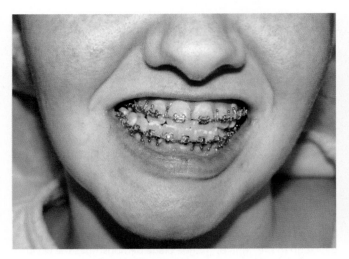

FIGURE 59-10. Occlusal analysis shows asymmetry and midline discrepancy of both jaws.

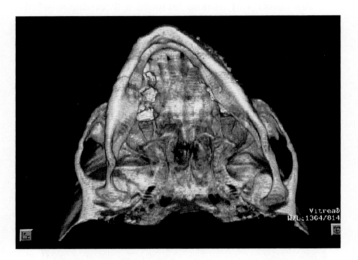

FIGURE 59-11. This three-dimensional CT clearly shows the asymmetry and deviation.

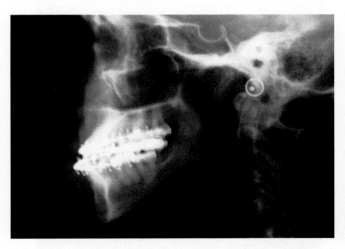

FIGURE 59-12. Lateral cephalogram shows relative mandibular prognathism despite the condylar fracture, although there is an inferior border discrepancy.

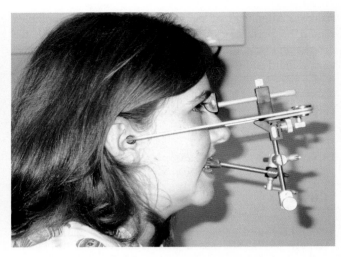

FIGURE 59-13. A facebow transfer is valuable but may be difficult in severe asymmetries with an abnormal ear and external auditory canal (EAC).

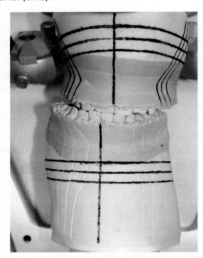

FIGURE 59-14. Mounted models on Erickson block with reference lines help determine surgical movements and splint fabrication. Note midline discrepancy in the midline reference lines on the bases of the casts.

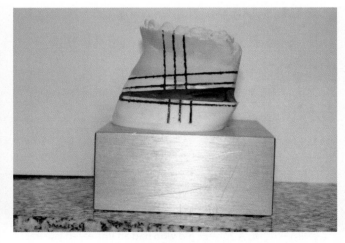

FIGURE 59-15. Lateral view of mounted models shows the planned asymmetrical maxillary osteotomy movement.

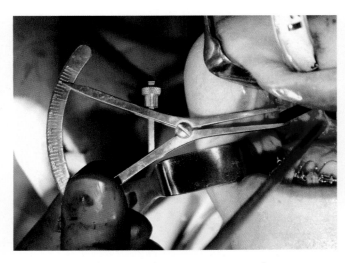

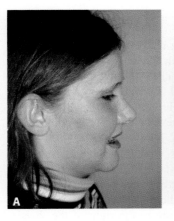
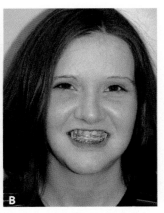

FIGURE 59-18.   **A,** Postoperative lateral view with animation. **B,** Postoperative frontal view with animation.

FIGURE 59-16.   Intraoperative measurement confirms correct positioning with the intermediate splint; compare maxillary gap to Figure 59-15.

side (Figure 59-16). The resultant maxillary osteotomy gap was grafted with allogeneic tibial bone that was mortised in place and fixated. This surgical plan was determined with model surgery to level the cant of the maxillary occlusal plane. A Steinmann pin was placed in the nasal bones as an external vertical reference point; in addition,

a Fox occlusal plane was used to evaluate the level of the maxilla in relation to the infraorbital rims during surgery (Figure 59-17). Multiple methods of evaluating symmetry are helpful in achieving a good result, and intermediate splints, internal and external reference landmarks, and careful clinical inspection from different views are all valuable surgical skills for bimaxillary jaw surgery in the patient with a facial asymmetry. The unsplit, intact mandible is also a key reference for determining any changes in maxillary position. In this case, after the maxilla was correctly positioned and the occlusal plane leveled, the mandible was split and repositioned to the corrected plane of occlusion. A bilateral SSO was cut before the Le Fort procedure but was not split, and as mentioned, this is a common sequence for most surgeons. Consideration was given toward a VRO on the left, but the rotation seemed favorable and the fixation was more stable than anticipated. Most patients with facial asymmetry have horizontal as well as vertical mandibular hypoplasia and require lower facial advancement more often than reduction. A genioplasty was performed to advance the chin point 4 mm and to level the deviation of the symphysis region. After the orthognathic phase of surgery, intraoperatively the endotracheal tube was switched from a nasal to oral intubation for the performance of a simultaneous rhinoplasty procedure. A standard internal rhinoplasty was performed to narrow the nose, refine the tip, and reduce the nasal dorsum. Often, facial asymmetry affects multiple facial subunits, and the nose may appear to be asymmetrical or deviated in relation to the maxilla, mandible, and chin, so attention to detail is required in order to create overall midface symmetry.

At 3-month follow-up, the postoperative results were satisfactory to the patient and surgeon (Figure 59-18), the occlusion was aligned and stable, and finishing orthodontics were completed without difficulty.

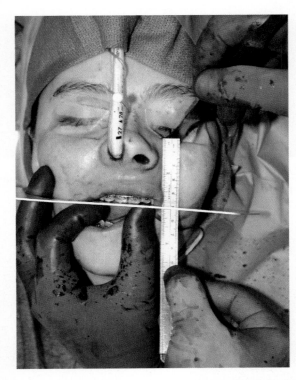

FIGURE 59-17.   A modified Fox plane can be used as a reference to evaluate leveling of the maxilla in reference to the infraorbital rims.

Case 2

This is a 17-year-old young man with a large open bite and right laterognathism, with posterior vertical maxillary excess, dental crowding, a class III molar relationship, dentofacial asymmetry, and a mandibular prognathism (Figures 59-19 to 59-22). He complained of lip incompetence; difficulty eating, chewing, and biting food; nasal obstruction; and xerostomia. His father had a history of mandibular prognathism as well. He denied previous facial trauma, and the orbital rims were symmetrical, but the right ear was slightly lower than the left. The TMJs articulated well and there was no facial pain. The mandibular midline was 6 mm to the right of the facial midline, and the chin was excessive vertically and 6 mm to the right of the mandibular midline. Also, there is a mild transverse deficiency of the posterior maxilla and a wide posterior mandibular dimension.

The treatment plan began with an extraction of teeth numbers 1, 16, 17, 18, 2, 4, 13, 21 and 28 before presurgical orthodontics, which was performed to level, align, and decompensate the dentition in preparation for a possible segmental Le Fort I osteotomy with posterior expansion, a bilateral SSO, genioplasty with vertical reduction and rotation, and possible midline mandibular osteotomy with mandibular narrowing. Presurgical records included

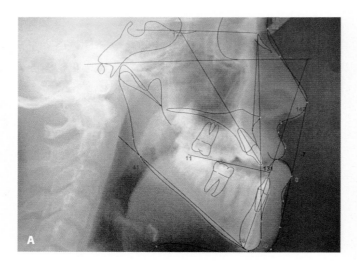

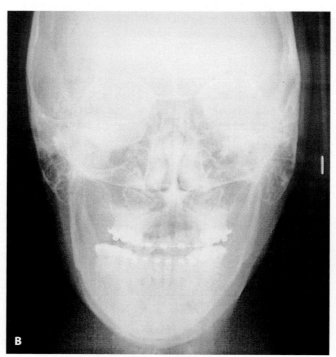

FIGURE 59-21.   **A,** Presurgical cephalometric analysis. **B,** Presurgical PA cephalogram.

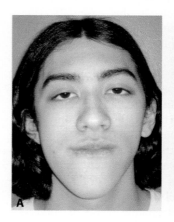
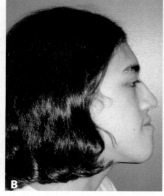

FIGURE 59-19.   **A,** Initial frontal view. **B,** Initial profile view.

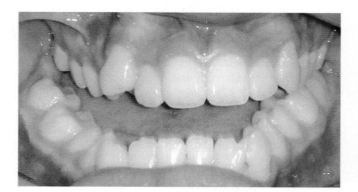

FIGURE 59-20.   Initial occlusion.

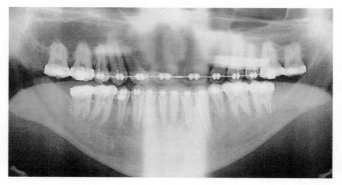

FIGURE 59-22.   Initial Panorex.

mounted dental models, a facebow transfer, and detailed radiographs. A three-dimensional CT scan would have also been valuable. The surgery consisted of a bilateral SSO that was cut, but not split until after the maxilla was positioned, and the anterior midline mandibular osteotomy was performed. The maxilla was advanced 6 mm, using an intermediate splint to position the maxilla, which was fixated rigidly with a 6-mm prebent advancement plate at the piriform rims, and two additional plates in the posterior maxillary buttress regions. During surgery, both internal and external references were used to properly position the maxilla vertically, and the use of prebent plates assisted in the proper AP positioning of the maxilla. Model surgery had been performed with a midline mandibular osteotomy with plans to narrow the excessive mandibular width and correct the mandibular asymmetry. The chin was also extremely long and deviated to the right side; therefore, a vestibular incision was used and vertical reference marks were made in the symphysis bone. A low geniotomy wedge resection was performed and a midline osteotomy was created between the mandibular central incisors (Figure 59-23). The SSO segments were then separated, and the mandible was secured into the customized splint. The occlusion was placed into intermaxillary fixation. The anterior midline osteotomy was first fixated with a four-hole noncompression titanium miniplate. These four screws were placed apical to the anterior tooth roots (Figure 59-24). A 5-mm wedge of bone was then removed and the chin point was repositioned with two cross-shaped titanium plates. The inferior chin point repositioned 5 mm to the left, and then the SSO was fixated with monocortical plates bilaterally. The teeth articulated into the splint well, and then the nasal septum was sutured to the anterior nasal spine and an alar base cinch suture technique was performed; finally, the anterior maxillary vestibular incision was closed in a V-Y fashion.

The postoperative course was without complication, and at 1 month, the splint was removed. The occlusion remained stable at 1 year follow-up, and the facial symmetry was excellent (Figures 59-25 to 59-29). This case is an example of severe developmental, nontraumatic orthognathic asymmetry, which can be challenging for the orthodontist and surgeon because the orthodontic preparation may be different for the left and right sides. If the asymmetry is mild, it is tempting to inappropriately manage the problem with single-jaw surgery. Many such facial asymmetries are often undertreated, when in fact they may require overcorrection to account for some relapse potential. In fact, each case must be treated as an individual because each asymmetry is unique and requires careful attention to detail in the diagnostic and treatment phases of management.

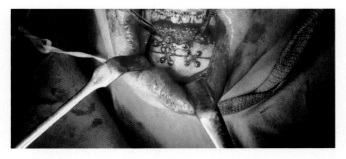

FIGURE 59-24.   Genioplasty fixation with plates and screws.

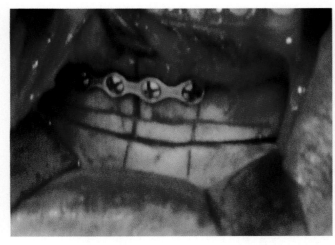

FIGURE 59-23.   Genioplasty with wedge excision and midline osteotomy.

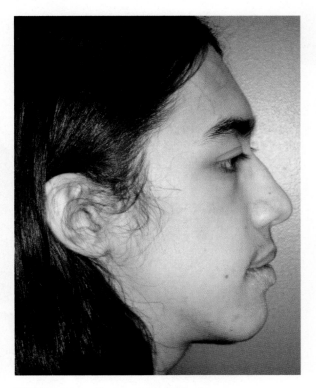

FIGURE 59-25.   Postsurgical profile view.

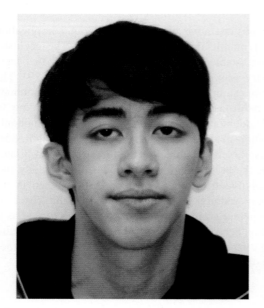

FIGURE 59-26.   Postsurgical frontal view.

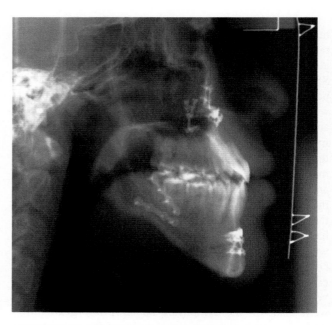

FIGURE 59-28.   Final lateral cephalometric view.

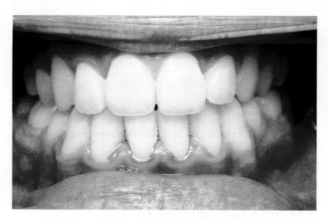

FIGURE 59-27.   Final occlusion.

CONCLUSIONS

Correction of asymmetrical orthognathic deformities often requires surgery of both the maxilla and the mandible. Combining osteotomies of the maxilla and the mandible is more complicated than single-jaw surgery and is perhaps associated with increased morbidity, but the surgical options are more extensive and the postoperative results are improved with less potential replase. Bimaxillary jaw surgery does not result in twice the morbidity of single-jaw surgery and is typically tolerated as well as single-jaw surgery with similar periods of postsurgical convalescence. The indications for bimaxillary surgery include severe facial asymmetries and deformities that cannot be adequately managed with one-jaw

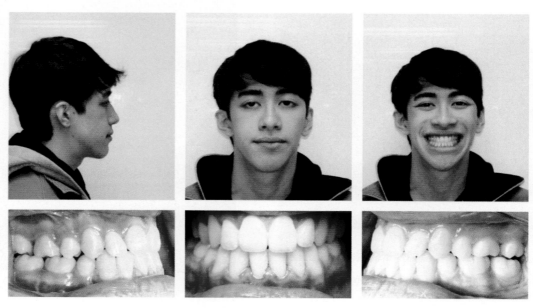

FIGURE 59-29.   One-year follow-up records.

surgery, skeletal deformities of both jaws, unfavorable planned surgical movements that are prone to relapse, and complex three-dimensional movements for which single-jaw surgery would represent a functional and cosmetic compromise. Skeletal dentofacial asymmetries may develop from a primary etiologic event but usually present with secondary compensations of both the hard and the soft tissues of the face; such an asymmetry is an excellent indication for bimaxillary surgery. Current surgical techniques have reduced the morbidity and hospital length of stay and have improved the overall functional and aesthetic surgical outcomes. In addition, the use of three-dimensional imaging and computerized treatment planning has recently been used to improve accuracy and predictability of the diagnosis and treatment plan; this reinforces the concept that comprehensive facial analysis and attention to detail in the treatment of facial asymmetries are critical to a successful outcome.

ACKNOWLEDGMENT

The authors would like to thank Dr. Andre Ferreira for the orthodontic support in these cases.

References

1. Proffit W, White R, Savers D, editors. Contemporary treatment of dentofacial Dentoformity. St. Louis: Mosby; 2003.
2. Bell WH, Condit CL. Surgical-orthodontic correction of adult bimaxillary protrusion. J Oral Surg 1970;28:578–590.
3. Connole PW, Small EW. Combined maxillary and mandibular osteotomies: discussion of three cases. J Oral Surg 1971;29:572–578.
4. Epker BN, Wolford LM. Middle third face osteotomies: their use in the correction of acquired and developmental dentofacial and craniofacial deformities. J Oral Surg 1975;33:491–514.
5. Turvey TA. Simultaneous mobilization of the maxilla and mandible: surgical technique and results. J Oral Maxillofac Surg 1981;40:96–99.
6. Gross BD, James AB. The surgical sequence of combined total maxillary and mandibular osteotomies. J Oral Surg 1978;36:513–522.
7. Shackleford TK, Larsen RJ. Facial asymmetry as an indicator of psychological, emotional, physiological distress. J Pers Soc Psychol 1997;72:456–466.
8. Cohen MM. Malformations, deformations and disruptions. In: The Child with Multiple Birth Defects. New York: Raven; 1982:1.
9. Cohen MM. Perspectives on craniofacial asymmetry 1. The biology of asymmetry. Int J Oral Maxillofac Surg 1995;24:2–7.
10. Gorlin RJ, Deformations and disruptions. In: Syndromes of the Head and Neck. 3rd ed. New York: Oxford University Press; 1990:1.
11. Johnston MC, Bronsky PT. Prenatal craniofacial development: new insights on normal and abnormal mechanisms. Crit Rev Oral Biol Med 1995;6:368–422.
12. Seow WK, Urban S, Vafaie N, Shusterman S. Morphometric analysis of the primary and permanent dentitions in hemifacial microsomia: a controlled study. J Dent Res 1998;77:27–38.
13. Poswillo DE. The pathogenesis of the first and second branchial arch syndrome. Oral Surg Oral Med Oral Pathol 1975;35:302–327.
14. Poswillo DE. Hemorrhage in development of the face. Birth Defects 1975;11:61.
15. Kearns GJ, Padwa BL, Kaban LB. Hemifacial microsomia: the disorder and its surgical management. In Booth PW, Schendel SA, editors. Maxillofacial Surgery. St. Louis: Churchill Livingstone; 1999; pp. 917–942.
16. Posnick JC. Hemifacial microsomia: evaluation and treatment. In: Craniofacial and maxillofacial surgery in children and young adults. Philadelphia: WB Saunders; 1999; pp. 419–445.
17. Pruzansky S. Not all dwarfed mandibles are alike. Birth Defects 1969;1:120.
18. Kaban LB, Moses MH, Mulliken JB. Surgical correction of hemifacial microsomia in the growing child. Plast Reconstr Surg 1988;82:9–19.
19. Cousley RR, Calvert ML. Current concepts in the understanding and management of hemifacial microsomia. Br J Plast Surg 1997;50:536–551.
20. Vargervik K, Hoffman W, Kaban LB. Comprehensive surgical and orthodontic management of hemifacial microsomia. In Turvey TA, Vig KW, Fonseca RJ, editors. Facial Clefts and Craniosynostosis: Principles and Management. Philadelphia: WB Saunders; 1996; pp. 537–564.
21. Stella JP, Chaisresoahurnpon N, Epker BN. Diagnostic criteria for midface deficiency [abstract]. Cleft Palate-Craniofac Assoc 1993;182:6.
22. Johnson GP. Craniofacial analysis of patients with complete clefts of the lip and palate. Cleft Palate J 1980;17:17–23.
23. Fonseca RJ, Turvey TA, Wolford LM. Orthognathic surgery on the cleft patient. In Fonseca RJ, Baker SB, Wolford LM, editors. Oral and Maxillofacial Surgery: Cleft/Craniofacial/Cosmetic surgery. Vol 6. Philadelphia: WB Saunders; 2000; pp. 87–146.
24. Bishara SE. Cephalometric evaluation of facial growth in operated and non-operated individuals with isolated clefts of the palate. Cleft Palate J 1973;10:239–246.
25. Bardach J. The influence of cleft repair on facial growth. Cleft Palate J 1990;27:76–78.
26. Shaw WC, Dahl E, Asher-McDade C, et al. A six-center international study of treatment outcome in patients with clefts of the lip and palate. Part 5. General discussion and conclusions. Cleft Palate Craniofac J 1992;29:413–418.
27. Semb G. A study of facial growth in patients with unilateral cleft lip and palate treated by Oslo CLP team. Cleft Palate Craniofac J 1991;28:1–21.
28. Ross RB. Treatment variables affecting facial growth in complete unilateral cleft lip and palate. Cleft Palate J 1987;24:5–77.
29. Shin JH, Persing J. Asymmetric skull shapes: diagnostic and therapeutic consideration. J Craniofacial Surg 2003;14:696–699.
30. Kane AA, Lo LJ, Vannier MW, Marsh JL. Mandibular dysmorphology in unicoronal synostosis and plagiocephaly without synostosis. Cleft Palate Craniofac J 1996;33:418–423.
31. Cohen MM. Perspectives on craniofacial asymmetry. IV. Hemiasymmetries. Int J Oral Maxillofac Surg 1995;24:134–141.
32. Pollock RA, Newman MH, Burdi AR, Condit DP. Congenital hemifacial hyperplasia: an embryonic hypothesis and case report. Cleft Palate J 1985;22:173–184.
33. Yoshimoto H, Yano H, Kobayushi K, et al. Increased proliferative activity of osteoblasts in congenital hemifacial hypertrophy. Plast Reconstr Surg 1998;102:1605–1610.
34. Parry CH. Collections from Unpublished Papers. Vol 1. London: Underwood; 1825.

SECTION 7

35. Romberg MH. Trophoneurosen. In Klinische Ergebnisse. Berlin: A Forstner; 1846; pp. 75–81.

36. Stone J. Parry-Romberg syndrome: a global survey of 205 patients using the Internet. Neurology 2003;61:674–676.

37. Shah JR, Juhasz C, Kupsky WJ, et al. Rasmussen encephalitis associated with Parry-Romberg syndrome. Neurology 2003;61:395–397.

38. Stern HS, Elliott LF, Beegle PH. Progressive hemifacial atrophy associated with Lyme disease. Plast Reconstr Surg 1992;90:479–483.

39. Moss ML, Crikelair GF. Progressive facial hemiatrophy following cervical sympathectomy in the rat. Arch Oral Biol 1959;1:254–258.

40. Rees TD. Facial atrophy. Clin Plast Surg 1976;3:637–646.

41. Roddi R, Riggio E, Gilbert PM, et al. Progressive hemifacial atrophy in a patient with lupus erythematosus. Plast Reconstr Surg 1994;93:1067–1072.

42. Franz FP, Blocksma R, Brudage SR, et al. Massive injection of liquid silicone for hemifacial atrophy. Ann Plast Surg 1988;20:140–145.

43. Roddi R, Riggio E, Gilbert PM, et al. Clinical evaluation of techniques used in the surgical treatment of progressive hemifacial atrophy. Craniomaxillofac Surg 1994;22:23–32.

44. Pisarek W. Reconstruction of craniofacial microsomia and hemifacial atrophy with free latissimus dorsi flap. Acta Chir Plast 1988;30:194–201.

45. Marchetti C, Cocchi R, Gentile L, Bianchi A. Hemimandibular hyperplasia: treatment strategies. J Craniofac Surg 2000;11: 46–53.

46. Obwegeser HL, Makek MS. Hemimandibular hyperplasia—hemimandibular elongation. J Maxillofac Surg 1986;14: 183–208.

47. Chen YR, Bendov-Samuel RL, Huang CS. Hemimandibular hyperplasia. Plast Reconstr Surg 1996;97:730–737.

48. Stassen LF, Kerwala CJ. New surgical technique for the correction of congenital muscular torticollis (wry neck). Br J Oral Maxillofac Surg 2000;38:142–147.

49. Chen CE, Ko JY. Surgical treatment of muscular torticollis for patients above 6 years of age. Arch Orthop Trauma Surg 2000;120:149–151.

50. Kiliaridis S, Katsaros C. The effects of myotonic dystrophy and Duchenne muscular dystrophy on the orofacial muscles and dento-facial morphology. Acta Odontol Scand 1998;56:369–374.

51. Proffit WR, Vig KW, Turvey TA. Fractures of the mandible condyle: frequently an unsuspected cause of facial asymmetry. Am J Orthod 1980;78:1–24.

52. Proffit WR, Turvey TA. Dentofacial asymmetry. In Proffit WR, White RP, Sarver DM, editors. Contemporary Treatment of Dentofacial Deformity. St. Louis: Mosby; 2003; pp. 574–644.

53. Demianczuk AN, Verchere C, Phillips JH. The effect on facial growth of pediatric mandibular fractures. J Craniofac Surg 1999;10:323–328.

54. Pirttiniemi PM. Associations of mandibular and facial asymmetries—a review. Am J Orthod Dentofacial Orthop 1994;106:191–200.

55. Stabrun AE. Impaired mandibular growth and micrognathic development in children with juvenile rheumatoid arthritis. Eur J Orthod 1991;13:423–434.

56. Bazan MT An overview of juvenile rheumatoid arthritis. J Pedod 1981;6:68–76.

57. Kjellberg H, Fasth A, Kiliaridis S, et al. Craniofacial structure in children with juvenile rheumatoid arthritis compared with healthy children with ideal or postnormal occlusion. Am J Orthod Dentofacial Orthop 1995;107:67–78.

58. Mericle PM, Wilson VK, Moore TL, et al. Effects of polyarticular and pauciarticular onset juvenile rheumatoid arthritis on facial and mandibular growth. J Rheumatol 1996;23: 159–165.

59. Stabrun AE, Larheim TA, Hoyeraal HM, Rosler M. Reduced mandibular dimensions and asymmetry in juvenile rheumatoid arthritis pathologic factors. Arthritis Rheum 1988;31:602–611.

60. Walton AG, Welburg RR, Thomason JM, Foster HE. Oral health and juvenile idiopathic arthritis: a review. Rheumatology 2000;39:550–555.

61. Ince DO, Ince A, Moore TL. Effect of methotrexate on the TM joint and facial morphology in juvenile rheumatoid arthritis patients. Am J Orthod Dentofacial Orthop 2000;118: 75–83.

62. Schellhas KP, Piper MA, Omlie MR. Facial skeletal remodeling due to temporomandibular joint degeneration: an imaging study of 100 patients. Cranio 1992;10:248–259.

63. Hegtvedt AK. Diagnosis and management of facial asymmetry. In: Peterson L, ed. Principles of Oral and Maxillofacial Surgery. Philadelphia: JB Lippincott; 1992; pp. 1400–1414.

64. Sailer HF, Haers PE, Zollikofer CP, et al. The value of stereolithographic models for preoperative diagnosis of craniofacial deformities and planning of surgical corrections. Int J Oral Maxillofac Surg 1998;27:327–333.

65. O'Mara RE. Role of bone scanning in dental and maxillofacial disorders. In Freeman M, Weissman HS, editors. Nuclear Medicine Annual. New York: Raven; 1985; pp. 265–284.

66. O'Mara RE. Scintigraphy of the facial skeleton. Oral Maxillofac Surg Clin North Am 1992;4:51–60.

67. Strumas N, Antonyshyn O, Caldwell CB, Mainprize J. Multimodality imaging for precise localization of craniofacial osteomylitis. J Craniofac Surg 2003;14:215–219.

68. Severt TR, Proffit WR. The prevalence of facial asymmetry in the dentofacial deformities population at the University of North Carolina. Int J Adult Orthod Orthognath Surg 1997;12:171–176.

69. Peck S, Peck L. Skeletal asymmetry in esthetically pleasing faces. Angle Orthod 1991;61:43–48.

70. Burk PH. Stereophotogrammetric measurement of normal asymmetry in children. Hum Biol 1971;43:536–548.

71. Sutton PR. Lateral facial asymmetry methods of assessment. Angle Orthod 1968;38:82–92.

72. Cheney EA. Dentofacial asymmetry and their clinical significance. Am J Orthod 1961; 47:814–829.

73. Harvold E. Cleft lip and palate: morphologic studies of facial skeleton. Am J Orthod 1954;40:493–506.

60

CHAPTER

Soft Tissue Changes Associated with Orthognathic Surgery

Stephen Schendel, MD, DDS, Richard Jacobson, DMD, MS, and Dror Aizenbud, DDS

The analysis of facial soft tissues and the associated aesthetic outcomes in orthognathic surgery is the most challenging and unpredictable component in the orthodontic-surgical treatment planning process. There remains a need for an ideal procedure capable of assessing and predicting accurately the entire soft tissue facial envelope in a three-dimensional manner. The final aesthetic facial appearance and the establishment of a functional and stable occlusion are both equal and important goals in orthognathic surgery. Soft tissue changes related to the skeletal maxillary and/or mandibular movements have been classically studied in the lateral profile view from cephalometric evaluation and comparative ratios of soft to hard tissue movements established based upon mean values of responses and on a simple correlation of one variable with another or using linear regression equations.[1-18] In addition, these ratios have been calculated from linear changes limited to specific two-dimensional cephalometric landmarks in the midsagittal plane. This method is restrictive, and its accuracy and reliability in predicting realistic profile changes is questionable because such an approach does not take into account the more complex geometric three-dimensional interactions of highly variable individual parameters such as soft tissue tension, thickness, muscle strain, posture, and tonus. In addition, such technical parameters as surgeon expertise and soft tissue closure are unpredictable variables that are difficult to account for in the predication of final outcomes.

Traditionally, several methods for the evaluation and prediction of facial soft tissue outcomes have been described in the literature and are separately reviewed in this chapter: (1) the lateral cephalometric "line drawing" tracing prediction (manual and computer-assisted),[19-21] (2) the photographic prediction,[22,23] (3) the computerized video (digital) imaging

(video-cephalometrics) prediction,[24-38] and (4) the three-dimensional computer-assisted prediction utilizing image fusion.[39-51]

LATERAL CEPHALOMETRIC PREDICTION (MANUAL AND COMPUTER-ASSISTED)

The cephalometric soft tissue and skeletal analysis for planning orthodontic treatment has been reported as early as the 1950s and rapidly became an irreplaceable tool in the evaluation and treatment planning process for patients who require orthognathic surgery.[52] The literature is replete with reports describing different methods of cephalometric analysis, planning and prediction based on specific landmarks repositioning in response to determined skeletal movements.[1-21,24-38] Three visual treatment objective methods have traditionally used: (1) the "cut-and-paste" technique, which involves manual cutting, moving, and repositioning of cephalometric acetate overlay tracings to obtain the desired aesthetic profile as well as a class I occlusal relationship,[19,21] (2) the computer-assisted technique, which generates soft tissue prediction profile tracings by using software programs from the lateral cephalometric radiograph,[20] (3) the computer-assisted photographic imaging technique, which integrates digital images of the patient with the lateral cephalogram to predict a two-dimensional image simulation of the suitable skeletal and soft tissue profile outcome.[24-38] In all three techniques, the soft tissue profile is adjusted and changes are planned according to previously reported soft tissue–to–bone ratios. Factors influencing accuracy of such a prediction tracing include understanding of profile planning, accuracy of surgery, degree of relapse, accuracy and reproducibility of tracings, soft–to–hard tissue ratio, reliability of cephalometrics and of photography, and variation in lip posture limitation of two-dimensional planning. Authors comparing the accuracy and predictability of the manual versus the computed technique have found quite similar values in mandibular advancement planning results with only a few points differing between prediction and outcomes of cephalometric tracings.[5,7] Conversely, the hand technique has been found more accurate in the maxillary and bimaxillary prediction of soft tissue changes, particularly in the lip area.[5]

Historically, the first studies on soft tissue changes after orthognathic surgery were directed to the lower lip and chin after mandibular procedures.[53] Conversely, it was not until the mid-1970s that the first reports on soft tissue changes associated with maxillary surgery (advancement, intrusion, retrusion, or bimaxillary) were published.[2,4,11,17] This correlates with the evolution of orthognathic surgery from the lower jaw to the upper with increasing knowledge and skill.

Mandibular Surgery

The lower lip, the mentolabial fold (MLF), and the neck-chin angle are the anatomic regions most strongly influenced by the anterior or posterior surgical repositioning of the mandible.

Mandibular Advancement

The main changes affect the lower lip with a global reduction in thickness, lengthening, and straightening, as well as the chin area, with a decrease in the lower labial sulcus or MLF depth, whereas changes on the upper lip (minor anterior movement) are usually negligible, temporary, and limited only to patients with class II deep-bite deformities. The lower lip also presents the most variable soft tissue–to–bone ratios, ranging from 0.38:1 to 0.80:1, contrary to the chin ratios, which are almost invariable in a 1:1 relationship, probably due to the tight attachment of the mental soft tissue to the underlying skeletal bases[1,8,11,13,14,54] (Table 60-1).

Mandibular Setback

With mandibular horizontal retropositioning, the lower lip has been found to become more everted and shorter, with a closure of the MLF, whereas the upper lip can sometimes be displaced posteriorly with a discrete opening of the nasolabial angle. The Li:L1 (labi inferiorus:lower incisor) ratio was approximately 0.6:1, and in the chin region, Pg' (pogonion') followed Pg and the B point in an almost 1:1 ratio. These ratios have been consistently identified in several studies regardless of the magnitude of the setback movement[1,20] (Table 60-2).

Genioplasty

The most unpredictable points when planning a genioplasty are the superior and inferior vermilion borders, as well as the Pg' and Me' (menton).[1,5,15] Also, studies have shown a difference, although slight, between the sliding genioplasty and the alloplastic genioplasty (Tables 60-3 and 60-4). The relationship between the soft tissue and the bone is worst with the

setback genioplasty in which about half of the bony movement is lost because of the soft tissue response, which often can lead to a less than desirable result or a flat lower lip–chin relationship lacking the normal S curve (Table 60-5). Vertical elongation of the chin also demonstrates a poor tissue-to-bone response (Table 60-6).

Maxillary Surgery

Soft tissue changes related to maxillary surgery have proved to be relatively more unpredictable than in the mandibular surgery, regardless of the type and the amount of skeletal movement produced. The nasolabial angle and the upper lip are the anatomic regions most strongly influenced and the most variable depending on the adjunctive soft tissue procedures and neuromuscular tone.

Maxillary Advancement

The main changes induced by maxillary advancement are located in the nasal region and the upper lip. The vermilion border of the upper lip (Ls) typically advances horizontally with a rotational and translational movement around the subnasale following the upper incisor (U1) in a soft tissue–to–bone ratio ranging from 0.33:1 to 0.9:1.[1,4,6–7,9,18,55] The latter high value has been reported when a V-Y technique and nasal cinch for the closure of the maxillary vestibular incision is utilized, which prevented the thinning and shortening of the upper lip and widening of the nose invariably associated with maxillary advancements.[3] The thinning of the upper lip may result in the loss of the visible vermilion border, which is aesthetically undesirable. The nasal effects imply a decreasing of the nasolabial angle, widening of the alar bases—which can be limited by using the alar base cinch suture procedure—deepening of the supratip break, and nasal tip elevation (1 mm for every 6 mm of superior movement of the U1).[56–58] In some patients, the tip elevation may produce positive aesthetic changes, such as the disappearance of the nasal hump that usually accompanies maxillary advancement or impaction[56–58] (Tables 60-7 and 60-8).

Maxillary Impaction

Surgical repositioning of the maxilla mainly affects the morphology of the nose and upper lip in both vertical and horizontal dimensions.[1,7,9,12,16,17] The decrease in the amount of the visible vermilion due to an inward rolling of the upper lip, a down-turning of the corners of the mouth, and a widening of the alar base of the nose are the main undesirable aesthetic effects associated with the decrease of the face height resulting from this procedure. Some authors have clinically observed that such changes are probably mainly related to postoperative muscular reorientation of the oronasal area rather than to the amount of skeletal movement. The ratios of vertical shortening in the upper lip related to the superior impaction of the maxilla have been reported to range from 0.2:1 to 0.4:1 by authors who did not perform an anatomic reorientation of the facial muscles around the

TABLE 60-1. **Soft Tissue Changes Associated with Mandibular Advancement**

Anatomic Structure	Landmarks	Ratio	Author(s)
Lower lip (H)	Li: li	0.62:1	Lines and Steinhauser[11]
		0.85:1	Talbott[72]
		0.38:1	Quast et al[73]
		0.56:1	Mommaerts and Marxer[14]
		0.43:1	Hernandez-Orsini et al[74]
		0.26:1	Dermaut and De Smit[75]
		0.66:1	Thuer et al[76]
		0.8:1	Ewing and Ross[77]
		0.6:1	Mobarak et al[78]
	ILS: B pt.	0.88:1	Keeling et al[79]
	Three-dimensional analysis	1.25:1	McCance et al[43,79]
Chin (H)	Pgs: Gn	1:1	Lines and Steinhauser[11]
	Pgs: Pg	0.94:1	Hernandez-Orsini et al[74]
		0.97:1	Quast et al[73]
		1:1	Thuer et al[76]
			Keeling et al[80]
			Ewing and Ross[77]
		1.03:1	Mommaerts and Marxer[14]
		1.04:1	Talbott[72]
		1.1:1	Dermaut and De Smit[75]
		1-1.1:1	Mobarak et al[78]
	Gns: Gn	0.95:1	Hernandez-Orsini et al[74]
		0.97:1	Quast et al[73]
	Mes: Me	0.87:1	
		0.97:1	Hernandez-Orsini et al[74]
	Three-dimensional analysis	1.25:1	McCance et al[43,79]
Chin (V)	Mes: Me	0.93:1	Mommaerts and Marxer[14]
Lower labial sulcus (H)	ILS: B pt.	0.86–0.95:1	Mobarak et al[78]
		0.88:1	Thuer et al[76]
		0.93:1	Hernandez-Orsini et al[74]
		0.97:1	Quast et al[73]
		1:1	Ewing and Ross[77]
		1.01:1	Talbott[72]
		1.06:1	Mommaerts and Marxer[14]
		1.19:1	Dermaut and De Smit[75]
Upper lip (H)	Ls: Li	−0.02:1	Hernandez-Orsini et al[74]
Menton	Mes: Me	0.92–1.04:1	Mobarak et al[78]

Gn=gonion, H=horizontal, ILS= inferior labial sulcus, Li= labi inferiorus, Ls= labi superiorus, Mes= soft tissue menton, Pgs= soft tissue pogonion, V=vertical.

oronasal area. Conversely, it was shown that when a functional orientation of the musculature is accomplished (V-Y closure of maxillary vestibular incision and alar base cinch suture),[4,100] the postsurgical lip closely approaches its preoperative morphology, presenting only a minimal and negligible shortening (10%).[15] This finding is of capital importance in planning and predicting the final suitable vertical maxillary impaction and the resultant lip-to-tooth relationship. After the posterior maxillary intrusion, the soft tissue chin (MLF and Pg') has been found to autorotate on the same arc as the bony chin on in a 1:1 ratio, with the MLF angle unfolded from the inferior labial sulcus[55] (Tables 60-9 and 60-10).

Maxillary Setback

The upper lip and the nasal soft tissues closely follow the skeletal movements posteriorly.[1,7,12] As observed in advancement and intrusion cases, there is also a widening of the alar

bases with a tendency for the tip of the nose to rotate downward, with a resulting opening of the nasolabial angle.[59] This may in some patients result in a parrot's-beak nasal appearance. The same deformity can also be found after inferior repositioning of the maxilla and down graft. There is also a tendency for the upper lip to thicken after the maxillary posterior movement (see Table 60-6).

Bimaxillary Surgery

Different studies have confirmed that the soft tissue response associated with double-jaw surgery is similar to those found in single-jaw procedures, with the exception of vertical movement of the lower lip and chin.[23,27,29]

Photographic Prediction

First described by Henderson in 1974,[22] the photographic soft tissue profile planning technique has been progressively

TABLE 60-2. **Soft Tissue Changes Associated with Mandibular Setback**

Anatomic Structure	Landmarks	Ratio	Author(s)
Lower lip (H)	Li: Li	−0.75:1	Lines and Steinhauser[11]
		−0.93:1	Gjorup and Athanasiou[81]
		−1.02:1	Mobarak et al[78]
	Li: Pg	−0.5:1	Enacar et al[82]
		−0.6:1	Hershey and Smith[83]
		−0.69:1	Aaronson[84]
		−0.8:1	Gaggl et al[85]
	Three-dimensional analysis	−1:1	McCance et al[43,79]
Chin (H)	Pgs: Gn	−1:1	Lines and Steinhauser[11]
	Pgs: Pg	−0.83:1	Gaggl et al[85]
		−0.9:1	Hershey and Smith[83]
		−0.91:1	Gjorup and Athanasiou[81]
		−1:1	Robinson et al[86]
		−1.04:1	Mobarak et al[78]
	Three-dimensional analysis	−1:1	Gaggl et al[85]
Lower labial sulcus (H)	ILS: B pt.	−0.03:1	Gjorup and Athanasiou[81]
		−1:1	Robinson et al[86]
		−1.09:1	Mobarak et al[78]
	ILS: Pg	−0.93:1	Aaronson[84]
Upper lip (H)	Ls: Li	−0.2:1	Lines and Steinhauser[11]
	Ls: Pg	−0.2:1	Hershey and Smith[83]
		−0.32:1	Gaggl et al[85]

Gn=gonion, H=horizontal, ILS= inferior labial sulcus, Li= labi inferiorus, Ls= labi superiorus, Pgs= soft tissue pogonion.

abandoned owing to the difficulty in correctly obtaining a satisfactory superimposition of an enlarged photograph on the cephlometric radiograph and the evolution of more sophisticated techniques. Other techniques have used Moiré stereophotogrammetry. In general, these techniques are little used today.

TABLE 60-3. **Soft Tissue Changes Associated with Advancement Genioplasty**

Anatomic Structure	Landmarks	Ratio	Author(s)
Chin (H)	Pgs: Pg	0.57:1	Bell and Dann[87]
		0.75:1	McDonnel et al[88]
		0.67:1	Proffit and Epker[89]
		0.85:1	Bell and Gallagher[90]
		0.81:1	Gallagher et al[91]
		0.93:1	
		0.7:1	Epker and Fish[92]
		1:1	Krekmanov and Kahnberg[93]
Lip (H)	Li: Pg	0.44:1	Busquets and Sassouni[94]

H=horizontal, Li=labi inferiorus, Pgs=soft tissue pogonion.

TABLE 60-4. **Soft Tissue Changes Associated with Alloplastic Chin Implants**

Anatomic Structure	Landmarks	Ratio	Author(s)
Chin (H)	Pgs: Pg Silicone	0.60:1	Bell and Dann[87]
	Pgs: Pg Proplast	0.90:1	Dann and Epker[95]
		1:1	Proffit and Epker[89]

H=horizontal, Pgs=soft tissue pogonion.

Computerized Digital Video Imaging

Visual Treatment Objective (VTO) has been done by manual creation of simulated treatment tracings based on cephalometric radiographs. The first computer-based cephalometric systems appeared in the late 1970s.[60,61] At present, a number

TABLE 60-5. **Soft Tissue Changes Associated with Setback Genioplasty**

Anatomic Structure	Landmarks	Ratio	Author(s)
Chin (H)	Pgs: Pg	−0.33:1	Hohl and Epker[96]
		−0.50:1	Krekmanov and Kahnberg[93]
		−0.58:1	Bell[97]
	Interpositional	−0.75:1	Wessberg et al98

H=horizontal, Pgs=soft tissue pogonion.

TABLE 60-6. **Soft Tissue Changes Associated with Vertical Augmentation or Reduction Genioplasty**

Anatomic Structure	Landmarks	Ratio	Author(s)
Augmentation			
Chin (V)	Interpositional	1:1	Wessberg et al[98]
Reduction			
Chin (V)	Pgs: Pg	−0.26:1	Park et al[99]
	Mes: Me	−0.25:1	Hohl and Epker[96]
		−0.35:1	Krekmanov and Kahnberg[93]
		−0.40:1	Ewing and Ross77

Mes=soft tissue menton, Pg=pogonion, V=vertical

TABLE 60-7. **Soft Tissue Changes Associated with Maxillary Advancement with Nasolabial Muscle Reconstruction**

Anatomic Structure	Landmarks	Ratio	Author(s)
Upper lip (H)	Ls: Incisor (vertical maxillary excess)	−0.76:1	Schendel et al[17]
	Ls: Incisor (bimaxillary protrusion)	−0.66:1	
Upper lip (H)			
	Ls: Is	-0.67:1	Radney and Jacobs[16]
Upper labial sulcus (H)	SLS: Is	−0.33:1	
Nose (H)	Sn: Is	−0.33:1	
Nasolabial angle	NLA	Increase	

H=horizontal, Is=inferior stomion, Ls=labi superiorus, NLA=naso-labial angle, SLS=superior labial sulcus, SN=soft tissue nasion

of two-dimensional computer-assisted imaging systems allow image fusion of photographs, tracings, and radiographs. These computer-assisted programs permit rapid measurement and treatment planning of the skeletal and soft tissue. The validity and reliability of these systems are limited by their two-dimensional nature when dealing with a three-dimensional object.[62] The first reports on the video imaging techniques in the late 1980s dramatically changed the concept and the approach of the treatment planning and counseling in orthognathic surgery. These techniques enabled the superimposition of the lateral cephalometric radiographs and/or tracings on a two-dimensional patient's digital profile image, thus allowing the visualization as well as the manipulation of parts of the image in order to simulate the suitable aesthetic results according to the movement of the underlying maxillary bone.[25–27,29] Moreover, computer imaging provides a more realistic and tangible image of the treatment compared with the traditional "line drawing" cephalometric profile tracings of the surgical simulation. The two main advantages in using this technique are (1) the facilitation and enhancement of the communication between the orthodontist and/or the surgeon and the patient and (2) the capability of helping in the preoperative treatment planning by manipulating the images until the desired soft tissue profile is achieved. Studies have shown that 89% of surgical candidates who underwent this technique found their two-dimensional image predictions realistic and considered that the desired result was achieved.[31,33] Moreover, 83% of

TABLE 60-8. **Soft Tissue Changes Associated with Maxillary Advancement**

Anatomic Structure	Landmarks	Ratio	Author(s)
Upper lip (H)	Ls: Is	0.5:1	Dann et al[4]; Proffit and Epker[89]; Radney and Jacobs[16]; Bundgaard et al[100]
		0.62:1	Mansour et al[12]
		0.65:1	Rosenberg et al[101]
		0.74:1	Lin and Kerr[102]
		0.82:1	Rosen[103]
		0.9:1	Carlotti et al[3]
	SLS: Is	0.66:1	Hack et al[7]
		0.91:1	
	Three-dimensional analysis	1:1	McCance et al[43,79]
Upper lip (V)	Ls: Is	0.3:1	Dann et al[4]
		−0.3:1	Bundgaard et al[100]
	Ss: Is	−0.32:1	Rosen[103]
Nasolabial angle	Nasolabial angle: Is	−1.2°:1	Dann et al[4]
Nasal tip (H)	Pn: Is	0.28:1	Dann et al[4]
		0.36:1	Hack et al[7]
	Pn: Ia	0.17:1	Proffit and Epker[89]
Nasal base (H)	Sn: A pt.	0.57:1	Freihofer[104]
		0.51:1	Rosen[103]
	Sn: A pt. (thick lip)	0.3:1	Stella et al[18]
	Sn: A pt. (thin lip)	0.46:1	
	Sn: Ia	0.24:1	Mansour et al[2]
	Sn: ANS	0.60:1	Hack et al[7]
	Three-dimensional analysis	1.25:1	Ewing and Ross[77]
Upper labial sulcus (H)	SLS: Ia	0.52:1	Mansour et al[12]
	SLS: A pt	0.38:1	Hack et al[7]
		0.76:1	Lin and Kerr[102]

ANS=anterior nasal spine, H=horizontal, Ia=incisor point, Is=inferior stomion, Ls=labi superiorus, Pn=pronasale, SLS=superior labial sulcus, Sn=soft tissue nasion, Ss=stomion superius, V=vertical.

TABLE 60-9. **Soft Tissue Changes Associated with Maxillary Impaction**

Anatomic Structure	Landmarks	Ratio	Author(s)
Upper lip (V)	Ls: Is	−0.38:1	Schendel et al[17]
		−0.51:1	
		−0.3:1	Radney and Jacobs[16]
	SS: Is	−0.4:1	
	SLS: Is	−0.42:1	Mansour et al[12]
	Ls: Pr	−0.31:1	
	Ls: ANS	−0.06:1	Sakima and Sachdeva[105]
	SS: ANS	−0.41:1	
Upper lip (H)	Ls: Ia	0.89:1	Mansour et al[12]
Upper labial sulcus (V)	SLS: Is	−0.25:1	Radney and Jacobs[16]
	SLS: ANS	0.12:1	Sakima and Sachdeva[105]
Upper labial sulcus (H)	SLS: Ia	0.76:1	Mansour et al[12]
Nose (V)	Sn: Is	−0.2:1	Radney and Jacobs[16]
	Pn: Is	−0.16:1	
	Pn: Pr	−0.15:1	Mansour et al[12]
Nasal base (V)	Sn: Pr	−0.28:1	
Full Face Evaluation			
Upper lip (middle) (H)	Three-dimensional analysis	1:1	McCance et al[43,79]
Alar Base (H)	Three-dimensional analysis	1.25:1	
Nasal base (V)	Sn: ANS	0.29:1	Hack et al[7]
Upper labial sulcus (V)	SLS: A pt	0.54:1	
Upper lip (V)	SLS: Is	0.72:1	

ANS=anterior nasal spine, H=horizontal, Ia=incisor point, Is=inferior stomion, Ss= stomion superius, Ls=labi superiorus, Pn=pronasale, Pr=porion, V=vertical.

patients found that this technique was useful in deciding whether or not to under-go orthognathic surgery.[31,33] The most problematic and challenging parameter to solve is to accurately calculate the postoperative soft-to-hard tissue changes, given the variability of the soft tissue thickness, tonicity as well as translations relative to bony changes and the two-dimensionality of the system. For the moment, the currently used commercial preprogrammed algorithms are based on clinically retrospective studies of stability of the soft tissues after bone and dental movements and use default soft-to-hard tissues ratios. The utilization of such default ratios accounts for some of the variability and inaccuracy in predicting the soft tissue outcome regardless of the technique, manual versus computed. Studies revealed several specifics concerning the accuracy and reliability of predictions regardless of the software program used: (1) upper and lower lips are the least accurately predictable regions, probably owing to a high individual variability in thickness and tonicity, (2) the vertical plane prediction changes are generally more accurate than in the sagittal plane, and (3) sagittal changes are more easily perceived than vertical changes.[27,33]

TABLE 60-10. **Soft Tissue Changes Associated with Mandibular Autorotation**

Anatomic Structure	Landmarks	Ratio	Author(s)
Lower lip (H)	Li: Ii	0.75:1	Mansour et al[12]
Lower lip (V)	Si: Is	−0.93:1	
	Si: Me	−1.03:1	Sakima and Sachdeva[105]
	Li: Me	−1.48:1	
Chin (H)	Pgs: Pg	0.86:1	Gaggl et al[85]
		1:1	Radney and Jacobs[16]
	Pgs: Me	0.79:1	Sakima and Sachdeva[105]
Chin (V)	Pgs: Gn	−0.8:1	Lines and Steinhauser[11]
	Pgs: Me	−0.98:1	Sakima and Sachdeva[105]
	Mes: Me	−1.2:1	Mansour et al[12]
Lower labial sulcus (H)	ILS: B pt.	0.9:1	Mansour et al[12]
		1:1	Radney and Jacobs[16]
Inferior labial sulcus (V)	ILS: Me	−1.05:1	Sakima and Sachdeva[105]
Inferior labial sulcus (H)	ILS: Me	0.61:1	

H=horizontal, Gn=gonion, Ii= lower incisor, ILS=inferior labial sulcus, Is=inferior stomion, Li= labi inferiorus, Me=menton, Pgs=soft tissue pogonion, Si= soft tissue incisor, V= vertical.

Mandibular Advancement

Dentofacial Planner Plus and *Quick Ceph Image* software programs have been found to be relatively accurate in predicting changes in the lower third of the face associated with mandibular advancement.[24,35] Changes of reference points between the computer's predicted and post-treatment tracings in the lower lip in the vertical plane are more predictable than in the sagittal plane, thus the final preoperative computed prediction usually tends to be more protrusive than the actual value, whereas the opposite is true in the chin area, with a soft tissue pogonion (Po') that tends to be more superior.[24,35] An overall predictability of more than 80% can be attained particularly in the lip area, whereas the least predictable region is the submental area.[24,35] On the contrary, authors who tested the *Prescription Planner/Portrait* software found that the computer-predicted lower lip was more retrusive and thinner than on the actual profile, and they found no differences between patients who underwent mandibular advancement alone versus associated with genioplasty.[36,37]

Mandibular Setback

The only available study used *Quick Ceph Image* and *Portrait Planner* software programs and showed that (1) the results were accurate enough for use in communication and patient education, (2) 30% of the sample showed significant errors greater than 2 mm and these errors were bigger in the vertical plane in the area of the lower lip, with a tendency to underestimate the amount of lip retraction, and also in the chin area, (3) the accuracy and predictability were not as good as in mandibular advancements, probably owing to the technique of image compression, and (4) both software programs showed similar results.[26]

Bimaxillary Surgery

Several studies evaluating the accuracy of computerized surgical prediction methods using the *Quick Ceph Image* software program showed that the most important discrepancies between the computer generated tracing versus the actual tracing were the following: (1) the lower lip tended to be predicted more inferior, shorter, and more protrusive than on the actual profile, (2) the upper lip tended to be shorter, with the superior labial sulcus located more posterior than on the actual profile, and (3) the soft tissue pogonion (Pg') was located more inferior than on the actual profile. These differences have been found to be probably related to the inaccuracy and variability of the default soft-to-hard tissue ratios used by the software rather than to the type of maxillary movement, association of mandibular or genioplasty procedure ,or type of closure of the Le Fort I incision (V-Y vs. non V-Y).[38]

Authors who have tested the *DentoFacial Planner* software in predicting changes in patients who underwent a Le Fort I procedure (advancement and intrusion) found that the nasal tip and the subnasale on the computer prediction were more posterior than on the actual profile.[28]

Maxillary Impaction

The utilization of *Orthognathic Treatment Planner (OPT)* and *Prescription Portrait* software programs have shown a good global accuracy and reliability to within 1.5 mm in the majority of the measurements, but better in the sagittal plane.[30]

Three-dimensional Computer-Assisted Prediction

The foremost critique, which could be addressed to the previous methods of prediction, is that the analyses were based on two-dimensional lateral cephalograms, whereas the actual soft tissue changes are of course always three-dimensional! For this reason, current efforts are all directed in developing as accurately as possible a reliable and easily usable three-dimensional computer treatment planning software to predict the facial soft tissue outcome in response to skeletal movements as close as possible to reality.

In the early 1980s, different authors, supported by the advances in three-dimensional computed tomography (CT) scanning techniques, pointed out the importance of the management of the third dimension in the evaluation and surgical planning of craniofacial surgery, inaugurating a new and exciting era.[40,45] The first rudimentary computer-assisted software programs were at the beginning elaborated only for planning osteotomies and bone relocation, without taking into account the soft tissue envelope changes.[40,45] In the mid-1990s, the need to improve the three-dimensional soft tissue representation and prediction gave rise to a tremendous impetus, which led to a plethora of more or less reliable and accurate computer systems.[39,43,46] One of the most used methods in assessing the three-dimensional details of the face is based on cone beam computed tomography (CBCT) scan data, which allows the separate visualization of the different constituents of the facial anatomy, thus enabling the surgeon to differentiate and separately manipulate the bone from the air and soft tissue surfaces.[39,41-44,46-50]

Even though the CBCT scan has the capacity of displaying both bone and soft tissue details, the three-dimensional reconstructed soft tissue images are generally incomplete and not lifelike. For this reason, some authors have recommended the simultaneous use of laser surface scanner images or photogrammetric images, which are merged with the scan images, in order to improve the quality and accuracy of the production of the three-dimensional facial morphology.[41,42]

Dolphin Imaging software can integrate and superimpose traditional two-dimensional photographs with digital two-dimensional lateral and frontal cephalometric radiographs. Two-dimensional photographs can also be imported and wrapped onto three-dimensional CBCT and CT images for presentation purposes (Figures 60-1 to 60-4). Dolphin Imaging allows the operator to use both orthogonal and perspective projection-type cephalometric renderings. Visualization filters can then be applied and transparency adjusted for viewing the soft and hard tissues. Virtual orientation of the face imaging space using the semitransparent filter allows the operator to rotate and orient the virtual patients, optimally matching bilateral and anatomic structures. Simulation of surgical results and soft tissue movement is possible only in the two-dimensional environment. Traditionally, in photogrammetry as seen previously, separate three-dimensional data sets (each containing its own coordinate system) are generated for each viewpoint, as a range map, and are subsequently stitched together to produce a new overall three-dimensional coordinate system. Stitching multiple sides together has historically worked well for data input of "inanimate objects" in which motion is not a factor. This technique does not work well when the subjects are animate, because "stitching" separate three-dimensional images together to generate a single three-dimensional model of the patient can compromise accuracy owing to the discontinuity of surface information. There is no guarantee that two separate images taken at different points of time with the movement factor will still match and can result in a fracture of information along the midline. This compromises accuracy. The preferable way to generate a three-dimensional surface image derived from multiple viewpoints is to generate a single unified and continuous coordinate system by selecting the best quality data for any given xyz coordinate from each of the viewpoints. For this to work, the reconstructive algorithms must be able to place a value on the quality of each point generated. This is the great advantage of using active photogrammetry and very fast capture time incorporated in systems such as the 3dMD system.

The importance of three-dimensional virtual surgical planning increases with the complexity of the deformity and reconstruction needed to correct it. Three-dimensional image fusion has further increased the importance and accuracy of virtual treatment planning and several systems are now available. At the center of the three-dimensional approach is the "**P**atient-**S**pecific **A**natomic **R**econstruction" (**PSAR**), which is an anatomically accurate record in which all of the patient's three-dimensional images are superimposed into one valid three-dimensional structure and combined with the relevant biomechanical properties and is called *Image Fusion*.[61,62] There are a number of potential advantages of registering anatomically accurate three-dimensional facial surface images to CT/CBCT data sets.

- Surface images may correct for CBCT surface artifacts of the soft tissue caused by patient movement.
- Independently acquired surface images compensate for soft tissue compression from upright CBCT device stabilization aids (i.e., chin rest, forehead restraint) or from supine soft tissue draping changes.
- Surface images most notably may supplement missing anatomical data (e.g., nose, chin).
- Surface images may provide a more accurate representation of the soft tissue that reflects the patient's natural head position for diagnosis and treatment planning.

In relation to surface three-dimensional construction, a surface image has two components, the geometry of the face and the color information, or texture map, that is mathematically applied to the shape information.

Stereo photogrammetry is the optical method of obtaining an image by means of one or more stereo pairs of photographs taken simultaneously. The concept was first applied to the face as early as 1967.[63] This technique differs from the other optics-based methods in that it requires no special pattern projection and the subject can be illuminated with regular photographic flash. Once the three-dimensional geometry of researchers have reported accurate identification of facial landmarks from 0.5 to 0.2 mm.[64–67]

In the early 2000s, studies were focused mainly on the generation of real-time and mathematical realistic modeling of nonlinear three-dimensional soft tissue deformations occurring simultaneously with the underlying bone movements, such as the CASP technique (computer-assisted three-dimensional virtual reality soft tissue planning and prediction for orthognathic surgery), which is based on three-dimensional reconstructed CT images combined with surface data as follows: processing of CT data using a specific algorithm and soft tissue and bone segmentation, generation of a three-dimensional color individualizing facial model by mixing digitized color photographs with the reconstructed three-dimensional soft tissue (color facial texture-mapping technique), and utilization of two separate algorithms to study the soft tissue model deformation.[48–51] The final result is a virtual reality workbench, which allows a real-time generation of individualized predicted and animated color

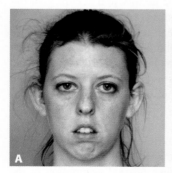 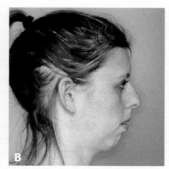 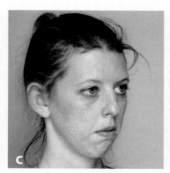 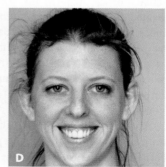

FIGURE 60-1. Preoperative views. Young woman with combined maxillary and mandibular deformity and muscle hyperfunction, class II malocclusion with vertical maxillary excess, and microgenia. **A,** Frontal. **B,** Lateral. **C,** Three-quarter view. **D,** Smiling.

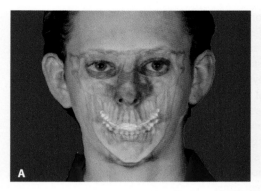
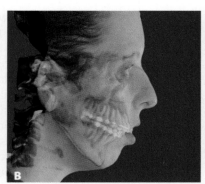
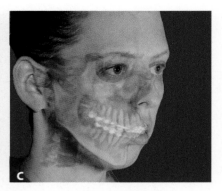

FIGURE 60-2. Preoperative dolphin views with semitransparent soft tissue. **A,** Frontal. **B,** Lateral. **C,** Three-quarter view.

facial models resulting from translation and rotation of the underlying bone.

Recent studies have described three-dimensional soft tissue prediction procedures using two different mathematical simulation models based on the finite element method (FEM) or mass spring. Studies have shown the sound superiority of the three-dimensional technique over the two-dimensional software programs in predicting the lower third of the face, especially in the lip and chin area.[41,42] This type of technique is seen in the 3dMDface,[68] Vultus System, which allow the capture of the face surface by using a multiple camera views synchronized in a single capture to produce a single three-dimensional polygon surface mesh. The surfaces images obtained with no radiation are then visualized and manipulated using a specific software platform.

Workup

Initiation of the patient *workup* requires collecting, cataloging, and archiving of all relevant three-dimensional image data sets related to one point in time, referred to as an *episode of care*. Registration of the data sets could be performed using fiducial markers, but there are considerable workflow and quality drawbacks to this method, including the additional time needed to place the markers themselves and image distortion. A more direct method is to do a best-fit scenario between the data sets. The first step in this registration process entails segmentation of the outer surface of the CBCT data to generate a separate object that represents the outer geometry keeping the original spatial relationship (*DICOM skin*). Next, the geometry of the three-dimensional optical surface image is registered to the DICOM skin, which acts as the reference object to ensure that the three-dimensional surface adopts the coordinate system of the DICOM upon completion. If the software is well designed and user-friendly, superimposition should only take less than 30 seconds to complete. After registration, numerous options allow interaction with the data sets by rendering the volumes either independently or separately including scrolling through the volume in three-dimensional or simultaneously in the coronal, sagittal, and axial planes.

Simulation refers to an imitation of a real-world process in a computer program using mathematical models to study

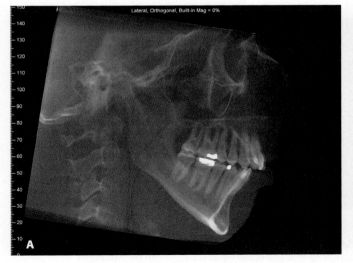
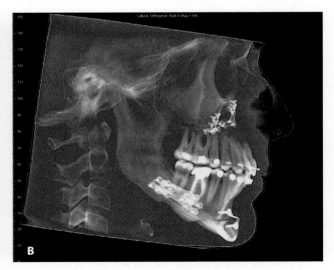

FIGURE 60-3. Cephalometric radiographs demonstrate maxillary impaction and slight advancement with larger mandibular advancement and associated chin advancement by sliding osteotomy. **A,** Preoperative. **B,** Postoperative.

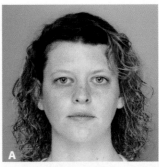
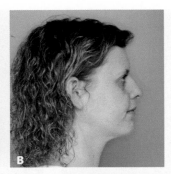
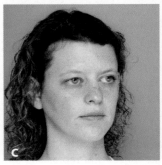
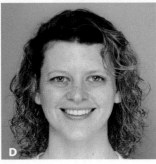

FIGURE 60-4. Postoperative facial views. Perioral muscle reconstruction was done per Schendel to prevent unaesthetic nasal and lip changes.[58, 59] **A,** Frontal. **B,** Lateral. **C,** Three quarter view. **D,** Smiling.

the effects of the changing parameters and conditions to make a decision. Computer-based simulation gives the clinician the opportunity to perform virtual surgery or treatment, increasing the possibility of a successful outcome with no risk to the patient.

The Mass-Spring Model technique of simulation involves implementing a biomechanical model that defines the relationship between the hard and the soft tissue with hundreds of thousands of nonlinear connector points. This generates three-dimensional deformable tissue models that include spring-based force computations to model the physical characteristics of real tissue reactions. This mechanism simulates deformable tissues, such as the soft tissue of the face. The models employ force computations from physical laws and study of facial surgery cases and apply these forces to the three-dimensional model components. The computations modeled include tissue deformation and relaxation; external forces such as gravity; and three-dimensional collision detection with force feedback. The advantage of this approach is that computations are well within the power of available PCs and occur in real time.

Results

Use of three-dimensional imaging and computer simulation for treatment occurs as the following patient demonstrates. Figure 60-5 shows the stages in treatment planning for a young woman with mandibular retrusion. The PSAR has been created by the 3dMD Vultus system and the profile and three-quarter views are visualized in Figure 60-5. Osteotomies are simulated for the mandibular advancement by the sagittal split ramus osteotomy technique and the resultant mandibular advancement done virtually. The result is displayed and altered until the aesthetic and functional result desired is achieved. The measurements in all three planes of space are then automatically generated (Figure 60-6). The soft tissue is simultaneously reconstructed and the final aesthetic result can be seen in the virtual environment (Figure 60-7). Surgery can then proceed along these guidelines (Figure 60-8). The actual soft tissue changes occurring with surgery can be visualized in a histogram with the actual spot measurements recorded (Figure 60-9). We have found this system to be accurate for advancement surgery of either the maxilla or the mandible (Figure 60-10). Inaccuracies in the soft tissue simulation arise when vertical movements are

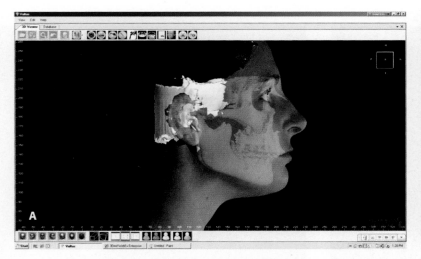
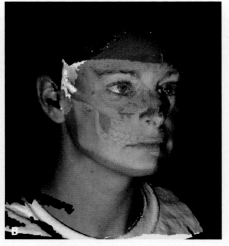

FIGURE 60-5. **A,** Patient-specific anatomic reconstruction (PSAR) of a case of a young woman with mandibular retrusion. The profile view is shown. The skin has been made semitransparent so that the underlying skeleton can be visualized. Only the bone, only the soft tissue, or a combined image with variable transparency can be visualized such as shown here. **B,** Three-quarter view.

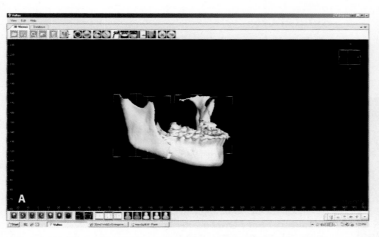
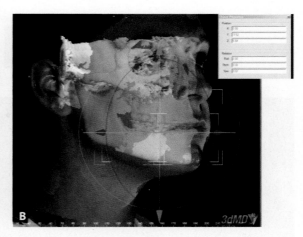

FIGURE 60-6. **A,** Osteotmies marked on the mandible only, which has been isolated. Note that the sagittal split osteotomies are anatomically correct and can be varied according to the need by the surgeon. **B,** Jaws repositioned on the PSAR of the skeleton and transparent soft tissue with actual surgical three-dimensional vectors shown.

undertaken or when there is preexisting soft tissue deformation from the device or muscle hyperfunction in the original data set. Also, soft tissue variations occur according to how each surgeon handles the soft tissues and what adjunctive techniques are performed. Because of these facts, the soft tissue simulation module should include the ability to rearrange the tissues based on the surgeon's experience. The Vultus system has such an option, and we have found it very accurate when this is done.

DISCUSSION

Correctly planning and accurately predicting surgical outcome is paramount in facial surgery. Gossett and coworkers[69] have outlined a three-fold purpose for computer-simulated predictions: (1) guide the treatment to the desired result, (2) give the patient a reasonable preview of the outcome; and (3) serve as a communication tool between orthodontist, surgeon, and patient. Advancements in computer imaging have revolu-

tionized the treatment of dentofacial deformities and specifically orthognathic surgery. Use of this image fusion technology now permits the creation of PSARs on a routine basis, and a more comprehensive diagnosis and treatment plan can, thus, be obtained. Both the skeletal and the associated soft tissue changes thus become more accurate and predictable. At this point, no system is fully automatic but the present systems provide a great improvement over the old two-dimensional soft tissue calculations. Surgeon experience and incite are still important parts of obtaining the desired functional and aesthetic result. In the end, treatment outcomes are improved. The ideal system would predict the soft tissue behavior resulting from the movements of the underlying bone and

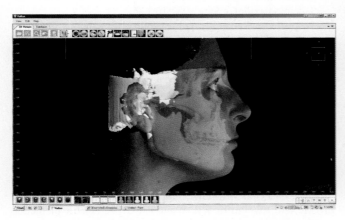

FIGURE 60-7. Reconstructed facial soft tissues in the virtual model of the profile after simulated surgery. Again, the overlying soft tissue has been made semitransparent to help with the visualization.

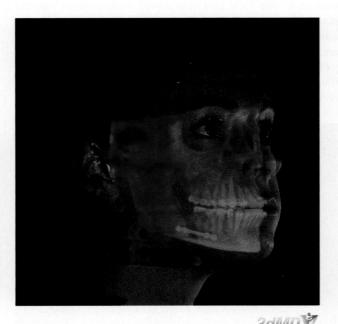

FIGURE 60-8. Actual postoperative result from mandibular advancement with transparent skin.

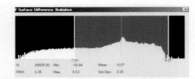

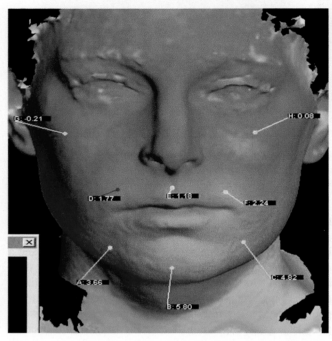

FIGURE 60-9. Histogram created shows the actual postoperative soft tissue changes. The areas with more change are indicated by *orange to red colors*. Spot measurements can be done as shown.

transfer of the ideal and customized computerized surgical plan to the operating room. In conclusion, it should be kept in mind that all the previously mentioned prediction techniques are strongly dependent on rapidly developing technology subject to daily improvements. Different studies have shown that the accuracy and reliability are far from perfect yet but are constantly improving.[70,71]

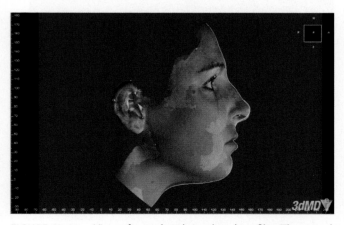

FIGURE 60-10. View of actual and simulated profiles. The actual profile is outlined in *green* for visualization. Note the good overall accuracy.

References

1. Betts N, Fonseca R. Soft tissue changes associated with orthognathic surgery. In Bell WH, editor. Modern Practice in Orthognathic and Reconstructive Surgery, Vol III. Philadelphia: WB Saunders; 1992.
2. Burstone CJ, James RB, Legan H, et al. Cephalometrics for orthognathic surgery. J Oral Surg 1978;36:269.
3. Carlotti AE Jr, Aschaffenburg PH, Schendel SA. Facial changes associated with surgical advancement of the lip and maxilla. J Oral Maxillofac Surg 1986;44:593.
4. Dann JJ 3rd, Fonseca RJ, Bell WH. Soft tissue changes associated with total maxillary advancement: a preliminary study. J Oral Surg 1976;34:19.
5. Eckhardt CE, Cunningham SJ. How predictable is orthognathic surgery? Eur J Orthod 2004;26:303.
6. Ewing M, Ross RB. Soft tissue response to orthognathic surgery in persons with unilateral cleft lip and palate. Cleft Palate Craniofac J 1993;30:320.
7. Hack GA, de Mol van Otterloo JJ, Nanda R. Long-term stability and prediction of soft tissue changes after Le Fort I surgery. Am J Orthod Dentofacial Orthop 1993;104:544.
8. Iizuka T, Eggensperger N, Smolka W, Thuer U. Analysis of soft tissue profile changes after mandibular advancement surgery. Oral Surg Oral Med Oral Pathol Oral Radiol Endod 2004;98:16.
9. Jensen AC, Sinclair PM, Wolford LM. Soft tissue changes associated with double jaw surgery. Am J Orthod Dentofacial Orthop 1992;101:266.
10. Legan HL, Burstone CJ. Soft tissue cephalometric analysis for orthognathic surgery. J Oral Surg 1980;38:744.
11. Lines P, Steinhauser W. Soft tissue changes in relationship of movement of hard structures in orthognathic surgery. J Oral Surg 1974;32:891.
12. Mansour S, Burstone C, Legan H. An evaluation of soft-tissue changes resulting from Le Fort I maxillary surgery. Am J Orthod 1983;84:37.
13. Mobarak KA, Espeland L, Krogstad O, Lyberg T. Soft tissue profile changes following mandibular advancement surgery: predictability and long-term outcome. Am J Orthod Dentofacial Orthop 2001;119:353.
14. Mommaerts MY, Marxer H. A cephalometric analysis of the long-term, soft tissue profile changes which accompany the advancement of the mandible by sagittal split ramus osteotomies. J Craniomaxillofac Surg 1987;15:127.
15. Pospisil OA. Reliability and feasibility of prediction tracing in orthognathic surgery. J Craniomaxillofac Surg 1987;15:79.
16. Radney LJ, Jacobs JD. Soft-tissue changes associated with surgical total maxillary intrusion. Am J Orthod 1981;80:191.
17. Schendel SA, Eisenfeld JH, Bell WH, Epker BN. Superior repositioning of the maxilla: stability and soft tissue osseous relations. Am J Orthod 1976;70:663.
18. Stella JP, Streater MR, Epker BN, Sinn DP. Predictability of upper lip soft tissue changes with maxillary advancement. J Oral Maxillofac Surg 1989;47:697.
19. Cohen MI. Mandibular prognathism. Am J Orthod 1965;51:368.
20. Hing NR. The accuracy of computer generated prediction tracings. Int J Oral Maxillofac Surg 1989;18:148.
21. McNeill RW, Proffit WR, White RP. Cephalometric prediction for orthodontic surgery. Angle Orthod 1972;42:154.
22. Henderson D. The assessment and management of bony deformities of the middle and lower face. Br J Plast Surg 1974;27:287.

23. Kinnebrew MC, Hoffman DR, Carlton DM. Projecting the soft-tissue outcome of surgical and orthodontic manipulation of the maxillofacial skeleton. Am J Orthod 1983;84:508.

24. Aharon PA, Eisig S, Cisneros GJ. Surgical prediction reliability: a comparison of two computer software systems. Int J Adult Orthod Orthognath Surg 1997;12:65.

25. Chunmaneechote P, Friede H. Mandibular setback osteotomy: facial soft tissue behavior and possibility to improve the accuracy of the soft tissue profile prediction with the use of a computerized cephalometric program: Quick Ceph Image Pro: v. 2.5. Clin Orthod Res 1999;2:85.

26. Kazandjian S, Sameshima GT, Champlin T, Sinclair PM. Accuracy of video imaging for predicting the soft tissue profile after mandibular set-back surgery. Am J Orthod Dentofacial Orthop 1999;115:382.

27. Koh CH, Chew MT. Predictability of soft tissue profile changes following bimaxillary surgery in skeletal class III Chinese patients. J Oral Maxillofac Surg 2004;62:1505.

28. Konstiantos KA, O'Reilly MT, Close J. The validity of the prediction of soft tissue profile changes after Le Fort I osteotomy using the dentofacial planner (computer software). Am J Orthod Dentofacial Orthop 1994;105:241.

29. Lu CH, Ko EW, Huang CS. The accuracy of video imaging prediction in soft tissue outcome after bimaxillary orthognathic surgery. J Oral Maxillofac Surg 2003;61:333.

30. Sameshima GT, Kawakami RK, Kaminishi RM, Sinclair PM. Predicting soft tissue changes in maxillary impaction surgery: a comparison of two video imaging systems. Angle Orthod 1997;67:347.

31. Sarver DM. Video imaging—a computer facilitated approach to communication and planning in orthognathic surgery. Br J Orthod 1993;20:187.

32. Sarver DM, Johnston MW. Video imaging: techniques for superimposition of cephalometric radiography and profile images. Int J Adult Orthod Orthognath Surg 1990;5:241.

33. Sarver DM, Johnston MW, Matukas VJ. Video imaging for planning and counseling in orthognathic surgery. J Oral Maxillofac Surg 1988;46:939.

34. Sarver DM, Weissman SM. Long-term soft tissue response to Le Fort I maxillary superior repositioning. Angle Orthod 1991;61:267.

35. Schultes G, Gaggl A, Karcher H. Accuracy of cephalometric and video imaging program Dentofacial Planner Plus in orthognathic surgical planning. Comput Aided Surg 1998;3:108.

36. Sinclair PM, Kilpelainen P, Phillips C, et al. The accuracy of video imaging in orthognathic surgery. Am J Orthod Dentofacial Orthop 1995;107:177.

37. Syliangco ST, Sameshima GT, Kaminishi RM, Sinclair PM. Predicting soft tissue changes in mandibular advancement surgery: a comparison of two video imaging systems. Angle Orthod 1997;67:337.

38. Upton PM, Sadowsky PL, Sarver DM, Heaven TJ. Evaluation of video imaging prediction in combined maxillary and mandibular orthognathic surgery. Am J Orthod Dentofacial Orthop 1997;112:656.

39. Altobelli DE, Kikinis R, Mulliken JB, et al. Computer-assisted three-dimensional planning in craniofacial surgery. Plast Reconstr Surg 1993;92:576–585; discussion 586.

40. Cutting C, Bookstein FL, Grayson B, et al. Three-dimensional computer-assisted design of craniofacial surgical procedures: optimization and interaction with cephalometric and CT-based models. Plast Reconstr Surg 1986;77:877.

41. Holberg C, Heine AK, Geis P, et al. Three-dimensional soft tissue prediction using finite elements. Part II: clinical application. J Orofac Orthop 2005;66:122.

42. Holberg C, Schwenzer K, Rudzki-Janson I. Three-dimensional soft tissue prediction using finite elements. Part I: implementation of a new procedure. J Orofac Orthop 2005;66:110.

43. McCance AM, Moss JP, Fright WR, et al. A three-dimensional analysis of soft and hard tissue changes following bimaxillary orthognathic surgery in skeletal III patients. Br J Oral Maxillofac Surg 1992;30:305.

44. Meller S, Nkenke E, Kalender WA. Statistical face models for the rediction of soft-tissue deformations after orthognathic osteotomies. Med Image Comput Comput Assist Interv 2005;8:443.

45. Moss JP, Grindrod SR, Linney AD, et al. A computer system for the interactive planning and prediction of maxillofacial surgery. Am J Orthod Dentofacial Orthop 1988;94:469.

46. Moss JP, McCance AM, Fright WR, et al. A three-dimensional soft tissue analysis of fifteen patients with class II, division 1 malocclusions after bimaxillary surgery. Am J Orthod Dentofacial Orthop 1994;105:430.

47. Westermark A, Zachow S, Eppley BL. Three-dimensional osteotomy planning in maxillofacial surgery including soft tissue prediction. J Craniofac Surg 2005;16:100.

48. Xia J, Ip HH, Samman N, et al. Three-dimensional virtual-reality surgical planning and soft-tissue prediction for orthognathic surgery. IEEE Trans Inf Technol Biomed 2001;5:97.

49. Xia J, Samman N, Yeung RW, et al. Computer-assisted three-dimensional surgical planing and simulation. 3D soft tissue planning and prediction. Int J Oral Maxillofac Surg 2000;29:250.

50. Xia J, Wang D, Samman N, et al. Computer-assisted three-dimensional surgical planning and simulation: 3D color facial model generation. Int J Oral Maxillofac Surg 2000;29:2.

51. Xia JJ, Gateno J, Teichgraeber JF. Three-dimensional computer-aided surgical simulation for maxillofacial surgery. Atlas Oral Maxillofac Surg Clin North Am 2005;13:25.

52. Broadbent B. A new technique and its application in orthodontics Angle Orthod 1931;2:45.

53. Trauner R, Obwegeser H. The surgical correction of mandibular prognathism and retrognathia with consideration of genioplasty. I. Surgical procedures to correct mandibular prognathism and reshaping of the chin. Oral Surg Oral Med Oral Pathol 1957;10:677.

54. Joss CU, Joss-Vassalli IM, Kiliaridis S, Kuijpers-Jagtman AM. Soft tissue profile changes after bilateral sagittal split osteotomy for mandibular advancement: a systematic review. J Oral Maxillofac Surg 2010;68:1260.

55. Carlotti AE Jr, Schendel SA. An analysis of factors influencing stability of surgical advancement of the maxilla by the Le Fort I osteotomy. J Oral Maxillofac Surg 1987;45:924.

56. O'Ryan F, Carlotti A. Nasal anatomy and maxillary surgery. III. Surgical techniques for correction of nasal deformities in patients undergoing maxillary surgery. Int J Adult Orthod Orthognath Surg 1989;4:157.

57. O'Ryan F, Schendel S. Nasal anatomy and maxillary surgery. I. Esthetic and anatomic principles. Int J Adult Orthod Orthognath Surg 1989;4:27.

58. O'Ryan F, Schendel S. Nasal anatomy and maxillary surgery. II. Unfavorable nasolabial esthetics following the Le Fort I osteotomy. Int J Adult Orthodon Orthognath Surg 1989;4:75.

59. Mason, M. and Schendel, S.A., "Perioral Procedures as an Adjunct to Orthognathic Surgery, Oral and Maxillofacial Surgery Clinics of North America, 8(1):95–110, 1996.

60. Schendel, S, Eisenfeld J, Bell WH, et al. The long face syndrome: vertical maxillary excess. Am J Orthod 1976;70:398–408.

61. Schendel SA, Lane C, Duncan K. 3D orthognathic simulation using image fusion. In Farmand A, editor. Seminars in Orthodontics. Vol 15. 2009; pp. 48–56.

62. Schendel SA, Jacobson R. Three-dimensional imaging and computer simulation for office based surgery. J Oral Maxfac Surg 2009;67:2107–2114.

63. Schendel S, Montgomery K, Sorokin A, Lionetti G. A surgical simulator for planning and performing repair of cleft lips. J Craniomaxillofac Surg 2005:33;223–228.

64. Burke PH, Beard FH. Stereophotogrammetry of the face. A preliminary investigation into the accuracy of a simplified system evolved for contour mapping by photography. Am J Orthod 1967;53:769–782.

65. Ayoub A, Garrahy A, Hood C, et al. Validation of a vision-based, three-dimensional facial imaging system. Cleft Palate Craniofac J 2003;40:523–529.

66. Ayoub AF, Wray D, Moos KF, et al. Three-dimensional modeling for modern diagnosis and planning in maxillofacial surgery. Int J Adult Orthod Orthognath Surg 1996;11:225–233.

67. Khambay B, Nairn N, Bell A, et al. Validation and reproducibility of a high-resolution three-dimensional facial imaging system. Br J Oral Maxillofac Surg. 2008;46:27–32.

68. 3dMDface System. Availible at www.3dmd.com

69. Gossett CB, Preston CB, Dunford R, et al. Prediction accuracy of computer-assisted surgical visual treatment objectives. J Oral Maxillofac Surg 2005;63:609.

70. Donatsky O, Bjorn-Jorgensen J, Hermund NU, et al. Accuracy of combined maxillary and mandibular repositioning and of soft tissue prediction in relation to maxillary antero-superior repositioning combined with mandibular set back A computerized cephalometric evaluation of the immediate postsurgical outcome using the TIOPS planning system. J Craniomaxillofac Surg 2009;37:279.

71. Jones RM, Khambay BS, McHugh S, Ayoub AF. The validity of a computer-assisted simulation system for orthognathic surgery (CASSOS) for planning the surgical correction of class III skeletal deformities: single-jaw versus bimaxillary surgery. Int J Oral Maxillofac Surg 2007;36:900.

72. Talbott J. Soft tissue response to mandibular advancement surgery [master's thesis]. Lexington: University of Kentucky; 1975.

73. Quast DC, Biggerstaff R, Haley JV. The short-term and long-term soft-tissue profile changes accompanying mandibular advancement surgery. Am J Orthod 1983;84:29–36.

74. Hernandez-Orsini R, Jacobson A, Sarver DM, et al. Short-term and long-term soft tissue profile changes after mandibular advancements using rigid fixation techniques. Int J Adult Orthod Orthognath Surg 1989;4:209–218.

75. Dermaut LR, De Smit A. Effects of sagittal split advancement osteotomy on facial profiles. Eur J Orthod 1989;11:366–374.

76. Thuer U, Ingervall B, Vuillemin T. Stability and effect on the soft tissue profile of mandibular advancement with sagittal split osteotomy and rigid internal fixation. Int J Adult Orthodon Orthognath Surg 1994;9:175–185.

77. Ewing M, Ross R. Soft tissue response to mandibular advancement and genioplasty. Am J Orthod Dentofacial Orthop 1992;101:550–555.

78. Mobarak KA, Krogstad O, Espeland L, Lyberg T. Factors influencing the predictability of soft tissue profile changes following mandibular setback surgery. Angle Orthod 2001;71:216–227.

79. McCance AM, Moss JP, Fright WR, et al. A three-dimensional soft tissue analysis of 16 skeletal class III patients following bimaxillary surgery. Br J Oral Maxillofac Surg 1992;30:221–227.

80. Keeling SD, Labanc J, Van Sickels JE, et al. Skeletal change at surgery as a predictor of long-term soft tissue profile change after mandibular advancement. J Oral Maxillofac Surg 1996;54:134–144.

81. Gjorup H, Athanasiou AE. Soft tissues and dentoskeletal profile changes associated with mandibular setback osteotomy. Am J Orthod Dentofac Orthop 1991;100:312–323.

82. Enacar A, Taner T, Toroglus S. Analysis of soft tissue profile changes associated with mandibular setback and double jaw surgeries. Int J Adult Orthod Orthognath Surg 1999;14:27–35.

83. Hershey HG, Smith L. Soft tissue profile change associated with surgical correction of the prognathic mandible. Am J Orthod 1974;65:483–503.

84. Aaronson S. A cephalometric investigation of the surgical correction of mandibular prognathism. Angle Orthod 1967;379:251.

85. Gaggl A, Schultes G, Karcher H. Changes in soft tissue profile after sagittal split ramus osteotomy and retropositioning of the mandible. J Oral Maxillofac Surg 1999;52:542–546.

86. Robinson SW, Speidel T, Isaacson RJ, et al. Soft tissue profile change produced by reduction of mandibular prognathism. Angle Orthod 1972;42:227.

87. Bell WH, Dann J III. Correction of dentofacial deformities by surgery in the anterior part of the jaws: a study of stability and soft tissue changes. Am J Orthod 1973;64:162–187.

88. McDonnel JP, McNeill R, West RA. Advancement genioplasty: a retrospective cephalometric analysis of osseous and soft tissue changes. J Oral Surg 1977;35:640.

89. Proffit WR, Epker B. Treatment planning for dentofacial deformities. In Bell WH, White RP, editors. Surgical Correction of Dentofacial Deformities. Philadelphia: WB Saunders; 1980; pp. 183–187.

90. Bell WH, Gallagher D. The versatility of the genioplasty using a broad pedicle. J Oral Maxillofac Surg 1983;41:763–769.

91. Gallagher DM, Bell W, Storum KA. Soft tissue changes associated with advancement genioplasty performed concomitantly with superior repositioning of the maxilla. J Oral Maxillofac Surg 1984;42:238–242.

92. Epker BN, Fish LC. Definitive immediate presurgical planning. In Epker BN, Fish LC, editors. Dentofacial Deformities: Integrated Orthodontic and Surgical Correction. Vol 1 St. Louis: CV Mosby; 1986; pp. 103–127.

93. Krekmanov L, Kahnberg K. Soft tissue response to genioplasty procedures. Br J Oral Maxillofac Surg 1992;30:87–91.

94. Busquets CJ, Sassouni V. Changes in the integumental profile of the chin and lower lip after genioplasty. J Oral Surg 1981;39:499–504.

95. Dann JJ, Epker B. Proplast genioplasty: A retrospective study with treatment recommendations Angle Orthod 1977;47:173–185.

96. Hohl TH, Epker B. Macrogenia: a study of treatment results, with surgical recommendations. Oral Surg Oral Med Oral Pathol Oral Radiol Endod 1976;41:545–567.

97. Bell W. Correction of mandibular prognathism by mandibular setback and advancement genioplasty. Int J Oral Surg 1981;10:221–229.

98. Wessberg GA, Wolford LM, Epker BN. Interpositional genioplasty for the short face. J Oral Surg 1980;38:584–590.

99. Park HS, Ellis E, Fonseca RJ, et al. A retrospective study of advancement genioplasty. Oral Surg Oral Med Oral Pathol Oral Radiol Endod 1989;67:481–489.

100. Bundgaard M, Melson B, Terp S. Changes during and following total maxillary osteotomy (Le Fort I procedure): a cephalometric study. Eur J Orthod 1986;8:21–29.

101. Rosenberg A, Muradin M, van der Bilt A. Nasolabial esthetics after Le Fort I osteotomy and V-Y closure: a statistical evaluation. Int J Adult Orthod Orthognath Surg 2002;17:29–39.

102. Lin SS, Kerr JS. Soft and hard tissue changes in class III patients treated by bimaxillary surgery. Eur J Orthod 1998;20:25–33.

103. Rosen H. Lip-nasal aesthetics following Le Fort I osteotomy. Plast Reconstr Surg 1988;81:171–182.

104. Freihofer HJ. Changes in nasal profile after maxillary advancement in cleft and non-cleft patients. J Maxillofac Surg 1977;5:20–27.

105. Sakima T, Sachdeva R. Soft tissue response to Le Fort I maxillary impaction surgery. Int J Adult Orthodon Orthognath Surg 1987;4:221–231.

Suggested Readings

Schouman T, Baralle MM, Ferri J. Facial morphology changes after total maxillary setback osteotomy. J Oral Maxillofac Surg 2010;68:1504.

Scolozzi P, Schendel S. Soft-tissue changes and predictions of orthognathic surgery. In Fonseca R, editor. Orthognathic Surgery. Amsterdam: Elsevier; 2009; pp. 372–381.

SECTION 7

Complications of Orthognathic Surgery

Joseph E. Van Sickels, DDS

Complications of elective orthognathic surgery may be minor or major, immediate or delayed, and can be divided into several broad and overlapping categories (Table 61-1). Several factors involved in the specific types of problems that may occur, including any significant patient medical history; the use of tobacco; the presence of oral habits; whether surgery includes the maxilla, mandible, or chin; the applied regional surgical anatomy; the magnitude of bony movement; the need for segmental jaw surgery; and the specific methods of fixation employed. The variey of morbidities encountered may fall into one or more of the following general areas: vascular problems, neural complications, infectious disorders, aberrant fracture of the osteotomy segments, occlusal discrepancies, temporomandibular joint (TMJ) dysfunction, dental injuries, and other miscellaneous complications. The approach to orthognathic complications addressed in this chapter is divided into two areas of clinical significance: prevention and management of these complications. In general, prevention focuses on the preoperative patient evaluation, data gathering, and treatment planning phases, whereas the intraoperative surgical management may result in complications that are not completely in the control of the surgeon and may also require immediate attention. Many of the undesirable results of orthognathic surgery are caused by errors in the preoperative clinical examination, dental model analysis and model surgery, or cephalometric analysis or computer planning for surgery. It should be remembered that the majority of patients with dentofacial deformities have altered or unusual craniofacial anatomy that may dictate the need for a departure, or variation, from usual established treatment protocols, but attention to detail is tantamount in the data gathering and treatment planning stages of care. Complications from elective surgery typically performed in young, healthy patients, even when minor in nature, may be devastating to the patient and family; therefore, a comprehensive understanding of the possible complications and prevention and management is critical for the oral and maxillofacial surgeon.

TABLE 61-1. Complications of Orthognathic Surgery

Diagnostic errors	Relapse
Treatment planning errors	Malocclusion
Errors in model surgery	Limited mouth opening
Vascular supply problems	Pain, edema
Bleeding	Sinus problems
Hematoma formation	Fistula formation
Nerve injuries	Lip shortening
Unfavorable osteotomies	Nasal septal deviation
Nonunion	Nasal airflow obstruction
Malunion	Alar base widening
Temporomandibular joint problems	Epiphora
Condylar resorption	Anosmia
Facial scarring	Dental injuries
Cosmetic deformities	Periodontal problems
Infection	Salivary gland injuries
Hardware failure	

VASCULAR COMPLICATIONS

Acute Maxillary Hemorrhage

Severe acute hemorrhage has been documented with both maxillary and mandibular surgery and can have both immediate and delayed effects.[1-7] In general, massive hemorrhage is rare both acutely and in the immediate postoperative period, but it is more likely to occur with maxillary versus mandibular surgery. The blood vessels that are most at risk of iatorogenic injury during maxillary surgery include the maxillary artery, posterior superior alveolar artery, and descending palatine arteries.

Massive blood loss can rarely occur secondary to injury to the internal carotid artery and the internal jugular vein, but more likely, it occurs from injury to the major branches of these blood vessels. During Le Fort surgery when separating the pterygoid plates from the maxilla, it is possible to fracture the base of the skull by vigorously manipulating chisels or directing chisels in an aberrant direction superiorly.[8,9] In fact, there is extreme variability in the location of the posterior portion of the Le Fort osteotomy; this may not be under the control of the surgeon and may result in high fractures near the skull base or low anterior fractures through the pterygoid plates or even further forward in the maxillary alveolus. This can result in direct or indirect damage to major vessels in the region of the posterior maxilla and skull base. When considering vascular injuries from maxillary surgery, it should remembered that blood vessels may be injured directly during osteotome placement (branches of the maxillary artery) or indirectly through shattering the pterygoid plates with bone edge shearing through the regional vasculature (descending palatine arteries, ptergoid venous plexus). Meticulous efforts should be made by the surgeon to properly direct osteotomes low and medial in the pterygoid plate region and to down-fracture the maxilla only when it is deemed possible to do so without the need to apply excessive forces. If the maxilla is extremely difficult to mobilize, the posterior osteotomy may be redirected into the tuberosity region and away from the pterygoid plates to avoid the vessels in the area (Figure 61-1).[10] Patients who are undergoing a maxillary osteotomy to correct malposition of their maxilla after trauma may present special considerations. The previous midface trauma may have resulted in fractures at the base of the skull as well as unpredicatble scar formation and

fusion of bony segments that do not fall along the usual natural suture lines or planes of cleavage. Therefore, excessive surgical manipulation in order to mobilize the maxilla may result in the direction of the osteotomy following the previous fracture lines and not along the usual intended path of induced fracture from Le Fort surgery.

Generally, when brisk bleeding is encountered during Le Fort surgery, the surgeon should follow the basic principles of completion of the osteotomy, with down-fracture of the maxilla, and assessment of the area for the bleeding source, at the specific site of hemorrhage. This may be difficult especially if the bleeding is brisk, so as an alternative, the region may need to be packed with gauze to limit blood loss and allow for some vasculature contraction and platelet aggregation in order to improve visualization. The surgeon should keep in mind that the best opportunity to identify and ligate a bleeding vessel is when it is first cut. Ligature clips may be applied or electrocautery may be used if the vessel is seen clearly. In the posterior aspect of the maxilla, placement of vascular suture would be difficult. When brisk hemorrhage obscures the surgical field, gauze packing, with thrombin impregnation, should be followed by attempts to directly occlude the bleeding vessel. Another option is to pack resorbable hemostatic materials, such as Surgicel (oxidized cellulose), Avitene (microfibrillar collagen), or Gelfoam (absorbable gelatin sponge), in the region under pressure, with expected tamponade of the source of bleeding.

The internal and external carotid arteries, or terminal branches, may be susceptible to both direct and indirect insult during the orthognathic surgery. Thrombosis of the internal carotid artery after orthognathic surgery may occur because of excessive neck extension with poor patient positioning.[11] Mortality associated with thrombosis of the internal carotid artery has been estimated to be 40%, with an additional 52% of patients sustaining a significant permanent neurologic deficit. Extension of the neck serves to stretch and partially fix the internal carotid artery against the cervical vertebrae

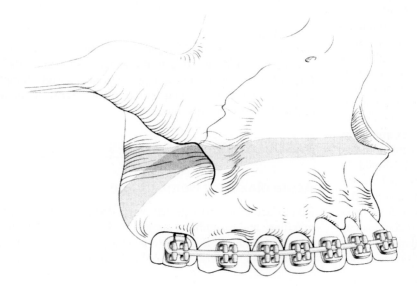

FIGURE 61-1. The posterior osteotomy is directed into the tuberosity region behind the second molar when the maxilla is difficult to mobilize.

during surgery, and contralateral rotation of the head results in further stretch of the artery. Malpositioning of the patient's head in this manner places the internal carotid artery at risk for both direct and indirect trauma and should be avoided.

Delayed Maxillary Hemorrhage

Delayed hemorrhage after a Le Fort I osteotomy may occur as early as several hours after surgery during the night of surgery to as late as 9 or 10 days postoperatively after surgery. The blood vessels most frequently involved are the descending palatine artery, the internal maxillary artery, and the pterygoid venous plexus of veins.[6] Typically, delayed hemorrhage is more likely venous in origin involving the pterygoid venous plexus of veins.

Recommendations to reduce these types of vascular injuries include careful placement and orientation of the pterygomaxillary osteotome in the pterygomaxillary suture with angulation of the osteotomy inferior from the zygomaticomaxillary crest toward the pterygoid plates.[12] The mean distance from the most inferior junction of the maxilla and the pterygoid plates to the position of the internal maxillary artery in the pterygopalatine fossa is 25 mm. With an average length of an osteotome of 15 mm, assuming normal vascular anatomy, the margin of safety in order to separate the entire pterygomaxillary junction is only 10 mm. However, as mentioned, patients with dentofacial and craniofacial anomalies may have anatomic variation from these normative values. The internal maxillary artery and its branches are most vulnerable to damage during their course through the pterygopalatine fossa and pterogomaxillary fissure, at the specific time when the maxillary tuberosity is separated from the pterygoid plates with the curved pterygomaxillary osteotome.

The posterior superior alveolar and the descending palatine arteries may be severed during the Le Fort I osteotomy procedure because they lie in close proximity to the bony walls, although the posterior superior alveolar artery does not usually present a significant concern for bleeding. It is generally recommended that the greater palatine arteries be preserved by gentle bone removal in the area of the posteromedial maxilla that surrounds these vessels. This should be performed with retraction and protection of the vessels, and a rotary instrument may be used to undermine the bone adjacent to the vessels; then a chisel could be used to fracture the bone away from the vessels (Figure 61-2). However, if bleeding is encountered, the descending palatine artery should be ligated or cauterized rather than allowing it to retract and continue to bleed, possibly resulting in delayed hemorrhage in the postoperative period. Preservation of the descending palatine vessels has been shown to have minimal effects on a single-piece Le Fort osteotomy owing to the extensive blood supply from the palatal and buccal soft tissues; however, consideration should be given toward preservation of these vessels during segmental maxillary surgery in order to maximize the blood supply to the maxillary segments and minimize neural deficits to the palatal mucosa and dentition.

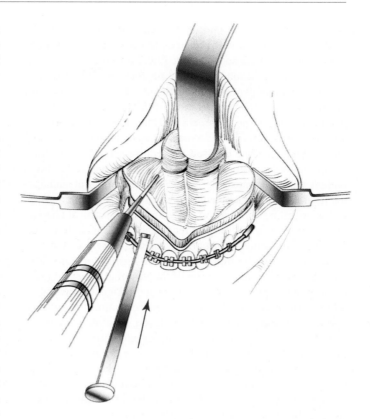

FIGURE 61-2.   A drill is used to create a groove both medially and laterally to the descending palatine artery; then a chisel is used to gently fracture the bone and preserve the vessel.

In general, when large magnitude advancements of the maxilla are necessary (>8 mm), it may be difficult to preserve the palatine vessels, and they may be stretched to the point of severance, or to the point of thrombosis, so routine sacrifice may be the most prudent option.

There are several treatment options for the patient with postoperative hemorrhage after maxillary surgery, and these vary with the degree and severity of the bleeding. The most obvious sign of this type of problem is hemorrhage eminating from both nares.[3] When a patient is initially seen with postoperative bleeding, intermaxillary fixation (IMF), if present, should be released. The patient's general physical status should be assessed, high blood pressure should be controlled, and appropriate complete blood count and bleeding and coagulation studies should be ordered. Abnormal coagulation parameters warrant prompt correction and possible hematologic consultation. It should be remembered that this surgery may be the first in a young patient and may disclose a previously undiagnosed bleeding disorder. With a good light source and suction for visualization, the nasal cavity should be examined to reveal whether a bleeding site is arterial or venous in nature. Most likely, in the immediate perioperative period, significant nasal bleeding may result from tears in the nasal mucosa that may not have been addressed during surgery and may have become more active after extubation with a nasal endotracheal tube (ETT). If adequate visualization and assessment are not possible, the nose should be anesthetized and decongested with a local anesthetic and a vasoconstrictor. Local anesthetic injections in the nose and around the palatine foramina are useful in decreasing postoperative hemorrhage, at least to allow for evaluation and definitive ligation. If the bleeding is minor in nature, it may be possible to treat the patient with bed rest and the use of anterior and posterior nasal packing for 3 to 5 days, which can also be used for recurrent bleeding or for a patient not responding to initial therapeutic measures. For a patient who does not respond to local attempts at management, or in whom the bleeding is severe or persistent, a return to the operating room for exploration of the surgical site and direct ligation or packing is recommended. As a preferred, less invasive option, angiography of the vessels in the area may be peformed promptly and with minimal morbidity. This will allow direct embolization of the vessel at the exact point of severance, providing that there is sufficent bleeding to allow visualization of contrast extravasation. Additional operative techniques may be employed depending upon the specific clinical examination or angiographic findings. These include packing of the maxillary sinus or, in extreme cases, ligation of the external carotid artery at the lingual/facial artery branch; however, with collateral circulation, persistent bleeding may still occur after the external carotid artery is ligated. In general, severe late postoperative hemorrhage is most effectively managed by an interventional radiologist with angiography and embolization.

Mandibular Hemorrhage

As with maxillary surgery, major vessels can be injured during mandibular orthognathic surgery. Occlusion of the internal carotid artery has been described after a mandibular bilateral sagittal split osteotomy (BSSO),[13] and major central nervous system morbidity may occur after this injury, as mentioned previously. The medical and surgical management of internal carotid artery thrombosis is beyond the scope of this chapter, and prevention is accomplished with appropriate patient head positioning. Typically, vascular injuries with mandibular surgery are due to indirect trauma either through forceful placement of a retractor on the lingual surface of the ramus of the mandible to retract the inferior alveolar neurovascular bundle or the use of a mallet and chisel on the medial aspect of the mandible, with severance of the inferior alveolar artery or vein. Placement of retractors and the use of chisels on the medial posterior aspect of the mandible should be performed with caution. It is preferable to limit dissection and subsequent chisel use to the area of the retrolingual fossa just distal to the area of the mandibular foramen.

Hemorrhage with Sagittal Split Osteotomy

Early reports noted numerous incidences of excessive bleeding with the sagittal split osteotomy (SSO).[14] The vessels most commonly injured are the internal maxillary artery, the facial artery, and the inferior alveolar artery. These injuries were attributed to inexperience, excessive soft tissue stripping and dissection, and lack of appropriate instrumentation for the specific procedure. With current surgical techniques and instrumentation, excessive hemorrhage during an SSO is not a major concern. In a series of 256 mandibular SSOs, the incidence of hemorrhage was 1.2% (3 cases)[15] and included 2 cases of inferior alveolar artery injury and 1 anterior facial artery injury. In a series of 1264 consecutive patients who underwent an SSO of the mandible, 15 patients (1.2%) had bleeding complications.[16] Of this group, the most common injury occurred to the retromandibular vein, and there was 1 case of bleeding from the facial artery. Four patients required reoperation owing to the development of a large expanding hematoma. It should be noted that the majority of the cases in this series were perfomed using the classic Obwegeser technique without modifications. Hemorrhage due to vascular injury on the medial or lateral aspects of the mandible during an SSO may be controlled in a number of ways. The simplest methods include gauze packing, using electrocautery, clamping with a hemostats or hemoclip if the severed vessel can be identified, or injecting epinephrine (1:100,000 or 1:50,000) into the vessel walls. Obviously, caution should be exercised when applying electrocautery in close proximity to neural tissues, such as the inferior alveolar nerve, and when indicated, bipolar cautery should be used. As with bleeding from maxillary surgery, extraoral cervical approaches to the carotid arterial system to control bleeding sources are seldom necessary, and in these rare cases, the involved vessel may be amenable to angiography and embolization.

Hemorrhage with Vertical Ramus Osteotomy

Vascular injury during a vertical ramus osteotomy (VRO) of the mandible could be divided into three regions of the ramus: superior, middle, and inferior. In the superior sigmoid notch region, the maxillary artery is at risk for injury and it should be protected with careful placement of a Bauer retractor in the sigmoid notch. In the midramus region, the inferior alveolar artery and vein enter the mandibular foramen, and surgeons use the antilingula as the anterior reference for placement of the vertical osteotomy just posterior to this landmark to avoid inferior alveolar neurovascular injury. The inferior aspect of the VRO places the facial artery and vein at risk for injury; this area should also be protected with a Bauer retractor. The posterior aspect of the VRO places the retromandibular vein at risk for injury, and careful subperiosteal dissection around the posterior border of the ramus should be followed by careful placement of a Merrill-Levaseur retractor. In consideration of these sites of potential bleeding and the need to access them surgically for control, the sequence of the VRO cuts should correspond to the surgeon's ability to access a bleeding vessel if severed after completion of the osteotomy. Note that the VRO should be "scored" through the lateral ramus first but not "completed" through to the medial ramus. Therefore, because the facial artery and retromandibular vessels may be controlled with extraoral pressure or retraction under or behind the mandible, the inferior cut should be completed first. Because the maxillary artery can be accessed with gauze packing to tamponade any bleeding in the sigmoid notch region, this superior cut should be performed second. Finally, because the inferior alveolar artery is inaccessible from a lateral approach, the middle of the VRO should be completed third or last, because the osteotomy could then be completed, the proximal segment retracted laterally, and the inferior alveolar artery accessed immediately for packing or ligation directly through the osteotomy site. In a study of intraoral VROs, there was a low incidence of damage to the maxillary artery.[17] The masseteric artery may be injured inadvertently by placing a saw or bur cut too far superior for the horizontal osteotomy on the medial aspect of the mandible into the region of the sigmoid notch. The inferior alveolar artery may also be injured during a VRO, which is usually caused by a vertical osteotomy of the ramus placed too far anterior, owing to variability of the position of the mandibular foramen with reference to the antilingula. This may result in severance of the inferior alveolar nerovascular bundle on the medial aspect of the ramus from the oscillating saw used laterally on the ramus for the vertical osteotomy. During a VRO, access to the bleeding inferior alveolar vessel is difficult, given the lateral approach. Fortunately, in most instances, intraoperative bleeding along the ramal cut or in the sigmoid notch can be controlled by gauze pressure tamponade, until completion of the osteotomy allows improved access for vessel ligation of electrocautery. Late vascular sequelae, such as the formation of an aneurysm, may require angiography and embolization.

Vascular Compromise (Avascular Necrosis)

The morbidity of vascular compromise or ischemic complications varies between maxillary and mandibular procedures. The long-term complications of loss of blood supply resulting from orthognathic surgery range from fibrosis of pulpal tissues and minor periodontal defects and gingival papillary necrosis to major loss of teeth, alveolus, or complete bony segments, and the more severe complications increase with increasing number of bone segments. The most frequent complication associated with segmental maxillary surgery is interruption of the blood supply.[18] The major risk factors include three or more segments, advanced age, co-morbid medical history including small vessel disease, immunocompromise, or poor wound healing (e.g.. diabetes mellitus), a smoking history, previous maxillary surgery, simultaneous premolar extraction with posteriorization of the maxilla and kinking of the palatal soft tissues, the inadvertent or prolonged use of Rowe disimpaction forceps for mobilization of the maxilla with palatal pressure, prolonged intraoperative hypotensive anesthesia, a severe skeletal abnormality with significant bony movements (>10 mm), superior maxillary movement (impaction), maxillary expansion with stretching or tearing of the palatal mucosa, pressure from a palatal cov-

erage splint, lack of segment stabilization, inadequate preoperative evaluation, and poor follow-up and lack of recognition of the early signs of the development of avascular necrosis (e.g., gray, dusky gingiva).[18] Several recommendations have been proposed to avoid vascular complications associated with segmental maxillary osteotomies. Preoperative planning is critical to ensure that adequate space exists between teeth for interdental osteotomies; careful examination of periapical radiographs before surgery should be done to confirm root divergence, and model surgery should simulate the surgical plan and minimize the amount of bone removal in the osteotomy sites. Intraoperative deails should include care during interdental osteotomies with the use of chisels and burs, or preferably saws (to prevent soft tissue damage despite contact of the cutting blade with the palatal mucosa), with copious irrigation for completion of the osteotomies. These steps will minimize the amount of heat generation and decrease the chance of creating necrotic bone or root defects. Release of soft tissues adjacent to osteotomy sites and gentle mobilization of segments to avoid tearing and cutting of flaps are essential. Splints with palatal bars used for stabilization should not impinge on the palatal pedicle that serves as the major blood supply to maxillary segments. Special consideration must be given to the patient who has had previous palatal surgery or multiple segmental procedures or has a cleft palate. In these instances, standard flap designs may not be adequate, and multiple small access incisions may be preferable to a standard bilateral circumvesticular incision. Complications such as periodontal defects, pulpal necrosis, and delayed union or nonunion are more commonly seen in the anterior region of the mandible but may be associated with any maxillary or mandibular segmental procedure. Mandibular segmental procedures require detailed planning of soft tissue incisions and careful elevation of soft tissue pedicles. In order to minimize intraoperative complications, the vascular supply to involved segments must be optimized by designing as large a soft tissue flap as possible to supply the involved segment(s), maintaining maximal soft tissue attachment to the segment(s) to be mobilized, avoiding stripping of the lingual mucoperiosteal pedicle, and making the bony osteotomies as apical as possible to include as much muscle tissue for blood supply as possible.

Avascular, or aseptic, necrosis or the major loss of soft and hard tissues of the maxilla is rare and is most often due to a compromised blood supply. As mentioned previously, this may be caused by a kinked vascular pedicle in the palatal mucosa or iatrogenic tearing of palatal flaps. Isolated cases of loss of the entire maxilla or individual segments have been reported (Figure 61-3).[18] More common and subtle complications secondary to vascular compromise range from flattening of the papilla and loss of the gingiva to periodontal defects in the areas of the osteotomies. The treatment of avascular necrosis may be divided into initial and delayed management strategies. Initially, the problem must be identified, and supportive care is provided, including irrigation, chlorhexidine rinses, and instruction on good oral hygiene practices. If

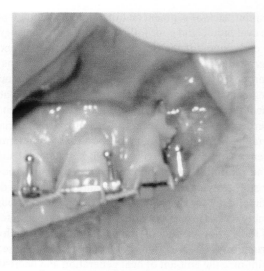

FIGURE 61-3. Avascular necrosis after a Le Fort I osteotomy.

mobility of the maxilla exists, attempts should be made to stabilize the mobile segments, with the possible need to return to the operating room. As mentioned, intermaxillary fixation should be released, if present, to allow for a comprehensive assessment. Prophylactic systemic antibiotics may be considered. The most appropriate initial management is prompt referral for hyperbaric oxygen (HBO) therapy. The problem with avascular necrosis is that by the time it is diagnosed, the damage has already occurred, and complete resolution, despite prompt HBO therapy, is unlikely. The delayed, or long-term, management of avascular necrosis includes allowing a sufficient period of time for demarcation of necrotic segments (months), then planning conservative removal of nonviable bone segments and teeth and repair of any associated oroantral and oronasal fistulae that may be present. Reconstructive options must include free flap bone graft options (fibula) with associated soft tissue transfer, owing to the compromised blood supply in the area, which will not provide an environment conducive to support healing of a standard iliac crest corticocancellous bone graft. After bone grafting, dental implant and prosthetic reconstruction may be considered.

Avascular necrosis of the proximal segment with an SSO is rare and has been attributed to excessive stripping of the segments.[19] Loss of bone secondary to aseptic necrosis has resulted in facial disfigurement with loss of the mandibular angle projection, or excessive antegonial notching. As early as 1974, Grammer and colleagues[20] noted that necrosis of large areas of bone in the proximal segment after mandibular SSO occurred secondary to wide lateral elevation of the mucoperiosteal pedicle in the animal model. They proposed that devitalized bone usually revascularized; however, when revascularization does not occur, a substantial loss of bone from the mandibular ramus can occur, especially in the gonial angle region. In 1977, Epker[21] presented modifications of the sagittal split and discussed a technique in which

the amount of lateral dissection of the masseter muscle and associated periosteum was greatly decreased. Adoption of this technique has greatly minimized the incidence of avascular necrosis after a mandibular SSO. In addition, rigid fixation of the bony segments, which permits early revascularization amd prevents segment mobility, has also minimized the incidence of avascular necrosis in the mandible.

Early publications suggested that an advancement genioplasty could be done successfully by repositioning the anterior inferior border of the mandible as a free, but pedicled, bone graft. However, after a horizontal osteotomy of the inferior border of the mandible with advancement, resorption of the advanced bone segment occurs to varying degrees and may result in slight, or almost complete, loss of the advanced genial segment. Preservation of the lingual pedicle (geniohyoid and genioglossus muscles) and the buccal pedicle (platysma and depressor anguli oris and depressor labii inferioris muscles) minimizes bone resorption and results in a more predictable soft and hard tissue chin contour. Larger magnitude genial advancements may require wider soft tissue dissection and release of lingual and buccal soft tissues to achieve the desired advancement, and suprahyoid myotomies were historically performed to allow greater chin advancement before the use of rigid fixation. However, with maintenance of an adequate labial soft tissue pedicle and the use of rigid internal fixation, bone loss should be negligible.

The intraoral vertical subcondylar osteotomy is the mandibular procedure in which the proximal segment is at most risk for avascular necrosis due to the wide release of periosteal attachments. One study reported 2 out of 42 patients with necrosis of the distal tip of the proximal segment.[22] The surgical technique involved stripping the entire lateral and medial surfaces of the mandible up to the neck of the condyle. With more recent modifications of the VRO technique in which a soft tissue pedicle of medial pterygoid muscle attached to the posterior and medial aspect of the proximal segment is maintained, aseptic necrosis of the tip of the proximal segment is generally not a major concern.[23]

NONUNION OF THE MAXILLA

Nonunion, delayed union, or fibrous union of the maxilla may be due to both local and systemic factors. The blood supply to the maxilla may be compromised by poor surgical planning or may be questionable because of scarring from previous surgery, such as in the previously operated cleft palate patient. The presence of palatal scarring with large maxillary advancements may make it difficult to passively reposition the maxilla and may worsen hyponasal or hypernasal speech abnormalities as well as velopharyngeal incompetence (VPI) in cleft patients, and consideration may be needed for distraction osteogenesis, although the data regarding these issues indicate no significant differences between Le Fort surgery and maxillary distraction regarding speech alterations and VPI. One of the major contributory factors to postoperative maxillary mobility is patients with parafunctional activity, excessive masticatory forces during function, or occlusal irregularities or interferences. In those patients in whom the maxilla has been moved in an anterior and inferior direction, there may be insufficient bony interfaces in the pillar regions (piriform rim and buttresses) to allow for complete osseous healing. Patients with systemic conditions that interfere with healing, such as diabetes mellitus, smoking, or an immunocompromised illness, require individualized case planning to minimize anticipated complications from poor bone healing. When an unstable maxillary movement (e.g., inferior repositioning) is anticipated, bone plates and screws may be combined with additional forms of stabilization, including skeletal suspension wires (circumzygomatic or piriform rim wires), as well as a period of intermaxillary fixation ranging from 1 to 6 weeks. With inferior repositioning of the maxilla, bone plates and bone grafts can be combined with adjustable pins for additional stability (Figure 61-4). When these methods are used, it may be acceptable to limit the use of intermaxillary fixation for a period of 1 week. In general, bone gaps of 5 to 6 mm or greater, resulting from large maxillary advancements, should receive allogeneic block bone grafting at the pillars of the maxilla, including the piriform rim and maxillary buttress regions. If the advanced maxilla has sufficient bone contacts in multiple regions, isolated defects may be filled with particulate allo-

geneic bone or alloplastic materials. In some cases, large bone gap defects in critical structural locations in the maxilla may require simultaneous autogenous block bone grafting with plate and screw fixation in order to provide for physical support.

After maxillary surgery, the primary physical finding that a nonunion exists is mobility of the maxilla during maximal intercuspation. The patient is generally able to move the maxilla superiorly by simply clenching the teeth together. Treatment of a mobile maxilla may be divided into early and late management. The use of short-term intermaxillary fixation is controversial and may not assist with bone healing across an established area of fibrous tissue interposition between bony segments and, in fact, may contribute to the nonunion by the constant pull of the mandible during attempted opening of the mouth. If maxillary mobility is noted in the early postoperative period, a short period of intermaxillary fixation may be beneficial to allow for neovascularization at the bone gap. Conversely, if the patient is already in intermaxillary fixation, removal may allow functional remodeling and bony consolidation. This is particularly important in the patient who has parafunctional occlusal activities, and selective occlusal adjustment after an occlusal analysis may be the most important means to allow bony union to occur. In addition, flat plane occlusal splints may be used to distribute occlusal forces more evenly and appropriately. Again, for minor occlusal discrepancies, selective occlusal equilibration

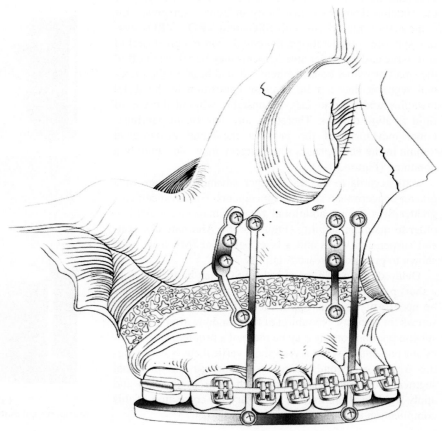

FIGURE 61-4. Inferior maxillary repositioning using bone grafts, plates, and adjustable pins.

may resolve premature contacts that may have contributed to mobility of the maxilla. Also, patients should be instructed on the use of a soft diet. Heavy intermaxillary elastics should be discontinued because, with function, they put intermittent strong forces on the maxilla by the attempts at opening of the mandible. For patients with posterior relapse, light short class III elastics can help prevent further movement and may allow osseous consolidation. However, all elastics must be used judiciously because they may aggravate the nonunion problem. Even if the final result is a minor class III malocclusion, this is usually easier to manage than a nonunion of the maxilla.

The late management of maxillary nonunion involves surgery for débridement of the fibrous tissue and either initial allogeneic bone grafting or autogenous bone block grafting and rigid stabilization of the maxilla at the buttress regions. This would include the use of bone plates and screws, particulate or corticocancellous allogeneic or autogenous bone grafts, auxiliary stabilization techniques, and possibly the use of alloplastic materials. The reoperation should be approached aggressively by completely mobilizing the maxilla and removing interpositional fibrous tissue to allow an osseous union.

NONUNION OF THE MANDIBLE

Nonunion or delayed union of the mandible may be due to avascular necrosis, insufficient bone contact, instability of the fixation devices, or instability of bone fragments. This complication may occur with SSOs and VROs. VROs warrant specific considerations, not only because a great deal of soft tissue and muscular attachements may be reflected off of the small proximal bone segment but also because the proximal segment may not lie in close apposition to the distal mandible and may, in fact, be unstable without the use of rigid fixation devices. Therefore, any significant parafunctional movement of the jaws or incidental postsurgical trauma in the early phases after surgery may contribute to a nonunion (Figure 61-5).

With regards to the SSO, larger advancements are of a greater concern than small advancements. For advancements greater than 7 mm, additional fixation may be required in order to maintain stability (Figure 61-6). Alternatively, skeletal suspension wires and a brief period of IMF have been shown to provide increased stability.[24]

Delayed union of a mandibular SSO may be treated with a short period of IMF. Alternatively, a second operation may be necessary with the application of additional plates and screws for stability. Nonunion of the mandible after a vertical subcondylar osteotomy may be more of a problem with edentulous patients or when a very short vertical cut is used (Figure 61-7). A second operation, to access the proximal segment from an extraoral approach to properly align and apply rigid fixation, may be necessary for correction of this complication.

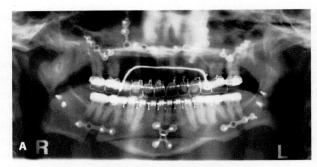

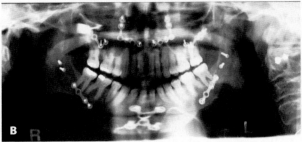

FIGURE 61-5.   **A** and **B,** Rigid fixation failure 2 weeks after bimaxillary surgery.

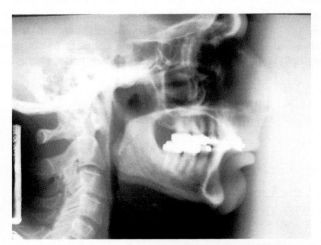

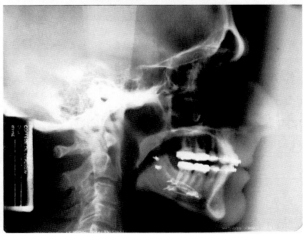

FIGURE 61-6.   Large mandibular advancement using both monocortical plates and bicortical screws.

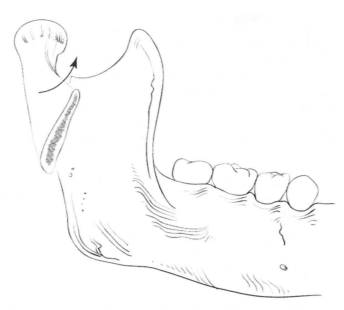

FIGURE 61-7.   Severe condylar rotation is common with a short subcondylar VRO.

DENTAL AND PERIODONTAL INJURIES

Dental and periodontal injuries can be secondary to both vascular and nonvascular causes and are most frequently related to treatment planning errors or technical errors made at the time of surgery (Figure 61-8). Segmental procedures in the maxilla and mandible may cause a number of problems, including injury to tooth roots, loss of teeth, need for postop-

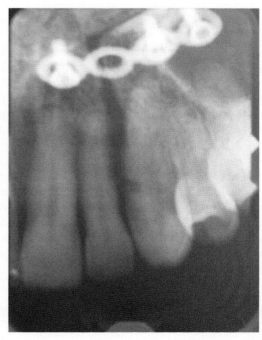

FIGURE 61-8.   Injured and exposed root surfaces adjacent to a segmental interdental osteotomy.

erative endodontic therapy, and the development of significant interdental periodontal defects.

Regarding sufficient space between teeth for interdental osteotomies, preoperative orthodontic mechanics with coils can be used to maximize the space between root apices in the area of the planned interdental osteotomy. Periapical radiographs should be assessed for the direction of the root apices, which should be divergent at the planned osteotomy site. A minimum space of 3.0 mm is advocated between teeth for interdental osteotomies (1.0 mm on each root surface and 1.0 mm for the osteotome), and 5.0 mm is recommended for subapical osteotomies above the root apices to avoid injury to dental branches of the nerves.[25] Precise model surgery can greatly reduce the frequency of dentoalveolar injuries. The segmental surgery should be planned so that a minimal amount of bone is removed between osseous segments. Excessive manipulation and torquing of the bony segments should avoided but, when necessary, should be performed toward the root apices rather than at the gingival margin to minimize mucosal lacerations and subsequent periodontal defects. Segments should be tipped apart while maintaining interproximal tooth contacts whenever possible. Copious irrigation of fine fissure burs or reciprocating saw should be used when cutting through the outer cortex of the maxilla. This should be followed by gentle and progressive chisel placement in the oseteotomy site to permit gentle separation of the bone segments. When a bony palatal island is maintained during segmental maxillary surgery, the release of palatal soft tissues should occur under the bony island rather than toward the dentoalveolar segments. After the bony segments are gently separated, small amounts of bone may be judiciously removed toward the root surfaces. When larger wedges of bone are planned for removal, less bone should be removed initially as a wedge than the amount that was treatment planned, with careful additional bone removal as required to approximate the segments. When the bone segments do not fit together passively, the bony interferences may be gently sequentially reduced, because large bony defects after excessive removal of bone usually fill with scar tissue rather than with an osseous union.

With regards to mandibular segmental surgery, it is usually necessary to separate both the buccal and the lingual cortical plates, leaving only a small amount of lingual cortical plate near the cervical portion of the roots to be separated by a fine chisel. The use of a reciprocating, or micro-oscillating, saw is recommended to cut through the mandible, with careful palpation on the lingual surface in order to avoid iatrogenic soft tissue injury. Owing to the dense lingual cortical bone, the use of chisels is more hazardous in the mandible than in the maxilla, where they could fragment the lingual cortex or tear through the lingual pedicle region by applying excessive force once the lingual cortex has been separated. Therefore, chisels and osteotomes should be used with caution after the osteotomy has been completed with a saw, and the bony segments should be separated with minimal tapping of the osteotome through to the lingual surface.

FISTULA FORMATION

Postoperative fistulas in the oronasal and oroantral regions generally result from soft tissue injury at the time of surgery. Fistulas have been reported with isolated segmental osteotomies as well as Le Fort osteotomies.[26] This complication may occur as a result of using rotary instruments or saws or performing osteotomies that perforate the palatal mucosa at the time the segmental osteotomies are completed. Impingement of soft tissue in the segmental osteotomy site during segment repositioning and fixation may also result in tissue necrosis and subsequent fistula formation. Iatrogenic tearing of the palatal mucosa at the time of attempted tissue stretching may also result in nonhealing defects with the potential for tissue necrosis and communication between the nasal cavity or maxillary sinus and the oral cavity. This may occur most commonly when an osteotomy is created in the midline of the maxilla, where the palatal mucosa is extremely thin, with maxillary segmental expansion movements that stretch the midpalatal tissue, leaving a resultant tissue deficiency and nasal communication (Figure 61-9).

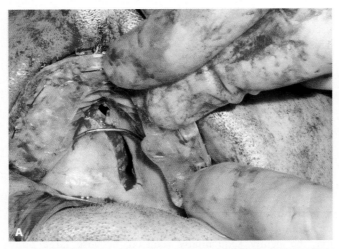

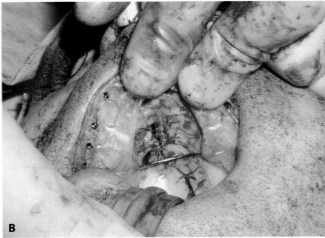

FIGURE 61-9.   **A,** Oronasal communication during a two-piece Le Fort I osteotomy. **B,** Palatal mucosal release and sutures with good oral hygiene led to spontaneous closure.

Despite alterations in the method of osteotomy, careful soft tissue manipulation at the time of surgery in an attempt to prevent tissue perforation is the best method for prevention of postoperative fistula formation. When expansion is required, the palatal mucosa can be incised with two parallel incisions just medial to the greater palatine foramen; bony separation then occurs in the midpalatal region.[26] The tissue can stretch and expand in an area removed from the location of bony separation in the midline. An alternative technique involves making paramedian osteotomies in the nasal floor immediately adjacent to the lateral nasal walls. The overlying palatal mucosa is thicker soft tissue and somewhat more elastic than the thin midline palatal mucosa.[27] If a small tear of the palatal mucosa is noted after a bony cut, care should be taken to release the palatal tissue from above before expansion of segments to allow laxity and closer approximation of the mucosa to prevent a large soft tissue defect.

When a fistula is noted postoperatively, several measures may be used to allow the fistula to close spontaneously, and the prevention of sinus and nasal infections is essential. This may include systemic antibiotic therapy, nasal decongestants, and consideration for the provision of nasal drainage, if necessary. It may be advisable to construct an appliance that will obturate the fistula without placing pressure on the surrounding tissues that can contribute to spontaneous closure by providing a scaffold for tissue migration and also by reducing food and bacterial contamination at the site. Care must be taken to ensure that there is not excessive pressure on the palatal mucosa from a palatal obturator splint that can result in decreased vascularity, with further loss of soft tissue and underlying bone, creating a larger hard and soft tissue defect to address with surgical correction. If local measures, appropriate medical therapy, and fistula obturation have been unsuccessful, surgical closure of the fistula is generally required.

When considering closure of a fistula associated with segmental maxillary surgery, it is recommended that at least 6 months have elapsed to allow for complete revascularization of the individual maxillary segments, because a fistula may continue to close for 8 to 12 weeks, leaving a smaller soft tissue defect to correct surgically. Initially, a soft tissue flap should be raised from an area farthest from the bony segments with the least potential for loss of vascularity in the transfer. Buccal advancement flaps or local palatal island flaps may be used; however, if a large segment of the maxilla was involved with a significant loss of soft tissue, distant flaps should be considered, including the buccal fat pad, temporalis myofascial flap, or a tongue flap to transfer a large amount of well-vascularized soft tissue to the area of vascular compromise.

MANAGEMENT OF VASCULAR COMPROMISE

Objective measures to assess vascular compromise are limited to Doppler flowmetry of the maxillary gingiva that can be used to detect subtle decreases in the maxillary gingival blood flow during and after a Le Fort I osteotomy[28]; however, its use is limited in the clinical setting and is usually reserved for research studies. The early clinical indications of vascular compromise after orthognathic surgery include blanching or a "dusky gray" color of the attached gingiva followed by a cyanotic appearance of the attached gingiva and adjacent unattached mucosa.[29] These overlying soft tissues can be an indicator of underlying bony involvement. Three typical vascular compromise scenarios are possible: (1) loss of vascularity to the soft tissues, with maintenance of bony perfusion; (2) loss of vascularity to the bone, with maintenance of soft tissue perfusion; and (3) loss of vascularity to both the bone and the soft tissues. If cyanosis is noted in the immediate postoperative period (hours to days after surgery), IMF, if present, should be released and the oral cavity should be inspected for stretching, kinking, or constriction of palatal soft tissues. Splints must be carefully evaluated to identify areas of excessive pressure on palatal soft tissues by the appliance and should be removed to evaluate the underlying tissues directly. If removal of IMF and recontouring or removal of palatal splints is not helpful or if the tissue is already necrotic, supportive care is necessary to attempt to minimize the amount of hard and soft tissue loss; however, eventual loss of the soft tissue and exposure of the underlying bone is an expected occurrence in these cases. In severe cases, any portion of a retained necrotic segment of palatal mucosa should be treated as an intraoral free graft or biologic dressing for the underlying bone, with meticulous daily irrigations with or without packing of the wound. As with all tissue grafts, this mucosa should be secured, because this stability may allow some degree of spontaneous revascularization. HBO therapy may be helpful to minimize bone loss while promoting neovascularization or at least limit the propagation of the area of necrosis. After sufficient time has elapsed to allow establishment of the specific zones of necrosis and dental injuries, débridement of the necrotic tissues and removal of nonvital teeth should be performed. In a delayed fashion, surgical reconstruction of the resultant hard and soft tissue defects varies based upon the size of the defects but may include autogenous bone grafting, free tissue transfer with a fibula flap and associated soft tissue, and prosthetic reconstruction with dental implants and implant-supported prostheses.

INFECTION

The incidence of postoperative infections after orthognathic surgery is low.[16,30–33] Chow and coworkers[30] reviewed 1294 consecutively treated patients who underwent one- and two-jaw orthognathic procedures, and the complication rate was 9.7% overall, with a 7.4% incidence of postoperative infections. They noted that those patients who received only a single preoperative dose of antibiotic had a higher rate of infection than those with longer duration of perioperative antibiotic management, and as expected, two-jaw procedures had a higher incidence of infection than single-jaw proce-

dures. The incidence of infection was almost equal between maxillary and mandibular osteotomies. In a series of 57 patients who underwent an SSO of the mandible, there was 1 case of infection, resulting in significant relapse of the orthognathic procedure.[31] Becelli and associates[32] had a 2.48% incidence of infection when examining 482 sides of patients who underwent a mandibular SSO. These occurred within the first month after surgery and were treated effectively with systemic oral antibiotics, although several of patients required screw removal and wound débridement. Bouwman and colleagues[33] reviewed 700 consecutive cases of a BSSO for advancement of the mandible, and in 15 cases, bicortical screws required removal owing to infection. Teltzrow and coworkers,[16] in a study of 1264 patients, noted a 2.8% incidence infection after a BSSO requiring extraoral incision and drainage, despite a protocol including a single dose of perioperative intravenous antibiotic.

As seen from this review, the incidence of infection with orthognathic surgery is low and varies from one study to another, with an overall incidence of perhaps 1% to 5% consistent with clean-contaminated wounds. In addition, most infections occur within the first few weeks after surgery because many of these are due to an infected hematoma, which are usually resolved with an intraoral incision and drainage procedure in the office. Infections due to loose hardware may occur early if there was insufficient stability at the time of surgery but also may be seen several months after the surgery following bony remodeling and resultant screw loosening.

Osteomyelitis after orthognathic surgery is especially rare. Teltzrow and coworkers[16] had one patient develop osteomyelitis after a BSSO, which resolved after decortication and long-term systemic antibiotic therapy.

NERVE INJURY

Maxillary Sensory Injuries

Sensory injuries in the maxilla after orthognathic surgery have not been studied as extensively as those seen with mandibular surgery. With a carefully placed low circumvestibular incision combined with gentle soft tissue retraction, nerve injury is generally inconsequential and limited to the terminal branches of the infraorbital nerve (V2). Spontanous recovery of sensation to the lip, cheeks, and nose usually occurs within 2 to 8 weeks after surgery. In contrast, paresthesias due to damage of the sensory nerve supply to the teeth, gingiva, and mucosa are more common. Decreased sensation to the mucosa is typically transient and normal sensation commonly returns within 6 to 12 months. On occasion, patients will experience permanent numbness intraorally on the palate and buccal gingiva, and therefore, in order to preserve sensation to the palate, some authors advocate preservation of the greater palatine neurovascular bundle whenever possible.[29] Also, failure of the teeth to respond to electric pulp stimulation may be temporary; however, permanent loss of response to electrical, hot, or cold stimulation is not unusual and does not necessarily represent a tooth that requires endodontic therapy. The clinician must differentiate between a nonvital tooth and one that does not respond to stimulation but still has an intact blood supply. Many studies have shown decreased blood flow to the maxillary teeth during and after Le Fort osteotomy with pulpal blood flow studies, with return to normal within several months. A tooth that shows periapical radiolucency or a parulis with fistula formation upon examination may be a candidate for root canal therapy.

Mandibular Sensory Injuries

Sagittal Split Osteotomy

Although traction injuries to the inferior alveolar nerve may occur commonly during SSOs, frank transections of the inferior alveolar nerve occur less commonly.[34] The most likely time for this to occur is during the actual splitting process of the osteotomy. When the segments are being separated, care should be taken to visualize and protect the nerve, when possible. If the nerve is in the distal segment or encased in cortical bone, appropriate steps should be taken to release it. This may be as simple as releasing the nerve with a periosteal elevator from a medullary bone, or it may require additional bone cuts to release it from cortical bone. Laborious efforts to release the nerve should be avoided because this may cause worse iatrogenic injury to the nerve. One study suggested that low mandibular corpus body height and inferior position of the nerve in the class II retrognathic patient population may increase the risk for injury.[34] With a transection injury, repair of the nerve with one or more nonresorbable 6-0 to 8-0 monofilament nylon sutures placed in the epineurium has been recommended.[35] It may be necessary to perform a decortication laterally to release the nerve to the mental foramen for mobilization, especially if the plan is for a significant mandibular advancement that will further separate the proximal and distal nerve stumps and prevent direct repair without tension. It should be noted that one large series had a 3.5% incidence of transection of the inferior alveolar nerve, which occurred anterior to, or in the third molar region, in all instances.[15] Certainly, this is the location where the inferior alveolar nerve is most lateral and the buccal cortex of the mandible is thinnest, making the nerve most vulnerable to injury in this location. Nerve endings were approximated in nine patients by positioning the segments in close proximity, but without the need for epineurial sutures. The length of follow-up for these patients was 2 to 5 years, and all of the patients had some return of sensation to the normal inferior alveolar nerve distribution. Whether this represented spontaneous regeneration or new growth from the cervical plexus is unknown.

Conversely, if the transection occurs at the vertical bony cut, immediate repair may be difficult, and as mentioned, it may be necessary to expose more of the nerve in the distal segment. When excessive tension on the nerve repair site is present, the nerve may have to be exposed distally to the mental foramen to allow a tension-free repair. The need for such an extensive procedure needs to be weighed against the primary goals of the orthognathic surgical procedure.

Injury to the inferior alveolar nerve, in the absence of a transection, is frequently associated with the SSO of the mandibular ramus. Risk factors for neurosensory disturbance include advanced patient age, a simultaneous genioplasty procedure, and an increased magnitude of advancement.[36,37] Multiple techniques have been suggested to prevent these injuries, including varying the osteotomy design, cautious chisel placement, meticulous dissection technique, decompression of the lateral fragment if indicated, and perioperative steroid use. Vigorous medial retraction of the neurovascular bundle inferiorly during the horizontal osteotomy may cause the inferior alveolar nerve to be compressed against the lingula, and decreased intraoperative nerve conduction has been demonstrated.[34,38] Retraction on the medial aspect of the mandible should be done carefully to avoid compression nerve injuries. The most ideal location to create the lateral buccal (vertical) cut is in the first and second molar region where the cortex is the thickest, the mandible is the thickest, and the nerve is farthest from the lateral cortex.[15,39] Other recommendations to prevent nerve injuries are based on clinical experience, but no controlled studies have been done to determine whether one way is preferable over another.

Injury to the lingual nerve during an SSO can occur, but it is unusual.[40,41] The lingual nerve may be injured by overpenetration of bicortical screws used to rigidly fixate the osteotomy. The course of the lingual nerve near the medial surface of the mandible varies; therefore, any dissection on the lingual aspect of the mandible in the third molar region may temporarily or permanently injure this nerve.[42] As with inferior alveolar nerve injuries, lingual nerve injuries should be carefully followed and documented. If the nerve is visualized and has been transected, it should be repaired at the time of surgery. In general, symptoms of lingual nerve injuries after an SSO are rare and typically resolve with time.

VRO and Other Ramus Procedures

Although the vertical oblique osteotomy (VRO) of the mandibular ramus is an alternative to the SSO for horizontal mandibular excess and mandibular setback, this procedure may also result in permanent injury to the inferior alveolar nerve. The incidence of permanent paresthesia after an intraoral vertical subcondylar osteotomy has ranged from 9% to 11%.[43,44] Endoscopic approaches to the ramus may have a different incidence of nerve injury, but experience with these techniques is limited.[45] The incidence of nerve injury with the VRO procedure is mostly associated with the imprecise location of the inferior alveolar nerve. Traditionally, it has been suggested that a bulge on the lateral surface of the mandible (the antilingula) corresponds to the position of the lingula on the medial aspect of the mandible. Therefore, creation of an osteotomy posterior to the antilingula should theoretically avoid injury to the inferior alveolar nerve medially. Hogan and Ellis[46] showed that the bulge on the lateral surface of the ramus corresponds to the insertion of muscles and tendons and had no relationship to the medial position of the inferior alveolar nerve. Aziz and associates[47] showed in a cadavaric study that, in most instances, the position of the lingula was located posteroinferior to the position of the antilingula. In only 33% of the cadaver specimens, the lingula was found anterior to the antilingula. They noted that if the osteotomy was made 5 mm posterior to the antilingula, there was no risk of damage to the neurovascular bundle. Therefore, to avoid an injury to the inferior alveolar nerve, the saw blade should parallel the posterior border of the ramus and be placed 5 mm posterior to the bulge of the antilingula on the lateral aspect of the mandible. If, despite these precautions, postoperative paresthesia occurs, it should be carefully followed, although microneurosurgical repair is usually not warranted nor is it technically feasible.

Motor Nerve Injury

Injury to the branches of the facial nerve is much more common with extraoral approaches to the mandible than with intraoral orthognathic surgery. However, there have also been multiple reports of facial nerve injuries resulting from SSOs and VROs.[48–51] In one series that studied 1747 cases of SSO procedures, the incidence of facial nerve injury was 0.26%.[50] The degree of injury can vary from partial loss of motor function to total facial paralysis and is more often seen after a setback of the mandible than with mandibular advancement.[49] The possible causes of facial nerve injury during SSO setback include impingement on the nerve when the distal segment is moved posteriorly, fracture of the styloid process and subsequent displacement, and introduction of retractors behind the ascending ramus with impingement on the nerve. Most of the reported cases of facial nerve injury occurred with mandibular setbacks without use of the Hunsuck modification,[52] so the horizontal osteotomy extending to the posterior border of the mandibular ramus may have caused direct facial nerve injury. However, the most likely cause of facial nerve injury is pressure on the nerve trunk, either by the posteriorization of the distal segment or by the inadvertent placement of retractors behind the posterior border of the mandible (Figure 61-10). To prevent this complication, the horizontal osteotomy should extend just distal to the inferior alveolar neurovascular bundle and lingula into the retrolingular fossa when an SSO is used for mandibular setback. If a horizontal osteotomy extends to the posterior border, bony recontouring should be performed proximal to the lingula to prevent posterior overlap of the distal segment in the region of the posterior border of the ramus and the facial nerve. Unfortunately, the magnitude of the mandibular setback that causes this problem is unknown (possibly > 8 mm) and probably varies owing to variations in individual patient anatomy. Also, care should be taken when any retractors are placed behind the mandibular posterior border during all ramus osteotomy procedures.

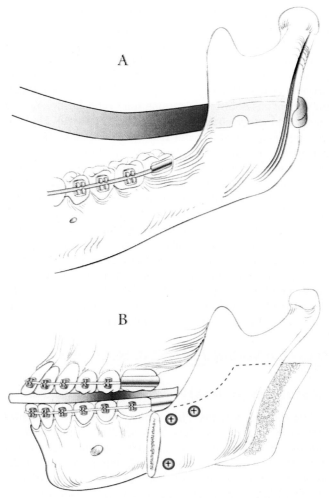

FIGURE 61-10. Causes of facial nerve injury with sagittal split osteotomy (SSO). **A,** Medial retraction behind ramus. **B,** Extension of the distal segment beyond the proximal segment posteriorly.

When a facial nerve paralysis occurs after surgery, a number of electrical tests can be used to determine the depth of injury and subsequent therapy. Electroneurography (ENOG), a study of peripheral nerve conduction, or electromyography (EMG), which is the detection and evaluation of electrical potentials from muscles, may be used diagnostically.[53,54] It is important to distinguish between an injury that causes segmental demyelination and one that causes distal wallerian degeneration. With axonal interruption, the ability to transmit a neuronal impulse is lost over a period of 5 to 7 days. When axonal degeneration occurs, the prognosis for complete spontaneous recovery is poor. When a high-grade nerve injury is noted, surgical exploration should be considered to rule out a partial or complete transection of the nerve. As long as the axon remains intact at the site of the conduction block, the nerve will continue to respond to electrical stimulation distal to the injury site even though paralysis may be present. Evoked electromyography (EEMG), a test in which the degree of muscle twitch elicited is recorded, has

SECTION 7

been used as a prognostic test.[55] If the response to EEMG remains greater than 25% at 5 days, the injury is considered mild and the prognosis for spontanous recovery is good.[55]

Clinical management of the patient during the recovery phases of the paralysis can vary depending on the specific nerve branches, and the type of nerve injury, involved. When the patient has difficulty obtaining full eyelid closure, an eye patch and methylcellulose eye drops may be useful. Physical therapy such as heat, facial massage, and facial exercises performed twice a day have been suggested for neurosensory reeducation. Facial cream should be massaged into the skin around the eyes and mouth and over the midface, ideally using an electrical vibrating device. Biofeedback neurosensory exercises may consist of raising the eyebrows, blowing the cheeks, and grinning while visualizing the attempts in a mirror. Even though no facial movement may be noted, intact nerve fibers will be activated and the exercise will help to maintain muscle tone through electrical and mechanical stimulation. Systemic corticosteroids had been used orally, intramuscularly, and intravenously for facial nerve paralysis in an attempt to decrease perineurial edema from the injury.

NASAL AND SINUS CONSIDERATIONS

Alterations in Nasal Form: Septal Deviation

Le Fort surgery with maxillary repositioning requires manipulation of nasal components, associated facial musculature, and the maxillary sinus. As a result, alterations can occur with the internal nasal anatomy including position of the turbinates, nasal septum, and internal nasal valve. Adverse effects of maxillary osteotomies on the alar bases, nasal tip, supratip depression, and upper lip may result in an unaesthetic postoperative facial appearance.[56-58] The bony and/or cartilaginous nasal septum may be deviated before surgery, at the time of surgery, or during extubation. Therefore, the septum should be inspected before and after surgery. During a Le Fort I osteotomy, it is possible to align the septum at its inferior anterior caudal end of the nasal crest of the maxilla posterior to the anterior nasal spine region. At surgery, the septum is disarticulated from the entire nasal crest of the maxilla, and most commonly with maxillary impaction, the maxilla will encroach upon the presurgical vertical dimension of the nasal septum. Owing to this expected change during maxillary impaction, attention must be given to careful positioning of the septum at the time of surgery. Failure to do so may result in septal deviation and nasal airflow obstruction, or the end result may be an abnormal position of the columella and nasal tip deviation.[57] Several techniques are used to avoid septal deviation during superior maxillary repositioning, including resection of an appropriate portion of the inferior aspect of the bony (vomer) and cartilaginous nasal septum or creating a deep groove in the superior aspect of the maxilla in order to prevent septal deviation as well as stabilize the septum in the midline. In segmental maxillary osteotomies, creating a bony island with parasagittal palatal

cuts may eliminate posterior superior pressure of the nasomaxillary crest on the nasal septum, although this will not eliminate pressure from the anterior portion of the maxilla on the nasal septum.

When septal deviation is recognized postoperatively, three choices for management should be considered (Figure 61-11), including immediate manipulation with manual repositioning, reoperation with reduction of the caudal septum, or septoplasty at a later surgical procedure, if indicated. If appropriate preventive measures for septal deviation were accomplished at the time of surgery, but the nasal septum appears to be asymmetrical, this may result from postoperative edema that may resolve spontaneously or may have occurred during extubation. In the early postoperative period, manipulation with a blunt instrument (e.g., Seldin elevator) placed within the nasal cavity on each side of the base of the nasal septum may allow for manual septal repositioning into a midline position (see Figure 61-11B and C). If rigid fixation has been used and the patient has no airway difficulties, short-term unilateral nasal packing on the side of the deviation may be considered. If septal deviation is due to lack of appropriate prevention during surgery, or if postoperative manipulation fails to result in correction, immediate reoperation with caudal septal resection, with or without the need to remove the rigid fixation for surgical access, may be indicated. If these approaches are not acceptable to either the patient or the surgeon, and the patient does not have significant airway difficulties or cosmetic concerns, the septal deviation may be reevaluated at a later date with consideration for a standard septoplasty procedure if necessary after complete resolution of edema and bony and soft tissue healing.

Alterations in Nasal Form: Internal Nasal Valve

An area of concern in maxillary surgery is alteration of the internal nasal anatomy, nasal airway resistance, and breathing patterns as a result of maxillary surgery. Expansion of the maxilla has shown little change in the nasal airway resistance, and many patients remain obligate mouth breathers even after maxillary expansion surgery.[59] Of greater concern is the possibility that superiorly repositioning the maxilla may decrease the normal nasal airflow owing to an overall decreased dimension of the nasal cavity. Several studies have documented that the reverse is true[60-62] and that superior maxillary repositioning increases the nasal cross-sectional area, decreases nasal airway resistance, and increases nasal breathing. The explanation for this decrease in nasal airway resistance and improved airflow is related to an alteration in configuration of the angulation of nasal valve area.[60-62] The internal nasal valve is formed by the junction of the nasal septum and the upper lateral nasal cartilages and the normal angle formed in this region is 10 to 15 degrees. In contrast, the "external" nasal valve is essentially formed by the nares, which are composed of the floor of the nose and the soft tissues within the nasal sill. The increase in alar base width that

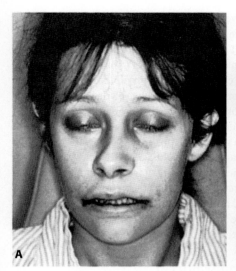
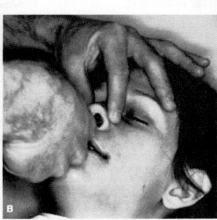
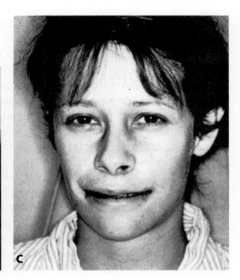

FIGURE 61-11. **A,** Deviated nasal septum postoperatively. **B,** Manual manipulation. **C,** Deviation correction.

results from elevating the soft tissues to expose the maxilla causes a slight widening of the internal nasal valve, increasing the angle of the internal nasal valve (>20 degrees), thereby reducing nasal airway resistance. Owing to the fact that this internal nasal valve is at the smallest cross-sectional area of the nose, slight alterations in this area have a significant effect on nasal breathing, whereas changes in larger intranasal areas have a much less effect on nasal airflow; this same phenomenon has been demonstrated in patients with cleft palates.[63] The effect of maxillary impaction on nasal airway resistance is determined preoperatively using the Cottle test, performed with lateral digital traction on the malar region to open the angle of the internal nasal valve while occluding the contralateral naris; an improvement in nasal airflow is typically expected with this maneuver.

Alterations in Nasal Form: Alar Base

In addition to the internal nasal changes, facial aesthetic changes in nasal morphology may result from maxillary surgery. Failure to properly manage the nasal septum, paranasal musculature, and labial mucosa may result in undesirable facial aesthetic results. Adverse changes in nasal and perioral configuration after maxillary surgery may include excessive alar base widening; increased prominence of the alar groove; upturning of the nasal tip (with an obtuse nasolabial angle); flattening, shortening, and thinning of the upper lip; and downturning of the labial commissures.[57] These complications may also be compounded by internal deviation of the nasal septum, or asymmetrical positioning of the columella and nasal tip due to septal deviation. These types of problems are difficult to manage and are best treated with prevention. The need to control alar base width and the necessity of reconstruction of paranasal and perioral musculature have been described previously.[56] It should be remembered that any maxillary movement results in alar base widening due to

musculature reflection off of the anterior maxilla, and maxillary advancement contributes to even further alar base expansion. Therefore, all Le Fort procedures should incorporate a closure technique that includes an alar base cinch suture to control the degree of alar base widening and attempt to reestablish the presurgical alar base width. Undesirable lower lip changes can be prevented by the use of a low vestibular incision, and the use of a V-to-Y or double V-to-Y closure when indicated to preserve or increase upper lip vermilion display.

Postoperative Sinus Disease

Postoperative complications related to the maxillary sinuses are primarily a result of sinus infections, alteration or interruption of the sinus drainage system, and the persistence of an oroantral fistula. Although many patients experience sinus discharge or excessive nasal drainage and other sinus symptoms in the immediate postoperative period, true perioperative infections of the sinus region and the development of chronic sinusitis after Le Fort surgery are rare.[64,65] Between 2 and 6 months after surgery, there will be normalization of the bony and soft tissue structures in over 55% of the patients,[65] although, at 6 months, as many as 30% of Le Ffort osteotomy patients will show some latent sinus mucosal edema and lack of normal mucociliary function.[65] The pseudociliated stratified ciliated columnar epithelium of the sinus mucosa may also undergo a squamous metaplasia after surgery that may lead to alterations in normal sinus function.

Despite the rarity of postoperative sinus infections, there are several potential causes of infections after maxillary orthognathic surgery. The formation and retention of substantial hematomas in the sinus cavity is an obvious source of potential infection. Perioperative intravenous antibiotic prophylaxis with continued postoperative oral systemic antibiotics will help to prevent the blood clot from becoming infected before resorption. Other potential causes of infection in the sinus include preexisting sinus disease, a history of smoking, dental infection due to trauma to the teeth during the surgery (segmental procedures), soft tissue ischemia and avascularity (again, with segmental surgery), and the presence of debris or retention of foreign bodies within the sinus. Foreign objects such as wires, bone plates, or screws are rarely the isolated cause of a sinus infection and do not appear to cause a significant increase in the incidence of infection after maxillary surgery.[64]

Preoperative assessment of patients presenting for maxillary surgery should include a history and clinical examination, with careful attention to symptoms of any preexisting maxillary sinus disease. Evaluation of preoperative radiographs may provide some information regarding the presence of occult sinus pathology. Postoperative management of sinus infections should include appropriate antibiotic therapy verified by culture and sensitivity, decongestants, intranasal vasoconstrictors, and irrigation of patent fistulae if present. Generally, sinus drainage can be managed to resolution within 10 to 14 days with these techniques. When a sinus infection is refractory to medical treatment, endoscopy, and possible surgical drainage of the sinus should be considered, and this sinus disease should be managed in a manner similar to treatment for patients with sinus disease who have not had Le Fort surgery with standard techniques.

UNANTICIPATED MANDIBULAR OSTEOTOMY FRACTURES

Management of Bad Splits

The intraoperative management of unusual osteotomy fragments (bad splits) is seen more frequently with mandibular procedures, especially the SSO, in which the osteotomy design has two right-angle turns to the ostetomy in which inadvertent splits in the bone may occur. The creation of additional osteotomy segments may occur on either the proximal or the distal bone fragments. The incidence of unfavorable fractures with a BSSO is 1.9% to 2.2%, with a slightly higher incidence when the third molars are present or have not been removed at least 9 months before surgery,[66,67] and depending upon the individual patient anatomy, these bad splits may occur in either the proximal or the distal segment. The standard method for intraoperative management of a bad split is to complete the separation of the proximal and distal segments and then assess the pattern of inappropriate fracture. Typically, bad splits can be addressed adequately via the same intraoral access used for the procedure, and transfacial access is rarely used to allow placement of additional fixation of bony segments. Management will vary depending on the size (small vs. large) as well as the specific location of the fragment, and some bad splits require no treatment. It must first be determined where the fracture deviated from the desired split, and of course, how to possibly prevent a similar occurrence on the other side or in the future. Often, it is

necessary to remove the free segment to gain access to the remaining mandible. A saw or a bur may be used to create a groove on the intact mandible or individual fracture segments so that the SSO can occur along the original planned lines of osteotomy; chisels can be used to complete the desired split. The key to management is to visualize the damage and determine the precise orientation of the problem geometrically. Once the split is successfully completed, the distal segment can be advanced to its desired position. The position and size of the remaining fragments may make positioning of the condylar segment difficult. Segments are sequentially stabilized with plates and screws or wires to the remaining bony fragments. An extraoral approach may be an option, but is usually not necessary. The following examples will illustrate the management of specific unanticipated osteotomy fractures.

Proximal Segment Buccal Plate Fracture, Partial

The difficulty in managing free bone segments depends on the location and size of the fractured pieces of bone. A fragment may shear off the lateral aspect of the proximal segment, thereby leaving the distal mandible intact. Whenever a buccal fragment shears off, the usual cause is an inadequate bone cut at the inferior border of the lateral vertical osteotomy. The split must then be completed, and as mentioned, this can be done by making a deep groove on the inferior border and connecting it with the previous osteotomy as it extends down the external oblique ridge. With gentle manipulation and prying, and when necessary, sectioning bone, the segments can be separated as originally planned. Stabilization of the distal segment with application of IMF will allow easier stabilization of the free buccal plate fragment with screws and plates. Figure 61-12 shows a buccal plate fracture

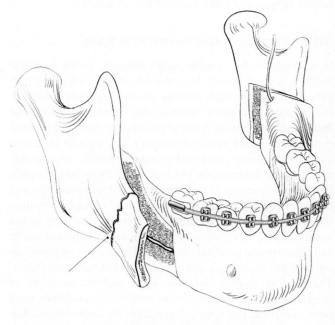

FIGURE 61-12. Proximal segment buccal plate fracture.

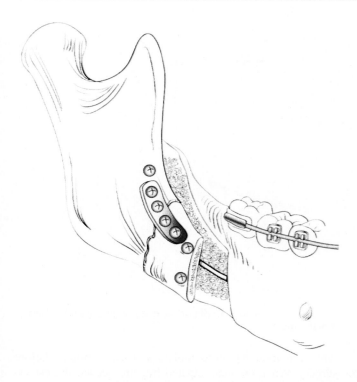

FIGURE 61-13. Rigid fixation used to stabilize the free fragment to the proximal segment; then bicortical fixation of the SSO.

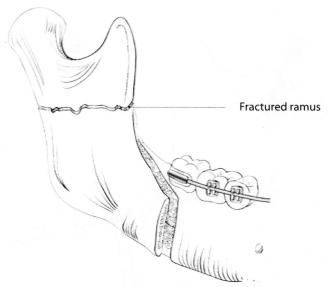

FIGURE 61-14. Horizontal fracture of the proximal segment.

and the main portion of the mandible is intact before completion of the split, so the free segment is stabilized with plate and screw osteosynthesis, as shown in Figure 61-13. Condylar position is not difficult to establish when a proximal segment is large enough to be positioned with adequate overlap and contact with the distal segment in its new position, and bicortical screws can be used, as usual, between the areas of contact of the two segments. With a small free buccal plate fragment, it is frequently easier to place a plate on the segment on the back table and then stabilize it to the proximal segment, although a very small buccal plate fracture segment may not need to be replaced, especially if it does not occur near the inferior border that might result in an unaesthetic postoperative result with excessive antegonial notching.

Proximal Segment Buccal Plate Fracture, Complete

When the buccal plate fracture occurs more superiorly, or there is a plan for a large mandibular advancement such that there will be no contact between the proximal and the distal segments when the occlusion is corrected (Figure 61-14), a different approach must be used. When the condyle and coronoid process are contained in the same proximal segment, owing to a horizontal osteotomy that is created too deeply on the medial ramus, and simulating a horizontal osteotomy of the mandible, control of condylar position is more difficult. The large proximal fragment should be stabilized with rigid fixation either in situ preferably or on the back table (but this

would require disarticulation); the fragment should be then stabilized to the remainder of proximal segment (Figure 61-15). This may requires a percutaneous transbuccal approach for screw placement or the use of right-angled instrumentation. At this point, the proximal segment is easier to manipulate as a complete unit, and it can be fixated to the distal segment into its planned position. This can be accomplished with the use of several plates or bicortical screws. Control of condylar position may be established by posterior, superior, and vertical pressure on the proximal segment, followed by the use of a proximal-distal clamp (e.g., Jeter-van

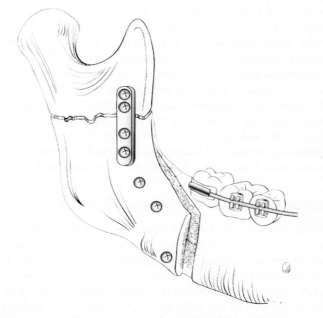

FIGURE 61-15. Fixation of the ascending ramus fracture with a plate and screws; then fixation of the SSO with bicortical screws.

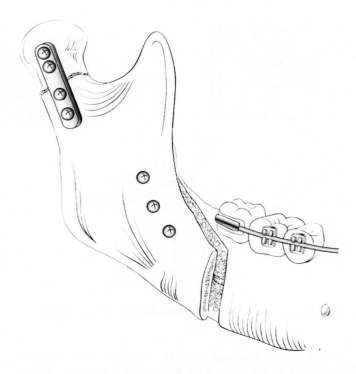

FIGURE 61-16. Fixation of the subcondylar osteotomy with a plate and screws; then bicortical SSO fixation.

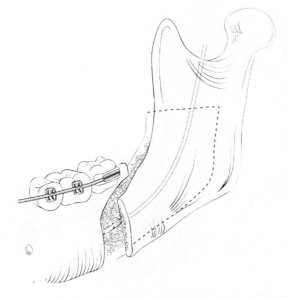

FIGURE 61-17. A lingual split of the distal segment in the third molar region.

Sickels) before placement of bicortical screws or by using the clamp on the coronoid process to stabilize the proximal fragment before screw placement.

Another bad split occurs with the creation of a subcondylar fracture with a condylar fragment separated from the proximal segment. In this case, the condyle must be rigidly fixated to the proximal segment to create a single proximal segment, and then the proximal and distal segments can be stabilized as usual for an SSO (Figure 61-16). Correct condylar positioning is extremely difficult to achieve in this setting, especially with a small condylar stump. The use of transbuccal percutaneous incisions may assist in the placement of a plate is placed on the condylar fragmant, and then the plate can be used as a handle to manipulate the condyle until holes can be drilled in the distal segment with screw placement and application of fixation. Alternatively, an endoscope-assisted technique can be used to improve visualization and application of fixation in this confined region.

Distal Segment Lingual Plate Fracture

Fortunately, fractures of the lingual plate of the distal segment occur less frequently than fractures of the buccal plate of the proximal segment. The underlying cause is frequently an impacted third molar, or it may be secondary to an incomplete ostetomy of the medial horizontal ramus or of the sagittal component of the SSO with the creation of a wedging effect on the medial aspect of the mandible (Figure 61-17). To prevent this type of inadvertant fracture, it is best to

remove mandibular third molars at least 9 months before surgery. When an unanticipated fracture occurs, the osteotomy must be completed along the original planned osteotomy lines. Because the resultant free lingual segment is not an obstruction when the osteotomy is completed, it generally maintains a substantial muscular and vascular pedicle attached to it from the mylohyoid muscle. The distal segment is then stabilized with the application of IMF, and the free lingual plate fragment is manipulated into an anterior position in contact with the distal segment and is fixated to the proximal segment with a lag screw technique using one or more bicortical screws. Then, one or more plates or a piece of titanium mesh may be used on the buccal aspect of the osteotomy site for fixation of the proximal and distal segments (Figure 61-18).

DISPLACEMENT OF THE PROXIMAL VRO SEGMENT

Excessive lateral displacement of the proximal segment can occur during a vertical subcondylar osteotomy. Depending on the geometry of the movement of the distal segment, the proximal, or condylar, segment may be displaced either laterally or medially. The desired position is to have the proximal segment in a lateral position to the distal segment of the mandible. Despite moderate flaring of the proximal segment, typically considerable remodeling occurs at the osteotomy site that allows accomodation of this position without any problems. Occasionally, however, the proximal segment will be flared excessively, especially with an asymmetrical movement of the mandible. This can be addressed intraoperatively by removing a second wedge at the sigmoid notch region to allow a more passive relationship of the proximal and distal segment without interferences that result in extreme lateral displacement of the proximal segment (Figure 61-19). Care

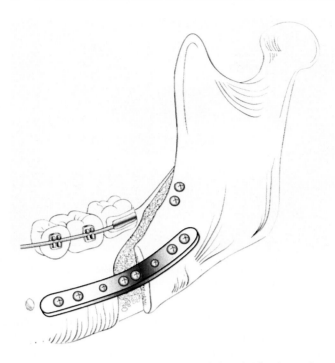

FIGURE 61-18. Two bicortical screws stabilize the free lingual segment to the proximal segment; then monocortical plate and screw fixation of the SSO.

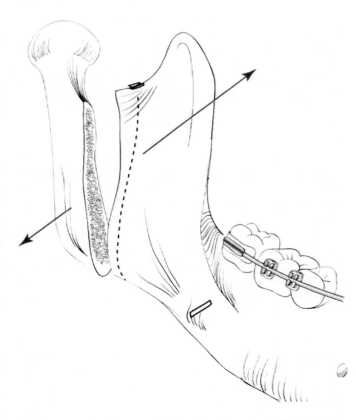

FIGURE 61-19. Excessive flaring of the proximal segment by premature contact at the sigmoid notch; correction by bone wedge removal from distal segment, wider at the sigmoid region than at the inferior border.

must be exercised when performin bony cuts in the sigmoid region because the masseteric branch, or the maxillary artery itself, can be injured iatrogenically. If excessive flaring is noted postoperatively either clinically or radiographically, the segment may be repositioned manually; but if this is not successful, reoperation with open repositioning may be necessary.

In some cases of asymmetry, the rotation of the distal mandible may cause the proximal condylar fragment to be displaced medial to the distal segment. There is a concern that this position may increase the incidence of nerve injury, but this has not been tested clinically, and in general, medial displacement of the proximal segment rarely causes a significant clinical problem. An uncommon patient complaint may be irritation of the posterior pharyngeal region due to contact from the proximal segment; if this occurs, the proximal segment should be repositioned or recontoured or a significant portion should be removed, likely in the inferior aspect of the proximal segment.

Finally, the relationship of the proximal and distal segments may form a butt joint with direct contact despite posterior repositioning of the distal segment. This would result in a clockwise rotation of the condyle that typically does not cause problems, but may contribute to short- and long-term relapse if there is significant tension on the posterior soft tissues with a tendency to displace the segments anteriorly.

PROXIMAL SEGMENT ROTATION

Lack of control of the proximal segment with an SSO can have several clinical effects with both aesthetic and functional consequences. The postoperative muscular influences are such that the proximal segment is pulled anteriorly and superiorly by the temporalis and masseter muscles, while the distal segment is pulled posteriorly and inferiorly by the mylohyoid, geniohyoid, genioglossus, and suprahyoid muscles (Figure 61-20). Therefore, this anterior and superior counterclockwise rotation of the proximal segment and clockwise rotation of the distal segment may result in an unpleasant cosmetic result with flattening of the gonial angle and notching the inferior border of the mandible in the antegonial notch region. This also may cause an unaesthetic protuberance in the cheek region secondary to the lateral positioning of the proximal segment. The type of fixation (wires vs. plates and screws) has been shown to affect the position of the proximal segment both during surgery as well as in the immediate postoperative period.[68]

The most ideal management of a rotated proximal segment is prevention of this complication. Several positioning appliances have been used to control the proximal segment during mandibular orthognathic surgery.[69-71] When rigid fixation is used, without positioning appliances, minimal insignificant rotation of the proximal segment may occur.[68] However, there is a tendency to rotate the proximal segment medially and superiorly as a result of large advancements.[72] This can lead to an unaesthetic result, especially if there was

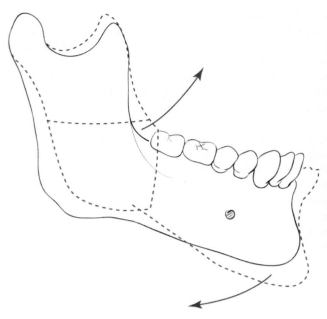

FIGURE 61-20. Diagram of relapse of mandibular orthognathic surgery, with counterclockwise rotation of the proximal segment and clockwise rotation of the distal segment.

any discrepancy in the height of the ramus before surgery (Figure 61-21).

The exact degree of rotation of the proximal segment that will cause clinically significant decreases in muscular bite forces or unaesthetic facial changes remains unknown; however, excessive rotation of the proximal segment should be assessed with regards to functional (decreased bite force generation or hypomobility) or aesthetic (loss of the gonial angle) problems, or both. An aesthetic problem in a patient with an acceptable occlusal result may be treated with the use of an alloplastic implant (e.g., high-molecular-weight porous polyethylene), customized for the specific defect based upon a stereolithography model. If the patient has an occlusal problem as well as aesthetic concerns, the SSO may need to be revised with surgery (Figure 61-22). When a malocclusion

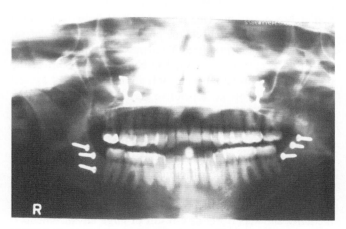

FIGURE 61-21. Radiograph of short mandibular ramus.

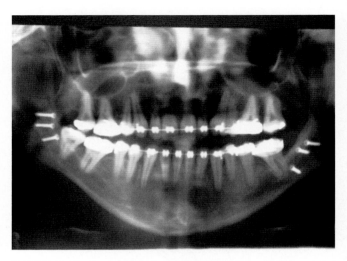

FIGURE 61-22. Occlusal discrepancy with a postoperative anterior open bite deformity.

and unaesthetic result are combined with a decrease in bite force and/or hypomobility of the mandible, reoperation with application of rigid fixation must be combined with an aggressive postoperative physiotherapy regimen.

After any orthognathic surgical procedure, most patients demonstrate a limitation in the degree of maximum interincisal opening. The most dramatic decreases are seen after BSSO procedures.[69] TMJ hypomobility should be restored with the use of postoperative physiotherapy. Ellis[73] examined the range of mandibular motion after an SSO advancement osteotomy in monkeys, when either IMF or rigid osseous fixation was used. Animals that did not have IMF maintained after surgery demonstrated a greater range of motion in the early postsurgical period and attained the preoperative level of mobility by 12 weeks after surgery. Animals that underwent 6 weeks of IMF showed significant decreases in range of motion when compared with the rigid fixation group at each time period after surgery. Several clinical studies have shown that regardless of whether IMF or rigid fixation is used, with postoperative physiotherapy, a normal, or near-normal, range of motion will typically return by 2 years after surgery.[67,74]

There are several potential causes of hypomobility in patients undergoing orthognathic surgery. Scar tissue induced by the surgery may play a major role in limited mouth opening. However, postoperative immobilization can compound the effects of surgical dissection and have adverse effects on the muscles, joints, and surrounding connective tissues. Immobilization by itself induces muscle atrophy with a marked decrease in muscle fiber diameter. This problem may be compounded if the muscle is immobilized in a position where the overall length of the muscle has been shortened. In addition, the use of IMF causes deleterious effects on the TMJ, with a series of degenerative changes in articular cartilage and synovial membranes, with decreased function of the synovium, decreased production of joint fluid, and intraarticular stasis leading to fibrous changes in the TMJ with hypomobility.

Techniques used to eliminate or minimize the period of immobilization will likely decrease postsurgical hypomobility. Despite this, it is strongly suggested that all patients have routine presurgical evaluation of muscle and joint function and a systematic rehabilitation regimen as part of their postsurgical program. Mandibular ramal procedures are potentially the most harmful to the surrounding connective tissues of the jaws. Mandibular advancements, in particular, are susceptible to postoperative hypomobility. If rigid fixation is used, mild self-directed physiotherapy beginning 1 to 2 weeks after surgery may suffice, consisting of either active or passive jaw exercises. When a patient's progress is limited or when surgery has been associated with longer periods of IMF, more aggressive physical therapy is often required. If this is unsuccessful, intra-articular pathology may be responsible for the problem and additional steps may need to be taken to restore a normal range of motion, such as arthroscopic lysis and lavage, if indicated.[75]

TMJ DYSFUNCTION

Short-Term Disorders

TMJ dysfunction in patients undergoing orthognathic surgery deserves careful preoperative examination. A number of patients presenting for orthognathic surgery will have preexisting muscular temporomandibular dysfunction.[76-78] Although a small percentage of patients will develop symptoms as a result of surgery, the large majority will improve after surgery. It is generally accepted that achieving a more appropriate functional relationship of the jaws can improve TMJ symptoms, but orthognathic surgery should not be offered as a primary cure for TMJ problems. It has been generally accepted that class II patients with preexisting anterior disk displacement may benefit from SSO surgery because the consdyle is placed in a different relationship to the glenoid fossa, and this may alleviate the internal derangement by creating additional joint space to allow the disk to assume a more normal position between the cobdyle and the glenoid fossa. However, patients should be advised that orthognathic surgery may have a positive effect, negative effect, or no effect on internal derangement of the TMJ. After surgery, patients may have acute or gradual increases in a variety of TMJ symptoms, and acute exacerbations may be treated with anti-inflammatory medications and physical therapy. Gradual increases or chronic manifestations of TMJ problems are managed with standard protocols for patients with TMJ symptoms, using nonsteroidal anti-inflammatory drugs, soft diet, moist heat, and a bite splint and physical therapy, when indicated. Concern exists that with rigid fixation, there will be a higher incidence of TMJ dysfunction compared with the use of wire osteosynthesis, because the condyle is rigidly stabilized in a new position that may or may not be tolerable or adaptable for the condyle, disk, or glenoid fossa; however, clinical experience and research studies that have compared wire to rigid fixation show that the condyle is capable of adapting functionally to the new position even when rigidly fixated.[74,77]

Long-Term Disorders

Condylar resorption may occur with or without orthognathic surgery and may be responsible for delayed relapse in the young female, class II, high-mandibular-plane-angle patient who undergoes a significant advancement of the mandible. Other causes of delayed relapse after SSO advancement may include preexisting or iatrogenically induced internal derangements of the disk, and class II patients may be more prone to having disk displacement than class I or class III patients. The incidence of condylar resorption or progressive condylar remodeling ranges from 5% to 10% of the patients who undergo orthognathic surgery[79-84] As mentioned, patients who require a large magnitude advancement of the mandible, and who have preoperative TMJ symptoms, are more likely to have this problem than those who have smaller magnitude SSO advancements and no preexisting symptoms.[79,81] Condylar resorption has been noted to occur as far as 12 to 17 months after surgery.[83] Management of this complex problem includes bite splint therapy, with a possible role for anti-inflammatory medications,[83,84] and some surgeons advocate open joint surgery with synovectomy to aggressively address the synovial inflammation and halt the progression of condylar resorption. Secondary surgery to treat resultant anterior open bite deformities using costochondral bone grafting is unpredictable, and the rib graft is susceptible to the same resorption as the condyle in as many as 50% of cases.[83]

UNANTICIPATED MAXILLARY FRACTURES

Whereas the literature has focused on the management of bad splits with mandibular osteotomies, little attention has been focused on inadvertant osteotomies encountered during maxillary orthognathic surgery. With modified cuts of the maxilla (e.g., stepped osteotomy), the bone leading to the zygomatic buttress may be thin and more easily prone to fracture (Figure 61-23). Management may be accomplished by using a plate and screws on either side of the gap, or fractured segment of bone, and then reinserting the fragment behind the plate if necessary (Figure 61-24). In many cases, a small free segment of the thin anterior maxillary wall may be sacrificed without any consequence, and this may be preferable to replacement as a free graft.

In addition, perhaps the most common unanticipated maxillary fracture with Le Fort surgery is the unpredictable fracture that occurs in the pterygoid plate region. Many studies using postoperative computed tomography scans have shown that the posterior osteotomy may occur in a variety of locations, including the maxillary alveolus in the area of the second molar, horizontally through the pterygoid plates, or even superiorly near the base of the skull. These inadvertent fractures may occur in these aberrant locations despite the appropriate use of the ptergoid plate osteotome in the

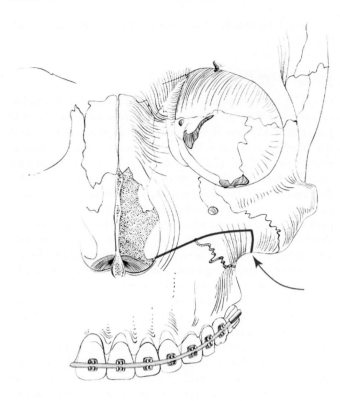

FIGURE 61-23. Fracture of the anterior wall of the maxillary sinus.

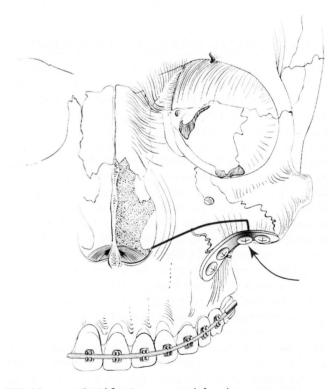

FIGURE 61-24. Rigid fixation to span defect; bone segment repositioned.

ptyerygomaxillary fissure, because access to the medial aspect of the pterygomaxillary junction is limited. Typically, these eccentric fractures have little clinical consequence in the majority of patients; however, the risks of neural and vascular injury, as well as the possibility of intracranial communication, do exist.

Despite careful preoperative treatment planning, either overimpaction or underimpaction of the maxilla may occur at the time of Le Fort surgery. This complication can be avoided with the use of internal, or preferably external, reference points. One option for external reference landmarks is to place a K-wire or Steinmann pin in the nasal bones at the nasion at the commencement of surgery and to take intraoperative measurements that will ensure that the maxilla is placed in the appropriate position at the end of surgery based upon the intended degree of impaction or downgrafting.[85] If the maxilla is found to be underimpacted afte surgery, very few options exist, although removal of plates and screws with placement of skeletal suspension wires in the outpatient setting has been advocated. Typically, a return to surgery to reposition and stabilize the maxilla into the correct position is warranted. When the maxilla is overimpacted, it is usually not possible to use multiple heavy vertical elastics in the early postoperative period to pull the maxilla inferiorly, and reoperation should be considered.

POSTOPERATIVE OCCLUSAL DISCREPANCIES

Occlusal abnormalities may be related to a number of factors in the preoperative, intraoperative, or postoperative phases of patient management. As a general rule, the majority of occlusal discrepancies between what was intended and what was obtained can be traced back to inaccuracies in preoperative patient records.[86]

Anterior Open Bite Malocclusions

Anterior open bites (apertognathia) after orthognathic surgery may be the result of technical difficulties seen with both the maxilla and the mandible at the time of surgery. With the maxilla, these include posterior interferences that are not recognized when IMF is applied during surgery; essentially, the IMF will attempt to close the "open bite" present due to posterior interferences and pull the condyles out of the glenoid fossa by doing so. If the maxilla is fixated with condyles not seated passively, with dislocation out of the glenoid fossa, when the IMF is released, there will be an immediate relapse with an open bite malocclusion. Occasionally, however, the open bite is not recognized until the next day owing to muscle relaxation and edema, and depending on the severity of the open bite, a return to the operating room for repositioning may be required.

Open bites that occur after orthodontic appliances have been removed may be due to relapse of surgically or orthodontically treated maxillary transverse discrepancies. Any molar interferences created after surgery may significantly affect the development of an open bite anteriorly. Surgical and orthodontic correction of severe maxillary transverse discrepancies have been noted to be unstable,[87] and when relapse of the transverse correction occurs, it is usually manifested by an anterior open bite malocclusion. Management of late open bites will depend on their severity; they typically respond to posterior occlusal equilibration with enameloplasty of the molar interferences and rarely require reoperation. In addition, the development of an open bite in the long-term postoperative period may be due to condylar resorption with large mandibular advancements, as described previously.

In addition, anterior open bites have been noted to recur years after initial treatment with both orthodontics and surgery.[87,88] The stability of orthodontic therapy varies depending upon the orthodontic techniques used to manage the open bite relationship.[89] Rotation of incisors that are flared with closure of an open bite may be no more problematic than for other tooth movements. When extrusion of teeth has occurred with orthodontic mechanics, the results are less predictable, and the mechanism of this phenomenon is somewhat controversial. Tooth extrusion may have caused an increased sensitivity to external factors, such as the tongue and circumoral musculature, which may predispose the occlusion to apertognathia. Lack of stability or recurrence of the open bite is, therefore, thought to be due to the continued presence of etiologic factors (e.g., tongue thrust habit) and failure of biologic and functional adaptation. A variety of measures may be taken to correct these problems including orthodontic cribs or appliances to decrease the influence of external factors or surgical techniques such as a partial glossectomy, although these are not commonly performed.

Relapse of the Mandible

Relapse of the mandible after a BSSO procedure has been well documented in the literature, especially with larger magnitude advancements,[90–93] although the use of rigid fixation over wire fixation, or no fixation, has resulted in a significant reduction in expected relapse after orthognathic surgery. However, occlusal discrepancies may occur secondary to several reasons, including errors in the technical aspects of application of rigid fixation. Occlusal changes seen with rigid fixation may be secondary to unpredictable condylar torque, condylar sag, or incorrect placement of the proximal segment at the time of SSO surgery. These condylar positional discrepancies may result in anterior or posterior open bites or lateral shifts of the occlusion. Severe occlusal discrepancies may require revision of the orthognathic procedure. Minor discrepancies can be treated by early aggressive orthodontics with orthopedic movement of the bony segments and teeth. Posterior open bites of less than 3 mm c an be treated with vertical elastics or other orthodontic mechanics. Larger posterior open bites may require maxillary repositioning, possibly using only a posterior segmental maxillary osteotomy for the specific posterior open bite region. Anterior open bites represent failure to properly place the condyle in the glenoid fossa or instability at the osteotomy site with loss of fixation. The use of IMF with heavy anterior elastic traction may prevent reoperation when the cause is noted to be instability at the osteotomy site with loose or ineffective hardware, whereas condylar malpositioning may require revision surgery.

The ideal time to initiate correction of occlusal discrepancies is as soon after surgery as the problem is noted. Removal of the plates and/or screws in an outpatient setting, with the application of elastic traction therapy, may occasionally correct some postoperative malocclusions. Failure to place the condyle in the fossa, either unilaterally or bilaterally, requires evaluation as to whether orthodontic therapy can correct the problem, or more likely, whether a second revision surgery is necessary. A lateral shift of the occlusion in which the midline is deviated to one side is usually due to condylar torque at the time of surgery. In fact, this is the most common complication after BSSO surgery with application of rigid fixation, because the plates and/or screws place the condyles in an unnatural position that is different on each side, with a tendency for a slight shift of the occlusion in the early postoperative period. If using a proximal-distal segment clamp for application of rigid fixation, the proximal segment should lie passively against the distal segemnt, and shifts or torque of the proximal segment may need to be addressed with recontouring or bone shimming, or the clamp can be repositioned in a different location. After surgery, a midline shift due to torque of the proximal segment may be treated with orthodontics if 1 to 2 mm; larger midline discrepancies may rarely require reoperation.

Relapse of a skeletal class III mandibuar setback surgery upon release of IMF has also been noted, especially with larger degrees of posterior mandibular movement.[94–96] Theoretically, this may be caused by pushing the proximal fragment back during surgery, especially with VRO as described previously, and with the release of IMF, the mandible rotates forward. To prevent this problem, it has been suggested that the inferior border of both the proximal and the distal segments be aligned and that the medial sling (medial pterygoid muscle) be released to allow a passive fit of the segments.[95] Others disagree and believe that clockwise rotation of the proximal segment is not responsible for the relapse.[96] In addition, the use of a monocortical plate and screws on the proximal and distal segments may provide a more stable occlusal result than that seen with the use of bicortical screws (Figure 61-25). When this occlusal discrepancy is seen after surgery, the short-term use of class III elastics can help to correct the problem (1–2 mm discrepancy). If the discrepancy is greater than 3 to 4 mm, orthodontic mechanics or interproximal reduction (IPR) may be effective, although a second revision operation may be necessary.

As discussed previously, an anterior open bite may be seen after BSSO with relapse (Figure 61-26). This is usually due to a failure of the plates and/or screws placed at the time of fixation, or technical difficulties incurred at the time of

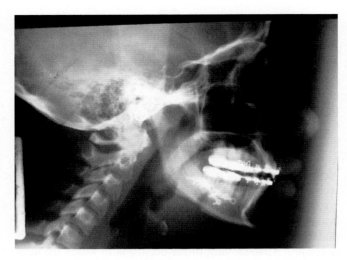

FIGURE 61-25. Monocortical plate and screws for SSO fixation.

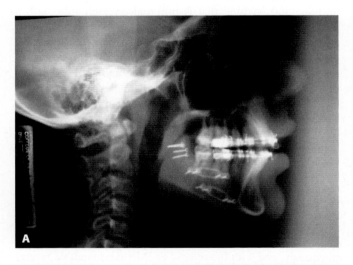

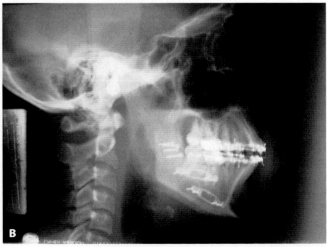

FIGURE 61-26. Postoperative open bite after bilateral sagittal split osteotomy (BSSO). **A,** At 24 hours. **B,** After 1 week of occlusal elastic therapy.

osteotomy with resulting edema in the joints that typically resolves with time. However, an anterior open bite is much more commonly seen in patients after an intraoral VRO upon release of IMF.[97,98] Recommendations to prevent this problem include removal of the coronoid process and temporalis muscle influence, the use of skeletal suspension wires for additional fixation, using modified osteotomy cuts of the ramus to maximize bony contacts, and extending the postoperative period of IMF to at least 8 weeks.[98] Also, postoperative guiding elastics have been used for an extended period of 2 to 6 weeks when open bites have been noted in the immediate postoperative period.

MISCELLANEOUS COMPLICATIONS

Owing to the proximity of the nasal ETT to the maxillary, ETTs may be injured from drills, saws, or osteotomes during maxillary orthognathic surgery, and in some cases reintubation is required, while in others packing around the ETT is sufficient. In order to avoid this complication, a wire-reinforced anode ETT may be preferable, although the rarity of this occurrence does not warrant major changes to routine.

Alar rim injuries, with alar necrosis, are due to pressure on the alar rim from an nasotracheal tube. Care should be taken when wrapping the head so that there is no pressure on the tip of the nose or the forehead or ears from the ETT or its components.

Soft tissue emphysema in the cervical and facial regions has been noted after a variety of procedures that may be unrelated to orthognathic surgery. However, there are several reports of air in the soft tissues of the head, neck, and chest after Le Fort I osteotomies.[99] Subcutaneous emphysema of the cheeks is likely due to forceful blowing of the nose postoperatively, which allows air to escape into the surrounding tissues through the maxillary sinus ostium. Forceful coughing can allow air to pass into the retropharyngeal space and into the mediastinum. Alternatively, rupture of a perivascular bleb or traumatic introduction of air through the cervical fascia is also possible. Subcutaneous emphysema may be managed by observation, heat, and systemic antibiotics. Therapy for pneumomediastinum consists of close observation, cardiac monitoring, intravenous fluids, and antibiotics. Chest tubes or drainage of the mediastinum may be necessary, but supplemental oxygen, as well as pulmonary physiotherapy, should be used.

Epiphora

Epiphora may be seen after Le Fort osteotomy and is frequently due to edema of the nasal mucosa. Alternatively, the nasolacrimal ductal drainage system may be injured when a concomitant partial inferior turbinectomy is performed with during maxillary osteotomy. Damage to the nasolacrimal apparatus may also occur if the bone cut for the Le Fort is placed too far superiorly along the medial wall of the sinus (i.e., lateral nasal wall). The incidence of nasolacrimal injury is infrequent and usually transient and resolves spontaneously. Meticulous soft tissue dissection and carefully placed osteotomies around the medial aspect of the piriform aperture may decrease the incidence of epiphora. Persistent excessive eye tearing that does not decrease after 3 weeks may need to be addressed with a dacryocystorhinostomy procedure.

Auriculotemporal Syndrome

The auriculotemporal syndrome, syndrome of gustatory sweating, or Frey's syndrome, is an unusual complication typically seen as a result of parotid gland surgery. After an injury to the auriculotemporal nerve, the symptoms are believed to be caused by a misdirected regeneration of parasympathetic fibers to denervated sweat glands, resulting in sweating of the cheek during mastication and salivation; this condition is diagnosed with an iodine-starch test. A number of authors have reported Frey's syndrome occurring after extraoral VRO and BSSO procedures,[100-103] with symptoms occurring between 3 months and 3 years after orthognathic surgery. Mild cases in which the patient may have symptoms only with spicy foods should be observed, because the symptoms may decrease with time. A variety of treatments have been suggested for more severe symptoms, including topical scopolamine patches and insertion of fascia lata or acellular human dermis matrix under the skin.[104] Because topical scopolamine has a number of undesirable side effects, there have been reports of the use of botulinum toxin as a successful treatment for this problem.[105,106]

Facial Scars

Although attempts are made to camouflage extraoral site incisions, unattractive facial scarring may occasionally occur. Egyedi and coworkers[107] noted 6 undesirable scars in a group of 100 patients with extraoral incisions for orthognathic surgery, although the criteria used to determine what was undesirable are unknown. Percutaneous incisions of 2 to 4 mm seldom leave significant scars, and the more common problem occurs when the epidermis adheres to the underlying fascia and muscle, with puckering or retraction of the skin. Scar revisions can improve the appearance of existing scars, although a scar will always be present. Other options for scar management include massage, injection of corticosteroids, and dermabrasion or laser resurfacing. With the use of intraoral techniques and endoscope-assisted surgery, most skin incisions can be avoided.

It should be noted that iatrogenic scarring of the cheek with skin retraction may occur during an SSO using bicortical screws placed with a transbuccal trocar approach. Whereas the majority of the skin puncture sites on the cheek heal without visible scars, there may be excessive scarring of the site, especially if the metal trocar becomes heated from the rotation of an eccentric drill bit during drilling the holes for the bicortical screws. The burn injury may require local wound care, intralesional steroid injections, or excision. Also, although the risk of salivary fistula exists through this trocar site, it would represent a rare occurrence.

Salivary Gland Injuries

Injuries to the parotid gland can occur with extraoral approaches for orthognathic surgical procedures. Painless swelling, parotid sialoceles, and fistulae have been reported in the first week after surgery.[108] The treatment of sialoceles or salivary fistulae may include the use of antisialogogue (anticholinergic) medications, pressure dressings, aspiration or drainage, and low-dose radiation to decrease salivary flow via induction of glandular atrophy. Sialography is not recommended in the acute phases of these injuries, because the contrast may extravasate into the soft tissues with inflammation or the procedure may create a larger fistula or increase the size of the current fistula. Resolution of a sialocele should be expected within 4 weeks with the appropriate use of nonsurgical therapies, and failure of these treatment options may require a more invasive surgical procedure.

Complications do occur during orthognathic surgery, and the clinician must be aware of the myriad of possible consequences in order to most appropriately manage or prevent these from occurring as well as to be able to adequately perform a detailed informed consent discussion with patients and families before orthognathic surgery. In most cases, complications from orthognathic surgery can be prevented with comprehensive diagnosis and treatment planning including a thorough history, clinical and radiographic examination, dental model and cephalometric analysis, and a meticulous attention to detail in the treatment planning phases for maxillary and mandibular surgery.

References

1. Panula K, Finne K, Oikarinen K. Incidence of complications and problems related to orthognathic surgery: a review of 655 patients. J Oral Maxillofac Surg 2001;59:1128–1136.
2. Bradley JP, Elahi M, Kawamoto HK. Delayed presentation of pseudoaneurysm after Le Fort I osteotomy. J Craniofac Surg 2002;13:746–750.
3. Lanigan DT, West RA. Management of postoperative hemorrhage following the Le Fort I maxillary osteotomy. J Oral Maxillofac Surg 1984;42:367–375.
4. Lanigan DT, Hey JH, West RA. Major vascular complications of orthognathic surgery: hemorrhage associated with Le Fort I osteotomies. J Oral Maxillofac Surg 1990;48:561–573.
5. Lanigan DT, Hey JH, West RA. Major vascular complications of orthognathic surgery: false aneurysms and arteriovenous fistulas following orthognathic surgery. J Oral Maxillofac Surg 1991;49:571–577.
6. Tiner BD, Van Sickels JE, Schmitz JP. Life threatening, delayed hemorrhage after Le Fort I osteotomy requiring surgical intervention: report of two cases. J Oral Maxillofac Surg 1997;55:91–93.
7. Lanigan DT, Hey J, West RA. Hemorrhage following mandibular osteotomies: a report of 21 cases. J Oral Maxillofac Surg 1991;49:713–724.

8. Girotto JA, Davidson J, Wheatly M, et al. Blindness as a complication of Le Fort osteotomies: role of atypical fracture patterns and distortion of the optic canal. Plast Reconstr Surg 1998;102:1409–1421.

9. Lanigan DT, Tubman DE. Carotid-cavernous fistula following Le Fort I osteotomy. J Oral Maxillofac Surg 1987;45:969–975.

10. Lanigan DT, Loewy J. Postoperative computed tomography scan study of the pterygomaxillary separation during the Le Fort I osteotomy using a micro-oscillating saw. J Oral Maxillofac Surg 1995;53:1161–1166.

11. Brady SC, Courtemanche AD, Steinbok P. Carotid artery thrombosis after elective mandibular and maxillary osteotomies. Ann Plast Surg 1981;6:121–126.

12. Turvey TA, Fonseca RJ. The anatomy of the internal maxillary artery in the pterygopalatine fossa: its relationship to maxillary surgery. J Oral Surg 1980;38:92–95.

13. Sanni KS, Campbell RL, Rosner MJ, Goyne WB. Internal carotid artery occlusion following mandibular osteotomy. J Oral Maxillofac Surg 1984;42:394–399.

14. Behrman SJ. Complications of sagittal osteotomy of the mandibular ramus. J Oral Surg 1972;30:554–561.

15. Turvey TA. Intraoperative complications of sagittal osteotomy of the mandibular ramus: incidence and management. J Oral Maxillofac Surg 1985;43:504–509.

16. Teltzrow T, Kramer F-J, Schulze A, et al. Perioperative complications following sagittal split osteotomy of the mandible. J Craniomaxillofac Surg 2005;33:307–313.

17. Tuinzing DB, Greebe RB. Complications related to the intraoral vertical ramus osteotomy. Int J Oral Surg 1985;14:319–324.

18. Lanigan DT, Hey JH, West RA. Aseptic necrosis following maxillary osteotomies: report of 36 cases. J Oral Maxillofac Surg 1990;48:142–156.

19. Lanigan DT, West RA. Aseptic necrosis of the mandible: report of two cases. J Oral Maxillofac Surg 1990;48:296–300.

20. Grammer FC, Meyer MW, Richter KJ. A radioisotope study of the vascular response to sagittal split osteotomy of the mandibular ramus. J Oral Surg 1974;32:578–582.

21. Epker BN. Modifications in the sagittal osteotomy of the mandible. J Oral Surg 1977;35:157–159.

22. Hall HD, Chase DC, Payor LG. Evaluation and refinement of the intraoral vertical subcondylar osteotomy. J Oral Surg 1975;33:333–341.

23. Hall HD, McKenna SJ. Further refinement and evaluation of the intraoral vertical sub-condylar osteotomy. J Oral Maxillofac Surg 1987;45:684–688.

24. Van Sickels JE. A comparative study of bicortical screws and suspension versus bicortical screws in large mandibular advancements. J Oral Maxillofac Surg 1991;49:1293–1298.

25. Dorfman HS, Turvey TA. Alterations in osseous crestal height following interdental osteotomies. Oral Surg Oral Med Oral Pathol 1979;48:120–125.

26. Wolford LM, Rieche-Fischel O, Mehara P. Soft tissue healing after parasagittal palatal incisions in segmental maxillary surgery: a review of 311 patients. J Oral Maxillofac Surg 2002;60:20–25.

27. Turvey TA. Management of the nasal apparatus in maxillary surgery. J Oral Surg 1980;38:331–335.

28. Dodson TB, Bays RA, Neuenschwander MC. Maxillary perfusion during Le Fort I osteotomy after ligation of the descending palatine artery. J Oral Maxillofac Surg 1997;55:51–55.

29. Epker BN. Vascular considerations in orthognathic surgery. II Maxillary osteotomies. Oral Surg Oral Med Oral Pathol 1984;57:473–478.

30. Chow LK, Singh B, Chiu WK, Samman N. Prevalence of postoperative complications after orthognathic surgery: A 15 year review. J Oral Maxillofac Surg 2007;984–992.

31. Ozdemir R, Baran CN, Karagoz MA, Dogan S. Place of sagittal osteotomy in mandibular surgery. J Craniofac Surg 2009;20:349–355.

32. Becelli R, Fini G, Renzi G, et al. Complications of bicortical screw fixation observed in 482 mandibular sagittal osteotomies. J Craniofac Surg 2004;15:64–68.

33. Bouwman JP, Husak A, Putnam GD, et al. Screw fixation following bilateral sagittal ramus osteotomy for mandibular advancement—complications in 700 consecutive cases. Br J Oral Maxillofac Surg 1995;33:231–234.

34. Teerijoki-Oksa T, Jaaskelainen SK, Forssell H, et al. Risk factors of nerve injury during a mandibular sagittal spit osteotomy. Int J Oral Maxillofac Surg 2002;31:33–39.

35. Ziccardi VB, Assael LA. Mechanism of trigeminal nerve injuries. Atlas Oral Maxillofac Surg Clin North Am 2001;9:1–11.

36. Van Sickels JE, Hatch JP, Dolce C, et al. Effects of age, amount of advancement, and genioplasty on neurosensory disturbance after a bilateral sagittal split osteotomy. J Oral Maxillofac Surg 2002;60:1012–1017.

37. Gianni AB, D'Orto O, Biglioli F, et al. Neurosensory alterations of the inferior alveolar and mental nerve after genioplasty alone or associated with sagittal osteotomy of the mandibular ramus. J Craniomaxillofac Surg 2002;30:295–303.

38. Jones DL, Wolford LM. Intraoperative recording of trigeminal evoked potential during orthognathic surgery. Int J Adult Orthodon Orthognath Surg 1990;5:163–174.

39. Rajchel J, Ellis E III, Fonseca RJ. The anatomic location of the mandibular canal: its relationship to the sagittal ramus osteotomy. Int J Adult Orthodon Orthognath Surg 1986;1:37–47.

40. Schendel SA, Epker BN. Results after mandibular advancement surgery: an analysis of 87 cases. J Oral Surg 1980;38:265–282.

41. Jacks SC, Zuniga JR, Turvey TA, Schalit C. A retrospective analysis of lingual nerve sensory changes after mandibular bilateral sagittal split. J Oral Maxillofac Surg 1998;56:700–704.

42. Miloro M, Halkias LE, Slone HW, Chakeres DW. Assessment of the lingual nerve in the third molar region using magnetic resonance imaging. J Oral Maxillofac Surg 1997;55:134–137.

43. Karas ND, Boyd SB, Sinn DP. Recovery of neurosensory function following orthognathic surgery. J Oral Maxillofac Surg 1990;48:124–134.

44. Westermark A, Bystedt H, von Konow L. Inferior alveolar nerve function after mandibular osteotomies. Br J Oral Maxillofac Surg 1998;36:425–428.

45. Troulis MJ, Kaban LB. Endoscopic approach to the ramus/condyle unit: clinical applications. J Oral Maxillofac Surg 2001;59:503–509.

46. Hogan G, Ellis E 3rd. The "antilingual"—fact or fiction? J Oral Maxillofac Surg 2006;64:1248–1254.

47. Aziz SR, Dorfman BJ, Ziccardi VB, Janal M. Accuracy of using the antilingual as a sole determinant of vertical ramus osteotomy position. J Oral Maxillofac Surg 2007;65:859–862.

48. Sakashita H, Miiyata M, Miyamoto H, Miyaji Y. Peripheral facial palsy after sagittal split ramus osteotomy for setback

of the mandible. A case report. Int J Oral Maxillofac Surg 1996;25:182–183.

49. Piecuch JF, Lewis RA. Facial nerve injury as a complication of sagittal split ramus osteotomy. J Oral Maxillofac Surg 1982;40:309–310.

50. de Vries K, Devriese PP, Hovinga J, van den Akker HP. Facial palsy after sagittal split osteotomies. A survey of 1747 sagittal split osteotomies. J Craniomaxillofac Surg 1993;21:50–53.

51. Motamedi MH. Transient temporal nerve palsy after intraoral subcondylar ramus osteotomy. J Oral Maxillofac Surg 1997;55:527–528.

52. Hunsuck EE. A modified intraoral sagittal splitting technic for correction of mandibular prognathism. J Oral Surg 1968;26:250–253.

53. Chow LC, Tam RC, Li MF. Use of electroneurography as a prognostic indicator of Bell's palsy in Chinese patients. Otol Neurotol 2002;23:598–601.

54. Gutmann L. Pearls and pitfalls in the use of electromyography and nerve conduction studies. Semin Neurol 2003;23:77–82.

55. May M, Klein SR, Blumenthal F. Evoked electromyography and idiopathic facial paralysis. Otolaryngol Head Neck Surg 1983;91:678–685.

56. O'Ryan F, Schendel S. Nasal anatomy and maxillary surgery. I. Esthetic and anatomic principles. Int J Adult Orthodon Orthognath Surg 1989;4:27–37.

57. O'Ryan F, Schendel S. Nasal anatomy and maxillary surgery. II. Unfavorable nasolabial esthetics following Le Fort I osteotomy. Int J Adult Orthodon Orthognath Surg 1989;4:75–84.

58. O'Ryan F, Carlotti A. Nasal anatomy and maxillary surgery. III. Surgical techniques for correction of nasal deformities in patients undergoing maxillary surgery. Int J Adult Orthodon Orthognath Surg 1989;4:157–174.

59. Warren DW, Hershey HG, Turvey TA, et al. The nasal airway following maxillary expansion. Am J Orthod Dentofacial Orthop 1987;91:111–116.

60. Walker DA, Turvey TA, Warren DW. Alterations in nasal respiration and nasal airway size following superior repositioning of the maxilla. J Oral Maxillofac Surg 1988;46:276–281.

61. Erbe M, Lehotay M, Gode U, et al. Nasal airway changes after Le Fort I impaction and advancement: anatomical and functional findings. Int J Oral Maxillofac Surg 2001;30:123–129.

62. Kunkel M, Hochban W. The influence of maxillary osteotomy on nasal airway patency and geometry. Mund Kiefer Gesichtschir 1997;1:194–198.

63. Gotzfried HF, Masing H. Improvement of nasal breathing in cleft patients following mid-face osteotomy. Int J Oral Maxillofac Surg 1988;17:41–44.

64. Bell CS, Thrash WJ, Zysset MK. Incidence of maxillary sinusitis following Le Fort I maxillary osteotomy. J Oral Maxillofac Surg 1986;44:100–103.

65. Kahnberg KE, Engstrom H. Recovery of maxillary sinus and tooth sensibility after Le Fort I osteotomy. Br J Oral Maxillofac Surg 1987;25:68–73.

66. Mehra P, Castro V, Freitas RZ, Wolford LM. Complications of the mandibular sagittal ramus osteotomy associated with the presence or absence of third molars. J Oral Maxillofac Surg 2001;59:854–858.

67. Precious DS, Lung KE, Pynn BR, Goodday RH. Presence of impacted teeth as a determining factor of unfavorable splits in 1256 sagittal split osteotomies. Oral Surg Oral Med Oral Pathol Oral Radiol Endod 1998;85:362–365.

68. Hatch JP, Van Sickels JE, Rugh JD, et al. Mandibular range of motion after bilateral sagittal split ramus osteotomy with wire osteosynthesis or rigid fixation. Oral Surg Oral Med Oral Pathol Oral Radiol Endod 2001;91:274–280.

69. Ellis E III. Condylar positioning devices for orthognathic surgery. Are they necessary? J Oral Maxillofac Surg 1994;52:536–552.

70. Helm G, Stepke MT. Maintenance of the preoperative condyle position in orthognathic surgery. J Craniomaxillofac Surg 1997;25:34–38.

71. Merten HA, Halling F. A new condylar positioning technique in orthognathic surgery. Technical note. J Craniomaxillofac Surg 1992;20:310–312.

72. Harris MD, Van Sickels JE, Alder M. Factors influencing condylar position after the bilateral sagittal split osteotomy fixed with bicortical screws. J Oral Maxillofac Surg 1999;57:650–654.

73. Ellis E III. Mobility of the mandible following mandibular advancement and maxillomandibular or rigid internal fixation: an experimental investigation in *Macaca mulatto*. J Oral Maxillofac Surg 1988;46:118–123.

74. Feinerman DM, Piecuch JF. Long-term effects of orthognathic surgery on the temporomandibular joint: comparison of rigid and non-rigid fixation methods. Int J Oral Maxillofac Surg 1995;24:268–272.

75. Van Sickels JE, Tiner BD, Alder ME. Condylar torque as a possible cause of hypomobility after sagittal split osteotomy. Report of three cases. J Oral Maxillofac Surg 1997;55:398–402.

76. De Boever AL, Keeling SD, Hilsenbeck S, et al. Signs of temporomandibular disorders in patients with horizontal mandibular deficiency. J Orofac Pain 1996;10:21–27.

77. Rodrigues-Garcia RC, Sakai S, Rugh JD, et al. Effects of major class II occlusal correction on temporomandibular signs and symptoms. J Orofac Pain 1998;12:185–192.

78. Panula K, Somppi M, Finne K, Oikarinen K. Effects of orthognathic surgery on temporomandibular joint dysfunction. A controlled prospective 4 year follow-up study. Int J Oral Maxillofac Surg 2000;29:183–187.

79. Cutbirth M, Van Sickels JE, Thrash WJ. Condylar resorption after bicortical screw fixation of mandibular advancement. J Oral Maxillofac Surg 1998;56:178–182.

80. Hwang SJ, Haers PE, Zimmermann A, et al. Surgical risk factors for condylar resorption after orthognathic surgery. Oral Surg Oral Med Oral Pathol Endod 2000;89:542–552.

81. Scheerlinck JP, Stoelinga PJ, Blijdorp PA, et al. Sagittal split advancement osteotomies stabilized with miniplates. A 2–5 year follow-up. Int J Oral Maxillofac Surg 1994;23:127–131.

82. Hoppenreijs TJ, Freihofer HP, Stoelinga PJ, et al. Condylar remodeling and resorption after Le Fort I and bimaxillary osteotomies in patients with anterior open bite. A clinical and radiological study. Int J Oral Maxillofac Surg 1998;27:81–91.

83. Hoppenreijs TJ, Stoelinga PJ, Grace KL, Robben CM. Long-term evaluation of patients with progressive condylar resorption following orthognathic surgery. Int J Oral Maxillofac Surg 1999;28:411–418.

84. Arnett GW, Milam SB, Gottesman L. Progressive mandibular retrusion-idiopathic condylar resorption. Part II. Am J Orthod Dentofac Orthop 1996;110:117–127.

85. Nishioka GJ, Van Sickels JE. Modified external reference measurement technique for vertical positioning of the maxilla. Oral Surg Oral Med Oral Pathol 1987;64:22–23.

86. Jacobson R, Sarver DM. The predictability of maxillary repositioning in Le Fort I orthognathic surgery. Am J Orthod Dentofac Orthop 2002;122:142–154.

87. Profitt WR, Turvey TA, Phillips C. Orthognathic surgery: a hierarchy of stability. Int J Adult Orthodon Orthognath Surg 1996;11:191–204.

88. Burford D, Noar JH. The causes, diagnosis and treatment of anterior open bite. Dent Update 2003;30:235–241.

89. Beane RA. Nonsurgical management of the anterior open bite: a review of options. Semin Orthod 1999;5:275–283.

90. Dolce C, Van Sickels JE, Bays RA, Rugh JD. Skeletal stability after mandibular advancement with rigid versus wire fixation. J Oral Maxillofac Surg 2000;58:1219–1228.

91. Dolce C, Hatch JP, Van Sickels JE, Rugh JD. Rigid versus wire fixation for mandibular advancement skeletal and dental changes after 5 years. Am J Orthod Dentofac Orthop 2002;121:638–649.

92. Blomqvist JE, Ahlborg G, Isaksson S, Svartz K. A comparison of skeletal stability after mandibular advancement and use of two rigid internal fixation techniques. J Oral Maxillofac Surg 1997;55:568–574.

93. Moenning JE, Bussard DA, Lapp TH, Garrision BT. Comparison of relapse in bilateral sagittal split osteotomies for mandibular advancement: rigid internal fixation (screws) versus inferior border wires with anterior skeletal fixation. Int J Adult Orthodon Orthognath Surg 1990;5:175–182.

94. Proffit WR, Phillips C, Turvery TA. Stability after surgical-orthodontic corrective of skeletal Class III malocclusion. 3. Combined maxillary and mandibular procedures. Int J Adult Orthodon Orthognath Surg 1991;6:211–225.

95. Franco JE, Van Sickels JE, Thrash WJ. Factors contributing to relapse in rigidly fixed mandibular setbacks. J Oral Maxillofac Surg 1989;47:451–456.

96. Costa F, Robiony M, Sembronio S, et al. Stability of skeletal Class III malocclusion after combined maxillary and mandibular procedures. Int J Adult Orthodon Orthognath Surg 2001;16:179–192.

97. Proffit WR, Phillips C, Dann C IV, Turvey TA. Stability after surgical orthodontic correction of skeletal Class III malocclusion. I. Mandibular setback. Int J Adult Orthodon Orthognath Surg 1991;6:7–18.

98. Tornes K, Wisth PJ. Stability after vertical subcondylar ramus osteotomy for correction of mandibular prognathism. Int J Oral Maxillofac Surg 1988;17:242–248.

99. Nannini V, Sachs SA. Mediastinal emphysema following Le Fort I osteotomy: report of a case. Oral Surg Oral Med Oral Pathol 1986;62:508–509.

100. Berrios RJ, Quinn PD. Frey's syndrome: a complication after orthognathic surgery. Int J Adult Orthodon Orthogn Surg 1986;1:219–224.

101. Kopp WK. Auriculotemporal syndrome secondary to vertical sliding osteotomy of the mandibular rami: report of a case. J Oral Surg 1968;26:295–296.

102. Tuinzing DB, van der Kwast WA. Frey's syndrome. A complication after sagittal splitting of the mandible. Int J Oral Surg 1982;11:197–200.

103. Guerrissi J, Stoyannoff J. Atypical Frey syndrome as a complication of Obwegeser osteotomy. J Craniofac Surg 1998;9:543–547.

104. Sinha UK, Saddat D, Doherty CM, Rice DH. Use of AlloDerm implant to prevent Frey syndrome after parotidectomy. Arch Facial Plast Surg 2003;5:109–112.

105. Eckardt A, Kuettner C. Treatment of gustatory sweating (Frey's syndrome) with botulinum toxin A. Head Neck 2003;25:624–628.

106. Restivo DA, Lanza S, Patti F, et al. Improvement of diabetic autonomic gustatory sweating by botulinum toxin type A. Neurology 2002;59:1971–1973.

107. Egyedi P, Houwing M, Juten E. The oblique subcondylar osteotomy: report of results of 100 cases. J Oral Surg 1981;39:871–873.

108. Dierks EJ, Granite EL. Parotid sialocele and fistula after mandibular osteotomy. J Oral Surg 1977;35:299–300.

Cleft Orthognathic Surgery

Kevin S. Smith, DDS

In treatment of children with cleft lip and palate facial anomalies, the use of an interdisciplinary team approach continues to be of primary importance throughout adolescence. The coordination of care between restorative dentistry, surgery, orthodontics, and prosthodontics is critically important during this phase of reconstruction of the cleft lip and palate patient. As stated by the American Cleft Palate Association (ACPA), the minimum requirements for a cleft lip and palate team include a surgeon (oral and maxillofacial surgeon, otorhinolaryngologist, or plastic surgeon), a speech and language pathologist, and an orthodontist. These minimum requirements may be inadequate if the team does not provide a consultation for the other members who are truly important in the care of cleft lip and palate patients, specifically restorative dentistry and psychological counseling. Many children with cleft lip and palate have malformed teeth, dental crowding, missing teeth, supernumerary teeth, and ectopic eruption that frequently require careful evaluation and treatment by pediatric or general dentists during the phases of mixed dentition and into the early permanent dentition. Many children have underdeveloped, or missing, maxillary lateral incisors and may be candidates for dental implants and/or other prosthetic reconstruction. Consequently, these professionals are of utmost importance to the team. Sometimes overlooked in interdisciplinary care of these patients is psychological counseling. A significant number of these children have self-esteem issues associated with their facial deformities, especially during the formative preteen years, and families need to maintain an open mind and discuss these social issues associated with their cleft lip and palate child. A thorough team discussion about the consultations that can be obtained, and the services that can be provided, must take place to ensure that each team member has access to all aspects of care and to ensure that patient expectations are reasonable and appropriate. On occasion, families become very complacent with follow-up and recall to the interdisciplinary cleft palate clinic owing to the fact that they have had their immediate

needs met once the cleft lip and cleft palate have been repaired surgically. If speech problems have been addressed, or do not exist, the family may be satisfied with the progress, and it is critical that the interdisciplinary team review the patient records to ensure that patients who have been noncompliant with regular team meetings attempt to reenter the regular team meetings, especially during late transitional dentition and early permanent dentition, to alleviate significant problems in treatment who may present late for treatment. When children are not followed routinely, and present late in the orthodontic and surgical sequencing for treatment of cleft lip and palate, the treatment becomes much more complex, social issues become much more significant, and the problems may increase exponentially (Figures 62-1 to 62-3).

Orthognathic care in the cleft lip and palate patient begins with development of the maxilla in the transitional dentition, and during this time, the orthodontist should take every opportunity to develop the transverse dimension of the maxilla. Expansion of the maxilla before alveolar cleft bone grafting will help to maintain the transverse dimensions of

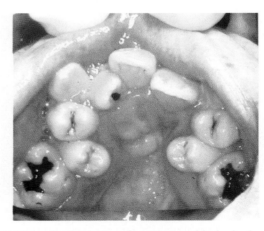

FIGURE 62-1. Occlusal view of an 18-year-old who had inappropriate management of cleft dentofacial anomaly.

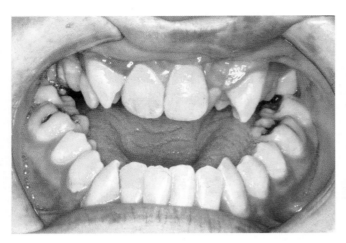

FIGURE 62-2. Anterior closed occlusal view of a patient with inappropriate cleft care. The patient was followed by a "cleft" surgeon, but without interaction from other cleft team members.

the maxilla and will alleviate potential transverse problems with orthognathic surgery once the child has reached adolescence. Before orthognathic surgery, orthodontists should be acutely aware of whether the child has a propensity for maxillary anteroposterior (AP) and/or vertical hypoplasia and should be careful not to treat these problems with extraction of teeth in the lower arch to try to maintain a class I occlusion. Early in the adolescent period, children who are treated in this manner have a greater problem later on once they have transitioned into a class III malocclusion and are missing significant lower arch dimension. The patient and family may initially think that the patient will not be a candidate for surgery, and this may have negative effects on the orthodontist-patient relationship if a surgery is recommended later. Statistically, the number of children who need to have orthognathic surgery and have had unilateral cleft lip and palate is approximately 25%.[1,2]

Other orthodontic considerations for the cleft patient requiring orthognathic surgery include preoperative orthodontic banding and bonding. It is critical to ensure that

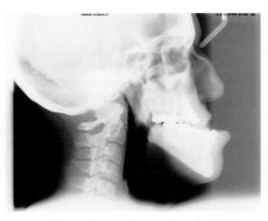

FIGURE 62-3. Lateral cephalogram of a cleft patient presenting for correction of a severe dentofacial anomaly.

surgical rectangular arch wires and adequate surgical lugs are in place before surgery to allow the surgeon to manipulate the maxilla during the surgical procedure. The surgeon will have a difficult enough time manipulating the maxilla without having additional problems associated with poorly bonded orthodontic appliances with small arch wires and without adequate surgical lugs for intraoperative intermaxillary fixation. These small issues can provide an increasingly frustrating surgical procedure that may result in inadequate treatment in fixation.

Maxillary hypoplasia in three planes of space is a common problem encountered in children with cleft lip and palate, and there is controversy regarding what degree of this restricted growth is surgically induced and what degree of hypoplasia is intrinsic.[3] Decisions must be made by the interdisciplinary team, with parental and patient input, regarding whether the patient will have early surgery, end-of-growth surgery, or both. Many children entering junior high school, grades 6 to 8, may be experiencing psychosocial issues owing to the negative aesthetic effects of severe maxillary hypoplasia, and these children may be candidates for early orthognathic surgery with maxillary advancement surgery (Figures 62-4 to 62-6). Discussions about early orthognathic surgery must include an understanding by the family and patient that, in most situations, the patient will require secondary surgery after the cessation of facial growth.

Early in the history of orthognathic surgery, the application to children with cleft lip and palate dentofacial anomalies proved to be difficult. Many institutions, both before and after the introduction of rigid fixation, employed a philosophy of "splitting the AP discrepancy" between the maxilla and the mandible or avoided treatment of the maxilla completely.[4,5] Patients with severe maxillary hypoplasia may have had a Le Fort I osteotomy performed, repositioning the maxilla as anterior as possible allowed by the scar tissue restriction. There is typically adjunctive bone grafting and some form of additional fixation utilized in these cases of large maxillary advancements in the cleft patient to prevent relapse. Subsequently, the mandible was then repositioned posteriorly to achieve a class I canine and molar relationship with the maxilla. In many patient situations, the projection of the mandible may be in a relatively normal position, and essentially, the technique of treating to the deformity was employed. Treating to the deformity has significant ramifications in the form of compromised facial aesthetics and possible iatrogenic obstructive sleep apnea due to narrowing of the posterior airway (Figures 62-7 and 62-8).

In contemporary orthognathic surgery of children with cleft deformities, if cephalometrically and clinically, the mandible is in a normal AP position, it should not be repositioned posteriorly to split the difference with the maxilla; this will allow increased projection of the maxilla, elevation of the nasal tip, increased lip support, and the establishment of stable occlusion. Maxillary advancement does not correct the lip scarring or retraction or compensate for an unaesthetic lip repair, and it does not normalize anatomic landmarks.[6] The

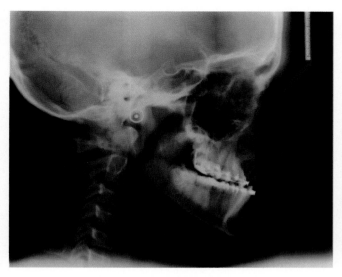

FIGURE 62-4.   Lateral cephalogram of a 12-year-old bilateral cleft lip and palate patient before orthognathic surgery.

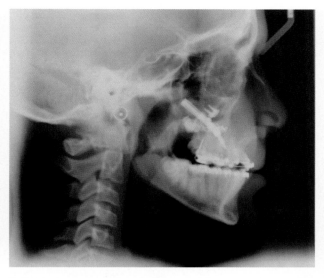

FIGURE 62-5.   Lateral cephalogram of the same 12-year-old with early intervention maxillary advancement. Secondary procedures were planned owing to continued growth.

skeletal surgery must occur before the final soft tissue revision, including any lip and nasal aesthetic procedures. The increased support provided by maxillary advancement for the nose and lip changes the cosmetic appearance without direct surgery on these structures. The judgment of the surgeon who performs the definitive lip and nasal surgery may be hindered if the skeletal deformity is not addressed before the final aesthetic soft tissue procedures.

Other presurgical orthognathic considerations for patients with bilateral cleft lip and palate include the use of palatal splints, especially in situations in which the bone graft is less than adequate in the alveolar cleft to help prevent fracture of

the bone graft in this area and after the down-fracture and manipulation of the maxilla. A palatal splint will help stabilize the bone of the lateral segments as well as the premaxilla so that the intersegment bone does not fracture and will allow stabilization of the entire complex so that additional bone grafting can be accomplished during the orthognathic procedure, if indicated. Occlusal splints must be fabricated before surgery with consideration of whether overcorrection of the jaw movements will be planned. Posnick and Ewing[7] showed that 24 patients without pharyngoplasty with mean maxillary advancements of 6.7 mm relapsed immediately after surgery with a mean relapse of 2.0 mm over a 2-year follow-up period. Planned overcorrection in the model surgery and

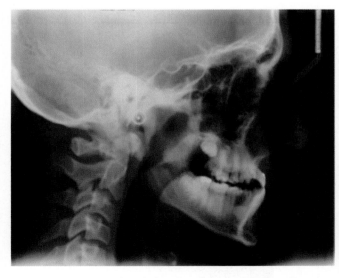

FIGURE 62-6.   Lateral cephalogram of the patient from Figures 62-4 and 62-5 at age 17. The patient asked the orthodontist for camouflage and did not want a second surgery. Note recurrent maxillary hypoplasia, not secondary to relapse, but continued mandibular growth.

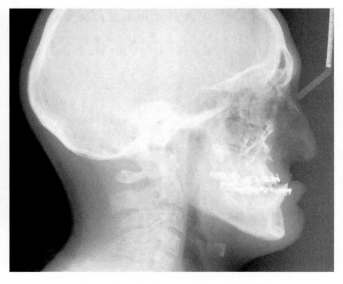

FIGURE 62-7.   Lateral cephalogram of a 17-year-old patient who had had early surgery for correction of maxillary hypoplasia.

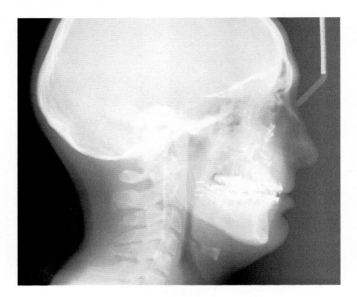

FIGURE 62-8. The patient in Figure 62-7 had surgery and, due to severe maxillary scarring and inadequate maxillary advancement, also had mandibular setback. "Splitting the difference" causes negative facial profile changes and narrowing of the airway with risk of obstructive sleep apnea (OSA). Note changes in the chin-neck-throat angle and narrowed posterior airway space.

splint fabrication will usually decrease or eliminate relapse potential. Cleft patients with relatively small maxillary AP discrepancies will usually have excellent results with minimal relapse after maxillary advancement with overcorrection (Figures 62-9 to 62-12).

The procedure for performing maxillary osteotomies is described elsewhere in this text, and the important aspects of differences in cleft patients are discussed. Cleft patients undergoing orthognathic surgery many times may have had a prior pharyngeal flap surgery to correct hypernasality and velopharyngeal incompetence (VPI). The anesthesiologist should be made aware of the presence of the pharyngeal flap and that plans for alteration from the usual intubation protocol may be necessary. The endotracheal tube should not be forced through the nasopharynx because it can track submucosally along the posterior pharyngeal wall. Using a small catheter or an endoscope first through the endotracheal tube then gently through the lateral ports of the pharyngeal flap will facilitate the intubation (Figure 62-13). Another technique is to use a gloved finger and digitally palpate the right or left lateral pharyngeal port, depending on which side of the nose the endotracheal tube is placed, through the mouth and contact the finger with the endotracheal tube, ensuring that it follows the finger through the intended port.

A cleft maxilla differs from an intact maxilla because of the absence of soft and hard tissues and multiple prior surgical procedures that were required to repair and close defects. Perfusion of the mobilized maxilla is dependent on vessels coming from the overlying soft tissues, predominantly involving the palatal tissues. In cleft patients, this tissue is commonly scarred and fibrotic; therefore, care must be exercised when designing the incision to perform the osteotomy in order to maximize preservation of blood supply. With few exceptions, almost all patients may be treated with a Le Fort I osteotomy via a circumvestibular incision and maxillary down-fracture approach. For those with severe palatal scarring, who have previously undergone an island palatal repair, and those with bilateral clefts of the maxilla, an anterior buccal soft tissue pedicle should be left intact on the mobilized maxilla to maintain adequate vascular perfusion. Technically, this is a more challenging operation. Almost all unilateral

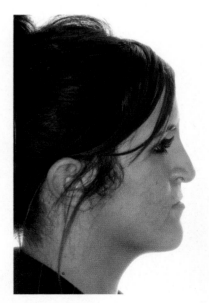

FIGURE 62-9. Unilateral cleft lip and palate patient before orthognathics. The patient is planned for only maxillary advancement with a 6-mm reverse overjet.

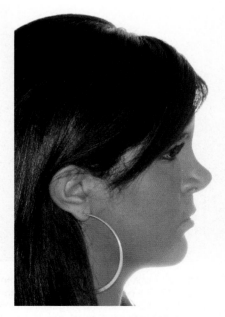

FIGURE 62-10. One year after maxillary advancement and rhinoplasty.

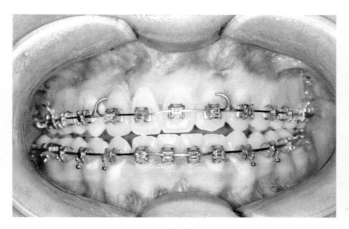

FIGURE 62-11.   Preoperative occlusal view of a unilateral cleft lip and palate patient before maxillary advancement.

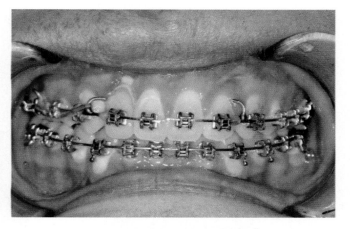

FIGURE 62-12.   Postoperative dental occlusal view 1 year after maxillary advancement.

cleft patients can be treated with a Le Fort I osteotomy via a circumvestibular approach. The circumvestibular incision is made from the zygomaticomaxillary buttress to the opposite side, high in the mucobuccal fold (Figure 62-14).

Subperiosteal dissection exposes the entire lateral wall of the maxilla from the piriform rims to the pterygoid plates and from the alveolus, above the roots of the teeth, to the inferior orbital rim. The broad exposure permits excellent visualization of all planned osteotomies. At the conclusion of maxillary mobilization, this incision permits the maxilla to be down-fractured and pedicled entirely based upon the palatal soft tissues and the remaining buccal soft tissues below the incision. Good visualization and ease of mobilization are the major advantages of this approach. Hemorrhage control is performed with direct visualization. With this in mind, the incision design for bilateral cleft lip and palate patient is different even if there is a well-healed alveolar cleft bone graft in place. A tunneling technique should be accomplished with a small vertical incision in the midline and horizontal incisions on the lateral segments with a tunneling technique in between the cuspid and the lateral incisor areas (Figure 62-15). When an anterior buccal pedicle remains, the operation is technically more difficult. This preservation of

labial soft tissues will prevent devascularization of the premaxillary bone segment and mucosa and can be accomplished in most cases without difficulty. For most patients with a cleft palate, the area of greatest resistance to mobilization of the posterior maxilla is the vertical portion of the palatine bone, located in the posteromedial aspect of the maxillary sinus. The bone is thick and access is limited, and this is the area of the descending palatine vessels that should be maintained, when possible. It is often desirable to segmentalize the maxilla of a cleft patient in order to improve occlusal relationships, but segmentation of the maxilla should be performed with caution, considering the compromised vascularity and scarring of the soft tissues.[8] The compromise of acceptance of a posterior cross-bite or other minor occlusal disharmonies may be preferred over the risk of avascular

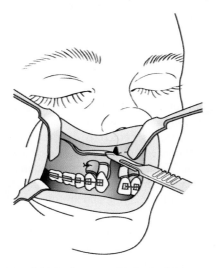

FIGURE 62-14.   A high circumvestibular incision ensures adequate perfusion to the anterior maxilla. Note that the attached gingiva on both sides of the cleft is reflected and preserved. The remaining tissue lining the cleft walls is later incised and reflected palatally or buccally, depending on where it is needed for closure.

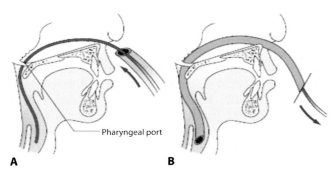

A   B

FIGURE 62-13.   A catheter passed nasally through the one of the velopharyngeal ports serves to guide the nasoendotracheal tube past the pharyngeal flap.

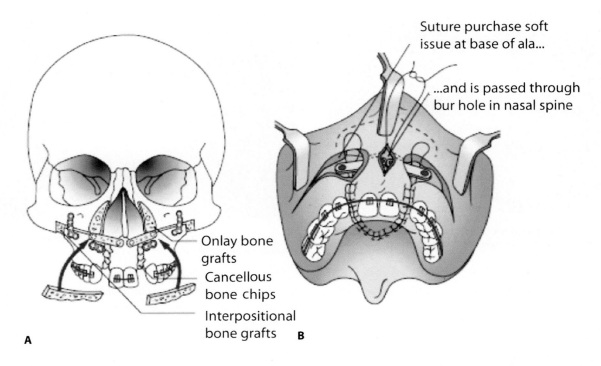

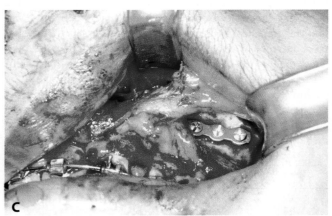

FIGURE 62-15. **A** and **B,** The premaxilla is secured with bone grafts, which are used to reconstruct the inferior piriform rim. These grafts are tunneled under the buccal flaps and secured to the anterior nasal spine anteriorly and to the lateral maxilla posteriorly. **C,** Intraoral view of the lateral maxillary incisions and medial incision with tunneling, providing an anterior pedicle to preserve blood supply to the premaxillary region. Note the rigid bone plates for osteotomy fixation.

necrosis of the soft and hard tissues after a segmental osteotomy. It is possible to close dental spaces with segmental osteotomies, and this is frequently done in residual alveolar clefts. During the osteotomy, closure of the nasal lining is of critical importance and, as stated earlier, requires bone grafting into the area to help stabilize the maxilla and to provide proper contours of the maxilla and alveolar bone.

General considerations in performing orthognathic surgery for cleft lip and palate patients include knowledge of differences in anatomy for children with and without cleft lip and palate deformities as compared with the typical skeletally mature adolescent orthognathic surgical patient. Patients with cleft maxillary deformities may have heavy buttressing of the maxilla, specifically at the piriform rim and pterygomaxillary buttress region of the posterior maxilla.[9] It is important to note this anatomic anomaly before orthognathic surgical procedures so that careful and thorough osteotomies can be completed in these regions to ensure that maxillary down-fracture can be completed without difficulty. Failure to weaken these buttress regions before mobilization may result in an unfavorable fracture, for example, in the pterygoid plate region extending to the skull base or orbit, and blindness has been reported after Le Fort I osteotomies in cleft patients.[9] Additional instrumentation that may help in down-fracturing and stretching of the soft tissue pedicle includes a modified Tessier rib-spreading forceps or a Smith sagittal split osteotomy–spreading forceps. These spreading forceps can easily fit posterior to the hard palate and allow slow controlled expansion of the scarred palatal soft tissue pedicle of the maxilla. This will increase the possible magnitude of down-grafting and advancement and improve the surgeon's ability to completely mobilize the maxilla.

Significant time must be taken to stretch the soft tissue pedicle in the vertical and AP dimensions to allow proper down-grafting and projection of the maxilla. Soft tissue handling is important after the down-fracture, and attempts at reconstruction of the nasal floor and closure of any residual fistulas will improve the final results of the surgery (Figure 62-16).

Residual bony defects can then be grafted to provide a better skeletal base for nasal aesthetic and alveolar and dental reconstruction in the future. The bone graft may be wedged into defects to help retain the proper maxillary position and promote osseous healing. Choices of bone augmentation range from iliac crest to the use of bone morphogenetic protein (BMP). Increasing clinical use of recombinant human bone morphogenetic protein-2 (rhBMP-2) has facilitated significant changes in maxillary bone grafting procedures within oral and maxillofacial surgery. Its use in cleft orthognathic surgery seems to be very appropriate. Consideration should be given to composite-type grafting scenarios where autogenous bone is used along with BMP. Bone grafts can be used for immediate stabilization with a membrane of BMP-impregnated collagen sponge over the site to help with enhanced bone formation in the region. Fixation of the cleft maxilla should be done with as heavy as fixation as possible for stabilization.[10,11] One consideration in the use of more

rigid fixation is that the weak link in maintaining the position of the maxilla is not the plate or screws but the bone and bony contacts. Therefore, the surgeon should attempt to maintain as much bone-to-bone contact as possible and use bone grafts at the buttress regions, when necessary. The relapse potential of the osteotomized cleft maxilla is clinically significant in many situations, and a slow posterior migration of the entire maxillary complex may still occur, regardless of the size of the plates and screws or the amount of bony contacts.

CLEFT DISTRACTION OSTEOGENESIS

Any discussion of orthognathic surgery in the cleft lip and palate patient must include consideration for the use of distraction osteogenesis (DO). As discussed in Chapter 63, children with severe class III malocclusions remain one of the very few indications for DO in facial bone reconstruction. Chapter 63 reviews the basic biologic principles and concepts of DO; however, it should be noted that in the mid-1990s at the First International Conference on Craniofacial Distraction Osteogenesis, DO was introduced in the opening ceremony as the panacea for facial bone osteotomies in all aspects of orthognathic surgery and other facial deformity correction.[12] As time and surgical experience have progressed, there are very few indications for DO in orthognathic surgery and/or the correction of facial deformities. Adolescents with severe maxillary hypoplasia due to cleft deformities are appropriately treated with DO owing to the fact that there is slow expansion of the scar that has restricted the growth of the maxilla and the most common level of the osteotomy for DO is at the Le Fort I level.[13]

Various DO techniques and devices are available for maxillary distraction in the cleft patient, but a common device used is an external head frame (halo) distraction device, in which traditional maxillary osteotomies are performed for the procedure. Care should be taken to completely mobilize the maxilla, because the distraction device will not overcome inadequate mobilization of the maxilla and hardware failure will likely occur. Specially made bone plates are secured to the maxilla with screws, and these plates have a large diameter rectangular wire looping around the upper lip to the external surface of the skin in the paranasal regions. This wire is attached to an adjustable activation bar that can be manipulated in the vertical, horizontal, and transverse planes of space. The activation bar is then attached to a vertical bar positioned at the midline of the face and connected to the head frame distraction device (Figures 62-17 and 62-18). One of the major advantages of an external head frame distraction device is that the vectors of distraction can be controlled in three planes of space easily during the distraction process. Also, there is ready access to the activation arms of the distraction device, and most of the mechanisms of the device are readily visible with only the interface at the bone being in a buried position. Large magnitude linear distraction movements are possible, with average reported AP distraction movements of 8 to 15 mm and vertical inferior

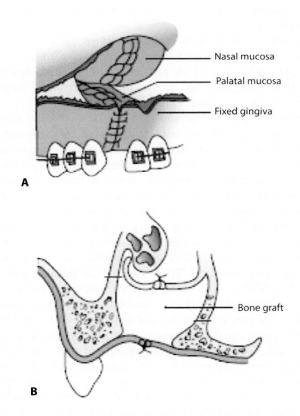

FIGURE 62-16. **A,** Buccal view shows the tissues lining the cleft elevated and sutured on the oral side. **B,** Deeper view into the cleft demonstrates closure of the oral and nasal tissues and the pocket for the bone graft.

Nasal mucosa

Palatal mucosa

Fixed gingiva

Bone graft

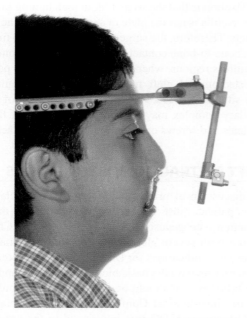

FIGURE 62-17. Lateral view of an external fixation distraction osteogenesis (DO) device. The cranial halo is fixated with multiple screws into the surface of the cranium. The vertical bar connects to the distraction arms, which are subsequently connected to the maxilla.

movements ranging from 1.6 to 13 mm.[13] Following the osteotomies and placement of the DO devices, the latency period is typically 5 days, and the distraction rate is usually 1 to 1.5 mm/day, depending upon the age of the cleft patient at the time of DO. Techniques that can aid in the proper final position of the maxilla with both internal and external DO appliances include occlusal splints and the use of intermaxillary elastics to guide the maxilla into the proper final location. During the DO activation period, alterations in the vector can be accomplished to allow the teeth to fit into the

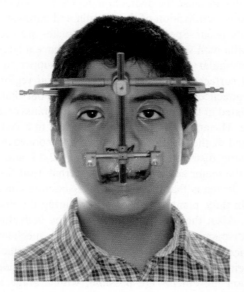

FIGURE 62-18. Frontal view of an external fixation DO device.

splint and the final resting position of the maxilla. The usual consolidation period, during which time the maxillary bone can heal, requires 2 to 3 months (8–12 wk). The removal of external frame distraction devices is simple and can be accomplished in the office with or without local anesthesia. The removal of the bone plates may be more complex and will require, at the minimum, local anesthesia and intravenous sedation. Patients may need to use a reverse-pull (protraction) headgear for night use for a period of 6 months after an external frame device has been removed to maintain the position of the maxilla and prevent relapse. Suzuki and colleagues[14] found a 22.3% horizontal relapse and a 53.7% vertical relapse during the first 6 months after DO surgery. Patients need to be prepared to wear the external head frame device for at least 3 to 4 months, and approximately 6 months of reverse-pull headgear in the postoperative period. Some have suggested that rigid fixation be accomplished after the distraction process, upon removal of the DO devices[15]; and these discussions should involve the orthodontist before surgery, but may serve to stabilize the maxilla further and prevent relapse. Disadvantages of external frame devices include the social appearance of the patient during treatment time, and other frequent complaints include difficulty finding a comfortable sleeping position and accidental trauma to the device from siblings, friends, and pets. The external frame device is large and bulky and may be easily caught on other objects or displaced by other people. Some patients decline the option of a head frame device owing to its appearance, especially if the child is in school. When using DO, the patient should be followed at regular intervals to ensure that the distraction process is proceeding as planned, and it should be recognized that the need for a reverse-pull headgear is also a disadvantage (Figures 62-19 to 62-21).

Internal distraction devices may also be used in the cleft patient and can work well and provide movement in the maxilla in the AP and yaw vector directions. Advantages of an internal device include increased patient acceptance, no visibility of the appliance externally, ability to remove the activation arms of the distractor once the distraction has been completed while leaving the distraction appliance in place for consolidation, and the ability to leave the extraction devices on for 6 to 9 months after the distraction process to allow for increased stability of the maxilla; this will eliminate the need for a post-DO reverse-pull headgear (Figures 62-22 to 62-26). Disadvantages of the internal devices are that the appliances are unidirectional in nature, they require a second surgery for removal, and they do not allow the surgeon to make significant changes once the appliances are in place and distraction is proceeding. In addition, placement of the devices in a parallel fashion bilaterally can be difficult for the surgeon. The surgical procedure includes typical osteotomies for the unilateral or bilateral cleft maxilla, downfracturing the maxilla to ensure adequate mobility of the maxilla, and then placement of the internal distraction devices and ensuring as close as possible paralleling bilaterally of the vector of distraction. Depending upon the need for

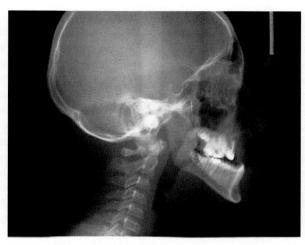

FIGURE 62-19. Lateral cephalogram of a patient with severe maxillary hypoplasia.

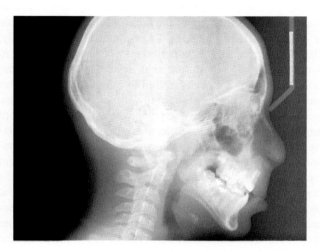

FIGURE 62-20. A patient after external frame DO with correction of the maxillary hypoplasia. The patient did not wear reverse-pull headgear in the postoperative phase.

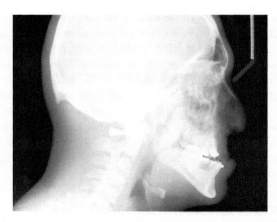

FIGURE 62-21. Lateral cephalogram of the same patient from Figures 62-19 and 62-20, who had maxillary relapse secondary to lack of reverse-pull headgear and class III elastics, shows significant maxillary relapse.

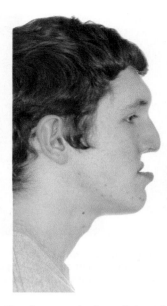

FIGURE 62-22. Preoperative lateral view of a bilateral cleft patient before internal maxillary distraction for maxillary advancement.

increasing the vertical dimension of the face, the angle of the distraction device can be changed to allow for a "ramping down" of the maxilla in a downward and forward vector. Essentially, changes in the vertical position of the maxilla can be effected with the angulation of the device at placement but cannot be altered during the course of the distraction process. Most internal distraction devices are secured with screws into the buttress of the zygoma and onto the body of the maxilla, and the activation arms are placed, if not already part of the devices, and the wounds are closed. Again, the latency period is 5 days, and the rate of distraction is 1 to 1.5 mm/day divided into a rhythm of two to three times per day. The

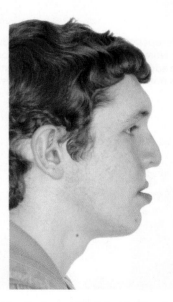

FIGURE 62-23. Postoperative lateral view of a bilateral cleft patient 1 year after 8.5-mm internal maxillary distraction.

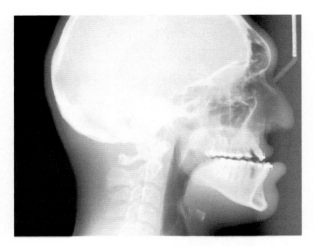

FIGURE 62-24. Preoperative lateral cephalogram shows the maxillary discrepancy in a bilateral cleft patient. The patient has severe palatal scarring, and internal maxillary advancement DO is planned.

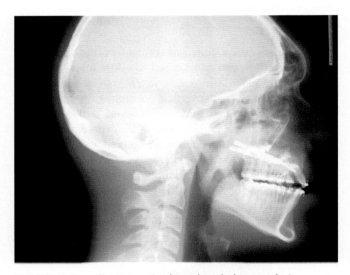

FIGURE 62-25. Postoperative lateral cephalogram during post-distraction healing. Note that, although the distraction devices are not parallel, the advancement proceeded without difficulty. Overcorrection was not done because the appliances remained for 6 months.

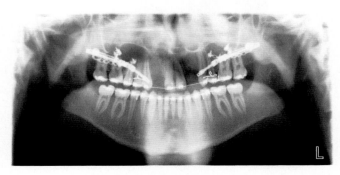

FIGURE 62-26. Postoperative Panorex at 1.5 weeks shows good position of the internal DO devices.

internal distraction devices can correct for midline asymmetries during distraction by adjusting the yaw during distraction via activation of one device more than the other so that midline changes occur as well. As with the external frame distraction device, the use of occlusal splints with good interdigitation of teeth into the splint can help guide the treatment path of the distracting maxilla, and as mentioned, as distraction progresses, changing the quantity of distraction on the right or left will change the midline position of the maxilla. Depending upon magnitude of the maxillary midline discrepancy, intermaxillary elastics can be used to settle the maxilla into its final occlusal resting place in the occlusal splint. The maximum possible distraction distance of the maxilla with currently available internal DO devices is 30 mm. For some internal distraction devices, once the distraction process has been completed, the activation arms that are visible in the oral cavity can be removed, leaving the rigid devices in place submucosally. At this point, there is nothing visible to the patient intraorally during the consolidation phase, and while healing of the bone is occurring, the device is typically left in place for 4 to 6 months postoperatively, although the consolidation period may be shorter in the 3- to 4-month period, as with external devices. After consolidation, local anesthesia can be used to remove the bone plates and distraction devices intraorally, although in some cases, bone may have healed over the plates, requiring a more aggressive approach for removal in an operating room setting. In most situations, by allowing additional time for consolidation with the distraction device in place, the patient usually avoids the need for a reverse-pull headgear in the post-DO period. Again, standard plates and screws may be used for additional stabilization when the buried DO devices are removed. If mandibular surgery is required for either internal or external distraction, it can be accomplished at the time of the initial surgery so that the mandible can be placed in any required position. Once the rigid fixation is accomplished in the mandible, the final splint is placed and the maxilla is distracted into the newly repositioned mandible.

During cleft orthognathic surgery, whether it is by traditional Le Fort techniques or DO, closure of fistulae should be accomplished whether they are palatal in nature or in the area of the alveolar cleft. Incisions should be made to account for the closure of the fistula. Careful attention should be made for manipulation of the nasal mucosa and closure with placement of a resorbable membrane in the area, and/or bone grafting, and then closure of the oral mucosa as a three-layer closure technique. If there is a significant bony defect in the alveolar cleft region or the piriform region, this should be augmented with bone, using the options discussed previously.

POSTSURGICAL CONSIDERATIONS

If at any time there is an early sign of relapse of the maxilla in the postoperative period, reverse-pull headgear should be applied along with vertical and class 3 elastics to help maintain the position of the maxilla in the healing phase and limit the amount of relapse. Patients and families must understand that there will be a secondary procedure to remove hardware, which may require general anesthesia in a hospital setting. The orthodontist provides a critical role in the postoperative management of these patients.

Velopharyngeal Considerations

It is possible for the cleft patient who has no VPI to develop VPI after maxillary advancement surgery. This is especially true in the cleft patient who has not had any form of pharyngeal flap for correction of speech problems.[16] Occasionally, it is necessary to section the pharyngeal flap to achieve the desired maxillary advancement; this may cause worsened hypernasality and should be discussed with patients and parents before maxillary surgical advancement. Although the literature is mixed, maxillary DO in the cleft patient has been reported to result in unchanged velopharyngeal function most commonly.. Many studies have shown no difference in worsening of hypernasality when comparing Le Fort to maxillary DO in the cleft patient. It should be remembered that worsening of hypernasality after maxillary surgery in the cleft patient, with or without DO, ranges from 6% to 17%, and in similar reports, 70% of children had an improvement in articulation after maxillary anterior repositioning.[13] Perhaps the most appropriate way to consider the effect of maxillary surgery on VPI is to classify the preoperative VPI status into mild, moderate, and severe. Maxillary advancement, with or without DO, may cause a worsening of one level, such that a mild VPI may progress to a moderate VPI that is well tolerated, whereas a severe VPI is certainly unlikely to change with maxillary surgery, and a pharyngeal flap may be required for correction. The concerning VPI status is the moderate VPI patient that may be tolerated presurgically but may become a severe VPI with significant symptoms postsurgically. This group should be the focus of future research in the area of VPI effects of Le Fort versus DO surgery in the cleft patient.

References

1. Ross RB. Treatment variables affecting facial growth in complete unilateral cleft lip and palate patients: an overview of treatment of facial growth. Cleft Palate J 1987;24:71.

2. DeLuke DM, Marchand A, Robles EC, et al. Facial growth and need for orthognathic surgery after cleft palate repair literature review and report of 28 cases. J Oral Maxillofac Surg 1997;55:694–697.

3. Maue-Dickson W. The craniofacial complex in cleft lip and palate: an updated review of anatomy and function. Cleft Palate J 1979;16:291–317.

4. Willmar K. On LeFort I osteotomy: a follow-up study of 106 operated patients with maxillofacial deformity. Scand J Plast Reconstr Surg 1974;12(Suppl):1–68.

5. Herber SC, Lehman JA. Orthognathic surgery in cleft lip and palate patient. Clin Plast Surg 1993;20:755–768.

6. Thongdee P, Samman N. Stability of maxillary surgical movement in unilateral cleft lip and palate with preceding alveolar bone grafting. Cleft Palate Craniofac J 2005;42:664–674.

7. Posnick J, Ewing M. Skeletal stability after LeFort I maxillary advancement in patients with unilateral cleft lip and palate. Plast Reconstr Surg 1990;85:706–710.

8. Drommer R. Selective angiographic studies prior to LeFort I osteotomy in patients with cleft lip and palate, J Maxillofac Surg 1979;7:264–269.

9. Turvey T, Vig KWL, Fonseca RJ. Maxillary advancement and contouring in the presence of cleft lip and palate. In: Turvey T, Big KWL, Fonseca RJ, eds. Facial Clefts and Craniosynostosis. Principles and Management Philadelphia: WB Saunders; 1996:452.

10. Posnick J, Dagys A. Skeletal stability and relapse patterns after Le Fort I maxillary osteotomy fixed with miniplates: the unilateral cleft lip and palate deformity. Plast Reconstr Surg 1994;94:924–932.

11. Posnick J, Tompson B. Cleft orthognathic surgery: complications and long-term results. Plast Reconstr Surg 1995;96:255–266.

12. Diner P, Vasquez, MP, editors. Transactions of the International Congress of Cranial and Facial Bone Distraction Osteogenesis. 1997;June 19–21; Paris, France.

13. Scolozzi P. Distraction osteogenesis in the management of severe maxillary hypoplasia in cleft lip and palate patients. J Craniofac Surg 2008;19:1199–1213.

14. Suzuki EY, Motohashi N, Ohyama K. Longitudinal dentoskeletal changes in UCLP patients following maxillary distraction osteogenesis using RED system. J Med Dent Sci 2004;51: 27–33.

15. Swennen G, Dujardin T, Goris A, et al. Maxillary distraction osteogenesis: a method with skeletal anchorage. J Craniofac Surg 2000;11:120–127.

16. Schendel, SA, Oeschlaeger M, Wolford LM, Epker BN. Velopharyngeal anatomy in maxillary advancement. J Maxillofac Surg 1979;7:116–124.

63

Distraction Osteogenesis of the Maxillofacial Skeleton

Michael Miloro, DMD, MD, FACS

Distraction osteogenesis (DO), osteodistraction, or callatosis, is a biologic process of new bone formation that occurs between bone segments that are separated by gradual incremental traction. This process commences when distraction forces are applied to the callous tissues that connect the divided bone segments and continues as long as these tissues are stretched by the applied forces. The traction generates tension that stimulates new bone formation in the gap parallel to the vector of distraction.[1] These factors are based upon the law of tension-stress that states that gradual traction on living tissues creates stresses that stimulate and maintain the regeneration and continued growth of both hard and soft tissues. DO is a surgical-orthopedic process, rather than an isolated surgical procedure, involving gradual separation of a fracture callous, which produces an unlimited quantity of new bone, with associated adaptive soft tissues changes, referred to as *distraction histogenesis*. Theoretically, the overlying soft tissue envelope, including the skin, subcutaneous tissues, muscles, fascia, and periosteum, respond favorably to the hard tissue movements with gradual elongation and accommodation and, therefore, a lower resistance and decreased overall bony relapse, although the clinical application of this theory has been questioned.[2] Although the principles of DO were developed many years ago, the application to the maxillofacial region began in the late 1980s and early 1990s.[3] Maxillofacial DO was applied to complex craniofacial deformities, including craniofacial microsomia, in an effort to grow bone and avoid grafting and to reduce bone resorption and relapse of surgical movements. In consideration of the evolutionary stages of surgery in general, these four stages include ablation, reconstruction, transplantation, and induction[4]; DO is classified within the most progressive stage of induction, or regeneration, in that bone is formed de novo as a type of endogenous tissue-engineered bone. In the 1990s, DO was welcomed with a major paradigm shift in the approach to the craniofacial asymmetry patient. Introduced as a new "disruptive technology" with wide applications in the maxillofacial region initially, DO was considered a panacea when, in fact, standard surgical techniques were perfectly adequate at the time. This overzealous enthusiasm has been followed by a period of intellectual reproach and a focus of the indications for this treatment scheme.[5] This reassessment phase has included a reappraisal of the myriad complications that may occur with DO as well as strategies for prevention and management.[6] In Ilizarov's opinion, ". . . there are no complications with the technique; there are only inexperienced surgeons causing problems for their patients,"[7] but perhaps the more important issue here is to define the indications for the use of maxillofacial DO. These indications include craniosynostosis and upper face deformities; maxillary and mandibular orthognathic discrepancies; mandibular condylar abnormalities including ankylosis; severe asymmetries of the maxillofacial region; maxillary alveolar cleft deformities; segmental defects of the jaws due to trauma or pathology; neonatal airway obstruction due to mandibular deficiency; and alveolar ridge deficiencies (Table 63-1). Despite the controversies surrounding the current indications for DO, the technique provides an additional arm in the treatment algorithm for congenital and acquired dentoskeletal deformities, with the advantages of no bone grafting or donor site morbidity and the ability to titrate the bony movements and grow an unlimited amount of new bone and with the disadvantages of a surgeon learning curve, vector control problems, and patient and parent cooperation during the entire DO process. With the application of maxillofacial DO to the appropriate clinical scenario, there are clear advan-

TABLE 63-1. **Indications for Maxillofacial Distraction Osteogenesis**

Severe maxillary deficiency
Severe mandibular deficiency
Transverse jaw deficiency
Temporomandibular joint ankylosis
Obstructive sleep apnea
Neonatal upper airway compromise
Hemifacial microsomia
Treacher Collins syndrome
Mandibular segmental defects
Craniosynostosis
Alveolar ridge deficiency
Alveolar cleft discontinuity
Alveolar cleft maxillary deficiency

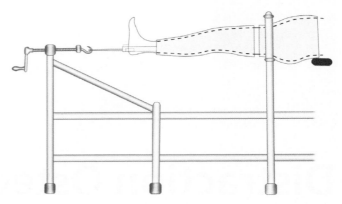

FIGURE 63-1. Early lower limb distraction osteogenesis (DO) traction device of Codivilla, 1905.

tages over conventional orthognathic and craniofacial surgical procedures, but it has become clear that DO will not replace standard surgical techniques, which can adequately accomplish the treatment goals in one surgical procedure, rather than through a process of gradual bone DO, which may take from weeks to months of treatment time.

HISTORY OF DO

DO was developed initially for orthopedic manipulation of long bones for a variety of problems. Although Ilizarov is generally credited with the concepts involved with distraction osteogenesis, it was Codivilla who first described the technique for femoral expansion in 1905[8] (Figure 63-1); and later, Abbott in 1927[9] used DO for tibial lengthening. In fact, Ilizarov is known as the "father of distraction osteogenesis," because he described the accepted principles of distraction osteogenesis in 1971.[10] 1951[C] that are still utilized clinically today. Ilizarov popularized the tension-stress effect by applying gradual traction to fractures and nonunions of endochondral long bones using large, external halo–type distraction devices (Figure 63-2) and recognizing that the increased cellular activity and metabolic response with neovascularization led to ossification of the site with bony union without the need for bone grafting. Ilizarov then realized that the mass or shape of these bones and joint articulations depends to a great extent on the available blood supply to the area as well as the functional burdens placed upon the bones (Wolff's law). Although orthodontists and oral and maxillofacial surgeons had been utilizing the principles of DO for years in the management of transverse maxillary deficiency, with both orthopedic sutural expansion in the growing patient and surgically assisted maxillary expansion in the adult, it was McCarthy who performed animal studies in the late 1980s that led to the clinical application of these principles to the maxillofacial region and the 1992 publication describing successful monofocal DO of the mandible in four children with craniofacial microsomia.[11] The average patient age was 6.5 years, with mandibular lengthening between 18 and 24 mm, with an 11- to 20-month follow-up period with minimal

morbidity or complications. Before McCarthy, Snyder in 1973[12] used external DO devices in the canine mandible, and in 1977, Michieli and Miotti[13] used intraoral mandibular DO devices in the dog model. Throughout the 1990s, there was an explosion of new ideas related to DO device design, including external (extraoral and rigid external [halo] devices), internal (intraoral, subperiosteal, or buried), semiburied devices, toothborne or hybrid devices, and monofocal, bifocal, multifocal, and transport vectors, as well as the clinical indications for DO, including maxillary and mandibular deficiencies in the vertical, anteroposterior, and transverse planes, temporomandibular joint (TMJ) ankylosis, obstructive sleep apnea, neonatal airway compromise, mandibular continuity defects after tumor ablation or trauma, craniosynostosis, vertical and horizontal alveolar ridge deficiency, alveolar cleft maxillary deficiency, and alveolar cleft discontinuity. Since the explosion of interest in maxillofacial DO in the 1990s, surgeons who have experience with DO have focused the clinical indications for this technique and

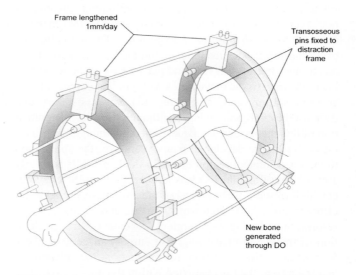

FIGURE 63-2. Lower limb lengthening halo DO apparatus of Ilizarov, 1951.

typically consider DO as an option only when conventional techniques for surgical correction are limited. In fact, only 4% of centers actively involved in performing DO on a regular basis have performed more than 100 cases of DO, making the designation of "experienced" a questionable misnomer. Even in the small number of known "DO centers," the reported incidence of complications with multivector DO is nearly 25%.[6] Therefore, in general, with other factors equal, the procedure with the lowest "cost" to the patient, in terms of finances, treatment time, and patient morbidity, should be used.

BIOLOGIC BASIS OF DO

Without a doubt, since the early 1990s, the unbridled enthusiasm about DO of the maxillofacial region has waned significantly since the resurgence of the technique and application to the maxillofacial region in the early 1990s.[5] Although the proposed benefits of DO that would allow it to replace traditional osteotomies for orthognathic surgery have not been borne out in clinical practice, DO maintains a place in the treatment of craniofacial malformations, specifically severe deformities in which there are poor conventional options for patient management. One of the major advantages of DO is the ability to lengthen bones to a greater degree than would be possible with orthognathic surgery, owing to the limitations based upon the envelope of discrepancy.[14] Unlike orthognathic surgery, the DO technique is not age-limited and could be applied not only to the skeletally immature child but also to the neonate with upper airway obstruction due to retrognathia in order to avoid a tracheostomy and permit normal speech and language development. DO is titratable, in that the clinician can continue to separate the bony segments until the desired results have been achieved (e.g., negative anterior overjet to account for some bony relapse or open airway at the tongue base in the Pierre Robin birth asphyxia patient). Also, the soft tissues are stretched slowly with DO so that they may gradually adapt to the bony movements and result in potentially less relapse than that achieved with conventional orthognathic surgery performed without rigid fixation techniques. In addition, regarding the TMJ, the mandibular condyle and disk position has additional time to adapt to any rotational changes that occur during distraction over a period of days or weeks, rather than acutely during orthognathic surgery in a period of minutes or hours. Also, with DO, there is no potential donor-site morbidity from the need for bone graft harvesting, which may be necessary, although uncommon, with orthognathic surgery. Both techniques are typically performed in the outpatient setting and, in fact, essentially in the same technical procedure, with application of distraction devices in lieu of plates and screws for orthognathic surgery. The cost of the DO procedure would typically be greater than orthognathic surgery because it usually requires two surgical procedures with general anesthesia in a hospital setting, and many more postoperative visits for the patient and family, as well as the

additional cost of the actual DO devices, which is much greater than the cost of plates and screws. The disadvantages of DO include the additional time required for the entire treatment process, potential surgeon inexperience with a highly technique-sensitive procedure, the need for parent and patient cooperation, low incidence of major infection with maxillofacial DO, nerve paresthesia (trigeminal, facial nerves), TMJ dysfunction, facial scarring (pin tracts) from external devices, premature fusion of segments, malunion, device hardware failure with screw loosening and plate fracture, and relapse with the need for initial overcorrection. In addition, the issue of growth of the craniofacial skeleton after DO is unpredictable. In general, it is believed that in the syndromic patient, the deficient bone, or involved side of the jaw (e.g., hemifacial microsomia) has less inherent growth potential and may not grow normally after surgical correction, despite Wolff's law. Functional remodeling is expected to play a role in the growing process, yet overcorrection of 25% to 33% is advocated to allow for some relapse of the bony consolidate and expected lack of continued "normal" growth. Because more patients who had DO in the 1990s as children are growing into adolescence in the new millennium and at the present time, an assessment of these growth issues may allow further clarification in the future.

Another controversial advantage of DO in the adolescent cleft patient undergoing maxillary advancement is the theoretical lower incidence of velopharyngeal incompetence (VPI) development, or worsening, than with a standard Le Fort advancement. Based upon the present available literature, there is no consensus on VPI or speech alterations when comparing DO with Le Fort osteotomies.[15] In assessing the magnitude of maxillary advancement on VPI, other studies have shown no significant improvement in speech hypernasality, or VPI, with DO movements less than 15 mm.[16] Perhaps the most appropriate manner in which to consider the issue of VPI is to classify the preoperative VPI status into mild, moderate, and severe VPI, and then evaluate the possible outcomes of either Le Fort osteotomy or DO. In most cases, mild or moderate VPI cases may progress to moderate to severe VPI, whereas severe VPI is not likely to improve after maxillary advancement with either form of surgery, and other surgical options are usually required to address this problem independently (e.g., pharyngeal flap procedure).

The potential complications of the DO process are many and variable, and the problem is that not many surgeons or surgical teams have extensive experience in managing patients who have undergone DO. Complications of DO may occur during the preoperative phase, intraoperative phase, distraction phase, or postdistraction phase of the treatment process. In the preoperative phase, patient selection and vector planning are critical, and application of DO to the inappropriate patient or for the wrong indication may be problematic. Intraoperatively, an inadequate corticotomy may be performed, and the DO devices may be placed with an improper vector or with lack of sufficient device stability. During the distraction phase, the device may malfunction, the vector may proceed in an improper fashion, and there may be dehiscence of the overlying soft tissues as well as facial scarring. In the postdistraction phase, there may be an inadequate total distraction distance, minor infections, a fibrous union, or malunion of the bone segments due to inadequate bony consolidation in the distraction gap resulting in potential bony relapse. Overall, many retrospective reviews[17] have shown that the most common complication with DO is nerve paresthesia (5% long-term), infection (<5%), condylar morphologic changes, incomplete osteotomy by the surgeon, device breakage, patient compliance problems, premature consolidation of bone, pin tract scarring, hypertrophic facial scarring, damage to teeth and roots, improper vector direction, TMJ ankylosis, hematoma at the distraction site, and periodontal problems. As expected, the more complex the DO device used (multivector vs. univector), the higher the incidence of complications, and patients of advanced age also have a higher incidence of complications, especially persistence of nerve paresthesia. In both animal[18] and clinical[19] studies, the incidence of prolonged paresthesia of the inferior alveolar nerve is variable, but generally remains low with mandibular DO corticotomies; and younger patients recover spontaneous neurosensory function more rapidly after nerve injury and to a greater degree or magnitude than older patients. With regards to the development of TMJ problems after DO, several reports have indicated the findings of hypomobility or fibrous ankylosis depend upon the specific direction and magnitude of mandibular movement, although more recent studies indicate that the TMJ accommodates to the DO process with no long-term functional TMJ abnormalities after mandibular DO.[20]

Regarding the overall process of new bone formation and transformation that occurs as a result of DO, this begins with the formation of a hematoma at the site of the corticotomy, or

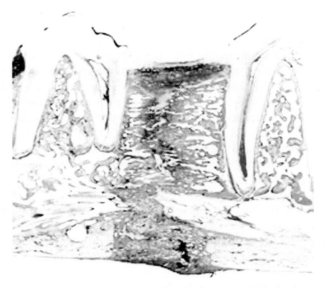

FIGURE 63-3. Healing of the distraction gap with four zones of bone formation (central, extending bone, bone remodeling, and mature bone zones).

bone fracture, as expected, with organization of the clot as functional stresses are introduced with DO. As the process of DO progresses, the histologic appearance of the bone in the distraction gap becomes organized into four distinct zones of varying bone maturation (Figure 63-3), including a central zone of fibrovascular granulation tissue composed of collagen fibrils and new capillaries that are oriented parallel to the vector of distraction. The next zone is that of extending bone formation, followed by the zone of bone remodeling, and finally, the zone of mature bone, which gradually transitions into the normal adjacent native cancellous bone. Throughout the latency, activation, and consolidation phases of distraction, this bone gradually transforms from immature, woven bone with neovascularization to a more mature lamellar bone end product with minimal callus formation (Figure 63-4). As the consolidation continues, the periosteum becomes proliferative and will re-form a cortical outline around the newly formed cancellous marrow; this cortex is responsible for the strength of the bony consolidate that will prevent relapse.

PRINCIPLES OF DO

Although the original description of the technique of DO by Ilizarov has been modified and should be adjusted based upon the specific clinical scenario and location of distraction, the basic principles remain unchanged (Table 63-2). The first principle involves the *surgical technique* used to create the separation between the bones. For long bones and the mandible, a corticotomy is performed, rather than a complete osteotomy, in order to preserve the endosteal continuity and blood supply in the distraction gap before the initiation of distraction in order to support the internal milieu of the ensuing distraction gap and provide the most conducive environment for bone formation (Figure 63-5). This has been referred to as "rotational osteoclasis." In most cases, a reciprocating or micro-oscillating saw, or rotary handpiece with a thin fissure bur, is used to perform the majority of the corticotomy, and a bone chisel and osteotome are used to complete the bony fracture. In the mandible, the location of the corticotomy is typically in the body, angle, or ramus region depending upon the intended distraction vector, horizontal (body), oblique (angle), or vertical (ramus), and a corticotomy will not section across the inferior alveolar canal or damage developing tooth buds that would occur if a complete osteotomy were performed. For the maxilla, a true corticotomy is not possible owing to the nature of the thin bone so, a standard Le Fort osteotomy is generally performed. At the same time as the corticotomy, the DO device is applied to the mandible, and the specific device and planned vector dictate the angulation of the corticotomy itself; so, in many cases, the device is applied before performing the corticotomy in order to visualize the area for the planned corticotomy and for placing a score mark in the midpoint between the stabilization plates and the screws of the DO device. Depending upon the specific DO device used, it may be secured to the mandible from an extraoral

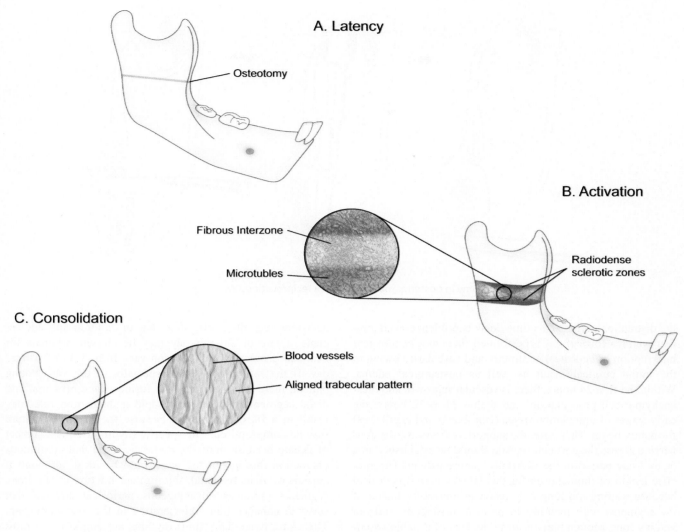

FIGURE 63-4.   Gap bone healing during latency, activation, and consolidation.

transfacial approach using transcutaneous pins that are then secured to the devices, or transoral DO devices may be secured to the mandible with standard bone screws. The extraoral pins should be placed parallel to each other and perpendicular to the distraction vector, and in order to minimize pin tract scarring, it is advisable to pinch the skin and

subcutaneous tissues together between the pins during transcutaneous pin placement. Before wound closure during surgery, the distraction devices must be activated to confirm that movement of the bone segments will proceed in an uninterrupted fashion, because failure to achieve segment distraction at the time of surgery must be corrected at this point in time during surgery. Many times, this maneuver will stretch the cancellous bone, but may also minimally convert the corticotomy to an osteotomy through physical separation of the bony segments. After activation of the devices at surgery, deactivation should occur in order to bring the bone edges in close proximity without compressive forces.

The second principle involves the *latency period,* defined as the interval between the initial surgical procedure (corticotomy and device application) and the device activation, typically ranging from 5 to 7 days (Table 63-3). The primary reason for the delay is to permit the establishment of a fibrovascular bridge across the endosteum of the bony segments that will act to support future bone formation during

TABLE 63-2.   **Principles of Distraction Osteogenesis (Ilizarov)[7]**

1. Surgical procedure
   a. Corticotomy
   b. Device application
2. Latency period (3–7 days)
3. Activation period
   a. Rate (1.0 mm/day)
   b. Rhythm (daily to four times/day)
4. Consolidation period (8–12 wk)
5. DO device removal

DO = distraction osteogenesis.

SECTION 7

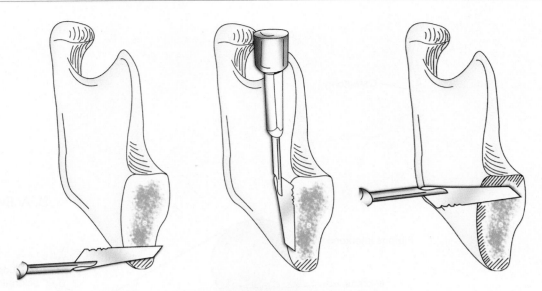

FIGURE 63-5.　Corticotomy in posterior mandible with a reciprocating saw.

the distraction period. This time delay is prudent considering that even if a corticotomy is performed, there may be transient interruption of endosteal continuity and vascularity owing to the initial surgical insult as well as postsurgical edema. Within the first 24 hours, there is vascular ingrowth and mesenchymal cell proliferation, and within 24 to 72 hours, the early stages of granulation tissue (fibroblasts and capillaries) formation begin. Therefore, the supportive fibrovascular connection across the corticotomy site should be established in a 5- to 7-day period in the skeletally mature patient. The specific length of time chosen for this latency period is critical because waiting too long may result in premature fusion of the segments with inability to perform distraction and not waiting long enough may result in the lack of a stable vasculature in the bony gap leading to a nonunion, or fibrous tissue interposed between the bony segments at the completion of distraction. The latency period is also age-adjusted, such that a shorter period is used for children (2- to 3-day latency) and neonates (zero-day latency), whereas a longer period is employed for elderly patients (7- to 10-day latency).

The third DO principle involves the *activation period,* which includes both the rate and the rhythm, or frequency, of distraction. For the typical adult patient, the usual rate of distraction is 1.0 mm/day in divided increments, generally 0.5 mm twice daily. Again, age plays a significant role in the

decisions regarding rate, such that in children and adolescents, a rate of 2.0 mm/day may be chosen, whereas for neonatal distraction, the rate can vary from 3.0 to 5.0 mm/day. If the rate is too slow, especially in the very young patient, there may be premature fusion of the proximal and distal segments, whereas too rapid a distraction rate may result in a fibrous nonunion because the microvasculature may be compromised. The specific rhythm used is a subject of debate because, initially, it was believed that continuous distraction throughout the day would be ideal, although it appears as if incremental, intermittent traction of the bony segments produces advantageous periosteal stresses that serve to enhance bone regeneration in the distraction gap. Therefore, twice-daily (bid) rhythms are employed in most patients for ease and patient compliance, so that distractions may occur at set times each day (e.g., 8:00 AM and 8:00 PM). If there is discomfort during the distraction activation, especially toward the end of the process when bone healing is advanced and consolidation is beginning, the rhythm may be adjusted to three times daily (tid) or four times daily (qid) schedules (e.g., 0.25 mm qid), and predistraction analgesics (nonsteroidal anti-inflammatory drugs [NSAIDs]) may be helpful for patient comfort. Typically, each specific distraction device is supplied with a screwdriver to activate the distraction, with an "arrow" inscribed on the screwdriver, as

TABLE 63-3.　**Distraction Protocols**

Location	Latency Period (days)	Rate (Total mm/day)	Rhythm	Consolidation Period (or 2 × Activation Period)
Mandible or maxilla: adult	5–7	1.0	bid	8 wk
Alveolar ridge	5–7	0.5–1.0	bid-tid	4 wk
Transport segment	5–7	1.0	bid-tid	4 wk
Mandible: neonatal	0	2.0–4.0	bid-qid	2 wk
Mandible: child	2–3	2.0	bid	3–4 wk
Mandible: elderly	7–10	0.5–1.0	qd-bid	10–12 wk

well as the distance of distraction achieved with one complete 360-degree turn of the screwdriver to ensure that patients or parents perform the turns correctly. Multivector devices may add confusion because there may be more than one movement performed during each activation of the device (x, y, and z axes). It should be remembered that the bony regenerate is "moldable" during this period, and it could be influenced by the use of orthodontic elastics, which can also affect the occlusal relationships of the dentition. This plasticity of the distraction bone can be used to bend the bone in cases in which vector correction is required (e.g., use of vertical anterior elastics for closure of an anterior open bite malocclusion).

The fourth principle of distraction involves the *consolidation period,* or period of neutral fixation, that has the greatest degree of variability based upon surgeon preference. This is the period of time for bony consolidation that occurs between the completion of distraction and the removal of the distraction device. In the adult patient, this is usually 8 to 12 weeks, whereas in the young patient, there may be sufficient strength in the bony regenerate immediately after completion of distraction to allow for removal of the DO devices immediately after distraction. It has been suggested that the consolidation period should equal twice the activation (distraction) period, so that the time is based upon total distraction distance; for example, if the activation period was 14 days, then the consolidation period should be approximately 28 days in length. During the consolidation period, a large, bulky extraoral multivector device may be replaced with a lightweight carbon fiber rod supplied by the companies for patient comfort. There is extreme variability in the length of the consolidation period because it is unclear exactly when device removal is appropriate and will not result in relapse owing to premature removal. An objective means of evaluating whether bony stability would exist if the DO devices were removed is limited to radiographic documentation that a bony cortex exists or that there is sufficient bone fill in the distraction gap. Because this period of the DO process is the least understood and adds the most time to the overall DO process, there has been a great deal of research interest in acceleration of the consolidation period by treating the distraction gap region with either chemical factors, such as growth factors, cytokines, insulin-like growth factor-I (IGF-I), fibroblast growth factor (FGF), transforming growth factor-beta-1 (TGF-β-1), and interleukin-6 (IL-6), as well as physical factors, including ultrasound stimulation, low-level laser stimulation[21] and electromagnetic therapy.

The fifth, and final, principle of distraction involves the *removal of the DO device.* Depending upon whether the devices are intraoral, extraoral, buried, or pin-retained, removal may be a simple procedure performed under local anesthesia or intravenous sedation in an outpatient clinic or it may require more extensive surgery performed under general anesthesia in an operating room setting. There are technical developments ongoing that may allow the foot plates of buried devices to remain attached to the bone, possibly with resorbable materials (e.g., oly-G-lactic acid [PGLA], poly-L-lactic acid [PLLA] co-polymers), which would make the removal of buried devices simpler without the need for extensive reexposure of the surgical site. Further refinements and technologic advances in materials may allow fabrication of completely resorbable DO devices in the future. It should be noted that, in some cases, surgeons may choose to place titanium bone plates and screws in a conventional orthognathic surgical manner at the time of DO device removal ("hybrid" DO-orthognathic procedure) to prevent relapse in specific circumstances in which relapse is a major concern (e.g., Le Fort advancement in the cleft patient).

PATIENT EVALUATION AND VECTOR PLANNING

A comprehensive history and clinical examination should be performed in a manner similar to that done for the orthognathic surgical patient with an asymmetry. Particular attention should be directed toward examining the patient in a natural head position (NHP), despite asymmetries in orbitozygomatic position, ear deformities, and occlusal cants. Frontal, profile, bird's-eye, and worm's-eye views are helpful to visualize both hard and soft tissue volume and landmarks. A functional TMJ examination should be performed, especially with mandibular asymmetries. The standard radiographic evaluation should be used, including periapical radiographs to plan for interdental osteotomies, if necessary, a panoramic radiograph to assess the dentition and condylar/ramus morphology, and a posteroanterior cephalometric radiograph to assess orbitozygomatic discrepancies and occlusal cants. Care must be taken to maintain the patient's head in the NHP during the cephalometric films, such that in cases of microtia, or melotia (low-set ears), the ear rod on the affected side is allowed to contact the scalp passively in the temporal region, and it is not placed within the external auditory canal as on the unaffected side. The use of three-dimensional computed tomography (CT) scanning and computer planning is becoming invaluable in the assessment and treatment planning of craniofacial asymmetries and also in DO device design and vector planning.

The choice of distraction device depends upon several variables including the specific anatomic abnormality, the desired distraction vector, the overall magnitude of bony movement, the planned surgical access as well as access for device activation, patient and parent preferences, and surgeon experience. The DO devices are classified according to several factors. In relation to the skin surface, DO devices may be external or internal, and these internal devices may be buried or semiburied and placed transorally or transfacially. Devices may also be classified according to the type of tissue that anchors the devices, including boneborne, toothborne, or hybrid (a combination of bone- and toothborne) devices. Lastly, devices are classified according to the number of potential vectors of movement (Figure 63-6) as monovector (or univector or unidirectional, one vector),

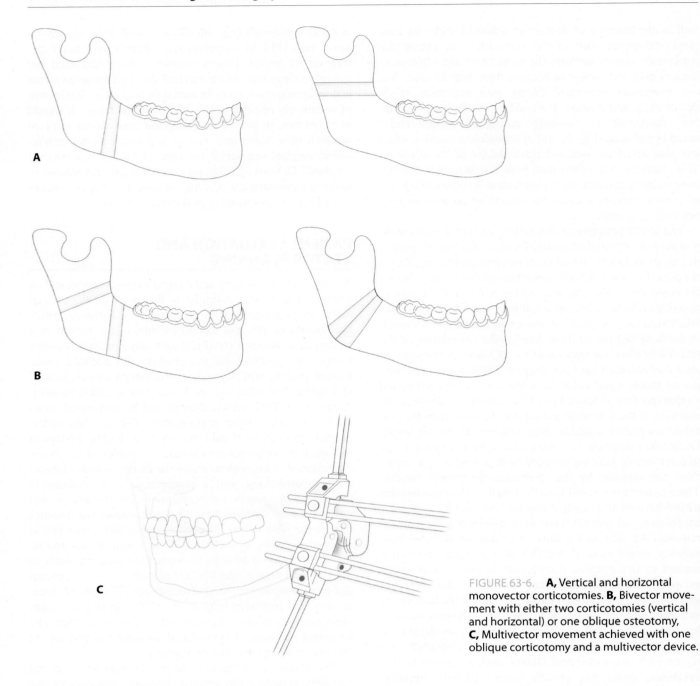

FIGURE 63-6. **A,** Vertical and horizontal monovector corticotomies. **B,** Bivector movement with either two corticotomies (vertical and horizontal) or one oblique osteotomy, **C,** Multivector movement achieved with one oblique corticotomy and a multivector device.

biplanar or bidirectional (two vectors), and multivector (or multiplanar, more than three vectors) devices. In general, the need to use a multivector device requires external placement with potential facial and pin tract scarring; but this problem should be balanced with the advantages of ease of access to the activation devices and the full control of multiplanar vectors in three planes of space (x, y, and z axes). Monovector devices usually require only one corticotomy and use a "straight screw" type device to achieve simple linear elongation of bone in a vertical, horizontal, or oblique vector. A bidirectional device may require two corticotomies performed perpendicular to each vector and the use of a specific device to achieve both vector movements, or a specialized

device may be used with only one corticotomy to achieve biplanar movement (Figure 63-7). For maxillary distraction, either internal or external devices may be used (Figure 63-8) and the RED (rigid external device), which uses a maxillary occlusal splint as well as an external multivector control arm, is used for maxillary and midface distraction in cleft and craniosynostosis cases.

The issue of distraction vector, or trajectory of movement of the bone segments, is important to consider for both the maxilla and the upper face as well as the mandible. However, most efforts have focused on distraction vector planning in the mandible (Figure 63-9). The three mandibular vectors are based upon the relationship of the direction of the corticot-

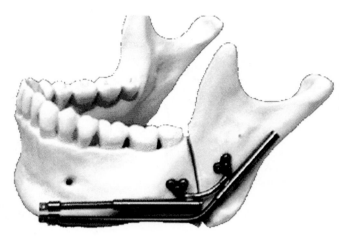

FIGURE 63-7. Oblique osteotomy with vertical and horizontal vector Wood distraction device.

omy to the occlusal plane. A vertical vector, perpendicular to the occlusal plane, is achieved with a horizontal osteotomy of the ramus, whereas a horizontal vector, parallel to the occlusal plane, results from a corticotomy performed vertically in the body or angle region of the mandible. An oblique vector, resulting in both vertical and horizontal elongation of the mandible, will result when the corticotomy is performed at an angle between zero degrees (the vertical vector) and 90 degrees (the horizontal vector) to the occlusal plane, generally in the angle region of the mandible. With regards to vector planning, it must be recognized that there are both biologic and mechanical forces that will significantly affect the direction of distraction (Figure 63-10). The biologic vectors result from the neuromuscular soft tissue envelope including the muscles of mastication and suprahyoid musculature. These forces may influence the distraction vector unpredictably, and the surgeon has little control over these factors. The mechanical vectors, conversely, are under full control of the surgeon and orthodontist involved in the care of the distraction patient. These mechanical forces include the distraction device itself, the intercuspation of the teeth, bone segment contact, the TMJ apparatus, and of course, the angulation of the corticotomy and DO device placement that determines the actual direction of vector movement. As an example of the result of the combined biologic and mechanical vector forces, a vertical distraction device in the ramus will result in counterclockwise rotation of the mandible with a posterior open bite occlusion, whereas a

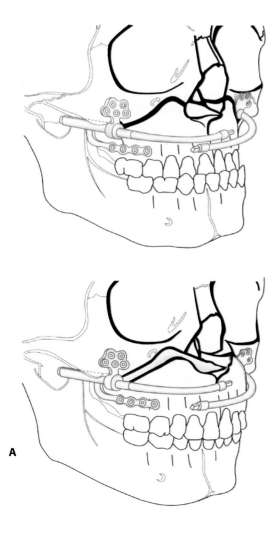

A

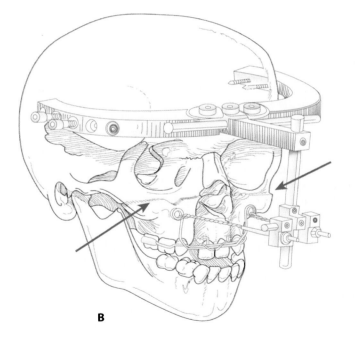

B

FIGURE 63-8. Maxillary distraction devices. **A,** Internal device. **B,** RED (rigid external device).

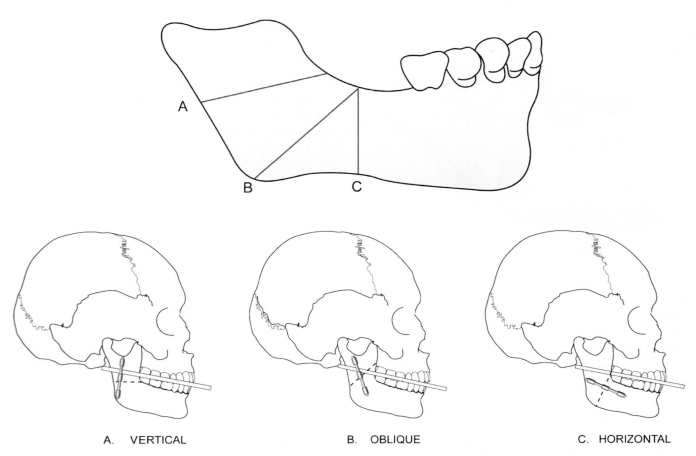

FIGURE 63-9. **A,** Osteotomy design for mandibular distraction. **a,** Horizontal osteotomy results in vertical vector. **b,** Oblique osteotomy results in oblique vector. **c,** Vertical osteotomy results in horizontal vector. **B,** Mandibular distraction vectors. **a,** Horizontal osteotomy *(dotted lines)* (parallel to occlusal plane) results in vertical vector. **b,** Vertical osteotomy (perpendicular to occlusal plane) results in horizontal vector. **c,** Oblique osteotomy results in oblique vector.

horizontal mandibular distraction vector has the tendency for clockwise rotation of the mandible with the development of an anterior open bite occlusion, due to the biologic vectors, including the suprahyoid musculature (Figure 63-11). Additional considerations in vector planning involve unilateral cases in which rotational forces also influence movement of the mandible (e.g., hemifacial microsomia). In an attempt to determine the precise placement of a distraction device to achieve the desired vector, a geometric formula may be used to allow proper positioning of the pins, or screws, of the distraction device. The pin (or screw) placement angle is determined by measuring the vertical and horizontal deficiencies in the mandible as well as the gonial angle of the mandible (condylion-gonion-menton), because this will dictate the intended vertical and horizontal movement of the mandible. The pin placement angle is determined (The formula is shown in Figure 63-11.): 180 subtracted by the gonial angle and multiplied by the product of the vertical deficiency (condylion-gonion distance) divided by the total deficiency (vertical plus horizontal [gonion-menton distance] deficiency). In the example shown with a 10-mm horizontal and a 10-mm vertical deficiency, with a gonial angle of 140 degrees, the pin placement angle is 20 degrees to the mandibular plane (gonion-menton). This formula can assist the surgeon if three-dimensional imaging and planning is not available. Remember that in the maxilla, the vector is mostly dependent upon the specific DO devices chosen (usually bilateral devices are necessary), including buried internal devices and REDs. There is generally a horizontal, or anteroposterior, vector in most maxillary distraction cases; however, vertical change may be achieved with intermaxillary vertical elastics or by variable adjustment of the external device and RED.

Regarding the technical aspects of distraction, the bone segments may be separated in a monofocal, bifocal, or trifocal fashion (Figure 63-12). The monofocal mode will separate two bone surfaces in a standard DO fashion, whereas a bifocal distraction will utilize a transport disk of bone that is moved through the soft tissues toward another segment of bone. The trifocal mode will move two segments of bone as transport disks toward each other, and specialized devices are available to assist with transport distraction. The bifocal and trifocal modes of transport distraction are typically used for reconstruction of segmental defects of the mandible

Biological Distraction Vectors

Mechanical Distraction Vectors

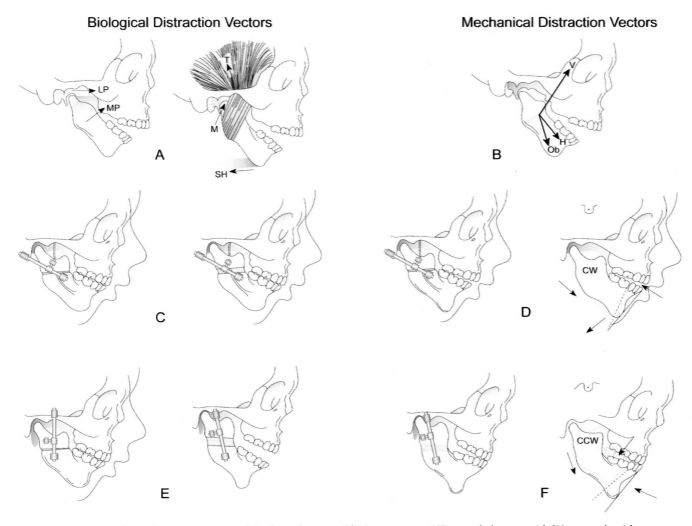

FIGURE 63-10. **A,** Biologic distraction vectors. LP = lateral pterygoid; M = masseter; MP = medial pterygoid; SH = suprahyoids; T = temporalis. **B,** Mechanical distraction vectors determined by corticotomy design and device placement. H = horizontal; O = oblique; V = vertical. Horizontal (H) vector **(C)** results in clockwise rotation (CW) **(D)** of the mandible with an anterior open bite occlusion. Vertical (V) vector **(E)** results in counterclockwise rotation (CCW) **(F)** of the mandible with a posterior open bite occlusion.

(Figure 63-13). With transport distraction, the transport disk of bone will develop a fibrocartilaginous cap on the advancing front of the bone segment as it moves through the subcutaneous soft tissues. When used for mandibular segmental defect reconstruction, this cartilage cap must be resected at the time of device removal and may require additional bone grafting at the junction site as well as the use of rigid fixation devices for stabilization. The formation of this cartilage cap can be used as an advantage in cases of TMJ reconstruction with DO (Figure 63-14). For example, in cases of TMJ ankylosis, after gap arthroplasty, a vertical ramus osteotomy (VRO; or variation) is performed with application of a distraction device with a vertical vector to distract the proximal bone segment into the newly created glenoid fossa. This particular transport disk will become the new condyle with a desirable cartilaginous cap to prevent future ankylosis, and it will function as a normal condyle as it assumes a more normal anatomic size, shape, and position.[22]

ORTHODONTICS FOR MAXILLOFACIAL DO

The orthodontist may play a critical role in the complex management of the patient undergoing DO as an integral member of the team for growth assessment, occlusal, and aesthetic evaluation and treatment planning.[23] The role of the orthodontist is in vector planning and modification, if necessary, during distraction, preparation of the dentition for DO, management of the dentition during active DO, and finalizing the occlusion at the completion of DO. The three phases of orthodontics for DO include predistraction, active distraction, and postdistraction treatment. Pre-DO orthodontics is similar to pre-orthognathic surgery preparation using fixed orthodontic appliances to eliminate dental compensations, coordinate arches, correct transverse deficiencies, correct occlusal disharmonies, eliminate crowding and potential dental interferences with distraction (e.g., retroclined maxillary incisors inhibiting forward mandibular movement), and

Vector Planning

Pin Placement Angle = 180 - gonial angle $\times$ $\dfrac{\text{vertical deficiency}}{\text{total deficiency}}$

180 - 140 x 10 / 20 = 40 x 1 / 2 = 20 degrees

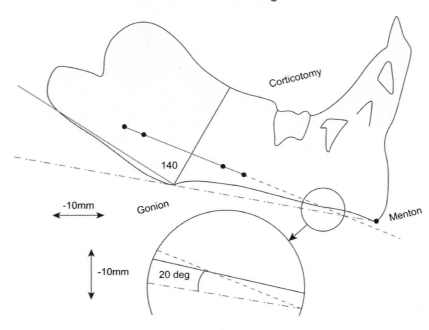

FIGURE 63-11. Vector planning formula for mandibular distraction. In the example, there is a 10-mm vertical and a 10-mm horizontal discrepancy that results in a pin placement angle of 20 degrees in reference to the mandibular plane (menton-gonion).

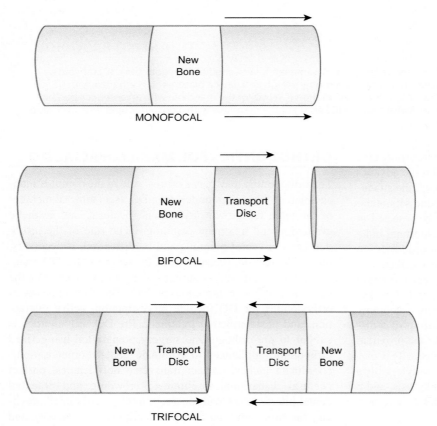

FIGURE 63-12. Monofocal, bifocal, and trifocal distraction schemes, based upon movement of the transport segment of bone.

Transport Distraction

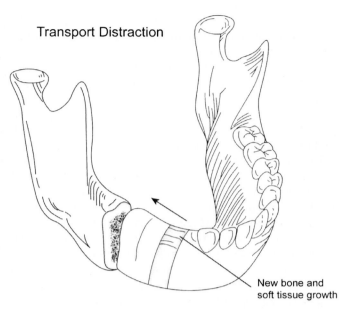

New bone and
soft tissue growth

FIGURE 63-13. Transport distraction for segmental defects of the mandible. As the transport segment advances through soft tissues, a fibrocartilaginous cap forms that requires resection after DO.

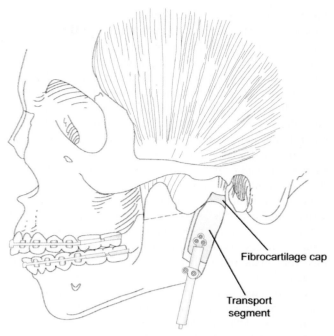

Fibrocartilage cap

Transport
segment

FIGURE 63-14. Condylar segment transport distraction. After condylectomy, a modified vertical ramus osteotomy with application of a DO device with vertical vector (and coronoidectomy). The transport segment moves toward the glenoid fossa with formation of a neocondyle with fibrocartilaginous cap.

creating root divergence at a tooth-bearing corticotomy site. As mentioned, orthodontic traction and occlusion is considered to be one of the mechanical vectors that is under the control of the clinician during active distraction. Dynamic changes are going on in the young patient with regards to the dentition and occlusion with transitioning from a primary to permanent dentition, vertical growth of the alveolar process and jaws, and possibly premature occlusal contacts that develop during distraction resulting in functional shifts that may affect the vector movement. Therefore, active DO ortho-

dontic intervention may include occlusal equilibration, the use of neutral occlusal bit plates, and fabrication of specific orthodontic stabilization devices to control mediolateral interarch relationships during distraction, especially with unilateral distraction vectors (Figure 63-15). For unilateral mandibular distraction, two concerns are control of developing laterognathism and contralateral cross-bite occlusion.

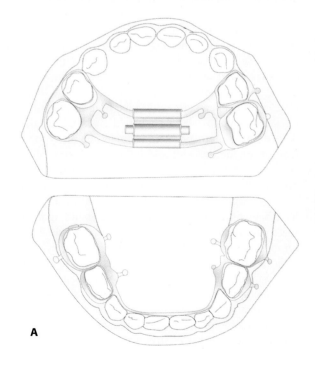

A

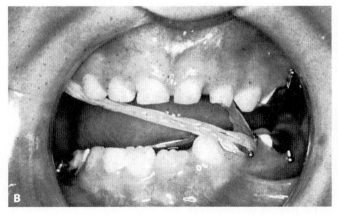

FIGURE 63-15. **A,** Orthodontic stabilization devices used for DO. **B,** Cross-arch elastics to control laterognathism and unilateral cross-bite elastics.

Laterognathism is the development of an asymmetrical habitual occlusion during DO that results in functional shifts toward the unaffected side, or in the direction of the distraction vector, that may limit the magnitude of distraction. Although functional appliances may be used, typically cross-arch elastics are used to control laterognathism, but these forces directly oppose the forces of DO, and therefore, overcorrection may be indicated. For contralateral cross-bite control, transpalatal and lingual arches with both intermaxillary cross-arch elastics and unilateral cross-bite elastics are used. Orthodontics with vertical elastics can also be used to decrease or eliminate developing open bites during distraction, by a combination of molding of the bony regenerate as well as tooth extrusion. Also, for vertical vectors in the ramus region to lengthen the ramus (e.g., hemifacial microsomia), it may be necessary to maintain the ipsilateral posterior open bite after mandibular plane leveling with a bite plate and sequential plate reduction to allow unimpeded maxillary growth. If active orthodontic intervention is used during distraction, then minimal postdistraction orthodontics may be required. Post-DO orthodontics must consider whether orthodontic finishing can be completed in the nongrowing patient or whether a planned malocclusion was performed with the expectation of future growth (e.g., a class III occlusion with anterior occlusal cross-bite expecting future maxillary growth). Again, functional appliances (e.g., bionator therapy) may be used for up to 6 months after DO, depending on patient age, to mold the regenerate during ossification. Finally, after bony consolidation, teeth may be moved orthodontically into the area of the distraction gap.

MANDIBULAR DISTRACTION

Mandibular anteroposterior hypoplasia constitutes the majority of dentoskeletal deformities that are treated with orthodontics and orthognathic surgery, and DO should not be considered in cases in which standard orthognathic surgical techniques can be employed (sagittal split osteotomy [SSO], VRO). When considering the indications for DO, the magnitude of the skeletal discrepancy must be severe enough to warrant distraction, and typically, these types of deformities are due to congenital craniofacial abnormalities that may be a component of a syndromic diagnosis, such as hemifacial (or craniofacial) microsomia, Pierre Robin sequence, Treacher Collins, Goldenhar's, or Nager's syndrome, or may also be associated with the myriad signs and symptoms of obstructive sleep apnea. In addition to congenital deformities, acquired mandibular retrognathis may result from condylar trauma or pathology that leads to TMJ ankylosis. In addition, DO can be applied to the mandible to correct transverse mandibular deficiency with mandibular widening via distraction as well as segmental mandibular defects managed with transport distraction osteogenesis. Typically, DO is considered for these severe deformities in which conventional orthognathic options are limited owing to the young age of the patient or the degree of bony movement, which may not allow application of rigid fixation, or in whom plates and screws may interfere with future growth, and the magnitude of soft tissue (skin, muscle, nerve) stretch that may not respond well to acute lengthening, and before the introduction of rigid fixation devices, may have contributed to relapse of the bony segments. As mentioned previously, a wide variety of distraction devices are available for mandibular DO procedures, and these include external, internal, semiburied, toothborne hybrid devices, with monofocal, bifocal, multifocal, and transport distraction vectors. In cases of severe horizontal and vertical ramus deficiency, either a multifocal multivector device or a combined distraction device may be used to accomplish both vertical and horizontal distraction vectors simultaneously (Figure 63-16). In cases of unilateral vertical ramus hypoplasia, for example with hemifacial microsomia, a stable univector distraction device can be used to level the mandibular occlusal plane and allow unimpeded future growth of the maxilla using a maxillary splint that is sequentially reduced during vertical maxillary growth (Figure 63-17). An alternative option for a patient with a unilateral vertical ramus deficiency (e.g., hemifacial microsomia) is to consider performing bimaxillary osteotomies, application of intermaxillary fixation (IMF), and the use of only a mandibular distraction device that will result in distraction of both the mandible and the maxilla owing to the use of IMF (Figure 63-18). Segmental defects of the mandible can be treated with the use of transport DO as mentioned previously, and ankylosis of the TMJ can also managed with the use of a transport segment of bone that is distracted toward the glenoid fossa in order to create a new condylar head with fibrocartilage. In a manner similar to surgically assisted maxillary expansion, mandibular expansion with distraction may be accomplished with a midline mandibular osteotomy and the use of an external or internal device (Figure 63-19).

A major indication for mandibular distraction has become popular as an alternative to tracheostomy or tongue-lip adhesion[24] in the neonate born with severe mandibular anteroposterior deficiency and airway obstruction with birth asphyxia due to isolated obstruction at the base of the tongue. Most often, this technique is considered for the Pierre-Robin (1923)[25] sequence patient with the triad of mandibular anteroposterior hypoplasia, a U-shaped cleft palate, glossoptosis due to an in utero problem of mandibular hypoplasia with lack of tongue descent, and failure of closure of the palatal shelves in the midline. The airway obstruction is present at birth in 70% of infants and results in a mortality rate of 2% to 26% even in experienced centers. A variety of methods have been used to address the airway, including the EXIT (ex utero intrapartum treatment) procedure in which immediate intubation is performed upon a staged delivery of the infant with the head delivered first for intubation. In general, for mild airway obstruction in the neonatal period, positional head therapy (prone, lateral, head extension positions) is usually effective to open the posterior pharynx, relieve the tongue obstruction, and maintain arterial oxygen saturation. For moderate airway obstruction, nasal stents can be placed

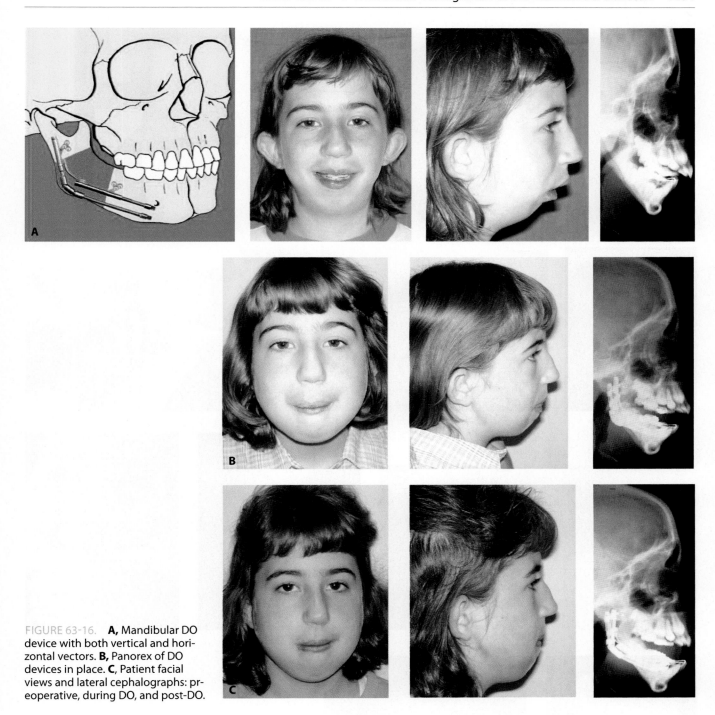

FIGURE 63-16.   **A,** Mandibular DO device with both vertical and horizontal vectors. **B,** Panorex of DO devices in place. **C,** Patient facial views and lateral cephalographs: preoperative, during DO, and post-DO.

using a 3.0 endotracheal tube or other nasal airway device, such as a nasal trumpet. For severe obstruction, with difficulty maintaining inspired oxygen concentrations above 90% most of the time, either an anterior glossopexy (tongue-lip adhesion) procedure can be used with a reported success rate less than 50%; a tracheostomy, which does not address the cause of the problem, can be performed with significant long-term morbidity including tracheostomy care, psychosocial issues, speech developmental delay, skin scarring, tracheal stenosis, and an average time of 18 to 36 months until

removal; or mandibular DO can be performed in order to correct the etiology of the problem and allow future mandibular growth, without significant morbidity. Among the few problems reported with neonatal mandibular distraction, alteration in the morphology of the condyle with reported cases of TMJ ankylosis has occurred,[26] although other reports show no ankylosis and an adaptation of the condyle to the distraction process.[27] The DO procedure will serve to advance the mandible, elevate the hyoid bone, and relieve the obstruction at the tongue base; one of the major benefits of

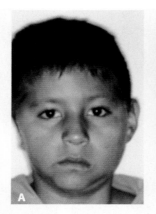
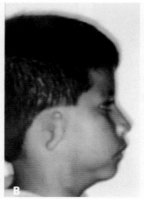
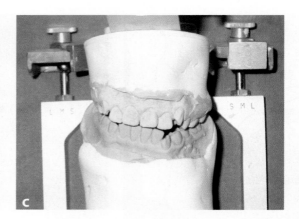

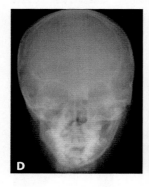
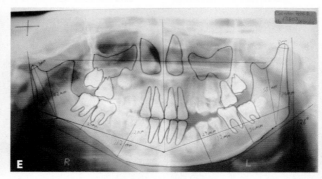
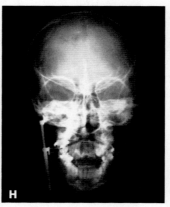

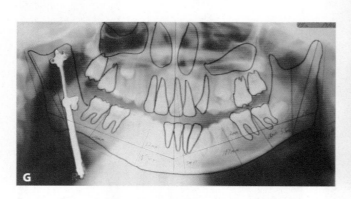
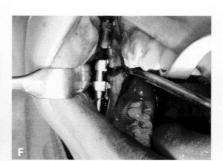
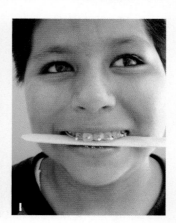

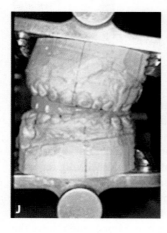
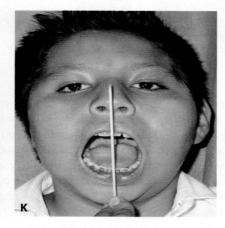

FIGURE 63-17. Mandibular DO for right hemifacial microsomia using a vertical vector device with creation of a posterior open bite on the affected side. **A–E,** Preoperative. **F,** Device activation during surgery. **G** and **H,** Post-DO films. **I** and **J,** Post-DO clinical with leveled mandibular occlusal plane, bite splint to allow maxillary growth, and **K,** excellent midline mouth opening.

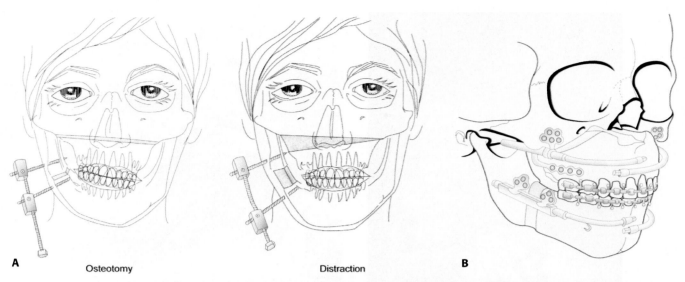

A
    Osteotomy   Distraction   **B**

FIGURE 63-18. **A,** Bimaxillary DO for hemifacial microsomia accomplished with unilateral mandibular corticotomy, Le Fort osteotomy, and placement of a mandibular DO device and use of intermaxillary fixation (IMF) to distract the mandible and maxilla simultaneously. **B,** Alternative technique for bimaxillary DO, requiring coordinated synchronous activation of each device.

DO is the ability to titrate the degree of mandibular forward movement and continue until the airway obstruction has been relieved and confirmed by laryngoscopy. Owing to expected relapse in the young patient, overcorrection is advocated, and creation of a reverse overjet class III jaw relationship is preferable at the time of DO completion. The presence of other abnormalities of the upper airway must be ruled out with direct laryngoscopy, because laryngomalacia or tracheomalacia would be contraindications to DO, and tracheostomy is warranted for severe airway obstruction. It is important to consider the distraction device options carefully for the very small mandible, and consideration should be given toward computer planning with SLA (stereolithography) and customized semiburied device fabrication when possible, in order to achieve the precise final position of the distal segment of the mandible (Figure 63-20). Conventional options for neonatal distraction include either internal plate and screw devices or external pin devices (Figure 63-21). Typically, the distraction rates in the neonate are accelerated over the typical adult rate of 1.0 mm/day to a 4.0-mm/day distrac-

tion rate in divided increments, and, in this manner, 2.0 cm of distraction may be accomplished within a period of 7 to 10 days while the patient is in the intensive care unit of the hospital. After a consolidation period of approximately twice the distraction period (14–30 days), the devices can be removed; resorbable devices are available and clinical research continues to determine efficacy.

MAXILLARY DISTRACTION

Maxillary DO has been performed for years by oral and maxillofacial surgeons and orthodontists using surgically assisted maxillary expansion techniques to address transverse maxillary deficiency. Similar considerations are made for maxillary DO as with mandibular DO in that DO should not be used in cases in which conventional orthognathic surgical procedures can be used. Maxillary DO at the Le Fort I level is typically reserved for cleft lip and palate patients, who have had numerous previous surgical procedures with severe maxillary anteroposterior hypoplasia, palatal scarring

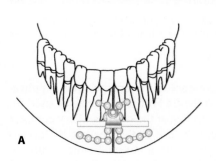
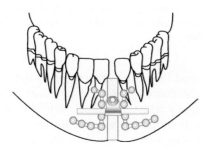
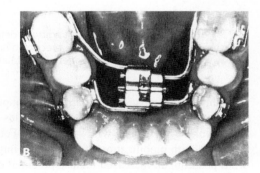

FIGURE 63-19. **A,** Mandibular widening by midline corticotomy and DO device placement. **B,** Midline osteotomy with a mandibular modified hyrax appliance.

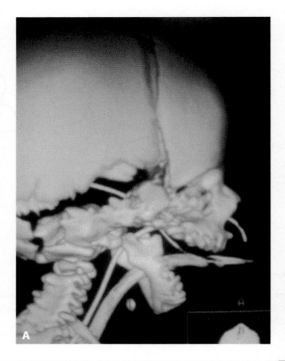

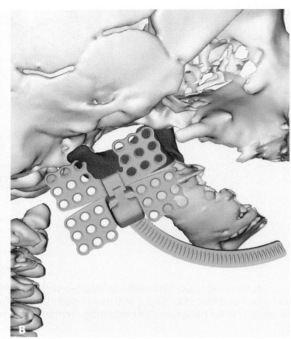

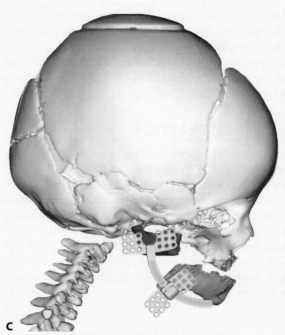

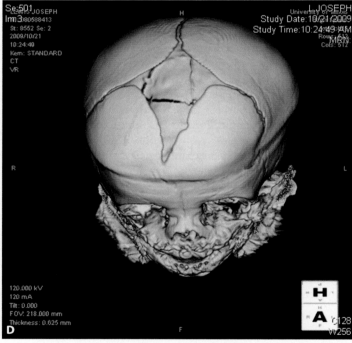

FIGURE 63-20.   Owing to unique mandibular deformity in this case of Pierre-Robin sequence **(A)**, a customized curvilinear DO device **(B)** was manufactured to achieve the precise advancement and rotation of the distal mandible with DO **(C)**, and DO continued until the airway was open and a reverse overjet was obtained **(D).**

(possibly with a pharyngeal flap), and compromised blood supply to the maxillary hard and soft tissues. These factors may result in difficulties with standard Le Fort surgery with problems with mobilization of the maxilla into the final forward position, an increased relapse potential compared with conventional orthognathic surgery even with rigid fixation, and worsening of speech and swallowing abnormalities or

VPI, especially in the presence of a pharyngeal flap. Application of maxillary DO at the Le Fort II level may be used for unusual midfacial deformities of the nasomaxillary complex such as Binder's syndrome; use at the Le Fort III level is generally for cases of syndromic or nonsyndromic craniosynostosis, such as Apert's, Crouzon's, and Pfeiffer's syndromes. In most cases of maxillary DO performed at the Le Fort I

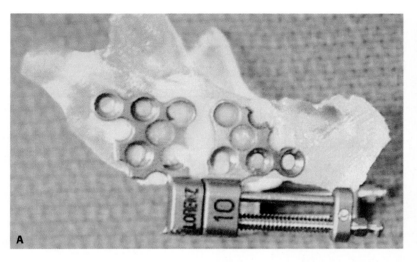

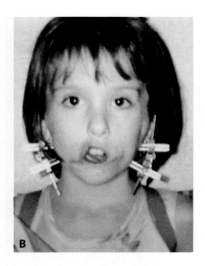

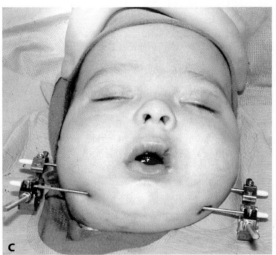

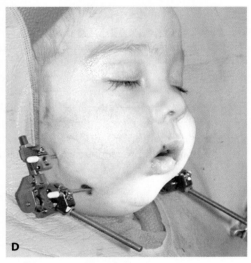

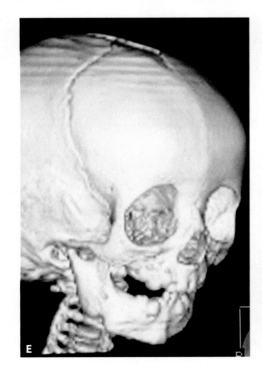

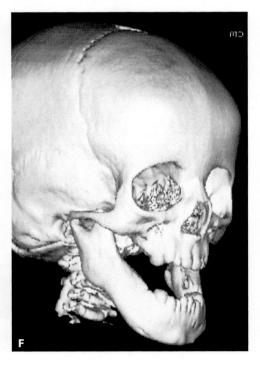

FIGURE 63-21.   Neonatal DO for airway management may include buried DO devices **(A)**, external devices stabilized with cortical pins **(B)**, or transfacial pins with external devices **(C and D)**. **E–F,** Pre- and post-DO computed tomography (CT) scans with mandibular advancement and airway improvement. *(Continued)*

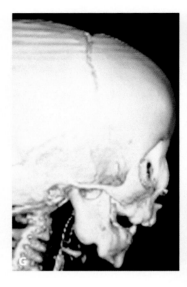
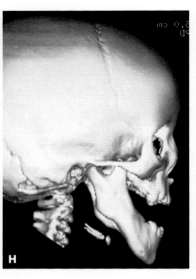

FIGURE 63-21. *(Continued)* **G–H,** Pre- and post-DO computed tomography (CT) scans with mandibular advancement and airway improvement.

level, semiburied intraoral devices are adequate (Figure 63-22), but for cases of more severe deformities in cleft patients in whom additional vector control is required, a RED may be used.

In a fashion similar to that used for mandibular transport DO, maxillary segmental distraction may be used, especially in the area of an alveolar cleft defect for closure without the need for bone graft procedures, using specialized distraction devices (Figure 63-23).

Maxillary distraction may also be used at the Le Fort III level for craniosynostosis cases, although the usual unidirectional vector of distraction fails to address the complex three-dimensional nature of the skull and cranial base abnormalities (Figure 63-24), and perhaps these deformities benefit from a one-stage surgical approach with cranial recontouring and application of small or resorbable fixation, without the need for DO device removal at a second surgical procedure, despite the potential DO advantages of maintenance of blood

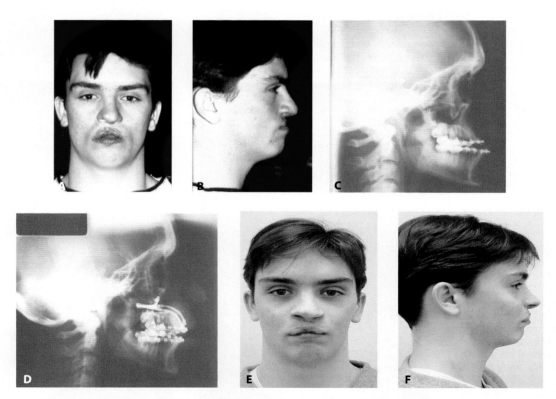

FIGURE 63-22. **A** and **B,** Maxillary DO in a cleft lip and palate patient using buried transmucosal DO devices. **C** and **D,** Pre- and postoperative lateral cephalographs. **E** and **F,** Post-DO facial and profile views.

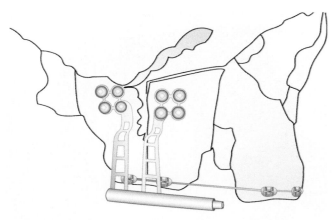

FIGURE 63-23.   DO device used for alveolar segment DO in a cleft alveolus to avoid bone grafting.

supply, less intraoperative blood loss, and lack of soft tissue limitation to cranial remodeling. Each patient must be evaluated independently to determine the most appropriate surgical procedure to achieve the desired result with the least patient morbidity.

ALVEOLAR RIDGE DISTRACTION

The subject of alveolar ridge distraction is covered in Chapters 11 and 12, but it deserves mention in this section on DO, because the indications and expected advantages of the technique are consistent with the other applications of DO to the craniomaxillofacial skeleton. The technique also represents an alternative form of transport DO that has been discussed previously, with the transport segment pedicled on the lingual periosteum and soft tissues for maintenance of blood supply, and a vertical vector of the planned bony distraction.

In areas of alveolar ridge deficiency, alveolar ridge DO offers an alternative option to autogenous or allogeneic or alloplastic bone grafting or guided bone regeneration, with the principal benefit being the soft tissue expansion of the attached and unattached gingiva during the process of distraction, in order to avoid a soft tissue dehiscence that frequently occurs with vertical alveolar ridge augmentation (Figure 63-25). Alevolar ridge DO is by no means a panacea for reconstruction of the alveolar ridge, because there may be several complications including poor vector control with an inadvertent lingual orientation or deviation of the transport segment due to the soft tissue pedicle, as well as unpredictable osseous healing in the distraction gap[28] (Figure 63-26), that may require bone grafting at the time of endosseous implant placement, thereby negating the expected benefit of avoidance of bone grafting.

THE FUTURE OF MAXILLOFACIAL DO

In the maxillofacial region, the application of DO maintains specific indications including severe skeletal deformities of the maxilla and mandible that are not amenable to correction by conventional orthodontic and orthognathic surgical treatment methods. Because one of the major limitations or disadvantages of the DO process is the length of the consolidation period, basic and clinical research will continue to focus on methods to shorten the consolidation period by accelerating the process of osseous healing in the distraction gap using both locally applied stem cells, growth factors, and cytokines, as well as the application of external sources of bone stimulation. Development of customized devices specifically designed with an exact vector for the individual patient is an option using three-dimensional computer treatment

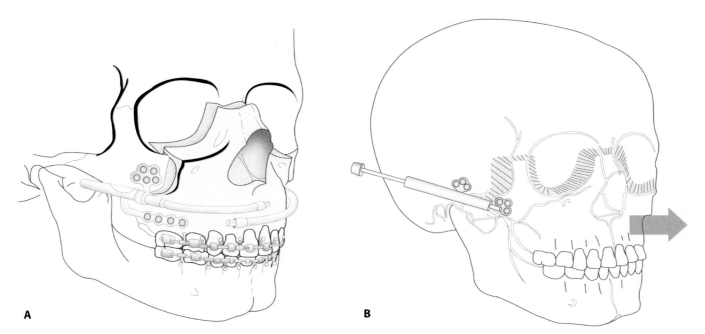

A   **B**

FIGURE 63-24.   DO at the Le Fort II **(A)** and Le Fort II **(B)** levels with semiburied devices.

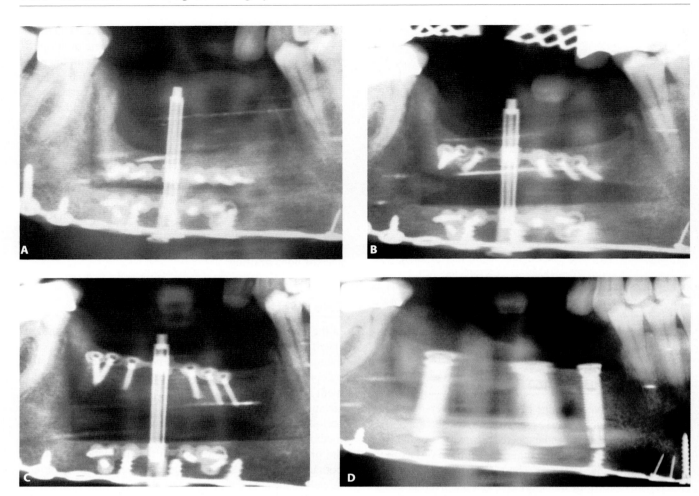

FIGURE 63-25. **A–D.** Alveolar DO with endosseous implant placement.

planning, and further developments may allow cost containment in the future. The development of automatic devices with internal preprogrammed daily incremental device activation will continue, as well as the refinement of resorbable materials that can be used for distraction, especially in the pediatric age group, that will provide sufficient rigidity to allow bony movement despite significant soft tissue restriction and then undergo spontaneous resorption at the appropriate time, in order to avoid the morbidity of an additional surgical procedure for device removal.

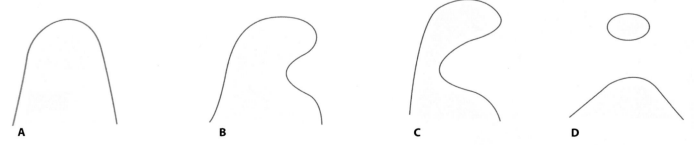

FIGURE 63-26. Possible final outcomes of alveolar DO. **A** shows a nearly normal alveolar ridge morphology. **B** shows a minor buccal concavity defect. **C** shows a major buccal defect, but with lingual/palatal bony continuity. **D** shows a complete separation of the transport segment from the native bone. B and C are most common.

References

1. Samchukov ML, Cope JB, Harper RP, Ross JD. Biomechanical considerations of mandibular lengthening and widening by gradual distraction using a computer model. J Oral Maxillofac Surg. 1998 Jan;56(1):51–9.
2. Ruiz RL, Turvey TA, Costello BJ. Mandibular distraction osteogenesis in children. Oral Maxillofac Surg Clin North Am. 2005 Nov;17(4):475–84.
3. McCarthy JG, Schreiber J, Karp N, Thorne CH, Grayson BH. Lengthening the human mandible by gradual distraction. Plast Reconstr Surg. 1992 Jan;89(1):1-8; discussion 9–10
4. Murray JE. The origins and consequences of organ transplantation. Excelsior Surgical Society/Edward D. Churchill Lecture. Bull Am Coll Surg. 1995 Aug;80(8):14–25.
5. Stoelinga PJ.Distraction from the ground rules? Int J Oral Maxillofac Surg. 1998 Dec;27(6):414–5.
6. Suhr MA, Kreusch T. Technical considerations in distraction osteogenesis. Int J Oral Maxillofac Surg. 2004 Jan;33(1):89–94.
7. Ilizarov GA. The principles of the Ilizarov method. Bull Hosp Joint Dis 1988;48:1–16.
8. Codivilla A. The classic: On the means of lengthening, in the lower limbs, the muscles and tissues which are shortened through deformity. 1905.Clin Orthop Relat Res. 2008 Dec; 466(12):2903–9.
9. Abbott LC. The operative lengthening of the tibia and fibula. J Bone Joint Surg 1927. 9:128.
10. Ilizarov GA. Basic principles of transosseous compression and distraction osteosynthesis. Ortop Travmatol Protez. 1971 Nov;32(11):7–15.
11. Karp NS, McCarthy JG, Schreiber JS, et al. Membranous bone lengthening: a serial histologic study. Ann Plast Surg 1992;29:2.
12. Snyder CC, Levine GA, Swanson HM, Browne EZ Jr. Mandibular lengthening by gradual distraction. Preliminary report. Plast Reconstr Surg. 1973 May;51(5):506–8.
13. Michieli S, Miotti B. Lengthening of mandibular body by gradual surgical-orthodontic distraction. J Oral Surg. 1977 Mar;35(3):187–92.
14. Profitt WR, White RP. Surgical-Orthodontic Treatment, Mosby Year Book, St. Louis, Missouri, 1991, pp. 4–5.
15. Pereira V, Sell D, Ponniah A, Evans R, Dunaway D. Midface osteotomy versus distraction: the effect on speech, nasality, and velopharyngeal function in craniofacial dysostosis. Cleft Palate Craniofac J. 2008 Jul;45(4):353–63.
16. Harada K, Ishii Y, Ishii M, Imaizumi H, Mibu M, Omura K. Effect of maxillary distraction osteogenesis on velopharyngeal function: a pilot study. Oral Surg Oral Med Oral Pathol Oral Radiol Endod. 2002 May;93(5):538–43.
17. van Strijen PJ, Breuning KH, Becking AG, Perdijk FB, Tuinzing DB. Complications in bilateral mandibular distraction osteogenesis using internal devices. Oral Surg Oral Med Oral Pathol Oral Radiol Endod. 2003 Oct;96(4):392–7.
18. Block MS, Daire J, Stover J, Matthews M. Changes in the inferior alveolar nerve following mandibular lengthening in the dog using distraction osteogenesis. J Oral Maxillofac Surg. 1993 Jun;51(6):652–60.
19. Whitesides LM, Meyer RA. Effect of distraction osteogenesis on the severely hypoplastic mandible and inferior alveolar nerve function. J Oral Maxillofac Surg. 2004 Mar;62(3):292–7.
20. Gunbay T, Akay MC, Aras A, Gomel M. Effects of transmandibular symphyseal distraction on teeth, bone, and temporomandibular joint. J Oral Maxillofac Surg. 2009 Oct; 67(10):2254–65.
21. Miloro M, Miller JJ, Stoner JA. Low-level laser effect on mandibular distraction osteogenesis. J Oral Maxillofac Surg 2007;65:168–176.
22. McCormick SU, McCarthy JG, Grayson BH, Staffenberg D, McCormick SA. Effect of mandibular distraction on the temporomandibular joint: Part 1, Canine study. J Craniofac Surg. 1995 Sep;6(5):358–63.
23. Grayson BH, Santiago PE. Treatment planning and biomechanics of distraction osteogenesis from an orthodontic perspective. Semin Orthod 1999;5:9–24.
24. Douglas B. The treatment of micrognathia associated with obstruction by a plastic procedure. Plast Reconstr Surg 1946; 1:300–308.
25. Le chute de la base de la langue consideree comme une nouvelle cause de gene dans la respiration naso-pharyngienne {Backward lowering of the root of the tongue causing respiratory disturbances}. Bull. Acad. Nat. Med (Paris) 89: 37, 1923.
26. Miloro M. Mandibular distraction osteogenesis for pediatric airway management. J Oral Maxillofac Surg. 2010 Jul; 68(7):1512–23.
27. McCormick SU, Grayson BH, McCarthy JG, Staffenberg D. Effect of mandibular distraction on the temporomandibular joint: Part 2, Clinical study. J Craniofac Surg. 1995 Sep;6(5): 364–7.
28. García García A, Somoza Martin M, Gandara Vila P, Gandara Rey JM. A preliminary morphologic classification of the alveolar ridge after distraction osteogenesis. J Oral Maxillofac Surg. 2004 May;62(5):563–6.

Suggested Readings

1. Herford A, Audia F, Stucki-McCormick SU. Alveolar distraction osteogenesis and vector control—a preliminary report. In Arnaud E, Diner PA, editors. Proceedings of the Third International Meeting on Craniofacial Distraction Osteogenesis. 2001;June 14–16; Paris, France. Bologna, Italy: Monduzzi; 2001.
2. Hoffmeister B, Marcks CH, Wolff KP. The floating bone concept in intraoral distraction. J Craniomaxillofac Surg 1998;26(Suppl 1):76–81.
3. Moses JJ. Sagittal distraction of the mandible: a technique for nerve preservation and condylar axis stability. Proceedings of the Fourth International Congress of Osteogenesis of the Facial Skeleton. 2003;July 2–5; Paris, France. Bologna, Italy: Monduzzi; 2003.
4. Watzinger F, Wanschitz F, Rasse M, et al. Computer-aided surgery in distraction osteogenesis of the maxilla and mandible. Int J Oral Maxillofac Surg 1999;28:171–175.
5. McCarthy JG, Stelnicki EJ, Grayson BH. Distraction osteogenesis of the mandible: a ten-year experience. Semin Orthod 1999;1:3–8.
6. Grayson BH, Stucki-McCormick SU, Santiago PE. Vector of device placement and trajectory of mandibular distraction. J Craniofac Surg 1998;8:473–480.
7. Stucki-McCormick SU, Fox R, Mizrahi R. Distraction osteogenesis for congenital mandibular deformities. Atlas Oral Maxillofac Surg Clin North Am 1999;7:85–110.
8. Perlyn CA, Schmelzer RE, Sutera SP, et al. Effect of distraction osteogenesis of the mandible on upper airway volume and

resistance in children with micrognathia. Plast Reconstr Surg 2002;109:1809–1818.

9. Denny A, Kalantarian B. Mandibular distraction in neonates: a strategy to avoid tracheostomy. Plast Reconstr Surg 2002;109:896–904.

10. Woodson BT, Hanson PR, Melugin MB, Gama AA. Sequential upper airway changes during mandibular distraction for obstructive sleep apnea. Otolaryngol Head Neck Surg 2003;128:142–144.

11. Smith KS. Pediatric sleep apnea and treatment with distraction osteogenesis. Ann R Australas Coll Dent Surg 2000;15:163–167.

12. Cope JB, Yamashita J, Healy S, et al. Force level and strain patterns during bilateral mandibular osteodistraction. J Oral Maxillofac Surg 2000;58:171–189.

13. Cope JB, Samchukov ML, Cherkashin AM, et al. Biomechanics of mandibular distractor orientation: an animal model analysis. J Oral Maxillofac Surg 1999;57:952–964.

14. Contasti G, Guerrero C, Rodriguez AM, Legan HL. Mandibular widening by distraction osteogenesis. J Clin Orthod 2001;35:165–173.

15. Bell WH, Gonzalez M, Samchukov ML, Guerrero CA. Intraoral widening and lengthening of the mandible in baboons by distraction osteogenesis. J Oral Maxillofac Surg 1999;57:548–563.

16. Kewitt GF, Van Sickels JE. Long-term effect of mandibular midline distraction osteogenesis on the status of the temporomandibular joint, teeth, periodontal structures, and neurosensory function. J Oral Maxillofac Surg 1999;57:1419–1426.

17. Guerrero CA, Bell WH, Contasti GI, Rodriguez AM. Intraoral mandibular distraction osteogenesis. Semin Orthod 1999;5:35–40.

18. Molina F. Combined maxillary and mandibular distraction osteogenesis. Semin Orthod 1999;5:41–45.

19. Padwa BL, Kearns GJ, Todd R, et al. Simultaneous maxillary and mandibular distraction osteogenesis with a semiburied device. Int J Oral Maxillofac Surg 1999;28:2–8.

20. Moses JJ, Vega L. Sagittal distraction of the mandible. In Arnaud E, Diner PA, editors. Proceedings of the Third International Meeting on Craniofacial Distraction Osteogenesis. 2001;June 14–16; Paris, France. Bologna; Italy: Monduzzi; 2001.

21. Polley JW, Figueroa AA. Rigid external distraction: its application in cleft maxillary deformities. Plast Reconstr Surg 1998;102:1360–1374.

22. Cohen SR. Midface distraction. Semin Orthod 1999;5:52–58.

23. Ahn JG, Figueroa AA, Braun S, Polley JW. Biomechanical considerations in distraction of the osteotomized dentomaxillary complex. Am J Orthod Dentofacial Orthop 1999;116:264–270.

24. Liou EJ, Chen PK, Huang CS, Chen YR. Interdental distraction osteogenesis and rapid orthodontic tooth movement: a novel approach to approximate a wide alveolar cleft or bony defect. Plast Reconstr Surg 2000;105:1262–1272.

25. Costantino PD, Buchbinder D. Mandibular distraction osteogenesis: types, applications, and indications. J Craniofac Surg 1996;7:404–407.

26. Guerrero CA, Gonzalez M. Intraoral bone transport by distraction osteogenesis in mandibular reconstruction. In Arnaud E, Diner PA, editors. Proceedings of the Fourth International Congress of Osteogenesis of the Facial Skeleton. 2003;July 2–5; Paris, France. Bologna, Italy: Monduzzi; 2003.

27. Herford AS. Use of a plate guided distraction device for transport distraction osteogenesis of the mandible. In Arnaud E, Diner PA, editors. Proceedings of the Fourth International Congress of Osteogenesis of the Facial Skeleton. 2003;July 2-5; Paris, France. Bologna, Italy: Monduzzi; 2003.

28. Stucki-McCormick SU, Fox R, Mizrahi R, Erickson M. Transport distraction: mandibular reconstruction. Atlas Oral Maxillofac Surg Clin North Am 1999;7:65–84.

29. Gantous A, Phillips JH, Catton P, Holmberg D. Distraction osteogenesis in the irradiated canine mandible. Plast Reconstr Surg 1994;93:164–168.

30. Aronson J. Temporal and special increases in blood flow during distraction osteogenesis. Clin Orthop Rel Res 1994;301:124–131.

31. Klesper B, Lazar F, Siessegger M, et al. Vertical distraction-osteogenesis of fibula transplants for mandibular reconstruction a preliminary study. J Craniomaxillofac Surg 2002;30:280–285.

32. McCarthy JG, Stelnicki EJ, Mehrara BJ, Longaker MT. Distraction osteogenesis of the craniofacial skeleton. Plast Reconstr Surg 2001;107:1812–1827.

33. Stucki-McCormick SU, Fox RM, Mizrahi RD. Reconstruction of a neocondyle using transport distraction osteogenesis. Semin Orthod 1999;5:59–63.

34. Piero C, Alessandro A, Giorgio S, et al. Combined surgical therapy of temporomandibular joint ankylosis and secondary deformity using intraoral distraction. J Craniofac Surg 2002;13:401–410.

35. Chin M. Distraction osteogenesis for dental implants. Atlas Oral Maxillofac Surg Clin North Am 1999;7:41–63.

36. Jensen OT, Cockrell R, Kuhike L, Reed C. Anterior maxillary alveolar distraction osteogenesis: a prospective 5-year clinical study. Int J Oral Maxillofac Implants 2002;17:52–68.

37. Block MS, Gardiner D, Almerico B, Neal C. Loaded hydroxylapatite-coated implants and uncoated titanium-threaded implants in distracted dog alveolar ridges. Oral Surg Oral Med Oral Pathol Oral Radiol Endod 2000;89:676–685.

38. Robiony M, Polini F, Costa F, Politi M. Osteogenesis distraction and platelet-rich plasma for bone restoration of the severely atrophic mandible: preliminary results. J Oral Maxillofac Surg 2002;60:630–635.

39. Millisi W, Millisi-Schobel G. Alveolar distraction osteogenesis of the mandible. In Arnaud E, Diner PA, editors. Proceedings of the Fourth International Congress of Osteogenesis of the Facial Skeleton. 2003;July 2–5; Paris, France. Bologna, Italy: Monduzzi; 2003.

40. Zechner W, Bernhart T, Zauza K, et al. Multi-dimensional osteodistraction for correction of implant malposition in edentulous segments. Clin Oral Implants Res 2001;12:531–538.

41. Stucki-McCormick SU, Moses JJ, Robinson R, et al. Alveolar distraction devices. In Jensen OT, editor. Alveolar Distraction Osteogenesis. Carol Stream, IL: Quintessence Publishing; 2002; pp. 41–58.

42. Chin M. Alveolar distraction osteogenesis with endosseous devices in 175 cases. In Arnaud E, Diner PA, editors. Proceedings of the Third International Meeting on Craniofacial Distraction Osteogenesis. 2001;Juny 14–16; Paris, France. Bologna, Italy: Monduzzi; 2001.

43. Stucki-McCormick SU, Moses JJ. Vertical alveolar distraction of the posterior mandible. In Jensen OT, editor. Alveolar Distraction Osteogenesis. Carol Stream, IL: Quintessence Publishing; 2002; pp. 89–94.

44. Millesi G, Klug C, Millesi W, et al. Vertical distraction osteogenesis in the mandible combined with L-shaped osteotomy and guided bone regeneration. Cranio-maxillo-facial distraction. Graz, Austria: University of Graz; 2002.

45. Hidding J, Lazar F, Zoller JE. The Cologne concept on vertical distraction osteogenesis. In Arnaud E, Diner PA, editors. Proceedings of the Third International Meeting on Craniofacial Distraction Osteogenesis. 2001;Juny 14–16; Paris, France. Bologna, Italy: Monduzzi; 2001.

46. Hidding J, Lazar F, Zoller JE. Initial outcome of vertical distraction osteogenesis of the atrophic alveolar ridge. Mund Kiefer Gesichtschir 1999;3(Suppl 1):79–83.

47. Garcia AG, Martin MS, Vila PG, Maceiras JL. Minor complications arising in alveolar distraction osteogenesis. J Oral Maxillofac Surg 2002;60:496–501.

48. Holzhauer DP, Larsen PE, Miloro M, Vig KWL. Distraction osteogenesis of the mandible with a modified intraoral appliance: a pilot study in miniature pigs. Int J Orthod Orthognath Surg 1998;13: 241–247.

Surgical and Nonsurgical Management of Obstructive Sleep Apnea

B. D. Tiner, DDS, MD, and Peter D. Waite, MPH, DDS, MD

Sleep and dreaming have been sources of mystery and fascination since biblical times. Sleep consists of inevitably recurring episodes of readily reversible relative disengagement from sensory and motor interaction with the environment.[1] The function of sleep remains a mystery, and only in recent years has there been research into specific symptom complexes and causes of sleep disorders. In 1979, the Association of Sleep Disorders Center and the Association for the Psychophysiological Study of Sleep published the first classification of sleep and arousal disorders.[2]

Modern sleep research became possible in 1924 when Hans Berger,[3] a German psychiatrist, described the recording of human electroencephalography. Loomis and colleagues in 1935[4,5] published a quantitative description of the four levels of sleep based on electroencephalogram (EEG) characteristics. The historic discovery of a cyclic phase of sleep characterized by rapid conjugate eye movements was made by Aserinsky and Kleitman in 1953.[6] Subsequent studies confirmed this to be a very active phase of sleep that correlated closely with dreaming.[7]

NORMAL SLEEP STAGES

Normal sleep architecture includes both quiet sleep (non–rapid eye movement [non-REM] sleep) and active sleep (rapid eye movement [REM] sleep). Non-REM sleep consists of four stages that are based largely on the original criteria of Loomis and colleagues.[4,5] Stage 2 predominates and accounts for 45% to 50% of total sleep time. The four stages of non-REM sleep represent progressively deeper sleep marked by the increasing appearance of high-amplitude slow waves in stages 3 and 4, which are collectively known as *delta sleep*. Non-REM sleep is characterized by a general slowing of all levels of activity. Progression through all four stages of non-REM sleep usually occurs rapidly after sleep onset. REM sleep occurs after non-REM sleep has been established, and the first REM period normally occurs after 70 to 90 minutes of non-REM sleep. The average duration of a period of REM sleep is approximately 20 minutes. The initial REM period of the night is usually very brief, but subsequent REM periods become longer. During an average night of REM/non-REM cycle progression, four to six REM periods normally occur at intervals of 60 to 90 minutes. REM sleep occupies about 20% to 25% of total sleep time in a healthy young adult. REM sleep EEG patterns look very similar to those seen during the wakeful state. Generalized skeletal muscle atonia (except for the ocular muscles) and absence of reflexive activity are other features unique to REM sleep. Marked physiologic changes also occur during REM sleep. Temperature, blood flow, and oxygen use in the brain are increased. Heart rate, blood pressure, and respiration show dramatic fluctuations and increase in average rate.

During sleep, the control of respiration is influenced by two systems: the metabolic control system and the behavioral control system.[8] The influences of hypoxia and hypercarbia on ventilation are the predominant components of the metabolic control system of respiration. This system predominantly controls respiration during non-REM sleep. The behavioral control system governs respiration during voluntary activities, such as swallowing or speaking, and may suppress the ventilatory response to metabolic stimuli. During REM sleep, the effects of hypoxia and hypercarbia on ventilation are much less than during non-REM sleep, and the behavioral control system may predominate. With a blunted response to hypoxia and hypercarbia, irregular respirations, and decreased skeletal muscle tone of the upper airway muscles during REM sleep, an episode of partial or complete airway obstruction with apnea or hypopnea may occur.

SLEEP APNEA SYNDROME

The sleep apnea syndrome is a disorder characterized by abnormal breathing in sleep and sleep fragmentation. At least 30 episodes of apnea occur during 7 hours of nocturnal sleep in these patients. *Apnea* is defined as the cessation of airflow from the nostrils and mouth for at least 10 seconds. These apneic episodes can result in hypoxemia, hypercarbia, systemic and pulmonary hypertension, polycythemia, cor pulmonale, bradycardia, and cardiac dysrhythmias. Sudden death has occurred in patients with sleep apnea. Throughout the night, the alternating episodes of apnea and arousal from sleep may occur as frequently as 400 to 600 times, with each typical apnea episode lasting 15 to 60 seconds. These episodes can amount to as much as 50% of a night's sleep. The frequent disruption results in symptoms similar to those of sleep deprivation. These include excessive daytime sleepiness, fatigue, depression, personality changes, and impotence. These dysfunctional symptoms are common primary complaints and are often the reason people seek treatment.

Epidemiologic data suggest that sleep apnea syndrome may be quite common, particularly in its milder forms. In fact, obstructive sleep apnea (OSA) is the second most common sleep disorder, insomnia being the most common. A 1993 Sleep Commission Report estimated that 20 million Americans have sleep apnea, with the majority being undiagnosed and untreated.[9] The exact prevalence is unknown, but sleep apnea syndrome may affect up to 2% to 3% of adult males.[8] In certain populations, the prevalence may be as high at 10%. Most patients are diagnosed after age 40, but sleep apnea can occur at any age. There is a strong male predilection, with men outnumbering women by up to 8:1 until menopause. This implies a hormonal influence. The cost for diagnosis and treatment of this sleep disorder accounts for over $50 million (U.S.) in hospital bills each year. Overall, sleep disorders and sleepiness cost the U.S. economy a minimum of $15.9 billion in direct costs each year.[10]

Classification

Central sleep apnea, OSA, and mixed sleep apnea are the variations of apnea that occur in the syndrome. In central sleep apnea, respiratory muscle activity ceases simultaneously with airflow at the mouth and nostrils.[11] This disorder is found in patients with central nervous system (CNS) insufficiency that affects the outflow of neural output from the respiratory center to the diaphragm and other muscles of

respiration. CNS disorders associated with central sleep apnea include brainstem neoplasms, brainstem infarctions, bulbar encephalitis, bulbar poliomyelitis, spinal surgery, cervical cordotomy, and primary idiopathic hypoventilation.

Patients with central sleep apnea have been treated with some success by using respiratory-stimulating drugs such as theophylline, progesterone, and acetazolamide. In severe central apnea, modalities of treatment have included phrenic nerve pacemaker implantation to ensure regular respiration during sleep and nocturnal mechanical ventilation with a negative-pressure ventilator for more severe cases. There are no simple and convenient methods of treatment for mild central apnea.

The most common type of sleep apnea by far is obstructive. This is characterized by sleep-induced obstruction of the upper airway that results in cessation of airflow with preservation of respiratory effort, respiratory center drive, and diaphragmatic contraction.[11]

Mixed sleep apnea is a combination of central and obstructive apnea. This pattern begins with an episode of central apnea with no airflow detectable at the mouth and nostrils and no respiratory muscle activity. The pattern ends with an episode of obstructive apnea with cessation of airflow only at the mouth and nostrils.[11]

Differential Diagnosis

Profound hypersomnolence is a characteristic feature of both sleep apnea and narcolepsy; hence, they are often confused. However, unlike sleep apnea, narcolepsy affects both sexes equally, with most patients experiencing the onset of symptoms around or shortly before puberty.[12] The first symptom to appear with narcolepsy is usually excessive daytime somnolence (EDS). The sleep attacks can range from mild to severe and are characterized by the sudden onset of overwhelming sleepiness that lasts 30 seconds to 20 minutes. After brief naps, the narcoleptic usually feels refreshed and relatively free from disturbing symptoms for up to 2 hours. Serious accidents, marital discord, and the inability to hold jobs frequently result from these sleep attacks. Another feature of narcolepsy is the abrupt loss of muscle control (cataplexy). Attacks can be particularly disabling because they are characteristically precipitated by emotional experiences such as laughter, anger, or excitement. Additional associated symptoms of narcolepsy include sleep paralysis and hypnagogic hallucinations. Sleep paralysis is the skeletal muscle atonia of REM sleep persisting into the awake state. Hypnagogic hallucinations are REM sleep imagery occurring while falling asleep. Patients are sometimes misdiagnosed as schizophrenic if hypnagogic hallucinations are prominent.

Diagnosis of narcolepsy is made by documenting sleep-onset REM periods during a nocturnal polysomnography.[12] In normal sleep, REM sleep is usually not seen until about 70 to 90 minutes into sleep. The clinical features of narcolepsy probably represent abnormal manifestations of REM sleep.

Treatment modalities for narcolepsy include behavioral therapies, CNS stimulants, tricyclic antidepressants, or monoamine oxidase inhibitors (only in resistant cases) and L-tryptophan.[13]

Other disorders that may be confused with sleep apnea syndrome include sleep-related abnormal swallowing syndrome, gastroesophageal reflux, depression, alcohol or drug dependence, and sleep-related nocturnal myoclonus.

History of OSA Syndrome

OSA has a remarkably short history, considering the incidence and disabling symptoms of the syndrome. Burwell and coworkers published the first description of the syndrome in 1956.[14] Their report compared an obese, somnolent, polycythemic patient with the sleepy red-faced boy, Joe, in the Charles Dickens novel *The Posthumous Papers of the Pickwick Club* (1837). However, Burwell and coworkers did not link their patient's excessive daytime sleepiness to nocturnal sleep fragmentation. In 1966, Gastaut and associates[15] were the first investigators to demonstrate repeated apneas in pickwickian patients during sleep. They correctly attributed the excessive daytime somnolence in these patients to nocturnal sleep fragmentation caused by repeated apneas.

The misdiagnosis of narcolepsy in patients with sleep apnea and the general skepticism of EDS as a valid clinical sign are the two main reasons sleep apnea syndrome was overlooked for so long.

Clinical Manifestations

Sleep apnea patients present with a variety of symptoms and clinical manifestations. Patients with OSA most often complain of EDS. The patients may experience serious social, economic, and emotional problems from the EDS associated with this disorder. The uncontrollable desire to sleep may predispose the patients to occupational or automobile accidents.

Almost all patients or their bed partners give a history of heavy, loud snoring that has usually been present for several years before the EDS was noted. The snoring is produced from the passage of air through the oropharynx causing vibrations of the soft palate. Typically, the snoring is interrupted periodically by apneic episodes that last 30 to 90 seconds. Bed partners usually describe an episode in which the snoring stops and the patient seems to stop breathing for a period of time. A loud snort followed by a hyperventilation usually signals an end to the apneic episode.

Other common presenting complaints are morning headaches and nausea that result from the hypercarbia that develops with the hypoventilatory episodes. Depression, personality changes, and intellectual deterioration may also develop.

The systemic hypertension that is a common finding in OSA may be related to the catecholamine release triggered by the systemic hypoxemia. In more advanced severe cases, pulmonary hypertension, polycythemia, and cor pulmonale may develop and become life-threatening. However, most patients do not manifest these disturbances because their ventilation during wakeful periods is sufficient to prevent these complications of chronic hypoxia.

A prominent sinus dysrhythmia is commonly associated with the apneic episodes. The extent of bradycardia is directly proportional to the severity of the oxygen desaturation. The greatest degree of cardiac slowing occurs in obstructive apneas in which a Müller maneuver is performed. Increased vagal efferent tone mediates the bradycardia.

The development of severe and life-threatening medical complications from the apneic events clearly depends on the frequency, duration, and degree of hypoxemia and associated hypertensive response.

Physical Findings

A major feature of OSA is obesity. The increased body weight correlates with increased frequency of apnea and the severity of hypoxemia. However, the morbidly obese, somnolent, hyperventilating patient with cor pulmonale represents only a small number of sleep apnea patients. Lower body mass index (BMI) patients with OSA often have more abnormal cephalometrics than obese people.[16,17]

Obstruction can occur at a number of points in the airway. Physical examination of these patients may reveal hypertrophy of the tonsils or adenoids, retrognathia, micrognathia, macroglossia, deviation of the nasal septum, a thick short neck, or tumors in the nasopharynx or hypopharynx. Both primary and secondary medical conditions are associated with OSA, owing to their effects on the upper airway anatomy. These may include temporomandibular joint disorders, myxedema, goiter, acromegaly, and lymphoma.

Most patients with classic OSA have no identifiable craniofacial anomaly. However, there does appear to be a significant subpopulation of sleep apnea patients with craniofacial anomalies.[18,19] Lowe and colleagues[20] found several alterations in craniofacial form in subjects with OSA that may reduce the dimensions of the upper airway and subsequently impair stability of the upper airway. A sample of 25 adult male patients with moderate to severe OSA showed a posteriorly positioned maxilla and mandible, a steep occlusal plane, overerupted maxillary and mandibular teeth, proclined incisors, a steep mandibular plane, a large gonial angle, increased upper and lower facial heights, a posteriorly placed pharyngeal wall, and an anterior open bite in association with a long tongue.[20] Bacon and coworkers[18] evaluated 32 patients with sleep apnea by cephalometry and demonstrated an anteroposterior shortening of the cranial base, a posterior facial compression with narrowing of the pharyngeal airway, and an increased lower facial height. Rivlin and associates[21] reported on nine OSA patients with posterior displacement of the mandible. The number of apneas correlated with the total posterior displacement.[21]

DIAGNOSIS

Physical Examination

A diagnostic evaluation includes a thorough history and physical examination, fiberoptic endoscopy, radiologic evaluation, and polysomnography. Little additional information can be gained from routine laboratory tests. Except in severe cases, pulmonary function tests, electrocardiogram (ECG), arterial blood gases, and chest radiographs are often normal during wakefulness in sleep apnea patients.

Other diagnostic tests that may aid in evaluating sleep apnea patients include a complete blood count (CBC), serum electrolytes, and thyroid function tests. Secondary polycythemia may be revealed by a CBC, and nocturnal carbon dioxide retention may be reflected by increased bicarbonate levels. Hypothyroidism, a contributing cause of sleep apnea, may be identified from thyroid function studies.

After a complete history is obtained from the patient and his or her bed partner, a complete clinical examination of the mouth, nasal, pharyngeal, and laryngeal areas is performed. The emphasis of the clinical examination should be the identification of anatomic abnormalities that may contribute to or produce obstruction during sleep. The nose is examined for a deviated nasal septum and enlargement of the turbinates. Micrognathia, retrognathia, and macroglossia may be noted in examination of the oral cavity. Occasionally, masses or tumors in the nasopharynx or hypopharynx may be noted. In the pharynx, adenotonsillary hypertrophy, a long soft palate, a large base of the tongue, and excess pharyngeal mucosa are potential causes of obstruction. The larynx is examined for vocal cord webs and paralysis of the vocal cords. OSA patients may present with any combination of these anatomic abnormalities.

After topically anesthetizing the nasal cavity and pharynx, a fiberoptic endoscope is introduced through the nose. In sequential fashion, the nasopharynx, oropharynx, hypopharynx, and larynx are examined. The appearance and position of the soft palate, base of tongue, and lateral pharyngeal walls are evaluated. Changes in the position of the base of the tongue such as forward movement with protrusion of the mandible are noted. The appearance of the pharyngeal airway and degree of pharyngeal wall collapse is noted while the patient performs a modified Müller maneuver. To accomplish this maneuver, the patient attempts to inspire with the mouth and nose closed. Increased negative pressure in the pharynx will demonstrate the point of collapse.

Cephalometric Examination

A lateral cephalogram is routinely obtained in the radiologic evaluation of sleep apnea patients (Figure 64-1). Cephalometric analysis is performed to identify any skeletal and soft tissue abnormalities that may exist. The advantages of cephalometry are its easy access, low cost, and minimal radiation exposure. However, it should be recognized that there are obvious limitations of evaluating a three-dimensional area with a two-dimensional lateral cephalometry.

Mandibular or maxillary position can be evaluated by a number of methods including the SNA (sella-nasion–A point) and SNB (sella-nasion–B point) angles. Patients with skeletal deficiencies are more likely to have obstruction at the base of the tongue or at the level of the soft palate. Riley and colleagues[22,23] determined that OSA patients had an inferiorly positioned hyoid bone, a longer-than-normal soft palate, and a narrowing at the base of the tongue. The position of the hyoid bone is determined by drawing a perpendicular line from the mandibular plane (MP) through the hyoid bone (H). The mean MP-H distance for normal subjects is 15.4 ± 3 mm (see Figure 64-1). The position of the hyoid bone is important because it serves as a central anchor for the muscles of the tongue and thereby partly determines tongue position. Soft palate length is measured from a line drawn from posterior nasal spine (PNS) to the tip of the soft palate shadow (P). The mean PNS-P distance in normal subjects is 37 ± 3 mm. Posterior airway space (PAS) is determined by a line drawn from point B through the gonion (Go) intersecting the base of the tongue and the posterior pharyngeal wall. Figure 64-2 demonstrates change in PASs after maxillomandibular advancement (MMA). Mean PAS in normal subjects was determined to be 11 ± 1 mm. Lower face height is measured from the anterior nasal spine (ANS) to the menton (Me).

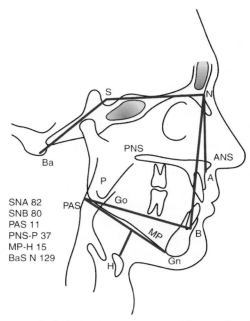

FIGURE 64-1. Cephalometric screening used for initial evaluation of patients with obstructive sleep apnea syndrome. A = A point; ANS = anterior nasal spine; B = B point; Ba = basion; Gn = gnathion; Go = gonion; H = hyoid; MP = mandibular plane; N = nasion; P = palate; PAS = posterior airway space; PNS = posterior nasal spine; S = sella; SNA = sella-nasion–A point; SNB = sella-nasion–B point. (Adapted from Tiner BD, Waite PD. Surgical and nonsurgical management of obstructive sleep apnea. In Peterson LJ, Indresano AT, Marciani RD, Roser SM, editors. Principles of Oral and Maxillofacial Surgery. Vol 3. Philadelphia: JB Lippincott; 1992; p. 1535.)

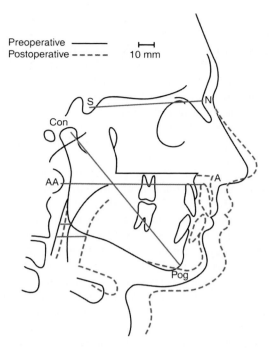

Preoperative ———
Postoperative ---- |—| 10 mm

FIGURE 64-2.   Change in posterior airway space after maxillary and mandibular advancement. A = A point; AA = anterior edge of atlas; Con = condylion; N = nasion; Pog = Pogonion; S = sella. (Adapted from Tiner BD, Waite PD. Surgical and nonsurgical management of obstructive sleep apnea. In Peterson LJ, Indresano AT, Marciani RD, Roser SM, editors. Principles of Oral and Maxillofacial Surgery. Vol 3. Philadelphia: JB Lippincott; 1992; p. 1536.)

There is no absolute value for this measurement in OSA patients. However, some studies have shown an increased lower face height and a shortened cranial base with OSA patients.[18]

Computed Tomography

Computed tomography (CT) is an alternative to cephalometry and has been used to provide a quantitative assessment of the upper airway at various levels. With three-dimensional CT reconstructions, Lowe and coworkers[24] found OSA patients with larger tongue surface areas and smaller airway surface areas. Haponik and associates[25] found significantly decreased cross-sectional areas of the nasopharynx, oropharynx, and hypopharynx in OSA patients when compared with control subjects by using CT scanning. Some authorities believe that the airway can be assessed only by a CT scan. However, Riley and colleagues[23,26] compared patients who had three-dimensional CT scans and found a statistically significant correlation between the PAS measured on the lateral cephalogram and the volume of the pharyngeal airway measured on CT scans. Waite and Villos[27] demonstrated by helical CT analysis that MMA increases both anteroposterior and lateral dimension of the airway at all levels from nasopharynx to hyoid. Many studies are currently being done to determine the effects of patient position and changes in airway. A cephalogram and a CT scan are static evaluations at a fixed time of a dynamic system and they should be viewed as only part of the overall evaluation of the patient.

Polysomnography

Nocturnal polysomnography remains the gold standard for establishing the diagnosis of sleep apnea, quantitating its severity, and determining the success of treatment modalities. The study is performed in a sleep laboratory and the patient's sleep is monitored overnight. At least 4 hours of total sleep time must be recorded for a diagnostic study. The components of the polysomnogram include the EEG, electrooculogram (EOG), electromyogram (EMG), and ECG (lead V2). Sleep staging and architecture are determined by the EEG, EOG, and EMG tracings. Potentially lethal cardiac dysrhythmias are detected by the ECG. Oxygen saturation is measured by ear oximetry. A 5% or greater decrease in arterial oxygen saturation from baseline is significant during episodes of apnea or hypopnea. Respiratory effort and breathing pattern are measured using respiratory inductive plethysmography or by measuring intrathoracic pressure changes with an esophageal balloon catheter. The distinction between an episode of central apnea and obstructive apnea is made by correlating airflow at the nose and mouth with movement of the abdominal and thoracic respiratory muscles. Central apnea occurs if both airflow and respiratory muscle movement stop simultaneously. An episode of obstructive apnea occurs when airflow at the mouth and nose ceases but respiratory muscles in the abdomen and thorax continue to move dysfunctionally.

Of particular interest are the number of respiratory events (apneas and hypopneas), the number of oxygen desaturations below 90%, and the lowest oxygen desaturation. The respiratory disturbance index (RDI) can be calculated from these data:

$$RDI = \frac{Apneas + Hypopneas}{Total\ sleep\ Time} \times 60$$

An RDI greater than 5 is considered abnormal and an RDI greater than 20 is considered clinically significant, because EDS usually does not occur below this level. OSA also becomes clinically significant when oxygen desaturation events fall below 85%.

Site of Obstruction

After a complete presurgical evaluation, each patient is grouped according to the site of obstruction: type I, oropharynx; type II, oropharynx and hypopharynx; and type III, hypopharynx. In a review of 40 OSA patients, Riley and coworkers[28] found the majority of patients had a type II obstruction (soft palate and base of tongue).

The mandible, base of tongue, hyoid, and pharyngeal wall are intimately related by their muscular and ligamentous attachments. The mandible is related to the base of the tongue by the genioglossus muscle. The tongue, through multiple muscular and connective tissue attachments, is related to the hyoid bone and to the mandible in such a way that retraction of the mandible results in a narrowing of the airway and posterior movement of the tongue. Compensatory mechanisms exist in non–sleep-apneic patients to prevent occlusion of the airway. However, in sleep-apneic patients, these mechanisms do not exist or are unable to compensate adequately.

Obstruction of the upper airway is primarily prevented by the action of the pharyngeal dilating muscles contracting in phase with respiration. Reduced muscle tone is normal and prominent during REM sleep. However, OSA patients may have a significant reduction in muscle activity during non-REM sleep so that the pharynx becomes narrower and airway resistance increases. In patients with abnormal skeletal development, the reduction in size of the resting airway may predispose them to upper airway obstruction during sleep.

The patency of the upper airway is determined by a balance between the pharyngeal musculature and the negative oropharyngeal pressures that are generated from resistance to airflow in the nasopharynx. Because the airway of OSA patients is unstable even at rest, any structural narrowing of the airway will eventually hinder the muscular component of the balance. Collapse of the airway in OSA is primarily a result of high intraluminal negative pressures associated with hypotonic pharyngeal wall musculature and disproportionate anatomy in either the oropharynx or the hypopharynx or both. Disproportionate anatomy includes any combination of large base of tongue, long soft palate, narrow mandibular arch, shallow palatal arch, or retrognathic mandible.

MEDICAL TREATMENT

Once the diagnosis has been confirmed, the treatment approach for sleep apnea is determined by the severity of the physiologic derangements and the predominant type of apnea. Regardless of the predominant type of apnea present, all patients should be cautioned that certain drugs may precipitate or exacerbate OSA. Alcohol and other CNS depressants have been shown to aggravate sleep apnea and even to precipitate apnea and oxygen desaturations in normal persons.[29]

Weight loss and nasal continuous positive airway pressure (CPAP) are the initial modes of therapy that should be initiated in obese patients with moderate OSA. A study of 16 patients who lost an average of 20 kg showed fewer apneas, reduced oxygen desaturations, and less daytime sleepiness than a control group of patients who did not lose weight.[30] Many patients can relate weight gain in preceding years to an increase in severity of their OSA symptoms. Unfortunately, weight loss by dietary measures is seldom sustained, and OSA symptoms recur with weight gain. Riley and associates[31] found that 47 of 50 OSA patients who were between 20% and 100% overweight at the time of diagnosis had regained all the weight they had initially lost 5 to 7 years later.

The role of oxygen therapy in the treatment of sleep apnea is controversial. In a study by Motta and Guilleminault,[32] the administration of oxygen increased the duration of apneic episodes and led to worsening of acidosis and hypercarbia during both REM and non-REM sleep. It is unknown how many of their patients had chronic obstructive lung disease. Other studies have shown that supplemental oxygen therapy consistently reduced the severity of oxygen desaturation and decreased the frequency of apnea.[33,34]

The combined experience of these reports suggests that oxygen therapy limited to a flow rate of 2 L/min can be used safely in most OSA patients and will produce beneficial effects on respiration. The dangers of profound hypoxemia are greater than the concerns of prolonged apnea, acidosis, and hypercarbia. The effects of oxygen therapy on a patient with severe airway obstruction or chronic respiratory acidosis should be monitored with oximetry or polysomnography.

Several drugs have been used in the treatment of OSA syndrome with variable results. The carbonic anhydrase inhibitor acetazolamide stimulates respiration by producing a metabolic acidosis. This drug reduced the number of apneas and decreased the severity of oxygen desaturations in a group of patients with central sleep apnea.[35] However, in several cases, acetazolamide given to patients with mild OSA produced more frequent OSAs of longer duration.[36] Therefore, acetazolamide is probably not indicated in the management of OSA syndrome.

Some patients with OSA benefit from the respiratory stimulant effect of progesterone, especially those with the obesity-hypoventilation syndrome.[37-40] Progesterone increases alveolar ventilation and improves oxygenation, but its effect on frequency of apnea is limited. Major side effects that limit its long-term use include decreased libido, alopecia, and impotence.

The tricyclic antidepressant protriptyline is the most effective and best studied drug for the treatment of OSA.[41] In a study of 12 patients, Smith and colleagues[42] showed a reduction in apnea frequency and oxygen desaturation during non-REM sleep, in addition to a decrease in REM sleep. Protriptyline produces its beneficial effect by a preferential stimulation of upper airway muscle tone and by decreasing the percentage of time spent in REM sleep, thereby reducing the more severe REM-related apneas. Anticholinergic side effects such as dry mouth, constipation, urinary retention, and impotence are frequent and limit its use.

Oral Appliances

The use of a variety of prosthetic devices is another approach to treatment. The nasopharynx and the posterior tongue are the two anatomic areas of concern. Insertion of a nasopharyngeal airway has been used to prevent upper airway occlusion at the level of the soft palate.[43] The American Sleep Disorders Association recommends that oral appliances may be used in patients with primary snoring, mild OSA, or in those with moderate to severe OSA who refuse or are intolerant of nasal CPAP. The U.S. Food and Drug Administration has granted market clearance for 32 oral appliances for snoring but only 14 of these have received market clearance for

TABLE 64-1.   Food and Drug Administration Approved Oral Appliances for the Treatment of Obstructive Sleep Apnea

Appliances	Manufacturer
Adjustable PM Positioner	Jonathan A. Parker, DDS
Elastic Mandibular Advancement, Triation (EMA-T)	Frantz Design, Inc.
Elastic Mandibular Advancement	Frantz Design, Inc.
Elastomeric Sleep Appliance	Village Park Orthodontics
Equalizer Airway Device	Sleep Renewal Inc.
Herbst	Orthodontics, SUNY at Buffalo
Klearway	Great Lakes Orthodontics, Ltd.
NAPA	Great Lakes Orthodontics, Ltd.
OSAP	Snorefree, Inc.
PM Positioner	Jonathan A. Parker, DDS
Silencer	Silent Knights Ventures, Inc.
Sleep-In Bone Screw System	Influence Inc.
SNOAR Open Airway Appliance	Kent J. Toone, DDS
Thornton Oral Appliance	W. Keith Thornton, DDS

treatment of snoring and OSA (Table 64-1).[44] Common side effects of oral appliance therapy include excessive salivation, xerostomia, soft tissue irritations, transient discomfort of the teeth and temporomandibular joint (TMJ), and temporary minor occlusal changes. Uncommon, more serious complications include permanent occlusal changes and significant TMJ discomfort.

Removable anterior repositioning splints have been used somewhat successfully to temporarily advance the mandible while passively bringing the tongue forward with it.[44–46] The optimal amount of forward movement is between 50% and 75% of the patient's maximum protrusive distance. An important design feature of these devices is that the appliance must maintain the mandible in the forward position while the patient is asleep. Bear and Priest[47] used a mandibular anterior repositioning splint to determine whether surgical advancement of the mandible would have any lasting and positive effect on a patient's OSA.

A tongue-retaining device (TRD) that pulls the tongue forward without moving the mandible forward has also been used successfully in some patients with mild to moderate OSA.[48,49] The TRD functions by placing the tongue into a cup or bubble positioned between the anterior teeth. Surface adhesion holds the tongue in place and the appliance requires that the patient's jaw remains partially open. One disadvantage of the TRD is that the tongue is not always held forward because surface tension of the tongue in the bubble is lost after a time. The TRD and mandibular anterior repositioning splints both force nasal breathing, which can be difficult for patients with inadequate nasal airways.

Arguably, the most researched oral appliance is the Klearway titratable appliance developed by Alan Lowe, DMD, PhD, at the University of British Columbia, Canada. It features a maxillary and mandibular component connected with an adjustable screw mechanism (Figure 64-3). The components are made of a thermoactive acrylic resin that is slightly soft at body temperatures and very compliant at high temperatures. This property decreases major tooth discomfort and considerably increases retention in those patients who have lost a significant number of teeth. A unique feature of the Klearway appliance is that it permits both lateral (1–3 mm) and vertical (1–5 mm) jaw movement during sleep, which reduces the risk of TMJ and jaw muscle discomfort. This movement also facilitates oral breathing in patients with nasal airway obstruction. The screw mechanism of the appliance allows for an 11-mm anterior movement of the mandible with a total of 44 incremental steps of 0.25 mm. In a study of 38 patients with moderate to severe OSA by Lowe and coworkers,[50] the Klearway appliance reduced the RDI to less than 15/hr in 80% of the moderate group and in 61% of the severe group. The Klearway appliance is marketed worldwide by Great Lakes Orthodontic Ltd., Tonawanda, NY).

Another commonly used and effective oral appliance is the Herbst appliance, which is an anterior mandibular positioning device. It consists of two full-coverage clear acrylic components snapped onto the maxillary and mandibular teeth connected with two rod and tube attachments that allow vertical opening, protrusion, limited lateral movement, and no retrusive movement. It is used only at night and advances the mandible 5 to 7 mm or at least 75% of the patient's maximum protrusive distance. A study by Clark and associates[51] on 24 patients with mild to severe OSA using the Herbst appliance showed a significant improvement in the RDI after 4 months of appliance use in 58% of the subjects on the postappliance polysomnogram.

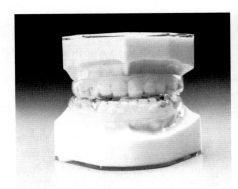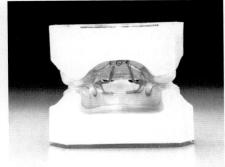

FIGURE 64-3.   Klearway oral appliance.

Another disadvantage of oral appliances is the need to wear them nightly. As with any device, compliance has been shown to be a problem with oral appliances. If appliance therapy is successful, further treatment options may include mandibular advancement surgery to achieve the same forward tongue position on a permanent basis.

Continuous Positive Airway Pressure

CPAP through the nose has been shown to be quite successful in treating a broad range of OSA patients and is at present the most successful nonsurgical treatment.[52–54] The nasal CPAP is administered while the patient is asleep by means of a tight-fitting mask that is connected to a compressor. A CPAP of 7 to 15 cmH$_2$O acts as a pneumatic splint of the upper airway and prevents passive collapse of soft tissues during respiration. Stimulation of mechanoreceptors of the genioglossus muscle leading to increased airway tone has also been suggested as a mechanism of action. Sullivan and colleagues were the first to report the successful treatment of sleep apnea with nasal CPAP in 1981.[55] In most cases, this therapy is effective in eliminating apneas and hypopneas, improving arterial oxygen saturations, reducing or eliminating excessive daytime sleepiness, and eliminating sleep disruption and fragmentation. CPAP may be combined with surgery and weight loss, or it may be used as a sole form of therapy. Although initially recommended for short-term relief of sleep apnea, the use of nasal CPAP for long-term care of patients has increased over the past few years. In recent years, bilevel positive airway pressure (BiPAP) systems that allow independent regulation of inspiratory and expiratory pressures and the newest modification in CPAP systems, auto-CPAP, have been used to more effectively treat OSA and increase tolerance and compliance.[56,57] Auto-CPAP units adjust the CPAP throughout the night rather than delivering one fixed pressure. Optimal CPAP is delivered to the patient adjusting for positional changes, alcohol or sedative effects, sleep-state–dependent changes (REM vs. non-REM), and the effects of upper airway infections or congestion. BiPAP ($2,500) and auto-CPAP ($1,600) systems are more expensive than traditional CPAP ($600–$800) systems.

Despite the uniform success of this therapy, patient compliance remains a problem. Compliance rates at 12 months have been reported as low as 54%.[58] The average nightly use of CPAP is 4.8 hours and the rate of use is usually determined in the first week of use. Overall, approximately one third of patients love CPAP, one third struggle with CPAP but eventually tolerate it, and one third hate CPAP and never use it. Patient dissatisfaction results from nasal dryness and congestion, sore throat, dryness of the skin and eyes, claustrophobia, and the inability to tolerate the noise, discomfort, or mask. Careful patient selection and follow-up are essential if nasal CPAP is selected as a treatment modality.

SURGICAL TREATMENT

Surgery has been the primary form of therapy for OSA. To be successful, the surgical procedure must either bypass the obstructive area or prevent collapse of the soft tissues in the upper airway at the obstruction. Many patients and surgeons tend to view surgical treatment of OSA as a quick and permanent cure. However, a clear definition of what constitutes a cure is lacking in the literature. This problem often makes a determination of the efficacy of individual surgical procedures difficult. Only objective data obtained from a postoperative polysomnogram can be accepted as proof of efficacy for surgical procedures. Currently, the procedures used in the surgical treatment of OSA include tracheostomy, nasal surgery, uvulopalatopharyngoplasty (UPPP), and several orthognathic surgical procedures. Selection of the individual procedure is determined by the severity of the sleep apnea, the presence of a maxillofacial skeletal deficiency, the site of the obstructive segment, and the presence of morbid obesity.

Tracheostomy

Tracheostomy was the first efficacious surgical procedure for treating OSA, performed by Kuhlo and coworkers in 1969.[59] It is almost 100% curative in relieving the signs and symptoms of OSA because it bypasses all the potential obstructive sites in the upper airway. After tracheostomy, there is a rapid and striking reduction in daytime somnolence and a marked improvement in sleep architecture owing to a major reduction in the frequency of arousals. Sinus dysrhythmias, bradycardia, pulmonary hypertension, hypoxemia, and apnea all improve dramatically with the procedure. Tracheostomy clearly is an effective surgical treatment for patients with OSA.

The disadvantages of a permanent tracheostomy can have a devastating effect on sleep apnea patients. Almost all patients experience psychological depression from the social and medical problems associated with a lifelong tracheostomy. The tracheostomy leaves the patient aesthetically disfigured and exposes the patient to common local complications such as bleeding, infection, pain, and granulation tissue formation. Patients are also at increased risk for the more serious complications of tracheal stenosis or erosion into an adjacent blood vessel. Because of these disadvantages and complications, a permanent tracheostomy should be reserved for severe cases of OSA with significant cardiovascular symptoms. Simmons and coworkers[60] have suggested that tracheostomy should be the primary therapy for all patients who spend substantial time in severe oxygen desaturations below 50% and for those who have life-threatening cardiac dysrhythmias during sleep apnea. Tracheostomy may also be used as an interim treatment until adjunctive procedures to reconstruct the upper airway are completed.

Nasal Surgery

Significant obstruction in the nasal cavity has been shown to cause excessive daytime sleepiness, sleep fragmentation, hypopneas, and periodic breathing during sleep.[61] In most patients with moderate to severe OSA, nasal obstruction is not the major contributing factor. The obstruction may be due to a deviated nasal septum, nasal polyps, or enlargement of the turbinates. In these patients, septoplasty, nasal polypectomy, or turbinectomies are usually helpful only as adjunctive surgical procedures in the treatment of OSA. Unless the obstruction in the nasal cavity is severe, surgical correction usually will not yield any significant improvement on a repeat polysomnography.

Uvulopalatopharyngoplasty

The oropharynx and soft palate can cause significant airway obstruction during sleep. At least 10% of persons older than 40 years snore regularly and significantly. Loud and intermittent snoring is found in almost all patients with OSA. In many cases, habitual snoring is present for many years before sleep apnea is diagnosed. Ikematsu[62] followed a large number of habitual snorers over several years and found that 91% of these patients had decreased oropharyngeal dimensions and longer soft palates and uvulas than normal subjects. He was able to eliminate their snoring by surgically excising the excessive soft tissue in the palatal folds and partially excising the uvula.

With minor modifications, Simmons and coworkers[60] and Fujita and associates[63] popularized the UPPP for the treatment of OSA. The procedure was designed to eliminate oropharyngeal obstruction by performing a tonsillectomy and adenoidectomy, excising the uvula, removing redundant lateral pharyngeal wall mucosa, and resecting 8 to 15 mm along the posterior margin of the soft palate.

The surgical technique of UPPP varies to some degree by patient and surgeon, but the basic goal is to shorten the palate and widen the PAS (Figure 64-4). A mucosal incision is created with electocautery on the anterior surface of the soft palate. The dissection is frequently carried laterally to include the palatine tonsil. The tonsillar bed is coagulated and hemostasis achieved. Palatal muscle is excised and mucosa from the nasopharynx is pulled forward for primary closure. Multiple interrupted resorbable sutures are placed. If the tonsil is removed, the mucosa of the anterior fauces pillar is closed to the posterior fauces pillar. This attempt to remove redundant pharyngeal tissue and stretch or tighten the posterior pharyngeal wall results in constriction. In addition, frequently by shortening the soft palate, the width of the soft palate is thickened, as demonstrated cephalometrically. Lymphoid tissue from the tonsillar fossa can be removed separately or in conjunction with the uvula (Figure 64-5). The amount of velum to be excised is determined by the location of palatal competence and closure of the nasopharynx. These can be estimated or identified during nasopharyngoscopy. Palatal incompetence can occur but usually is of minimal concern if the patient swallows carefully. Pain with swallowing usually lasts for several weeks.

UPPP results in symptomatic improvement in the patient and eliminates habitual snoring in almost all cases. However, reports show that significant objective improvement on the postoperative polysomnogram ranges only from 41% to 66%.[58,60,64,65] This procedure only eliminates the obstruction at the level of the soft palate and does not address

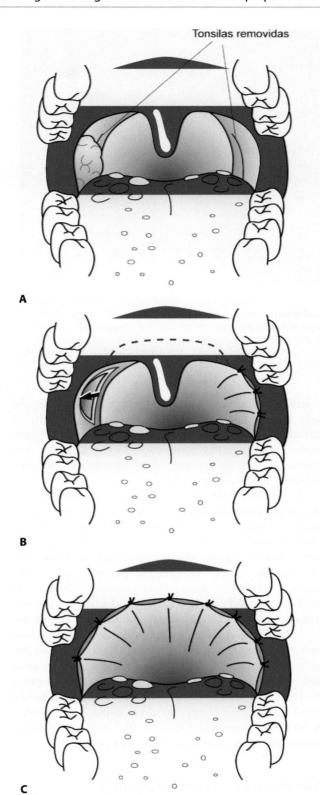

FIGURE 64-4.   **A–C,** Uvulopalatopharyngoplasty. Tonsils and uvula are removed and the anterior pillar is closed to the posterior pillar. (Adapted from Tiner BD, Waite PD. Surgical and nonsurgical management of obstructive sleep apnea. In Peterson LJ, Indresano AT, Marciani RD, Roser SM, editors. Principles of Oral and Maxillofacial Surgery. Vol 3. Philadelphia: JB Lippincott; 1992; p. 1540.)

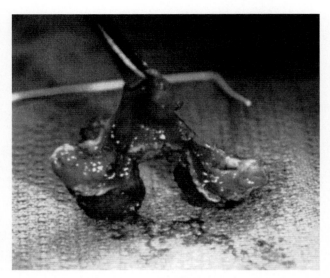

FIGURE 64-5. Surgical specimen of tonsils and uvula. (Reproduced with permission from Tiner BD, Waite PD. Surgical and nonsurgical management of obstructive sleep apnea. In Peterson LJ, Indresano AT, Marciani RD, Roser SM, editors. Principles of Oral and Maxillofacial Surgery. Vol 3. Philadelphia: JB Lippincott; 1992; p. 1541.)

obstructions occurring in the hypopharyngeal and base of tongue areas. Many patients have more than one site of obstruction. If UPPP is performed when the presurgical evaluation demonstrates obstruction localized to the soft palate–tonsil area, the success rate of the surgical procedure approaches 90% treating OSA.[23,26]

Complications from UPPP are related to changes in palatal function. Permanent velopharyngeal incompetence occurs in approximately 5% of patients and is more common during the first 2 months postoperatively. Patients experience occasional reflux of liquids into the nose and mild nasal air escape during speech. However, hypernasal speech and changes in the quality of the patient's speech are usually not seen. Simmons and colleagues[64] reported a 5% to 10% rate of minor wound infections that resolved with antibiotics. Palatal stenosis is definitely a risk with this operation and occurs in approximately 1% of patients. It occurs more frequently with excessive resections of the posterior tonsillar pillars and injudicious use of electrocautery. Postoperative pain after UPPP is significant, and narcotic analgesia should be used with caution to prevent sedation-induced exacerbation of OSA. Postsurgical deaths have resulted from the combination of pharyngeal edema and narcotic use.

Laser-Assisted Uvulopalatoplasty

In the late 1980s, Dr. Yves-Victor Kamami (Paris, France) designed a procedure to reshape and recontour the soft palate under local anesthesia with a CO_2 laser to treat snoring and selected patients with OSA syndrome.[66] He originally named the procedure "laser resection of the palatopharynx" (LRPP). Initially, the procedure was accomplished in four or five ses-

sions spaced at monthly intervals. Over time, the procedure evolved into a one-stage technique for most patients. It consisted of two paramedian vertical incisions placed lateral to the uvula extending up toward the junction of the hard and soft palates for 2 to 3 cm. A second horizontal incision was placed just under the roof of the uvula, leaving a small uvula to prevent centripetal scar formation. Over a 5-year period, Kamami[66] treated 63 OSA patients with this technique. The RDI was reduced by more than 50% in 55 patients that were classified as successful responders. The RDI improved from 41.5 to 16.9 for the average responder, and for the entire group, the average RDI improved from 41.3 to 20.3.

In the early 1990s in the United States, Dr. Yosef Krespi modified the procedure and renamed it "laser-assisted uvulopalatoplasty" (LAUP). He initially used the procedure to treat loud habitual snoring. In a study of 280 patients treated in the office under local anesthesia, 84% were cured with an average of 2.7 sessions.[67] Overall results for OSA patients treated with LAUP are far less encouraging, with an average successful surgical response of 52.2%.[68] Based on these findings, the current main indications for LAUP include loud habitual snoring, upper airway resistance syndrome, and mild OSA (apnea index < 20). All snoring patients who elect to undergo LAUP should be evaluated for OSA preoperatively and again postoperatively if OSA was previously diagnosed. If not, then the patient and surgeon may be lulled into a false sense of security by eliminating the snoring without eliminating the undiagnosed OSA, potentially increasing patient morbidity and mortality.[69]

The most common complication after LAUP is a moderate to severe sore throat. Patients experience pain 8 to 10 days after surgery and reach their peak pain intensity on the fourth or fifth postoperative day. Pain control is achieved with oral analgesics and anesthetic gels. The risk for velopharyngeal insufficiency is low because the procedure is frequently done in stages and the surgeon has the opportunity to evaluate speech and soft palate function after each session. Patients are also at low risk for bleeding and infection. The great majority of patients can eat, drink, and speak almost immediately and can resume full activities the following day.

Orthognathic Surgery Procedures

Various orthognathic surgical procedures have been described for the treatment of OSA. The majority of patients have airway obstruction at the level of the soft palate and at the base of the tongue (type II obstruction). Orthognathic surgical procedures can change the size of the airway in several regions. Mandibular advancement and genial advancement probably work by changing the position of the mandible and hyoid bone with subsequent effects on the genioglossus and hyoglossus muscles. OSA patients with identifiable craniofacial anomalies can clearly benefit from a variety of these procedures.

Mandibular Advancement

Total mandibular advancement was the first orthognathic surgical procedure used in the treatment of OSA. Kuo and colleagues in 1979[70] and Bear and Priest in 1980[47] reported complete reversal of sleep apnea symptoms in patients with horizontal mandibular deficiency treated by mandibular advancement. More recently, Alvarez and coworkers[71] reported the successful treatment of an edentulous patient with sleep apnea by mandibular and genial advancement.

A bilateral sagittal ramus osteotomy is usually the procedure of choice for total mandibular advancement. The amount of advancement is determined preoperatively from the orthognathic surgery database. Adjunctive orthodontic treatment is frequently necessary to obtain the desired occlusion and to eliminate dental compensations that would otherwise limit the amount of advancement. After advancement with the standard surgical technique, the fragments are rigidly fixed with screws or bone plates. For large advancements of 7 mm or more, long-term stability is enhanced with a 5- to 7-day course of maxillomandibular fixation and skeletal suspension wires. In advancements of 6 mm or less, maxillomandibular fixation is usually not necessary.

The exact reason for how mandibular advancement improves OSA is not clearly known, but the suspected effect is the pulling of the tongue forward off the pharyngeal wall. This effect is created by anteriorly moving the insertion of the genioglossus and geniohyoid muscles. If this were the only factor, anterior chin procedures would be equally effective as total mandibular procedures. Variations of geniotomies have been designed to maximally pull the tongue muscles forward.

Genial Advancement

A rectangular osteotomy apical to the teeth but maintaining the inferior border of the mandible allows the genial tubercles with their muscular attachments to be maximally advanced with minimal cosmetic change (Figure 64-6). A modified vestibular mucosal incision is made in the anterior mandible. Periosteum is reflected down to the inferior border. An oscillating saw is used to make parallel horizontal cuts that include the genial tubercle. The osteotomy is designed in a shape similar to a drawer so that it can be pulled outward with the genial muscles. The bone must be broad enough cuspid tocuspid to be rotated 90 degrees and set on top of the buccal cortex. The outer cortical and cancellous bone of the rectangle can then be removed and the inner cortex rigidly fixed with bone screws. Any hemorrhage from the cancellous bone should be controlled.

This procedure does not change the aesthetic chin or advance the anterior belly of the digastric muscle, which may be helpful in suspending the hyoid. In contrast to this procedure, a horizontal sliding geniotomy does advance the genial tubercles and the anterior belly of the digastric muscle.

Genial Advancement with Hyoid Myotomy and Suspension

In 1984, Riley and associates[72] described an alternative technique in which an inferior mandibular osteotomy and an associated hyoid myotomy and suspension were used in the

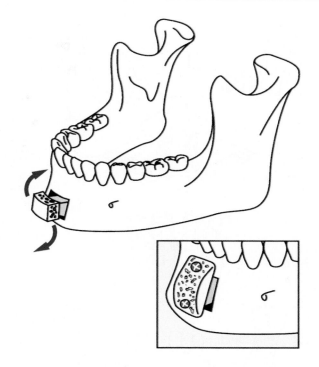

FIGURE 64-6. Genial tubercle advancement. The outer table of the symphysis is removed and the inner table is secured with 2-mm screws. (Adapted from Tiner BD, Waite PD. Surgical and nonsurgical management of obstructive sleep apnea. In Peterson LJ, Indresano AT, Marciani RD, Roser SM, editors. Principles of Oral and Maxillofacial Surgery. Vol 3. Philadelphia: JB Lippincott; 1992; p. 1542.)

treatment of OSA (Figure 64-7). This technique is similar to a horizontal mandibular osteotomy, which is commonly used for advancement genioplasty. The osteotomy is designed to include the genial tubercle on the inner cortex of the anterior mandible where the genioglossus muscle attaches. Repositioning the anteroinferior segment of the mandible forward with the attached genioglossus muscle theoretically pulls the tongue forward and improves the hypopharyngeal airway. In conjunction with the osteotomy, the body and greater cornu of the hyoid are isolated through a submental incision. The infrahyoid muscles are transected, taking care to remain on the hyoid bone at all times to avoid injury to the superior laryngeal nerves (see Figure 64-7A). This allows the hyoid bone to be pulled anteriorly and superiorly. Strips of fascia or nonresorbable suture are passed around the body of the hyoid and attached to the intact portion of the anterior mandible to complete the hyoid suspension.

In 1989, Riley and colleagues[73] published a review of 55 patients with OSA who were treated with inferior mandibular osteotomy and hyoid suspension. Forty-two patients had obstruction at both the oropharynx and the hypopharynx and received concomitant UPPP and inferior mandibular osteotomy with hyoid myotomy and suspension. The remaining 6 patients were determined to have obstruction localized to the base of the tongue and underwent the osteotomy and hyoid suspension only. All patients were reevaluated by polysom-

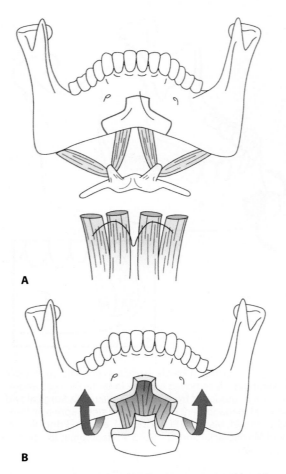

FIGURE 64-7.　Inferior mandibular osteotomy and hyoid myotomy. **A,** Omohyoid, sternohyoid, and thyrohyoid muscles released (see Figure 64-8 for more detail on muscular relationships). **B,** Inferior segment is advanced anteriorly and locked on the anterior mandible. (**A** and **B,** Adapted from Tiner BD, Waite PD. Surgical and nonsurgical management of obstructive sleep apnea. In Peterson LJ, Indresano AT, Marciani RD, Roser SM, editors. Principles of Oral and Maxillofacial Surgery. Vol 3. Philadelphia: JB Lippincott; 1992; p. 1543.)

nography 6 months after surgery. Thirty-seven patients (67%) were considered to be responders to surgery based on the polysomnogram results. Genioglossus advancement ranged from 8 to 18 mm with a mean of 13 mm. All responders to surgery showed significant improvement in their RDI and oxygen desaturation events. Eighteen patients (33%) were considered nonresponders and failed to show significant improvement by polysomnography. The presence of preexisting chronic obstructive pulmonary disease (COPD) was found to be a determining factor in increasing the risk of failure.

In 1994, Riley and colleagues[74] reported on a new modified technique for hyoid suspension that fixed the hyoid to the thyroid cartilage instead of the anterior margin of the mandible. When this modified technique was performed with inferior mandibular osteotomy, in lieu of the original hyoid suspension technique, the surgical response rate (with or without UPPP) was raised to 79.2%. The 5 nonresponders in this study of 24 patients achieved postoperative RDI values close to levels at which they would have been considered surgical responders.

Long-term follow-up of these patients has shown that the indication for this procedure is limited. Patients with normal pulmonary function, normal skeletal mandibular development, the absence of obesity, and moderate OSA are candidates for treatment with inferior mandibular osteotomy with hyoid myotomy and suspension.

The most serious reported complication from a hyoid suspension has been severe aspiration in one patient, in which the thyrohyoid membrane was totally sectioned.[28] Other complications have included wound infections, transient sensory disturbances of the mental nerve, and mandibular fracture. An advantage to hyoid suspension is that it circumvents the need for maxillomandibular fixation and does not affect the occlusion.

Maxillomandibular Advancement

Combined advancement of the maxilla and mandible with or without hyoid suspension is the most recent and efficacious surgical procedure for the treatment of OSA. The surgical technique includes a standard Le Fort I osteotomy in combination with a mandibular sagittal split osteotomy for advancement of the maxilla and mandible. A concomitant inferior mandibular osteotomy with or without hyoid myotomy and suspension, as previously described, is also performed. This surgery may result in a significant facial change, which is most often favorable (Figures 64-8 and 64-9). Several authors have described the use of MMA in treating large series of OSA patients.[75-80] In a series of 23 patients, Waite and coworkers[75] performed a high sliding horizontal geniotomy without the hyoid myotomy and suspension. All patients were reevaluated by polysomnography at 6 weeks postoperatively. The surgical success with MMA was 65% based on a postsurgical RDI of less than 10. Riley and associates[76] reported the largest series of OSA patients treated with MMA in which 98% (89 of 91) were successfully treated based on a postoperative RDI of less than 20 with at least a 50% reduction in the RDI compared with the preoperative study. It should be noted that 67 of the 91 patients (74%) did not receive phase 1 therapy based on their two-phase protocol for reconstruction of the upper airway. Despite this, the MMA was labeled a phase 2 procedure. In 1997, Hochban and colleagues[77] reported a 98% success rate on 38 OSA patients consecutively treated with a 10-mm MMA as the primary surgery, without any adjunctive procedures. Their criteria for success were based on the more rigid postoperative RDI of less than 10. Patient selection for MMA was based on subjective symptoms of excessive daytime sleepiness, an RDI of greater than 20, and specific craniofacial characteristics determined cephalometrically Only 2 patients who were morbidly obese were treated surgically. Based on their excellent results, the authors concluded that a stepwise algorithm of staged surgical procedures was not justified. In

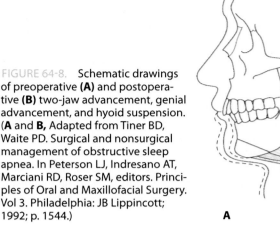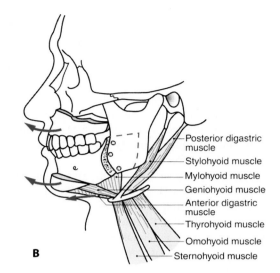

FIGURE 64-8.   Schematic drawings of preoperative **(A)** and postoperative **(B)** two-jaw advancement, genial advancement, and hyoid suspension. (**A** and **B,** Adapted from Tiner BD, Waite PD. Surgical and nonsurgical management of obstructive sleep apnea. In Peterson LJ, Indresano AT, Marciani RD, Roser SM, editors. Principles of Oral and Maxillofacial Surgery. Vol 3. Philadelphia: JB Lippincott; 1992; p. 1544.)

Posterior digastric muscle
Stylohyoid muscle
Mylohyoid muscle
Geniohyoid muscle
Anterior digastric muscle
Thyrohyoid muscle
Omohyoid muscle
Sternohyoid muscle

a series of 50 OSA patients consecutively treated with MMA, Prinsell[78] reported a 100% success rate based on a postoperative RDI of less than 15, an apnea index (AI) of less than 5, or a reduction in the RDI and AI of greater than 60%. In this series, occasional concomitant nonpharyngeal procedures and an anterior interior mandibular osteotomy were accomplished with the MMA as a single-stage operation. In 1999, Lee and coworkers[79] proposed a three-stage protocol for the surgical treatment of OSA patients. All 35 patients in their series had type II obstruction with collapse at the oropharyngeal and hypopharyngeal areas. Stage 1 reconstruction consisted of a UPPP and inferior sagittal osteotomy with genioglossus muscle advancement, or an anterior mandibular osteotomy. If stage 1 was unsuccessful, patients advanced to stage 2, which consisted of MMA with rigid fixation. A hyoid myotomy and suspension was the sole component of stage 3 reconstruction. Based on postoperative polysomnography, 69% (24 of 35) were considered surgical respondents based on an RDI of less than 20. Of the 11 stage 1 failures, 3 elected to proceed to stage 2 reconstruction with MMA. All patients who underwent MMA had a postoperative RDI of less than 10, indicating a 100% response rate. No patient

required stage 3 reconstruction. Bettega and associates[80] treated 51 consecutive OSA patients according to the Stanford two-step surgical procedure. Forty-four patients had phase 1 surgery with a success rate of 22.7% (10 of 44). Twenty patients underwent MMA as part of phase 2 in the protocol. Of these, 75% (15 of 20) were considered to be surgical responders based on a postoperative RDI of less than 15 and at least a 50% reduction in the RDI. Of the 5 failures, 3 had postoperative RDIs of less than 20.

The PAS consistently increases with MMA. However, there is no direct relationship between the gain in PAS and the remission of sleep apnea. MMA is effective for patients who have obstruction at the base of the tongue. This surgical treatment is the most efficacious procedure for expanding the pharyngeal airway and improving or eliminating OSA. It remains the best current alternative to tracheostomy.[81] Indications for this procedure include severe mandibular deficiency (SNB < 74 degrees), morbid obesity, severe OSA (RDI > 50, oxygen desaturations < 70%), hypopharyngeal narrowing, and failure of other forms of treatment.[82] The success rate of MMA appears to increase when adjunctive procedures such as UPPP, partial glossectomy, septoplasty, or turbinectomies are

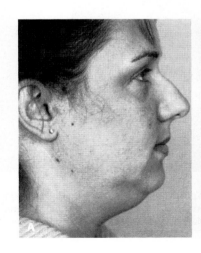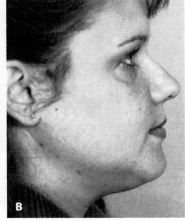

FIGURE 64-9.   Preoperative **(A)** and postoperative **(B)** photographs of a patient with obstructive sleep apnea syndrome who underwent two-jaw surgery with a genial advancement. (**A** and **B,** Reproduced with permission from Tiner BD, Waite PD. Surgical and nonsurgical management of obstructive sleep apnea. In Peterson LJ, Indresano AT, Marciani RD, Roser SM, editors. Principles of Oral and Maxillofacial Surgery. Vol 3. Philadelphia: JB Lippincott; 1992; p. 1545.)

included in the treatment plan. This lends support to the theory that most OSA patients have multiple levels of obstruction.

Adjunctive orthodontic therapy is usually indicated in patients selected for MMA. Presurgical orthodontics improves the postoperative occlusion and eliminates pre-existing dental compensations that would otherwise limit the amount of advancement. Maximum advancement of the facial skeleton and maintenance of a functional occlusion and acceptable aesthetics are the goals of surgical-orthodontic correction.

The osteotomies are rigidly fixed with miniplates and bicortical screws (Figure 64-10). With large advancements (>7 mm), skeleton suspension wires and a short course of maxillomandibular fixation (1 wk) can be used to reduce surgical relapse. Potential complications of MMA include surgical relapse, nonunion, bleeding, malocclusion, infection, unfavorable changes in facial appearance, and permanent or temporary sensory disturbances of the inferior alveolar and infraorbital nerves.

The long-term skeletal stability of MMA has been shown to be quite good. Louis and colleagues[83] showed a mean relapse of 0.9 ±1.8 mm among 20 maxillary advancement patients who underwent MMA for OSA. The mean follow-up period was 18.5 months (range 6–29 mo). When the patients were divided into three groups reflecting small (≤6 mm), medium (7–9 mm), and large (≥10 mm) advancements, there was no statistical difference in the measured relapse among the groups. Rigid fixation was achieved with four miniplates and no bone grafts were used in any of the maxillary advancements. Nimkarn and coworkers[84] reported on 19 OSA patients who underwent MMA with simultaneous genioplasty and found relatively stable long-term (>12 mo) surgical stability of the maxilla and mandible. Maxillary and mandibular advancement was stable over the long term in both the vertical and the horizontal planes. With the exception of gonion in the vertical plane, there was no statistically significant correlation between the amount of surgical advancement and the amount of postsurgical instability.

Mandibular Setbacks

In a small number of patients, a mandibular setback procedure can be the initiating factor in the development of OSA. Riley and associates[85] reported on two women who developed OSA syndrome after mandibular osteotomies for correction of class III malocclusion and skeletal prognathism. Neither patient had any symptoms of sleep apnea before surgery. Postoperatively, both patients began to snore loudly. Evaluation by polysomnography confirmed the presence of OSA syndrome. A comparative examination of the preoperative and postoperative lateral cephalograms of each patient showed a more inferiorly positioned hyoid bone and a narrowing of the pharyngeal airway as a result of the mandibular setback procedure.

In an attempt to identify those patients potentially at risk for OSA, all patients who are planned for mandibular setback procedures should be questioned preoperatively and postoperatively about the presence or absence of snoring, excessive daytime sleepiness, or observed apneas during sleep. Although the vast majority of patients who undergo mandibular setbacks are able to adapt to the changes in the skeletal and muscular apparatus, a subset of patients may be at risk for developing overt signs of OSA after mandibular setbacks.

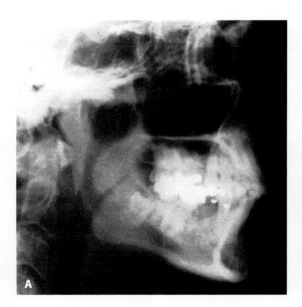 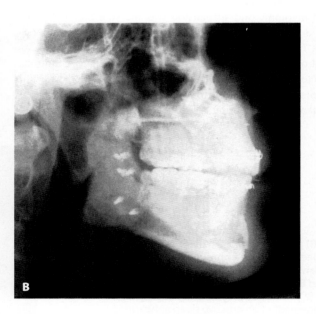

FIGURE 64-10.   Preoperative (**A**) and postoperative (**B**) radiographs of a two-jaw surgery and genial tubercle advancement for sleep apnea. (**A** and **B,** Reproduced with permission from Tiner BD, Waite PD. Surgical and nonsurgical management of obstructive sleep apnea. In Peterson LJ, Indresano AT, Marciani RD, Roser SM, editors. Principles of Oral and Maxillofacial Surgery. Vol 3. Philadelphia: JB Lippincott; 1992; p. 1546.)

COMPLICATIONS

Surgical complications in treatment of OSA may be severe and different from those related to routine orthognathic surgery. Sleep apnea patients are often older and more obese and, by the nature of their disease, have difficult airways. Obesity is a known co-morbidity associated with multiple medical issues such as hypertension, diabetes, heart disease, pulmonary dysfunction, poor intravenous access, and difficult airway management.

Respiratory failure is the major complication of airway surgery. Respiratory obstruction is a common cause of death in sleep apnea, especially after UPPP. Anesthesia protocols exist for management of the sleep apnea patient owing to physical characteristics such as obesity, short neck, small jaw, large tongue, difficult laryngoscopy, and poor mask ventilation. Jet ventilation and fiberoptic intubation are valuable techniques.[86]

Obesity, hypertension, COPD, myocardial infarction, and stroke are more common in the patient with OSA.[87] The surgeon should anticipate these medical problems and be prepared to manage appropriately. Standard intravenous access and central lines are much more difficult to obtain in the obese patient. Large obese surgical patients are more difficult owing to intraoral access, and obesity is often associated with increased infection and poor healing. Hypotensive anesthesia may be contraindicated and postoperative blood pressure management more complicated in the presence of pain control. Renal perfusion is often reduced in this group and antihypertensive medication will complicate fluid management. Older patients with hypertension and poor cardiac function need closer management of fluid status than the routine healthy orthognathic patient. People with COPD and low baseline oxygen saturations may desaturate quickly if oversedated postoperatively, and poor oxygen saturation may contribute to poor healing, dehiscence, and bone nonunion. Coronary artery disease especially stents, arrhythmias and strokes is often treated with anticoagulation or antiplatelet therapy. Extensive upper airway surgery such as MMA or tongue base or palate surgery is at a great risk for hemorrhage.

Patient positioning on the operating room table for large obese patient is clearly a challenge. Many sleep apnea patients just do not fit the average operating room table and careful positioning with padded support must be provided. Aggressive arm slings that wrap the shoulder upward often produce chronic pain and postoperative musculoskeletal pain.

Deep venous thrombosis has a higher association with extended surgery time, abdominal girth, and obesity. Sequential compression devices should be used on all OSA patients and maintained until adequate ambulation.[88,89] Antiplatelet therapy or low-dose heparin is not recommended owing to the continued bleeding in the maxilla, sinus, and nasal area. Soft tissue ecchymosis may create airway obstruction.

Malocclusion and inferior alveolar nerve paresthesia are the two most common postoperative complaints. MMA surgery is much different than orthognathic surgery because the intention is to maintain the same occlusion but move both the upper and the lower dentition forward, thereby increasing the upper airway space. Large skeletal changes are often necessary to open the airway but also pose greater challenges in maintaining the intricate relationship of intercuspation. Even a small percentage of relapse in a large advancement will result in a nonfunctional malocclusion. Patients with presurgical abnormal occlusion but good dentition should be considered for presurgical orthodontics. Patients must know in advance the risk of malocclusion and realize orthodontics is not considered medically necessary. Because the magnitude of skeletal change is greater than with orthognathic surgery, the skeletal fixation techniques must be modified.

Paresthesia may be more problematic in this patient subset owing to the greater skeletal change and the age distribution. Older age groups typically do not adjust to nerve injury as well as younger patients. Most nerve injuries improve slowly with time, but low-dose medical therapy with clonazapam, amitriptyline, or gabapentin can be very beneficial. Microneurosurgery in this patient group is unknown. Even complaints of paresthesia in the maxilla are reported that may be due to larger Le Fort advancements causing delayed infraorbital re-innervation and/or larger defects in the lateral wall of the sinus associated with chronic sinusitis. Most patients will tolerate mild paresthesia for the benefit of better breathing.

Typical patients that present for MMA are middle aged and, therefore, often have unique dental considerations, such as periodontal disease, missing teeth, impacted teeth, implants, and special prosthodontic factors. These factors may prevent presurgical orthodontics but also complicate treatment. Dental implants and extensive bridges do not behave like independent teeth with physiologic movement (Figure 64-11). Sometimes, malocclusion can be corrected by equilibration, new restorations, or even simple

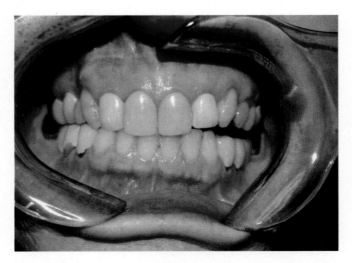

FIGURE 64-11. Postoperative malocclusion of the posterior dentition due to a deep curve of Spee and an extensive prosthetic bridge.

extractions. Periodontal disease, bone loss, and calculus can often be the cause of surgical wound infections. The geniotomy incision is the most likely to dehisce and become infected, perhaps owing to age-related periodontal factors.

Skeletal relapse is a common problem in all surgery, but in orthognathic surgery, this is often corrected by the orthodontist. Up to 20% relapse is reported in orthognathic surgery, which would be only 1 mm if the skeletal change was 5 mm. But in MMA surgery, the skeletal change is often 10 mm and a 20% relapse would be 2 mm, which may be beyond the envelope of treatment in orthodontics or equilibration. Larger skeletal changes imply larger bone gaps and less bone contact. Larger bone gaps also imply longer bone plates with greater flexibility. Therefore, the surgeon must use techniques that reduce relapse such as bone grafting and reinforced plating materials.

Hardware failure and plate fracture are not uncommon in skeletal surgery (Figure 64-12). Routine fixation systems are not designed for MMA surgery, and thin flexible plates used in larger bone defects will bend and flex, ultimately leading to stress fractures. This can be worsened by the surgeon bending and work-hardening the plate to fit an osteotomy gap. Large maxillary advancements anatomically do not have good bone apposition, and chronic movement with mastication will cause delayed healing, nonunion, or stress fracture of the plating system. Prebent OSA plates are stronger in the gap area and control the amount of advancement. Prebent OSA plates do not require the surgeon to bend the plate to fit the osteotomy step and are, therefore, stronger. Bone grafting the lateral wall of the maxilla is advisable owing to the limited bone contact and prevention of soft tissue ingrowth. This will improve stability, increase healing, and reduce relapse.[90]

Mandibular fixation of the sagittal split osteotomy can be done in several different ways. Bicortical position screws are probably the strongest, but when they fail, the entire construct is lost. Bicortical screws may compress the inferior alveolar nerve, and if rotation of the segments occurs, there

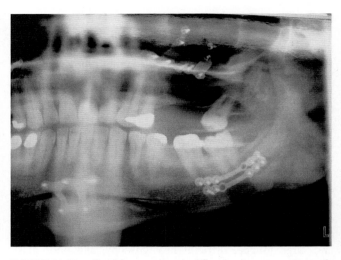

FIGURE 64-13. Double monocortical fixation increases strength in large advancements.

will be poor adaptation of the proximal and distal segments. Monocortical plates are perhaps kinder to the TMJ and nerve but more flexible. Stronger, stiffer alloys are available that improve the flexibility of the plate. Mandibular fixation in OSA patients usually requires a modification because the advancement is greater, there is less bone apposition, and the patients are stronger and larger. Double monocortical plate per side or superior bicortical position screws with a monocortical plate will increase the engineering support (Figures 64-13 and 64-14). Fixation of the osteotomy is ultimately the surgeon's choice based on multiple factors.

SUMMARY

Because the OSA syndrome is a complex disorder, the type of treatment selected should be tailored to the individual patient based on the relative risks and benefits of the therapy and the

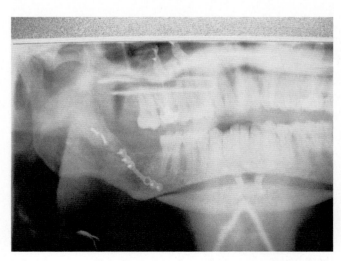

FIGURE 64-12. Plate fracture in the early postoperative period.

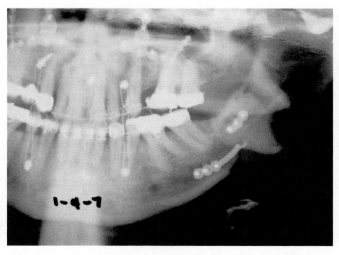

FIGURE 64-14. Combination of both monocortical and bicortical fixation screws.

TABLE 64-2. **Results of Maxillomandibular Advancement for Obstructive Sleep Apnea*****

Results	RDI	Desaturation[†]	Patients (N)	Percent of Total
Excellent	≤10	0	20	28.2
Good	≤10	≤20	26	36.6
Satisfactory	≤10	>20	15	21.1
Poor	>20	>20	10	14.1

RDI = respiratory disturbance index.
*Maxillomandibular advancement surgery results for 71 obstructive sleep apnea syndrome patients classified by polysomnography.
[†]Number of oxygen desaturations < 90%.

severity of the disease. Although a subset of the patients who present with OSA has an identifiable craniofacial anomaly, care must be used in choosing a simple mechanistic therapy. The success of the chosen therapy should be evaluated both subjectively and objectively. There is no clear agreement on what constitutes a cure of sleep apnea. Most authors use the RDI in assessing severity of disease and success of treatment. However, all agree that the potentially significant physiologic consequences that can be life-threatening result from hypoxemia. In some cases, patients after treatment have no oxygen desaturations below 90%, but in terms of RDI, they are considered not cured and are deemed treatment failures.

A more reasonable approach would be to define the concept of success in terms of "excellent," "good" "fair," and "poor" and to avoid using the term "cured" in assessing treatment outcomes. These terms could be quantitatively approached assigning lowest oxygen desaturation and RDI parameters to each one. In Table 64-2, the results of 71 patients treated by MMA are assessed by these criteria. In managing patients with severe sleep apnea, a "cure" is seldom achieved with a single surgical or medical treatment (tracheostomies excluded). However, MMA may significantly improve a patient to the point that nonsurgical therapies are more efficacious, if needed at all.

References

1. Schmidt HS. Disorders of sleep and arousal. In Gregory I, Smeltzer DJ, editors. Psychiatry Essentials of Clinical Practice. Boston: Little, Brown; 1983; p. 343.
2. Association of Sleep Disorders Center. Diagnostic classification of sleep and arousal disorders. 1st ed. Prepared by the Sleep Disorders Classification Committee. Sleep 1979;2:1.
3. Berger H. Uber das elektrenkephalogramm des menschen. Arch Psychiatr Nervenkr 1929;87:527.
4. Loomis AL, Harvey EN, Hobart GA. Potential rhythms of the cerebral cortex during sleep. Science 1935;81:597.
5. Loomis AL, Harvey EN, Hobart GA. Further observations on the potential rhythms of the cerebral cortex during sleep. Science 1935;82:199.
6. Aserinsky E, Kleitman N. Regularly occurring periods of eye motility and concomitant phenomena during sleep. Science 1953;118:273.
7. Freemon FR, editor. Sleep Research: A Critical Review. Springfield, IL: Charles C. Thomas; 1972.
8. Waldhorn RE. Sleep apnea syndrome. Am Fam Physician 1985;32:149.
9. National Commission on Sleep Disorders Research. Wake Up America: A National Sleep Alert. Washington, DC: Government Printing Office; 1993.
10. Sher AE. Treating obstructive sleep apnea syndrome: a complex task [editorial]. West J Med 1995;162:170–172.
11. Bornstein SK. Respiration during sleep: polysomnography. In Guilleminault C, editor. Sleep and Waking Disorders: Indications and Techniques. Menlo Park, CA: Addison-Wesley; 1982; p. 183.
12. Baker TL. Introduction to sleep and sleep disorders. Med Clin North Am 1985;69:1123.
13. Roth B, editor. Narcolepsy and Hypersomnia. Basel: S. Karger AG; 1980.
14. Burwell CS, Rubin ED, Whaley RD, et al. Extreme obesity associated with alveolar hypoventilation: a pickwickian syndrome. Am J Med 1956;21:811.
15. Gastaut H, Tassinari CA, Duron B. Polygraphic study of the episodic diurnal and nocturnal (hypnic and respiratory) manifestations of the pickwick syndrome. Brain Res 1966;2:167.
16. Partinen M, Quera-Salva MA, Jamieson A. Obstructive sleep apnea and cephalometric roentgenograms: the role of anatomic upper airway abnormalities in the definition of abnormal breathing during sleep. Chest 1988;93:1199–1205.
17. Tsuchiya M, Lowe AA, Pae EK, Fleetham JA. Obstructive sleep apnea subtypes by cluster analysis. Am J Orthod Dentofacial Orthop 1992;101:533–542.
18. Bacon WH, Krieger J, Turlot J-C, Stierle JL. Craniofacial characteristics in patients with obstructive sleep apnea syndrome. Cleft Palate J 1988;25:374.
19. Lyberg T, Kogstad O, Ojupesland G. Cephalometric analysis in patients with obstructive sleep apnea syndrome. J Laryngol Otol 1989;103:287.
20. Lowe AA, Santamaria JD, Fleetham JA, Price C. Facial morphology and obstructive sleep apnea. Am J Orthod 1986; 90:484.
21. Rivlin J, Hofstein V, Kalbfleisch J, et al. Upper airway morphology in patients with idiopathic obstructive sleep apnea. Am Rev Respir Dis 1984;129:355.
22. Riley R, Guilleminault C, Herran J, Powell N. Cephalometric analyses and flow-volume loops in obstructive sleep apnea patients. Sleep 1983;6:303.
23. Riley R, Guilleminault C, Powell N, Simmons FB. Palatopharyngoplasty failure, cephalometric roentgenograms, and obstructive sleep apnea. Otolaryngol Head Neck Surg 1985;93:240.
24. Lowe AA, Gionhaku N, Takeuchi K, Fleetham JA. Three-dimensional CT reconstruction of tongue and airway in adult subjects with obstructive sleep apnea. Am J Orthod Dentofacial Orthop 1986;90:364.
25. Haponik EF, Smith PL, Bohlman ME, et al. Computerized tomography in obstructive sleep apnea. Am Rev Respir Dis 1983;127:221.
26. Riley RW, Powell N, Guilleminault C. Current surgical concepts for treating obstructive sleep apnea syndrome. J Oral Maxillofac Surg 1987;45:149.
27. Waite RD, Villos G. Surgical changes of posterior airway spaces in obstructive sleep apnea. Oral Maxillofac Surg Clin North Am 2002;August.
28. Riley RW, Powell NB, Guilleminault C. Maxillary, mandibular, and hyoid advancement for treatment of obstructive sleep apnea: a review of 40 patients. J Oral Maxillofac Surg 1990;48:20.

29. Wiggins RV, Schmidt-Nowara WW. Treatment of the obstructive sleep apnea syndrome. West J Med 1987;147:561.
30. Smith PL, Gold AR, Meyers DA. Weight Loss in mild to moderately obese patients with obstructive sleep apnea. Ann Intern Med 1985;103:850.
31. Riley RW, Powell NB, Guilleminault C, NinoMucia G. Maxillary, mandibular, hyoid advancement: an alternative to tracheostomy in obstructive sleep apnea syndrome. Otolaryngol Head Neck Surg 1986;94:584.
32. Motta J, Guilleminault C. Effects of oxygen administration in sleep-induced apneas. In Guilleminault C, Dement WC, editors. Sleep Apnea Syndrome. New York: Alan R. Liss; 1978; p. 137.
33. Martin RJ, Sanders MH, Gray BA, et al. Acute and long-term ventilatory effects of hyperoxia in the adult sleep apnea syndrome. Am Rev Respir Dis 1982;125:175.
34. Smith PL, Haponik EF, Bleecker ER. The effects of oxygen in patients with sleep apnea. Am Rev Respir Dis 1984;130:958.
35. White DP, Zwillich CW, Pickett CK, et al. Central sleep apnea: improvement with acetazolamide therapy. Arch Intern Med 1982;142:1816.
36. Sharp JT, Druz WS, D'Souza V, et al. Effect of metabolic acidosis upon sleep apnea. Chest 1985;87:619.
37. Lyons HA, Huang CT. Therapeutic use of progesterone in alveolar hypoventilation associated with obesity. Am J Med 1968;44:881.
38. Sutton FD, Zwillich CW, Creagh CE, et al. Progesterone for outpatient treatment of pickwickian syndrome. Ann Intern Med 1975;83:476.
39. Orr WC, Imes MK, Martin RJ. Progesterone therapy in obese patients with sleep apnea. Arch Intern Med 1979;139:109.
40. Strohl KP, Hensley MJ, Saunders NA, et al. Progesterone administration and progressive sleep apneas. JAMA 1981;245:1230.
41. Brownell LG, West P, Sweatman P, et al. Protriptyline in obstructive sleep apnea: a double-blind trial. N Engl J Med 1982;307:1037.
42. Smith PL, Haponik EF, Allen RP, et al. The effects of protriptyline in sleep-disordered breathing. Am Rev Respir Dis 1983;127:8.
43. Afzelius LE, Elmquist D, Hougaard K, et al. Sleep apnea syndrome: an alternative to tracheostomy. Laryngoscope 1981;91:285.
44. Lowe AA. Oral appliances for sleep breathing disorders. In Kryger M, Roth T, Dement W, editors. Principles and Practice of Sleep Medicine. 3rd ed. Philadelphia: WB Saunders; 2000; pp. 929–931.
45. Clark GT. Management of obstructive sleep apnea with dental appliances. Calif Dent Assoc J 1988;16:26.
46. Soll BA, George PT. Treatment of obstructive sleep apnea with a nocturnal airway-patency appliance. N Engl J Med 1985;313:386.
47. Bear SE, Priest JH. Sleep apnea syndrome: correction with surgical advancement of the mandible. J Oral Surg 1980;38:543.
48. Cartwright RD, Samelson CF. The effects of a nonsurgical treatment for obstructive sleep apnea: the tongue-retaining device. JAMA 1982;248:705.
49. Clark GT, Nakano M. Dental appliances for the treatment of obstructive sleep apnea. J Am Dent Assoc 1989;118:611.
50. Lowe AA, Sjoholm CF, Ryan JA, et al. Treatment, airway and compliance effects of a titratable oral appliance. Sleep 2000;23:172–178.
51. Clark GT, Arand D, Chung E, Tong D. Effect of anterior mandibular positioning on obstructive sleep apnea. Am Rev Respir Dis 1993;147:624–629.
52. Sullivan CE, Issa FG, Berthon-Jones M, et al. Home treatment of obstructive sleep apnea with continuous positive airway pressure applied through a nose-mask. Bull Eur Physiopathol Respir 1984;20:49.
53. Issa FG, Sullivan CE. The immediate effects of continuous positive airway pressure treatment on sleep pattern in patients with obstructive sleep apnea syndrome. Electroencephalogr Clin Neurophysiol 1986;63:10.
54. Klein M, Reynolds LG. Relief of sleep-related oropharyngeal airway obstruction by continuous insufflation of the pharynx. Lancet 1986;1:935.
55. Sullivan CE, Issa FG, Berthon-Jones M, et al. Reversal of obstructive sleep apnea by continuous positive airway pressure applied through the nares. Lancet 1981;1:862.
56. Laursen SB, Dreijer B, Hemmingsen C, Jacobsen E. Bi-level positive airway pressure treatment of obstructive sleep apnea syndrome. Respiration 1998;65:114–119.
57. Meurice J, Marc I, Series F. Efficacy of auto-CPAP in the treatment of obstructive sleep apnea/hypopnea syndrome. Am J Respir Crit Care Med 1996;153:794–798.
58. Katsantonis GP, Schweitzer PK, Branham GH, et al. Management of obstructive sleep apnea: comparison of various treatment modalities. Laryngoscope 1988;98:304.
59. Kuhlo W, Doll E, Franck MD. Erfolgreiche behandlung eines pickwick-syndroms ddurch eine dauertrachealkanuele. Dtsch Med Wochenschr 1969;94:1286.
60. Simmons FB, Guilleminault C, Silvestri R. Snoring, and some obstructive sleep apnea, can be cured by oropharyngeal surgery. Arch Otolaryngol 1983;109:503.
61. Heimer D, Scharf S, Lieberman A, et al. Sleep apnea syndrome treated by repair of deviated nasal septum. Chest 1983;84:184.
62. Ikematsu T. Study of snoring, 4th report: therapy. J Jap Otorhinolaryngol 1964;64:434.
63. Fujita S, Conway W, Zorick F, et al. Surgical correction of anatomic abnormalities in obstructive sleep apnea syndrome: uvulopalatopharyngoplasty. Otolaryngol Head Neck Surg 1981;89:923.
64. Simmons FB, Guilleminault C, Miles LE. The palataopharyngoplasty operation for snoring and sleep apnea: an interim report. Otolaryngol Head Neck Surg 1984;92:375.
65. Guilleminault C, Hayes B, Smith L, et al. Palatopharyngoplasty in obstructive sleep apnea syndrome. Bull Eur Physiopathol Res 1983;19:595.
66. Kamami YV. Outpatient treatment of sleep apnea syndrome with CO_2 laser: laser-assisted UPPP. J Otolaryngol 1994;23:395–398.
67. Krespi YP, Pearlman SJ, Keidar A. Laser-assisted uvula-palatoplasty for snoring. J Otolaryngol 1994;23:328–334.
68. Terris DJ, Wang MZ. Laser-assisted uvulopalatoplasty in mild obstructive sleep apnea. Arch Otolaryngol Head Neck Surg 1998;124:718–720.
69. Sher AE. Update on upper airway surgery for obstructive sleep apnea. Curr Opin Pulm Med 1995;1:504–511.
70. Kuo PC, West RA, Bloomquist DS, et al. The effect of mandibular osteotomy in three patients with hypersomnia sleep apnea. Oral Surg 1979;48:385.
71. Alvarez CM, Lessin ME, Gross PD. Mandibular advancement combined with horizontal advancement genioplasty for the

treatment of obstructive sleep apnea in an edentulous patient. Oral Surg 1987;64:402.

72. Riley R, Guilleminault C, Powell N, et al. Mandibular osteotomy and hyoid bone advancement for obstructive sleep apnea: a case report. Sleep 1984;7:79.

73. Riley RW, Powell NB, Guilleminault C. Inferior mandibular osteotomy and hyoid myotomy suspension for obstructive sleep apnea: a review of 55 patients. J Oral Maxillofac Surg 1989;47:159.

74. Riley RW, Powell NB, Guilleminault C. Obstructive sleep apnea and the hyoid: a revised surgical procedure. Otolaryngol Head Neck Surg 1994;111:717–721.

75. Waite PD, Wooten V, Lachner J, et al. Maxillomandibular advancement surgery in 23 patients with obstructive sleep apnea syndrome. J Oral Maxillofac Surg 1989;47:1256.

76. Riley RW, Powell NB, Guilleminault C. Obstructive sleep apnea syndrome: a review of 306 consecutively treated surgical patients. Otolaryngol Head Neck Surg 1993;108:117–125.

77. Hochban W, Conradt R, Brandenburg U, et al. Surgical maxillofacial treatment of obstructive sleep apnea. Plast Reconstr Surg 1997;99:619–626.

78. Prinsell JR. Maxillomandibular advancement surgery in a site-specific treatment approach for obstructive sleep apnea in 50 consecutive patients. Chest 1999;116:1519–1529.

79. Lee NR, Givens CD, Wilson J, Robins RB. Staged surgical treatment of obstructive sleep apnea syndrome: a review of 35 patients. J Oral Maxillofac Surg 1999;57:382–385.

80. Bettega G, Pepin JL, Veale D, et al. Obstructive sleep apnea syndrome fifty-one consecutive patients treated by maxillofacial surgery. Am J Respir Crit Care Med 2000;162:641–649.

81. Riley RW, Powell NB, Guilleminault C. Obstructive sleep apnea syndrome: a surgical protocol for dynamic upper airway reconstruction. J Oral Maxillofac Surg 1993;51:742–747.

82. Prinsell JR. Maxillomandibular advancement surgery for obstructive sleep apnea syndrome. J Am Dent Assoc 2002;133:1489–1497.

83. Louis PJ, Waite PD, Austin RB. Long-term skeletal stability after rigid fixation of Lefort I osteotomies with advancements. Int J Oral Maxillofac Surg 1993;22:82–86.

84. Nimkarn Y, Miles PG, Waite PD. Maxillomandibular advancement surgery in obstructive sleep apnea syndrome patients: long-term surgical stability. J Oral Maxillofac Surg 1995;53:1414–1418.

85. Riley RW, Powell NB, Guilleminault C, Ware W. Obstructive sleep apnea syndrome following surgery for mandibular prognathism. J Oral Maxillofac Surg 1987;45:450–452.

86. Boyce JR, Waite PD, Louis PJ, Ness TJ. Transnasal jet ventilation is a useful adjunct to teach fibreoptic intubation: a preliminary report. Can J Anaesth 2003;50:1056–1060.

87. He J, Kryger MH, Zorick FJ, et al. Mortality and apnea index in obstructive sleep apnea. Experience in 385 male patients. Chest 1988;94:9–14.

88. Hersi AS. Obstructive sleep apnea and cardiac arrhythmias. Ann Thorac Med 2010;5:10–17.

89. Muntz J. Duration of DVT prophylaxis in the surgical patient and its relation to quality issues. Am J Surg 2010;200:413–421.

90. Lye KW, Waite PD, Wang D, Sittitavornwong S. Predictability of prebent advancement plates for use in maxillomandibular advancement surgery. J Oral Maxillofac Surg 2008;66:1625–1629.

Facial Aesthetic Surgery

Blepharoplasty

Tirbod Fattahi, DDS, MD, FACS

INTRODUCTION

Blepharoplasty, commonly referred to "eyelid lift," is a widely accepted and utilized aesthetic surgical procedure. According to a recent survey, blepharoplasty of upper and lower lids was the third most commonly performed cosmetic procedure in United States in 2008, trailing body liposuction and breast enhancement.[1] Contributing to its popularity is its relative ease of performance, ability to be done in an office setting with minimal anesthesia, and lack of a prolonged recovery period

The history of blepharoplasty to correct "lid disorders" dates all the way back to the first century A.D. in Rome when Aulus Cornelius Celsus described excision of eyelid skin.[2] Since then, multiple refinements and modifications have been proposed.

Eyes are the "windows to the soul"; attractive eyes are one of the main features of an aesthetic and balanced face (Figure 65-1).[3] In order to achieve an excellent result, blepharoplasty

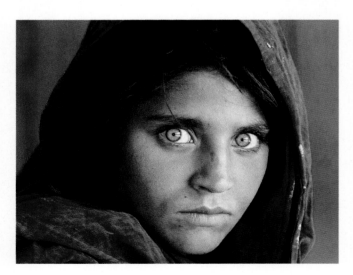

FIGURE 65-1. Open, attractive, youthful eyes. (From McCurry S. National Geographic, June 1985; 167: cover photo.)

of upper and lower lids demands a clear understanding of the appropriate preoperative diagnosis, regional anatomy, surgical execution, and management of any postoperative complications. Perhaps more important than the aforementioned concepts, it is paramount to remember that any cosmetic surgical procedure requires an appreciation of what the patient wants. Discrepancies between what the practitioner wants to treat and what the patient wants to have treated can lead to suboptimal results. Often times, patients will present to the clinician's office with a specific complaint regarding the appearance of the periorbital region. Based on the vast amount of information available on the internet, most patients can be quite focused about their concerns. Considering the complex anatomy of the periorbital region, the clinician must formulate a clear diagnosis and treatment plan that corresponds to the patient's concerns. For example, a patient may not be satisfied with the appearance of the upper eyelids and complain that she has difficulty applying makeup to the upper lids simply because they are so "sagging." This patient may present for what she perceives as an eyelid issue. Often times, however, these patients suffer from brow ptosis and actually need brow elevation in order to address the "sagging" eyelids (Figure 65-2). Therefore, proper preoperative communication and treatment planning is absolutely necessary in order to obtain satisfactory results and a "happy" patient. The purpose of this chapter is to familiarize the reader with commonly used nomenclature, surgical anatomy, patient selection, surgical execution, and potential complications associated with upper and lower lid blepharoplasty.

NOMENCLATURE

As is common with many aesthetic procedures, multiple "phrases" and "terms" are used to describe the appearance of the upper and lower lids. This can sometimes lead to confusion for the novice surgeon. A list of commonly used diagnoses follows:

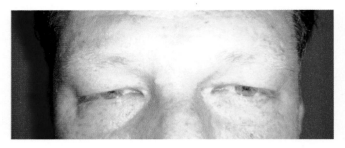

FIGURE 65-2. Patient complaining of "heavy eyelids." Examination revealed brow ptosis in addition to dermatochalasia of eye lid skin.

- **Dermatochalasia:** This is a nonspecific term implying excess skin; this is applicable to any part of the facial skin; typically due to a weak bony foundation (hypoplastic infraorbital rim in case of the lower lids), aging process, exposure to sunlight, genetics, and environmental causes (Figure 65-3).
- **Blepharochalasia:** This is a more specific term implying an inflammatory component to redundant skin of the lids. This is often related to angioedema and episodic swelling and edema of the periorbital region.
- **Blepharoptosis:** This acquired or congenital condition relates to drooping of upper lids. This is usually secondary to disinsertion of the levator palpebral superioris aponeurosis (LPS) from the upper tarsal plate (Figure 65-4). This condition is different from brow ptosis, which often causes excess upper lid skin. Blepharoptosis can occur simultaneously with dermatochalasis and blepharochalasis of lids and requires repair of LPS dysfunction.
- **Pseudoptosis:** This term should not be confused with blepharoptosis; this "ptosis," albeit not a true ptosis, is due to the appearance of "drooping" upper eyelid skin without any levator dysfunction. This is simply excessive, heavy lid skin causing a "drooping appearance." There is no indication for ptosis surgery in these patients.
- **Prolapsed fat pads:** Prominent lower lid fat pads or the medial fat pad of the upper lid can present as a "bulge" secondary to weakening of the orbital septum. The term "prolapsed" is more accurate than "herniated" because the septum is still intact, albeit weak, as opposed to a herniation in which there is a distinct opening through which fat bulges (Figure 65-5).
- **Hypertrophic orbicularis oculi:** This is a distinct and hypertrophic portion of the pretarsal component of the

orbicularis oculi in the lower lid. Although this can be considered aesthetic in many individuals, in some patients, this condition may exacerbate the "bulge" in the lower lid.
- **Prolapsed lacrimal gland:** This infrequent occurrence is due to the weakness of the septum of the upper lid, causing a unilateral or bilateral fullness in the lateral aspect of the upper lids due to the descent of the lacrimal gland.
- **Lower lid malposition:** This general term applies to any degree of abnormality associated with the lower lid. This could encompass frank ectropion, entropion, lower lid rounding or shortness, and lateral canthal dystopia (Figure 65-6).

ANATOMY

Surgical anatomy of the eye lids is rather complex.[4–10] There are numerous structures in both upper and lower lids with similar functions, but different names (Figure 65-7). Also, it

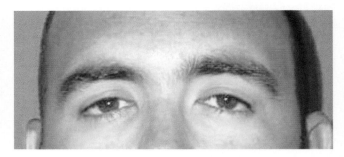

FIGURE 65-4. Patient with congenital ptosis of the upper lids and down-slanting of the lateral canthal angle.

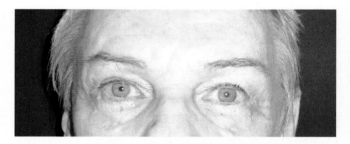

FIGURE 65-5. Patient with prolapsed fat pads of the lower lids and dermatochalasia of all four lids.

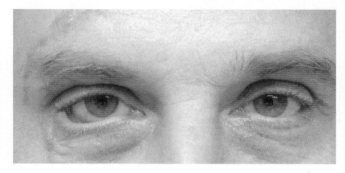

FIGURE 65-6. Right side lower eyelid rounding and frank ectropion.

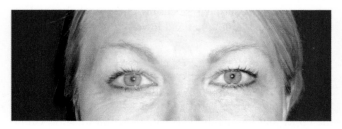

FIGURE 65-3. Patient with dermatochalasia of the eyelids and normal brow position.

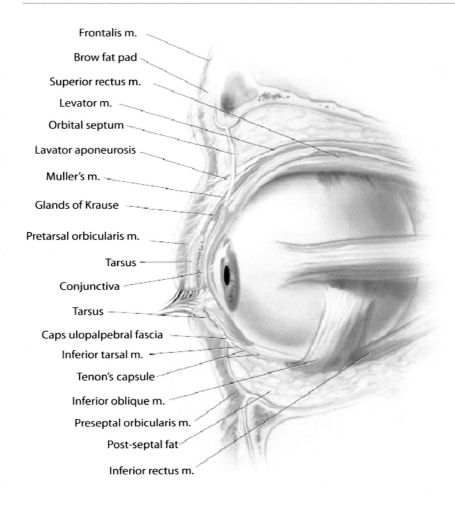

Frontalis m.
Brow fat pad
Superior rectus m.
Levator m.
Orbital septum
Lavator aponeurosis
Muller's m.
Glands of Krause
Pretarsal orbicularis m.
Tarsus
Conjunctiva
Tarsus
Caps ulopalpebral fascia
Inferior tarsal m.
Tenon's capsule
Inferior oblique m.
Preseptal orbicularis m.
Post-septal fat
Inferior rectus m.

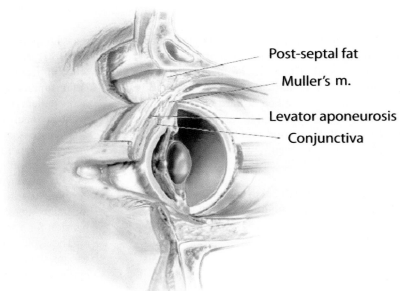

Post-septal fat
Muller's m.
Levator aponeurosis
Conjunctiva

FIGURE 65-7.   Anatomic details for upper and lower eye lids.
(From Fattahi T. Blepharoplasty. In Fonseca RJ, ed. Oral and
Maxillofacial Surgery, 2nd ed. St. Louis, Mo.: Elsevier; 2009: 579–594.)

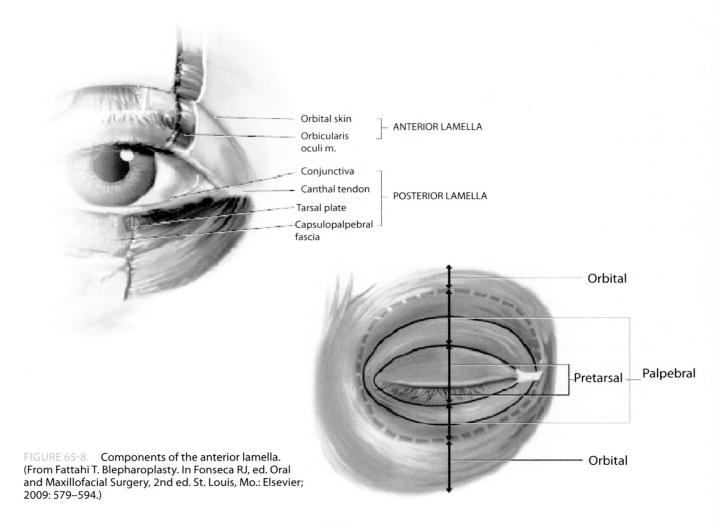

FIGURE 65-8. Components of the anterior lamella. (From Fattahi T. Blepharoplasty. In Fonseca RJ, ed. Oral and Maxillofacial Surgery, 2nd ed. St. Louis, Mo.: Elsevier; 2009: 579–594.)

is imperative to remember that, at times, surgical alterations of the lid anatomy may involve alteration of the brow or midface structures as well. Therefore, an understanding of the surgical anatomy of those particular areas is also helpful.

The most consistent method toward understanding the surgical anatomy of the upper and lower lids is to divide each lid into three lamellae: anterior, middle, and posterior. Each lamella has several components, which are discussed individually.

- Anterior lamella: skin, orbicularis oculi
- Middle lamella: orbital septum, orbital fat pads
- Posterior lamella: lid retractors, suspensory system, tarsus, conjunctiva

Anterior Lamella

The anterior lamella includes the eyelid skin and the orbicularis oculi muscle (Figure 65-8). Upper and lower lid skins are the thinnest skin on the body; the average thickness of the epidermis complex in the adult lid is about 130 μm.[11] This thinness can be considered both an attribute and a disadvantage to the surgeon; although the lid skin is amenable to

massaging after surgery if necessary, it is also quite susceptible to scarring if handled improperly during surgery.

A clinically significant region of the skin of the upper lid is the supratarsal crease. This crease (two distinct creases in many patients) is the point of attachment of the upper septum to the aponeurosis of the levator palpebral superioris muscle. This crease is usually found approximately 8 to 10 mm cephalad to the upper lid margin. There are no well-defined creases in the lower lid in most patients; however, with age and exposure to the environment, lower lid creases/rhytids begin to develop just inferior to the lashes. These creases run in a medial to lateral direction and can be utilized for placement of incision for a transcutaneous lower lid blepharoplasty.

The orbicularis oculi is a circular skeletal muscle encompassing the lids and adjacent tissues. The muscle is innervated by the facial nerve (seventh cranial nerve) and has two major components: palpebral and orbital. The palpebral portion is further subdivided into pretarsal and preseptal. The orbital portion originates from the superomedial and inferomedial orbital rim, the maxillary process of the frontal bone, the frontal process of maxilla, and the medial canthal tendon. The fibers sweep across the eyelids, onto the forehead and the cheek regions, respectively. The orbital portion covers the corrugator supercilii muscle. This portion of the orbicularis oculi is rarely encountered during blepharoplasty. Only involuntary movements are associated with the orbital portion of the muscle.

The preseptal and pretarsal components of the palpebral portion of the muscle have voluntary and involuntary movements. The pretarsal portion is firmly attached to the tarsal plates; the preseptal component is anchored medially to the medial canthal tendon and laterally attach to the lateral canthal region. The palpebral components of the orbicularis oculi are responsible for the blink reflex and moving the marginal tear film toward the lacrimal puncta.

Middle Lamella

The middle lamella comprises the orbital septum and the orbital fat pads (Figure 65-9). The septum is essentially a fascial membrane separating the eyelids from the deeper orbital contents. The septum maintains the orbital fat pads on its posterior surface. In both lids, the septum originates from the arcus marginalis, the confluence of the periorbital periosteum and the periosteum of the facial bones. In the upper lid, the septum attaches to the levator aponeurosis, approximately 2 to 5 mm above the superior edge of the tarsal plate; this fusion represents the clinically significant supratarsal crease. This crease may not be present in approximately 50% of the Asian population. In this group of patients, the septum attaches directly to the superior aspect of the upper tarsus (Figure 65-10). In the lower lid, the septum attaches directly on the inferior aspect of the tarsal plate. The orbital septa of the lower and upper lids actually meet each other medially just deep to the orbicularis oculi muscle around the posterior lacrimal crest. Laterally, the septum fuses with the lateral canthal tendon region.

Just deep to the septum, one finds the preaponeurotic orbital fat pads and the lacrimal gland (Figure 65-11). In the upper lids, there are two fat pads: nasal and middle. The lacrimal gland occupies the space laterally. These two fat pads separate the septum from the underlying levator aponeurosis. The tendon of the superior oblique muscle separates the central fat from the nasal fat compartment. In the lower lids, there are three fat pads: medial, central and temporal. The medial fat pad is the most vascular; this is of clinical significance during fat removal in blepharoplasty in order to prevent postoperative retrobulbar bleed. The inferior oblique muscle separates the medial from the central fat pad. The temporal fat pad may have more than one component.

Posterior Lamella

Lid retractors, suspensory system, tarsus, and the conjunctiva make up the posterior lamella of the lids (Figure 65-12). Lid retractors oppose the action of the orbicularis oculi. In the upper lid, the retractors include the levator aponeurosis (fascial condensation of the levator palpebral aponeurosis [LPS]), and Müller's muscle. LPS is a parasympathetically innervated muscle (cranial nerve III); from the lesser wing of the sphenoid bone, it travels superior to the superior rectus muscle and becomes aponeurotic as it attaches to the lower two thirds of the anterior surface of the upper tarsal plate. Müller's muscle is a sympathetically innervated (superior cervical chain) muscle originating from the inner surface of the LPS and inserting on the superior edge of the upper tarsal plate. Both muscles are elevators of the upper lid. In the lower lid, the lid retractors include the capsulopalpebral fascia and a lesser defined muscle known as the

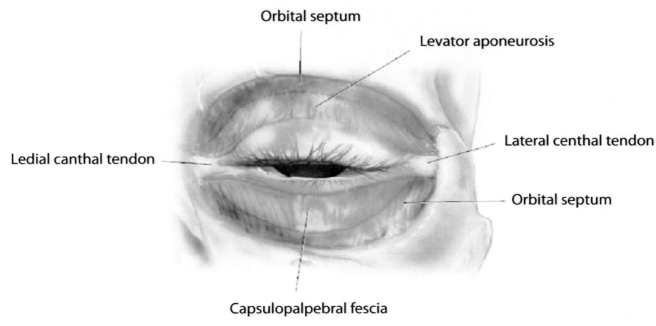

FIGURE 65-9.   Components of the middle lamella. (From Fattahi T. Blepharoplasty. In Fonseca RJ, ed. Oral and Maxillofacial Surgery, 2nd ed. St. Louis, Mo.: Elsevier; 2009: 579–594.)

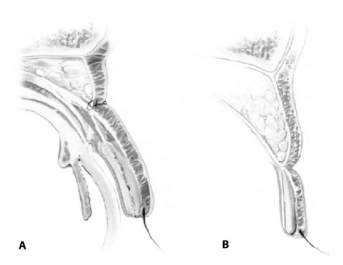

FIGURE 65-10. Differences in the attachment of levator aponeurosis in Asians **(A)** and non-Asians **(B)**. (**A** and **B,** From Fattahi T. Blepharoplasty. In Fonseca RJ, ed. Oral and Maxillofacial Surgery, 2nd ed. St. Louis, Mo.: Elsevier; 2009: 579–594.)

inferior tarsal or *palpebral muscle,* also known as *Horner's muscle.* The capsulopalpebral fascia is an extension of the inferior rectus muscle attaching to the inferior edge of the lower tarsal plate. Horner's muscle is a portion of the deep head of the orbicularis oculi muscle. These two lower lid retractors are analogous to the levator aponeurosis of the LPS and Müller's muscle of the upper lid, respectively.

The two hammock-like suspensory systems of the upper and lower lids include Whitnall's ligament and Lockwood's ligament, respectively. They are also known as the *superior* and *inferior transverse suspensory ligaments.* They prevent the globe from craniocaudal movement. Whitnall's ligament is a fascial condensation originating from the trochlea and attaching to the orbital lobe of the lacrimal gland. This ligament is found just superior to the LPS, but deep to the septum. Lockwood's suspensory ligament is a fascial condensation of Tenon's capsule (bulbar fascia) running between the medial orbital walls and attaching to the lateral retinaculum. Lockwood's suspensory system is just anterior to the capsulopalpebral fascia.

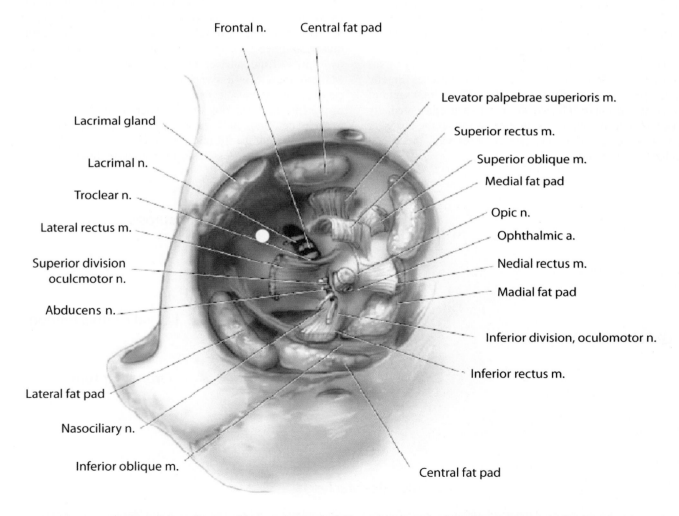

FIGURE 65-11. Anatomy of the right eye with septum removed. (From Fattahi T. Blepharoplasty. In Fonseca RJ, ed. Oral and Maxillofacial Surgery, 2nd ed. St. Louis, Mo.: Elsevier; 2009: 579–594.)

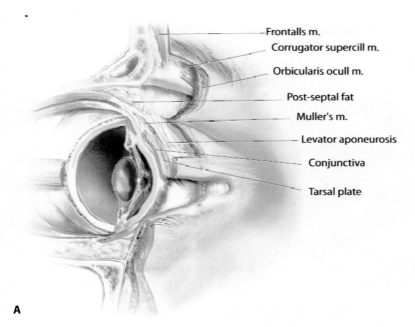

A

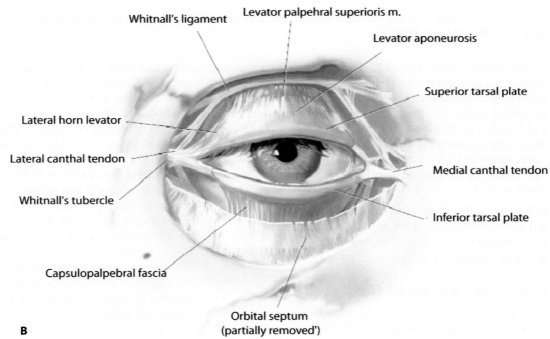

B

FIGURE 65-12.   **A** and **B,** Components of the posterior lamella (**A** and **B,** From Fattahi T. Blepharoplasty. In Fonseca RJ, ed. Oral and Maxillofacial Surgery, 2nd ed. St. Louis, Mo.: Elsevier; 2009: 579–594.)

Tarsal plates provide the main skeletal support to the upper and lower lids. They are made of dense fibroelastic tissue lined with meibomian glands. In the lower lid, the tarsal plate is only 4 to 6 mm in height; in the upper lid, the plate is 8 to 10 mm in height.

Conjunctiva makes up the last component of the posterior lamella. It lines the most inner aspect of the lids (palpebral conjunctiva), forms the fornix, and then turns onto the globe and covers the anteriormost aspect of the cornea (bulbar conjunctiva).

Although not specifically components of the posterior lamella, the lateral and medial canthi play a significant role in the transverse and spatial relationship of the lower and upper lids. Lateral and medial canthi are lateral and medial fibrous extensions of the tarsal plates. Both canthi have two heads: superficial and deep (anterior and posterior). The anterior limb of the medial canthus and the posterior limb of the lateral canthus are thicker than their counterparts. The two limbs of the medial canthal tendon cover the lacrimal sac; the two limbs of the lateral canthal tendon cover Eisler's fat pad.

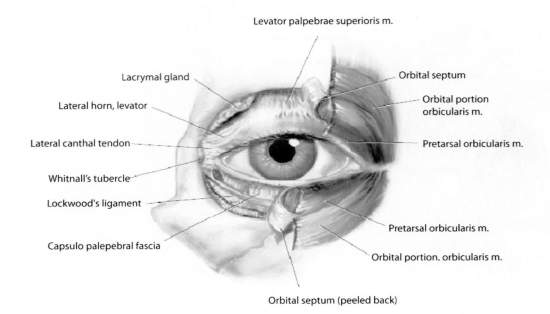

Levator palpebrae superioris m.

Lacrymal gland

Lateral horn, levator

Lateral canthal tendon

Whitnall's tubercle

Lockwood's ligament

Capsulo palepebral fascia

Orbital septum

Orbital portion orbicularis m.

Pretarsal orbicularis m.

Pretarsal orbicularis m.

Orbital portion. orbicularis m.

Orbital septum (peeled back)

FIGURE 65-13. Components of the lateral retinaculum. (From Fattahi T. Blepharoplasty. In Fonseca RJ, ed. Oral and Maxillofacial Surgery, 2nd ed. St. Louis, Mo.: Elsevier; 2009: 579–594.)

The lateral retinaculum (LR) is a clinically significant structure in the lateral orbital rim (Figure 65-13).[12–14] LR is essentially a labyrinth of connective tissue anchored within the lateral orbital rim that maintains the position, integrity, and function of the globe. It is attached to Whitnall's tubercle, a bony protuberance 10 mm inferior to the zygomaticofrontal suture and 3 mm posterior (deep) to lateral orbital wall rim within the zygomatic bone. The following structures attach to the LR:

- Lateral canthal tendon (posterior limb).
- Lateral horn of LPS aponeurosis.
- Lockwood's ligament of the lower lid.
- Check ligament of lateral rectus muscle.

Innervation and Blood Supply

Sensory innervation of the eye lids is provided by the fifth cranial nerve (trigeminal); specifically, the first and second divisions (ophthalmic and maxillary). The lacrimal nerve travels in a superior and lateral direction providing sensation to the lacrimal gland, upper lid, and brow region. The frontal nerve divides into the supraorbital (centrally) and supratrochlear (medially) to provide sensation to the upper lid, midbrow, forehead, scalp, and nasal bridge. The nasociliary nerve gives off branches to provide sensation to the globe. The infraorbital nerve emerges from its foramen to provide sensation to the lower lid, midcheek, and upper lip and anterior maxillary teeth. The zygomatic nerve divides into the zygomaticotemporal and zygomaticofacial nerve to provide sensation to the temple and lateral brow and lateral aspect of lower lid and cheek respectively.

The blood supply to the eyelids is provided by the internal and external carotid systems. The ophthalmic artery, facial artery, and infraorbital artery are the main arteries in this region. The ophthalmic artery is a branch of the internal carotid system and has multiple branches (supraorbital, supratrochlear, ethmoidal, marginal, and external nasal). The facial artery becomes the angular artery in the medial canthal region and anastomoses with the branches of the ophthalmic artery medial to the lacrimal sac. The infraorbital artery emerges from the maxillary artery and supplies the lower lid region. The marginal and peripheral cascades (anastomoses between the internal and the external carotid systems) within the lid proper are responsible for the blood supply to the lashes and tarsus (marginal) and the conjunctiva and lid muscles (peripheral).

The venous system mirrors that of the arterial system, although deep anastomoses with the pterygoid plexus of veins and the superior ophthalmic vein exist that may lead to a retrograde infection.

Lacrimal System

The lacrimal system begins with the lacrimal gland sitting in the lacrimal fossa. Tears are produced in the gland and then travel in a lateral to medial direction toward the lacrimal puncta by the blink reflex. Accessory lacrimal glands within the upper and lower fornices are known as *glands of Kraus* and *Wolfring*. Tears enter the upper and lower canaliculi, approximately 8 to 10 mm away from the lacrimal sac. Both canaliculi have a 2-mm vertical component before making a 90-degree turn to form the common canaliculus. The common canaliculis runs deep to the pretarsal orbicularis oculi to empty into the nasolacrimal duct, which then travels into the inferior meatus approximately 15 mm from the nasal floor.

PATIENT EVALUATION

Perhaps the most significant component of any aesthetic surgery is a thorough understanding of the patient's needs and desires. The surgeon must recognize the patient's complaint and then determine whether the patient's expectations are realistic. Patients seeking blepharoplasty usually complain of "bags under the eyes," "excess skin in the upper lids," "always looking tired," "deceased vision laterally," and "inability to apply makeup to the upper lids."[15–17] It is important to establish the exact reason a patient is seeking to have surgery. This is facilitated by giving the patient a hand mirror and asking him or her to point to the areas of concern.

Once the chief complaint has been elicited, a complete medical history must be obtained. Medical conditions such as thyroid disease, heart disease, liver dysfunction, bleeding disorders, and seasonal allergy and edema must be ruled out. Many of these conditions may interfere with the proper diagnosis and surgical execution of blepharoplasty. It is particularly important to determine whether a patient has had LASIK (laser-assisted in situ keratomileusis) surgery in the past 6 months because the conjunctiva can become anesthetic after this procedure and mask symptoms associated with dry eyes.

Once the history has been completed, a step-by-step approach must be undertaken to evaluate the lids. With all aesthetic procedures, one must first gauge an overall view of the *entire* face before focusing on the specific area of concern. This overall image often provides a tremendous amount of information about the aging process that can then be relayed to the patient during the evaluation of the face.

After this overall assessment, the clinician must evaluate the position of the brows and forehead. If a patient appears to have dermatochalasia of the upper lids, one must ascertain that the dermatochalasia is not due to brow ptosis. Performing an upper blepharoplasty in the presence of brow ptosis will only cause further descent of the brow and lead to an unaesthetic result. If the brow appears ptotic, the patient may need to have a brow elevation (e.g., endoscopic, open, browpexy) *before* upper blepharoplasty.[18] There are specific measurements for an ideal brow for males and females. Generally, there are three parts to an eyebrow: medial, apex, and tail. In a male, all three regions should be aligned with the supraorbital rim. A masculine brow is one with little elevation in its apex or tail. Conversely, a female brow should have a slight elevation medially (0–2 mm compared with the underlying supraorbital rim), elevate to 10 mm at the apex (compared with the underlying supraorbital rim), and then slightly descend toward the tail aspect. A complete evaluation of the brow and forehead is described in Chapter 68.

Next, attention should be directed toward the upper lids. Determination of the presence or absence of a supratarsal crease must be made. Typically, the supratarsal crease is approximately 9 to 11 mm above the lid margin. This can be measured with a ruler while elevating the brow with one hand and asking the patient to look downward. If the supratarsal crease is significantly greater than 9 to 11 mm, one must consider the possibility of levator disinsertion from the septum. With the brow kept in its normal position, excess upper lid skin must be pinched between two fingers to determine the amount of dermatochalasis. This can be subjectively graded from 0 to 3, with 3 being significant hooding in which excess lid skin is sitting on top of the lashes to 0 being no redundant tissue. Assessment of the upper lid fat pads must also be done. Usually, one finds prolapsed medial fat pad in the upper lid, especially in an older patient. Another important consideration is the presence of lid ptosis (blepharoptosis).[7,19] This can be determined in two ways. The first method is to measure the palpebral fissure. This is the distance between the central aspect of the upper lid and the central aspect of the lower lid with the patient gazing in a primary position. This width should be almost 10 mm bilaterally. A significant decrease in palpebral fissure width should raise the suspicion for upper lid ptosis. The other method is the margin reflex distance-1 (MRD-1). This is the distance between the light reflex in the patient's cornea and the central upper lid margin with the patient's eyes in the primary position of gaze. The upper lid usually covers 2 mm of the superior limbus of the iris (Figure 65-14). The normal MRD-1 is approximately 4 to 5 mm; a smaller number may indicate upper lid ptosis. The MRD-1 is more accurate than the

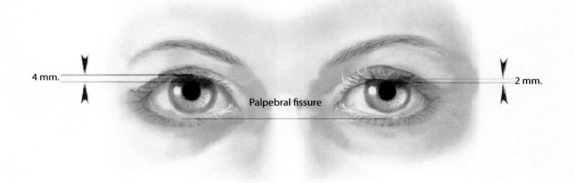

4 mm.   Palpebral fissure   2 mm.

FIGURE 65-14. Normal margin reflex distance-1 (MRD-1) of the right eye and abnormal MRD-1 of the left eye denote left upper eyelid ptosis.

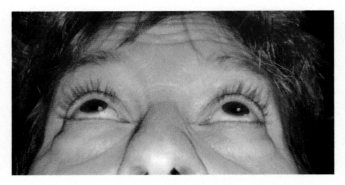

FIGURE 65-15.   Asking the patient to look up will accentuate the borders of the lower eyelid fat prolapse.

palpebral fissure width because the latter can be altered by lower lid malposition (rounding, ectropion).

After the upper lid, focus should be directed at the lower lids. The presence of the fine rhytids just inferior to the lashes should be noted. Any excess skin in the lower lid subunit should be assessed. One can usually find prolapsed fat pads along the lower lids. The presence of prolapsed lower lid fat pads can be assessed by asking the patient to look upward or by gently pushing on the upper lids (while the eye is closed) to determine any lower lid "bulges" (Figure 65-15). A hypertrophic orbicularis oculi muscle can be differentiated from a lower lid prolapsed fat pad by asking the patient to smile; animation of the muscles of facial expression emphasizes hypertrophy of the orbicularis oculi muscle. Lower lid retraction can be assessed by measuring the distance from the inferior limbus to the central portion of the lower lid. Usually, the lower eye lid is at the level of the inferior limbus. Another method is the MRD-2, the distance from the light reflex of the cornea to the central aspect of the lower eyelid with the patient's eyes in primary gaze. This distance should be approximately 5 to 5.5 mm.[20] This distance is increased in lower lid retraction.

Lower lid laxity should also be determined by the snap and distraction test (Figure 65-16). The snap test is performed by pulling the lower lid downward and then releasing it to determine how quickly the lid "snaps" back into place. This should occur in less than 1 second or with one or two blinks. The lid distraction test is performed by pulling the lid away from the globe in an anterior and inferior direction. If the lid is distracted more than 7 mm, the lid is considered abnormally loose. If the snap or distraction tests are positive, the surgeon should consider a lid-tightening procedure at the time of blepharoplasty in order to prevent postoperative lid malposition.

Consideration should also be given to the midface region. If there is evidence of midface ptosis (e.g., prominent nasolabial fold, nasojugal fold), the patient should be advised about other indicated procedures such as midface lift or fat repositioning.

Other components of the physical examination should include a visual acuity examination. If there is diminished vision due to excessive hooding of the upper lids or to other intrinsic globe issues, a formal visual field test by an ophthalmologist or optometrist should be done. Many times, insurance companies will require such a test before authorizing upper blepharoplasty. Extraocular movements should be recorded preoperatively to ensure full and unrestricted movement of each periorbital muscle. Bell's phenomenon should also be assessed to prevent corneal exposure and desiccation in case of a residual lagophthalmos after surgery. The patient is asked to close her or his eyes tightly; the clinician then opens the lid to assess position of the cornea. A normal Bell's phenomenon will roll the globe and cornea in an upward position upon forceful closure of the lids (Figure 65-17).

If the patient has reported symptoms of dry eyes, a Schirmer test should be done to evaluate tear secretions. After drying the inferior fornix of the lower lid, a Schirmer strip is bent and inserted in the lateral aspect of the lower fornix. Room lights may need to be dimmed to prevent reflex

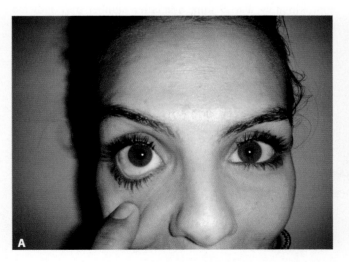
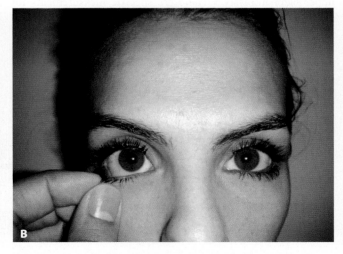

FIGURE 65-16.   Snap and distraction test. **A,** In the snap test, the lower eyelid is pulled inferiorly to assess how quickly it resumes its normal position next to the globe. **B,** In the distraction test, the lid is pulled in an anterior direction to assess its laxity.

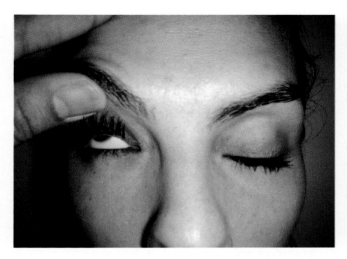

FIGURE 65-17. Normal Bell's phenomenon. Note the upward rotation of the iris as the lids are forcefully opened.

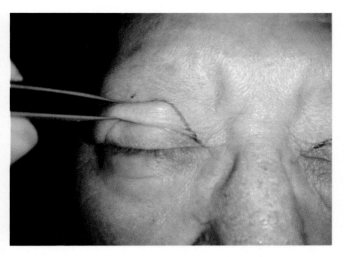

FIGURE 65-18. Fine forceps grasps the excess upper lid skin until the lashes evert.

blinking. A normal Schirmer test is 15 mm of wetness on the strip after 5 minutes. Five to 10 mm of wetness suggests hyposecretion, whereas less than 5 mm is highly indicative of dry eyes. If the Schirmer test is abnormal, further investigation is warranted. These patients will definitely require a very "conservative" blepharoplasty and may need frequent eye lubricants postoperatively.

A complete set of photographs is an absolute necessity in any aesthetic surgery. For blepharoplasty, frontal repose, frontal animated (smile), three quarters, profile, and a photograph with the patient looking in an upward gaze are sufficient.

SURGICAL PROCEDURES

Upper lid blepharoplasty is begun by marking the patient in the preoperative area.[21–24] The patient should be in a sitting position facing the surgeon. Most patients have a supratarsal crease. This crease can be used as the inferior aspect of the incision if the crease is in a normal position. The brow is elevated with the nondominant hand. A fine-tipped marker is used to outline the crease. The incision is marked just above the superior punctum and extends laterally and fades into one of the crow's feet. It is important to maintain the incision within the eyelid subunit and not extend too far laterally. The upper portion of the incision is determined by pinching the excess upper lid skin by a fine blunt forceps until the eyelashes began to evert (Figure 65-18). This position is marked at its highest position. This will serve at the superior incision once it is connected medially and laterally to the inferior incision. The basic shape of the incision is nearly an ellipse or oval (Figure 65-19). Although a skin/muscle flap can be elevated simultaneously, the easiest method of flap elevation is a skin-only flap. This is done quite easily after administration of local anesthetic with a vasoconstrictor for hemostasis purposes. The skin flap is incised and undermined by iris scissors. Hemostasis is obtained by electrocautery. At this

point, hypertrophic or ptotic orbicularis oculi can be excised cautiously. This will further expose the orbital septum, which will need to be incised if preaponeurotic fat pads (usually the nasal fat pad) need to be removed. A transverse incision through the orbital septum will expose the underlying medial and central upper lid fat pads (Figure 65-20). The prolapsed portion of the fat pads are then grasped with hemostats, and cut with scissors; electrocautery is applied to the cut edges of fat pads to ensure complete hemostasis before releasing the clamp and allowing the fat pads to retract posteriorly. Closure is not done until both sides are performed to ensure equal amount of skin, muscle, and fat resection. A slight lagophthlmos (<1–2 mm) is desirable at this point (Figure 65-21). This resolves within a few days. Skin closure is with 6-0 sutures. If a supratarsal crease does not exist, a skin-muscle flap can be elevated simultaneously. The inferior edge of the incision in this situation would be approximately 9 to 10 mm above the lashes. A skin-muscle flap will allow creation of a new supratarsal crease by attaching the levator aponeurosis directly to the inferior edge of the incision.

For lower lid blepharoplasty, the first decision to be made is whether a transconjunctival or transcutaneous blepharo-

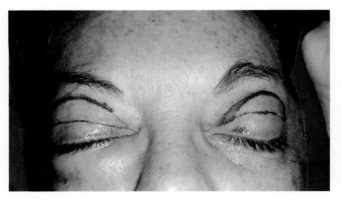

FIGURE 65-19. Typical markings for upper eyelid blepharoplasty.

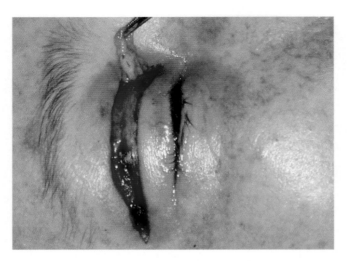

Exposure of the nasal fat pad after incising the septum.

plasty is to be performed. If the patient has prolapsed lower fat without excess skin, a transconjunctival lower lid blepharoplasty is indicated. Of note, it is also possible to "reposition" the fat in the nasojugal area via a transconjunctival approach if needed. If however, excess skin is present in the lower lid, the surgeon has three choices: (1) a transcutaneous lower lid blepharoplasty with removal of fat and skin, (2) a transconjunctival lower lid blepharoplasty to remove the fat with a skin-tightening procedure at the same time or later time (i.e., chemical peel, CO_2 laser resurfacing). and (3) a lower eyelid "pinch" blepharoplasty.[25–33] This decision must be made preoperatively and discussed with the patient at length. If a transcutaneous lower lid blepharoplasty is considered, a lid-tightening procedure must be strongly considered at the same time to prevent postoperative lid malposition, especially if the patient has preoperative lid laxity (i.e., positive snap or distraction tests, previous lower lid blepharoplasty).

For transconjunctival lower lid blepharoplasty, the patient is marked in the preoperative area by gently pushing on the globe or asking the patient to look up and determining the areas of prolapsed fat. These regions are marked with a marking pen. A transconjunctival lower lid blepharoplasty is performed by gentle retraction of the globe with a globe retractor, followed by incising the palpebral conjunctiva and

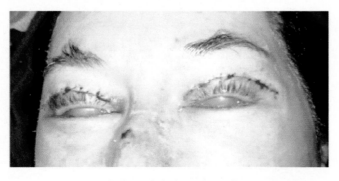

Slight lagophthalmos (metallic eye shields in place) after upper eyelid blepharoplasty

capsulopalpebral fascia with electrocautery (Figure 65-22). The incision is approximately 5 to 6 mm inferior to the lid margin. This will allow easy access into the three lower lid fat pads without disrupting the orbital septum. With gentle pressure on the globe, fat is easily protruded into the surgical field.[34] Each prolapsed fat pad is clamped with a hemostat, excess fat is trimmed, and electrocautery is used to cauterize the clamp before release to ensure hemostasis. It is prudent to ensure that no muscle is attached to the fat before resection. Both sides are then evaluated simultaneously to ensure equal removal of fat. The incision is closed with resorbable , and if a skin-tightening procedure is to be done at the same time, the surgeon proceeds as appropriate.

A transcutaneous lower lid blepharoplasty is initiated with skin markings for the ideal incision. Preoperative marking for the location of prolapsed fat pads is done as described previously. The ideal location of a transcutaneous lower lid blepharoplasty incision is within 3 to 4 mm of the lower lashes (Figure 65-23). The incision is started medially just below the punctum and extends laterally. At the lateral canthal region, the incision should rise, following the upward curve of the lower lid, and then gently descend and blend in with one of the crow's feet. A skin-only flap is first elevated. Once the skin flap is retracted inferiorly, a muscle flap is blunted dissected and elevated in a steplike fashion. This step should decrease the incidence of lower lid retraction because the skin incision and muscle incision will not be at the same location. Once the muscle has been elevated, the orbital septum can be clearly seen. A transverse incision is made through the orbital septum, exposing the underlying fat pads. Each fat pad is approached individually. Excess fat is clamped and removed and hemostasis obtained as previously described. Once the fat has been removed, attention is directed toward the lateral aspect of the incision where the lateralmost portion of the preseptal orbicularis muscle flap (off the inferior aspect of the incision) is suspended to the lateral retinaculum with a 4-0 suture. This pexing of the muscle to the thick fascial condensation of the lateral orbital wall will significantly reduce the risk of lower lid malposition postoperatively.[35] Once this has been done, the inferior skin flap is grasped at its lateral edge and pulled cephalad; excess skin is then removed with scissors. Next, the muscle flap is closed, followed by closure of the skin incision using 6-0 sutures.

A "pinch" lower eyelid blepharoplasty is indicated in patients with no fat prolapse but with excess eye lid skin. This procedure begins with "pinching" the excess skin with fine forceps in a cephalad direction toward the lashes; then the "rolled" lower eyelid skin is simply excised with the incision being placed 3 to 4 mm below the lashes. There is no muscle or fat excision in this maneuver (Figure 65-24). Closure of the skin incision is performed using 6-0 sutures.

POSTOPERATIVE CARE

Because upper and lower lid blepharoplasty is considered a "clean" surgical wound, perioperative antibiotic coverage for

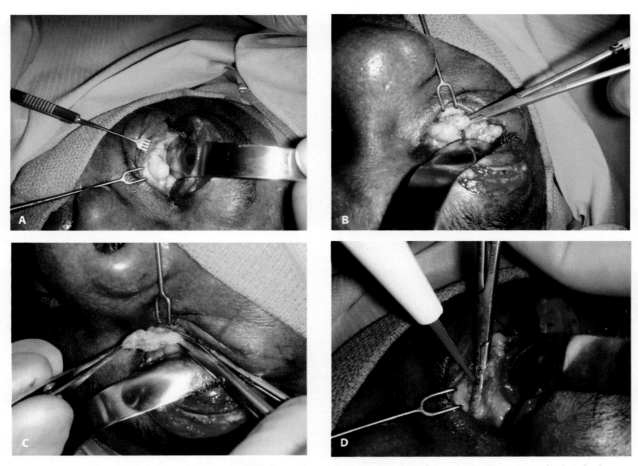

FIGURE 65-22.   Lower eye lid transconjunctival blepharoplasty. **A,** Exposure of the fat pads. **B,** Clamp is applied at the base of each fat pad. **C,** Scissors are used to cut the excess fat. **D,** Electrocautery is utilized on the clamped fat pad for hemostasis before releasing the fat pad.

greater than 24 hours is not recommended. All patients should have ice cold compresses applied to the surgical site in the recovery room and for the first 48 hours postoperatively. No contact lenses should be worn for the first few days after surgery. Patients are instructed to avoid exercise and heavy lifting for the first 2 weeks postoperatively to decrease the chance of capillary tears and bruising.

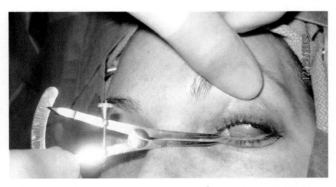

FIGURE 65-23.   Placement of lower eyelid transcutaneous blepharoplasty. The incision is approximately 4 mm inferior to the lower lashes.

Ophthalmic steroid eyedrops may be used to decrease chemosis. All nonresorbable sutures are removed in 5 days. Steri-Strips can be used to support the incision if necessary (Figure 65-25).

COMPLICATIONS AND MANAGEMENT

There are minor and major complications associated with blepharoplasty.[2,7,36–39] Fortunately, the major problems are rare. Minor issues include chemosis, bruising, subconjunctival hemorrhage, and blurred vision. All of these issues are transient and will resolve within the first 7 to 14 days after surgery.

More major complications include those associated with aesthetics, lid position, and function of the eyes. Aesthetic complications involve persistence of orbital fat pads, excess or redundant skin, and asymmetry between the two sides. This can be prevented by precise preoperative assessment. The lateral fat pad of the lower lid is usually the most difficult to access. Most underresections are associated with this particular pad. Persistent excess skin postoperatively can be prevented by measuring the patient while the patient is sitting. When the patient lies supine, the brows raise;

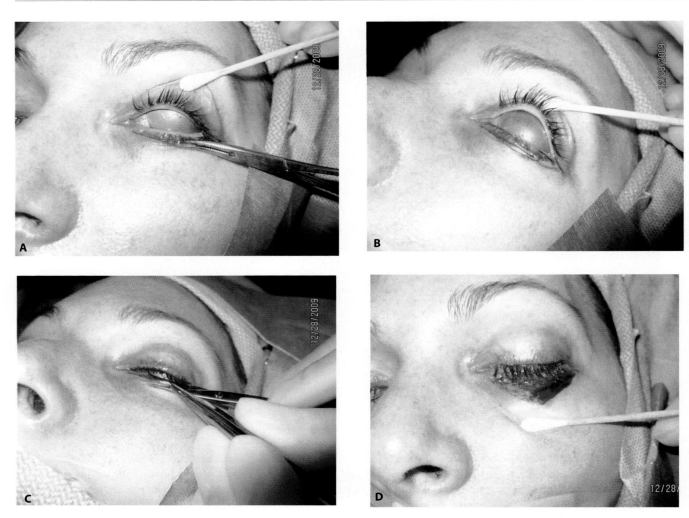

FIGURE 65-24. Pinch blepharoplasty. **A,** Excess skin is pinched with forceps. **B,** Appearance of pinched skin before excision. **C,** Excision of skin only. **D,** Underlying orbicularis oculi muscle. Note amount of skin resection

this can remove some of the dermatochalasia and lead to underremoval of excess skin. Asymmetries usually occur owing to unequal removal of fat and skin from both sides. All fat and excised skin should be kept and labeled throughout the procedure to ensure equal amount of resection (assuming there were no asymmetries preoperatively). Asymmetries can also be due to the position of the supratarsal crease or incision. It is imperative to measure the distance between the

lashes and the crease (incision) if any doubt exists regarding potential asymmetries between two sides.

Lid malposition can occur if excess skin was removed or if there was lid laxity preoperatively, or both. After a conservative transcutaneous lower lid blepharoplasty, a minor rounding (<1 mm) of the lower lid can occur without any adverse sequela. This is usually amenable to massage. However, if the rounding is greater, or if there is frank ectro-

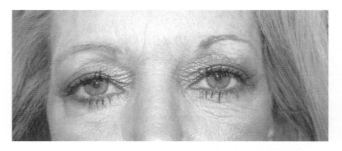

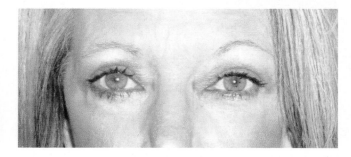

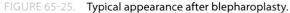

FIGURE 65-25. Typical appearance after blepharoplasty.

pion, this will need surgical repair in most cases. Although massage and taping of the lids can help, most patients will need a lid-tightening procedure, mucosal graft for posterior lamella lengthening, tarsorrhaphy, or skin graft for anterior lamella lengthening. This is the main reason the author advocates pexing of the preseptal orbicularis muscle to the lateral retinaculum in every transcutaneous lower lid blepharoplasty.

Perhaps the biggest complications after blepharoplasty are related to functional issues. Dry eyes after blepharoplasty are usually due to a preexisting condition or excessive skin resection leading to a persistent lagophthalmos or both. This requires application of artificial tears, taping of the lids, and massage. Referral to an ophthalmologist or oculoplastic surgeon may be warranted if the condition persists. Diplopia after blepharoplasty can occur if the superior oblique or the inferior oblique muscles are injured during surgery. Care must be taken during fat removal to ensure that all muscle and fascia have been removed from the fat pads before excision. Electrocautery near these muscles can also cause disturbances of vision. Persistent diplopia can be a serious problem and must be referred to an ophthalmologist. Retrobulbar bleeds and blindness are the gravest complications of upper and lower blepharoplasty. Meticulous hemostasis is mandatory during surgery to decrease the chance of postoperative bleeding. Intense, unilateral pain, and progressive proptosis and chemosis are hallmarks of a retrobulbar bleed; this requires emergent attention by an inferior canthotomy and cantholysis to decrease the intraocular pressure and evacuate any clots. If this pressure is allowed to increase, optic nerve ischemia can occur that will cause irreversible visual disturbance. The canthotomy and cantholysis should be kept open for 24 to 48 hours. Once the situation has been resolved, the lateral canthal tendon can be repaired.

References

1. Cosmetic Surgery National Data Bank, 2008. American Society for Aesthetic Plastic Surgery (ASAPS), New York. www.surgery.org.
2. Pastorek N, Bustillo A. Blepharoplasty. In Azizzadeh B, editor. Master Techniques in Facial Rejuvenation. 1st ed. Philadelphia: Elsevier; 2007.
3. McCurdy JA. Beautiful eyes: characteristics and application to aesthetic surgery. Facial Plast Surg 2006;22:204.
4. Tremblay JF, Anatomical considerations for blepharoplasty. In: Moy RL, Fincher EF, editors. Blepharoplasty. 1st ed. Philadelphia: Elsevier; 2006:1–9.
5. Zide BM, Jelks GW, The eyelids. In: Zide BM and Jelks GW, editors. Surgical Anatomy of the Orbit. 1st ed. New York: Raven Press; 1985:21–32.
6. Spinelli HM, Anatomy. In: Spinelli HM, editor. Atlas of Aesthetic Eyelid and Periocular Surgery. 1st ed. Philadelphia: Saunders; 2004:2–27.
7. Harris P, Mendelson B. Eyelid and midcheek anatomy. In: Putterman AM, editor. Cosmetic Oculoplastic Surgery. 3rd ed. Philadelphia: WB Saunders; 1999:45–63.
8. Yousif JN, Sonderman P, Dzwierzynski WW, et al. Anatomic considerations in transconjunctival blepharoplasty. Plast Reconstr Surg 1995;96:1271.
9. Wilhelmi BJ, Mowlavi A, Neumeister MW. Upper blepharoplasty with bony anatomical landmarks to avoid injury to trochlea and superior oblique muscle tendon with fat resection. Plast Reconstr Surg 2001;108:2137.
10. Ullmann Y, Levi Y, Ben-Izhak O, et al. The surgical anatomy of the fat in the upper eyelid medial compartment. Plast Reconstr Surg 1997;99:658.
11. Gonzales-Ulloa M, Castillo A, Stevens E, et al. Preliminary study of the total restoration of the facial skin. Plast Reconstr Surg 1954;13:151.
12. Gelks GW, Glat PM, Jelks EB, et al. The inferior retinacular lateral canthoplasty: a new technique. Plast Reconstr Surg 1997;100:1262.
13. Turk JB, Goldman A. Soof lift and lateral retinacular canthoplasty. Facial Plast Surg 2001;17:37.
14. Knize DM. The superficial lateral canthal tendon: anatomic study and clinical application to lateral canthopexy. Plast Reconstr Surg 2002;109:1149.
15. Furnas DW. Festoons, mounds, and bags of the eyelids and cheek. Clin Plast Surg 1993;20:367.
16. Jelks GW, Jelks EB. Preoperative evaluation of the blepharoplasty patient. Clin Plast Surg 1993;20:213.
17. Fincher EF, Moy RL. Cosmetic blepharoplasty. Dermatol Clin 2005;23:431.
18. Hoenig JA. Comprehensive management of eyebrow and forehead ptosis. Otolaryngol Clin North Am 2005;38:947.
19. Clauser L, Tieghi R, Galie M. Palpebral ptosis: clinical classification, differential diagnosis, and surgical guidelines: an overview. J Craniofac Surg 2006;17:246.
20. Karesh JW. Blepharoplasty. Atlas Oral Maxillofac Surg Clin North Am 1998;6:87.
21. Ross AT, Neal JG. Rejuvenation of the aging eyelid. Facial Plast Surg 2006;22:97.
22. Morgan JM, Gentile RD, Farrior E. Rejuvenation of the forehead and eyelid complex. Facial Plast Surg 2005;21:271.
23. Purewal BK, Bosniak S. Theories of upper eyelid blepharoplasty. Ophthalmol Clin North Am 2005;18:271.
24. Rohrick RJ, Coberly DM, Fagien S, et al. Current concepts in aesthetic upper blepharoplasty. Plast Reconstr Surg 2004;113:32e.
25. Perkins SW, Batniji RK. Rejuvenation of the lower eyelid complex. Facial Plast Surg 2005;21:279.
26. Lee AS, Thomas JR. Lower lid blepharoplasty and canthal surgery. Facial Plast Surg Clin North Am 2005;13:541.
27. Murakami CS, Orcutt JC. Treatment of lower eyelid laxity. Facial Plast Surg 11994;0:42.
28. Mommaerts MY, De Rui G. Prevention of lid retraction after lower lid blepharoplasties: an overview. J Craniomaxillofac Surg 2000;28:189.
29. Garcia RE, McCollough EG. Transcutaneous lower eyelid blepharoplasty with fat excision. Arch Facial Plast Surg 2006;8:374.
30. Pacella SJ, Nahai FR, Nahai F. Transconjunctival blepharoplasty for upper and lower eyelids. Plast Reconstr Surg 2010;125:384–392.

31. Korn BS, Kikkawa DO, Cohen SR. Transcutaneous lower eyelid blepharoplasty with orbitomalar suspension: retrospective review of 212 consecutive cases. Plast Reconstr Surg 2010; 125:315–323.

32. Niamtu J III. Surgical treatment options for lower eyelid aging. Cosmetic Dermatol 2008;21:652–657.

33. Kim EM, Bucky LP. Power of the pinch: pinch lower lid blepharoplasty. Ann Plast Surg 2008;60:532–537.

34. Oh CS, Chung IH, Kim YS, et al. Anatomic variations of the infraorbital fat compartment. Br J Plast Surg 2006;59:376.

35. Flowers RS. Canthopexy as a routine blepharoplasty component. Clin Plast Surg 1993;20:351.

36. Ghabrial R, Lisman RD, Kane MA. Diplopia following transconjunctival blepharoplasty. Plast Reconstr Surg 1998;102: 1219.

37. Wolfort FG, Vaughan TE, Wolfort SF, et al. Retrobulbar hematoma and blepharoplasty. Plast Reconstr Surg 1999;104: 2154.

38. Lelli GJ, Lisman RD. Blepharoplasty complications. Plast Reconstr Surg 2010;125:1007–1017.

39. Pacella SJ, Codner MA. Minor complications after blepharoplasty: dry eyes, chemosis, granulomas, ptosis, and sclera show. Plast Reconstr Surg 2010;125:709–718.

Basic Principles of Rhinoplasty

James Koehler, DDS, MD, and Peter D. Waite, MPH, DDS, MD

For many cosmetic surgeons, rhinoplasty is one of the most challenging surgical procedures. A clear understanding of nasal anatomy is critical in order to provide an aesthetic result that does not compromise nasal function. Developing a pattern of analysis of the nose is vital for proper diagnosis and for determining the most appropriate treatment plan. Numerous rhinoplastic techniques have been described. Some surgeons favor an endonasal approach whereas others believe that an external approach is more desirable. Each surgeon must become familiar with all technique options in order to address the wide variety of challenges of rhinoplasty surgery.

The goal of this chapter is to give a broad overview of the diagnosis and treatment of nasal deformities. It is by no means exhaustive because multiple textbook volumes have been written on this subject. The reader should gain an understanding of nasal anatomy and determine how to systematically analyze the nose. Both endonasal and external rhinoplasty are described.

NASAL ANATOMY

A clear understanding of nasal anatomy is important to successfully perform nasal procedures and decrease the incidence of complications.

Surface Anatomy

The terms used to describe the surface anatomy of the nose are important in nasal form analysis and for treatment plan formulation (Table 66-1). For descriptive purposes, the spatial relationships are described as cephalic, caudal, dorsal, basal, anterior, posterior, superior, and inferior (Figure 66-1).

Skin and Soft Tissue

The soft tissue that overlies the bone and cartilage may influence the final result of rhinoplasty. The thickness of the skin will determine how it will redrape after performing a rhinoplasty. The skin thickness varies along the dorsum of the nose. The skin is fairly thick and mobile in the region of the nasion. It quickly thins over the nasal dorsum and is generally thinnest and most mobile in the middorsal region (rhinion). In the distal third of the nose, the skin tends to be more thick and adherent and has an increased sebaceous content.

A patient with thin skin will show dramatic changes with alteration of the underlying bone and cartilage, and this limits room for error because little is camouflaged by the thickness of the skin. Conversely, for thick-skinned individuals, more aggressive sculpturing of the nasal skeleton must be performed in order to effect significant changes. Although thick skin may mask imperfections, it does not redrape as well and can result in underlying fibrosis and formation of a polybeak deformity (supratip scarring). Better results are possible with thin-skinned patients; however, the margin for

TABLE 66-1. **Surface Anatomy of the Nose**

Glabella: the most forward projecting point of the forehead in the midline at the level of the supraorbital ridges.

Radix: the junction between the frontal bone and the dorsum of the nose.

Rhinion: the anterior tip at the end of the suture of the nasal bones.

Dorsum: the anterior surface of the nose formed by the nasal bones and the upper lateral cartilages.

Supratip break: the slight depression in the nasal profile at the point where the nasal dorsum joins the lobule of the nasal tip.

Infratip lobule: the portion of the tip lobule that is found between the tip-defining points and the columellar-lobular angle.

Tip-defining points: there are four tip defining points: the supratip break, the columellar-lobular angle, and the most projected area on each side of the nasal tip formed by the lower lateral cartilages.

Alar sidewall: the rounded eminence forming the lateral nostril wall.

Alar-facial junction: the depressed groove formed on the face where the ala joins the face.

Columella: the skin that separates the nostrils at the base of the nose.

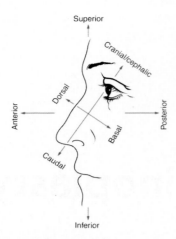

error is smaller. The surgeon must sometimes modify the technique depending on the type of skin of the patient.

Superficial Musculoaponeurotic System and Nasal Musculature

The muscles of the nose are encased in the nasal superficial musculoaponeurotic system (SMAS). This is a fibromuscular layer that separates the skin and subcutaneous tissue from the nasal cartilage and bone. The SMAS of the nose is in continuity with the SMAS of the face. During rhinoplastic surgery, the dissection is performed beneath the SMAS. Violating the SMAS will often result in increased bleeding, scarring, and postoperative edema.

The muscles of the nose can be divided into four categories: the elevators, the depressors, the compressors, and the dilators (Figure 66-2). The muscles of significance are the paired depressor septi nasi. These muscles can result in drooping of the nasal tip during smiling. This added tension on the nasal tip must be recognized preoperatively and addressed by resection in order to achieve a cosmetic result.[1]

Blood Supply

There is a rich blood supply to the subdermal vascular plexus of the nose that arises from branches of both the internal and the external carotid arteries. The blood supply from the internal carotid artery that supplies the external nose includes the dorsal nasal artery and the external nasal artery. The dorsal nasal artery is a branch of the ophthalmic artery. The external nasal artery is a branch of the anterior ethmoid artery.

The external nose is also supplied by branches of the facial artery and the internal maxillary artery, which originate from the external carotid artery. The facial artery branches include the angular artery, lateral nasal artery, alar artery, septal artery, and superior labial artery (Figure 66-3).

The internal nose is supplied by the internal and external carotid branches. The ophthalmic artery, a branch of the internal carotid, branches into the anterior and posterior

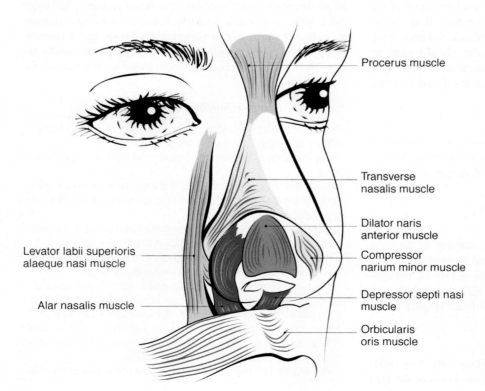

Procerus muscle

Transverse nasalis muscle

Dilator naris anterior muscle

Compressor narium minor muscle

Depressor septi nasi muscle

Orbicularis oris muscle

Levator labii superioris alaeque nasi muscle

Alar nasalis muscle

FIGURE 66-2. Nasal musculature. The muscles of the nose are grouped into the elevators (light blue), the depressors (dark blue), the compressors (light gray), and the dilators (dark gray). (Adapted from Jewett B. Anatomic considerations. In Baker SR, editor. Principles of Nasal Reconstruction. St. Louis: Mosby; 2002; p. 17.)

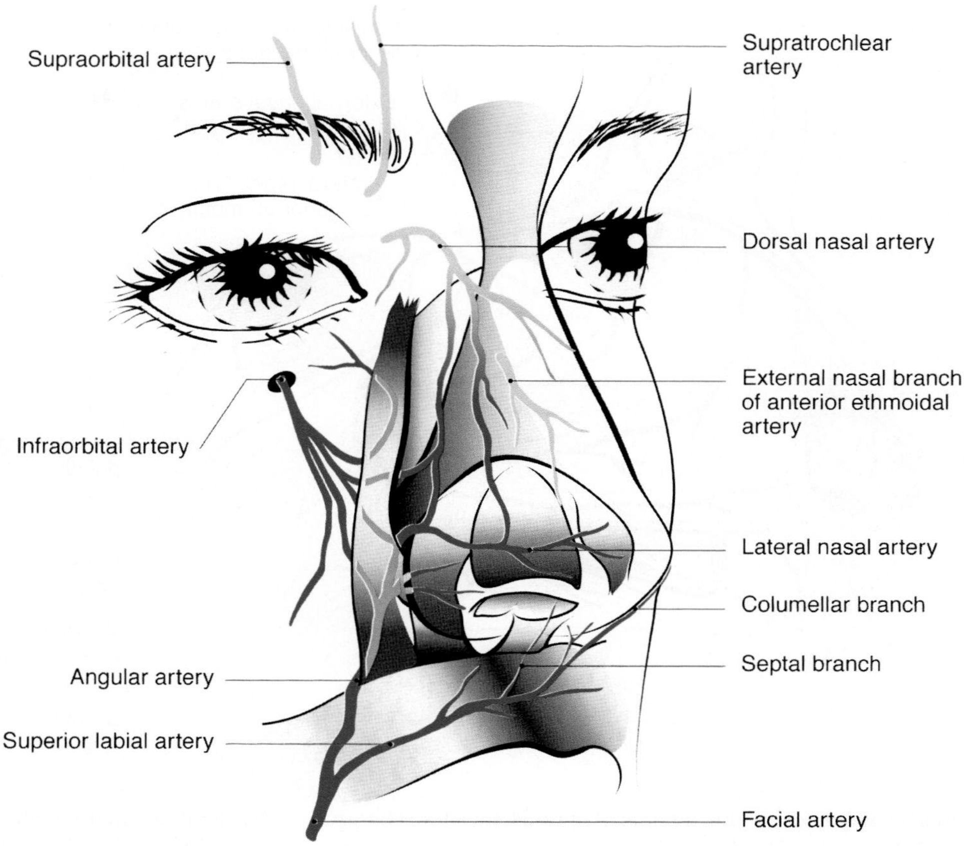

FIGURE 66-3. Arteries of the external nose. The arterial supply of the external nose comes from branches of the external carotid artery *(dark blue)* and the internal carotid artery *(light blue)*. (Adapted from Jewett B. Anatomic considerations. In Baker SR, editor. Principles of Nasal Reconstruction. St. Louis: Mosby; 2002; p. 18.)

ethmoidal arteries. The anterior ethmoidal artery supplies the anterosuperior part of the septum and the lateral nasal wall. The posterior ethmoid artery supplies the septum, lateral nasal wall, and superior turbinate.[2]

The internal maxillary artery branches include the sphenopalatine artery and the greater palatine artery. The sphenopalatine artery supplies most of the posterior part of the nasal septum, lateral wall of the nose, roof, and part of the nasal floor. The greater palatine artery supplies a portion of the anterior and inferior portion of the nasal septum (Figure 66-4).[2]

The surgically significant area for internal nasal bleeding is known as *Kiesselbach's plexus* (also termed *Little's area)*. This is the area in the anteroinferior part of the nasal septum that is a common site of epistaxis. It is where the sphenopalatine, greater palatine, superior labial artery, and anterior ethmoid arteries anastamose (Figure 66-5).[2] The venous drainage of the nose is primarily from the facial and ophthalmic veins.

One concern during nasal surgery is the possibility of compromised blood flow to the nasal tip if the surgeon performs an external rhinoplasty. The blood supply to the nasal tip has been analyzed by lymphoscintigraphic studies, cadaver dissections, and histologic sections.[3,4] The conclusion is that the primary blood supply to the nasal tip comes from the bilateral lateral nasal arteries that course in a plane superficial to the alar cartilages in the subdermal plexus approximately 2 to 3 mm above the alar groove. Thus, a

columellar incision does not compromise tip blood supply. Also, there are no significant veins and minimal lymphatics in the columellar region.[3,4] Some surgeons believe that external rhinoplasty remains more edematous for longer postoperative periods than an endonasal rhinoplasty.

Bone and Cartilage

The structure of the nose consists of the paired nasal bones as well as the frontal process of the maxilla. The bone is thickest near the junction with the frontal bone and tapers as it joins with the upper lateral cartilages.

The upper lateral cartilages are in intimate contact with the nasal bones and underlie the nasal bones for approximately 6 to 8 mm. The connection between the nasal bones and the upper lateral cartilages should not be violated because this may disrupt the internal nasal valve, causing nasal obstruction and asymmetry. The internal nasal valve is formed by the junction of the upper lateral cartilages and the nasal septum.

The lower lateral cartilages compose the lower third of the nose and connect to the upper lateral cartilages in a union described as the *scroll*. There are various configurations of the scroll.[5,6] The scroll is described as interlocked (52%), overlapping (20%), end to end (17%), or opposed (11%) (Figure 66-6). The scroll provides significant support to the nasal tip. When performing an endonasal rhinoplasty, this

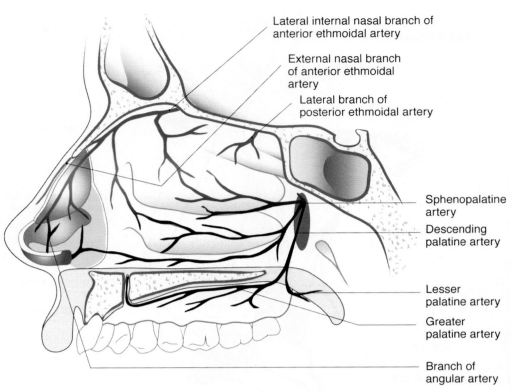

Lateral internal nasal branch of anterior ethmoidal artery

External nasal branch of anterior ethmoidal artery

Lateral branch of posterior ethmoidal artery

Sphenopalatine artery

Descending palatine artery

Lesser palatine artery

Greater palatine artery

Branch of angular artery

FIGURE 66-4. Arteries of the lateral nasal wall. The arterial supply of the lateral nasal wall arises from branches of the external carotid artery *(black)* and the internal carotid artery *(blue)*. (Adapted from Jewett B. Anatomic considerations. In Baker SR, editor. Principles of Nasal Reconstruction. St. Louis: Mosby; 2002; p. 23.)

area is violated by the intercartilaginous incision (Figures 66-7 to 66-9). The lower lateral cartilage is divided into medial and lateral crura. The medial crura are in intimate contact with the nasal septum and provide tip support. The lateral crura extend superiorly and form dense fibroareolar tissue attachments with the pyriform aperture. The intermediate crus is the diverging of the medial crus before turning to become the lateral crus proper. The highest point of the intermediate crus is an important surgical landmark known as the *tip-defining point* (Figure 66-10).

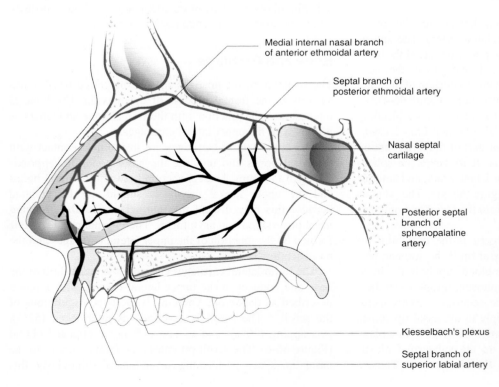

Medial internal nasal branch of anterior ethmoidal artery

Septal branch of posterior ethmoidal artery

Nasal septal cartilage

Posterior septal branch of sphenopalatine artery

Kiesselbach's plexus

Septal branch of superior labial artery

FIGURE 66-5. Arteries of the nasal septum. The arterial supply of the nasal septum arises from branches of the external carotid artery *(black)* and the internal carotid artery *(blue)*. Kiesselbach's plexus is formed by the sphenopalatine artery, greater palatine artery, superior labial artery, and anterior ethmoid arteries. It is a common site of epistaxis. (Adapted from Jewett B. Anatomic considerations. In Baker SR, editor. Principles of Nasal Reconstruction. St. Louis: Mosby; 2002; p. 23.)

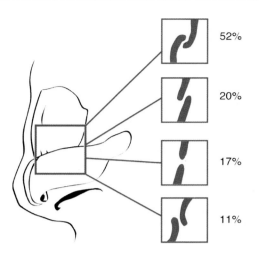

52%

20%

17%

11%

Various configurations of the scroll

FIGURE 66-6. Configurations of the scroll. The relationship of the upper lateral and lower lateral cartilages is termed the scroll. Anatomic studies have identified four common configurations: interlocked (52%), overlapping (20%), end to end (17%), and opposed (11%). (Adapted from Lam SM, Williams LE. Anatomic considerations in aesthetic rhinoplasty. Facial Plast Surg 2002;18:209–214.)

The nasal septum is formed by both bone and cartilage. The ethmoid and vomer provide bony support posteriorly. The quadrangular cartilage provides support anteriorly (Figure 66-11).

Support for the nasal tip is classified into major and minor divisions. The major tip support comes from the size, shape, and strength of the lower lateral cartilages, the attachment of the medial crura of the lower lateral cartilage to the caudal septum, and the fibrous attachment of the lower lateral cartilage to the upper lateral cartilage. The minor tip support comes from the nasal spine, the membranous septum, the

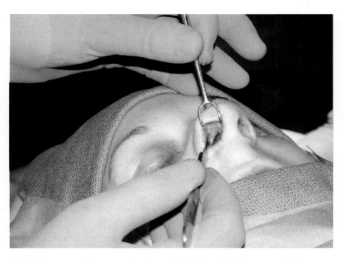

FIGURE 66-8. Intercartilaginous incision. The intercartilaginous incision, between the upper and the lower cartilage, allows access to the nasal dorsum. Note the incision does not violate the nasal valve.

cartilaginous dorsum, the sesamoid complexes, the interdomal ligaments, and the alar attachments to the skin (Table 66-2).[5]

Nerves

The sensory nerve supply to the skin of the external nose is provided by the ophthalmic and maxillary divisions of the trigeminal nerve. Branches of the supratrochlear and infratrochlear nerves supply the skin in the region of the radix and rhinion. The lower half of the nose is supplied by the infraorbital nerve and the external nasal branch of the anterior ethmoidal nerve (a branch of the nasociliary nerve that arises

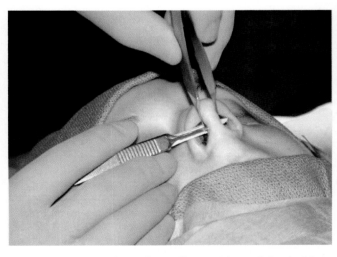

FIGURE 66-7. Partial transfixion. The partial transfixion incision through the membranous septum and short of the medial crural foot pads.

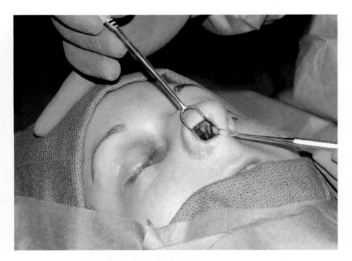

FIGURE 66-9. Connecting intercartilaginous and partial transfixion incisions. The intercartilaginous incision extends along the upper edge of the lateral crus to connect with the transfixion incision. This will provide access for a septoplasty during internal rhinoplasty.

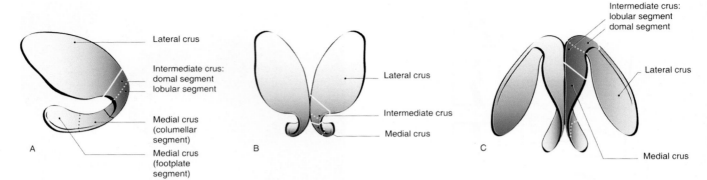

FIGURE 66-10. **A–C,** Anatomy of the lower lateral cartilages. The lower lateral cartilages are often described as having a lateral crus, a medial crus, and an intermediate crus. The intermediate crus is the most projected portion of the lower lateral cartilages and these form two of the tip-defining points seen on nasal tip analysis. **(A–C,** Adapted from Jewett B. Anatomic considerations. In: Baker SR, editor. Principles of Nasal Reconstruction. St. Louis: Mosby; 2002; p. 21.)

from the ophthalmic branch of the trigeminal nerve) (Figure 66-12).

The main sensory nerve supply to the nasal septum comes from the internal nasal nerve (a branch of the anterior ethmoidal nerve) and the nasopalatine nerve (Figure 66-13). The lateral nasal wall sensation is supplied by the anterior ethmoidal nerve, branches of the pterygopalatine ganglion, branches of the greater palatine nerve, the infraorbital nerve, and the anterior superior alveolar nerve.

Parasympathetic innervation is derived from branches of the pterygopalatine ganglion, which are derived from cranial nerve VII. Some sympathetic branches reach the nasal cavity via the nasociliary nerve.[2,7]

Nasal Valve

The airflow through the nose is regulated by the internal and external nasal valves. The external nasal valve comprises the lower lateral cartilage and the nasal septum and floor. Collapse of the external nasal valve can sometimes be noted when the nares become occluded on even gentle inspiration. This problem is seen in patients with narrow nostrils, a projecting nasal tip, and thin alar sidewalls. External nasal valve collapse is usually seen in patients who have had previous rhinoplasty surgery and excessive trimming of the cephalic portion of the lower lateral cartilages. It is also seen with increased age and in facial nerve paralysis. The external nasal valve collapse can be corrected by deprojecting the overprojected nose, realigning the lateral crura into a more caudal orientation, and placing alar batten grafts to provide structural support and prevent collapse.[8]

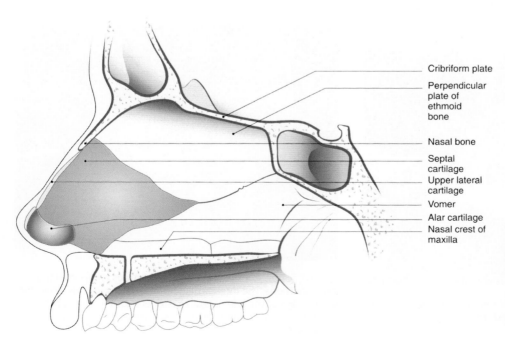

FIGURE 66-11. Anatomy of the nasal septum. The nasal septum is composed of the perpendicular plate of the ethmoid, the vomer, and the quadrangular cartilage. (Adapted from Jewett B. Anatomic considerations. In Baker SR, editor. Principles of Nasal Reconstruction. St. Louis: Mosby; 2002; p. 22.)

TABLE 66-2. **Tip Support Mechanisms**

The three major tip support mechanisms are
1. The size, shape, and strength of the lower lateral cartilages.
2. The attachment of the medial crura to the caudal septum..
3. The attachment of the lower lateral cartilages to the upper lateral cartilages.

The minor tip support mechanisms are

1. The interdomal ligament.
2. The sesamoid complex extending the support of the lateral crura to the piriform aperture.
3. The attachment of the alar cartilages to the overlying skin.
4. Cartilaginous septal dorsum.
5. Nasal spine.
6. The membranous septum.

The internal nasal valve is formed by the junction of the septum with the upper lateral cartilages. The angle formed should be a minimum of 10 to 15 degrees to maintain patency. Deviation of the nasal septum or separation of the upper lateral cartilages from the nasal bones can lead to obstruction. This problem is also seen after rhinoplasty if the patient has had weakening of the upper and lower lateral cartilages. These patients often have a pinched appearance in the supra-alar region. The Cottle test is used to evaluate obstruction at the internal valve by using a finger to distract the check and lateral wall of the nose, thereby opening the valve. If nasal airflow is dramatically improved, then the internal valve may require correction. These patients often have symptomatic relief by the use of external taping devices. Surgical correction involves the placement of spreader grafts

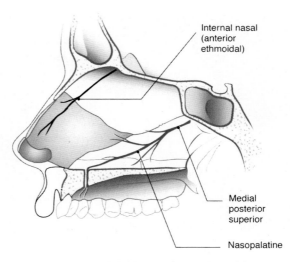

FIGURE 66-13. Sensory nerves of the nasal septum. The main sensory nerve supply comes from the internal nasal nerve (a branch of the anterior ethmoidal nerve V1 *(black)* and the nasopalatine nerve V2 *(blue)*. (Adapted from Jewett B. Anatomic considerations. In Baker SR, editor. Principles of Nasal Reconstruction. St. Louis: Mosby; 2002; p. 19.)

between the septum and the upper lateral cartilages to increase the angle at this junction.[8–10]

COSMETIC EVALUATION

The cosmetic evaluation begins in the same way as with any examination, by eliciting the chief complaint of the patient. The patient should be given a mirror and a cotton-tipped applicator to point out specific cosmetic concerns. Following this, a thorough medical history should be obtained. Specific attention should be directed toward obtaining a history of nasal trauma, nasal obstruction, previous nasal surgery, and medications (including over-the-counter and herbal medications).

Psychiatric Stability

In addition to analyzing the nose, the surgeon needs to assess whether the patient is psychologically prepared for a cosmetic procedure. Patients should have realistic expectations and motivations. A patient who is internally motivated (e.g., wishes to improve self-esteem) to have the procedure is a better candidate than one who desires the procedure for external reasons (e.g., spouse wants them to have it done).[11,12]

The surgeon should beware of patients who are indecisive, rude, uncooperative, or depressed, who have unrealistic expectations, or who have significant personality disorders because they may never be satisfied. Other warning signs of poor patients are those who overly flatter, are talkative, consider themselves to be a very important patient, have minimal or no deformity, are surgeon shoppers, are price hagglers, or are involved in litigation. Most importantly, do not operate on a patient that you do not like.[11–14]

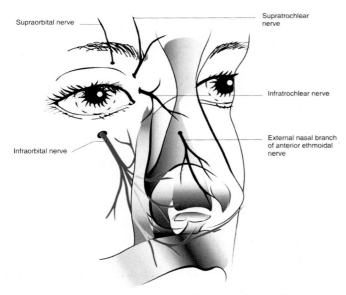

FIGURE 66-12. Sensory nerves of the external nose. The sensory innervation of the nose is derived from the V1 (ophthalmic: *black)* and from V2 (maxillary: *blue)* divisions of the trigeminal nerve. (Adapted from Jewett B. Anatomic considerations. In Baker SR, editor. Principles of Nasal Reconstruction. St. Louis: Mosby; 2002; p. 19.)

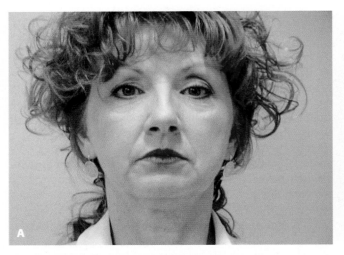
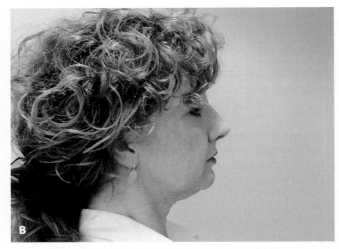
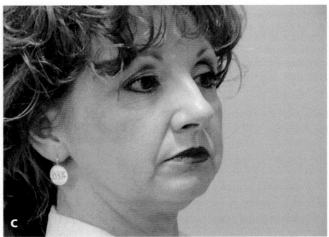
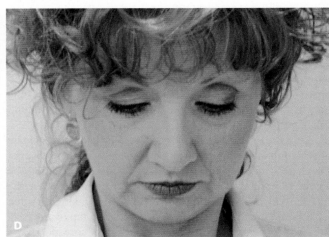

FIGURE 66-14.   Preoperative rhinoplasty. **A,** Preoperative frontal view shows the width of the nose and alar base. **B,** Preoperative lateral view shows the nasal profile and dorsum in relation to the nasofrontal angle and nasolabial angle. **C,** Preoperative three quarter, or oblique, view is most natural and often revealing for harmony of the orbital rims and gull wings that flow into the nasal dorsum. **D,** Preoperative basal view is taken either from above or from below the patient and is a good view of tip and base morphology.

General Facial Analysis

Before performing a specific analysis of the nose, a global assessment of the face and its proportions should be done. Refer to Chapter 53 for additional information on facial analysis in orthognathic surgery.

Nasal Analysis

The nasal examination should be performed in a systematic manner so that the proper diagnosis is obtained (Figures 66-14 and 66-15).

GENERAL ASSESSMENT

Skin

The skin should be assessed for its thickness, mobility, and sebaceous gland content. Any pigmentations or scars should also be noted. Thick skin does not redrape well after rhinoplasty.

Symmetry

Any gross asymmetries in all views should be noted.

Lateral View
NASOFRONTAL ANGLE

The *nasofrontal angle* is defined as the angle formed by lines that are tangential to the glabella and the nasal dorsum and intersect through the radix as seen on a profile view. The normal angle is between 125 and 135 degrees (Figure 66-16).

The position of the radix should then be assessed in terms of its anteroposterior and vertical positions from a profile view. The radix should lie in a vertical plane somewhere between the lash line and the supratarsal folds. In addition, it should be 4 to 9 mm anterior to the corneal plane (see Figure 66-16).

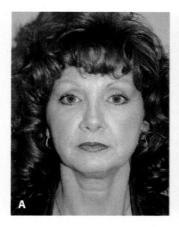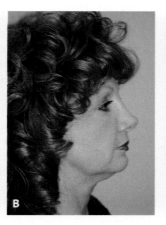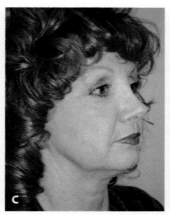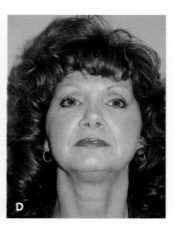

FIGURE 66-15. Postoperative rhinoplasty. **A,** Postoperative frontal view shows the change in the width of the nose. This is the patient's most critical analysis. **B,** Postoperative lateral view shows the change in dorsal reduction and tip position. **C,** Postoperative three quarter, or oblique, view demonstrates the symmetry and graceful balance of the nose with the face. **D,** Postoperative basal view shows the width of the nose and any tip deviation from the dorsal midline.

NASAL DORSUM

In women, the nasal dorsum should lie approximately 2 mm posterior to a line drawn from the radix to the nasal tip. In men, the nasal dorsum should lie on this line or slightly in front of it (see Figure 66-16).

The length of the nose (radix to tip) can be measured clinically or on photographs taken during the initial examination. The ideal nasal length should approximate the distance from stomion to menton if the lower facial height is proportionate to the middle facial height (glabella to subnasale). If the lower face height is not proportionate, it is best to estimate the nasal length as 0.67 times the middle facial height.

NASAL TIP DEFINITION

The nose should have four tip-defining points that when drawn on the nose in the frontal view appear as two equilateral triangles (Figure 66-17). These points include the

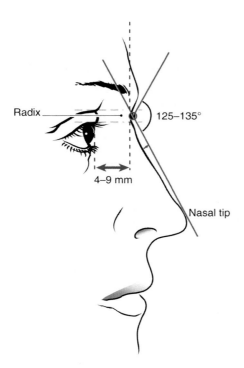

FIGURE 66-16. Position of the nasal dorsum and radix. The nasal dorsum is typically 2 mm behind a line drawn from the radix to nasal tip in women. In men, the nasal dorsum typically lies on this line. The radix should lie between the upper eyelid margin and the supratarsal folds in a vertical plane and approximately 4 to 9 mm anterior to the corneal plane. (Adapted from Austermann K. Rhinoplasty: planning techniques and complications. In Booth PW, Hausamen JE, editors. Maxillofacial Surgery. New York: Churchill Livingstone; 1999; p. 1380.)

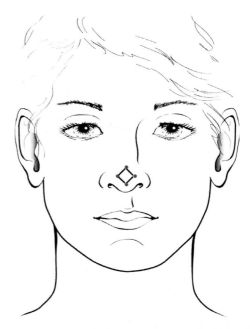

FIGURE 66-17. Nasal tip-defining points. A nose should have four tip-defining points. These are defined by the supratip, columellar-lobular angle, and the tip-defining points of each intermediate crus of the lower lateral cartilages.

SECTION 8

supratip break, the columellar-lobular angle, and the two tip-defining points (the most projected portion of the nasal tip).

NASAL TIP PROJECTION

Nasal tip projection can be defined as the distance that the tip (pronasale) projects anterior in the facial plane.[15] Perception of nasal tip projection can be influenced by may factors: upper lip length, nasolabial angle, nasofrontal angle, dorsal hump, and chin projection. There are several methods to determine whether the nasal tip projection is adequate. Most cosmetic rhinoplasty procedures are designed to preserve tip projection.

The simplest method to remember is Simons' method, which states that the lip-to-tip ratio is 1:1. Essentially the length of the upper lip (from subnasale to labrale superioris) should equal the nasal projection (measured from subnasale to pronasale). This method may be invalid because of the wide variation in lip lengths.[16]

The Goode method is another way of determining nasal projection. Using the Goode method, a line is drawn from the radix to the nasal tip. A second line is drawn from the radix to the alar columellar junction. A third line is drawn perpendicular to this and passes through the nasal tip. Goode's analysis states that if the nasofacial angle is between 36 and 40 degrees, then the length of the perpendicular line passing through the nasal tip should be 0.55 to 0.6 of the length of the nasal dorsum (Figure 66-18).[16]

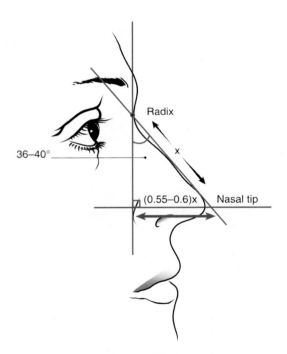

FIGURE 66-18. Goode's method of nasal projection. This method is sometimes used to determine adequacy of nasal projection. If the nasofrontal angle is between 36 degrees and 40 degrees, then the length of a perpendicular line through the nasal tip should be 0.55 to 0.6 the length of the nasal dorsum. x = nasal length. (Adapted from Austermann K, Rhinoplasty: planning techniques and complications. In Booth PW, Hausamen JE, editors. Maxillofacial Surgery. New York: Churchill Livingstone; 1999; p. 1380.)

Gunter and Rohrich[17] describe another technique of assessing nasal tip projection. If the nasal dorsal length is appropriate, the tip projection should be 0.67 times the ideal nasal length. The ideal nasal length should be equal to the distance from stomion to menton or 1.6 times the distance from the nasal tip to stomion. The tip projection is measured from the alar facial junction to the nasal tip.[17] This method is subject to a great deal of facial variation.

In addition, a vertical line drawn from the most projected portion of the upper lip should divide the nose in two equal halves between the alar facial groove and the nasal tip. If the anterior portion is greater than 60%, then the nose is likely to be overprojected (Figure 66-19).[17]

NASAL TIP ROTATION

The nasal tip rotation is evaluated by the nasolabial angle and the columellar-lobular angle. *Nasolabial angle* is defined as the angle formed by lines that are tangential to the columella of the nose and the philtrum of the lip and intersect at the subnasale. In women, this should be approximately 95 to 110 degrees, whereas in men, this should be 90 to 95 degrees. Lip position may be dependent on tooth position. The *columellar-lobular angle* is defined as the angle formed by the intersection of a line tangential to the columella and a line tangential to the infratip lobule. This angle is normally between 30 and 45 degrees.

TIP SUPPORT

The strength of the cartilage in the tip of the nose is apparent when one presses on the tip. A nose with poor support may require cartilaginous struts to counteract the inherently weakened tip from the rhinoplasty. The effect of facial animation

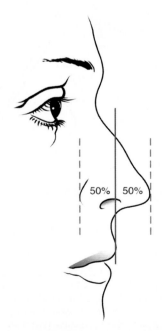

FIGURE 66-19. Nasal projection. A vertical line through the most projected part of the upper lip should divide the nose into two equal parts. If the nasal tip is greater than 60%, then the nose may be overprojected.

should also be noted. Some patients have overactive depressor septi nasi muscles, which result in a drooping nasal tip on smiling. The columella show on a lateral view should be 3 to 4 mm below the inferior alar rim.[13]

Frontal View

WIDTH OF NASAL DORSUM

The width of the nasal body and tip should be approximately 80% of the alar base width. This is assuming that the alar base is in proper anatomic proportions. The alar base width should approximate the intercanthal distance. If the width of the nasal dorsum is significantly greater than 80%, then lateral nasal osteotomies should be considered. The eyebrows should gracefully flow into the nasal dorsum analogous to a gull wing in flight.

The alar rims and columella should also be a gently curving line that appears as a bird in flight.

ALAR WIDTH

The alar base width should approximate the intercanthal distance. Seldom is the nasal width less than the intercanthal dimension.

Basal View

From a basal view, the columella-to-lobule ratio should be 2:1. Nostril size and shape should also be noted. An aesthetic nostril is teardrop-shaped, but there is a great amount of ethnic variation (Figure 66-20).

Oblique View

The oblique view is most natural and sometimes more revealing than standard photographs. It demonstrates the flow of subunits and facial harmony. The three-quarters view is how we usually see each other in routine interaction.

Functional Considerations

Although the patient desires cosmetic correction of the nose, the functional significance of the nose should be closely

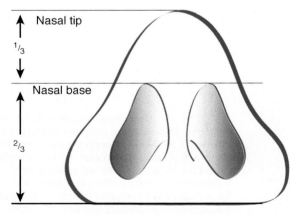

FIGURE 66-20.   Columella-to-lobule ratio. The columella-to-lobule ratio should be 2:1.

considered. Nasal airflow through both the internal and the external nasal valves should be evaluated. The septum should be evaluated for deviation and perforations. The septum is often a good site for harvesting autogenous cartilage for grafting. The turbinates should be evaluated for hypertrophy. Rhinoscopy with a nasal speculum can be performed both before and after the administration of a topical decongestant.

Photographs

The examination is not complete without standardized facial photographs. The standard facial photographs should include frontal, right, and left lateral views; right and left oblique views; and a high and low basal view. Close-up views are taken if warranted. The photographs are beneficial from a medicolegal standpoint, and they also allow the surgeon to study the nose in more detail and to develop a surgical plan.

ANESTHESIA

Proper anesthesia of the nose is important to ensure minimal distortion of the tissues as well as to provide adequate hemostasis. Before injecting the nose, cottonoids or cotton-tipped applicators soaked in 4% cocaine or oxymetazoline are placed in each nostril to constrict the mucous membranes of the turbinates. If the rhinoplasty is to be performed under sedation, cocaine is preferred because of its anesthetic properties. If the procedure is performed under general anesthesia, oxymetazoline is sufficient.

Three cottonoids are placed in each nostril: one along the middle turbinate, one along the superior nasal vault, and one along the inferomedial septum.

Local anesthesia is achieved with 2% lidocaine with 1:100,000 epinephrine. In an endonasal rhinoplasty, the following areas are injected:

- 0.5 mL deposited at the junction of each upper and lower lateral cartilage (intercartilaginous area)
- 0.5 mL deposited in the region of each marginal incision
- 3 mL along the nasal dorsum and lateral nasal bones (hugging periosteum)
- 1 mL along the nasal septum
- 0.5 mL at each alar base
- 1 mL at each infraorbital nerve
- 1 mL at the nasal tip

For external rhinoplasty, the following additional area is injected:

- 1 mL to the columella

INCISIONS/SEQUENCING

Multiple incision techniques are used to gain access to the cartilage and bone support of the nose.

Complete Transfixion

This incision provides access to the caudal septum, medial crura, and nasal spine. The incision is made with a no. 15 blade, beginning just caudal to the superior caudal end of the nasal septum. The incision extends inferiorly through the membranous septum, following the cephalic margin of the medial crura (Figure 66-21A; see also Figure 66-7). It results in ptosis and deprojection of the nose.

Partial Transfixion

This incision is similar to the complete transfixion incision except that it stops at the level of the medial footpads of the lower lateral cartilages. The advantage of this incision is that the attachments of the medial footpads of the lower lateral cartilages to the caudal septum are not disrupted (see Figures 66-7 and 66-21B).

Hemitransfixion

This incision is a complete transfixion incision that is performed on only one side of the membranous septum. It does not traverse both mucosal surfaces, and therefore, some attachments of the medial crura to the caudal septum are maintained. Access to the nasal septum is good with this incision; however, delivery of the lower lateral cartilage on the side opposite to the incision is difficult (see Figures 66-7 and 66-21C).

Killian Incision

This incision is seldom used in rhinoplasty. It is a useful incision to gain access to the nasal septum if only a septoplasty is to be performed. The incision is made several millimeters cephalad to the caudal edge of the septum. It can be extended onto the nasal floor if needed.

Intercartilaginous Incision

This incision is made at the junction of the upper and lower lateral cartilages. The nare is elevated superiorly with a double skin hook. A no. 15 blade should pass below the lower lateral cartilage and above the upper lateral cartilages. This incision is typically made after a transfixion incision. The

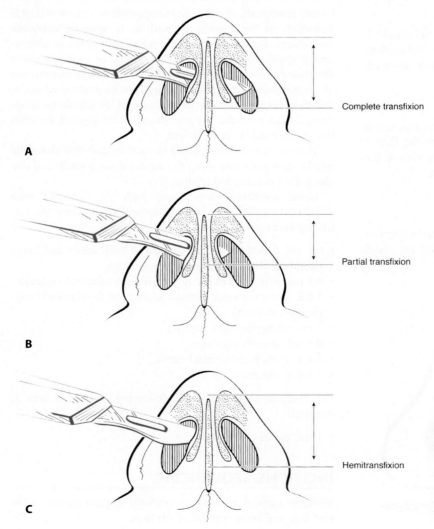

A

Complete transfixion

B

Partial transfixion

C

Hemitransfixion

FIGURE 66-21. Transfixion incisions. **A,** A complete transfixion incision is made caudal to both the medial crura and through the membranous septum. **B,** A partial transfixion incision is similar except the incision stops short of the medial footpads of the medial crura. **C,** A hemitransfixion incision is a complete transfixion incision that is performed on only one side; therefore, the other medial crura and footpad are not violated.

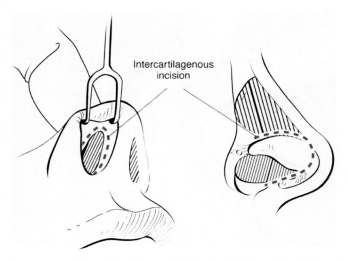

FIGURE 66-22.   Intercartilaginous incisions. The intercartilaginous incision is made at the junction of the upper and lower lateral cartilages. The blade should pass below the lower lateral and above the upper lateral cartilage. (Adapted from Alexander R. Fundamental terms, considerations, and approaches in rhinoplasty. In Waite PD, editor. Atlas of the Oral and Maxillofacial Surgery Clinics of North America: Rhinoplasty. Philadelphia: WB Saunders; 1995; p. 19.)

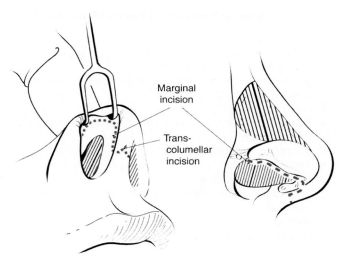

FIGURE 66-23.   Marginal incision. This incision is made parallel to the caudal edge of the lower lateral cartilage. This incision can be combined with bilateral intercartilaginous incisions for a cartilage delivery technique in endonasal rhinoplasty or combined with a transcolumellar incision for an external rhinoplasty. (Adapted from Alexander R. Fundamental terms, considerations, and approaches in rhinoplasty. In Waite PD, editor. Atlas of the Oral and Maxillofacial Surgery Clinics of North America: Rhinoplasty. Philadelphia: WB Saunders; 1995; p. 19.)

intercartilaginous incision is then connected to the transfixion incision (Figure 66-22; see also Figures 66-8 and 66-9).

Intracartilaginous Incision

This incision is made through both the vestibular nasal mucosa and a portion of the lower lateral cartilages. This incision is similar to the intercartilaginous incision except that it is made 3 to 5 mm posterior to the junction of the upper and lower lateral cartilages. This incision in effect performs a complete cephalic strip of the lower lateral cartilages without the need for delivering the cartilage. The disadvantage is that the lower lateral cartilage is not directly visualized and it may, therefore, be difficul to achieve symmetry between the right and the left sides.

Rim/Marginal Incision

This incision parallels the caudal edges of the lower lateral cartilages. The incision is used in combination with an intercartilaginous incision in an endonasal rhinoplasty. The two incisions allow the lower lateral cartilage to be delivered and visualized. This allows the surgeon to more accurately trim the cartilage if needed. In an open rhinoplasty, this incision is combined with a transcolumellar incision in order to gain access to the lower lateral cartilage and nasal dorsum (Figure 66-23).

Transcolumellar Incision

This incision is made through the thinnest portion of the columella at a level just superior to the flaring of the medial

crura. The incision can be made with a notched V in the center of the columella or as a "stair step." This will break up the scar and assist in closure. This incision is connected with a marginal incision bilaterally for open rhinoplasty (see Figure 66-23).

The two principle techniques are the endonasal and external rhinoplasty. Each of these techniques are described in general terms, in the order in which the authors perform them. Other surgeons may perform the sequence in a different order (Tables 66-3 and 66-4).

SEPTOPLASTY

In rhinoplasty surgery, there are several reasons to access the nasal septum: (1) to correct nasal airflow obstruction, (2) to

TABLE 66-3. **Surgical Sequence for Endonasal Rhinoplasty**

1. Local anesthesia
2. Partial transfixion incision (see Figure 66-7)
3. Intercartilaginous incision (join with partial transfixion) (see Figures 66-8, 66-9, 66-21, and 66-22)
4. Septoplasty (if needed) (see Figures 66-24 and 66-25)
5. Dorsal reduction (see Figures 66-28 to 66-30)
6. Lateral nasal osteotomies (see Figure 66-31)
7. Marginal incision (see Figure 66-23)
8. Delivery of lower lateral cartilages (see Figure 66-37)
9. Tip modification (i.e., cephalic strips/cartilage grafting/suture techniques)
10. Alar base modification (see Figure 66-41)
11. Closure, taping, and splinting

TABLE 66-4. **Surgical Sequence for External Rhinoplasty**

1. Local anesthesia
2. Bilateral marginal incisions (see Figure 66-23)
3. Columellar incision (see Figure 66-23)
4. Skeletonization of upper and lower lateral cartilages and nasal dorsum
5. Dorsal reduction
6. Dome division if access is needed to the septum for septoplasty or graft harvest
7. Septoplasty (if needed)
8. Turbinate reduction
9. Lateral nasal osteotomies
10. Tip modification (i.e., cephalic strips/cartilage grafting/suture techniques)
11. Alar base modification
12. Closure, taping, and splinting

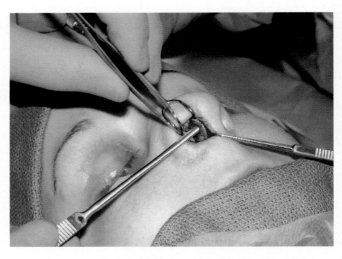

FIGURE 66-25.   Elevation of mucoperichondrium. The Cottle elevator is specifically designed to elevate the nasal envelope without perforation.

assist in the correction of asymmetries, and (3) to harvest cartilage for tip grafting.

Access to the nasal septum in an endonasal approach is through a partial-transfixion incision, which is connected to bilateral intercartilaginous incisions. The partial-transfixion incision can be extended to the nasal floor on the side on which the septoplasty is to be performed. After completing the incisions, the caudal aspect of the nasal septum is exposed by dissecting the mucoperichondrium from one side. Two tunnels will be developed, one superior and the other inferior, that will ultimately be joined so that wide exposure of the septum is obtained.[18] Intially sharp dissection is done with a no. 15 blade or scissors to expose a portion of the caudal septum. The perichondrium is gently scored using a no. 15 blade. A dental amalgam condenser is then used in a sweeping motion to develop a plane between the perichondrium and the nasal septum (Figure 66-24). Once this plane of dissection is started, a Freer or Cottle elevator can be used to complete the septal envelope (Figure 66-25). The muco-

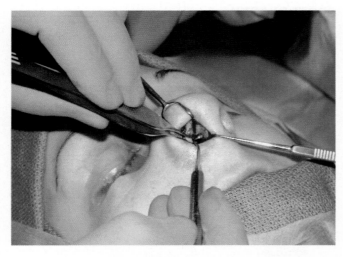

FIGURE 66-24.   Identifying perichondrium. The perichondrium is elevated with a dental amalgam condenser. One will notice a slight blue-gray cartilage and a distinct plane of dissection.

perichondrium is tightly bound at the junction of the septum and the maxillary crest.

Once the septum is exposed, it can be treated in one of four ways: (1) resection, (2) morselization, (3) segmental transection, and (4) swinging door flaps.[18] Submucosal resection allows a significant portion of cartilage to be harvested for grafting. At least 1 cm should be maintained superiorly and anteriorly in an L-shaped configuration to provide support for the nose (Figure 66-26). In order to resect the cartilage, a Cottle elevator is used to cut the cartilage. Fomon scissors may be used to make the superior and inferior cuts through the bony septum. The cartilage can also be removed with a Ballenger swivel blade. If no cartilage is needed for the rhinoplasty, the resected cartilage can be morselized and replaced. Morselization can be performed in situ. Another technique for aligning the septum is through a segmental transection. In this technique, the mucoperichondrium is elevated on one side of the septum. Cross-hatching with a no. 15 blade is performed to weaken the cartilage (Figure 66-27). The mucoperichondrium on the other side of the septum provides support. Some 4-0 gut mattress sutures can be positioned through the septum to assist in realignment. A septal splint is placed for 1 week. Finally, a swinging door type flap can be used to reposition a large segment of flat cartilage that is improperly angulated. The mucoperichondrium is elevated on one side. Through and through incisions are made on either side of the deviated cartilage. The cartilage is also separated from the maxillary crest so that it can hinge into a more normal position. Septal splints may be required for 1 week. In all septal procedures, a 4-0 gut on a straight needle is routinely used to perform a mattress suture through the septum and mucosa. This decreases the likelihood of a septal hematoma formation and circumvents the need for nasal packs.

Tears in the septal mucosa are not uncommon. However, it is not problematic as long as the tears are only on one side of the septum. Unilateral tears require no elaborate closure.

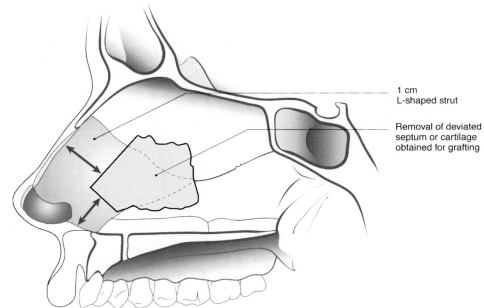

1 cm
L-shaped strut

Removal of deviated
septum or cartilage
obtained for grafting

FIGURE 66-26.   Resection of cartilage/bone from the nasal septum. This may be done to harvest cartilage for grafting procedures or for removal of grossly deviated septum. It is important to maintain 1 cm dorsally and caudally for nasal support.

If the tear is through and through, at least one side should be closed. This is best done with a 5-0 chromic gut suture.

TURBINECTOMY

Although the focus of this chapter is the cosmetic rhinoplasty, some mention needs to be made on maintaining function. Inferior turbinate hypertrophy is a problem that can result in nasal obstruction after cosmetic rhinoplasty, if the problem is not recognized preoperatively Hypertrophy of the inferior turbinates is the most common cause of nasal airway obstruction.[19,20] Hypertrophy can be caused by numerous factors. Most commonly, it is related to allergic symptoms. Hypertrophy caused by allergy should be managed medically with antihistamines and topical corticosteroids. If this fails, surgical management can be considered.[21] In cases of a

deviated nasal septum, the turbinate on the side at which the nasal passage is enlarged can become hypertrophic with time. In patients with anatomic enlargement of the turbinate, the problem needs to be recognized so that the nasal passage does not become obstructed when the septum is straightened.

Management of inferior turbinate hypertrophy is controversial and outside the scope of this chapter. The surgical procedures used to treat this problem have included corticosteroid injection, turbinate outfracture, electrocautery, cryosurgery, laser reduction, partial turbinate resection, total turbinate resection, submucous turbinate resection, and vidian neurectomy[20-24] Each of these procedures has various advantages and disadvantages; the procedure chosen depends on the patient. The most common complications from turbinate surgery are hemorrhage, atrophic rhinitis, and ozena.

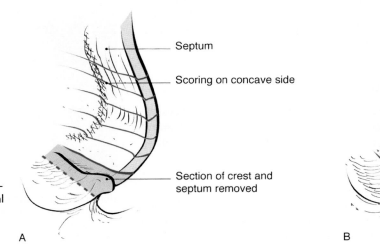

Septum

Scoring on concave side

Section of crest and
septum removed

FIGURE 66-27.   Septal repositioning. A deviated nasal septum can be repositioned by removing the obstruction inferiorly (A) and cross-hatching the cartilage to allow the deviated portion to be repositioned (B). (A and B, Adapted from Robinson RC. Functional septorhinoplasty. In Waite PD, editor. Atlas of the Oral and Maxillofacial Surgery Clinics of North America: Rhinoplasty. Philadelphia: WB Saunders; 1995; p. 35.)

A

B

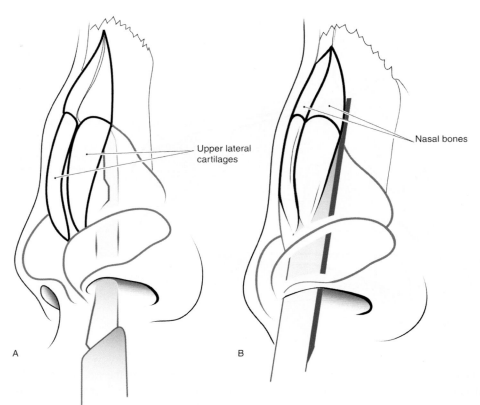

A   B

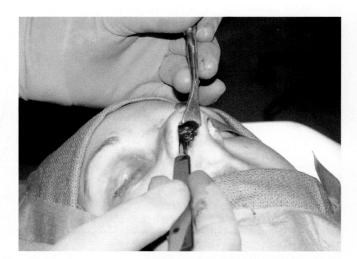

FIGURE 66-28. Removal of a dorsal hump. **A,** The dorsal hump is removed by first using a scalpel to incise through the upper lateral cartilages. **B,** Next, a Rubin osteotome is used to reduce the bony prominence. Care is needed to keep the osteotome from being directed too far posteriorly thereby overreducing the dorsum. **(A** and **B,** Adapted from Austermann K, Rhinoplasty: planning techniques and complications. In Booth PW, Hausamen JE, editors. Maxillofacial Surgery. New York: Churchill Livingstone; 1999; p. 1389.)

NASAL DORSUM

Reduction

One of the most dramatic changes that can be achieved in rhinoplasty surgery is correction of a dorsal hump. There are many ways to remove the hump. Some surgeons use a scalpel and osteotome; others use rasps; and a few use power rasps. The authors recommend to first incise the cartilaginous convexity below the nasal bones and then to use a Rubin osteotome to remove the bony hump (Figures 66-28 to 66-31). Care must be taken to keep the osteotome directed superficially, because it can deflect downward and result in overreduction. After removing the gross hump, sequential rasping can be used for refinement. After removal of any significant dorsal hump, the patient is left with an open roof deformity. This must be closed with lateral nasal osteotomies (see Figure 66-31).

Augmentation

Augmentation is indicated when there has been excessive reduction from previous rhinoplasty or from a post-traumatic defect. Several techniques are used to augment the nasal dorsum.

Autogenous Augmentation

In the setting of acute trauma, cranial bone grafts can be used to provide support. These are cantilevered off the frontal bone with a miniplate. The graft must be properly shaped so that it provides support but does not distort the shape of the nose.[25–27] Rib cartilage can also be harvested for augmentation of the nasal dorsum. Silicone sizers can be used to estimate the size and shape of graft needed. Once the graft is harvested, a 0.035-inch K-wire can be placed in the center of the graft to stabilize it. Rib grafts have a tendency to distort with time and the K-wire may help limit this tendency.[28]

FIGURE 66-29. Dorsal reduction. An Aufricht retractor lifts the dorsal drape and can protect the skin during hump reduction. A no. 15 blade is used to incise the cartilaginous dorsum. Working through this incision, an osteotome or rasp is used to reduce the bone of the dorsum.

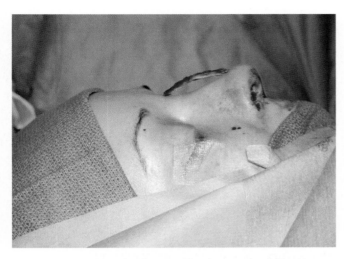

FIGURE 66-30.   Dorsal reduction. The dorsum should be about two thirds of the cartilage and one third of the bone.

For a less aggressive augmentation, autogenous cartilage harvested from the nasal septum can be used. This can be layered and sutured together. It is then placed through traditional rhinoplasty incisions.[29–31]

Alloplastic Augmentation

Another technique is to use cadaveric dermis along the nasal dorsum. The advantage here is that no harvesting is required and the material is pliable. However, the resorption of this material is unpredictable. Other implantable materials include silicone and expanded polytetrafluoroethylene (ePTFE) implants. These can be contoured to the appropriate size intraoperatively. The issue with implants is that the grafts can extrude or become infected. Meticulous placement is essential.[31–34]

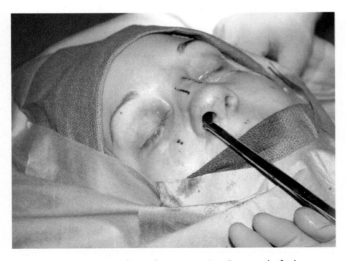

FIGURE 66-31.   Lateral nasal osteotomies. Removal of a large dorsal hump will often leave a flat open roof deformity; this can be reduced by lateral nasal osteotomies with an invert chisel saw, or rasp.

Osteotomies

Osteotomies are performed after the nasal reduction has been performed. The purposes of lateral nasal osteotomies include reduction of the open nasal roof, correction of deviated nasal bones, and narrowing of a wide nasal base (see Figure 66-31).

The two principal types of nasal osteotomy are lateral and medial. The lateral nasal osteotomy can be performed at different levels. It typically begins low on the piriform rim and can end either high or low in its relationship to the nasal bones. Thus, the osteotomy is often termed a *low-to-low osteotomy* or a *low-to-high osteotomy*. These osteotomies can be performed via an internal or external technique. Regardless of which technique is used, limited periosteal dissection is favored so that support is provided to the nasal bones. Medial osteotomies are seldom needed but can be used to obtain a controlled fracture in patients with thick nasal bones or when a low-to-low technique is used. Also, regardless of the osteotomy technique, the osteotomies should not be carried above the intercanthal line. The bone above this point becomes much thicker and mobilization becomes difficult. Care should be taken when performing medial osteotomies, because the thicker portion of the nasal bone can be included in the lateral osteotomy segment and result in widening of the upper nasal dorsum. This is termed a *rocker deformity.*

Lateral nasal osteotomies are not always required to close an open roof deformity after dorsal hump reduction. Some surgeons believe it is better to place spreader grafts in those patients with short nasal bones so that compromise of the internal nasal valve does not occur. If an osteotomy is performed in a patient with shorter nasal bones, a low-to-high technique is preferred.

NASAL TIP

Understanding the mechanisms of nasal tip support is critical when performing rhinoplasty. The surgeon must understand both the desired and the undesired changes that occur from the surgical approach or technique.[35]

The three major tip support mechanisms include

1. The size, shape, and strength of the lower lateral cartilages.
2. The attachment of the medial crura to the caudal septum.
3. The attachment of the lower lateral cartilages to the upper lateral cartilages.

The minor tip support mechanisms include

1. The interdomal ligament.
2. The sesamoid complex, extending the support of the lateral crura to the piriform aperture.
3. The attachment of the alar cartilages to the overlying skin.
4. The cartilaginous septal dorsum.
5. The nasal spine.
6. The membranous septum.[36,37]

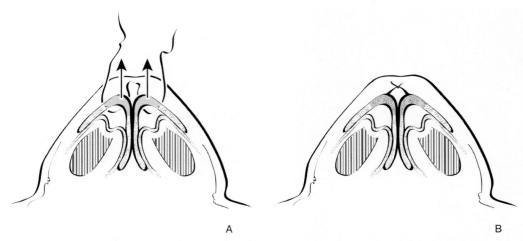

A   B

FIGURE 66-32. Lateral crural steal. **A** and **B,** A horizontal mattress suture is placed in the lateral crura in order to increase nasal projection and narrow the nasal tip. (**A** and **B,** Adapted from Taylor CO. Surgery of the nasal tip. In Waite PD, editor. Atlas of the Oral and Maxillofacial Surgery Clinics of North America: Rhinoplasty. Philadelphia: WB Saunders; 1995; p. 61.)

Certain surgical procedures can affect tip support. For example, a complete transfixion incision will disrupt the fibrous attachments of the caudal septum to the medial crura, thus leaving little support for the nasal tip. Suturing techniques and cartilage strut grafts may be necessary to reestablish support if this incision is performed. Intercartilaginous incisions, which are useful to gain access to the nasal dorsum, interrupt the ligamentous connections of the upper and lower lateral cartilages. This can result in cephalic tip rotation, which may or may not be desirable. A cephalic strip procedure creates even further disruption and rotation of the lower lateral cartilages. Most often, tip rhinoplasty is designed to refine and decrease the tip lobule while maintaining or even increasing rotation and projection.

The cartilaginous support of the nasal tip is often described in terms of a tripod concept.[38,39] The medial crura of both the lower lateral cartilages together form one strut of the tripod, and each of the lateral crura of the lower lateral cartilages forms a strut. By selectively shortening or lengthening any of these struts, the tip position can be altered.

The tip position changes are referred to in terms of both projection and rotation. *Tip projection* is the distance from the tip of the nose to the alar-facial junction. Increasing tip projection is one of the most difficult procedures to perform in rhinoplasty surgery. Nasal tip projection can be increased by both grafting and nongrafting techniques.

Tip Projection

INCREASING TIP PROJECTION

Nongrafting techniques to increase nasal projection include

1. Suturing of divergent medial crura: For this technique to be effective, there must be diverging medial crura. Intervening soft tissue may require excision before suturing with mattress sutures.[40]
2. Lateral crural steal: The lower lateral cartilage is skeletonized and the lateral crura cartilages are sutured with a

mattress suture so that the lateral crura now contributes to the medial crura (Figure 66-32). This results in increased projection and some rotation as well.[41,42]

Grafting techniques to increase projection include

1. Collumellar strut: This technique involves the placement of a strut of septal cartilage between the feet of the medial crura and abutted against the nasal spine. The medial crura are elevated superiorly with double skin hooks and the cartilage strut is sutured to the medial crura via mattress sutures. Only a minor amount of tip projection can be increased with this method.
2. Peck graft: This is an onlay graft in the region of the nasal tip. Layers of cartilage are placed in the domal region to increase projection. The graft material is either conchal or septal cartilage. The cartilage is secured to the dome by sutures. This technique can increase projection by 2 to 6 mm (Figure 66-33).

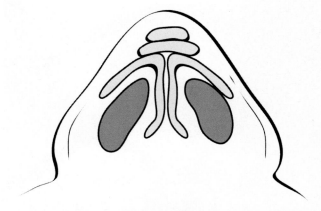

FIGURE 66-33.   Peck graft. This involves the placement of layers of cartilage grafts in the region of the nasal tip to increase nasal projection. (Adapted from Taylor CO. Surgery of the nasal tip. In Waite PD, editor. Atlas of the Oral and Maxillofacial Surgery Clinics of North America: Rhinoplasty. Philadelphia: WB Saunders; 1995; p. 62.)

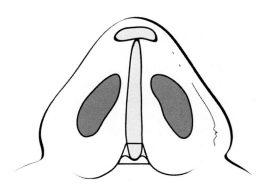

FIGURE 66-34. Umbrella graft. This is essentially a columellar strut graft placed between the medial crura combined with a tip graft. This technique improves support of the medial crura as well as increases nasal projection. (Adapted from Taylor CO. Surgery of the nasal tip. In Waite PD, editor. Atlas of the Oral and Maxillofacial Surgery Clinics of North America: Rhinoplasty. Philadelphia: WB Saunders; 1995; p. 61.)

3. Umbrella graft: This technique involves the creation of a cartilaginous structure that resembles the appearance of an umbrella. It is useful when both tip projection and support of weak medial crura are required. The umbrella graft is constructed from harvested septal, ear, or rib cartilage. It is then sutured in position so that the "handle" of the umbrella is between the medial crura and the "canopy" of the umbrella rests atop the dome. The canopy portion can be modified to incorporate the Peck graft technique by stacking layers of cartilage (Figure 66-34).[43]

4. Shield graft: This graft was first described by Sheen.[30] A piece of septal cartilage is shaped to form a trapezoidal configuration measuring 6 to 8 mm superiorly and 5 mm inferiorly The graft is usually 10 to 12 mm long and is beveled so that the corners are blunted. The graft is placed in a pocket through an endonasal approach or sutured in position via an open approach. The superior and lateral aspect of the graft forms the tip-defining points (Figure 66-35).[30]

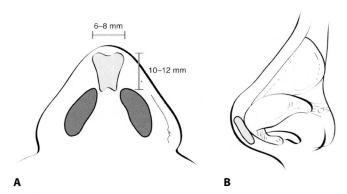

A **B**

FIGURE 66-35. Shield graft. **A** and **B,** This is a grafting technique used to redefine the tip-defining points of the nose. The graft is typically 6 to 8 mm wide superiorly, 5 mm wide inferiorly, and 10 to 12 mm long. (**A** and **B,** Adapted from Taylor CO. Surgery of the nasal tip. In Waite PD, editor. Atlas of the Oral and Maxillofacial Surgery Clinics of North America: Rhinoplasty. Philadelphia: WB Saunders; 1995; p. 62.)

DECREASING TIP PROJECTION

Decreasing tip projection involves reduction of the tip-supporting mechanisms. Achieving acceptable results when decreasing projection can be difficult because nasal definition can be lost.[44] If the nasal projection needs to be decreased, be certain to first confirm that the problem is not the result of an optical illusion caused by a low radix position. If the problem is a low radix, a dorsal radix graft is the appropriate treatment.

Methods to decrease projection include

1. Complete transfixion incision: As discussed previously, a complete transfixion incision will decrease tip support. Intercartilaginous incisions or cephalic strips will also weaken the tip support but will increase tip rotation.
2. Lower the septal angle: If the septum is providing significant support for the nasal tip, the septal angle must be lowered. This is done by excision of a portion of the caudal septum. In addition, the medial crura can be separated from the caudal septum to decrease projection.
3. Crural excision: To dramatically decrease tip projection, the medial and lateral crura may need to be sectioned, overlapped, and sutured into a new position with less projection. This technique maintains the natural shape of the tip at the domes (Figure 66-36). Excision of a segment cartilage in the domes and suturing them back together can be done, but it will change the shape of the nasal tip.

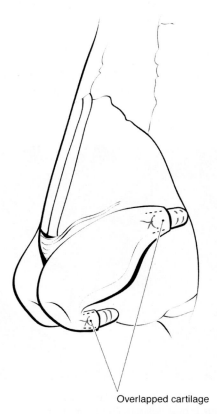

Overlapped cartilage

FIGURE 66-36. Crural excision. This is used when the nasal tip needs dramatic deprojection. A portion of the lateral crura is excised and the ends are sutured back together.

Sometimes, after decreasing the nasal projection, the patient may have flaring of the ala and increased infratip columellar show. This can be treated with an alar base resection but this should be used judiciously.

Tip Rotation

INCREASING TIP ROTATION

Understanding the tripod concept and tip-supporting mechanisms is important when determining which of the following methods to use to increase tip rotation.

1. Removal of dorsal hump: A subtle way to increase rotation of the tip is to reduce a dorsal hump if present.
2. Resection of the caudal septum: A small triangular piece of caudal septum can be removed. The base of this triangular shape is at the nasal dorsum.
3. Cephalic strips from lower lateral cartilages: A complete strip of cephalic cartilage from the lower lateral cartilages will result in increased tip rotation. Even an intercartilaginous incision will result in some tip rotation (Figure 66-37).
4. Shorten the lateral crura.
5. Shield graft: A shield graft gives the illusion of increased tip rotation.
6. Augmentation of premaxilla: Placement of cartilage or ePTFE in the premaxilla region below the anterior nasal spine will also give the illusion of increased tip rotation.

DECREASING TIP ROTATION

Decreasing tip rotation is done by two methods:

1. Trim the caudal septum near the anterior nasal spine.
2. Augment the nasal dorsum: this creates the illusion of decreased tip rotation.

Tip Shape

In addition to changing the tip position, the tip shape must also be considered. Historically, changes to the nasal tip were performed by selective cartilage excision and reapproximation. The Goldman tip is an example of such a technique. The current trend is to preserve and reorient existing cartilage and place cartilaginous grafts if required.[45] Excessive grafting can be unpredictable in the long run.

Although cartilage preservation is emphasized, there is still sometimes a need to remove cartilage. There are three principal techniques of cartilage excision in the nasal tip region: a complete strip technique, a weakened complete strip technique, and an interrupted strip technique. A greater resection generally results in more dramatic tip narrowing and rotation.

Complete strip techniques involve the removal of a complete piece of cartilage from the cephalic end of the lower lateral cartilages (Figure 66-38; see also Figure 66-37). This procedure is thought to be more stable because it leaves an intact strip of the inferior border of the lower lateral cartilage. Aggressive resection can result in loss of tip support, alar notching, alar retraction, and the appearance of increased collumellar show. Most surgeons feel that a minimum width of 6 mm is required to maintain the structural integrity of the lower lateral cartilage.

The weakened complete strip technique involves the removal of a complete cephalic strip followed by weakening of the cartilage by selective morselization of the medial and lateral crura with a scalpel blade.

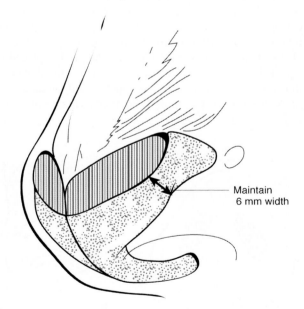

FIGURE 66-38. Complete strip technique. This involves the excision of a strip of cartilage on the cephalic portion of the lower lateral cartilage. This will result in increased tip rotation. It is important to maintain a minimum of 6 mm width of cartilage for structural support of the nose. (Adapted from Taylor CO. Surgery of the nasal tip. In Waite PD, editor. Atlas of the Oral and Maxillofacial Surgery Clinics of North America: Rhinoplasty. Philadelphia: WB Saunders; 1995; p. 58.)

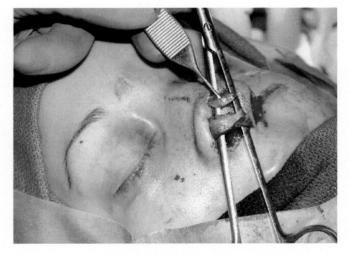

FIGURE 66-37. Delivery of lower lateral cartilage. The lower lateral cartilage is best delivered by a marginal incision or exposed through an open rhinoplasty for direct visualization and surgical manipulation. Tip refinement is improved in this case by complete tip reduction to reduce the volume of the tip.

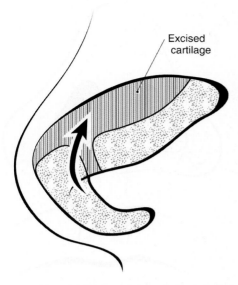

FIGURE 66-39.   Interrupted strip technique. This is similar to the complete strip except the remaining cartilage is also divided in a vertical fashion. This allows for even greater tip rotation, as indicated by the *arrow;* however, it can result in a pinched nasal tip and functional problems. The cartilage can be weakened by scoring it in a vertical fashion and this is termed a *weakened complete strip technique.* (Adapted from Taylor CO. Surgery of the nasal tip. In Waite PD, editor. Atlas of the Oral and Maxillofacial Surgery Clinics of North America: Rhinoplasty. Philadelphia: WB Saunders; 1995; p. 59.)

An interrupted strip involves division of the lateral crura from the dome (Figure 66-39). This technique provides greater rotation than a complete strip but can also result in complications, including loss of tip support, alar notching, and alar retraction. In addition, the nasal tip can develop a pinched appearance. The classic Goldman tip is an example of an interrupted strip technique (Figure 66-40). In this technique, the lateral crura are divided lateral to the tip-defining

points. The medial segments are sutured together, which results initially in increased tip projection. The lateral crural segments are left alone as independent units. This procedure is no longer commonly used because of problems with tip asymmetry, pinched appearance of the nasal tip, and long-term tip ptosis.

For patients with a broad nasal tip, transdomal suturing techniques are often used to narrow the tip. Volume reduction is performed first if needed by cartilage excision as described previously. Next, excision of excessive interdomal soft tissue is performed. A 4-0 polydioxanone transdomal suture is placed in a horizontal mattress fashion to narrow and reorient the alar cartilages. The advantage of this technique is that the suturing can be done multiple times until the surgeon is satisfied with the result. In addition, the long-term results of this technique have been favorable.[46–48]

NASAL BASE ALAR REDUCTION

The alar base should approximate the intercanthal distance and be no more than 1 to 2 mm wider than this. The nostrils should have a symmetrical appearance. Asymmetry of the nostril is often due to a deviated nasal septum and this should be reevaluated before consideration of an alar base resection.

The primary procedure to reduce the alar base width is an alar base resection. Alar modification is often considered in cases in which the nose has to be deprojected or to balance the anatomy in certain ethnic types. It is mandatory to be conservative when performing alar reduction because it is difficult to correct an overreduction. If there is any doubt, the surgeon should delay the alar base reduction until a later date.[49]

The procedure is performed by excising a small wedge of vestibular mucosa and skin. The angulation can be adjusted so that greater reduction of the outer perimeter of the ala is reduced and only limited reduction of the internal perimeter is performed.[49] The excision should be conservative and will rarely be greater than 3 mm in width (Figure 66-41).

POSTOPERATIVE MANAGEMENT

After performing the rhinoplasty, the surgeon must decide whether intranasal stents or packing is necessary. We generally do not place nasal packing. If the septum requires additional support during healing, silicone stents are placed. These stents are also used if there are mucosal tears or if a turbinectomy was performed. The stents help reduce the incidence of synechiae formation. The stents are secured to each other by a 3-0 silk suture passed through the columella and are typically left in place for 1 week.

Next, the nasal dorsum is splinted. Benzoin or mastisol is painted on the nasal dorsum and #fr1/4>-inch brown paper tape is applied. After placement of the tape, the splint is applied. A metal Denver splint or thermoplastic splint is contoured and applied. Additional paper tape can be placed over the splint.

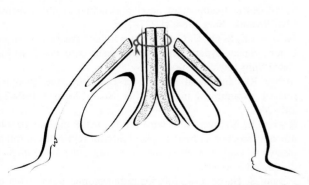

FIGURE 66-40. Goldman tip. This is an interrupted strip technique in which the lateral crura are divided lateral to the tip-defining points. The medial segments are then sutured together to increase nasal tip projection and to narrow the nasal tip. (Adapted from Willis AE, Costa LE. Surgical management of the nasal base. In Waite PD, editor. Atlas of the Oral and Maxillofacial Surgery Clinics of North America: Rhinoplasty. Philadelphia: WB Saunders; 1995; p. 61.)

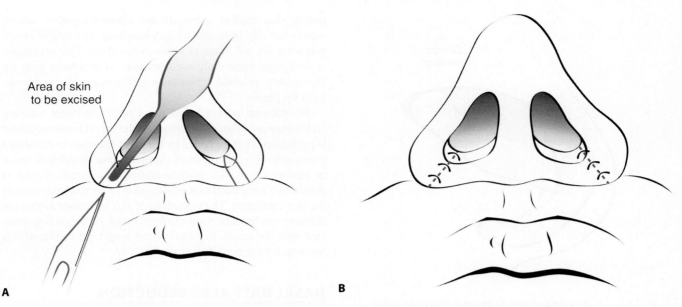

FIGURE 66-41. Alar base reduction (Weir's excision). **A,** This is used to narrow an overly wide nostril. **B,** A small amount of vestibular mucosa and skin is excised and sutured together. The excision is usually 1 to 2 mm wide.

References

1. Rohrich RJ, Huyn B, Muzaffar AR, et al. Importance of the depressor septi nasi muscle in rhinoplasty: anatomic study and clinical application. Plast Reconstr Surg 2000;105:376–383; discussion 384–388.

2. Rosse C, Gaddum-Rosse P, eds. Hollinshead's Textbook of Anatomy Ear, Orbit, Nose. 5th ed. Philadelphia: Lippincott-Raven; 1982:730–739.

3. Rohrich RJ, Muzaffar AR, Gunter JP. Nasal tip blood supply: confirming the safety of the transcolumellar incision in rhinoplasty. Plast Reconstr Surg 2000;106:1640–1641.

4. Toriumi DM, Mueller R, Grosch T, et al. Vascular anatomy of the nose and the external rhinoplasty approach. Arch Otolaryngol Head Neck Surg 1996;122:24–34.

5. Lam SM, Williams LE. Anatomic considerations in aesthetic rhinoplasty. Facial Plast Surg 2002;18:209–214.

6. Dion MC, Jafek BW, Tobin CE. The anatomy of the nose. External support. Arch Otolaryngol 1978;104:145–150.

7. Janfaza P, Nadol JB, Galla R, et al. Surgical Anatomy of the Head and Neck. 1st ed. Philadelphia: Lippincott Williams & Wilkins; 2001; p. 908.

8. Toriumi DM, Josen J, Weinberger M, et al. Use of alar batten grafts for correction of nasal valve collapse. Arch Otolaryngol Head Neck Surg 1997;123:802–808.

9. Sheen JH. Spreader graft: a method of reconstructing the roof of the middle nasal vault following rhinoplasty. Plast Reconstr Surg 1984;73:230–239.

10. Gunter JP, Rohrich DR, William P. Dallas Rhinoplasty. 1st ed. Vol.1. St. Louis: Quality Medical; 2002; pp. 654–656.

11. Correa AJ, Sykes JM, Ries WR. Considerations before rhinoplasty. Otolaryngol Clin North Am 1999;32:7–14.

12. Meyer L, Jacobsson S. The predictive validity of psychosocial factors for patients' acceptance of rhinoplasty. Ann Plast Surg 1986;17:513–520.

13. Tardy ME Jr, Dayan S, Hecht D. Preoperative rhinoplasty: evaluation and analysis. Otolaryngol Clin North Am 2002;35:1–27, v.

14. Rohrich RJ. The who, what, when, and why of cosmetic surgery: do our patients need a preoperative psychiatric evaluation? Plast Reconstr Surg 2000;106:1605–1607.

15. Petroff MA, McCollough EG, Hom D, et al. Nasal tip projection. Quantitative changes following rhinoplasty. Arch Otolaryngol Head Neck Surg 1991;117:783–788.

16. Crumley RL, Lanser M. Quantitative analysis of nasal tip projection. Laryngoscope 1988;98:202–208.

17. Gunter JP, Rohrich DR, William P. Dallas Rhinoplasty. 1st ed. Vol. 1. St. Louis: Quality Medical; 2002; p. 65.

18. Gunter JP, Rohrich RJ. Management of the deviated nose. The importance of septal reconstruction. Clin Plast Surg 1988;15:43–55.

19. Courtiss EH, Goldwyn RM, O'Brien JJ. Resection of obstructing inferior nasal turbinates. Plast Reconstr Surg 1978;62:249–257.

20. Pollock RA, Rohrich RJ. Inferior turbinate surgery: an adjunct to successful treatment of nasal obstruction in 408 patients. Plast Reconstr Surg 1984;74:227–236.

21. Jackson LE, Koch RJ. Controversies in the management of inferior turbinate hypertrophy: a comprehensive review. Plast Reconstr Surg 1999;103:300–312.

22. Mabry RL. Intranasal steroids in rhinology: the changing role of intraturbinal injection. Ear Nose Throat J 1994;73:242–246.

23. Rohrich RJ, Kreuger JK, Adams WP Jr, et al. Rationale for submucous resection of hypertrophied inferior turbinates in rhinoplasty: an evolution. Plast Reconstr Surg 2001;108:536–544; discussion 545–546.

24. Elwany S, Harrison R. Inferior turbinectomy: comparison of four techniques. J Laryngol Otol 1990;104:206–209.

25. Posnick JC, Seagle MB, Armstrong D. Nasal reconstruction with full-thickness cranial bone grafts and rigid internal skeleton fixation through a coronal incision. Plast Reconstr Surg 1990;86:894–902; discussion 903–904.

26. Jackson IT, Choi HY, Clay R, et al. Long-term follow-up of cranial bone graft in dorsal nasal augmentation. Plast Reconstr Surg 1998;102:1869–1873.

27. Celik M, Tuncer S. Nasal reconstruction using both cranial bone and ear cartilage. Plast Reconstr Surg 2000;105:1624–1627.
28. Gunter JP, Clark CP, Friedman RM. Internal stabilization of autogenous rib cartilage grafts in rhinoplasty: a barrier to cartilage warping. Plast Reconstr Surg 1997;100:161–169.
29. Sancho BV, Molina AR. Use of septal cartilage homografts in rhinoplasty. Aesthetic Plast Surg 2000;24:357–363.
30. Sheen JH. Achieving more nasal tip projection by the use of a small autogenous vomer or septal cartilage graft. A preliminary report. Plast Reconstr Surg 1975;56:35–40.
31. Toriumi DM. Autogenous grafts are worth the extra time. Arch Otolaryngol Head Neck Surg 2000;126:562–564.
32. Parker Porter J. Grafts in rhinoplasty: alloplastic vs. autogenous. Arch Otolaryngol Head Neck Surg 2000;126:558–561.
33. Adamson PA. Grafts in rhinoplasty: autogenous grafts are superior to alloplastic. Arch Otolaryngol Head Neck Surg 2000;126:561–562.
34. Romo T 3rd, Sclafani AP, Jacono AA. Nasal reconstruction using porous polyethylene implants. Facial Plast Surg 2000;16:55–61.
35. Adams WP Jr, Rohrich RJ, Hollier LH, et al. Anatomic basis and clinical implications for nasal tip support in open versus closed rhinoplasty. Plast Reconstr Surg 1999;103:255–261; discussion 262–264.
36. Tardy ME Jr, Cheng EY, Jernstrom V. Misadventures in nasal tip surgery. Analysis and repair. Otolaryngol Clin North Am 1987;20:797–823.
37. Thomas JR, Tardy ME Jr. Complications of rhinoplasty. Ear Nose Throat J 1986;65:19–34.
38. McCollough EG, Mangat D. Systematic approach to correction of the nasal tip in rhinoplasty. Arch Otolaryngol 1981;107:12–16.
39. Anderson JR. New approach to rhinoplasty. A five-year reappraisal. Arch Otolaryngol 1971;93:284–291.
40. Tebbetts JB. Shaping and positioning the nasal tip without structural disruption: a new, systematic approach. Plast Reconstr Surg 1994;94:61–77.
41. Foda HM, Kridel RW. Lateral crural steal and lateral crural overlay: an objective evaluation. Arch Otolaryngol Head Neck Surg 1999;125:1365–1370.
42. Kridel RW, Konior RJ, Shumrick KA, et al. Advances in nasal tip surgery. The lateral crural steal. Arch Otolaryngol Head Neck Surg 1989;115:1206–1212.
43. Mavili ME, Safak T. Use of umbrella graft for nasal tip projection. Aesthetic Plast Surg 1993;17:163–166.
44. Tardy ME Jr, Walter MA, Patt BS. The overprojecting nose: anatomic component analysis and repair. Facial Plast Surg 1993;9:306–316.
45. Tebbetts JB. Rethinking the logic and techniques of primary tip rhinoplasty: a perspective of the evolution of surgery of the nasal tip. Otolaryngol Clin North Am 1999;32:741–754.
46. Tardy ME Jr, Patt BS, Walter MA. Transdomal suture refinement of the nasal tip: long-term outcomes. Facial Plast Surg 1993;9:275–284.
47. Daniel RK. Rhinoplasty: a simplified, three-stitch, open tip suture technique. Part I: primary rhinoplasty. Plast Reconstr Surg 1999;103:1491–1502.
48. Daniel RK. Rhinoplasty: a simplified, three-stitch, open tip suture technique. Part II: secondary rhinoplasty. Plast Reconstr Surg 1999;103:1503–1512.
49. Tardy ME Jr, Patt BS, Walter MA. Alar reduction and sculpture: anatomic concepts. Facial Plast Surg 1993;9:295–305.

67

CHAPTER

Rhytidectomy

G. E. Ghali, DDS, MD, and Andrew R. Banker, DDS, MD

Face-lifting has received significant attention over the past several decades owing to increasing patient demands for a more youthful appearance. The face undergoes harmonious changes in the facial skeleton, deep soft tissue elements, and skin texture during the aging process. Dissection of cadavers has identified facial ligaments, muscle expansions, and dissection planes that give us a better understanding of facial aging and rejuvenation. Perhaps more important, it has also been the catalyst for the evolution of a variety of face-lifting techniques. The goal of facial rejuvenation should be to address all components of aging, leaving the patient with a younger-appearing face and a long-lasting result. If this is accomplished, the patient's face and neck will continue to age harmoniously.[1]

Critical evaluation of early techniques and a clear understanding of surgical anatomy have provided insight into the perils and pitfalls of surgical rejuvenation of the face and have resulted in the complexity of various rhytidectomy techniques. Today, rhytidectomy is one of the most frequently performed aesthetic surgical procedures in the United States.

Numerous techniques are currently used for performing face-lifts but no general agreement as to which of these techniques is most effective[2]; facial aesthetic surgeons have discussed the advantages and disadvantages of superficial and deep face-lifts for many years. A clear consensus is difficult because patient variables such as past medical history, anatomy, genetic background, social history (e.g., smoking, alcohol), motivation to have aesthetic surgery, and environment make it virtually impossible to perform a blinded long-term prospective clinical study. Evaluation of facial aesthetic surgery is also difficult because most procedures yield satisfactory results initially, often producing enough improvement to be accepted as a good result.

HISTORY

Although doubt still exists as to who performed the first face-lift, most authorities date the procedure to the early part of the 20th century[3-13] Historically, rhytidectomy procedures may be divided into three main categories: skin excision, subcutaneous undermining, and superficial musculoaponeurotic system (SMAS) manipulation. Early rhytidectomy procedures were limited to skin excision and wound closure without any appreciable subcutaneous undermining.[3,4,8-10,14] Beginning in the late 1920s, the conventional face-lift operation, consisting of skin dissection with subcutaneous undermining, was established.[13]

The subcutaneous rhytidectomy was the preferred technique for many years. A small amount of subcutaneous tissue is elevated with the skin and is simply redraped, leaving the patient with less redundancy. However, this technique does not address underlying skeletal deformities, ptotic deep soft tissue structures, or changes in skin texture. Therefore, it usually results in a more unnatural look and increases the likelihood of complications, particularly skin slough.

In an attempt to improve the results obtained with the subcutaneous face-lift, several clinicians described techniques to correct platysmal banding and submental lipomatosis.[15-18] The third historic category came with the advent of SMAS manipulation. Multiple surgeons have described various techniques involving the SMAS and platysma to enhance cervicofacial rhytidectomy.[1,19-35] In 1974, Skoog[19] described a procedure based on surgical anatomy. At that time, the subdermal plane was accepted by most to be the anatomic limit for face-lifting and rejuvenation. Skoog's technique redraped the skin and platysma together, leaving the patient with a more youthful jaw line.

Subsequently Mitz and Peyronie's description of the SMAS[21] provided an anatomic basis for restoration of

TABLE 67-1. **Generations of Rhytidectomy**

I Subcutaneous dissection only with variable skin undermining
II Subcutaneous dissection + SMAS plication or imbrication
III Subcutaneous dissection + SMAS plication or imbrication + deep midface section dissection
IV Composite dissection

SMAS = superficial musculoaponeurotic system.

the face. Hamra[35] (initially with the deep-plane and later with the composite rhytidectomy) and, later, Owsley[36] (with the multiplanar/multivector approach) modified and improved Skoog's technique by performing a more complete release of the nasolabial fold. Ramirez[37] showed that after subperiosteal release, the soft tissues of the cheek, forehead, jowls, lateral canthus, and eyebrows can be restored to their youthful relationship with the underlying skeleton. Finally, Watson and colleagues[38] described a technique similar to that of Owsley but combined it with laser resurfacing. This technique involved a larger plane of subdermal or subcutaneous undermining than that described by Hamra.

Four generations of rhytidectomy techniques are recognized (Table 67-1).[39] Current literature has popularized more complex procedures including the deep-plane and composite rhytidectomies.[1,34,35,40] These methods have incorporated multiplanar dissections and craniofacial techniques in an attempt to gain better control of the midface soft tissues. Whether these techniques provide longer-lasting results remains to be shown.[1,34,35,39–42] Multiple authors have cautioned that the more complex deep-plane and composite rhytidectomies typically carry increased morbidity.[1,41,43–49]

PATIENT EVALUATION

When a rhytidectomy is being contemplated, the treatment requirements of the surgeon must be balanced with the desires of the patient (Table 67-2).[50] These requirements are critical for proper patient selection. The patient evaluation must include general medical and psychological considerations in addition to physical facial features. Neglect of any aspect of the patient evaluation can lead to future problems.[51]

A thorough medical evaluation must be completed before surgery. Medical illnesses such as diabetes, hypertension, hypothyroidism, and asthma must be appropriately treated

TABLE 67-2. **Rhytidectomy Requirements**

Patient	Surgeon
Minimal morbidity risk	Safe and predictably consistent outcomes
Long-lasting results	
Quick recovery	Reasonable operative time
Affordable	Reasonable cost to patients
Performed on outpatient basis; will be ambulatory	Reasonable postoperative recovery period
	Adaptable for revision procedures
	Teachable to residents and fellows

and controlled preoperatively. Medical evaluation is essential for detecting conditions that may adversely affect a patient's ability to tolerate an anesthetic or that may compromise the final surgical result. Appropriate consultations regarding cardiovascular disease, pulmonary disease, coagulopathies, and other active medical problems should be obtained preoperatively. Current medication profiles should be elicited, including aspirin and aspirin-containing compounds, nonsteroidal anti-inflammatory drugs, and herbal drugs, as well as high doses of vitamin E. Examination of prior surgical incisions, such as those resulting from previous thyroidectomies or parotidectomies, is useful in evaluating the wound-healing capacity.

Tobacco and alcohol use, as well as the use of illicit substances, may increase the incidence of surgical complications. Cigarette smoking, diabetes mellitus, and previous head and neck radiation therapy may also impede healing and should be recognized preoperatively. Patients should be told that cigarette smoking significantly increases the likelihood of skin flap necrosis, poor healing, and unsightly scars.[52,53] Studies have demonstrated a 12-fold greater risk of skin slough in smokers than in nonsmokers.[54,55] Animal studies involving skin flap experiments have also supported this conclusion.[56,57]

A review of the patient's psychological history should focus on motivation for surgery and outcome expectations. Patients seeking surgery based on recent emotional events or with unrealistic expectations should be further counseled and the procedure postponed or cancelled.[58,59]

The goal of face-lifting is to correct anatomic changes to the face and neck that have occurred as a result of the normal aging process. Patients considered for rhytidectomy present with various degrees of age-related alterations to the facial soft tissues. Ideally, face-lift candidates are 45 to 55 years of age, are in good health, are of normal weight, possess a good bone structure, and possess a thin neck and a deep cervicomental angle. Physical examination of the patient includes a detailed regional evaluation of the face. A face-lift is capable of correcting specific anatomic regions, and a complete and detailed description of the patient's physical characteristics is important. A systematic evaluation allows the surgeon to assess the areas that can be improved with an isolated rhytidectomy and to determine whether other ancillary procedures will be beneficial. In addition, a detailed regional evaluation provides an opportunity for the surgeon and the patient to understand the limitations of the rhytidectomy; the surgeon can refer to the evaluation when explaining the expected outcome.

Evaluation of the upper facial one third includes the forehead and upper and lower eyelids. In general, these areas are not affected by the standard rhytidectomy and are, therefore, not addressed in this review. Evaluation of the middle facial one third includes the face and ears. The quality of the skin should be noted, including thickness, redundancy, previous scarring, fine or coarse rhytids, and the location of the hairline. Patients with significant elastosis or actinic damage do

TABLE 67-3. **Dedo Classification of Facial Profiles**

Classification	Comments
I. Normal	Well-defined cervicomental angle. Good muscle tone No submental fat
II. Cervical skin laxity	Obtuse cervicomental angle owing to relaxed skin
III. Submental fat accumulation	Requires submental lipectomy
IV. Platysma muscle banding	Requires muscle clipping, plication, or imbrication
V. Retrognathia/ microgenia	Requires genioplasty or orthognathic surgery
VI. Low hyoid	Difficult to alter Important to inform patient of limitation

Adapted from Dedo DD. A preoperative classification of the neck for cervicofacial rhytidectomy. Laryngoscope 1980;90:1894–1896.

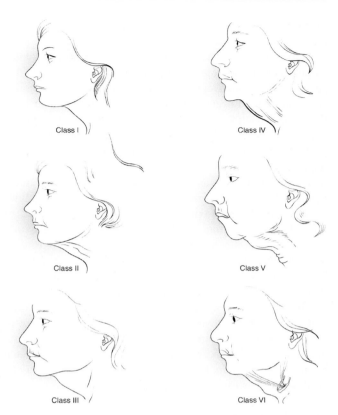

FIGURE 67-1. Six classes of facial profiles by Dedo. (Adapted from Dedo DD. A preoperative classification of the neck for cervicofacial rhytidectomy. Laryngoscope 1980;90:1894–1896.)

not obtain and retain the same quality of results as do patients possessing good skin quality. Assessment of the earlobe shape and position is critical, and any deviations from normality should be pointed out to the patient preoperatively. Documentation of the nasolabial folds, including length, depth, and symmetry, as well as an assessment of the degree of jowls should be noted. Presence of perioral rhytids is important because they are not corrected with rhytidectomy procedures.

The evaluation of the lower facial one third includes the chin, jaw line, and neck. A useful preoperative classification of the neck for cervicofacial rhytidectomy divides the neck profile into six distinct classes (Table 67-3).[60] Using this classification, the clinician can identify each patient's specific abnormality and choose the most appropriate procedure for optimal results (Figure 67-1). Skin redundancy, platysmal banding, cervicomental angle, and submental fat accumulation are important to note in this region. In addition, the degree of ptosis of the submandibular glands should be assessed and recorded at this time.

Preoperative photographs provide invaluable medicolegal documentation as well as an opportunity to review patient characteristics before and during surgery. The surgeon should obtain the photographs of the full face in repose and smiling, right and left profiles, and right and left three-quarter views. Closeups of the forehead, eyebrows, and periorbital and perioral regions should be taken, depending on the particular deformity.

An essential component of the patient evaluation includes the preoperative visit. It is an excellent opportunity to educate the patient regarding various aspects of the procedure, postoperative care, and expectations. It is wise to review any and all patient instructions during the preoperative visit including medications, skin cleaning, and makeup. Patients must discontinue all aspirin-containing compounds, nonsteroidal anti-inflammatory medications, and vitamin E at least 2 weeks before surgery. Germicidal shampoo and skin cleaners are used several days before the scheduled date of the

procedure to reduce bacterial counts. The patient should wash his or her hair and face and remove all makeup the night before surgery. A written copy of postoperative instructions should be given to and reviewed with the patient (see Appendix).

A description of the expected convalescence is appropriate during the preoperative visit. In general, 10 to 14 days is a reasonable time period to wait for ecchymosis to resolve sufficiently to allow camouflage with makeup. Patients should not expect to return to work or social activities before this time. They should be educated regarding expectations in the early postoperative period because those unaware of the slow evolution of results will quickly become frustrated. It should be clearly explained that appearance will continue to improve over a period of several months.

SURGICAL TECHNIQUE

Superficial-Plane Rhytidectomy

Once appropriate monitors are placed and the patient is adequately sedated, proposed incision lines and anticipated areas of undermining are marked with a skin marker while the patient is seated in an upright position. The face, neck, and hair are prepared with an appropriate antiseptic surgical scrub. Skin preparations should include the full length of the planned incision and all exposed skin within the surgical field.

Our preference is to perform rhytidectomies under local anesthesia with appropriate sedation and analgesia. Suitable agents include intravenous fentanyl, midazolam, ketamine, and/or propofol. Local anesthesia is provided along the incision line with a 2% lidocaine solution with 1:100,000 epinephrine via a dental syringe. Hydrodissection is performed within the planned plane of dissection with a tumescent anesthetic technique (Figure 67-2).[61-66]

Although multiple techniques exist for mixing the tumescent solution, our preference is to mix 20 mL of a 2% lidocaine with 1:100,000 epinephrine solution with 180 mL of normal saline, creating a solution of 0.2% lidocaine with a 1:1,000,000 epinephrine concentration. This mixture is administered through four trocar sites: temporal, infralobular, mastoid, and submental (Figure 67-3). The solution is deposited subcutaneously in the supra-SMAS plane.

Hydrodissection should extend 1 cm beyond the proposed undermining mark that delineates the anticipated extent of flap development. Approximately 75 mL of the tumescent anesthetic solution is deposited per side, with an additional 50 mL deposited in the submental region. The anesthetic is allowed to work for 8 to 10 minutes before proceeding.

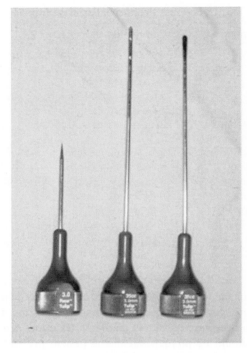

FIGURE 67-2. From left to right: procar/trocar, infiltrator, and dissector used for the tumescent technique.

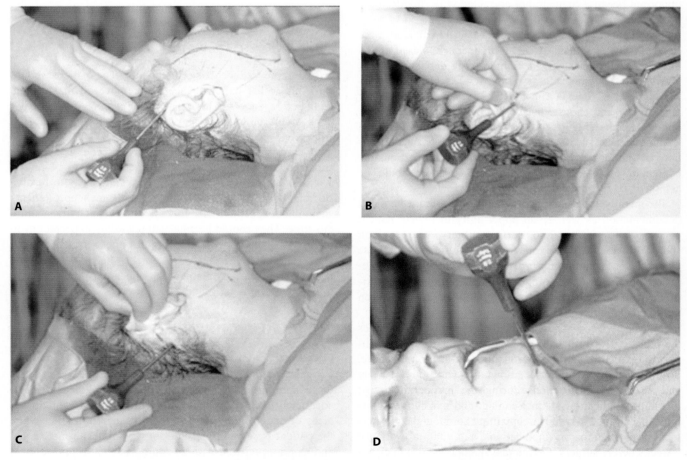

FIGURE 67-3. Four trocar sites are typically used. **A,** Temporal. **B,** Infralobular. **C,** Mastoid. **D,** Submental.

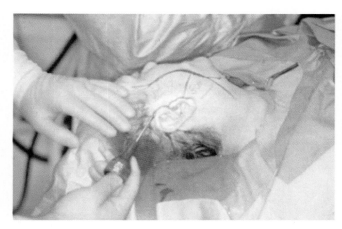

FIGURE 67-4.   Cervicofacial dissection in the supra-SMAS (superficial musculoaponeurotic system) plane without suction.

Typically, the contralateral side is not infiltrated until just before initiating closure on the first side.

Following deposition of the anesthetic solution, blunt cannula dissection of the cervicofacial and submental regions is performed. The cervicofacial dissection is generally performed without suction (Figure 67-4), whereas the submental dissection is performed under suction (Figure 67-5). The submental dissection, using the blunt cannula, is accomplished before the initiation of the cervicofacial dissection. As previously mentioned, the planned incisions should be marked with the patient seated in an upright position, and before administration of the local anesthetic, to prevent distortion of local anatomy. Numerous modifications of the standard face-lift incision are available, but several general principles should be followed closely.[67–70]

It is not necessary to shave the hair in the incision area. If necessary, the hair may be braided along the proposed incision, with the temporal extension placed no more than 2 cm within the hair and parallel to the hairline. Some surgeons recommend a pretrichial incision to prevent the posterosuperior migration of the temporal line.

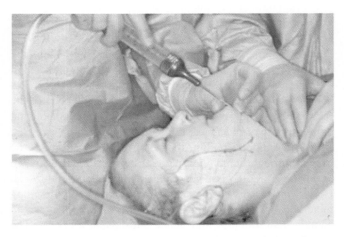

FIGURE 67-5.   Submental dissection in the supraplatysmal plane under suction.

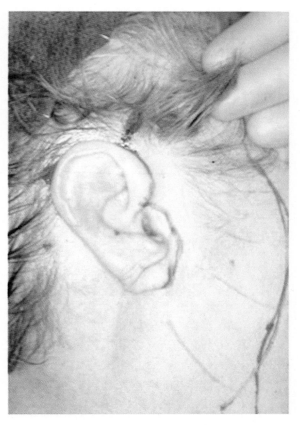

FIGURE 67-6.   Temporal, preauricular, and infralobular components of the typical rhytidectomy incision.

The incision should be extended inferiorly toward the root of the helix, anterior to the curve of the crus helicis, following the margin of the tragus, and proceed anteriorly just above the base of the incisura intertragica (Figure 67-6). Preservation of the incisura helps to prevent distortion of the tragus postoperatively, providing a more aesthetic scar. The incision curves inferiorly 1 to 2 mm below the junction of the lobule with the cheek, rising superiorly onto the back of the conchal bowl approximately 3 to 5 mm and reaching the level of the postauricular sulcus or superior crus of the antihelix. The incision is then directed posteroinferiorly approximately 4 to 5 cm into the scalp of the retromastoid region (Figure 67-7).

If significant cervical skin redundancy is noted, the incision may parallel the posterior hairline for several centimeters before being directed into the hair-bearing skin. This maneuver can prevent a step deformity in the posterior hairline when significant cervical skin is excised. Care must be taken to maintain approximately a 90-degree angle at the reflection of the posterior flap to prevent skin slough at the tip of the flap.

Several considerations for incision design are important in the male patient.[18,71] In the temporal region, the planned incision is affected by the patient's hair pattern. Individuals with thick temporal hair can tolerate a standard incision. Those with thinning hair, temporal recession, or significant male pattern baldness require a modification of the incision design.

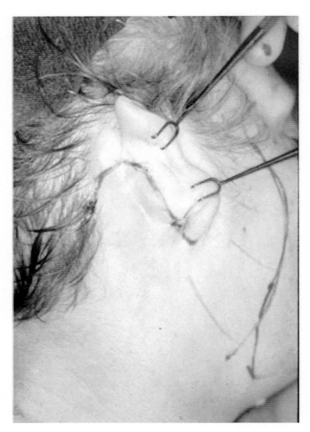

FIGURE 67-7.   Postauricular and mastoid components of the typical rhytidectomy incision.

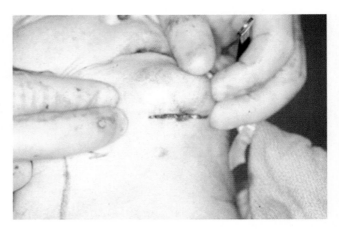

FIGURE 67-8.   Submental incision placed to address platysmal banding.

In the preauricular region, the male sideburn must be taken into consideration and the non–hair-bearing skin anterior to the ear must be left intact to prevent an unnatural appearance. Therefore, the incision should extend in a linear fashion, following a natural skin crease adjacent and parallel to the sideburn. This is in contrast to the curved incision used in female patients.

Last, the posterior extension of the incision is placed along the margin of the postauricular hairline. Although this placement has the potential to be slightly more noticeable, the importance of preventing posterior displacement or a step deformity to the hairline must be taken into account. A final consideration in the male patient is the inevitable transfer of hair-bearing skin into the postauricular region or into the ear canal itself.

Management of the cervical region, if indicated, is begun with the placement of a transverse incision in a submental skin crease as an extension of the submental trocar puncture (Figure 67-8). This incision should not be placed in the dominant crease of the "double-chinned" deformity, because scarring may result during the healing process and accentuate the crease. The incision should be approximately 2 cm in length and placed just inferior to the dominant crease.

Dissection in the submental region proceeds in a subcutaneous plane and joins the lateral subcutaneous neck planes subsequent to the submental dissection. Excess subcutaneous fat may be excised with sharp scissors or a cannula, if indicated. Lipectomy in the submental region should be done cautiously. Overly enthusiastic removal of fat in this region can lead to an atrophic appearance of the cervical facial tissues or a "cobra" neck deformity.[17]

Next, the anterior borders of the platysma bands are identified, and excess subcutaneous tissue is removed. The medial borders should be released along their deep surface from the submental region inferiorly to the level of the thyroid cartilage. The medial borders are then repositioned in the midline, and any overlapping tissue is excised. Plication of the medial platysma borders proceeds from the submental region to the level of the thyroid cartilage with a 2-0 slow-resorbing suture (Figure 67-9).

A horizontal myotomy of the inferior aspect of the platysma may be beneficial in accentuating the cervicomental angle and relieving tension along the anterior surface of the neck. Partial horizontal transection is frequently all that is required and can be performed with sharp scissors at the inferiormost aspect of the dissection of the medial borders. If complete transection is indicated, the lateral aspect of the platysma can be excised through the lateral neck face-lift flap.[72–75]

Flap Development

Flap development is initiated by undermining 1 cm along the entire length of the face-lift incision. This is accomplished in a subdermal plane with a blade or sharp scissors, using skin hooks for retraction (Figure 67-10). On the underside of the flap, maintain approximately 3 to 4 mm of subcutaneous fat to preserve the subdermal vasculature.

In the temporal region, the depth of the flap should be carried through the temporoparietal fascia (subgaleal) down to the loose areolar tissue overlying the deep temporal fascia. Dissection in this plane creates a thicker flap, providing increased protection from any ischemic injury that would damage hair follicles and create subsequent alopecia. The temporal dissection is extended in this plane using a combination of blunt and sharp dissection.

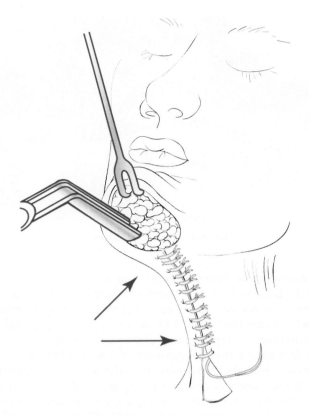

FIGURE 67-9.   Platysmal plication accomplished.

Blunt-tipped scissors should be used in a push-cutting motion into the residual tunnels that were developed secondary to the previous blunt cannula dissection (Figure 67-11). Rees T-clamps are used for countertraction and aid in the dissection. Undermining in this plane can be safely carried superiorly to the level of the lateral canthus.

At this point, the dissection is carried inferiorly and medially across the cheek in the subcutaneous plane. This zone of transition from the sub-SMAS (deep to the temporoparietal fascia) to the subcutaneous plane of dissection corresponds

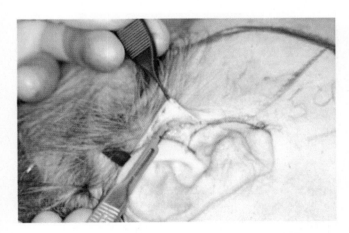

FIGURE 67-10.   Flap development initiated by 1 cm undermining via a blade or sharp dissection scissors.

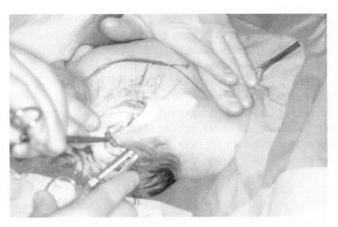

FIGURE 67-11.   Scissors are used in a push-cutting motion with the tips up.

to the mesotemporalis that contains the superficial temporal artery and the frontal branch of the facial nerve.[76–79] The facial nerve is located anterior and inferior to the frontal branch of the superficial temporal artery, so preservation of this vessel during dissection helps to protect this important nerve.

The extent of undermining necessary depends on the patient. Younger patients without excessive laxity of the skin require only 4 to 5 cm of undermining, but older patients with redundant tissue and severe jowling may require undermining to within 1 cm of the oral commissure. When platysma banding is present, the cervical dissection is carried inferiorly to the level of the thyroid cartilage and should communicate with the dissection from the contralateral side.

In the postauricular region, the flap should be developed in the subcutaneous plane below the earlobe to protect the great auricular nerve. This nerve is the one most commonly injured during rhytidectomy procedures (Figure 67-12).[80,81] The great auricular nerve runs just deep to the superficial fascia overlying the sternocleidomastoid muscle and supplies sensation below and behind the ear. With the head turned 45 degrees toward the contralateral side, the great auricular

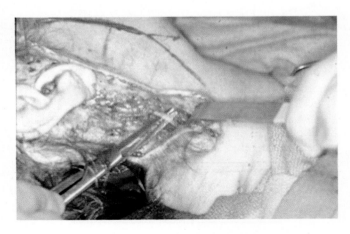

FIGURE 67-12.   Great auricular nerve demonstrated.

nerve consistently crosses the middle of the sternocleidomastoid muscle at a level 6.5 cm below the caudal edge of the bony external auditory canal (Erb's point).[80] Maintaining subcutaneous dissection below the earlobe helps protect the great auricular nerve, but above the level of the earlobe, the greater auricular is not at risk and dissection may be carried deeper.[81] Meticulous hemostasis is then accomplished with bipolar cautery. Overzealous use of electrocautery should be avoided on the skin-flap side to reduce the risk of ischemic injury and flap necrosis.

Next, the underlying SMAS in the cheek region is manipulated. Many of the age-related changes in the facial region are due to ptosis of the underlying fat. Correction of these changes is best obtained by repositioning this tissue along direction lines (vectors) different from those used for the skin flap. Independent bidirectional suspension of the SMAS and the skin flap reposition the ptotic facial tissues, providing longer-lasting results and reducing an unnatural appearance.

SMAS manipulation can be by plication, imbrication, or a combination of these techniques; there are proponents of each method. *Plication* is a technique whereby the SMAS is folded upon itself to obtain the desired repositioning, and *imbrication* is a technique in which the SMAS is incised or excised so that the distal portion is repositioned to overlap the proximal tissue (Figure 67-13).

SMAS plication is accomplished with a 2-0 slow-resorbing suture on a tapered needle (Figure 67-14). All knots are buried to prevent irritation to the skin flap or palpability. Two key sutures are placed initially, with the first extending from the fascia overlying the angle of the mandible to the fascia immediately inferior to the tragus. The second

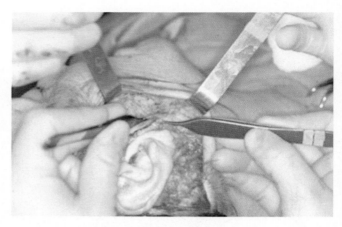

FIGURE 67-14.   The area of plication is assessed.

suture is placed from the fascia lateral to the oral commissure to the fascia immediately superior to the tragus. Several additional sutures may be placed, if needed, in the preauricular and postauricular areas. This suture placement provides a posterosuperior repositioning of the ptotic tissues.

Imbrication requires elevation of a sub-SMAS flap. An incision is made horizontally just inferior to the zygomatic arch and vertically posterior to the angle of the mandible. Landmarks for the incision include the zygomatic arch, tragus, platysma muscle, and mandible (Figure 67-15). The horizontal incision is made approximately 1 cm below and parallel to the zygomatic arch to prevent damage to the frontal branch of the facial nerve. The middle portion of the tragus may be used as a reference for staying below the zygomatic arch.

The incision is carried forward 2 to 3 cm. The vertical incision descends inferiorly along the posterior border of the platysma several centimeters below the angle of the mandible. It is important to keep the incision posterior to the angle of the mandible to prevent damage to the marginal mandibular branch of the facial nerve. The SMAS is then elevated for 2 to 3 cm in a sub-SMAS plane (Figure 67-16). The flap is

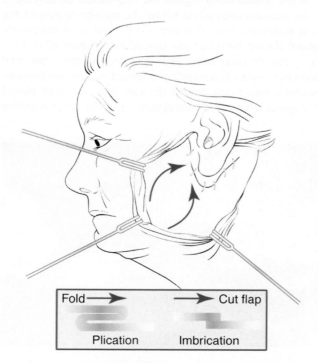

FIGURE 67-13.   Illustration of plication versus imbrication.

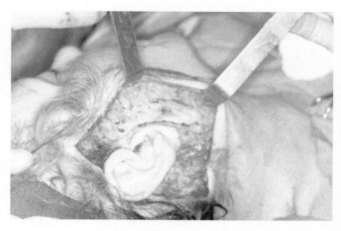

FIGURE 67-15.   The area of proposed resection in preparation for imbrication is marked.

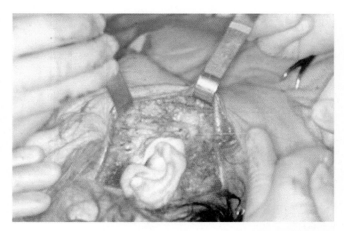

FIGURE 67-16. After SMAS flap elevation, 2-0 resorbable suture on a tapered needle is used for buried knots to secure the imbrication.

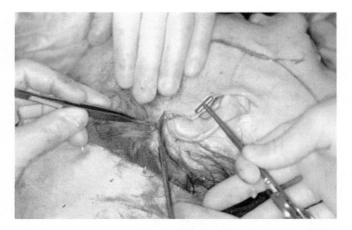

FIGURE 67-17. After the placement of key staples, flap trimming is accomplished with a blade or Iris scissors.

redraped posterosuperiorly and sutured using the technique previously described for plication.

Redraping of the skin flap is performed with the patient's head in a neutral position. Extension or flexion of the neck influences the amount of skin excised and may adversely affect the outcome. Key suspension staples or sutures are placed before trimming the skin flap. In general, the skin flap is redraped in a posterosuperior direction with an emphasis on the posterior direction. The majority of the needed superior suspension is accomplished by SMAS manipulation. Care should be taken to prevent a misdirection of facial rhytids and a distortion of the temporal hairline. Careful assessment of appearance should be made before suturing the flap in place.[82]

The first key skin-suspension suture (or staple) is placed in the temporal region just above the ear. The flap is then grasped, and the appropriate vector is determined and held in place while the flap is trimmed and the staple placed. The second staple is placed in the postauricular region at the most posterior and superior aspect of the flap. Careful attention should be given to proper inset of the ear. In a nonoperated ear, the long axis of the ear lobe hangs 10 to 15 degrees posterior to the long axis of the ear proper. This relationship must be maintained to prevent obvious deformities of the ear.

Skin Closure

Trimming of excess skin is performed with a blade or Iris scissors (Figure 67-17). It is important to be aware of the amount of skin to be excised in the temporal region to prevent distortion of the hairline. The distance from the lateral canthus to the anterior margin of the temporal hairline should be recorded preoperatively to serve as a reference for skin excision. Skin closure in the hair-bearing scalp (i.e., temporal and mastoid regions) is performed with subdermal 3-0 resorbable sutures. Staples may be used to approximate skin margins of the temporal and mastoid scalp. Our preference is to provide a layered closure to minimize tension on the most superficial aspect of the skin.[82] The immediate postauricular

region is closed with a 4-0 plain gut suture, without the need for deep sutures. In the preauricular region, a 4-0 resorbable suture is placed followed by approximation of the skin edges with a 6-0 or 7-0 nylon running suture. The deep layers of the submental incision are closed with 4-0 resorbable suture, and 6-0 nylon is used for the skin edges.

The decision of whether to place drains must be made on an individual basis, depending on how much oozing or edema is present. In our experience, drains are rarely needed. Antibacterial ointment and gauze dressings should be placed along the incision lines. Gauze is also placed preauricularly and postauricularly as well as in the submental region. The entire face should then be wrapped, taking care to prevent excessive tightness of the dressing because it can lead to ischemia of the flaps. In addition, the appropriate positioning of the ears under the dressing should be noted. Dressings should not be manipulated for evaluation until the first postoperative day. Most complications in rhytidectomy occur early in the postoperative period (i.e., 24–36 hr); close follow-up is, therefore, essential.[83–87] Some surgeons prefer to use no dressings postoperatively.[88] The degree of edema and ecchymosis postoperatively is frequently underestimated and can be quite shocking to the patient, despite the surgeon's best attempts to educate her or him. The patient's hair should be gently cleansed and rinsed for additional comfort. Incision lines should be cleansed daily with a 1:1 solution of hydrogen peroxide and water. Antibacterial ointment should be used until all sutures are removed.

The preauricular sutures are removed after 4 to 5 days, as are the staples in the temporal and mastoid regions after 10 days. Patients should be instructed not to wash their hair until all sutures have been removed and then to wash only gently with baby shampoo. Written suggestions for the avoidance of ultraviolet light and high heat from hair dryers and for the use of sunblock and incision massage should be given to the patient and repeated orally in the early postoperative visits. The effects of the procedure are still striking for years after surgery (Figure 67-18).

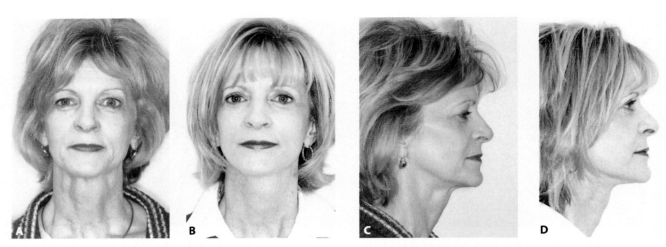

FIGURE 67-18. Typical result achieved with a superficial-plane rhytidectomy including SMAS imbrications and upper blepharoplasties. **A** and **B,** Preoperative photographs. **C** and **D,** Photographs taken 2 years postoperatively.

COMPLICATIONS

Based on the literature, complication rates tend to be lower for superficial rhytidectomy techniques than for the more complex composite and deep-plane techniques.[1,34,35,39,46,47,49,50] Major types of surgical complications include hematoma, facial nerve injury, skin loss, scarring, alopecia, auricular deformities, and temporal hairline deformities.

Major Complications

Hematoma

Hematoma formation is the most common major complication that results from rhytidectomy. It occurs postoperatively in roughly 2% to 4% of patients within the first 48 hours; the cause varies.[89] Early recognition is essential because untreated hematomas are associated with an increased risk of skin slough (Figure 67-19). Typical signs and symptoms of hematoma include increased facial pain, tightening of dressings, ecchymosis of the buccal mucosa and lips, and bulging of the lips. Hematomas are best treated with early exploration of the wound, with the most common finding being diffuse oozing under the skin flap. Removal of clots is indicated, followed rarely by bipolar cautery or suture ligation of larger vessels (Figure 67-20). Pressure dressings and drains may be used to complement these techniques but are no substitute for meticulous hemostasis. Factors associated with increased risk of

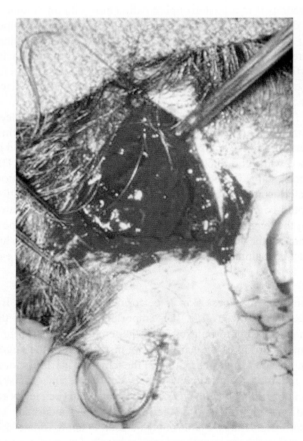

FIGURE 67-20. Early exploration and clot evacuation are essential in preventing skin slough. Clot being removed from left temporal region.

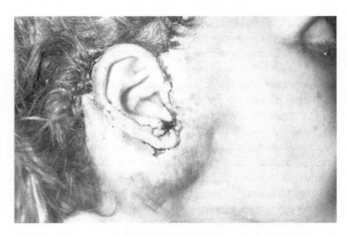

FIGURE 67-19. Hematoma present in early postoperative period.

hematoma formation include preoperative hypertension, intraoperative hypotension, and postoperative hypertension.

A review of 500 face-lifts demonstrated a 2.6% incidence of hematoma formation; however, in this same population, patients with preoperative hypertension had a 9.2% incidence of hematoma formation.[90] Preoperative hypertension in this review was associated with a 2.6-fold increase in the risk of hematoma formation. Conversely, intraoperative hypotension was associated with increased hematoma formation, probably as a result of rebound hypertension. In a review of 806 face-lifts, Rees and Aston[91] reported 23 hematomas (2.8%), with 20 of the 23 associated with controlled intraoperative hypotension. Maintenance of a normotensive state during surgery was associated with a decreased incidence of hematomas.

In another review of 1236 face lifts by Rees and coworkers,[92] a 1.9% incidence of hematoma formation was noted. The incidence drops to approximately 1% in normotensive general anesthetic states. Postoperative hypertension also has been associated with an increased risk of hematoma formation.[93] The average maximum blood pressure postoperatively in the preceding study was 152/98, a relatively minor elevation in blood pressure. Kamer and Kushnick[94] described an increase in hematoma formation when using propofol as the intraoperative anesthetic agent. With propofol, the overall incidence of hematoma formation was 4.2%. A combination of valium, demerol, and brevital had only a 2% incidence of hematoma formation, however. Finally, recent studies show a decrease in the incidence of hematoma formation with the use of fibrin glue sprayed under the flap before closure.[95]

Patient cooperation is helpful in the prevention of hematomas. Instructions for the reduction of hematoma formation include eliminating aspirin, aspirin-containing compounds, nonsteroidal anti-inflammatory drugs, and vitamin E for at least 2 weeks preoperatively and avoiding exertion and bending for 2 weeks postoperatively. The importance of patient compliance should be stressed in the preoperative visits.

Facial Nerve Injury

The facial nerve branch injured most often varies with different reports in the literature.[85,96] In the author's experience, the marginal mandibular and temporal (frontal) branches of the facial nerve are injured most often. These two branches are the most superficial and have less crossover anastomosis than other branches of the facial nerve. Injury to the marginal mandibular branch invariably occurs during extension of the subcutaneous dissection anteriorly to the lateral chin region, where the nerve courses superficial to the depressors of the mouth. Less commonly, it may be damaged during dissection in the region of the mandibular angle (Figure 67-21). Injury to the temporal branch frequently occurs during temporal dissection because the plane is in transition from subgaleal to subcutaneous levels. Damage to these structures may result in temporary or permanent motor deficits to the respective muscles of facial expression.

Compiled reviews of face-lifting have demonstrated a 0.7% (50 of 6500) incidence of temporary injury and a 0.1%

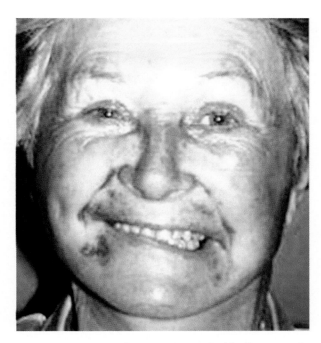

FIGURE 67-21.   Patient demonstrates typical findings associated with unilateral injury to the marginal mandibular branch of the facial nerve.

(7 of 6500) incidence of permanent injury.[76] Facial nerve injury is less likely with SMAS placation techniques versus SMAS imbrication or more complex composite and deep-plane techniques.[48,82] Rates of facial nerve injury with sub-SMAS dissections have been reported as high as 16%.[97] Prevention of facial nerve injury is achieved through a complete understanding of face-lift anatomy and the usual course and common variations of the facial nerve and meticulous attention to detail during the procedure. Most surgeons would agree that injury to the facial nerve is the most devastating complication associated with rhytidectomy; fortunately, permanent injury to the facial nerve is rare.[1,39,44,46,47,48,76,97]

Skin Slough

Skin slough is the result of vascular compromise to the involved soft tissue flap. It most commonly occurs in the post-auricular and mastoid regions because of the thinness of the skin and it being farthest from the blood supply of the cervicofacial skin flap (Figure 67-22). Fortunately, small sloughs in this region are concealed by the hair and ear. The incidence of postoperative skin slough is approximately 2% to 3%.[85]

Delay in the evacuation of hematomas is a major cause of skin slough and underlies the importance of early detection. Hematomas of significant size prevent the reestablishment of nutrient flow to the skin flap from the richly vascularized underlying tissues and cause tension within the flap, which creates further ischemia. When skin necrosis does occur, a black eschar forms that separates at approximately 1 week, and the wound then heals by secondary intention. Reassurance should be given to the patient because most areas of minor skin necrosis heal without major sequelae. A minimum of 3 to

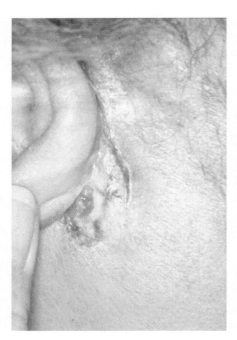

FIGURE 67-22. Most common site for skin slough located in the postauricular region.

6 months should elapse before any major surgical revision is undertaken.

Local ischemia may result from various factors including diabetes mellitus and tobacco use. Without a doubt, cigarette smoking increases the risk of skin slough.[52–57] Nicotine has been implicated as a factor that predisposes patients to skin necrosis by affecting several aspects of wound healing, including alteration of epithelialization, impairment of the inflammatory phase of healing, and compromise of small blood vessel flow.[98] In evaluating the effects of tobacco on face-lifts, Rees and associates[52] demonstrated a 12-fold greater risk of skin slough in smokers compared with non-smokers. Webster and colleagues[53] advocated a more conservative undermining (short flap technique) in face-lift patients who smoke. It is the author's opinion that abstinence from smoking for at least 2 weeks—and preferably 1 month—is recommended before operating on a patient who has not stopped smoking. Improper tissue manipulation and flap design are easily preventable causes of skin slough that result from inexperience. Delicate handling of skin flaps is essential during elevation to prevent a compromised result. Skin flaps should be designed to maintain an adequate thickness of subcutaneous tissue on their deep surface (3–4 mm) and, in the postauricular region, to maintain a 90-degree angle at the tip of the flap.

Neurosensory Disturbances

Neurosensory disturbances, particularly transient numbness or hypesthesia, are common in the early postoperative period as a result of elevation of the skin flap and interruption of small sensory nerves. As a result, a temporary, diffuse cutaneous numbness that lasts 4 to 6 weeks is not uncommon.

During this time, patients should be warned about possible injury to numb skin from razors, curling irons, and hair dryers. The most common nerve injured during rhytidectomy is the great auricular nerve. Injury to this nerve is the result of an improper plane of dissection over the sternocleidomastoid muscle. Studies have shown the great auricular nerve to cross the middle portion of the sternocleidomastoid muscle approximately 6.5 cm below the caudal edge of the bony external auditory canal, which courses cephalad just deep to the SMAS.[80,81] Injury to the great auricular nerve occurs when the postauricular dissection is carried too deep, thereby violating the strict subcutaneous plane in this region.

Minor Complications

The significance of a complication may vary according to the patient's ability to deal with the complication. A particular patient may be frantic over a mild postauricular skin slough, whereas another patient may demonstrate minimal to no anxiety associated with marginal mandibular nerve weakness. Although the authors do not discuss minor complications in detail, complications that occur after rhytidectomy may include widened scars, auricular deformities, edema or ecchymosis, loss of temporal hair tuft or temporal alopecia, and sialoceles.[89,96,99] When complications occur, the surgeon must acknowledge them to the patient and take appropriate measures to correct the problem. Availability of the surgeon in the postoperative period is the key to successful management of most postoperative complications.

SUMMARY

Since the early 1980s, numerous rhytidectomy techniques have been described to improve the results of facial rejuvenation. When contemplating facial rejuvenation surgery, the treatment requirements of the surgeon must be balanced with the desires of the patient. These requirements are critical in defining the advantages of one technique of face-lifting over another. As we prepare our patients for aesthetic surgery, we must consider all the variables discussed and individualize each treatment plan. Not all patients should undergo a deep-plane face-lift; however, many will benefit from release of the retaining ligaments and a repositioning of tissues in multiple vectors.

In the realm of oral and maxillofacial surgery, the rhytidectomy procedure finds great application as an adjunct to traditional skeletal surgery. It seeks to reverse the effects of gravity and relaxation of the facial skin and fascia by resuspending the facial units and eliminating excess skin and subcutaneous tissue. Although a wide variety of techniques are reported for face-lifting, this chapter has attempted to provide a broad overview of the superficial-plane rhytidectomy technique. By tailoring the approach to the specific needs of each patient, based on a thorough knowledge of surgical anatomy, the maxillofacial surgeon should achieve consistently good results with minimum morbidity.

References

1. Hamra ST. Composite rhytidectomy. Plast Reconstr Surg 1992; 90:1–13.
2. Miller TA. Face-lift: which technique? Plast Reconstr Surg 1997;100:501.
3. Joseph J. Hangewangenplastik (Melomio-plastik). Dtsch Med Wochenschr 1921;47:287.
4. Lexer E. Die Gesamte Wiederherstellungschiurgie. Vol 2. Leipzig: JA Barth; 1931:548.
5. Rogers BO. A brief history of cosmetic surgery. Surg Clin North Am 1971;51:265–288.
6. Rogers BO. The development of aesthetic plastic surgery: a history. Aesthetic Plast Surg 1976;1:3.
7. Rogers BO. A chronologic history of cosmetic surgery. Bull N Y Acad Med 1977;47:265–302.
8. Passot R. La chirirgie esthetique des rides du visage. Presse Med 1919;27:258.
9. Bourguet J. La disparipion chirurgicale des rides et plis du visage. Bull Acad Med (Paris) 1919;82:183.
10. Bettman AG. Plastic and cosmetic surgery of the face. Northwest Med 1920;19:205.
11. Kolle FS. Plastic and Cosmetic. New York: Appleton; 1911; pp. 116–117.
12. Miller CC. Semilunar excision of the skin at the outer canthus for the eradication of crow's feet. Am J Dermatol 1907;11:483.
13. Barnes H. Truth and fallacies of face peeling and face lifting. Med J Reconstr 1927;126:86.
14. Hollander E. Cosmetic surgery. In Joseph M, editor. Handbuch der Kosmetik. Leipzig: Verlag von Veit; 1912.
15. Aufricht G. Surgery for excess skin of the face and neck. In Wallace EB, editor. Transactions of the International Society of Plastic Surgeons. Second Congress. London: Livingstone; 1960; pp. 495–502.
16. Adamson JE, Horton CE, Crawford HH. The surgical correction of the "turkey gobbler" deformity. Plast Reconstr Surg 1964;34:598–605.
17. Millard DR, The Aging face. In Pigott RW, Hedo A. Submandibular lipectomy. Plast Reconstr Surg 1968;41:513–522.
18. Baker TJ, Gordon HL. Rhytidectomy in males. Plast Reconstr Surg 1969;44:219–222.
19. Skoog T, editor. The Aging Face. In Plastic Surgery—New Methods and Refinements. Philadelphia: WB Saunders; 1974:308-323.
20. Guerro-Santos J, Espaillat L, Morales F. Muscular lift in cervical rhytidoplasty. Plast Reconstr Surg 1974;54:127–130.
21. Mitz V, Peyronie M. The superficial musculoaponeurotic system (SMAS) in the parotid and cheek area. Plast Reconstr Surg 1976;58:80–88.
22. Owsley JQ. Platysma-fascial rhytidectomy: a preliminary report. Plast Reconstr Surg 1977;60:843–850.
23. Owsley JQ. SMAS-platysma face lift. Plast Reconstr Surg 1983;71:573–576.
24. Connell BF. Cervical lifts: the value of plastyma muscle flaps. Ann Plast Surg 1978;1:32–43.
25. Connell BF. Contouring the neck in rhytidectomy by lipectomy and a muscle sling. Plast Reconstr Surg 1978;61:376–383.
26. Gerro-Santos J. The role of the platysma muscle in rhytidoplasty. Clin Plast Surg 1978;5:29–49.
27. Guerro-Santos J. Surgical correction of the fatty fallen neck. Ann Plast Surg 1979;2:389–396.
28. Aston SJ. Platysma muscle in rhytidoplasty. Ann Plast Surg 1979;3:529–539.
29. Lemmon ML, Hamra ST. Skoog rhytidectomy: a five year experience with 577 patients. Plast Reconstr Surg 1980;65:283–297.
30. Lemmon ML. Superficial fascia rhytidectomy. A restoration of the SMAS with control of the cervicomental angle. Clin Plast Surg 1983;10:449–478.
31. Kaye BL. The extended neck lift: the "bottom line." Plast Reconstr Surg 1980;65:429–435.
32. Kaye BL. The extended face-lift with ancillary procedures. Ann Plast Surg 1981;6:335–346.
33. Teimourian B. Face and neck suction-assisted lipectomy associated with rhytidectomy. Plast Reconstr Surg 1983;72:627–633.
34. Hamra ST. The tri-plane facelift dissection. Ann Plast Surg 1984;12:268–274.
35. Hamra ST. The deep-plane rhytidectomy. Plast Reconstr Surg 1990;86:51–61.
36. Owsley JQ. Lifting the malar fat pad for correction of prominent nasolabial folds. Plast Reconstr Surg 1993;91:463–474.
37. Ramirez OM. The subperiosteal rhytidectomy: the third-generation facelift. Ann Plast Surg 1998;28:218–232.
38. Watson SW, Stone TL, Sinn DP. The four dimensional rhytidoplasty. Am J Cosmet Surg 2001;18:5–13.
39. Duffy MJ, Friedland JA. The superficial-plane rhytidectomy revisited. Plast Reconstr Surg 1994;93:1392–1403.
40. Adamson PA, Dahiya R, Litner J. Midface effects of the deep-plane vs the superficial musculoaponeurotic system plication face-lift. Arch Facial Plast Surg 2007;9:9–11.
41. De la Plaza R, Valiente E, Arroyo JM. Supraperiosteal lifting of the upper two-thirds of the face. Br J Plast Surg 1991;44:325–332.
42. Ramirez OM, Maillard GF, Musolas A. The extended subperiosteal facelift: a definitive soft-tissue remodeling for facial rejuvenation. Plast Reconstr Surg 1991;88:227–236.
43. Keller GS. KTP laser rhytidectomy. Facial Plast Surg Clin North Am 1993;1:157.
44. Beeson WH. Extended posterior rhytidectomy. Facial Plast Surg Clin North Am 1993;1:215.
45. Binder WJ. A comprehensive approach for aesthetic contouring of the midface in rhytidectomy. Facial Plast Surg Clin North Am 1993;1:253.
46. Rubin LR, Simpson RL. The new deep plane face lift dissections versus the old superficial techniques: a comparison of neurologic complications [editorial]. Plast Reconstr Surg 1996; 97:1461–1465.
47. Baker DC. Deep dissection rhytidectomy: a plea for caution [editorial]. Plast Reconstr Surg 1994;93:1498–1499.
48. Adamson PA, Moran ML. Complications of cervicofacial rhytidectomy. Facial Plast Surg Clin North Am 1993;1:133–142.
49. Kaye BL. The superficial-plane rhytidectomy revisited [discussion]. Plast Reconstr Surg 1994;93:1404–1405.
50. Ghali GE, Smith BR. A case for superficial rhytidectomy. J Oral Maxillofac Surg 1998;56:349–351.
51. Caplin DA, Perlyn CA. Rejuvenation of the aging neck: current principles, techniques, and newer modifications. Facial Plast Surg Clin North Am 2009;17:589–601, vi–vii.
52. Rees TD, Liverett DM, Guy CL. The effect of cigarette smoking on skin-flap survival in the facelift patient. Plast Reconstr Surg 1984;73:911–913.
53. Webster RC, Kazda G, Hamden US, et al. Cigarette smoking and facelift: conservative versus wide undermining. Plast Reconstr Surg 1986;77:596–604.
54. Lawrence WT, Murphy RC, Robson MC, et al. The detrimental effect of cigarette smoking on flap survival: an experimental study in the rat. Br J Plast Surg 1984;37:216–219.

55. Kaufman T, Eichenlaub EH, Levin M, et al. Tobacco smoking: impairment of the experimental flap survival. Ann Plast Surg 1984;13:468–472.

56. Craig S, Rees TD. The effects of smoking on experimental skin flaps in hamsters. Plast Reconstr Surg 1985;78:842–846.

57. Nolen J, Jenkins RA, Kurihara K, et al. The acute effects of cigarette smoke exposure on experimental skin flaps. Plast Reconstr Surg 1985;75:544–551.

58. Edgerton MT, Webb WL, Slaughter R, et al. Surgical results and psychosocial changes following rhytidectomy. Plast Reconstr Surg 1964;33:503–521.

59. Goin MK, Burgoyne RW, Goin JM, et al. Prospective psychologic study of 50 female facelift patients. Plast Reconstr Surg 1980;65:436–442.

60. Dedo DD. A preoperative classification of the neck for cervicofacial rhytidectomy. Laryngoscope 1980;90:1894–1896.

61. Schoen SA, Taylor CO, Owsley TG. Tumescent technique in cervicofacial rhytidectomy. J Oral Maxillofac Surg 1994;52:344–347.

62. Klein JA. The tumescent technique for liposuction surgery. Am J Cosmet Surg 1987;4:263.

63. Lillis PJ. Liposuction surgery under local anesthesia: limited blood loss and minimal lidocaine absorption. J Dermatol Surg Oncol 1988;14:1145–1148.

64. Klein JA. Tumescent technique for regional anesthesia permits lidocaine doses of 35 mg/kg for liposuction: peak plasma lidocaine levels are diminished and delayed 12 hours. J Dermatol Surg Oncol 1990;16:248–263.

65. Klein JA. The tumescent technique anesthesia and modified liposuction technique. Dermatol Clin 1990;8:425–437.

66. Lillis PJ. The tumescent technique for liposuction surgery. Dermatol Clin 1990;8:439–450.

67. Talamas I. A nondeforming rhytidectomy incision. Aesthetic Plast Surg 1999;23:228–232.

68. Stuzin JM, Baker TJ, Baker TM. Refinements in face lifting: enhanced facial contour using Vicryl mesh incorporated into SMAS fixation. Plast Reconstr Surg 2000;105:290–301.

69. Knize DM. Periauricular facelift incisions and the auricular anchor. Plast Reconstr Surg 1999;104:1508–1520.

70. Little JW. Hiding the posterior scar in rhytidectomy: the omega incision. Plast Reconstr Surg 1999;104:259–272.

71. Baker DC, Aston SJ, Guy CL, et al. The male rhytidectomy. Plast Reconstr Surg 1977;60:514–522.

72. Peterson R. The role of the platysma muscle in cervical lifts. In Symposium on Surgery of the Aging Face. St. Louis: Mosby; 1978; pp. 115–124.

73. Connell BF. Contouring the neck in rhytidectomy by lipectomy and a muscle sling. Plast Reconstr Surg 1978;61:376–383.

74. Aston SJ. Platysma muscle in rhytidoplasty. Ann Plast Surg 1979;3:529–539.

75. Henderson J, O'Neill T, Logan A. Direct anterior neck skin excision for cervicomental laxity. Aesthetic Plast Surg 2010;34:299–305.

76. Baker DC, Conley J. Avoiding facial nerve injuries in rhytidectomy. Anatomical variation and pitfalls. Plast Reconstr Surg 1979;64:781–795.

77. Liebman EP, Webster RC, Berger AS, et al. The frontalis nerve in the temporal brow lift. Arch Otolaryngol 1982;108:232–235.

78. Stuzin JM, Wagstrom L, Kawamoto HK, et al. Anatomy of the frontal branch of the facial nerve: the significance of the temporal fat pad. Plast Reconstr Surg 1989;83:265–271.

79. Trussler AP, Stephan P, Hatef D, et al. The frontal branch of the facial nerve across the zygomatic arch: anatomical relevance of the high-SMAS technique. Plast Reconstr Surg 2010;125:1230–1231.

80. McKinney P, Katrana DJ. Prevention of injury to the greater auricular nerve during rhytidectomy. Plast Reconstr Surg 1980;66:675–679.

81. McKinney P, Gottlieb J. The relationship of the great auricular nerve to the superficial musculoaponeurotic system. Ann Plast Surg 1985;14:310–314.

82. Webster RC, Smith RC, Karolow WW, et al. Comparison of SMAS plication with SMAS imbrication in face-lifting. Laryngoscope 1982;92:901–912.

83. Webster R, Smith R, Hall B. Facelift—better results with safer surgery of the head and neck. In Ward P, Berman W, editors. Plastic and Reconstructive Surgery of the Head and Neck. St. Louis: CV Mosby; 1984; pp. 321–323.

84. Gordon HL. Rhytidectomy. Clin Plast Surg 1978; 5:97–107.

85. Baker DC. Complications of cervicofacial rhytidectomy. Clin Plast Surg 1983;10:543–562.

86. Rees TD, Baker DC. Complications of aesthetic facial surgery. In Conley J, editor. Complications of Head and Neck Surgery. Philadelphia: WB Saunders; 1980.

87. Lindsey JT. Five-year retrospective review of the extended SMAS: critical landmarks and technical refinements. Ann Plast Surg 2009;62:492–496.

88. Aston SJ. Problems and complications in platysma-SMAS cervicofacial rhytidectomy. In Kaye B, Gradinger G, editors. Symposium on Problems and Complications in Aesthetic Plastic Surgery of the Face. St. Louis: CV Mosby; 1983.

89. Griffin JE, Jo C. Complications after superficial plane cervicofacial rhytidectomy: a retrospective analysis of 178 consecutive facelifts and review of the literature. J Oral Maxillofac Surg 2007;65:2227–2234.

90. Straith RE, Raju D, Hipps C. The study of hematomas in 500 consecutive facelifts. Plast Reconstr Surg 1977;59:694–698.

91. Rees TD, Aston SJ. Complications of rhytidectomy. Clin Plast Surg 1978;5:109–119.

92. Rees TD, Barone CM, Valaur FA, et al. Hematomas requiring surgical evacuation following face lift surgery. Plast Reconstr Surg 1994;93:1185–1190.

93. Berner RE, Morain WD, Noe JM. Postoperative hypertension as an etiological factor in hematoma after rhytidectomy. Plast Reconstr Surg 1976;57:314.

94. Kamer FM, Kushnick SD. The effect of propofol on hematoma formation in rhytidectomy. Arch Otolaryngol Head Neck Surg 1995;121:658–661.

95. Zoumalan R, Rizk SS. Hematoma rates in drainless deep-plane face-lift surgery with and without the use of fibrin glue. Arch Facial Plast Surg 2008;10:103–107.

96. Niamtu J 3rd. Complications in facelift surgery and their prevention. Oral Maxillofac Surg Clin North Am 2009;21:59–80, vi.

97. Barton FE. Rhytidectomy and the nasolabial fold. Plast Reconstr Surg 1992;90:601–607.

98. Mosley LH, Finseth F, Goody M. Nicotine and its effect on wound healing. Plast Reconstr Surg 1978; 61:570–575.

99. Clevens RA. Avoiding patient dissatisfaction and complications in facelift surgery. Facial Plast Surg Clin North Am 2009; 17:515–530, v.

Appendix Postoperative Rhytidectomy Instructions

IMMEDIATELY UPON ARRIVING HOME

Head elevation: Lie down with your head and back elevated on two pillows. You must sleep in this position for 1 week.

Dressings: Do not remove bandages. These will be removed at the office on your first postsurgery visit.

Ice packs: Place ice packs (ice in freezer bags or packages of frozen peas) over the cheek areas on and off over a period of 24 hours. *Do not* put ice on after 24 hours unless you are told to do so.

Swelling: Ice packs will keep swelling and bruising to a minimum.

Bruising: Bruising often lasts 7 to 14 days.

Medication: Take pain medication *only if needed* and with food or crackers.

Diet: Upon arriving home from surgery, begin with clear liquids until fully awake; then begin regular food intake with soft foods.

Suture care: Keep all sutures clean with a peroxide-water solution. Keep sutures covered with antibiotic ointment at all times. Clean three to five times per day.

ONE DAY OR MORE AFTER SURGERY

Moist heat: Ice packs are to be discontinued 24 hours after surgery. *Wait 12 hours;* then you may begin moist heat. Use a moist washcloth between an electric heating pad and your face. Do not use heat continuously; for example, use for 30 minutes and then off for 30 minutes. *Do not* set the heating pad higher than *medium* at any time, regardless of how cool it feels to you.

Activity: Stay up as much as possible. Avoid bending over or lifting heavy objects for 1 week. Strenuous activities should be limited for 2 to 3 weeks.

Work: Most people plan to return to work in 2 weeks. This depends on how you feel about being seen with bruising. Most of the bruising can be masked with makeup if you prefer to return earlier.

Makeup: Cosmetics may be applied on the sixth day. Ask about special coverup products for bruising. Mint green coverstick followed by a flesh-tone foundation will cover most bruises.

Bathing: You may bathe or shower, but keep the bandages dry. When bandages are removed, gently wash the facial areas.

Hair care: You may wash your hair on the fifth day after surgery. *Do not bend over* to wash your hair; this may cause bleeding or swelling to occur. Use medium heat on your hair dryer. High heat or hot rollers should not be used for 7 to 10 days. You may use color on your hair in 3 weeks.

Diet: Eat regular but soft meals. You will need to take vitamins and minerals to help with the healing. We will be glad to give you vitamin and mineral information.

Sun: Protect your facial skin from excessive sun exposure for 1 month after surgery.

PLEASE REPORT ANY OF THE FOLLOWING TO OUR OFFICE

Excessive pain or bleeding
Itching or rash around stitches
Oral temperature > 100°F (37.8°C)
Excessive swelling/bruising, fatigue, or depression

Forehead and Brow Procedures

Angelo Cuzalina, MD, DDS

Upper facial cosmetic surgery has enjoyed an unprecedented increase in popularity over the past decade. The yearning of baby boomers to look and feel rejuvenated has led to new endoscopic techniques aimed at creating a more youthful and natural appearance with shorter recovery periods than existed in past decades.[1–3] Yet some older techniques, such as an open coronal browlift, are still used routinely by some surgeons with wonderful results. Variations on the hairline or trichophytic open brow lift may be the perfect treatment for a patient with an extremely high highline and brow ptosis. The ultimate goal of improving a person's appearance remains unchanged. Society shapes our views of what looks attractive, and no mathematical formula can ever be used to determine an ideal eyebrow position (Figure 68-1). Each individual has his or her own unique perception of facial beauty. For most people, the upper face and eyes impart more emotion than does any other part of the human body; it is clear that rejuvenation of this vital area can provide an aesthetically pleasing result.

Aesthetic concerns of the forehead and brow regions of the face affect a wide range of age groups. Unlike the standard lower face and neck rhytidectomy, which more commonly affects patients after the age of 45 years, cosmetic concerns in the upper third of the face may be evident for patients in their 20s and 30s owing to genetic predisposition. The forehead and brow area must be entirely evaluated for a wide range of interlacing diagnoses. Matching the problem(s) to the ideal rejuvenation technique(s) is essential for maximum aesthetic benefits. Thinning skin and laxity due to age and gravity encompass only a portion of the forehead and brow dilemmas that must be addressed when planning rejuvenation procedures (Figure 68-2).

The aging process typically leads to forehead and brow ptosis on almost every patient; however, it is important to distinguish whether the ptosis in the forehead and brow region is owing to problems with brow position, upper eyelid laxity, or a combination of the two (Figure 68-3). Other problems such as dynamic lines caused by muscle activity in the glabellar region, variable hairline patterns, bony abnormalities, and asymmetries, as well as skin texture itself, must also be assessed in relation to one another. Achieving the patient's desired expectation depends not only on sound surgical skill and judgment but also critically on communication between the surgeon and the patient. Truthful disclosure of what can reasonably be attained is prudent and helps to prevent patient dissatisfaction.

Rejuvenation of the upper third of the face is one of the most rewarding and fulfilling procedures a surgeon can offer to select patients. Specific elevation and correction of lateral hooding can be appear natural and still impart a tremendous improvement in the patient's overall beauty and youthful appearance (Figure 68-4). The goal of this chapter is to review the upper third of facial anatomy specific to forehead and brow rejuvenation techniques and to discuss a variety of the most common techniques for rejuvenating the forehead and brow region.

ANATOMIC AND AESTHETIC CONSIDERATIONS

It is generally accepted that a youthful forehead is roughly one third of the overall facial height.[4–9] Essentially, the distance from the hairline to the glabella is equal to the distance from the glabella to the point at the base of the columella or subnasale (Figure 68-5). A youthful-appearing eyebrow is different for men and women. The female eyebrow should be arched with the highest point of the brow on a sagittal line from the lateral canthus.[10,11] The entire brow itself should be above the orbital rim. In general, the medial brow of the female is located ideally 1 to 3 mm above the orbital rim and the lateral third of the brow 5 to 10 mm above the rim.[12] This is in contrast to a typical male eyebrow that should lie at or only slightly above the orbital rim in a more horizontal or uniform arch fashion (Figure 68-6). Elevating the lateral

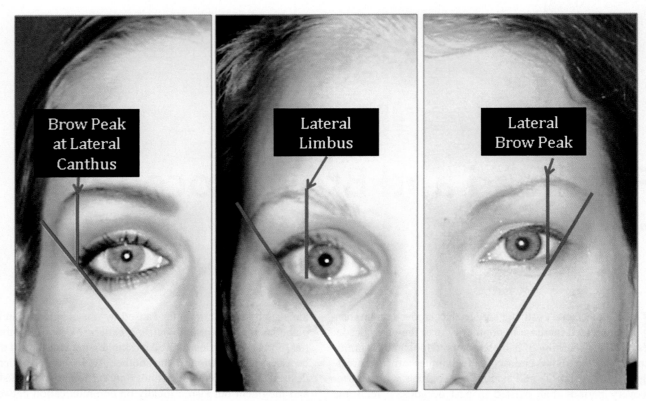

FIGURE 68-1. Three different types of aesthetically pleasing foreheads and eyebrow position. The tail of the eyebrow is located along the alar-canthal line. The greatest brow arch is seen in the lateral third between the lateral limbus and the canthus of the eye. The outer half of the brow is "ideally" located 5 to 10 mm above the orbital rim in females.

third of the male eyebrow disproportionately more than the remaining brow will create a feminine appearance.

The detailed anatomy of individual areas has been well described in the literature and often relates to the specific procedure being performed.[13–25] Therefore, the following anatomic discussion is simplified by separating the specific regions into bony landmarks, muscle and fascial anatomy, vessel and nerve anatomy, and specific endoscopic anatomy; each anatomic region is addressed individually as it relates to specific surgical procedures.

Bony Landmarks

Bony landmarks of the forehead and brow region can be focused all around the frontal bone, which makes up the highest percentage of the upper third of the face. The connections (suture lines such as the nasofrontal, zygomaticofrontal, and coronal) are important landmarks because they can be clinically relevant for limits of dissection and can help surgeons determine their location during dissection. For instance, the zygomaticofrontal suture line is an ideal location to end most basic brow lift dissections (Figure 68-7). Additional dissection can be performed if midface lifting is also planned or if the patient desires more elevation at the lateral canthal region. Overaggressive dissection here in many patients can create an unnatural cat's-eye appearance,

particularly if too much tissue is elevated medially along the suture line and lateral canthus. Likewise, the nasofrontal suture line is a nice landmark to note during dissection for a few reasons. First, dissection usually needs to proceed only a few millimeters below this suture level onto the nasal bones for adequate release. Second, the paired procerus muscles can be identified here and transection performed if required. Third, depending on the level of horizontal transection in this area, the nasofrontal angle point of take-off can be altered slightly if desired. Last, nasal tip rotation can be achieved if wanted, especially with significant dissection below the nasofrontal suture line.

Another general bony landmark is the orbital rim, which limits inferior dissection but must be well visualized and free of periosteal attachments to lift the brow and brow fat pads for long-term results. Important muscle and fascial attachments are also located at the level of the orbital rim medially and laterally. The tenacious temporal fusion line (zone of fixation) that exists along the temporal ridge must be identified during dissection.[26,27] It is also important to know its location preoperatively so that proper incision placement can be made to facilitate a clean dissection under this area that enhances visualization endoscopically (Figure 68-8).

Bony thickness varies in different areas of the skull. In addition, venous lakes present on the inside surface of the skull tend to be more centralized around the sagittal suture

Youthful brow   Aging brow

Galeal fat pad

Orbicularis oculi

Fusion at orbital rim

Preseptal fat pad

Frontalis

Frontal bone

Levator aponeurosis

Orbital septum

Preaponeurotic fat pad

A   **B**

Periosteum

Subgaleal areolar fascia

Deep fascia

Arcus marginalis

Eyelid fat pad

Levator palpebrae superioris

Whitnall's ligament

Orbitalis

Frontalis

Brow fat pad

Orbicularis oculi

Orbital septum

Levator aponeurosis

C

FIGURE 68-2. **A,** The youthful brow is elevated proportionately and has densely adherent periorbital fascia and muscle. **B,** Brow descent due to aging and the associated loss of fascial integrity, along with orbital fat prolapse. **C,** Cross-section of the brow near the midpupillary position.

line. If bone tunnels or screws are planned for fixation purposes, the midline should be avoided, if possible, because of the sagittal sinus as well as higher-density venous lakes in this area (Figure 68-9). Thickness does increase posteriorly near the occiput, but screw or bone tunnel fixation here is more challenging and is not required. Caution must be taken also to avoid lateral placement because of thinness of the lateral skull and the middle meningeal arteries. Knowledge of average thickness for a given location and internal anatomy indicates that the safest location for bone tunnels or screws is located along a parasagittal line approximately at the midpupil or lateral limbus line and just anterior to the coronal suture (see Figure 68-9).

Muscle and Fascial Anatomy

Paired muscles of the forehead and brow region are often thought of as elevators and depressors. Although several depressor muscles can pull the brow down or obliquely, the only true elevator of the forehead, the frontalis, moves upward to raise the brow. This movement, along with some static tone, maintains brow position but also can lead to horizontal creases over time. The frontalis originates from the deep galeal plane (galea aponeurotica that connects to the occipitalis posteriorly). It inserts into the orbital portion of the orbicularis oculi, which inserts into the dermis immediately below the eyebrow. Its lateral extension fuses into the dense collection of fascia almost 1 cm wide, called the *zone of adherence,* which extends along the superior temporal line and ends inferiorly just above the zygomaticofrontal suture.

The fascial attachments, known as the *orbital ligament* (see Figure 68-7), are the inferior termination point of the zone of adherence near the orbital rim where connective tissue fibers of the temporoparietal fascia are fixated to the bone at the superolateral orbital rim (Figure 68-10). Lateral

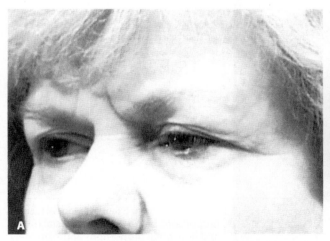 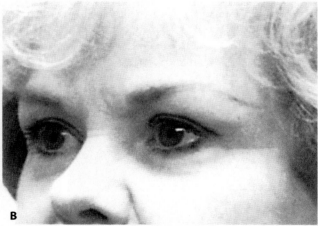

FIGURE 68-3. **A,** Rejuvenation of the upper third of the face must address whether the problem is limited to brow ptosis, eyelid ptosis, or a combination of both, as seen in the patient on the left. Skin texture must also be evaluated. **B,** One month after a coronal brow lift, upper blepharoplasties, and full-face laser resurfacing.

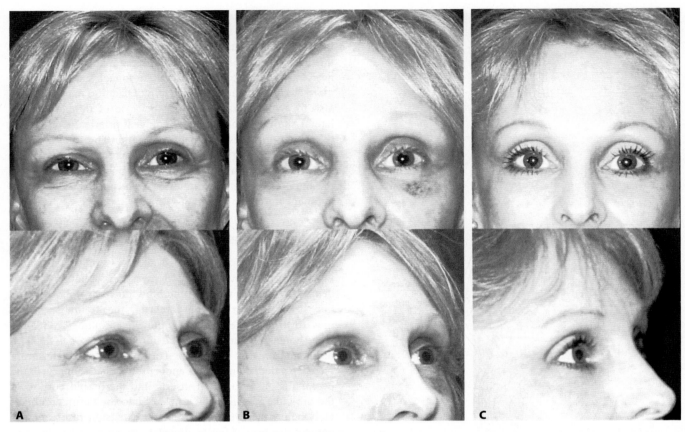

FIGURE 68-4.   **A,** Preoperative view of patient with classic lateral hooding brow ptosis and only "pseudo" upper eyelid laxity or ptosis. **B,** One week after endoscopic forehead and brow lift only. (Slight overcorrection is noted in this early period.) **C,** Correction of lateral hooding with isolated brow lift after 1 month.

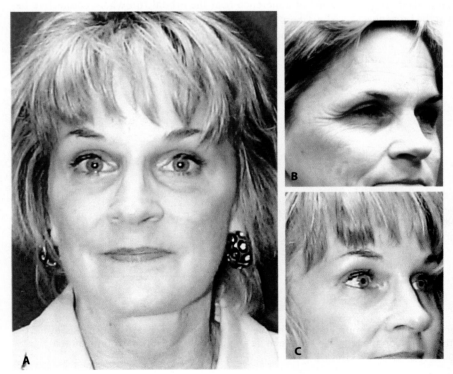

FIGURE 68-5.   **A,** Example of ideal facial proportions based on vertical facial thirds and horizontal proportions approximately the width of the eye or one fifth of the facial width. **B,** Preoperative. **C,** Six weeks after endoscopic forehead and brow lift along with laser skin resurfacing.

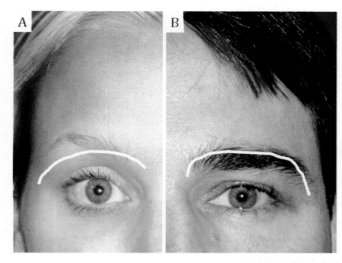

FIGURE 68-6.   **A,** Female brow shown with a nicely accentuated arch in the lateral third well above the orbital rim. **B,** The average male brow position is level with the orbital rim with a symmetrical arch form.

and posterior along a near-horizontal line from the orbital ligament is the orbicularis-temporal ligament, which is the transverse fusion zone of fibers from the lateral orbicularis, the temporoparietal fascia, and the temporalis fascia. These are important clinical anatomic areas because freeing the zones of adherence is necessary to achieve long-term results with lift procedures. However, care is required in this region to avoid overzealous stretching and injury to the facial nerve.

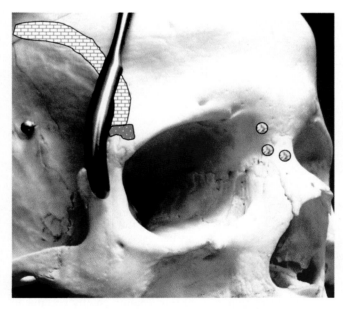

FIGURE 68-7.   Periosteal elevator shown at a more aggressive level of dissection to elevate the lateral canthus slightly, if desired. Fascial and muscle attachments are labeled. Elevation at this level detaches only the superficial layer of the lateral canthal tendon. (The deep portion of the lateral canthus is 5 mm within the orbital rim attached to Whitnall's tubercle.)

The acronym *SCALP* applies for the standard layers in the forehead: *s*kin, sub*c*utaneous tissue, *a*poneurosis (the thick galeal fascia), *l*oose areolar (subgaleal) plane, and *p*eriosteum[28–30]; however, the galeal fascia fuses into the frontalis muscle and its midline fascial attachments at this level. This allows a sliding movement over the scalp with contraction of the muscle. The frontalis and galea together can also be thought of as an extension of the temporoparietal fascia in the temporal region as well as the superficial musculoaponeurotic system (SMAS) below the level of the zygomatic arch.[31–33] The temporoparietal fascia appears somewhat loose or spongy clinically and houses the temporal nerve within its undersurface.

Many other paired forehead and brow muscles thought of as depressors are present along the brow to facilitate facial expression.[34–41] The two most well known are the procerus and the corrugator supercilii, which are present in the glabella (Figure 68-11). The procerus muscles are paired superiorly but fuse inferiorly into one muscle belly that originates from the nasal bones and cartilage. Superiorly, procerus fibers insert into the medial frontalis and the overlying dermis. The procerus is responsible for depression and frowning in the midline, which often creates a horizontal crease ("bunny lines") across the upper portion of the nose. The corrugator supercilii are depressors that act obliquely across the glabella and produce the classic vertical lines seen when squinting (Figure 68-12). The corrugator originates from the frontal bone just above the nasal bones and inserts in the dermis of the medial brow. The corrugator has two heads, the oblique and the transverse, that act to pull the medial brow in respective locations. Together, the paired procerus muscles and corrugator are the main depressors of the medial brow and are the most common muscles treated with botulinum toxin type A to help alleviate frown lines in the glabella. These same two muscles are also most often transected during a brow or forehead lift to achieve a smoother and longer-lasting result (Figure 68-13).

Another depressor muscle of importance is the depressor supercilii, which originates on the frontal process of the maxilla just below the corrugator supercilii and inserts in the medial frontalis fibers and dermis just above the medial brow. Because it lies superficial to the corrugator, it can be easily paralyzed inadvertently by botulinum toxin. It is also important to note because it lies behind the corrugator and can be transected by aggressive dissection through the corrugator during a brow lift. Although patients with a very low medial brow position may occasionally benefit from this maneuver, it often gives rise to overelevation of the medial brow after surgery, which causes the patient to look somewhat surprised (Figure 68-14). Superficial to the depressor supercilii is the orbital portion of the orbicularis oculi that inserts into portions of the adjacent depressors, the superficial surface of the inferior frontalis, as well as the dermis below the brow.[42,43] The orbital portion of the orbicularis muscle originates in part from the medial canthal tendon and adjacent bone. Deep to all the depressors is the galeal fat pad,

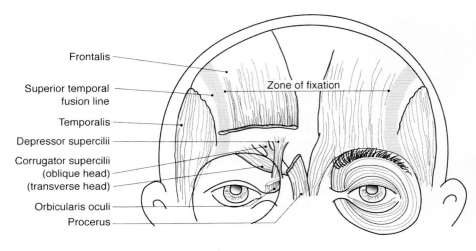

Frontalis
Superior temporal fusion line
Temporalis
Depressor supercilii
Corrugator supercilii (oblique head) (transverse head)
Orbicularis oculi
Procerus
Zone of fixation

FIGURE 68-8.   Cutaway portions of the frontalis muscles, procerus, and orbicularis oculi on one side demonstrate the relationship to the deeper depressors of the brow (corrugator supercilii and depressor supercilii). The zone of fixation *(blue)* runs medial to the superior temporal fusion line.

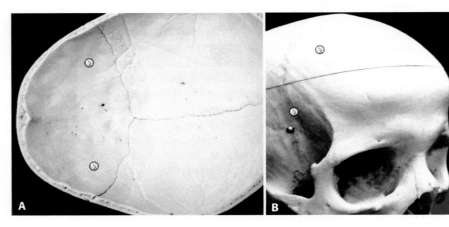

FIGURE 68-9.   **A,** Inside view of the calvarium of the skull demonstrates the high density of venous lakes near the midline and associated structures. **B,** The ideal location placement for bone screws or tunnels based on ideal vector of lift and anatomic limitations.

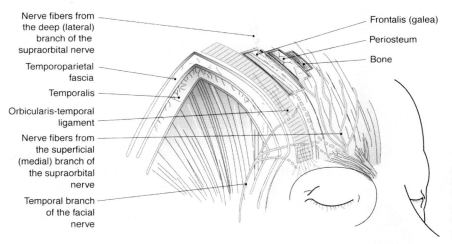

Nerve fibers from the deep (lateral) branch of the supraorbital nerve
Temporoparietal fascia
Temporalis
Orbicularis-temporal ligament
Nerve fibers from the superficial (medial) branch of the supraorbital nerve
Temporal branch of the facial nerve
Frontalis (galea)
Periosteum
Bone

FIGURE 68-10.   Layers of fascia are seen on each side of the zone of fixation *(blue).* The layers must be elevated and connected to a uniform sliding plane surgically to achieve pleasing and long-lasting brow lift results while not damaging the associated motor and sensory nerves.

which lies immediately below the transverse head of the corrugator and helps in identification of muscular landmarks.[44] The galeal fat is usually exposed clinically instantly after transection through the periosteum along the orbital rim (Figure 68-15).

Finally, paired temporalis muscles are located in each temporal fossa, where they originate and then insert on the coronoid process of the mandible. The importance of these muscles during upper facial rejuvenation chiefly pertains to their overlying fascia, which can be used to delineate surgical planes and aid in fixation. The spongy temporoparietal fascia is superficial to the dense and shiny white temporalis fascia. The temporalis fascia adheres to the temporalis muscles below and splits into a superficial and deep layer in the lower

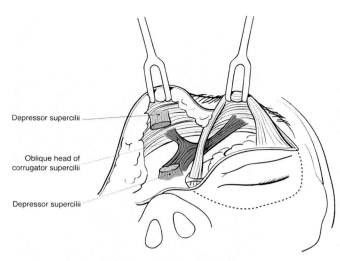

FIGURE 68-11.   The oblique and transverse heads of the corrugator supercilii are seen behind the stump of the depressor supercilii. Both heads of the corrugator muscles and the orbicularis oculi insert into the dermis below the brow.

half of the fossa. For consistency, the superficial layer of deep temporalis fascia (which really describes only that portion of deep temporalis fascia at the level of the split and below) is subsequently referred to simply as *temporalis fascia*. In essence, this term will be used to describe any of this deep thick fascial layer that is seen clinically from the temporal crest down to the zygomatic arch (Figure 68-16).

One method of fixation during brow lifting is the use of suture to fixate the temporoparietal fascia from below a skin incision to the dense and adherent temporalis fascia above the incision to elevate the lateral brow. Some surgeons advocate removing a window of temporalis fascia and exposing the underlying temporalis muscle in hopes of creating scarification in this region and improving fixation longevity.[12]

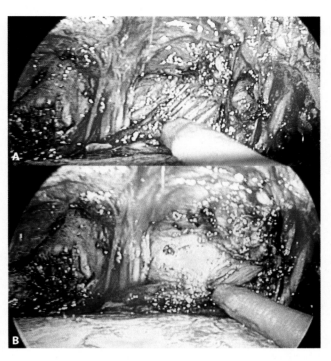

FIGURE 68-13.   Endoscopic views of the right side of the forehead. **A,** Location of the corrugator supercilii relative to the supraorbital nerve immediately before it is transected with a needle tip cautery. **B,** Following transection through the belly of the corrugator supercilii.

Vessel and Nerve Anatomy

Blood supply to the upper face and scalp is plentiful and comes from multiple sources. Several major vessels of the

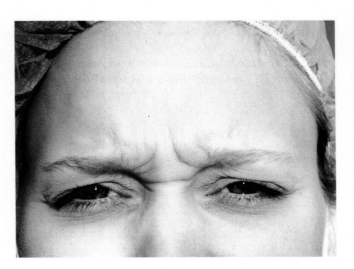

FIGURE 68-12.   Frown lines of the glabella are produced by the actions of the corrugator supercilii to produce the classic vertical wrinkles, whereas the actions of the more vertically arranged fibers of the procerus muscle produce the horizontal wrinkles seen across the bridge of the nose.

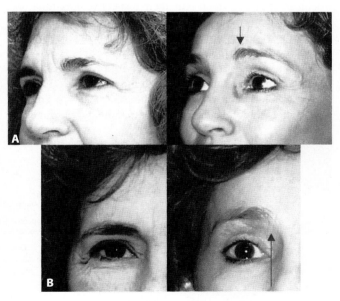

FIGURE 68-14.   Before **(A)** and after **(B)** photos following endoscopic forehead and brow lifting demonstrate good elevation of the lateral hooding but overresection of the medial depressors in the area indicated *(arrow)*. This can result in a surprised look, especially when the patient elevates the brow, as shown.

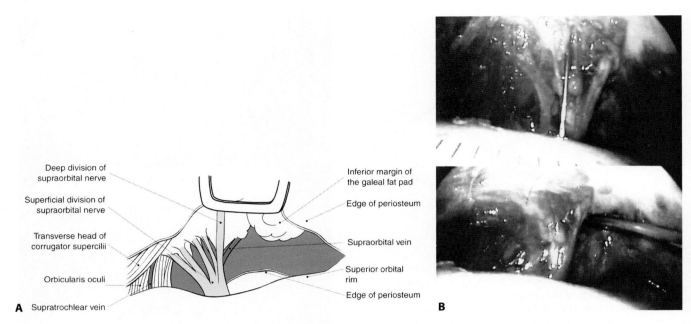

FIGURE 68-15. **A,** Right-sided forehead landmarks. **B,** Endoscopic view of the right supraorbital nerve and vessels. The first view is seen with a 27-gauge needle over the nerve trunk after it is placed through the skin of the brow level with the patient's medial limbus (iris).

upper face originate from the external carotid artery including the superficial temporal artery and the facial artery. These give rise to the blood supply in the medial canthal region via the angular artery and in the lateral canthal region by way of the frontal or anterior branch of the superficial temporal artery. The internal carotid artery gives way to the middle meningeal artery and the ophthalmic artery. The ophthalmic artery then gives rise to the supraorbital and supratrochlear arteries, which exit their respective foramina and supply the majority of the forehead and midscalp with blood. The terminal arterial branches of the upper face have major anastomoses with adjacent vessels (Figure 68-17).

Venous drainage of the upper face follows the respective arterial supply but can be somewhat more variable. However, one particular vein, known as the *sentinel vein* (medial zygomaticotemporal vein), runs perpendicular through the temporalis fascia connecting the superficial and middle temporal veins (Figure 68-18).[45] The sentinel vein can most often be found approximately 1 cm lateral or posterior to the zygomaticofrontal suture line (Figures 68-19 and 68-20). It is clinically significant during endoscopic procedures because, if injured, it can result in impaired field visualization and significant bruising.

Nerve supply parallels arterial supply to some degree. The supratrochlear and supraorbital nerves, which are responsible for the majority of sensation in the forehead, exit via the same foramina or general location as the supraorbital and supratrochlear blood vessels. The sensory nerves originate from the first division of the trigeminal nerve. The supraorbital nerve has two divisions after exiting its foramen: the deep (or lateral) division supplies the more lateral and posterior portion of the forehead and scalp and the superficial

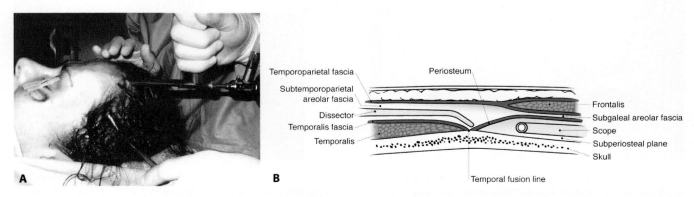

FIGURE 68-16. **A** and **B,** Endoscopic dissection must connect the tissue planes on each side of the temporal crest. Various approaches may be used as long as the anatomic planes seen here are sufficiently understood to allow proper tissue release, a clean endoscopic view, and protection of the facial nerve.

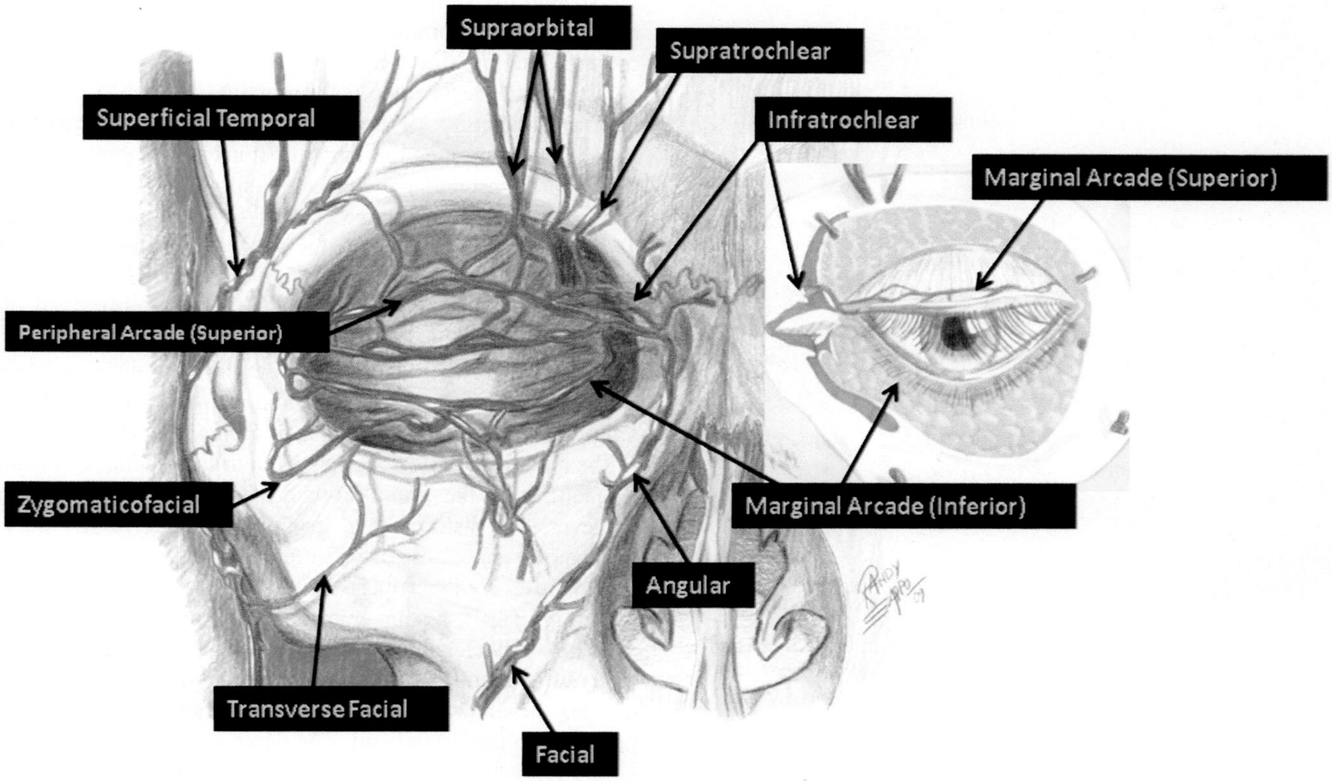

FIGURE 68-17. Periorbital arterial vessels demonstrate the excellent anastomotic blood supply for the periorbital and forehead regions. Most of the vessels have accompanying sensory or motor nerves running parallel with their course.

(or medial) division pierces the frontalis and runs superficially to the muscle, supplying sensation to the forehead along the midpupil line (Figure 68-21). The location of the supraorbital nerve's exit is relatively consistent. The supraorbital foramen or notch is typically found within 1 mm of a line drawn in a sagittal plane tangential to the medial limbus (Figure 68-22).[46] The deep division has been known to exit as often as 10% from another foramen that can be as high as 1.5 cm above the orbital rim. However, this was may be inaccurate. A review of 300 endoscopic brow lifts did not demonstrate any obvious supraorbital nerve over 0.5 cm from the rim. Further study of 40 cadaveric head dissections also failed to demonstrate any significant size foramen beyond

0.5 cm above the orbital rim at the level of the supraorbital notch or foramen. Microsize foramen can be seen in various locations on the forehead skull but are most consistent with tiny perforating vessels and would not support any notable sensation.

The supratrochlear nerves exit from around the orbital rim at an average of 9 mm medial to the exit of the supraorbital nerve.[46] The nerves supply sensation to the midforehead with some overlap from the supraorbital nerves. Infratrochlear nerves, also from division I of the trigeminal nerve, exit just below the supratrochlear nerves around the medial orbital rim to supply sensation to the upper nose and medial orbit. Zygomaticofrontal and zygomaticotemporal nerves are from

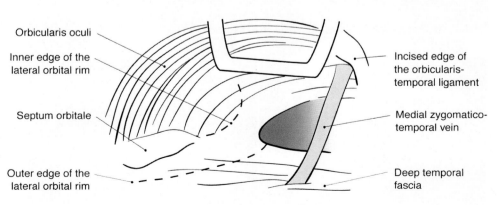

FIGURE 68-18. Dissection below the patient's right temporal crest with release of the orbicularis-temporal ligament. The medial zygomaticotemporal (sentinel) vein seen here pierces the temporalis fascia approximately 1 cm posterior to the zygomaticofrontal suture line.

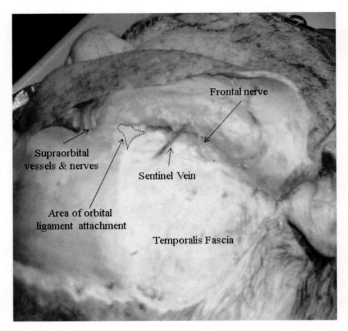

FIGURE 68-19. The sentinel vein, show here in *blue latex*, runs perpendicular to the temporalis fascia. The cadaver dissection also demonstrates the location of the temporal nerve, which runs obliquely just superficially to the sentinel vein in the deep temporoparietal fascia.

the orbital rim and zygomatic arch. Elevation of the deep tissues in this "safe zone" is essentially performed blindly through each of the small scalp incisions. Incisions and specific tissue release and fixation techniques are highly variable among surgeons.[52–59] The author prefers to dissect within

the second division of the trigeminal nerve. They exit their respective small foramina and supply sensation to the lateral orbit and temporal regions of the face.

The facial nerve supplies motor innervation to the forehead and glabella.[47–51] The frontal (or temporal) branch of the facial nerve supplies the frontalis muscle, the superior portion of the orbicularis oculi, the superior portion of the procerus, and the transverse head of the corrugator supercilii. The zygomatic branch of the facial nerve supplies the medial head of the orbicularis oculi, the oblique head of the corrugator supercilii, the inferior portion of the procerus, and the depressor supercilii (Figure 68-23).

The auriculotemporal nerve, from the third division of the trigeminal nerve, supplies sensation in front of the ear to the temporal skin above the zygomatic arch and along the course of the superficial artery. It may be confused clinically during a facelift with the frontal branch of the facial nerve. It can, however, be distinguished from the facial motor nerve because it runs within 1 cm anterior to the tragus of the ear and parallel to the superficial temporal artery. The much more significant frontal branch of the facial nerve runs an average of 2 cm anterior to the tragus when crossing the zygomatic arch. The temporal branch of the facial nerve crosses the arch at an oblique angle at an average of 2 cm posterior to the orbital rim. The depth of the temporal nerve is just below the SMAS at the arch and below the temporoparietal fascia immediately above the arch (Figure 68-24).

Initial dissection must be performed to gain adequate space for the endoscopic equipment. This early dissection is performed in the posterior forehead and temporal regions; endoscopy-guided dissection is used for the last 1 cm above

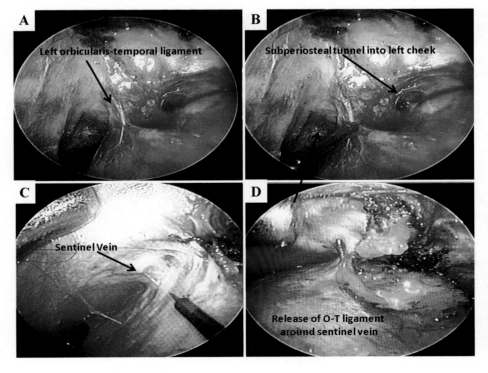

FIGURE 68-20. **A** and **B,** The left orbicularis-temporal (O-T) ligament, also known as the *orbital ligament,* immediately before release via needle tip cautery. Medial to O-T is a subperiosteal tunnel created by a larger elevator past the zygomaticofrontal suture and down into the left cheek. The orbicularis oculi muscle can be severed inside the tunnel. **C** and **D,** Exposure of the sentinel vein before and after complete release or the orbital ligament.

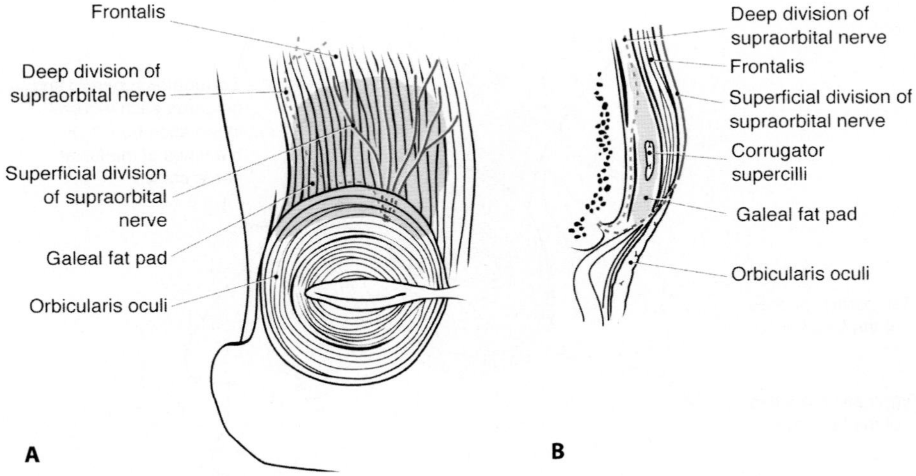

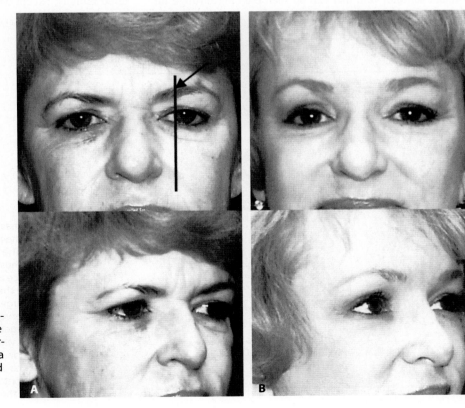

Frontalis

Deep division of
supraorbital nerve

Superficial division
of supraorbital
nerve

Galeal fat pad

Orbicularis oculi

Deep division of
supraorbital nerve

Frontalis

Superficial division of
supraorbital nerve

Corrugator
supercilli

Galeal fat pad

Orbicularis oculi

A   **B**

FIGURE 68-21.   **A** and **B,** Distribution of the superficial (medial) and deep (lateral) divisions of the supraorbital nerve.

a completely subperiosteal plane medially to the temporal crest and in the plane immediately above the temporalis fascia below the temporal line on each side. Subperiosteal dissection in the lateral forehead helps to avoid injury to the deep or lateral division of the supraorbital nerve, which runs in the subgaleal plane near the zone of fixation. Some surgeons begin their dissection in a subgaleal plane in the posterior scalp.[59,60] Regardless, a space is created in the safer posterior areas of the scalp to allow room for placement of an endoscope, which aids dissection in the more risky areas of the forehead.

The first anatomic landmark the surgeon must consider is the zone of fixation along the superior temporal crest. Its inferior edge is found near the superior lateral orbital rim. A convergence of fibers from the periosteum, galea, temporalis, and temporoparietal fascia interlace and fuse to form the zone of adherence, in much the same way the layers of tissue planes come together at the level of the zygomatic arch. The zone of fixation can be elevated bluntly at the hairline level and a couple of centimeters below, but as the surgeon approaches the lateral brow beginning approximately 1 cm above brow level, use of an endoscope aids dissection. At this point, the ligament has branches of the temporal nerve within it, and care must be taken to remain against the bone and temporalis fascia below to avoid nerve injury. Another fibrous attachment, the orbicularis-temporal ligament, is also

FIGURE 68-22.   **A,** Preoperative photograph demonstrates the location of the supraorbital vessels by a line drawn vertically from the medial iris. **B,** One and a half years after an endoscopic forehead and brow lift. No blepharoplasty was ever performed.

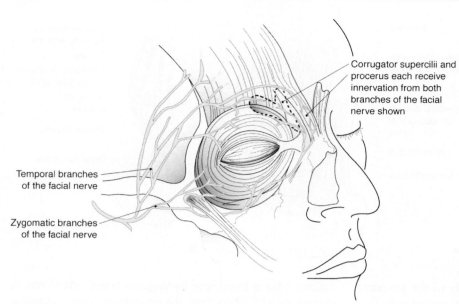

Corrugator supercilii and procerus each receive innervation from both branches of the facial nerve shown

Temporal branches of the facial nerve

Zygomatic branches of the facial nerve

FIGURE 68-23. Motor nerve supply to the forehead depressor muscle comes from both the temporal and the zygomatic branches of the facial nerve.

present here and contains motor nerve fibers (see Figure 68-18); it is the decussation of fibers from the temporoparietal fascia and of the temporal fascia that extends laterally from the orbital ligament. The zone of adherence becomes even more tenacious as the orbital ligament (see Figure 68-7) at the orbital rim level is approached. Slow meticulous dissection is required at this point to avoid nerve injury as well as injury to the sentinel vein that is located within the orbicularis-temporal ligament approximately 1 cm laterally to the zygomaticofrontal suture. Careful dissection exposes an intact sentinel vein that can be seen piercing through the

temporal fascia at a perpendicular angle and entering the temporoparietal fascia above (see Figure 68-18).

Dissection above the orbital rims in the subperiosteal plane should expose the entire superior orbital rim from each zygomaticofrontal suture. The curvature of the rims should be visualized so that transection through the periosteum can be made at the level of the rims. The nasofrontal suture may not always be seen but can be felt by the periosteal elevator used to lift tissue. When transecting through the periosteum across the entire orbital rim, subgaleal fat is often encountered initially, except when the transection is directly behind

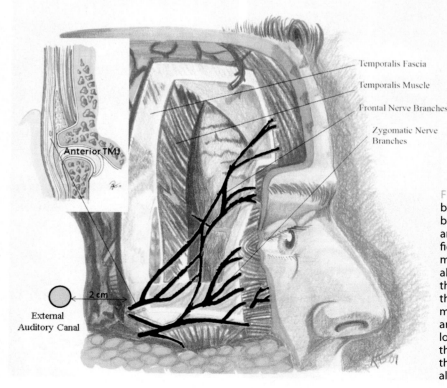

Temporalis Fascia

Temporalis Muscle

Frontal Nerve Branches

Zygomatic Nerve Branches

Anterior TMJ

2 cm

External Auditory Canal

FIGURE 68-24. The temporal and zygomatic branches of the facial nerve divide into multiple branches by the time they reach the zygomatic arch. The nerve branches are deep to the superficial musculoaponeurotic system (SMAS) in the midface and deep to the temporoparietal fascia above the arch. In facelift and forehead lifting, the surgeon must be either above or below the nerve branches and be most careful in the midzygomatic arch region because the tissues are all very condensed around the nerve in this location. Typically, there is a relatively safe area the first 2 cm in front of the ear canal because the frontal nerve is not found in this region along the arch.

the supraorbital nerve at the rim level where the deep (or lateral) division of the nerve is closely adherent to periosteum (see Figure 68-15). Preoperatively marking a point on the brow at a level tangential to the medial limbus iris helps the surgeon to easily identify the location of the supraorbital vessels and nerves.[46] Dissection through the periosteum in this region should be performed slowly and superficially to avoid injury to these structures (Figure 68-25). The transverse head of the corrugator supercilii is seen at the orbital rim level behind the supraorbital vessels and nerves. The corrugator supercilii can be carefully transected or partially excised.[61] Medially, the oblique head of the corrugator is encountered, and by a transection through this portion of muscle, the supratrochlear nerve and depressor supercilii muscle may be seen and protected from injury. Medially, in the glabella, the procerus muscle, which is variable in thickness, is seen. Care should be taken to avoid overaggressive muscle resection in thin patients because this can result in an atrophic defect in the glabella. Deeper dissection toward the skin level under the brow will lead to the orbicularis oculi but is typically not necessary to gain the desired effect (except with regard to the lateral orbicularis, where limited transection may improve lateral brow elevation).[62,63] In addition, one or more incisions through the periosteum at higher levels under the frontalis muscle in the midline can be performed but this is required only if deep horizontal lines are present.[64] It is more important to gain complete release of the retaining lateral ligaments, transection of those muscles causing glabellar lines, and adequate separation of the periosteum along the orbital rim to get the elevation of brow and forehead tissues for the most pleasing and long-term aesthetic result.[65-75]

PREOPERATIVE EVALUATION AND SURGICAL PREPARATION

Determining whether a patient will benefit from a brow or forehead lift and which procedure will work best is critical to avoid disappointing the patient. Commonly, the novice surgeon notices only horizontal forehead lines as an indication for a brow lift. Unfortunately, this is much less of a problem for most patients than is a low lateral brow position (hooding) or glabellar crease (see Figure 68-3). As discussed previously, the ideal female brow position is above the orbital rim at a level that varies among individuals. An average distance of 5 to 10 mm of brow elevation above the rim in the lateral third generally looks most pleasing. Men require a straight-up elevation of the entire brow to avoid feminizing their appearance by overelevation of the lateral brow. In addition, men may benefit more from a standard upper blepharoplasty and local transpalpebral brow lift if the brow ptosis is minimal. As with any cosmetic surgery, a decision regarding the risks and benefits must be made and must conform to the patient's desires. Patient education is required so that they know the risks as well as what can *realistically* be achieved (Figure 68-26). Even with fairly aggressive muscle resection and forehead elevation, patients often form new dynamic lines in the upper face after surgery. A *subcutaneous browlift,* which maintains a surgical plane above the frontalis muscle, may be required if heavy horizontal forehead lines exist and the patient wants them significantly reduced in appearance. Comparatively, subgaleal and subperiosteal dissection planes during forehead and brow lifting allow treatment of the depressors muscles but do not allow major affective treatment of the frontalis muscle and horizontal forehead creases

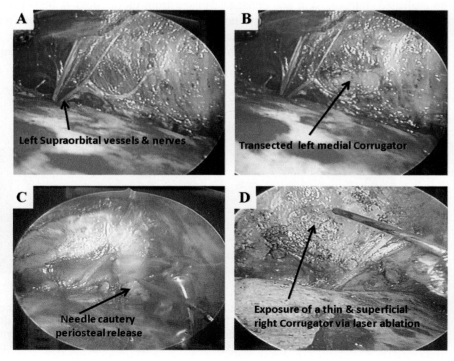

FIGURE 68-25. **A** and **B,** The left supraorbital vessels and nerves immediately adjacent to the medial portion of the oblique head of the corrugator muscle. **A,** An intact, large corrugator. **B,** The same muscle immediately after needle tip cautery has transected the midbelly of this muscle. **C,** Periosteal release is made 1.5 cm above the rim at the supraorbital neurovascular belly to prevent accidental trunk transection. All other regions of the brow are released directly at the arcus marginalis. **D,** The right corrugator muscle is thin and very superficial. Laser ablation of periosteum and brow fat medial to the nerve is performed to locate this sometimes small muscle for treatment.

Left Supraorbital vessels & nerves

Transected left medial Corrugator

Needle cautery periosteal release

Exposure of a thin & superficial right Corrugator via laser ablation

SECTION 8

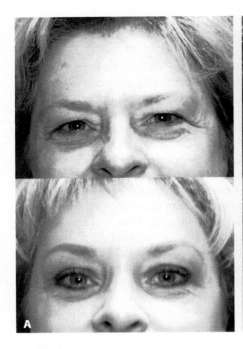

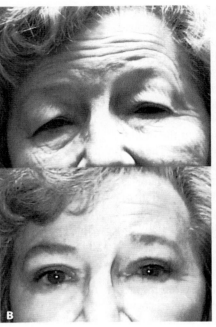

FIGURE 68-26. **A,** Because of both brow ptosis and upper eyelid laxity, the patient required upper blepharoplasties as well as endoscopic forehead and brow lifting to achieve the results she desired. **B,** The patient before and after only blepharoplasty and full-face laser skin resurfacing. She has multiple problems including asymmetry of the brows due to a blepharospasm on the left side, eyelid asymmetry and severe laxity, pseudoelevation of the brows due to frontalis compensation for severe eyelid ptosis, and severe actinic skin damage. She is not a good candidate for simultaneous brow lifting because a change in brow position will likely occur after the removal of the eyelid ptosis. She is a good candidate for botulinum toxin therapy on her left side.

(Figure 68-27). The depressor muscles and their resulting creases in the glabellar region can be adequately treated from a subperiosteal, subgaleal, or subcutaneous plane. Lateral crow's-feet owing to the action of the orbicularis oculi when smiling may appear improved after a brow lift because the muscle is unfolded. However, they are not completely eliminated by brow lifting alone, and the patient must understand that botulinum toxin therapy may be required to treat these particular lines on an ongoing basis.[76]

In addition to lines on the forehead, lines in the glabella, brow ptosis, and the condition of the patient's skin must also be evaluated. Intrinsic skin and collagen damage from the effects of sun, age, and smoking are not treated by lifting alone. Topical skin care (e.g., retinoic acid, microdermabrasion, pulsed-light therapy, sunblocks) along with possible surgical resurfacing must be considered.[77–79] In general, the forehead can be treated safely with chemical peels or laser skin resurfacing into the dermal level simultaneously with brow lifting procedures, provided the lifting is performed with a subgaleal or subperiosteal technique rather than a subcutaneous one. Finally, bony irregularities or hypertrophic bony orbital rims can be evaluated for treatment by means of a cephalometric radiograph or computed tomography (CT) scan as required. Bony contouring can be performed on a limited basis endoscopically, but a major reduction for significant bone hypertrophy such as a frontal boss is best treated with an open (coronal) approach. The amount of bone reduction is limited by the pneumatization of the frontal sinus, which is best evaluated by CT. Although treatment planning for placement of bone tunnels does not

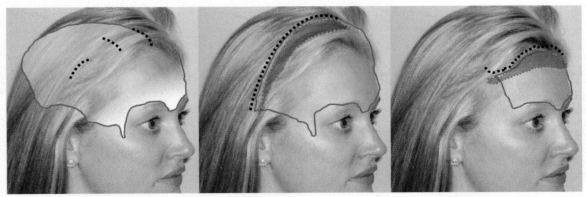

Endoscopic Brow Lift   Coronal Brow Lift   Trichophytic Brow Lift

FIGURE 68-27. The three most classic forms of brow lifting are presented using *dashed lines* to demonstrate the incision used for each technique. The *shaded areas* demonstrate the extent of dissection typically required for each technique. Interestingly, the endoscopic brow lift actually requires more undermining to allow tissue redraping because no direct scalp excision is performed compared with the other techniques.

require a preoperative CT, a standard cephalometric radiograph may help to reassure the surgeon regarding the thickness of corticocancellous bone available.

As with any surgical procedure, appropriate preoperative laboratory and other indicated tests must be performed. Written instructions are given to the patient regarding pre- and postoperative care, including instructions for shampooing hair with antibacterial soap or other antiseptic shampoo and avoidance of the use of hair spray or other hair products immediately before surgery. The patient should be thoroughly instructed on the critical need to avoid all medications that may cause platelet dysfunction 10 days before surgery (including aspirin and other nonsteroidal anti-inflammatory drugs, vitamin E, and many over-the-counter herbal supplements). Endoscopic techniques require a very dry operating field that necessitates strict avoidance of these medications as well as proper preoperative injection of vasoconstrictive agents.

Before induction of anesthesia, photographs are taken and the patient is marked while awake and sitting up. Following the introduction of general anesthesia or intravenous sedation, the patient is prepared and carefully injected with local anesthetic with epinephrine. The author prefers to use a local anesthetic with 1:100,000 epinephrine along the entire orbital rim and a tumescent anesthesia solution (250 mL of normal saline mixed with 1 mL of 1:1,000 epinephrine and 20 mL of 2% lidocaine) in the remaining upper forehead, temple, and posterior scalp. Careful injection in the desired tissue planes helps to avoid the formation of a hematoma during the injection and allows for a nearly bloodless procedure. Minor shaving of hair along the marked incision lines is performed if desired immediately before the final preparation and draping of the area.

CORONAL FOREHEAD AND BROW LIFT

Still one of the most common approaches for forehead and brow lifting, the classic coronal lift involves an incision across the entire forehead from ear to ear, staying well behind the hairline.[80-88] Dissection is typically in the subgaleal or subperiosteal plane and then connects to the subtemporoparietal plane laterally. This gives great exposure of the entire orbital rims for bony osteoplasty, if required, and treatment of muscles that require resection including the depressors (corrugator and procerus) as well as the frontalis. Heavy horizontal forehead creases can be addressed with this technique by way of either midline myotomies or minor midline thinning of the frontalis. Major resection of the frontalis should be avoided to prevent postoperative irregularities and strange facial expressions during frontalis movement. The lateral frontalis should be avoided to prevent nerve damage, ptosis, and other irregularities.

Regrettably, the coronal lift also has the disadvantages of a long incision and a significant elevation of the hairline. Patients with a high hairline are not good candidates for this technique because a significant amount of scalp excision is required. Many surgeons believe this scalp excision is a rea-

sonable trade-off because they feel that the technique gives a more lasting approach than do newer endoscopic techniques. If performed correctly, the endoscopic technique can be as long-lasting and possibly more precise than open brow lifting techniques. Care must be taken with the coronal lift to avoid elevating the medial brow too much and creating a very high hairline. Roughly, to gain 1 cm of brow elevation, 1.5 to 2 cm of scalp must be excised with this technique. The amount of tissue excised is not a precise determinant of the amount of brow elevation obtained. Scoring of the underlying fascia and muscle resection can cause the tissue to stretch oddly, making prediction of the exact brow elevation difficult.

The benefits of the coronal lift include great exposure and relatively easy dissection. It can also be used to extend the procedure into a deep-plane facelift by dissection over the zygomatic arches and onto the zygoma and masseter. This much more aggressive lift gives excellent elevation of the midface but greatly increases postoperative edema and the potential for motor nerve damage. The extended technique should be attempted only by an experienced surgeon,[89-93] and careful consideration should be given to alternative treatments. Comparatively, the basic coronal lift is an easier procedure for the novice surgeon. When selecting this tried-and-true method, one should take into account the disadvantages, including the lengthy scar and possible hair loss, significant scalp anesthesia, and a significantly elevated hairline.

TRICHOPHYTIC OR PRETRICHIAL FOREHEAD AND BROW LIFT

Although trichophytic and pretrichial lifts are sometimes thought to be the same procedure, the *pretrichial* lift actually involves an incision in front of the hairline. With this procedure, hair does not grow anterior to the incision, leaving a visible scar in front of the hairline. In contrast, in the *trichophytic* lift, although still at the frontal hairline, the incision is placed just behind the hairline. This incision is beveled so that follicles in front of the initial skin incision survive and hair grows anterior to the incision to better camouflage the resulting scar. It should be noted that many surgeons use these terms interchangeably. Even better than the trichophytic lift is the irregular trichophytic hairline, which not only employs a beveled incision but also creates a wavy pattern along the hairline for a more natural postoperative appearance compared with a straight-line scar.

Regardless of the specific incision design, the ultimate advantages of the trichophytic forehead and brow lift include great exposure (similar to that with the coronal approach) and the ability to lower a high forehead. Unlike the classic coronal lift, bare forehead skin is excised from the hairline. In addition, lateral incisions and dissection are usually limited with this technique unless required. Incision design can even improve hair thinning in the temporoparietal areas by excising the area of hair loss and bringing forward areas of dense hair-bearing scalp. The posterior scalp and hairline can be brought forward to lower a high forehead by almost any amount. The more lowering that is desired, the more posterior is the dissection and release. Limited or no posterior dissection can be performed if the hairline is to remain at the same level.

The forward dissection is the technique that varies the most among surgeons. A totally subperiosteal technique versus a subgaleal technique is an option. A subcutaneous technique has become more popular, particularly when the depressors in the lower brow are less concerning than the horizontal forehead creases.[94] Staying superficial to the frontalis breaks the dermal insertions that create deep horizontal rhytids. The subcutaneous lift is occasionally combined with deep dissection to treat glabellar lines as well as horizontal lines in the forehead.

Overall, the trichophytic technique of forehead and brow lifting is an invaluable tool for any surgeon performing facial cosmetic surgery. When a patient presents with a high forehead and low brow position, the trichophytic approach is the procedure of choice to correct both problems. The main disadvantage is the potential for a visible incision despite best efforts. All prospective patients considering this technique must be informed of the chance that there may be a visible scar at the hairline. Surprisingly, when presented with the potential problems and given the choice, many patients prefer to undergo an endoscopic approach with a slight elevation in hairline rather than risk a visible hairline scar. Still, the patient with an extremely high hairline is often thrilled with the lower hairline obtainable only with the trichophytic approach. Attention to detail and gentle soft tissue management are essential to attaining a natural hairline and hidden scar with this popular technique.

ENDOSCOPIC FOREHEAD AND BROW LIFT

Early attempts at endoscopic surgery began over a century ago with Nietze's description of a crude cystoscope. A few decades ago, endoscopic surgery progressed through use in upper gastrointestinal examinations and then intra-abdominal surgery. However, facial endoscopic cosmetic surgery did not blossom until the early 1990s. Over the past decade, the endoscopic forehead and brow lift procedure has

been considered by many to be the state-of-the-art technique for upper facial rejuvenation.[95–97] It is versatile and can be combined with many other procedures. The most noted benefits of the endoscopic technique are the smaller scars hidden in the hairline and selective brow elevation without the need for removal of any hair or skin (Figure 68-28).

The technique involves several incisions placed strategically behind the hairline to gain access for early blunt dissection and insertion of the endoscope and tissue retractor. Other incisions can be used as ports for dissecting tools such as periosteal elevators, electrocautery, lasers, tissue graspers, and suction instruments. Among surgeons a variety of incision (port) designs are used. Fixation points are usually placed at these incision sites; therefore, the author prefers five separate 2.5-cm-long incisions placed for easy access but mostly for ideal fixation placement. Each of the five incisions begins approximately 1 cm posterior to the hairline. One is placed in the midline in the sagittal plane and two in the parasagittal plane tangential to the lateral third of the brow (where maximum lift is typically desired in females). This same incision can be moved slightly medially in male patients to give a more even brow elevation. The midline incision plus the two parasagittal incisions are aligned vertically to avoid unnecessary transection of sensory nerves originating from the supraorbital nerves below. The two parasagittal incisions are placed medial to the temporal crest to gain access to skull bone rather than the more lateral temporalis fascia. Bone is the strongest fixation tissue available and ideally should be used thus.[98–100]

It is important to access the subperiosteal plane easily for a clean future endoscopic view. Accidental placement of the parasagittal incisions too far laterally over the zone of fixation or temporalis muscle makes pocket development difficult and obscures future endoscopic visualization. Moreover, the parasagittal incisions are located in a thick area of the frontal bone where there is a low density of venous lakes. Placing the incision here helps to prevent accidental intracranial injury during bone tunnel creation or placement of bone screws.

Lastly, two temporal incisions are made, one on each side of the head, for direct access to the thick temporal fascia. These incisions are placed perpendicular to the desired

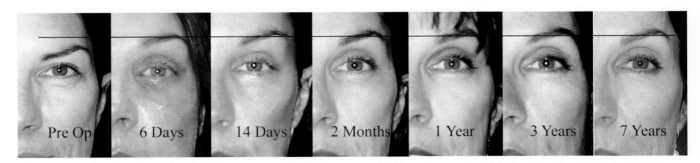

Pre Op   6 Days   14 Days   2 Months   1 Year   3 Years   7 Years

FIGURE 68-28. Sequential appearance after endoscopic forehead and brow lifting (eyelid and skin resurfacing procedures were also performed). Slight overelevation of the brow is noted for 6 days after surgery, as expected. The brow position remains very stable from 2 weeks to 7 years after the surgery. Adequate tissue release is the key to long-term stability of brow lifting.

elevation vector from the lateral canthal region. Coincidentally, the temporal incision parallels the course of the temporal branch of the facial nerve that is located 2 to 3 cm inferior to this incision. It also parallels the superficial temporal artery and vein. Arranging the three medial incisions on a vertical axis and the two temporal incisions in an oblique position to parallel the nerve and blood supply in each area can reduce interference with sensation and vascular supply to the scalp.

Dissection is performed through the above incisions down through periosteum medial to the temporal crest and down to the temporalis fascia lateral to the crest. Some surgeons may elect to use a subgaleal rather than a subperiosteal placement of the incision medially. Total subperiosteal dissection medial to the temporal lines rather than subgaleal dissection leads to better fixation and long-term stabilization (see Figure 68-28).

Blunt and blind dissection can be carried out after reaching the subperiosteal and subtemporoparietal planes through the five incisions. Finger dissection and long curved endoscopic periosteal elevators are used to lift the tissue anteriorly to a point 2 cm above the orbital rims and zygomatic arch. Posteriorly, blunt dissection should elevate the temporal tissues a few centimeters behind the ear, where the temporal fossa becomes self-limiting. The subperiosteal dissection above needs to elevate the scalp at least 10 cm posteriorly but can extend as far back as the lambdoid suture. Once these areas are freed, a connection can be made from the temporal region to the subperiosteal dissection through the upper portion of the zone of fixation at the temporal crest by finger

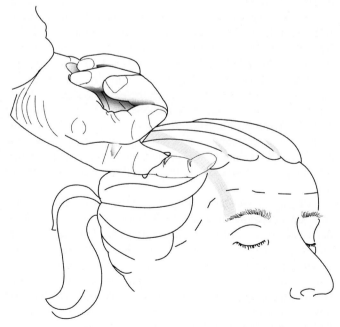

FIGURE 68-29. Blind finger dissection is performed initially, avoiding overzealous dissection inferiorly. Dissection proceeds from the subtemporoparietal plane laterally to the already elevated subperiosteal plane medially. The opposite direction of elevation (medial to lateral) may produce false tunnels in the temporoparietal tissue, which impair future endoscopic vision.

dissection (Figure 68-29). Blind release of the more inferior portion of the temporal line where the facial nerve crosses should be avoided. Endoscope-guided dissection here helps to prevent nerve injury. Using finger dissection, the upper zone of fixation is broken through, proceeding from the temporal incision toward the medial scalp, rather than vice versa, to prevent creation of a false tunnel in the spongy or foamy temporoparietal fascia. False tunnels along the temporal crest create problems when the endoscope is inserted through the parasagittal port to visualize the lateral forehead; the tunnels force the placement of the endoscope in a more superficial plane within the temporoparietal fascia, which greatly increases the chance of nerve injury. Therefore, it is critical to stay firmly against the periosteum and the temporalis fascia when initially elevating the scalp and forehead.

Following blunt elevation of the scalp from each incision for complete flap elevation, the endoscope is normally inserted through one of the three more medial incisions. Poor initial blunt dissection makes the initial endoscopic dissection feel very tight, and care must be taken not to perforate the skin by excessive retraction. Medial dissection over the nasofrontal suture and orbital rims is performed under direct endoscopic vision with a curved and smooth elevator to avoid inadvertent tearing of the periosteum. The periosteum may be thin in some patients in whom a straighter elevator may be used to transect the periosteum at the level of the rim (arcus marginalis). However, the entire rolled edge of the orbital rim must be visualized before proceeding with periosteal incision (Figure 68-30). Typically, the periosteum is more precisely incised with a needle tip cautery or laser set at low power. The supraorbital nerves and vessels as described earlier are at a level tangential to the medial limbus and are immediately behind (superficial to) the periosteum from the internal endoscopic view.[46,101] This necessitates meticulous cautery dissection here to avoid injury to these structures (see Figure 66-25). Suction placed by an assistant from another port is required to maintain a clear view when using cautery or laser. Temporal incisions work well for suction ports during dissection over the rims because the endoscope and cautery take up most of the room through any of the middle three incision sites. With clear and near bloodless dissection at this point, transection can be performed through the corrugator supercilii and procerus. If unwanted bleeding is encountered and cannot be controlled easily with pinpoint accurate cautery, pressure should be applied externally over the rim until improved visualization allows for control of bleeding without nerve damage.

Vertical rhytids in the glabella created by the corrugators can be improved greatly by transection through these muscles. Likewise, horizontal glabellar lines are treated by transection of the procerus muscle that creates these particular facial wrinkles. Some surgeons advocate more aggressive surgical avulsion of these muscles with endoscopic biopsy forceps. Aggressive muscle removal may lead to a more permanent treatment of glabellar lines compared with isolated transection only, but it should be avoided in most cases owing

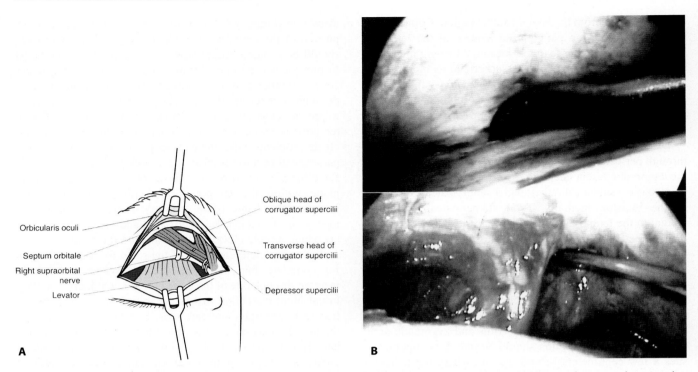

A

B

FIGURE 68-30.   **A,** The orbital rim and local depressor muscle as seen from a transblepharoplasty incision. **B,** Endoscopic photographs show the rolled border of orbital rim before periosteal release in the first view and the supraorbital nerve and vein in the next view after excising through the periosteum.

to an increased risk of significant postoperative irregularities and abnormal facial expression. As a rule, patients prefer a more natural appearance with some minor return of frown lines to risking a bizarre facial expression and glabellar depression.

Once the periosteum is completely freed across the orbital rims and appropriate muscles have been treated, the cut periosteal edges are spread apart (periosteal elevators work well for this) by at least 1 cm to aid the release at the arcus marginalis. This allows significant and long-term brow elevation. Next, the lateral orbital rim must be exposed in the subperiosteal plane after careful release below the zone of fixation and orbital ligament. Dissection along the anterior and inferior aspects of the temporal crest must be performed cautiously to avoid temporal nerve injury. Overzealous retraction of the dense tissue here that contains the nerve can result in nerve damage. Staying snuggly against periosteum and the temporalis fascia helps to prevent nerve damage and produces a much cleaner dissection. Slowly creating a distinct plane of dissection down to the zygomaticofrontal suture line and avoiding excess retraction help to prevent unwanted bleeding from the sentinel vein (zygomaticotemporal vein), which needs not be sacrificed for a standard endoscopic forehead and brow lift.

Dissection for a standard endoscopic brow lift should not proceed all the way to the zygomatic arch but should stop approximately 1 cm above this level. If an extended midface lift is planned and there is a desire to elevate tissue over the zygomatic arch itself, dissection must go below the superfi-

cial layer of deep temporal fascia just above the arch. Abbreviated midface lifts performed simultaneously with endoscopic brow lifts may simply stay in the subperiosteal plane along the lateral orbital rim and avoid the more risky full-arch release. The beauty of the classic endoscopic brow lift is its versatility and the ease with which additional procedures can be combined simultaneously with this elegant cosmetic surgery. For instance, the temporal incision of an endoscopic forehead lift can easily be extended inferiorly to meet up with the preauricular incision from a standard lower facelift. Also, midfacelifting (with intraoral dissection) can connect the intraoral subperiosteal dissection over the zygoma to the subperiosteal plane from the endoscopic brow lift through a tunnel near the lateral orbital rim (Figure 68-31).

After all dissection is complete, appropriate elevation and fixation is required (Figure 68-32). Many techniques have been described such as tissue suture only, bone screws and plates, resorbable screws, bone tunnels, local skin excision, temporalis muscle exposure for added scarification, tissue glue, and tight head wraps.[102] Regardless of any specific fixation technique, the key to long-term fixation is adequate lower forehead tissue release during endoscopic dissection. Failure to adequately release internal tissue results in a relapse of brow ptosis, even with heavy fixation and the appearance of a "nice" lift during surgery.

Once complete internal release of the forehead is obtained, the specific lifting vectors must be determined for the most pleasing aesthetic effect. The lateral third of the female brow

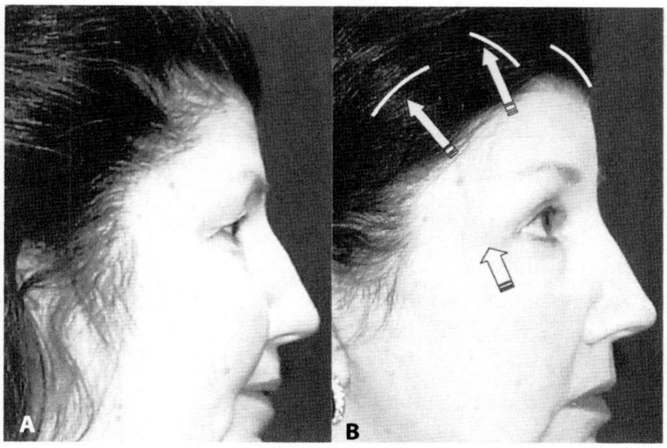

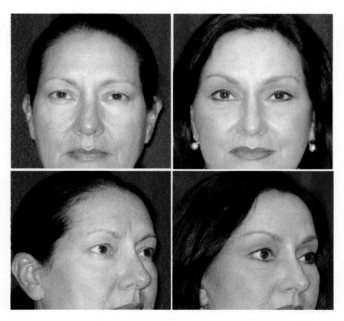

FIGURE 68-31. Before **(A)** and after **(B)** an endoscopic forehead, brow, and midface lift. *Arrows* represent vectors of lift. Fixation is performed at the level of the hairline through the temporal and parasagittal incisions shown.

is elevated to the greatest extent, which is up to 1 cm above the orbital rim. The medial brow should be only slightly above the rim level and definitely below the middle and lateral brow levels to avoid a surprised or bewildered expression (see Figure 68-14). Typically, the glabellar region is elevated on its own without the need for midline fixation, which helps to avoid overelevation medially. The lateral third of the brow is lifted straight up and fixated at the level of the hairline. The galeal tissue is typically secured to bone at this point, while the lateral brow is held at the desired height or 1 to 2 mm above the desired level.[12] Very little relapse occurs with proper technique and averages only 1 to 2 mm after 2 weeks. Measurements can also be made with clear circular templates from the pupil to the brow to help improve symmetry. The brow position remains very stable after this early recovery period (see Figure 68-28). A question remains as to

the time required for complete fixation of the periosteum. Some animal studies suggest a full 12 weeks are required for what is termed *full histologic periosteal refixation.*[103] However, some clinical evidence suggests that adequate fixation occurs in as little as 7 days. An example is the common fixation technique used by many surgeons who place a single transcutaneous bone screw at each parasagittal incision, which is removed after only 1 week. The 1-week fixation technique has been used with success for many years. It has been suggested that longer bony fixation may provide longer-term retention and less early relapse that some have considered normal. The key to long-term fixation seems for now to be determined usually by proper tissue dissection and release (Figure 68-33).

Although there are many fixation techniques, the use of bone tunnels at the parasagittal incisions appears to be one of the best methods for fixating the galea and periosteum near the hairline to a bone tunnel created posteriorly under the incision using a single heavy suture (see Figure 68-32). Fixation of the lateral tail of the brow is performed at each temporal incision, where an isolated heavy suture plicates the temporoparietal fascia in a posterior and superior vector to the thick temporalis fascia. Optional creation of a small window of exposed temporalis muscle in this area may aid in internal scar formation and fixation. The vector of lift at this outer tail of the brow follows a line drawn at an angle from the outer nasal ala that passes just beside the lateral canthus (see Figure 68-31).

Final closure of the hair-bearing scalp incisions can be performed with skin staples only with excellent scar formation because no skin is excised and no pressure exists at the

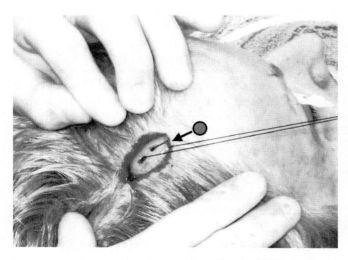

FIGURE 68-32. Example of bone tunnel fixation shown at the site of the right parasagittal incision. The *anterior circle* represents the position of suture placement through the galea, which elevates the lateral brow toward the bone tunnel.

FIGURE 68-33. The patient before an endoscopic brow lift **(left)** and 3 years after the lift **(right).** Extensive release of internal tissues was performed along the entire orbital rims superiorly with transection of the depressor muscles to obtain a very stable lift over time.

incision sites. Redundant tissue (forehead skin) created by an average of 1 cm of brow elevation is easily distributed evenly over the posterior 15 to 20 cm of elevated scalp, which essentially absorbs or redistributes this excess tissue with few to no signs of bunching. Because of this phenomenon, the endoscopic forehead and brow lift tends to elevate the hairline only a very small amount compared with the open skin excising coronal technique.

Interestingly, in a survey performed in 1998 of American Society of Plastic Surgeons members, of the total 6951 brow lifts performed by 570 members who returned the questionnaire, 3534 involved a coronal technique and incision and 3417 were performed endoscopically The most noted difference was the higher risk of hair loss with the coronal technique; however, both techniques enjoyed very low overall complication rates.

TEMPORAL LIFT

The rationale for lifting from a temporal approach alone is the potential to lift the outer brow and midface through a relatively conservative incision and with minimal dissection. Realistically, the procedure has a few potential problems that have kept the procedure from becoming extremely popular. The most worriesome problem is that the vector of dissection runs precisely perpendicular to the path of the frontal nerve making the potential for motor nerve injury possibly higher than other techniques. Also, the attempt to achieve significant lift in this tenacious area of tissue adhesion can be challenging and result in early relapse or inadequate lifting. Albeit challenging, a well-performed temporal lift may be the ideal procedure for the right patient.

The ideal patient for an isolate temporal brow lift has lateral brow hooding and mild midface ptosis but very little problems in the forehead or glabellar regions. For this patient, a temporal incision is made perpendicular to the desired vector of lift followed by dissection directly on top of temporalis fascia or in a very superficial subcutaneous plane (Figure 68-34A). Deep dissection below the nerve is inherently safer but requires more release of retaining ligament to obtain adequate lateral brow and ckeek lift. A subcutaneous flap above the frontal nerve is more likely to damage hair follicles or nerves, but obtaining adequate release for brow elevation is much easier and can be performed with the use of endoscopes or lighted retractors. Selection of the specific technique is operator dependent and based on the surgeon's comfort level. If adequate tissue release is achieved through the compact surgical region, good results can be obtained (see Figure 68-34B).

DIRECT BROW LIFT

The direct brow lift involves excision of an ellipse of skin adjacent to and just above the eyebrow (see Figure 68-34). A beveled incision is used to parallel the hair follicles of the brow or so that some follicles remain at the base of the bevel

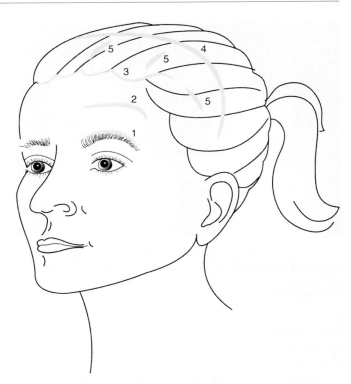

FIGURE 68-34. Representative incisions for typical brow lifting procedures: (1) direct brow lift, (2) midforehead lift, (3) trichophytic brow lift, (4) coronal brow lift, and (5) endoscopic brow lift.

to grow later above the scar. The dissection remains in the subcutaneous plane to avoid muscle or nerve injury.

Advantages of the direct brow lift are that it is a simple procedure (with an easy two-layer closure), it can be performed under local anesthesia, and it can treat brow position asymmetries. It remains a good alternative technique that may be an excellent option for an elderly patient who has severe brow ptosis and heavy wrinkles but cannot tolerate more extensive surgery and would benefit from a short procedure under local anesthesia. The main disadvantage is the potentially visible scar immediately above the brow.

MIDFOREHEAD AND BROW LIFT

Incisions made in the middle or upper forehead regions have similar advantages and disadvantages to the direct brow lift.[104–107] The incisions are made on each side of the forehead in an elliptical fashion so that the resulting scar follows a horizontal line already present in the forehead. Although this is probably the least used of all the techniques described, it may be a practical alternative for the elderly patient with thin eyebrows and deep horizontal rhytids who requires a short procedure under local anesthesia.

TRANSPALPEBRAL AND OTHER LOCAL BROW PROCEDURES

There has been a significant increase in the movement toward minimally invasive techniques to perform cosmetic surgery. New techniques for forehead and brow rejuvenation fill the literature and offer potentially exciting methods to gain aesthetic improvement with less risk than with current procedures. A few such procedures include lateral brow lifting with temporal incisions only, denervation techniques through small punctures around the brow, and direct approaches through an upper blepharoplasty incision. It should be noted that, although procedures such as making small punctures to destroy medial portions of facial nerve innervating medial depressors may seem minimally invasive, they are certainly not without risk.

Many of the "minimally invasive" procedures take advantage of the proximity of the local depressor muscle. For instance, the transpalpebral or transblepharoplasty approach for forehead rejuvenation gains access to the local depressors through an upper eyelid incision.[108] Dissection through this incision involves a short distance to the corrugator supercilii, the procerus, and depressor supercilii of the glabella, which can each be selectively transected from this incision to reduced unwanted wrinkles and elevate the medial brow (see Figure 68-11). Likewise, the orbicularis can be incised and subperiosteal dissection performed above the orbital rim to elevate the lateral brow through this same local incision. Suture plication of the periosteum above the rim may further elevate the lateral brow.

Another adjunctive technique in the upper third of the face is that of fat grafting in areas of age-related fat atrophy. Fat can essentially be grafted anywhere; however, caution is required in the glabellar region where occasional local necrosis can occur from fat infiltration. This also occurs occasionally after collagen injections in the same region.[109] There are a great number of alternative techniques, and each must be evaluated for safety, efficacy, and longevity on an individual basis.

BOTULINUM TOXIN–ASSISTED BROW LIFT

Botulinum toxin has been used for nearly 2 decades to improve the aesthetic appearance of the upper third of the face by reducing wrinkles of the forehead (horizontal lines), glabella (frown and bunny lines), and lateral orbital crow's-feet (laugh lines).[110] More recently, it has been used specifically to elevate certain regions of the brow to obtain a "chemical brow lift."[111] The depressor muscles are paralyzed with botulinum toxin not only to reduce the wrinkles they create but also to allow the frontalis muscle to elevate the brow farther because of the decrease in muscular antagonism. By decreasing the tone and downward pull of the orbicularis immediately below the brow, the lateral third of the eyebrow elevates approximately 2 to 4 mm from the result of botulinum toxin placed in the upper crow's-feet area. Such treatment of depressor muscles in the glabellar region can help elevate the medial brow. Of course, as with surgical brow lifting, overcorrection in the medial brow may result in an abnormal facial expression.

Dosages used vary with individuals. Botox comes in a 100-unit vial to be mixed with 1 to 10 mL normal saline. The more dilute solutions (6–10 mL/100 units) begin to lose efficacy and can distort the tissue, whereas high concentration mixtures (1–2 mL/100 units) may be wasteful and imprecise. Regardless of dilution, the total dosage in units of botulinum toxin and its proper placement determine the outcome. For most individuals, 5 to 10 units is all that is required for each lateral crow's-foot region. However, the larger muscles of the glabella (procerus and corrugators) require at least 15 units of the toxin and up to 50 units for maximum results. Appropriate dosage in the glabella is the most variable. Treatment of horizontal forehead lines typically requires between 15 and 25 units. It should be noted that simultaneous treatment of horizontal forehead lines from the frontalis may decrease or eliminate brow elevation that otherwise may have been created by botulinum toxin treatment of the depressor muscles. Moreover, excessive toxin treatment of horizontal lines close to the eyebrows (within 1 cm) should often be avoided owing to the risk of true ptosis of the forehead, brow, and upper eyelids.

Botulinum toxin has also been recommended to aid long-term stability of the surgical forehead and brow lift. The theory involved is that control of the downward pull of the depressors (by temporarily paralyzing them chemically) gives the periosteum time to attach securely in an elevated position. The injection can be done during surgery, but there is an increased risk of eyelid ptosis and an unwanted delay because botulinum toxin typically takes 3 to 5 days to take full effect. Therefore, ideally botulinum toxin is injected 1 to 2 weeks before surgery. Regardless of any benefit this may give to long-term surgical fixation, the resulting reduction in wrinkles of the forehead and glabella and in crow's-feet is almost always popular with patients, even though the results last for only 3 to 6 months.

ADJUNCTIVE PROCEDURES: SKIN CARE AND MICROPIGMENTATION

A variety of procedures can be used for the superficial treatment of poor skin texture and are covered more completely in Chapter 70. For complete rejuvenation of the upper third of the face, skin resurfacing techniques may be required to address aging problems, especially those related to sun exposure, that cannot be adequately treated with lifting methods alone.

Prior to any resurfacing procedure such as laser skin resurfacing, chemical peels, or dermabrasion, the patient should be treated with topical skin medications to decrease the risk of scarring and pigment problems. Retinoic acid–type preparations used for ideally 6 weeks before resurfacing and 4% hydroquinone for patients with darker skin tones (Fitzpatrick 3 or higher) are two possibilities (see Chapter 70). Simultaneous resurfacing procedures can be accomplished with brow lifting, provided the surgical plane of dissection is subperiosteal or subgaleal and not subcutaneous.

Another adjunctive procedure growing in popularity is medical micropigmentation. The use of new skin pigments that do not contain iron oxide has improved the appearance of tattoos placed to enhance a thin eyebrow or as permanently applied eyeliner. The ink is relatively permanent but often requires touch-ups owing to some fading over the first 3 to 5 years. Patients who have poor hand motor skills can greatly benefit from this procedure. A certified technician under a doctor's supervision usually performs the micropigmentation. However, consultation with a surgeon before micropigmentation is important because placement of a permanent brow tattoo in a more elevated position may create problems if the patient desires a surgical brow lift later. Therefore, if a patient is seeking brow lifting in addition to the micropigmentation, it is advisable to perform the surgical brow lift before the permanent makeup if feasible.

POSTOPERATIVE CARE

Following surgical forehead and brow lifting, a compression bandage is applied using a material such as Coban or Coflex. The pressure helps to limit edema and hematoma formation while possibly improving fixation. Typically, a drain is not required if a very dry field has been maintained. The patient should be instructed to limit activity and to use cold compresses over the eyes and brows. Head elevation is also recommended for the first several days. Avoidance of antiplatelet drugs preoperatively, a careful surgical technique, and the immediate postoperative use of cold compresses, elevation, and limited strenuous activity significantly decrease postoperative healing time.

The relatively snug postoperative dressing may be removed on postoperative day 1 to visually inspect the surgical site for any problems. A less constrictive Velcro-type head wrap can then be used to allow patient comfort and easy removal for showering. Patients are allowed to gently shampoo their hair after 24 hours but must be cautioned to avoid water pressure directly over any incision sites. Each incision is then cleaned twice a day with a dilute peroxide solution, and a thin layer of antibiotic ointment is applied for the first week. Staples are removed at the end of 1 week. Chemical treatments of hair such as "perms" should be delayed for at least 2 weeks to avoid possible hair loss as a reaction to the harsh chemicals. Hot curling irons or other similar devices must be used with caution because areas of scalp anesthesia may be present for months and can predispose a patient to an accidental self-inflicted burn.

COMPLICATIONS

Fortunately, major complications are rare with properly performed forehead and brow rejuvenation procedures. Good patient selection, diligent preoperative planning, meticulous surgical technique, and thorough postoperative care are all required to help limit the chance for complications.[112–115] Minor complications can always occur despite a surgeon's best efforts. No matter how minor the problem, the patient must be treated with concern and compassion. Typically,

patients who undergo cosmetic surgery are expecting to look better as soon as possible and are not always as tolerant of perioperative problems as are trauma patients. Extensive edema and ecchymoses are not normally considered complications but may warrant appropriate reassurance and even simple suggestions to hasten recovery when feasible. Suggestions regarding makeup from a well-trained staff member may greatly improve a postoperative patient's mood when shown how to better hide persistent erythema or ecchymosis.

True complications include poor scar appearance, wound dehiscence, hematoma, skin sloughs or perforations, asymmetries, sensory disturbances, facial paralysis, eyelid ptosis, corneal abrasions, dry eye syndrome, hair loss (alopecia), infection, relapse, irregular facial expressions, and contour irregularities. Of all these potential problems, permanent facial paralysis and major tissue loss are the most devastating. Fortunately, these particular complications are rare (<0.3%, which is less than that for a standard lower facelift). Regardless, it is critical to know the precise anatomy and to avoid improper or excessive retraction, overzealous cautery, and overthinning of the flaps when transecting the depressors. In addition, hematomas must be diagnosed and treated without delay.

Some problems such as corneal abrasions can be very concerning to the patient owing to the severe pain and can be nearly eliminated by proper technique and perioperative attention to detail. For instance, an eye lubricant should always be used. Also, thought should be given to the placement of temporary tape strips, such as Steri-Strips, over the eyelids or a tarsorrhaphy suture to help prevent inadvertent scratching of the cornea by gauze or tubing, for example, during the procedure (see Figure 68-16). All severe pain requires immediate evaluation, and suspected abrasion should be treated by appropriate ophthalmic drops for pain and patching of the affected eye for 12 to 24 hours. Appropriate ophthalmologic consultation is required for persistent or uncontrollable eye pain, persistent dry eye symptoms, or unusual changes in vision. Minor blurred vision for the first 12 hours is not unusual owing to chemosis and use of ophthalmic ointments.

Alopecia and sensory disturbances can be bothersome to the patient and often are not permanent. The problem is the inability to predict whether the numbness a patient has will partially, fully, or not go away, and just how soon it might be alleviated. With proper technique, an endoscopic forehead and brow lift has a high rate of sensory nerve recovery, but full recovery may take several months and require patient reassurance. Although exact numbers are not known, empirical observation of the last 300 endoscopic brow lifts suggests that sensory disturbances are an occasional early concern but an unusual complaint after 6 to 12 months. Most patients have early sensation of the forehead but numbness in the posterior scalp supplied by the deep branch of the supraorbital nerve. This is typically not a major concern to the patient and slowly improves over a period of 8 months. Alopecia, connversely, is a significant concern, especially if it persists longer than 6 to

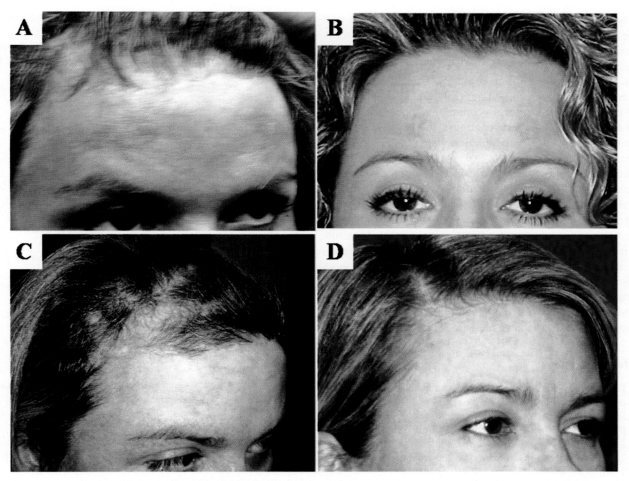

FIGURE 68-35. The patient 3 months after a trichophytic brow lift. She hoped to lift her brows and at the same time lower her high hairline. **A** and **C,** She developed severe telogen affluvium type alopecia with hair loss in a very sporadic pattern. **B** and **D,** Fortunately, she had complete hair regrowth, by 1 year postoperative, as seen on the right with hair growth in front of the beveled incision to create a nice scar behind the hairline.

12 months. Hair may return after an average 4- to 8-month dormancy period of the hair follicle. (Figure 68-35). The "shock" period of hair loss is called *telogen affluvium* and can be dramatic, but fortunately, it is temporary. However, excessive tension on the flaps, rough handling of wound margins, or excessive use of cautery near follicles may lead to permanent hair loss that requires treatment.[116]

Proper planning, technique, and postoperative care helps to reduce the incidence of complications. Immediate and appropriate treatment along with sincere concern for the patient's well-being should help to reduce the chance of the situation worsening or the patient being dissatisfied.

SUMMARY AND CONCLUSIONS

An explosion in the number of rejuvenation techniques for the upper face in the past decade, lead by the use of endoscopes and botulinum toxin, has revolutionized the treatment of aging in this area. Cosmetic surgery treatment of the upper third of the face is frequently an essential component for complete facial rejuvenation. Procedures are highly variable

and can offer improvement to both young and old. Matching the problems to the ideal rejuvenation techniques is essential for maximum aesthetic benefits. Even the best surgical technique can result in inadequate or even poor results if improper patient selection or incorrect diagnoses are made; for this reason, the forehead and brow area must be evaluated critically for a wide range of interlacing diagnoses.

Specific skin problems vary with a patient's age and sex, but gravity remains consistent and nonselective; therefore, the only issues regarding the occurrence of brow ptosis are when it will occur and how severe it will be. Wrinkles are also inevitable but may be dynamic or static in nature. Thanks to botulinum toxin, the previously difficult treatment of dynamic upper facial lines can be effected at low risk with a simple injection. The common and consistent finding of brow ptosis, especially in the lateral third of the brow, may now be selectively treated endoscopically to achieve a more youthful appearance. Society's idea of beauty at any one moment in time will ultimately help to guide the patient and surgeon to choose where the brow should be placed as opposed to merely raising it higher. True rejuvenation is likely more complex and involves multiple modalities and even tissue replacement such as fat grafting. Fat grafting is poised to be one of the most rejuvenating procedures of the face if more consistent techniques develop. The use of stem cells to enhance fat grafting results will likely become the norm at some point in the future. Only time and persistence will prove what best restores youth to the upper face.

Facial cosmetic surgery continues to rise in popularity exponentially. The aging population wants to feel and look more youthful but nonetheless demands to remain natural looking. Today's discerning patient is often very knowledgeable on the subject of the cosmetic surgery options and may insist on a specific technique. The advice of a well-trained surgeon and diagnostician may make or break the ultimate result and prevent a cosmetic disaster. It is vital that the surgeon refuse to perform treatment that is not in the best interest of the patient. Cosmetic surgery is a luxury and is an optional procedure, no matter how much of an emergency it seems to the patient. At the end of the day, it is the surgeon's responsibility to provide the patient with the best and safest options available to achieve realistic goals.

References

1. Ramirez OM. Endoscopic techniques in facial rejuvenation. An overview. Part 1. Aesthetic Plast Surg 1994;8:141–147.
2. Isse NG. Endoscopic facial rejuvenation. Endoforehead, the functional lift. Case reports. Aesthetic Plast Surg 1994;18:21–29.
3. Tessier P. Ridectomie frontale. [Lifting frontale.] Gaz Méd Fr 1968;75:55–65.
4. Becker FF, Johnson CM. Surgical treatment of the upper third of the aging face. In Cummings CW, Fredrickson JM, Harker LA, editors. Otolaryngology—Head and Neck Surgery. St. Louis: Mosby; 1986; p. 475.
5. Zide BM, Jelks GW. Surgical Anatomy of the Orbit. New York: Raven; 1985.
6. Fagien S. Eyebrow analysis after blepharoplasty in patients with brow ptosis. Ophthal Plast Reconstr Surg 1992;8:210.
7. Ellis DAF, Ward D. The aging face. J Otolaryngol 1986;15:217–223.
8. Johnson JD, Hadley RC. The aging face. In Converse JM, editor. Reconstructive Plastic Surgery. Philadelphia: WB Sanders; 1964; pp. 1306–1342.
9. Powell H, Humphrieys B. Proportions of the Aesthetic Face. New York: Thieme-Stratton; 1984.
10. Huntley HE. The Divine Proportion. New York: Dover; 1970.
11. Rickets RM. Divine proportion of facial aesthetics. Clin Plast Surg 1982;9:401.
12. Evans TW. Browlift. Atlas of Oral Maxilofac Surg Clin North Am 1998;6:111–133.
13. Ellis DAF, Bakala CD. Anatomy of the motor innervation of the corrugator supercilii muscle: clinical significance and development of a new surgical technique for frowning. J Otolaryngol 1998;27:222–227.
14. Larrabee WF, Mahielski KH. Surgical Anatomy of the Face. New York: Raven; 1993.
15. Gonzalez-Ulloa M. Facial wrinkles, integral elimination. Plast Reconstr Surg 1962;29:658.
16. Bostwick J, Eaves F, Nahai F. Endoscopic Plastic Surgery. St. Louis: Quality Medical; 1995.
17. Hiatt JL, Gartner LP. In Gardner J, editor. Textbook of Head and Neck Anatomy. 2nd ed. Baltimore: Williams & Wilkins; 1987; pp. 156–245, 373–345.
18. Hamas RS. Reducing the subconscious frown by endoscopic resection of the corrugator muscles. Aesthetic Plast Surg 1995;19:21–25.
19. Salasche SJ, Bernstein G, Senkarik. Surgical Anatomy of the Skin. Appleton & Lange; 1988.
20. Edwards BF. Bilateral neurotomy for the frontalis hypermotility. Plast Reconstr Surg 1957;19:341–344.
21. Ellis DAF, Masri H. The effect of facial animation on the aging upper half of the face. Arch Otolaryngol Head Neck Surg 1989;115:710–712.
22. Brennan HG. The forehead lift. Otolaryngol Clin North Am 1980;13:209.
23. Rafaty FM, Brennan HG. Current concepts in brow pexy. Arch Otolaryngol Head Neck Surg 1983;109:152.
24. Rafaty FM, Goode RL. The browlift operation in a man. Arch Otolaryngol Head Neck Surg 1978;104:69.
25. Rafaty FM, Goode RL, Fee WE. The browlift operation. Arch Otolaryngol Head Neck Surg 1975;101:467.
26. Knize DM. Reassessment of the coronal incision and subgaleal dissection for foreheadplasty. Plast Reconstr Surg 1998;102:478.
27. Grant JCB, editor. Grant's Atlas of Anatomy. 6th ed. Baltimore: Williams & Wilkins, 1972.
28. Tolhurst DE, Carstens MH, Greco RJ, et al. The surgical anatomy of the scalp. Plast Reconstr Surg 1991;87:603.
29. Tremolada C, Candiani P, Signorini M, et al. The surgical anatomy of the subcutaneous fascial system of the scalp. Ann Plast Surg 1994;32:8.
30. Carstens MH, Greco RJ, Hurwitz DJ, et al. Clinical applications of the subgaleal fascia. Plast Reconstr Surg 1991;87:615.
31. Waite PD, Cuzalina LA. Rhytidectomy. In Fonseca RJ, editor. Oral and Maxillofacial Surgery: Cleft/Craniofacial/Cosmetic surgery. Vol. 6. Philadelphia: WB Saunders; 1998; pp. 365–381.
32. Tobin HA, Cuzalina LA, Tharanon W, Sinn DP. The biplane face lift: an opportunistic approach. J Oral Maxillofac Surg 2000;58:76–85.
33. Tobin HA, Cuzalina LA. SMAS surgery versus deep-plane rhytidectomy. In Pensak ML, editor. Controversies in Otolaryngology. New York: Thieme; 2001; pp. 148–155.
34. Knize DM. Transpalpebral approach to the corrugator supercilii and procerus muscles. Plast Reconstr Surg 1995;95:52–60.
35. Aiache AE. Transblepharoplasty brow-lift. Presented at the American Society of Aesthetic Plastic Surgery. 1995;May; San Francisco.
36. Boyd B, Caminer D, Moon HK. Innervation of the procerus and corrugator muscles and its significance in facial surgery. Paper presented at the annual meeting of the ASPRS. 1997;September; San Francisco.
37. Knize DM. A study of the supraorbital nerve. Plast Reconstr Surg 1997;99:1224.
38. Knize DM. Muscles that act on glabellar skin: a closer look. Plast Reconstr Surg 2000;105:350.
39. Netter FM. Atlas of Human Anatomy. Summit, NJ: Ciba-Geigy; 1989.
40. Knize DM. An anatomically based study of the mechanism of eyebrow ptosis. Plast Reconstr Surg 1996;97:1321.

41. De la Plaza R, De la Cruz L. A new concept in blepharoplasty. Aesthetic Plast Surg 1996;20:221.

42. Lemke BN, Stasior OG. The anatomy of eyebrow ptosis. Arch Ophthalmol 1982;100:981.

43. Meyer DR, Linberg JV, Wobig JL, et al. Anatomy of the orbital septum and associated eyelid connective tissues. Ophthal Plast Reconstr Surg 1991;7:104.

44. Aiache AE, Ramirez OM. The suborbicularis oculi fat pads: an anatomic and clinical study. Plast Reconstr Surg 1995;95:37.

45. Trinei FA, Januszkiewicz J, Nahai F. The sentinel vein: an important reference point for surgery in the temporal region. Plast Reconstr Surg 1998;101:27.

46. Cuzalina LA, Holmes J. A simple and reliable landmark for identification of the supraorbital nerve in surgery of the forehead: an in vivo anatomical study. J Oral Maxillofac Surg 2005;63:25–27.

47. Gosain AK, Sewall SR, Yousif NJ. The temporal branch of the temporal nerve: how reliably can we predict its path? Plast Reconstr Surg 1997;99:1224.

48. Ellis E, Zide MF, editors. Surgical Approaches to the Facial Skeleton. Baltimore: Williams & Wilkins; 1995; pp. 59–169.

49. Liebman E, Webster R, Berger A, et al. The frontalis nerve in the temporal brow lift. Arch Otolaryngol Head Neck Surg 1982;108:232–235.

50. Furnas DW. Landmarks for the trunk and the temporofacial division of the facial nerve. Br J Surg 1965;52:694.

51. Correia P, Zani R. Surgical anatomy of the facial nerve as related to ancillary operations in rhytidoplasty. Plast Reconstr Surg 1973;52:549–552.

52. Isse NG. Endoscopic forehead lift. Clin Plast Surg 1995;22:661.

53. Isse NG. The endoscopic approach to forehead and brow lifting. Aesthetic Plast Surg 1998;18.

54. Vasconez LO, Core GB, Gamboa-Bobadilla M, et al. Endoscopic techniques in coronal brow lifting. Plast Reconstr Surg 1994;94:788.

55. Morselli PG. Fixation for forehead endoscopic lifting: a simple, easy, no-cost procedure. Plast Reconstr Surg 1996;97:1309.

56. Marchac D, Ascherman J, Arnaud E. Fibrin glue fixation in forehead endoscopy: evaluation of our experience with 206 cases. Plast Reconstr Surg 1997;100:704.

57. Hoeing JF. Rigid anchoring of the forehead to the frontal bone in endoscopic facelifting: a new technique. Aesthetic Plast Surg 1996;20:213.

58. De la Fuente A, Santamaria AB. Facial rejuvenation: a combined conventional and endoscopic assisted lift. Aesthetic Plast Surg 1996;20:471.

59. Isse NG. Endoscopic forehead lift, evolution and update. Clin Plast Surg 1995;2:661.

60. Adamson PA, Johnson CM, Anderson JR, et al. The forehead lift: a review. Arch Otolaryngol Head Neck Surg 1985;111:325–329.

61. Liang M, Narayaman K. Endoscopic oblation of the frontalis and corrugator muscles: a clinical study. Plast Surg Forum 1992;XV:54.

62. Su CT. Technique for division and suspension of the orbicularis oculi muscle. Clin Plast Surg 1981;8:673.

63. Byrd HS, Andochick SE. The deep temporal lift: a multiplanar lateral brow, temporal, and upper face lift. Plast Reconstr Surg 1996;97:928.

64. Kerth JD, Triumi DM. Management of the aging forehead. Arch Otolaryngol Head Neck Surg 1990;116:1137–1142.

65. Chierici G, Miller A. Experimental study of muscle reattachment following surgical detachment. J Oral Maxillofac Surg 1984;42:485.

66. Ramirez OM. Endoscopic subperiosteal browlift and facelift. Clin Plast Surg 1995; 22:639–660.

67. Tobin HA. The extended subperiosteal coronal lift. Am J Cosmet Surg 1993;10:47–57.

68. Psillakis JM, Rummley TO, Camargos A. Subperiosteal approach in an improved concept for correction of the aging face. Plast Reconstr Surg 1988;82:383–392.

69. Maillard GF, Cornette de St Cyr B, Scheflan M. The subperiosteal bicoronal approach to total face lifting: the SMAS-deep musculoaponeurotic system. Aesthetic Plast Surg 1991;15:285–291.

70. Ramirez OM. Endoscopic techniques in facial rejuvenation: an overview. Aesthetic Plast Surg 1994;18:141–371.

71. Daniel RK, Ramirez OM. Endoscopic assisted aesthetic surgery. Aesthetic Plast Surg 1994;14:18–20.

72. Toledo LS. Facial rejuvenation: technique and rationale. In Fodar P, Isse N, editors. Endoscopically Assisted Aesthetic Plastic Surgery. St. Louis: Mosby; 1996; pp. 91–105.

73. Psillakis JM. Subperiosteal approach for surgical rejuvenation of the upper face. In Psillakis J, editor. Deep face-lifting techniques. New York: Thieme; 1994; pp. 51–63.

74. Hinderer UT. The sub SMAS and subperiosteal rhytidectomy of the forehead and middle third of the face: a new approach to the aging face. Facial Plast Surg Clin North Am 1992;8:18–32.

75. Dempsey PD, Oneal RM, Izenberg PH. Subperiosteal brow and midface lifts. Aesthetic Plast Surg 1995;19:59–68.

76. Blitzer A, Brin MF, Keen MS, et al. Botulinum toxin for the treatment of hyperfunctional lines of the face. Arch Otolaryngol Head Neck Surg 1993;119:1018–1022.

77. Ruess WR, Owsley JQ. The anatomy of the skin and fascial layers of the face in aesthetic surgery. Clin Plast Surg 1987;14:677–682.

78. McCollough EG, Langsdon PR. Dermabrasion and chemical peel. New York: Thieme; 1998.

79. Buzzell RA. Effects of solar radiation on the skin. Otolaryngol Clin North Am 1993;26:1–11.

80. Ortiz-Monasterio FG, Olmedo A. The coronal incision in rhytidectomy: the brow lift. Clin Plast Surg 1978;5:167.

81. Ellenbogen R. Transcoronal eyebrow lift with concomitant upper blepharoplasty. Plast Reconstr Surg 1983;71:490.

82. Wojtanowski MH. Bicoronal forehead lift. Aesthetic Plast Surg 1994;18:33.

83. Abul-Hassan HS, Van Drasek Ascher G, Acland RD. Surgical anatomy and blood supply for the fascial layers of the temporal regions. Plast Reconstr Surg 1986;77:17.

84. Stuzin JM, Wagstrom L, Kawamoto HK, et al. Anatomy of the frontal branch of the facial nerve: the significance of the temporal fat pad. Plast Reconstr Surg 1989;83:265.

85. Savani A. Physiopathology of the aging face. In Psillakis JM, editor. Deep face-lifting techniques. New York: Thieme; 1994; pp. 11–23.

86. De la Plaza R, Valiente E, Arroya JM. Supraperiosteal lifting of the upper two thirds of the face. Br J Plast Surg 1991;4:325–332.

87. Wassef M. Superficial fascial and muscular layers in the face and neck: a histologic study. Aesthetic Plast Surg 1987;11:171.

88. Tirkanits B, Daniel RK. The biplanar forehead lift. Aesthetic Plast Surg 1990;14:111.

89. Ramirex OM, Maillard GF, Musolas A. The extended subperiosteal face lift: a definitive soft-tissue remodeling for facial rejuvenation. Plast Reconstr Surg 1991:88:227–236.

90. Psillakis JM. Embryology and anatomy review of the superficial fascia or SMAS. In Psillakis JM, editor. Deep face-lifting techniques. New York: Thieme; 1994; pp. 1–11.

91. Bosse JP, Papillon J, editors. Surgical anatomy of the SMAS at the malar region. In Transactions of the Ninth International Congress of Plastic and Reconstructive Surgery. New York: McGraw-Hill; 1987.

92. Owsley JQ. Aesthetic Facial Surgery. Philadelphia: WB Saunders; 1994.

93. Yousif NJ, Mendelson BC. Anatomy of the mid-face. Clin Plast Surg 1995;22:227–241.

94. Guyuron B, Davies B. Subcutaneous anterior hairline forehead rhytidectomy. Aesthetic Plast Surg 1988;12:77.

95. Aiache AE. Endoscopic face-lift. Aesthetic Plast Surg 1994;18:275.

96. Ramirez OM. Endoscopic forehead and facelift: step-by-step. Open Tech Plast Reconstr Surg 1995;2:116–26.

97. Matarasso A, Terino EO. Forehead-brow rhytidoplasty: reassessing the goals. Plast Reconstr Surg 1994;93:1378.

98. Newman JP, LaFerriere KA, Koch RJ, et al. Transcalvarial suture fixation for endoscopic brow and forehead lifts. Arch Otolaryngol Head Neck Surg 1997;123:313.

99. Kim SK. Endoscopic forehead scalp flap fixation with K-wire. Aesthetic Plast Surg 1996;20:217.

100. Pakkanen M, Salisbury AV, Ersek RA. Biodegradable positive fixation for endoscopic browlift. Plast Reconstr Surg 1996;98:1087.

101. Knize DM. A study of the supraorbital nerve. Plast Reconstr Surg 1995;96:564.

102. Loomis MG. Endoscopic brow fixation without bolsters or miniscrews. Plast Reconstr Surg 1996;98:373.

103. Dyer WK, Yung RT. Botulinum toxin-assisted brow lift. In Larrabee WF, Thomas JR, editors. Facial Plastic Surgery Clinics of North America: Rejuvenation of the Upper Face. Vol. 8, Number 3. Philadelphia: WB Saunders; 2000; pp. 343–354.

104. Brennan HG, Rafty FM. Midforehead incisions in treatment of the aging face. Arch Otolaryngol Head Neck Surg 1982;108:732–734.

105. Johnson CM, Waldman SR. Midforehead lift. Arch Otolaryngol Head Neck Surg 1983;109:155–159.

106. Cook TA, Brownrigg PJ, Wang TD, et al. The versatile midforehead browlift. Arch Otolaryngol Head Neck Surg 1989;115:163.

107. Johnson CM, Walman SR. Midforehead lift. Arch Otolaryngol Head Neck Surg 1983;109:155.

108. Guyuron B, Michelow BJ, Thomas T. Corrugator supercilii muscle resection through a blepharoplasty incision. Plast Reconstr Surg 1995;95:691–696.

109. Stegman SJ, Chu S, Armstrong RC. Adverse reactions to bovine collagen implant: clinical and histologic features. J Dermatol Surg Oncol 1988;14:39–47.

110. Keen MS, Khosh MM. The role of botulinum toxin A in facial plastic surgery. In Willet JM, editor. Facial Plastic Surgery. Upper Saddle River, NJ: Prentice Hall; 1997; pp. 323–329.

111. Frankel AS, Kamer FM. Chemical browlift. Arch Otolaryngol Head Neck Surg 1998;124:321.

112. Beeson WH, McCollough EG. Complications of the forehead lift. Ear Nose Throat J 1985;64:27.

113. Connell BF, Lambros VS, Neurohr GH. The forehead lift: techniques to avoid complications and produce optimal results. Aesthetic Plast Surg 1989;13:217.

114. Matarasso A. Endoscopic assisted foreheadbrow rhytidoplasty: theory and practice. Aesthetic Plast Surg 1995;19:141.

115. Daniel RK, Tirkantis B. Endoscopic forehead lift, aesthetics and analysis. Clin Plast Surg 1995;22:605–18.

116. Mayer TG, Fleming RW. Management of alopecia. In Cummings CW, Fredrickson JM, Harker LA, et al, editors. Otolaryngology—Head Neck Surgery. St. Louis: Mosby; 1986; p. 429.

Otoplastic Surgery for the Protruding Ear

Todd G. Owsley, DDS, MD

Auricular deformities, in particular prominent or protruding ears, are a common congenital anomaly, affecting nearly 5% of the white population.[1] Congenital in nature, children are most likely to suffer the consequences of the deformity in the form of ridicule by their peers. Protruding ears, commonly referred to as *prominauris,* can be predictably treated for children before they enter grade school and, thus, help them avoid the emotional trauma caused by the ridicule. Otoplastic surgery is primarily performed on children and can be a valuable service for the patient and satisfying for the surgeon.

It is important for the surgeon to understand the history of various surgical techniques to develop a predictable and successful technique to address the problem of protruding ears. Dieffenbach, in 1845, is credited with the first otoplastic technique to correct a prominent auricle.[2] Ely, in 1881,[3] authored the first case report describing correction of prominent ears in a 12-year-old boy who was being teased at school. Since that report, over 180 surgical techniques have been described in the literature for the correction of protruding ears.

When clinically evaluating the facial complex, the ears are often overlooked. If protruding ears are present, reduction otoplasty as an adjunctive or isolated procedure can be performed predictably and often with satisfying results. A thorough understanding of the embryology and development of the human auricle along with the resultant external anatomy of the ear is of paramount importance in developing a predictable and stable technique to deal with the common auricular deformities.

EMBRYOLOGY OF THE AURICLE

Malformations of the auricle are common, occurring in 1 out of 12,500 births.[4] They can occur alone or in combination with a syndrome affecting the head and neck structures. The embryogenesis of the auricle exemplifies in miniature the precise and logical progression so characteristic of the developing human form. The external ear development during the 3rd to 12th weeks of embryonic life is complex. The precursors to the auricle present in days 36 to 38 of intrauterine life, developing first from the first branchial groove where the first (mandibular) and second (hyoid) branchial arches are present (Figure 69-1). Both arches give rise to the auricular hillocks often referred to as the *auricular tubercles of His.*[4] Numbers 1, 2, and 3 arise from the caudal border of the mandibular arch, and numbers 4, 5, and 6 are formed from the cephalic border of the hyoid arch. The auricular hillocks present in their most prominent and characteristic form by intrauterine day 41. During this same stage, the groove between the mandibular and the hyoid arches (hyomandibular groove) widens and deepens by the increased growth of the hillocks. This groove eventually forms the external auditory canal and concha. By days 43 to 45, the hillocks have migrated and coalesced to form the auricle.[4] During this union, the mesenchyme of the hyoid arch increases substantially relative to the mandibular arch to contribute 85% of the external adult ear. Hillocks 2 and 3 from the mandibular arch lose their individuality and fuse to form the helical crus. Later, hillocks 4 and 5 from the hyoid arch merge and alter their configuration as they give rise to the helix and antihelical fold. Hillock 1 remains prominent and becomes the tragus, and hillock 6 becomes the antitragus.[4]

SURGICAL ANATOMY

The majority of the growth of the pinna is completed by an early age. The average child has 85% ear development by 3 years of age. The ear is nearly fully grown by the age of

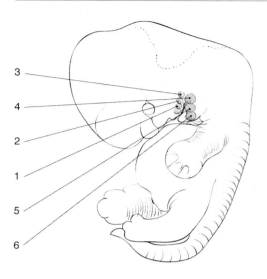

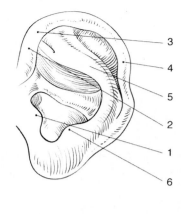

FIGURE 69-1. Development of the auricle from the first and second branchial arches. The *numbers in the left diagram* correspond to the structures in the right diagram. (Adapted from Owsley T. Otoplastic surgery for the protruding ear. In Fonseca RJ, editor. Oral and Maxillofacial Surgery. Vol 6. Philadelphia: WB Saunders; 2000; pp. 408–418.)

7 to 8 years. The ear height continues to grow into adulthood, but the width and distance of the ear from the scalp change little after 10 years of age. It is important to note that each individual's ears often vary in size and shape.[5] The average adult ear is approximately 6.5 cm in length and 3.5 cm in width. In the normal ear, the auricle lies between horizontal lines drawn from the upper rim of the orbit and the nasal spine. The normal posterior wall of the conchal bowl is set at an angle of approximately 90 degree to the mastoid.[6] A second 90-degree angle is formed as the antihelical fold and is called the *scaphaconchal angle.* These two angles in combination with the curvature of the helix set the auricle adjacent to the scalp at approximately 25 to 35 degrees and is called the *auriculocephalic angle* (Figure 69-2).[7] In otoplastic surgery, when correcting prominent ears, three important anatomic pearls can be used intraoperatively to assess the final result. The helical rim should be seen just lateral to the most lateral presence of the antihelix from the frontal view. The distance measured between the helical rim and the mastoid area is slightly less than 2 cm. Finally, the distance between the skull and the uppermost aspect of the helix is approximately 1 cm (Figure 69-3).

The auricular cartilage is a unique and delicate structure that is intricately shaped with multiple elevations and depressions providing both skeletal support and form to the adult ear. The cartilage of the auricle is a single piece of yellow (elastic) fibrocartilage with a complicated relief on the anterior, concave side and a smooth, posterior convex side. Cartilage thickness is fairly uniform throughout. The cartilage is covered on both surfaces by a thin, firm, adherent layer of perichondrium. The anterior lateral surface of the cartilage is covered with a fine, thin skin, closely adherent to the cartilaginous framework. Subcutaneous fat is practically nonexistent, but a diffuse subdermal vascular plane exists that supports flap viability.[8] The posterior surface of the cartilage framework is draped with a less adherent skin that contains two layers of fat and a larger subdermal plexus of arteries, veins, and nerves.

A helical border terminates anteriorly in a crus, commonly called the *radix,* which lies almost horizontally above the external auditory meatus. The antihelix crowning the posterior conchal wall separates and diverges into both a superior and an anterior crus enclosing the triangularis fossa. Between the helix and the antihelix lies a long, deep furrow called the *scaphoid fossa.* The conchal cavity, composed of the cymba (superior) and cavum (inferior) concha, arises from the floor, which is approximately 8 mm deeper than

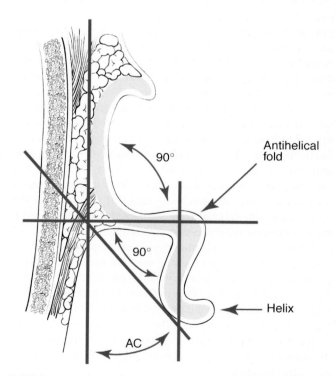

FIGURE 69-2. An axial section at the level of the helical crus demonstrates the ideal auriculocephalic angle (AC) of 30 degrees. (Adapted from Tanzer RC. Congenital deformities. In Converse J, editor. Reconstructive Plastic Surgery. Vol 4. 2nd ed. Philadelphia: WB Saunders; 1977.)

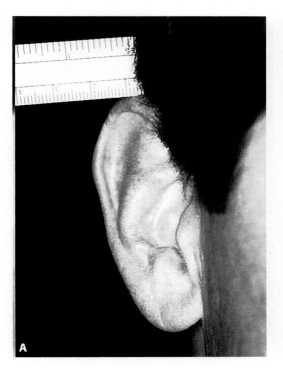
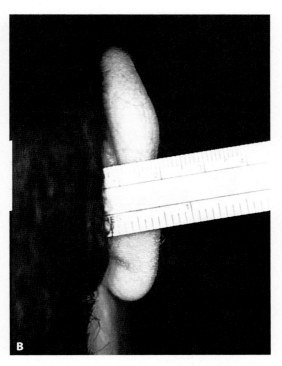

FIGURE 69-3.   **A** and **B,** Anatomic "pearls," useful intraoperatively. (**A** and **B,** Reproduced with permission from Owsley T. Otoplastic surgery for the protruding ear. In Fonseca RJ, editor. Oral and Maxillofacial Surgery. Vol 6. Philadelphia: WB Saunders; 2000; pp. 408–418.)

the overlying tragus and antitragus. The inferior tip of the helical cartilage is referred to as the *cauda* or *tail.* Extending from this inferiorly is the lobule, hanging devoid of skeleton (Figure 69-4).

BLOOD SUPPLY

The arterial blood supply to the ear is derived principally from two main branches of the external carotid artery: superficial temporal artery and posterior auricular artery. The superficial temporal artery emerges from the parotid capsule, 1 cm in front of the ear deep to the veins and below the anterior auricular muscle. It gives off the superior, medial, and inferior branches supplying the anterior and anterolateral surface of the auricle (Figure 69-5A). The posterior surface is dominantly supplied by the posterior auricular artery, which travels parallel to the postauricular crease upward crossing below the great auricular nerve and under the posterior auricular muscle. Awareness of this relationship is important to avoid damage to the artery or nerve during surgery. The posterior auricular artery gives off three branches—superior, medial, and inferior—providing a greater volume of blood to the postauricular ear than its anterior counterparts. These same vessels perforate the auricular cartilage over a large surface of the anterior ear and anastomose with the branches of the superficial temporal artery. The external ears have a tremendous blood supply, allowing multiple surgical approaches or salvage of the ear after traumatic avulsion.

Venous drainage of the ear via the complementary veins is into the external jugular vein. Lymphatic drainage is into three surrounding areas via the complex and extensive fine network of lymphatic vessels.

NERVE SUPPLY

The sensory nerve supply is primarily from the anterior and posterior branches of the great auricular nerve. The nerve is an important surgical landmark traveling 8 mm posterior to the postauricular crease. When dissecting in this area, care must be taken to avoid damage to the nerve that can result in near-complete anesthesia to the ear. Less important contributions of sensation are made by the auriculotemporal and lesser occipital nerves to the conchal cavity and external auditory meatus (see Figure 69-5B). Regional anesthesia of the auricle is readily accomplished by instilling anesthetic solution along its base anteriorly and posteriorly. Supplemental anesthesia may be needed at the posterior wall of the external auditory meatus supplied by the auricular branches of the vagus nerve (Arnold's nerve).

DEFORMITIES

Ear deformities are common and variable owing to the complex embryologic engineering that takes place in the development of the auricle, as described previously. Many classification systems of ear deformities have been attempted.

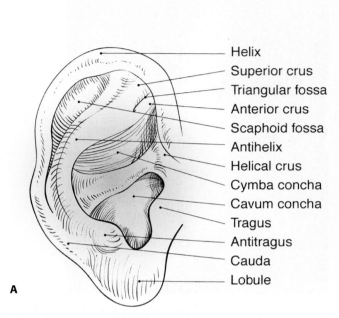

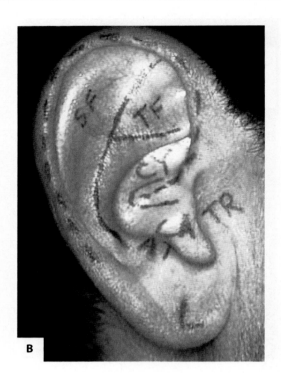

Helix
Superior crus
Triangular fossa
Anterior crus
Scaphoid fossa
Antihelix
Helical crus
Cymba concha
Cavum concha
Tragus
Antitragus
Cauda
Lobule

A

B

FIGURE 69-4. **A** and **B,** Anatomy of the external ear.

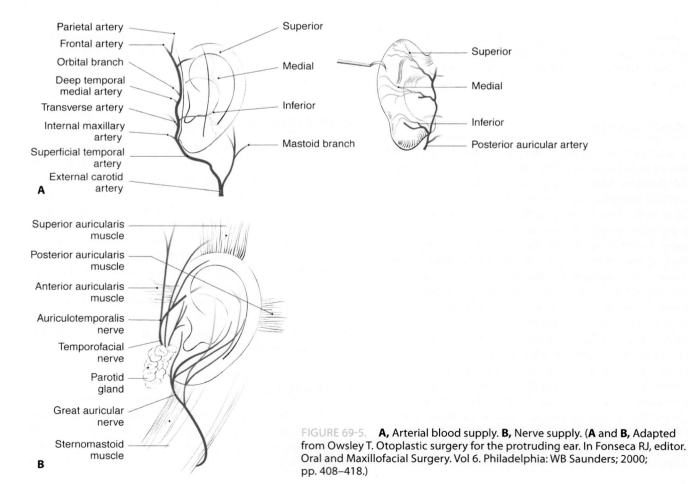

Parietal artery
Frontal artery
Orbital branch
Deep temporal medial artery
Transverse artery
Internal maxillary artery
Superficial temporal artery
External carotid artery

Superior
Medial
Inferior
Mastoid branch

Superior
Medial
Inferior
Posterior auricular artery

A

Superior auricularis muscle
Posterior auricularis muscle
Anterior auricularis muscle
Auriculotemporalis nerve
Temporofacial nerve
Parotid gland
Great auricular nerve
Sternomastoid muscle

B

FIGURE 69-5. **A,** Arterial blood supply. **B,** Nerve supply. (**A** and **B,** Adapted from Owsley T. Otoplastic surgery for the protruding ear. In Fonseca RJ, editor. Oral and Maxillofacial Surgery. Vol 6. Philadelphia: WB Saunders; 2000; pp. 408–418.)

Tanzer[9] classifies congenital ear defects, correlating embryologic development with a surgical approach for correction of the deformity. Marx[10] has a well-accepted classification system subdividing microtia into three groups according to severity. Rogers[6] simplifies classification of congenital ear defects, dividing them into four groups according to various stages of arrested development: microtia, lop ear, cup ear, and protruding ear. In this chapter addressing the prominent ear, the term *protruding* is used as a general term to refer to any ear that is more prominent than is considered "normal." It is beyond the scope of this chapter to classify other congenital abnormalities and their correction.

Protruding Ear

In patients with protruding ears, there are two major deformities that individually or in combination account for the majority of the abnormalities. Several lesser deformities are seen that can accentuate the abnormality as well. The most common is a poorly developed antihelical fold that can involve both the superior and the anterior crura. This eliminates a definition between the conchal cavity and the scapha, resulting in the lateral projection of the upper portion of the helix. The second abnormality is the formation of excessive conchal cartilage, in particular the posterior conchal wall. This causes significant protrusion of the auricle. It is not uncommon to recognize some degree of both abnormalities present producing the protruding auricle.

Other potential deformities are a protruding earlobe, irregularities along the helix including an unrolled margin of the helical rim, and more recently described, an anteromedially displaced insertion of the postauricular muscle. Of importance, this deformity is often bilateral and can be associated with ossicular deformities and a hearing deficit.[11]

Obviously, precise recognition of the cause or causes of the protruding ear is crucial in formulating the surgical technique to be employed in correction of the abnormality.

SURGICAL CORRECTION

Perhaps the most important indication for surgical correction of prominent ears is to eliminate the psychosocial effects that the ear defect produces. Macgregor[12] and others have well documented the irreversible social and psychological consequences that facial anomalies, especially of the ears, can inflict. The ridicule by peers begins as early as age 4 to 5 years during development, described as the body image concept. This leads to problems with social adjustment, self-image deficit, and ultimately, behavioral disorders. Therefore, most patients present at an early age for surgical correction. Most surgeons agree that surgical correction of the ear can be performed safely between 4 years of age and the beginning of school attendance to avoid the ridicule, becoming one of the most common elective procedures performed in young children. Adults also present to correct a life-long cosmetic defect.

SURGICAL TECHNIQUES

Many otoplasty techniques described in the surgical literature are similar and have evolved over an 80-year experience. Many techniques address only the conchal hypertrophy without mention of the antihelical fold. The described techniques generally can be subdivided into a "suture-only" technique, a cartilage splitting or weakening technique, or a combination of the two.

Furnas, in 1968,[13] described his suture-only technique for the correction of the prominent ear deformity. This technique consisted of a postauricular approach, removing the skin, connective tissue, and vestigial posterior auricular muscle and its ligament down to the underlying mastoid fascia. A total of two or three nonresorbable sutures are placed through conchal cartilage and mastoid fascia and tightened to the new desired retracted position of the ears. This remains a commonly used technique to set back the ears in patients with conchal hypertrophy alone. Problems associated with this technique have been relapse secondary to the cartilaginous memory, a shallow conchal bowl, and irregularities created in folding the conchal floor. Another difficult problem is displacing the conchal bowl anteriorly, creating narrowing of the external auditory canal.

The Converse–Wood-Smith technique[14] is used to correct and create an antihelical fold using a cartilage cutting and suture method. Several full-thickness cuts through cartilage are placed in the scaphoid fossa. The cartilage is then folded on itself, described as "tubing," and permanent horizontal mattress sutures are placed, forming the new antihelical fold. In addition, if excessive conchal cartilage is present, it can be addressed with a cartilage incision added at the rim of the bowl to reduce the bowl and retract the ear. A new antihelical fold is formed, however, typically with sharp cartilaginous ridges seen through the thin anterior auricular skin.

This chapter describes two techniques that address the two fundamental abnormalities in protruding ears and have produced consistent, satisfying cosmetic results, essentially eliminating the fear of relapse. The Davis method addresses the protruding ear caused by a hypertrophic posterior wall of the conchal bowl.[15] The Mustarde method is used to create a new antihelical fold[16] (Figure 69-6).

The refinement of other abnormalities such as the prominent earlobe are also discussed.

Davis Method

The Davis method, for the correction of conchal hypertrophy, is a cartilage excision technique performed in a step-wise fashion.[8,15]

1. Marking the cartilage excision: Initially, the area of cartilage to be removed is marked on the skin of the anterior surface of the conchal bowl. Methylene blue transfixion tattoos are preferred to mark the posterior surface of the conchal cavity. The line lies just below the lower crus border, carries forward into the cymbal fossa, and continues around as an "arrowhead" to preserve a well-defined

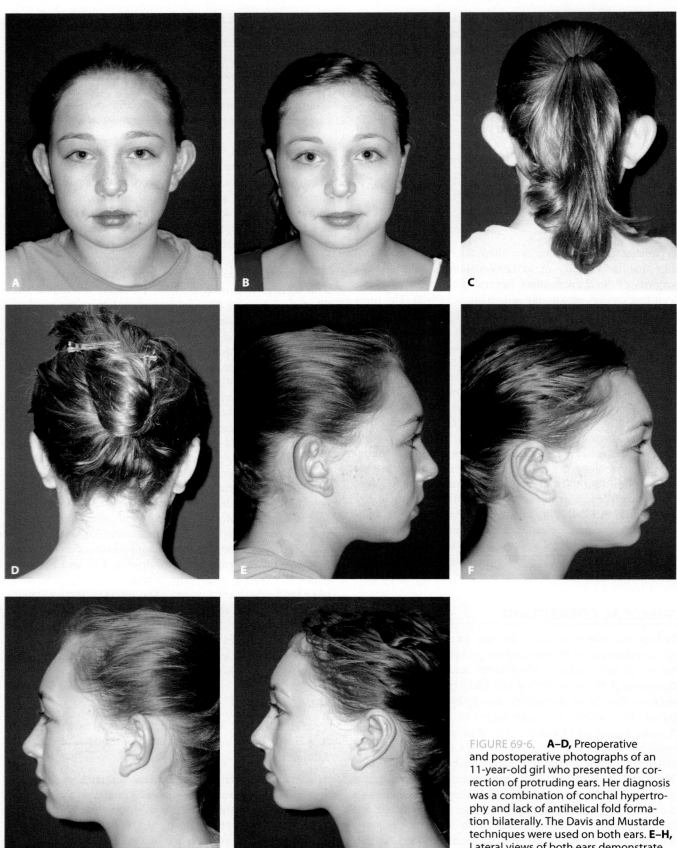

FIGURE 69-6.　**A–D,** Preoperative and postoperative photographs of an 11-year-old girl who presented for correction of protruding ears. Her diagnosis was a combination of conchal hypertrophy and lack of antihelical fold formation bilaterally. The Davis and Mustarde techniques were used on both ears. **E–H,** Lateral views of both ears demonstrate a natural-appearing, new antihelical fold and a deepened conchal bowl.

helical radix. The tracing should continue forward against the posterior edge of the external auditory canal. From that location, it curves posteriorly into the cavum concha, continuing onto the posterior conchal wall, leaving 8 mm of posterior conchal wall height measured from the conchal scaphal junction. This should complete the circle, which should appear "kidney bean" shaped including the entire conchal bowl. The exact height of the posterior wall is important and must be measured for each case individually (Figure 69-7A-C).

2. Removal of skin and cartilage: Before beginning the actual surgical procedure, local anesthesia is used for hydrodissection of the tightly adhered anterior auricular skin along the conchal bowl. This simplifies the dissection of cartilage from the overlying skin. The concha is exposed through a postauricular elliptical skin excision. The width of the ellipse is only to remove the predicted excess skin that is produced with ear retropositioning. The closure of the incision should be passive. This area is predisposed to hypertrophic or keloidal scarring when closed under tension. Once having removed the postauricular skin, the conchal cartilage is visualized along with the previously placed tattoo marks. The marks are used as a guide for incising through the cartilage, taking care to avoid perforation of the anterior skin. The dissection is then carried onto the anterior conchal cartilage surface subperichondrially. The hydrodissection along with a small, sharp Freer elevator allows separation between the skin and the cartilage. The cartilage is then removed, which includes the entire conchal bowl with the exception of the 8 mm left along the posterior conchal wall. The ear is then placed passively onto the mastoid surface, and the new projection of the helical rim is observed and carefully measured. Any defective prominence can be revised with further cartilage removal. The postauricular muscle and underlying connective tissue are removed down to the underlying mastoid fascia to allow for passive skin draping of the conchal floor, producing a natural-appearing, deepened conchal bowl. Any excessive postauricular skin can be removed at this time (see Figure 69-7D–F).

3. Ear fixation: The ear is fixed in its new position with three or four mattress transfixion sutures of 3-0 silk that perforate the skin anteriorly, anchor deeply into the postauricular muscle stump, and pass back through the anterior skin. The mattress sutures are then gently tied over a dental cotton roll, moistened with a triple antibiotic ointment, which has been placed into the cymbal and caval fossa, making sure to place one end of the cotton roll into the external auditory canal to avoid postoperative stenosis. The sutures and cotton roll hold the ear in place during healing, stretch and flatten the skin uniformly over the conchal floor, and give depth to the conchal bowl. The postauricular incision is then closed in a running fashion with a resorbable suture, leaving a small opening inferiorly for drainage. The cotton roll dressing is left in place for a minimum of 1 week for optimal healing (see Figure 69-7G–I)

Mustarde Method

The Mustarde method, first described in 1959, is indicated for the prominent ear with a poorly formed or lack of an antihelical fold.[16] This cartilage weakening technique relies on precisely placed horizontal mattress sutures, creating a new antihelical fold. It is rarely performed alone and used commonly in combination with the Davis method described previously.

1. Antihelical fold markings: The scapha is folded back against the underlying scalp by applying digital pressure on the superior helical rim, which creates an antihelical fold. The crest of the fold is marked with a surgical marker. To prepare for placement of the mattress sutures, marks are placed parallel to the crest at least 7 mm apart to avoid creating too narrow a fold. The lateral marks placed on the skin are transferred to the underlying cartilage with a hypodermic needle dipped in methylene blue (Figure 69-8A and B).

2. Dissection and cartilage weakening: Local anesthetic solution is infiltrated along the scaphal fossa beneath the anterior auricular skin, hydrodissecting the skin from the underlying cartilage. This is to facilitate the anterior dissection and mattress suture placement. The postauricular skin is then removed in an identical fashion as that described with the Davis method. Once having identified the marks placed on the posterior surface of the scaphoid cartilage, a Freer elevator is passed through a small horizontal incision created through the cartilage at the most inferior aspect of the new antihelical fold. The anterior auricular skin is then dissected from the underlying cartilage corresponding to the crest of the new antihelical fold. Through the tunnel dissected along the anterior surface of the cartilage, the body of the new antihelical fold is weakened to facilitate folding and remove the inherent memory. Many methods have been described; however, cartilage weakening can be performed adequately using a Brown-Adson forceps, a nasal rasp, or a dermabrader with a small diamond fraise (see Figure 69-8C–E).

3. Suture placement: Nonresorbable, horizontal mattress sutures (4-0 Mersilene) are placed. The sutures are all placed through the medial perichondrium, cartilage, and lateral perichondrium, being careful not to include the anterior skin. The sutures should be placed perpendicularly across the antihelical fold, so that upon tightening, a well-rounded, antihelical fold will be created. The sutures are tightened under direct observation and adjusted accordingly to form the new antihelical fold (see Figure 69-8F and G).

4. Dressing: The dressing is important and is placed to provide adequate pressure to obliterate dead space and avoid a postoperative hematoma formation. A carefully layered dressing is placed over the anterior and opposing posterior surfaces of the scaphoid region with a $\frac{1}{4}$-inch petrolatum gauze, followed by 4 × 4-inch fluffs, held secure with a pressure-type facial dressing (see Figure 69-8H and I).

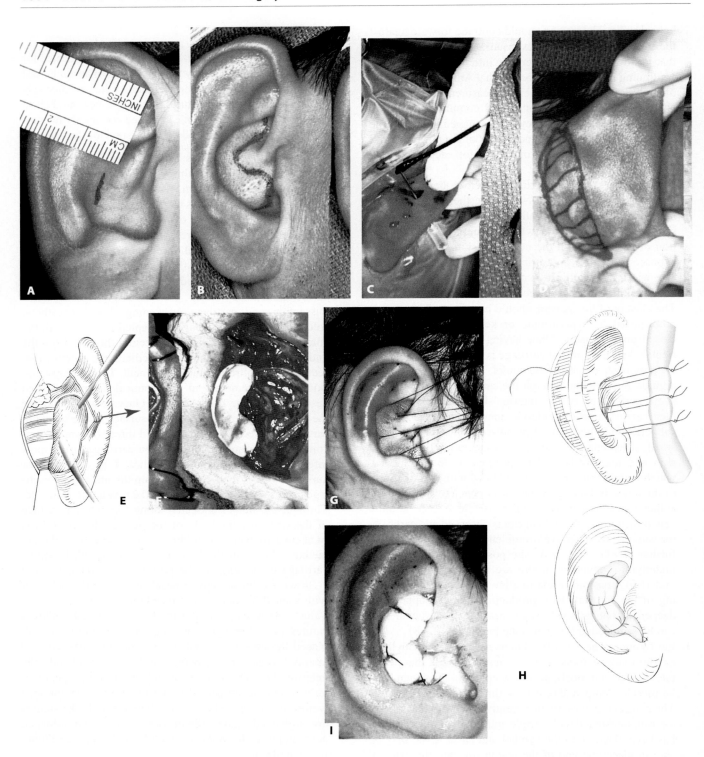

FIGURE 69-7.   Davis method. **A,** Marking the height of the posterior conchal wall that will remain. **B,** Marking the conchal bowl to be excised. **C,** Transferring the marking to the underlying cartilage with methylene blue. **D,** Initial amount of skin to be removed in an elliptical fashion. **E** and **F,** Postauricular view of excised cartilage. **G–I,** Through-and-through fixation sutures anchored to the postauricular muscle and mastoid fascia used to secure the cotton bolster. (**A–D, F, G,** and **I,** Reproduced with permission from Owsley T. Otoplastic surgery for the protruding ear. In Fonseca RJ, editor. Oral and Maxillofacial Surgery. Vol 6. Philadelphia: WB Saunders; 2000; pp. 408–418; **E** and **H,** adapted from Owsley T. Otoplastic surgery for the protruding ear. In Fonseca RJ, editor. Oral and Maxillofacial Surgery. Vol 6. Philadelphia: WB Saunders; 2000; pp. 408–418.)

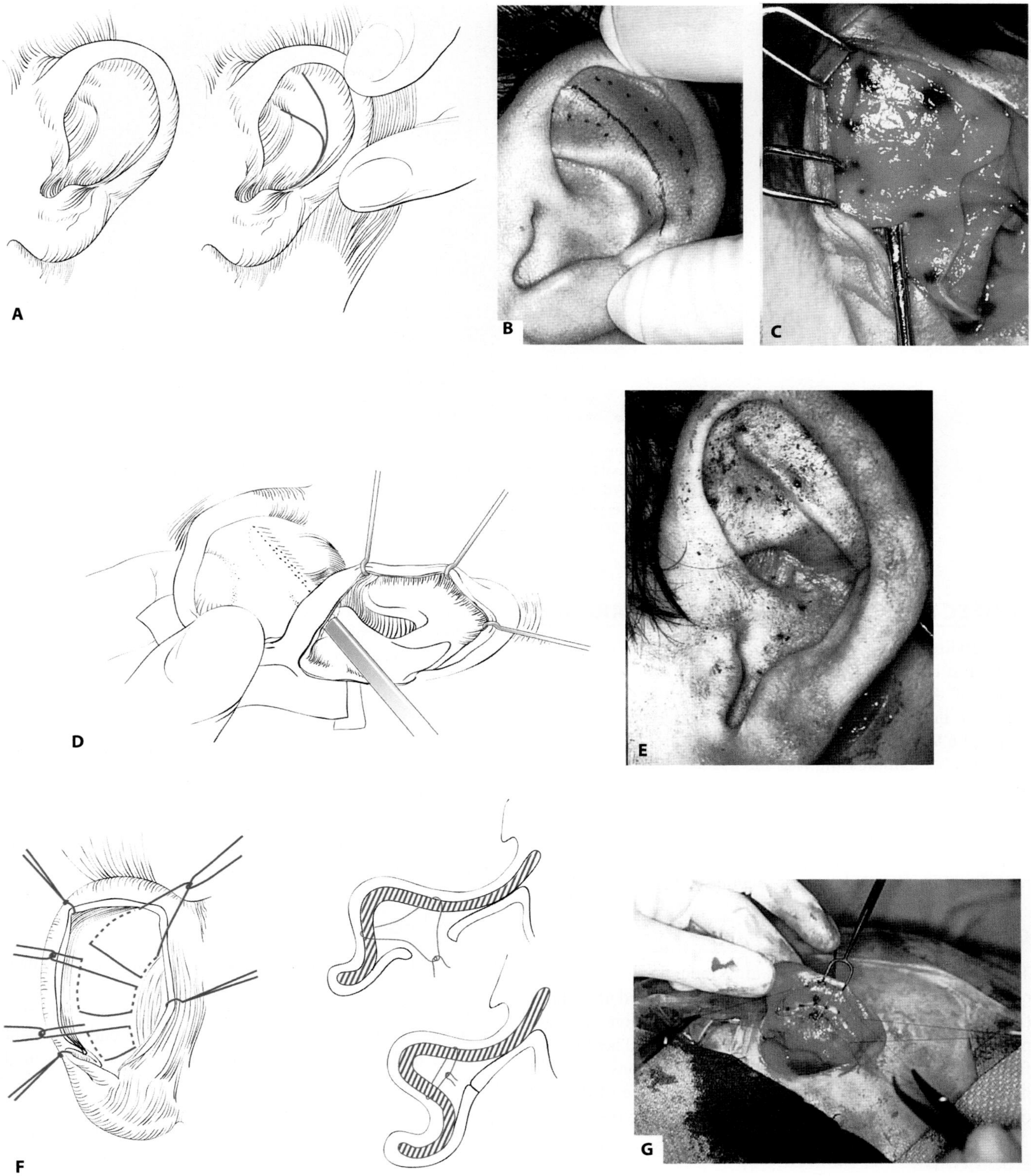

FIGURE 69-8.   Mustarde technique. **A** and **B,** Creating and marking the desired antihelical fold by folding back the helix with digital pressure. Lines, parallel to the crest of the fold, are marked and transferred to the underlying cartilage and used for suture placement. **C–E,** Dissection of the scaphoid fossa beneath the anterior skin for weakening and creation of the desired antihelical fold. **F** and **G,** Placement of the horizontal mattress sutures to create a new antihelical fold. *(continued)*

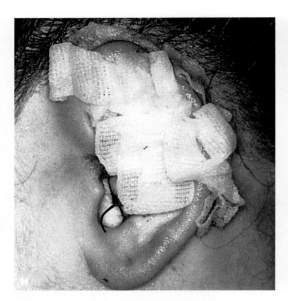
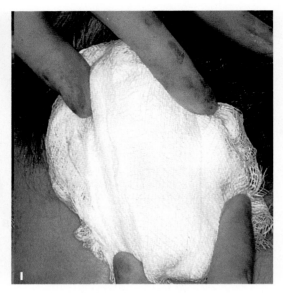

FIGURE 69-8. *(continued)* **H** and **I,** Placement of petrolatum gauze and fluffs as an important pressure dressing. (**A, D,** and **F,** Adapted from Owsley T. Otoplastic surgery for the protruding ear. In Fonseca RJ, editor. Oral and Maxillofacial Surgery. Vol 6. Philadelphia: WB Saunders; 2000; pp. 408–418; **B, C, E,** and **G–I,** reproduced with permission from Owsley T. Otoplastic surgery for the protruding ear. In Fonseca RJ, editor. Oral and Maxillofacial Surgery. Vol 6. Philadelphia: WB Saunders; 2000; pp. 408–418.)

CORRECTION OF THE PROTRUDING EARLOBE

A protruding earlobe often accompanies a protruding ear. If so, it must be identified and corrected simultaneously. If the lobule of the ear protrudes, an extension of the posterior auricular incision is drawn with a surgical marker in the shape of a V onto the earlobe. Finger pressure on the freshly marked lobe, compressing it to the mastoid skin, produces a mirror image imprint forming a W-shaped (fish-tail) portion of skin to be excised. After this portion is excised and hemostasis achieved, closure is accomplished with a 4-0 plain gut suture. The two V-shaped incisions are brought together, reducing the protruded state of the lobule (Figure 69-9).[14]

COMPLICATIONS

The incidence of complications after reduction otoplasty is quite low.[17] The major complications to be avoided are infection and keloid formation. Immediate complications include pressure necrosis from an overly tight dressing and hematoma formation. Delayed or long-term complications include hypertrophic or keloid scar formation, recurrence of the ear deformity, neurosensory deficits, and unaesthetic results.

Hematoma

Postoperative hematoma formation, with an incidence of 2% to 4%, is the most common problem that requires immediate and aggressive intervention.[17] It is most often related to inadequate hemostasis achieved at the time of surgery. Other factors in hematoma formation include an overly tight wound closure without drainage at the base of the wound, postoperative trauma, hypertension, and a preexisting bleeding dyscrasia. Persistent pain beneath the dressing or significant bleeding through and around the dressing suggests hematoma formation and demands prompt inspection. The presence of a hematoma is indicated by a tense and bluish swelling beneath the auricular skin, most often in the retroauricular space. Management includes suture removal, blood clot evacuation, hemostasis, and reclosure of the wound with a large pressure dressing reapplied. Large doses of antibiotics are advisable to prevent perichondritis. If this problem remains untreated, it can result in fibrosis, perichondritis, and cauliflower ear deformity.

Perichondritis

Wound infection in otoplasty occurs in the early postoperative period and is usually a sequela to an undetected or inadequately treated hematoma. Symptoms include pain, erythema, fever, and discharge that may or may not be present. Treatment includes high doses of antibiotics after appropriate wound cultures. Common bacteria include *Staphylococcus aureus, Escherichia coli,* and *Pseudomonas aeruginosa.* Adequate drainage is achieved by opening all sutures and carefully irrigating necrotic debris from the wound. All correction sutures must be removed and the cosmetic deformity addressed at a later date. The complication can be devastating, causing massive cartilage destruction with a severe deformity resulting, even with aggressive therapy. Prophylactic antibiotics have not been scientifically proved to be beneficial but are often used in the preoperative and postoperative period to avoid this devastating complication.

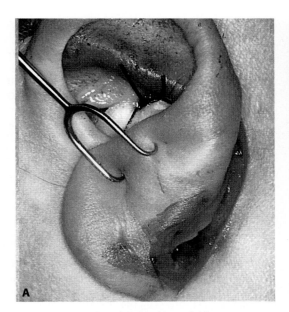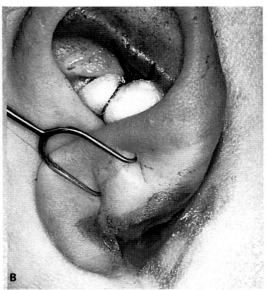

FIGURE 69-9.   **A** and **B,** Marking of skin to correct a protruding lobule. Areas marked are excised in "fishtail" fashion and closed. (**A** and **B,** Reproduced with permission from Owsley T. Otoplastic surgery for the protruding ear. In Fonseca RJ, editor. Oral and Maxillofacial Surgery. Vol 6. Philadelphia: WB Saunders; 2000; pp. 408–418.)

Keloid and Hypertrophic Scar Formation

The closure line of the skin incision in the postauricular region is susceptible to scar formation, especially closed under tension. It is most commonly seen in younger patients and patients with deeply pigmented skin. Keloid formation, one of the most frustrating of all postoperative complications, requires aggressive therapy. In the early stages of keloid formation, intralesional triamcinolone acetonide is injected weekly until regression or significant improvement is evident. Most hypertrophic scars improve with steroid infiltration, but some keloids can progress into significant unaesthetic lesions. Low-dose radiation, although potentially dangerous, may provide the only effective means of control of some keloids. The more advanced lesions require surgical excision combined with radiation and delayed skin grafting of the irradiated area, with final aid from intralesional triamcinolone. The risk can be minimized by ensuring that the skin incision is closed passively.

Aesthetic Complications

Inadequate correction of the ear deformity is the most common untoward result of otoplasty, often more obvious to the surgeon than to the patient. Calder and Nassan[18] described at least one complication or residual deformity in 16.6% of all the patients who underwent otoplasty using all techniques. Recurrence of the ear deformity is a more common complication of reduction otoplasty, but is less likely to happen after excising a portion of the cartilage as well as a segment of skin, as described in the Davis method.

Depending on sutures alone for achieving correction carries a greater risk of recurrence.

Telephone Ear Deformity

Telephone ear deformity occurs when the root of the helix and the ear lobule remain protruded while the middle half or third of the ear is set back against the head. This is more common in a large ear with a wide scapha. The incidence has been reported to be 3%.[19] Reverse telephone ear reveals a pronounced conchal bowl with respect to the lower and upper poles. These deformities can be avoided by carefully checking the position of the helical root, the upper helical rim, and the lobule at the completion of surgery.

Scapha Buckling

Scapha buckling or a transverse fold can develop in the Mustarde technique. This deformity can be avoided by placing the horizontal mattress sutures closer together where the scapha is widest, combined with adequate anterior scoring or weakening.

Narrowed Meatus

A constricted external auditory meatus can occur if the conchal bowl is rotated anteriorly in setting the ear back in any technique in which the conchal bowl is not excised. This problem is eliminated in the Davis method in which the floor of the conchal bowl is excised. Care must also be taken in placing the inferior end of the cotton roll bolster dressing into the external auditory canal to avoid stenosis.

SUMMARY

Reduction otoplasty carries few complications and can provide satisfying results for both the patient and the surgeon in the majority of cases. As in all cosmetic procedures, proper patient selection is imperative. Accurate preoperative assessment of the individual deformities and the appropriate choice of a surgical correction will minimize unfavorable aesthetic results. The single greatest cause of an unfavorable result in this procedure is inaccurate diagnosis.

The surgeon must understand the normal external anatomy of the ear and learn to recognize the pathologic characteristics of the abnormal ear. Having accurately assessed the deformity, the surgeon needs to be familiar with the various surgical approaches available to correct them. Finally, it is important to have a working knowledge of the potential complications of otoplasty and their prevention and treatment.

References

1. Ellis DA, Keohone JD. A simplified approach to otoplasty. J Otolaryngol 1992;21:66.
2. Deiffenbach JF. Die operative chirurgie. Leipzig: Brockhaus; 1845. Cited by Tanzer RC. Deformities of the auricle. In Converse JM, editor. Plastic and Reconstructive Surgery. 2nd ed. Philadelphia: WB Saunders; 1997; p. 1710.
3. Ely ET. An operation for prominence of the auricles. Arch Ophthalmol Otolaryngol 1881;10:97.
4. Karmody CS, Annino DJ Jr. Embryology and anomalies of the external ear. Facial Plast Surg 1995;11:251–256.
5. Strenstrom SJ. Cosmetic deformities of the ears. In Grabb W, Smith JW, editors. Plastic Surgery. Boston: Little Brown; 1968; p. 595.
6. Rogers BO. Microtic, lop, cup and protruding ears: four directly inheritable deformities? Plast Reconstr Surg 1968;41:208.
7. Allison GR. Anatomy of the external ear. Clin Plast Surg 1978; 5:419–422.
8. Davis JE. Aesthetics and Reconstructive Otoplasty. New York: Springer-Verlag; 1987; p. 77–87.
9. Tanzer RC. Congenital deformities. Deformities of the auricle. In Converse JM, editor. Reconstructive Plastic Surgery. 2nd ed. Philadelphia: WB Saunders; 1997; p. 1671.
10. Marx H. Die Missbildungen des Ohres. Sekundare Ohrmissbildingen. In Handke F, Lubarsch O, editors. Hanbush der Speziellen Pathologischen Anatomie und Histologie. Vol 12. Berlin: Springer-Verlag; 1926; p. 697.
11. Guyuron B, DeLuca L. Ear projection and the posterior auricular muscle insertion. Plast Reconstr Surg 1997;100:457–460.
12. Macgregor FC. Ear deformities: social and psychological implications. Clin Plast Surg 1978;5:347–350.
13. Furnas DW. Correction of prominent ears by concha-mastoid sutures. Plast Reconst Surg 1968;42:189–193.
14. Converse SM, Wood-Smith D. Corrective and reconstructive surgery in deformities of the auricle. In Papasella MM, Shumrick DA, editors. Otolaryngology. Vol 3: Head and Neck. Philadelphia: WB Saunders; 1973; pp. 500–527.
15. Davis J. Prominent ears. Clin Plast Surg 1978;5:471–477.
16. Mustarde JC. The correction of prominent ears using simple mattress sutures. Br J Plast Surg 1963;5:170.
17. Adamson PA, Strecker HD. Otoplasty techniques. Facial Plast Surg 1995;11:284–300.
18. Calder JC, Nassan A. Morbidity of otoplasty: a review of 562 consecutive cases. Br J Plast Surg 1994;47:170–174.
19. Lavy J, Sterns M. Otoplasty: techniques, results and complications—a review. Clin Otolaryngol 1997;22:390–393.
20. Tanzer RC. Congenital deformities. In Converse J, editor. Reconstructive Plastic Surgery. Vol 4. 2nd ed. Philadelphia: WB Saunders; 1977.
21. Davis JE. Anatomy of the ear. In Stark R, editor. Surgery of the Head and Neck. New York: Churchill Livingstone; 1987.

70

Adjunctive Facial Aesthetic Procedures

Joseph Niamtu, DMD

In the lifetime of almost everybody reading this book, there has been a significant paradigm shift in cosmetic facial surgery and it is a minimally invasive revolution. Since the mid-1990s, cosmetic facial surgery has ushered in "lunchtime" procedures such as neurotoxins, facial fillers, fractional lasers, and anatomic facial implants. Advances and refinement of chemical peeling, fat transfer, and skin care have also been made. Although many surgical practices perform these procedures, many clinicians from various specialties perform minimally invasive procedures (MIPs) as the bulk of their practices. MIPs interface well with all aspects and ages of cosmetic patients. Younger patients can benefit solely from MIPs, middle-aged patients may stave off surgery for a number of years with MIPs, and older patients can amplify surgical results with MIPs.

Another reason for this popularity is the fact that cosmetic facial surgery involves primarily females. Many females are in the workplace and have expendable income from employment, but cannot take off extended time for recovery; hence, they demand MIPs. MIPs have very distinct advantages and disadvantages. Neurotoxins and fillers, for instance, are very predictable and efficient. Other MIPs such as radiofrequency skin tightening and fractional lasers are frequently overmarketed by industry and the media, and the expectations often outweigh the results. The adage "if it sounds too good to be true, it probably is" must always be kept in mind with MIPs. In general, you get what you pay for, in terms of recovery. Many procedures that promise maximal effect with minimal recovery are often disappointing.

NEUROTOXINS

If there is a "real deal" in MIPs, it is neurotoxin technology. Before the mid-1990s, no predictable procedures existed to stop unwanted mimetic muscular movement and associated skin rhytids. Botulinum toxin A (BTA) is one of the seven serotypes of toxins produced by *Clostridia botulinum*. This toxin was originally used in humans to treat blepharospasm and strabismus. Treated patients coincidently noticed rhytid effacement on the treated side. This led to experimentation with these toxins for purely cosmetic use, and by the early 1980s, off-label cosmetic use of BTA was well under way. By 2002, Botox (BTA) was U.S. Food and Drug Administration (FDA) approved for glabellar wrinkles but was also used for numerous off-label wrinkle and medical treatments. In 2009, Dysport, another formulation of BTA, was FDA approved for glabellar wrinkles. At the time of the writing of this text, numerous other BTA preparations are in the pipeline for FDA approval and will surely become part of the armamentarium of the oral and maxillofacial surgeon (OMS). With their years of training in facial anatomy and experience with facial injections, OMSs can easily incorporate the cosmetic use of BTA in their practice.

BTA produces temporary muscle paralysis by preventing the release of acetylcholine at the neuromuscular junction. When selectively injected into the muscles of the head and neck, various cosmetic and functional changes are predictably achieved.

The most common regions for BTA injection are the glabella, frontalis, and lateral canthal regions. Additional muscles treated for cosmetic or functional reasons include the nasalis, levator labia superioris ala que nasi, orbicularis oculi, orbicularis oris, masseter, mentalis, and platysma.[1]

Because BTA will exert a temporary paralysis on any voluntary muscle, precise dosage and injection are paramount. In the upper face, levator palpebrae superioris injection remains the most feared complication. Keeping the toxin injections 10 mm above the bony orbital rim is a requisite to

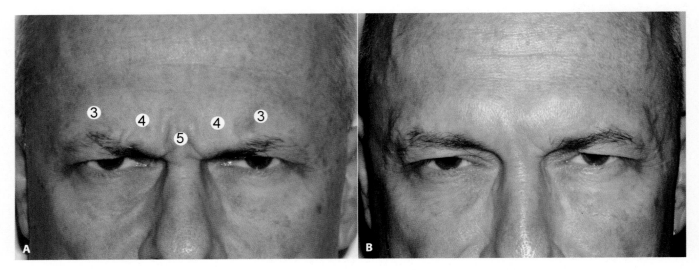

FIGURE 70-1. **A,** The *white dots* indicate common injection points for glabellar treatment with the respective number of Botox units for each area. **B,** The author 10 days after 20 units of Botox was injected into the glabella.

prevent upper eyelid ptosis. Novice injectors should actually measure and mark injection points on the brow and lateral canthal regions to remain 10 mm away from the orbital rim as not to inadvertently affect the levator palpebrae superioris or lateral extraocular musculature.

Although variable in some patients, most injection patterns and dosages are similar. Figure 70-1 shows the common injection points for the glabella, Figure 70-2 for the frontalis, and Figure 70-3 for the lateral canthal regions. For optimum treatment in females, the author recommend 5 Botox units or 15 Dysport units for each glabellar injection point. The frontalis, being a thinner muscle, is generally adequately treated with 3-unit injections, as is the lateral canthus regions. Males and patients older than 65 years old frequently require more units per area and the treatment may have a shorter longevity. After injection, BTA generally exerts its effects within

72 hours and paralysis averages 90 days. The glabellar region includes injection in the procerus muscle, both corrugator supercilii muscles, and the lateral orbicularis oculi regions.

INJECTABLE FACIAL FILLERS

Another paradigm shift has occurred since the turn of the last century with injectable fillers. Since the year 2000, bovine collagen was the most popular and only FDA-approved facial filler. Being from an animal source, allergy testing was required and results were very transient, often 2 to 3 months. Our European colleagues during this time had numerous choices of safe and predictable fillers. In 2003, Restylane (nonanimal stabilized hyaluronic acid) was approved by the FDA for the treatment of nasolabial folds. This natural polysaccharide was not only nonanimal but, owing to cross-linking

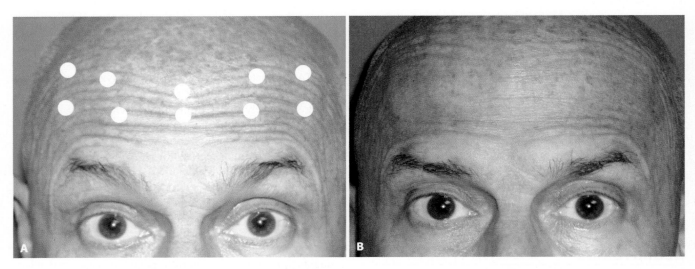

FIGURE 70-2. **A,** The *dots* show injection points on the author's frontalis region. The dose and position vary from patient to patient, but generally 2 to 3 units per injection point is adequate. **B,** The author 10 days after 25 units was injected into the frontalis region.

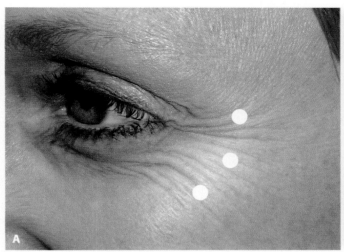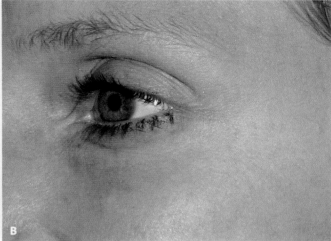

FIGURE 70-3.   **A,** Common injection points for the lateral canthal region. Generally, 3 units of Botox is injected at three regions in a semilunar shape with care to stay 1 cm lateral to the lateral orbital rim. **B,** The same patient 1 week after injection of 10 units of Botox on that side.

technology, lasted much longer that bovine collagen. Also, allergy testing was not required, which had been a major drawback for impetuous cosmetic patients and the "I want it now" generation.

The most common regions for filler injection in the author's practice are nasolabial folds, lips, vertical lipstick lines, perioral regions, and various skin wrinkles, in decreasing order.

Choice of Filler

Numerous FDA fillers are approved for on- and off-label use. The hyaluronic acid fillers (Juvederm Ultra, Juvederm Ultra Plus, Restylane, and Perlane) are far and away the most commonly injected products. These hyaluronic acid fillers are clear gels and can persist from 6 to 12 months, depending upon the injection site. Other common FDA-approved temporary fillers include hydroxylapatite (Radiesse), and porcine collagen (Evolence). L-Polylactic acid (Sculprta) and silicone oil (Silikon 1000) are stimulatory fillers in that they induce a foreign body reaction that induces collagen encapsulation and, hence, further augmentation. Sculptra may persist for up to 2 years and silicone can be permanent. Artefil is a filler consisting of polymethylmethacrylate microspheres in a collagen matrix and is also considered permanent filler. At the time of this publication, both Evolence and Artefil have closed operations in the United States, but will more than likely reappear under a new company.

Injecting the Nasolabial Folds

This author most frequently injects hyaluronic acid fillers in the nasolabial folds. It is easy to inject, feels natural, and can be reversed with hyaluronidase. The author's technique involves the intradermal placement of the filler in the depth of the nasolabial fold (NLF) from the alar base to the oral

commissure (or end of the fold).[2] Care must used to make sure the filler does not migrate laterally upon injection or the fold can be made larger. If the filler appears to be migrating laterally, the needle is removed and placed in a more medial position. It is imperative that the injector see the actual improvement of the wrinkle or fold while injecting. If the wrinkle is not improving as it is being injected, the needle is likely too deep and the filler is lateralizing. Figure 70-4 shows a hyaluronic acid filler being injected in the dermis of the nasolabial fold. Figure 70-5 shows a before and 14-day after injection picture on a patient treated with two syringes of Juvederm Ultra.

Injecting the Lips

Lip augmentation is more technique-sensitive and more difficult to learn than treating skin folds or wrinkles. Younger

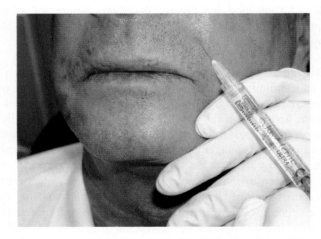

FIGURE 70-4.   An intradermal injection of hyaluronic acid filler is shown on the nasolabial fold.

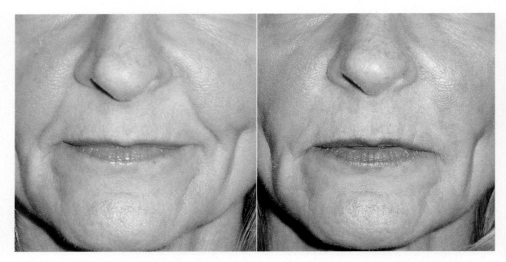

FIGURE 70-5. This patient is shown before and 2 weeks after injection of 0.8 mL of hyaluronic acid filler to each nasolabial fold.

patients can benefit with simple volumization of the deep lip. Older patients may require "white roll" outline, deep volumization, and vertical lipstick line fill, which presents a greater challenge.

Deep Lip Augmentation for Volume and Pout

Many young patients and virtually all females older than 40 can benefit from lip volumization. "Putting some air in the tires" can enhance facial beauty by a simple procedure. The lips are first anesthetized with intraoral perisulcular local anesthetic infiltration.[3] Next, the filler is injected at the level of the wet/dry line with the needle positioned in the mid lip. Filler is injected as the needle is withdrawn and the treatment is tapered to augment the center of the lip more than the lateral portions. Most younger patients can benefit from 0.4 to 0.5 mL of hyaluronic acid filler per lip, whereas older patients may require up to 1 mL per lip. Massage is performed with petroleum jelly to smooth and contour the gel to a smooth and homogenous state. Figure 70-6 shows deep lip injection and Figure 70-7 shows before and after images of deep lip volume augmentation using 0.8 mL of hyaluronic acid filler in each lip.

Defining the White Roll

The configuration of the vermilion/cutaneous junction is referred to as *Cupid's bow*. A light reflex exists in the aesthetic lip known as the "white roll." This treatment is usually imperative in older patients who have lost definition and outline and in younger patients with underdeveloped lip border anatomy.

Injection of the white roll involves the augmentation or reconstruction of Cupid's bow and its angular anatomy in the upper lip. The white roll of the lower lip is curvilinear in nature. In either lip, this area is injected by placing the needle in the potential space that exists between the mucosa and the orbicularis oris muscle. In the correct plane, the filler will flow freely and the filler is injected while withdrawing the needle. White roll augmentation in younger patients may involve only the central two thirds of the lip and gently tapers laterally. In older patients with loss of vertical dimension, the white roll may require extension to the commissures. Figure 70-8 shows hyaluronic acid filler being injected in the white roll region of the lip. Figure 70-9 shows a patient treated with white roll and deep volume injection.

In addition to the aforementioned areas, augmentation of the philtral columns, oral commissures, and vertical rhytids is also commonly performed.

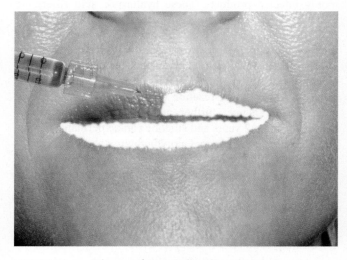

FIGURE 70-6. When performing deep lip volumization, the needle is inserted into the middle of the lip at the level of the wet/dry line and the filler is injected upon withdrawal. The injection is bilaterally tapered so the center of the lip has more volume than the lateral portions. The same procedure is repeated in the lower lip.

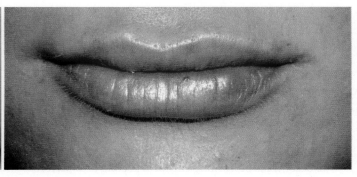

FIGURE 70-7.   This patient is shown before and after deep injection volumization of the upper and lower lips.

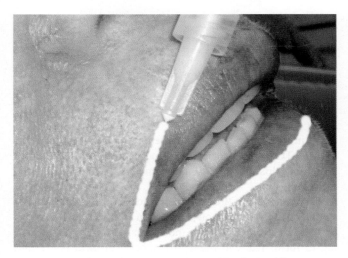

FIGURE 70-8.   White roll augmentation is performed by injecting a line of filler in the potential space between the mucosa and the orbicularis oris muscle to re-create or enhance the Cupid's bow effect.

CHEMICAL PEEL

Although laser resurfacing has changed the face (no pun intended) of treating wrinkles and dyschromias, chemical peel is a time-honored method for facial skin rejuvenation.

Chemical peeling is safe when performed with adequate training, is inexpensive, and has a moderate recovery of up to 1 week.

Chemical peels are performed with a myriad of acids, and deep or aggressive peels can cause problems with burns, scars, and hypopigmentation. The depth of the peel is dependent upon the peeling agent used, the concentration of the agent, the number of coats applied, and the physical properties of the skin. This section deals exclusively with trichloroacetic acid (TCA) chemical peeling. Peels can be classified into superficial, medium, and deep depending on how deeply the acid penetrates the skin. Superficial chemical peels are limited to the epidermis. Medium-depth peels are generally considered to be those that penetrate to the level of the papillary dermis; deep peels penetrate into the reticular dermis.

TCA exerts its actions by coagulating skin proteins. The author purchases TCA that is 30% compounded by the weight/volume method. Although the author will in some applications use this directly out of the bottle, most frequently the author dilutes it to 20% or 30%. To prepare a 20% solution of TCA, 4 mL of 30% TCA is diluted with 2 mL of water. To compound a 15% TCA solution, 2 mL of 30% TCA is mixed with 2 mL of water.

The novice peeler should gain expertise with 15% TCA and light peels without anesthesia before attempting more aggressive peeling with sedation.

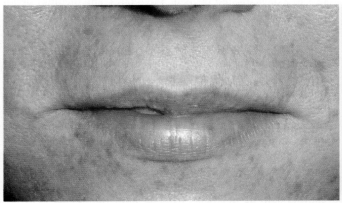 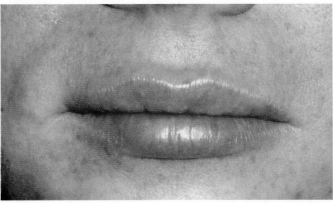

FIGURE 70-9.   This patient is shown before and after hyaluronic acid augmentation of the deep lip and vermilion/cutaneous junction.

All peel patients should be pretreated with Retin-A and hydroquinone 4% for 2 to 4 weeks before the peel. Darker skin types require longer prepeel skin priming.[4] Prepeel priming allows more efficient absorption of the acid into the skin, faster reepithelialization, and decreased postinflammatory hyperpigmentation. All peel patients are covered with an antiviral and antibiotic medication beginning the day before surgery and for the next 5 to 7 days. Superficial peels do not require this premedication unless the patient has a history of recurring herpes simplex infection.

The best means of learning chemical peeling is to perform superficial procedures on a patient such as an employee or friend who can be observed every day for the first week. It is imperative to learn the various stages of peeling and healing. A single coat of 15% (2 mL of 30% TCA and 2 mL of water) can be applied with minimal discomfort. The 4 mL of mixture is applied to the skin using a makeup sponge, cotton ball, Q-tips, or gloved finger. As the 15% solution is applied, the skin will tingle and slightly burn, but the discomfort is tolerable. This should be the treatment on one's first patient. The skin will develop a patchy white frost in some areas that will disappear in 5 to 10 minutes (Figure 70-10). After the procedure, the patient can apply hypoallergenic moisturizer multiple times a day. There will not be much peeling, only a little flaking, and there will not be a significant visible clinical result.

After experience with doing this several times, the same procedure can be performed, but a second coat applied this time. The second coat will burn more than the first, but two coats of 15% TCA are generally tolerable. The second coat will produce a more distinct patchy frost that the pervious single-coat 15% TCA treatments. With this treatment, it is advisable to apply Vaseline to the face for the first 48 hours, then moisturizer for the next several days. The goal is to keep

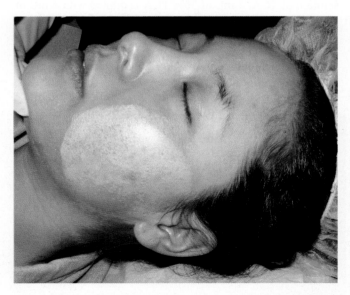

FIGURE 70-10. This patient is shown 5 minutes after a single application of 15% trichloroacetic acid (TCA) to the cheeks and has a patchy white frost.

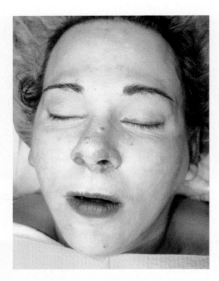

FIGURE 70-11. This patient has been treated with two or three coats of 30%; a homogenous white frost is evident 20 minutes into the procedure. The level of skin wounding with this extent of peel is the papillary dermis.

the skin moist continuously. Patients treated with two coats of 15% TCA will experience some distinct peeling at days 3 to 5, but this will be minimal compared with more aggressive peels.

Generally, the entire volume of the mixture is applied as a single coat. The surgeon must then wait several minutes before the next coat to allow the action to ensue and the frosting to form. The end point of a superficial peel is a scant, patchy, white frost. The end point of a basal layer peel is a light white frost with a pink background, and the end point of the medium (or deeper level) peel is a dense homogenous white frost (Figure 70-11).

The surgeon should not allow ego or desire to overtake common sense in learning these procedures. Begin with very conservative peels and after doing 5 or 6 patients, move on to the next level. It should take, in the author's opinion, at least 10 cases of superficial peeling before the surgeon begins using three- or four-coat treatments. The time of healing will coincide with the depth of injury. Superficial peels will heal in 1 to 2 days, basilar peels in 3 to 4 days, and medium-depth peels to the papillary dermis will heal in about 7 days.

Although some patients can be treated without sedation with three and four coats of 15% TCA, it can become very uncomfortable, and with the intense anesthesia training of our specialty, there is no reason for any surgical patient to be uncomfortable. Again, the author strongly recommends that before attempting three- and four-coat 15% TCA peels, practitioners perform multiple cases with one- and two-coat treatments to completely understand the peeling and wounding and healing process. Thinner tissues such as the upper eyelids must be treated more judiciously. In addition, because the neck has far less pilosebaceous units, it is never peeled as aggressively as the face. Patients with pigmented skin are also treated with caution and, therefore, less aggressive peels.

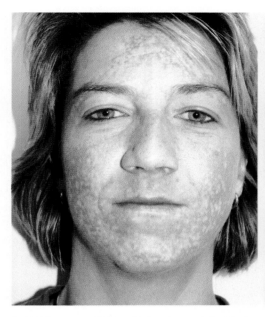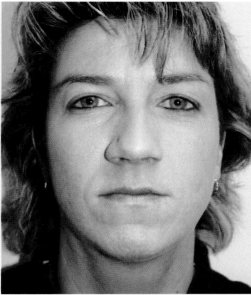

FIGURE 70-12. This patient was treated with three coats of 20% TCA to improve her melasma. She is shown before and 1 month after peel.

Resurfacing pigmented or ethnic skin is an advanced procedure and should not be performed by the novice.[5]

After the practitioner is experienced with multiple-coat 15% TCA peels, advanced treatments can be done with two or three coats of 20% TCA or straight 30% TCA (Figure 70-12). Chemical peeling is very technique sensitive and more of an art form than a science; extreme caution must be used with higher concentrations of acid because disfiguring burn and scarring can occur. Purchasing a dedicated text on chemical peeling and observing and mentoring cases is the safest and most effective means of learning chemical peeling. The Obagi Blue Peel is also a safe and effective way to perform TCA peels and is good for the novice peeler.[6]

MIDFACE IMPLANTS

For years, some cosmetic surgeons make patients tighter but not younger. Much of this has to do with pulling excess skin over an atrophic skeleton. Contemporary cosmetic surgeons realize the importance of volume replacement as an integral part of cosmetic facial surgery.[7,8] Many options exist to augment the midface including cheek lifts, injectable fillers, fat transfer, and alloplastic implants. Midface lifting has a reputation for being transient, fat and fillers resorb, but cheek implants are a permanent, three-dimensional means of volumizing the midface. When discussing implants with prospective patients, it is reassuring to tell a patient that the result will be permanent, but if they are unhappy, the implant can be removed in 5 minutes.

The youthful face is replete with volumizing fat in the right places. Older patients undergo fat atrophy as well as skeletal and cutaneous changes and the cheeks at some point become the jowls, leaving an atrophic hollow in their place. Almost any patient older than 45 years can benefit from some type of midface augmentation, and younger patients with developmental midfacial deformities are also excellent candidates.

A myriad of implant sizes and shapes are available and this can be confusing for the inexperienced facial surgeon. The author basically categorizes the regions of midfacial volume deficiency to the submalar region, the malar region, or a combination of both. Patients with otherwise normally developed midface features will lose fat in the infraorbital and submalar regions. This is very common in both males and females. This is the earliest and most common cosmetic problem, and therefore, the majority of implants (90%) the author places are silicone submalar implants. The implants run a bit small, so the average female will require medium to large submalar implants and males may require extra large submalar implants.

For the patient who has adequate submalar fill, but requests solely malar augmentation, the malar shell implant configuration is convenient. This implant lies more superior and lateral and produces the "high cheekbone look." The author uses this implant the least, because most of the author's patients have submalar atrophy.

The second most common facial implant is the combined submalar shell implant. This implant is a hybrid of the submalar implant and the malar shell implant and serves to augment both regions simultaneously. The author probably uses this on 5% of his patients. These implants actually run large and the author frequently uses a medium or large combined submalar shell but almost always trims the borders to customize the implant. Figure 70-13 shows typical patients in need of the three types of implants mentioned; Figure 70-14 shows the three types of implants the author most commonly uses to treat the aging midface.

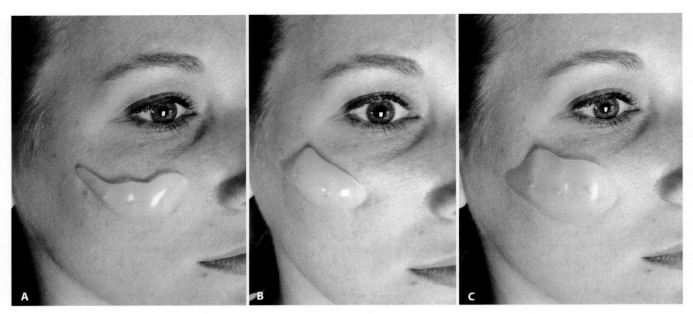

FIGURE 70-13. **A,** A patient with submalar deficiency. **B,** A patient with malar deficiency. **C,** A patient with deficiency in both the submalar and the malar regions.

The author prefers silicone implants because they are biocompatible, are easy to trim, will adapt to irregular contours, will not fracture with screw placement, and most important, are extremely easy to remove. Porous polyethylene implants can be a nightmare to remove owing to the extreme level of tissue ingrowth and frequently fracture and can cause much localized tissue damage when being removed.

Midface Implant Placement

Cheek implants can be placed with local anesthesia, although generally with intravenous sedation. The vast majority of cheek implants are concomitantly placed with face-lift surgery, although they are frequently placed as a stand-alone procedure.

About 5 mL of 2% lidocaine with 1:100,000 epinephrine is infiltrated percutaneously to the level of the periosteum along and slightly past the anticipated location of the implant. Another several milliliters of the anesthetic solution

is infiltrated intraorally around the sulcus and the anticipated implant position.

A 1-cm horizontal incision is made in the sulcus above the canine tooth to the level of the periosteum. Subperiosteal dissection is then performed superiorly with care to preserve the infraorbital nerve. At this point, the dissection proceeds in an oblique direction and tapers off over the zygomatic arch. Submalar implants require the smallest amount of dissection, whereas the malar shell and combined submalar shell implants require more extensive dissection. It is not uncommon to dissect over the masseter tendon at its zygomatic attachment. The tendon is not disturbed because the implant can safely lie over the tendon. It is important that the entire dissection remains subperiosteal and the dissection pocket needs to be only slightly larger than the size of the implant. Larger dissections are unnecessary, encourage implant mobility, and extend recovery. Figure 70-15 shows the incision, maxillary and malar dissection, implant placement, and the implant in position.

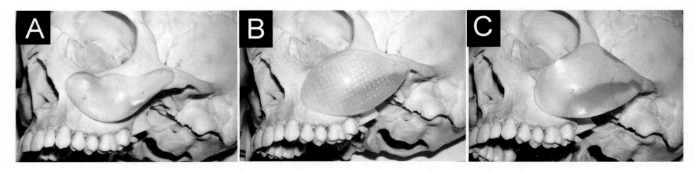

FIGURE 70-14. **Left** to **right,** A submalar implant **(A)**, a malar shell implant **(B)**, and a submalar shell implant **(C)**.

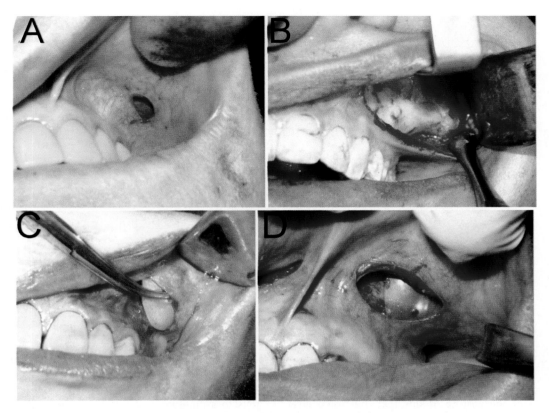

FIGURE 70-15.   A 1-cm incision **(A)** is used to perform a subperiosteal dissection over the anterior maxilla and the malar region and tapering over the zygomatic area **(B)**. The implant is then inserted into the dissection pocket **(C)** and should lie passively in place **(D)**.

Most of these implants will lie somewhere in line with the second premolar tooth, and this can be used as an index point to position both sides equally. After the proper position is achieved, the implant is secured with a single fixation screw. The screw is preferably placed over the denser buttress bone. At this point, the pocket is irrigated with antibiotic solution and the incision closed with 4-0 gut suture.

Postoperatively, no dressing is required. The patient is asked to refrain from excessive oral function and animation, and the recovery is generally approximately 1 week, although some patients may have residual swelling for several more days. Owing to the disruption of the lip elevators during the dissection, the patient will exhibit a weak smile or pucker that returns over a 10- to 14-day period. These patients are generally covered with antibiotics beginning intraoperatively and for the next 5 days. Figures 70-16 and 70-17 show before and after cases of patients treated with silicone cheek implants.

FRACTIONAL LASER RESURFACING

The mid 1990s ushered in another cosmetic facial surgery paradigm shift—laser skin resurfacing (LSR). Before predictable laser technology, dermabrasion and deep chemical peel were the common treatment options, both of which were difficult to control and art ruled over science. Laser technol-

ogy allowed precise ablation of tissue that was controllable in terms of microns, and each pass produced a controlled amount of damage. As with all new technology, many hard lessons were learned with LSR. Overtreatment and treatment of questionable areas produced significant scarring and hypopigmentation. The other drawback of LSR is the extended recovery. The recovery is formidable because the patient must heal with a raw face and reepithelialization can take up to 2 weeks. Extended erythema is also a drawback that can last for several months. The results, however, were unrivaled by any previous therapy, and to date, LSR treatment has overtaken the ability of aggressive CO_2 laser to simultaneously improve dyschromias, tighten deep wrinkles, and make new collagen. In terms of recovery, "you get what you pay for." If patients desire dramatic results, then 2 weeks of recovery is not too much to ask for the reversal of decades of aging. This author performs a high volume of traditional high fluence, high density, multipass CO_2 LSR; it remains one of the most dramatic procedures.

Owing to the demanding recovery and extended erythema associated with aggressive CO_2 laser, researchers have continued to look for a "friendlier" means of LSR. The erbium:yttrium-aluminum-garnet (Er:YAG) laser gained popularity in the mid-1990s and, although it enabled an easier recovery, the results were not as impressive as with traditional CO_2.

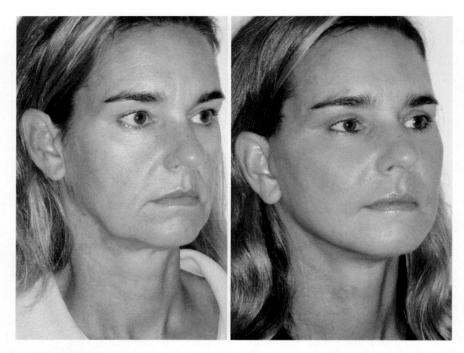

FIGURE 70-16. This patient underwent upper blepharoplasty, mini–face-lift, and bilateral silicone submalar cheek implants .

At the time of the writing of this text, fractional laser technology has become a popular option for facial rejuvenation. Fractional laser technology is very different from any previous laser treatment. Whereas traditional LSR treats the entire skin surface, fractional lasers do not treat the entire surface, but instead the laser beam is spaced and the result is treated microcolumns of lasered skin surrounded by untreated regions[9,10] (Figures 70-18 and 70-19). Traditional full-coverage ablative CO_2 laser treatment would be analo-

gous to a painting a wall with a paint roller, in which the entire surface is "treated." Fractional laser resurfacing would be like painting a wall with polka dots, in which some of the wall is painted and the remainder is untouched. Because a portion of the skin is not treated, the healing is easier and faster than with ablative LSR.

The push for a gentler laser has been demanded not only by patients, who want noticeable results with shorter recovery, but also by doctors, who want a laser procedure that can

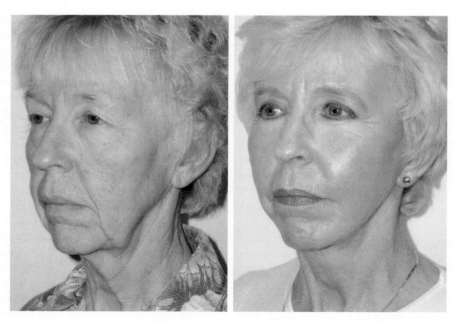

FIGURE 70-17. This patient was treated with a face-lift and medium submalar cheek implants and full-face CO_2 laser resurfacing.

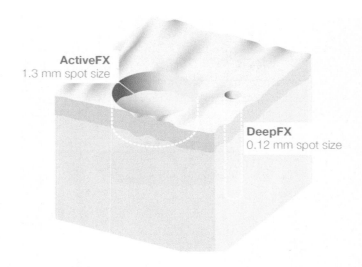

DeepFX™ - Variable Density
- 120 μm spot size   • 5-25% ablation

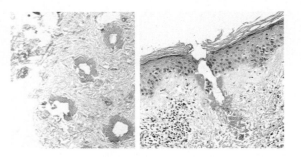

FIGURE 70-18. The effect of fractional laser skin resurfacing (LSR) in which laser microcolumns are surrounded by untreated areas of skin.

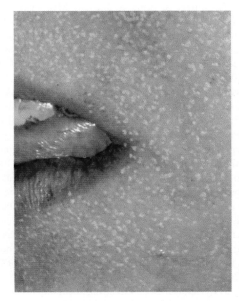

FIGURE 70-19. This patient is shown with the spaced treatment of nonablative CO_2 LSR known as Active FX (Lumenis Inc., Santa Clara, CA). The treated microcolumns of skin and the untreated areas are visible.

be performed without intravenous anesthesia or general anesthesia. This has been a good thing and a bad thing. It has been a good thing because fractional LSR has given us the ability to decrease recovery and prolonged erythema. It has, again in the author's opinion, been a bad thing because the results are not even close to those of traditional CO_2 LSR. Most practitioners who favor fractional LSR will perform three to five procedures to obtain significant results. The main theme of the newer technology was to decrease recovery; this has been done with most fractional LSR patients healing within 3 to 5 days. Having to do this three or four times, however, actually extends recovery time when compared with those of traditional LSR. For some surgeons, this may be a workable formula, but many patients expect bigger results. Some nonsurgical disciplines claim patients are very satisfied with the small changes seen from fractional LSR. Success with any procedure equals happy patients and low complications. Each type of surgeon has a different type of practice and what works in some practices may not be sufficient in others. Active FX fractional resurfacing is indicated for patients who will be satisfied with minor but noticeable results with a more user-friendly recovery. Figure 70-20 shows a patient treated with a single pass of Active FX fractional LSR. The areas of deeper pigmentation were treated with two or three passes.

Deep Fractional LSR

In the continuing search for a better laser treatment, deep fractional LSR is a newer technology. Similar to the Active FX treatment, the Deep FX (Lumenis, Inc., Santa Clara, CA) is a fractional laser with subtotal skin coverage. The difference is that the Active FX treatment penetrates the skin much deeper and can induce much more collagen production and, hence, more dramatic results. The spot size of the Deep FX is much smaller and the laser "drills" the microcolumns of energy from 400 to 900 μm into the dermis (Figure 70-21).

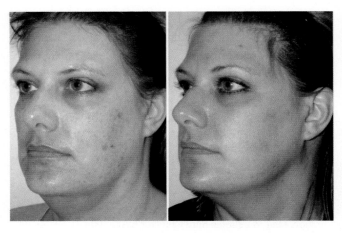

FIGURE 70-20. This patient was treated with a single pass of Active FX fractional LSR and the lentigos on the cheeks were treated with two additional passes.

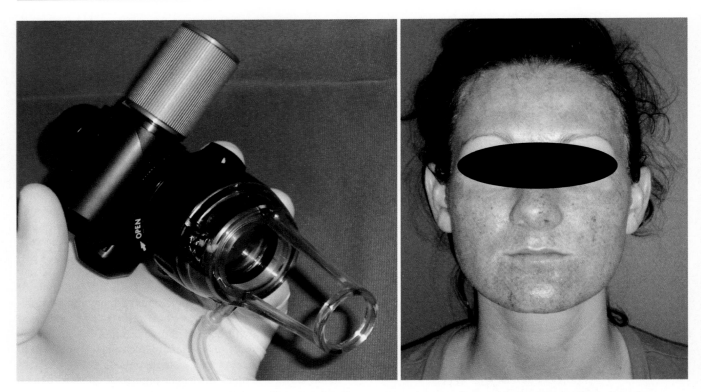

FIGURE 70-21.   The Deep FX is a more powerful and deeper-penetrating CO_2 treatment that enables treatment deeper into the dermis. Shown are the Deep FX laser handpiece and a patient 24 hours after a single pass of Deep FX resurfacing at 10 J/cm² and a density of 2.

Numerous clinicians are touting Deep FX's ability to improve wrinkles and acne scars, and encouraging work has been done with the treatment of burn scars using Deep FX laser technology. When performing Deep FX, the face is treated with one pass and areas of deeper wrinkling are treated with additional passes. Finally, a single pass of Active FX laser is performed over the entire face to blend the result. The Fraxel laser (Solta Medical, Heyward, CA) is another brand of laser that uses an erbium-doped system instead of CO_2.

CONCLUSION

OMSs are well positioned to incorporate cosmetic facial surgical procedures in their practices. Although traditional surgical procedures have been the mainstay of cosmetic facial surgery, MIPs have sprinted to the forefront of cosmetic treatment. The contemporary OMS understands the importance of MIPs, and they are a welcome and fun addition to our surgical practices.

References

1. Niamtu J 3rd. Complications in facelift surgery and their prevention. Oral Maxillofac Surg Clin North Am 2009;21:59–80, vi.

2. Niamtu J 3rd. New lip and wrinkle fillers. Oral Maxillofac Surg Clin North Am 2005;17:17–28, v.

3. Niamtu J 3rd. Simple technique for lip and nasolabial fold anesthesia for injectable fillers. Dermatol Surg 2005;31:1330–1332.

4. Obagi ZE, Obagi S, Alaiti S, Stevens MB. TCA-based blue peel: a standardized procedure with depth control. Dermatol Surg 1999;25:773–780.

5. Zhang AY, Obagi S. Diagnosis and management of skin resurfacing-related complications. Oral Maxillofac Surg Clin North Am 2009;21:1—12, v.

6. Johnson JB, Ichinose H, Obagi ZE, Laub DR. Obagi's modified trichloroacetic acid (TCA)–controlled variable-depth peel: a study of clinical signs correlating with histological findings. Ann Plast Surg 1996;36:225–237.

7. Binder WJ, Azizzadeh B. Malar and submalar augmentation. Facial Plast Surg Clin North Am 2008;16:11–32, v.

8. Terino EO, Edward M. The magic of mid-face three-dimensional contour alterations combining alloplastic and soft tissue suspension technologies. Clin Plast Surg 2008;35:419–50; discussion 417.

9. Sasaki GH, Travis HM, Tucker B. Fractional CO_2 laser resurfacing of photoaged facial and non-facial skin: histologic and clinical results and side effects. J Cosmet Laser Ther 2009;11:190–201.

10. Reddy BY, Hantash BM. Emerging technologies in aesthetic medicine. Dermatol Clin 2009;27:521–527, vii–viii.

Index

Information in figures and tables is indicated by *f* and *t*.

A

Abducens nerve, 1520*f*
Abdomen assessment, in trauma, 352–353
Abrasions, 362
Abutments
  in craniofacial implants, 313–314, 319–320
  in dental implants, 208–209
    connection, flap management and, 284, 285*f*
    fracture of, 225
    osseointegration and position of, 249–250
Achondroplasia, 1203*f*
Acid etching, of implant surfaces, 233–234
Acinic cell adenocarcinoma, 789
Activity status index, 18, 18*t*
Acupressure, for temporomandibular disorder, 1058
Acupuncture, for temporomandibular disorder, 1058
Acute suppurative sialoadenitis, 783
Adenoid cystic carcinoma, 788–789
Adenomatoid odontogenic tumor, 648–649
ADHD. *See* Attention deficit hyperactivity disorder (ADHD)
Adrenal disease, 34
Advancement flaps, 879–880
Aesthetic subunits, of face, 877–878
  frontoforehead, in dysostosis syndromes, 998–999
  maxillary-nasal base, in dysostosis syndromes, 1000
  orbitonasozygomatic, in dysostosis syndromes, 1000
  posterior cranial vault, in dysostosis syndromes, 999–1000
Aesthetic zone
  fixed partial dentures in, 212–214
  single-tooth replacement and, 210–211
Afterload, 18
Age. *See also* Geriatric patients; Pediatric patients
  as surgical comorbidity, 39–40, 69–74
  dental *vs.* chronologic, in alveolar cleft grafting, 967
  mandibular condyle fracture and, 450
  wound healing and, 11–12
AICD. *See* Automatic implantable cardioverter defibrillators (AICD)
Airway
  assessment, 26, 64–66
  in dysostosis syndromes, 997–998
  in gunshot wound management, 551–552
  in maxillofacial infection, 845–846
  in panfacial fractures, 599
  in pediatric facial trauma evaluation, 566

  in pediatric facial trauma, injury to, 567–568
  maintenance, in trauma, 328–330
  pediatric, 70–71
Alar nasalis muscle, 1532*f*
ALARA principle, 180
Alcohol abuse
  as surgical comorbidity, 38, 68
  oral cancer and, 698
Alfentanil, 46*f*, 48*f*, 49
Allantois, 1190*f*
Alpha 2 agonists, 58
Alveolar bone
  in edentulous patient, 123–124
  preservation of, in preprosthetic surgery, 134–136
Alveolar cleft repair
  grafting in
    allogenic bone for, 970
    bone morphogenic protein in, 970
    bone sources in, 969–972
    dental *vs.* chronologic age in, 967
    lateral incisors and, 967
    orthodontics and, pre- *vs.* postsurgical, 970–972
    patient size and, 968
    primary, 966
    rationale for, 965
    secondary, 966–969
    social issues with, 968
    surgical technique for, 972–974
    timing of, 966–969
  outcome measurement in, 965–966
  team dynamic and, 968
Alveolar development, 1207–1209
Alveolar distraction osteogenesis, 153–155, 1487, 1488*f*
Alveolar fracture
  classification of, 390–392
  Ellis classification, 392*f*
  etiology of, 388
  history in, 388–389
  history of, 387
  incidence of, 388
  maxillofacial examination for, 389–390
  physical examination for, 388–389
  radiography for, 390
  treatment of, 400–403

Alveolar osteitis, after third molar extraction, 114–115
Alveolar ridge
    discrepancies, in preprosthetic surgery, 150–151
    extension of, in preprosthetic surgery, 142–147
Alveoloplasty, in preprosthetic surgery, 136
Alveolus, oral cancer in, 708–709
Ameloblastic carcinoma, 642, 643f
Ameloblastic fibro-odontoma, 644
Ameloblastic fibroma, 644
Ameloblastoma, 637–641
    malignant, 642
    multicystic, 637–639
    peripheral, 640–641
    solid, 637–639
    unicystic, 639–640
American Society of Anesthesiologists (ASA) classification, 17t
Aminosteroids, 59t
Ammunition. See also Gunshot wounds
    classification of, 548–549
    velocities and muzzle energy of, 547t
Amnion, 1190f, 1191f
Amphetamine abuse, 68
Analgesic medications, perioperative, 57–58
Anemia, 28–29
    iron-deficiency, 29
    normocytic, 29
    sickle cell, 29
Anesthesia. See also Sedation
    alfentanil as, 49
    attention deficit hyperactivity disorder and, 87
    autism and, 87
    benzodiazepines in, 45–47
    cerebral palsy and, 88
    diazepam as, 46–47
    Down syndrome and, 88
    fentanyl as, 49
    fluids in, 75–76
    flumazenil as, 47
    general, definition of, 63t
    hydromorphone, 49
    in geriatric patients, 72–74
    in pediatric patients, 69–72
    in preprosthetic surgery, 130
    induction agents for, 50–52
    inhalation, 54–57
        in pediatric patients, 77–78
    laryngospasm and, 84–86
    lorazepam as, 47
    meperidine as, 49
    midazolam as, 47
    monitoring in, 74–75
    morphine as, 48–49
    muscular dystrophy and, 88–89
    nalbuphine as, 50
    naloxone as, 50
    opioids in, 47–50
    patient positioning and, 76
    perioperative complications, 84–86
    pharmacodynamics in, 43–44
    pharmacokinetics in, 44–45
    recovery from, 86–87
    remifentanil as, 49
    sedation in
        level of, 63
    sufentanil as, 49
    triazolam as, 47
Aneurysmal bone cyst, 663, 832
Angina, 18t

Angiogenesis, in wound healing, 5
Angiolysis, 63t
Angiosarcoma, 816
Angular artery, 1533f, 1534f, 1579f
Animal bites, 363
Ankylosing spondylitis, temporomandibular hypomobility and, 1159
Antagonists
    competitive, 44
    noncompetitive, 44
Anterior auricularis muscle, 1600f
Anterior crus, 1600f
Anterior ethmoidal artery, 1534f
Anterior lamella, 1518–1519
Anterior repositioning appliance, for temporomandibular
    disorder, 1060
Anterior table fracture, 528
Anterolateral thigh flap, 903–904
Antibiotic(s)
    after temporomandibular arthroscopy, 1116
    for maxillofacial infections, 852–853
    in pediatric facial trauma, ointment, 580–581
    in third molar extraction, 112–113
Anticholinergic medications, 59–60
Anticholinesterases, 59
Antidepressants, for temporomandibular disorder, 1053–1054
Antiemetic medications, 60–61, 85–86
Antihelix, 1600f
Antihistamines, for temporomandibular disorder, 1053
Antineoplastic agents, wound healing and, 11
Antitragus, 1600f
Anxiolytics, for temporomandibular disorder, 1053
Aortic regurgitation (AR), 20
Aortic stenosis (AS), 18t, 20
Apert's syndrome, 996, 1014–1022. See also Dysostosis syndromes
Apertognathia, after orthognathic surgery, 1448–1449
AR. See Aortic regurgitation (AR)
Arch length, 1263–1264
Arch symmetry, 1267
Arch width analysis, 1265–1266
Arm free flap, lateral, 905–906
Arrhythmias, cardiac, 21–22
Arthritis
    juvenile idiopathic, facial asymmetry in, 1397
    osteoarthritis, in temporomandibular joint, 1102
    rheumatoid, in temporomandibular joint, 1100–1101, 1159
    septic, in temporomandibular joint, 1043–1044
Arthroscope, 1079–1080
Arthroscopy, of temporomandibular joint
    abraders in, 1085
    advantages of, 1070
    anatomy in, 1087–1090
    anterior recess in, 1099–1100
    anti-inflammatory management after, 1116
    antibiotics after, 1116
    armamentarium for, 1082–1085
    articular disk in, 1095–1098
    biopsy forceps in, 1082, 1084f
    cannulas in, 1082
    chondromalacia grading in, 1102–1104
    complications of, 1118–1121
    contraindications, 1070
    danger zones in, 1086–1087
    diagnostic sweep in, 1092–1100
    diet after, 1116
    disk reduction for, 1109
    electrosurgery in, 1085–1086
    facial nerve trauma in, 1118–1119
    fibrocartilage scuffing in, 1119

for anterior release, 1108–1109
for botulinum toxin A delivery, 1107
for débridement, 1107
for diskopexy, 1109–1116
for hyaluronic acid delivery, 1107
for lysis and lavage, 1105–1107
for medication delivery, 1107
for posterior scarification/cauterization, 1109
for second puncture, 1104–1105
for steroid delivery, 1107
for synovectomy, 1108
fossa puncture in, 1090–1091
full-radius shaver in, 1085
glenoid fossa perforation in, 1120
goals of, 1069
hemarthrosis in, 1120
history of, 1069
immediate preoperative steps for, 1090
indications for, 1070
infection from, 1120–1121
instrument failure in, 1121
insufflation in, 1090
intermediate zone in, 1098–1099
laser in, 1086
maxillary artery damage in, 1120
medial synovial drape in, 1092–1093
meniscus mender in, 1082–1083, 1084f
nerve injury in, 1118–1119
On Point system for, 1081–1082
operative procedures in, 1104–1116
outflow needle puncture in, 1091
pain management after, 1116
palpation of anatomy in, 1090
patient evaluation for, 1070–1072
physical examination for, 1072–1078
physiotherapy after, 1117–1118
portals of entry for, 1086
postoperative patient management in, 1116
postoperative rehabilitation for, 1117–1118
probes in, 1082, 1084f
pterygoid shadow in, 1093–1094
retrodiskal synovium in, 1094
shavers in, 1083
Smith-Nephew system for, 1082, 1083f
technique for, 1090–1102
trigeminal nerve trauma in, 1119
vestibulocochlear trauma in, 1119
video, 1080–1082
whisker shaver in, 1085
Articular cartilage, in temporomandibular joint, 1035
Articular fossa, 1033–1034
AS. *See* Aortic stenosis (AS)
Asthma, 24
Asymmetry
    facial
        acquired, 1396–1397
        bone scans in evaluation of, 1398–1399
        case examples, 1403–1409
        clinical patient assessment in, 1397–1399
        congenital anomalies in, 1394–1395
        CT assessment of, 1398
        delayed treatment approach to, 1399
        developmental, 1395–1396
        etiology of, 1393–1394
        in condylar trauma, 1396–1397
        in congenital hemifacial hyperplasia, 1395
        in degenerative joint disease, 1397
        in facial hemiatrophy, 1395–1396

in hemifacial microsomia, 1394, 1395f
in hemimandibular hyperplasia, 1396
in juvenile idiopathic arthritis, 1397
in plagiocephaly, 1395
orthodontic considerations in, 1399–1401
overview of, 1393
radiographic assessment in, 1397–1398
stereolithographic modeling of, 1398
surgical treatment of, 1399–1409
mandibular, 1251
maxillomandibular, 1252
Atelectasis, 26
Atracurium, 59t
Atrial flutter, 21
Atropine, 60t, 61f
Attention deficit hyperactivity disorder (ADHD), 87
Auricle, embryology of, 1597
Auricular prostheses, 316–317
Auricular templates, 318
Auriculocephalic angle, 1598
Auriculotemporal nerve, 1600f
    in forehead anatomy, 1580
    in temporomandibular joint derangement surgery, 1130
    injury, in temporomandibular arthrocentesis, 1119
Auriculotemporal syndrome, after orthognathic surgery, 1451
Autism, 87
Autoimmune blistering disease, 806–809
Autoimmune disease, as surgical comorbidity, 36–37
Automatic implantable cardioverter defibrillators (AICD), 23
Avulsive injury
    dentoalveolar, 397–400
    maxillary fracture in, 461
    soft tissue, 362–363
Axonotmesis, 6, 925, 926f, 926t, 943

B
Ballistics, of gunshot wounds, 546
Barbiturates, 52–54
Basal cell carcinoma, 746
Basic multicellular unit (BMU), 7
Beare-Stevenson syndrome, 996. *See also* Dysostosis syndromes
Benign fibro-osseous disease, 653–6556
Benign mesenchymal tumors, 826–829
Benign migratory glossitis, 802
Benzamides, 86
Benzodiazepines, as outpatient anesthesia, 45–47
Benzylisoquinolones, 59t
Bilateral sagittal split osteotomy, 1331–1343, 1430, 1438, 1445–1446, 1449–1450
Biofeedback, for temporomandibular disorder, 1058
Biomechanics
    implants and, 201–209
    mandible fracture and, 410
    of osseointegration, 238–248
    of temporomandibular joint, 1040
    skin, 758
Biopsy
    in oral disease diagnosis, 619–620
    oral cancer, 687–688
    sentinel node, 716–717
Bisphosphonates
    implant treatment with, 238
    jaw osteonecrosis and, 870–873
Bite depth, 1258
Bites, 363, 581
Blasting, of implant surfaces, 233, 234
Bleeding control, in trauma, 338–339, 340f, 341f
Blepharochalasia, 1516

Blepharoplasty
  anatomy in, 1516–1522
  complications in, 1527–1529
  dry eyes after, 1529
  nomenclature in, 1515–1516
  overview of, 1515
  patient evaluation for, 1523–1525
  postoperative care for, 1526–1527, 1528f
  surgical procedures in, 1525–1526
Blepharoptosis, 1516
Blood disorders, 28–32
Blood pressure, in pediatric patients, 72
BMI. See Body mass index (BMI)
BMPs. See Bone morphogenic proteins (BMPs)
BMU. See Basic multicellular unit (BMU)
Body mass index (BMI), 38, 38t
Bolton's analysis, 1264–1265
Bonding, of impacted teeth, 103–105
Bone
  alveolar, characteristics of, in edentulous patient, 123–124
  calvarial, as grafting source, 969–970
  healing of, 6–7, 7f, 375f, 376f
  load-deformation relationship in, 240
  regeneration, principles of, 131–132
  Stafne's defect, 668–669
Bone cyst, traumatic, 667–668
Bone grafts
  calvarial bone for, 969–970
  cone beam CT in augmentation assessment, 187–191
  cranial, 909
  for gunshot wounds, 559–561
  for panfacial fractures, 599
  for temporomandibular joint disease, end-stage, 1174–1176
  iliac crest for, 907–909, 969
  in alveolar cleft repair
    allogenic bone for, 970
    bone morphogenic protein in, 970
    bone sources in, 969–972
    dental vs. chronologic age in, 967
    lateral incisors and, 967
    orthodontics and, pre- vs. postsurgical, 970–972
    patient size and, 968
    primary, 966
    rationale for, 965
    secondary, 966–969
    social issues with, 968
    surgical technique for, 972–974
    timing of, 966–969
  in zygomatic complex fractures, 477
  nonvascular, 906–909
  preprosthetic surgery and, 132–134, 149–150
    inlay, 149–150
    interpositional, 149, 150f, 152, 153f
    onlay, 149
  rib for, 969t
  tibial, 909, 969t
Bone loss, implants and, 239–246
Bone morphogenic proteins (BMPs)
  alveolar cleft grafting and, 970
  implant surface treatment with, 237–238
Bone scans, in facial asymmetry evaluation, 1398–1399
Botulinum toxin type A, 1609–1610
  for temporomandibular disorder, 1107
  in brow lift, 1591
Brain, development of, craniosynostosis and, 980
Branchial arches, 833t
Branchial cleft cyst, 833
Breastfeeding, in cleft lip and palate, 949–950

Breathing, in primary trauma survey, 330–336
  for pediatric patients, 566
Bronchitis, chronic, 24–25
Brow cosmetic surgery
  adjunctive procedures in, 1591–1592
  aesthetic considerations in, 1571–1583
  anatomic considerations in, 1571–1583
  botulinum toxin-assisted, 1591
  complications of, 1592–1593
  coronal lift, 1585
  direct lift, 1590
  endoscopic, 1586–1590
  micropigmentation in, 1591–1592
  midforehead lift, 1590
  postoperative care for, 1592
  preoperative evaluation for, 1583–1585
  pretrichial lift, 1585–1586
  skin resurfacing in, 1591
  surgical preparation for, 1583–1585
  temporal lift, 1590
  trichophytic lift, 1585–1586
Brown tumors, 826–827
Bruxism
  dental implants and, 202
  mandibular condyle fracture and, 451
  temporomandibular joint derangement and, 1124
Buccal branch, of facial nerve, 358f, 359f
Buccal mucosa, oral cancer in, 705
Bulbous pemphigoid, 809
Bullets. See also Gunshot wounds
  classification of, 548–549
  velocities and muzzle energy of, 547t
Burkitt's lymphoma, 829
Buttresses, of face, 594

C
C ramus osteotomy, 1328–1331
CAD. See Coronary artery disease (CAD)
Calcifying odontogenic cyst, 633–635
Calcium phosphate, implant surface treatment of, 237
Caldwell's view, 469
Calvarial bone, as grafting source, 969–970
Camouflage, orthodontic, 1228–1229
Cancer
  in temporomandibular joint, 1045
  lip
    anatomic considerations in, 728–729
    cervical lymphadenectomy in, 736–737
    epidemiology of, 727–728
    etiology of, 727–728
    evaluation of, 729–730
    management of, 729–737
    reconstruction in, 732–736
    surgical treatment of, 730–732
    treatment results in, 737–738
  oral
    alcohol and, 698
    biopsy of, 687–688
    cervical lymph node levels in, 685–686
    cervical lymph nodes in, 711–713
    chemoprevention for, 704
    chemotherapy for, 701–704
    deep venous thrombosis and, 698
    diagnosis, 687–688
    distant metastasis assessment in, 687
    ethnicity and, 677t
    etiology of, 678–679
    follow-up surveillance, 717–719

future treatments for, 719
histology of, 693–694
in alveolus, 708–709
in buccal mucosa, 705
in floor of mouth, 708
in gingiva, 708–709
in lip, 704–705
in palate, 709
in retromolar trigone, 706
in tongue, 706–708
mandible in, 709–710
MRI in, 686–687
neck dissection in, 713–716
    therapeutic, 717
overview of, 677–678
panendoscopy in, 695–696
perioperative issues with, 698–699
PET in, 687
premalignant disease in, 679–683, 694–695
primary lesion assessment, 684–685
radiation for, 699–701
recurrence of, 717–719
regional metastasis assessment in, 685–687
risk factors, 678
sentinel node biopsy in, 716–717
staging, 687
surgery for, 696–699
treatment choice for, 696
ultrasound in, 687
salivary gland, 788–789
skin
    lasers for, 756
    melanoma, 749–751, 814–815
        biopsy strategies, 751t
        clinical description, 749–751
        histologic description, 749–751
        risk factors, 749
        survival rates, 751t
    nonmelanoma, 743–749
        basal cell carcinoma, 746
        chemotherapy for, 756
        cryosurgery for, 755
        curettage and electrodesiccation for, 755–756
        environmental factors, 745
        epidemiology of, 743
        etiology of, 743–746
        grafting in, 757–768
        immunologic factors, 744
        interferons for, 756
        management of, 751–768
        Mohs' micrographic surgery for, 753–755
        photodynamic therapy for, 756
        predisposing lesions, 744
        prevention of, 745–746
        radiation therapy for, 755
        retinoids for, 756
        squamous cell carcinoma, 746–749
        standard excision of, 752
        syndromes in, 744
Candidosis, 798–801
Canine
    alveolar cleft grafting and, 969
    mandibular, site preparation for correction of single missing, 271
    maxillary, impaction of
        cone beam CT of, 181–183
        in pediatric patients, 160–163
Canker sores, 801–802
Cantilevered fixed partial dentures, 215–216

Cantilevers, osseointegration and, 251–252
Capsulopalpebral fascia, 1517f, 1519f
Carbon dioxide laser, 1086
Cardiac arrhythmias, 21–22
Cardiac dysrhythmia, 18t
Cardiac output, in pediatric patients, 71–72
Cardiovascular disease, 18–26
Cardiovascular system
    in geriatric patients, 73
    in pediatric patients, 71–72
Caries, dental, impacted third molar and, 101
Carpenter's syndrome, 1025. See also Dysostosis syndromes
Cauda, 1600f
Caudal neuropore, 1191f
Cavum concha, 1600f
Cawood classification, 127f
CBCT. See Cone beam computed tomography (CBCT)
Cementifying fibroma, 825
Cemento-osseous dysplasia, 655–656
Cementoblastoma, 825
Cementoma, 825
Central giant cell granuloma, 660–662
Centric relation bite registration, 1297–1298
Cephalometric analysis, in dysostosis syndromes, 1000
Cephalometric prediction, computerized, 1260–1261, 1411–1421
Cerebral palsy, 88
Cerebrospinal fluid (CSF), 523t
Cerebrovascular accident (CVA), 35
Cervical branch, of facial nerve, 358f, 359f
Cervical spine control, in trauma, 328–330
Champy method, 375f
Cheek, in pediatric facial trauma, 577–579, 580f
Chemical peel, 1613–1615
Chemoprevention, for oral cancer, 704
Chemotherapy
    for oral cancer, 701–704
    for skin cancer, topical, 756
Cherubism, 662–663
Chest assessment, in trauma, 348–349
CHF. See Congestive heart failure (CHF)
Children. See Pediatric patients
Chin asymmetry, 1251–1252
Chondrocalcinosis, in temporomandibular joint, 1101
Chondroma, 657
Chondromalacia, in temporomandibular joint, 1102–1104
Chondromatosis, in temporomandibular joint, 1045
Chronic bronchitis, 24–25
Chronic obstructive pulmonary disease (COPD), 24–25
Chronic ulcerative stomatitis, 806
Cicatricial pemphigoid, 808–809
Circulation, in primary trauma assessment, 336–343
    in pediatric patients, 566
Cisatracurium, 59t
Clear cell odontogenic carcinoma, 643
Cleft lip and palate
    classification of, 948
    embryology of, 947
    etiology of, 947–948
    facial asymmetry in, 1395
    feeding concerns with, 949–950
    genetics in, 947–948
    goals of repair, 945
    history of, 946–947
    management of children with, 945
    orthognathic surgery for
        distraction osteogenesis in, 1461–1464, 1469
        history of, 1456
        maxilla development in, 1454–1456

maxillary hyperplasia in, 1456
maxillary osteotomies in, 1458–1459
orthodontics and, 1454–1456
palatal splints and, 1457–1458
postsurgical considerations in, 1464–1465
surgical considerations in, 1460–1461
velopharyngeal considerations in, 1465
prenatal counseling for, 948–949
repair, 951–959
for bilateral cleft lip, 954–955
for cleft palate, 955–959
for complex facial clefting, 959–960
for unilateral cleft lip, 952–953
lip adhesion in, 952
outcome assessment, 960
presurgical orthopedics in, 951–952
presurgical taping in, 951–952
treatment planning and timing in, 950–951
Clenching, osseointegration and, 252–253
Clinical neurosensory testing, 925–929
Cloacal membrane, 1190*f*
Cloverleaf skull anomaly, 1025–1026. *See also* Dysostosis syndromes
Coagulopathy, 30
Cocaine, 68
Color, of craniofacial prostheses, 319
Comorbidities
autoimmune, 36–37
blood disorders, 28–32
cardiovascular disease, 18–26
endocrine, 32–34
immunodeficiency, 37–38
liver disease, 28
neurologic, 34–36
obesity, 38–39, 66
pregnancy, 40–41
renal disease, 27–28
respiratory disease, 23–26
smoking, 65
substance abuse, 38, 67–69
Competitive antagonists, 44
Compressor narium minor muscle, 1532*f*
Computed tomography (CT)
cone beam
advantages of, 179
conventional CT *vs.*, 179
for mandibular diagnostics, 191–197, 198*f*
for maxillary canine impaction, 181–183
implant evaluation with, 184–187, 187–191, 191–197, 198*f*, 203–204
in graft augmentation assessment, 187–191
in oral disease diagnosis, 618
machine factors in, 180
processing in, 180
radiation risks in, 179–180
conventional *vs.* cone beam, 179
for nasal fracture, 540–541
for preprosthetic surgery, 129–130
history of, 179
in obstructive sleep apnea, 1497
in oral disease diagnosis, 618
machine factors in, 180
of orbital fracture, 492
processing in, 180
radiation risks in, 179–180
Computerized cephalometric prediction, 1260–1261
Conchal cavity, 1598
Concussion, periodontal, 395
Cone beam computed tomography (CBCT)

advantages of, 179
conventional CT *vs.*, 179
for mandibular diagnostics, 191–197, 198*f*
for maxillary canine impaction, 181–183
implant evaluation with, 184–187, 187–191, 191–197, 198*f*, 203–204
in graft augmentation assessment, 187–191
in oral disease diagnosis, 618
machine factors in, 180
processing in, 180
radiation risks in, 179–180
Congenital epulis, 830
Congenital gingival granular cell tumor, 830
Congenital hemifacial hyperplasia, 1395
Congestive heart failure (CHF), 18*t*, 19–20
Conjunctiva, 1517*f*
Connective tissue graft, subepithelial, for dental implants, 290–295
Conscious sedation, 63*t*
Contamination, of gunshot wounds, 558
Context-sensitive half-time, 45, 46*f*
Continuous positive airway pressure (CPAP), 1500
Contractility, 18–19
Contusions, 362
COPD. *See* Chronic obstructive pulmonary disease (COPD)
Coronal forehead and brow lift, 1585
Coronary artery disease (CAD), 19
Corrugator supercilii, 1575
Corticosteroids, for temporomandibular disorder, 1052–1053
Cosmetic surgery
adjunctive procedures in, 1609–1620
blepharoplasty
anatomy in, 1516–1522
complications in, 1527–1529
dry eyes after, 1529
nomenclature in, 1515–1516
overview of, 1515
patient evaluation for, 1523–1525
postoperative care for, 1526–1527, 1528*f*
surgical procedures in, 1525–1526
forehead and brow
adjunctive procedures in, 1591–1592
aesthetic considerations in, 1571–1583
anatomic considerations in, 1571–1583
botulinum toxin-assisted, 1591
complications of, 1592–1593
coronal lift, 1585
direct lift, 1590
endoscopic, 1586–1590
micropigmentation in, 1591–1592
midforehead lift, 1590
postoperative care for, 1592
preoperative evaluation for, 1583–1585
pretrichial lift, 1585–1586
skin resurfacing in, 1591
surgical preparation for, 1583–1585
temporal lift, 1590
trichophytic lift, 1585–1586
otoplasty
aesthetic complications in, 1607
anatomy in, 1597–1599
complications of, 1606–1607
Davis method for, 1601–1603, 1604*f*
hematoma in, 1606
keloid formation in, 1607
Mustarde method for, 1603–1606
narrowed meatus after, 1607
perichondritis in, 1606
scapha buckling after, 1607

scarring in, hypertrophic, 1607
surgical techniques in, 1601–1606
telephone ear deformity after, 1607
rhinoplasty
  alar base reduction in, 1551, 1552f
  alar width in, 1541
  anatomy in, 1531–1537
  anesthesia for, 1541
  complete transfixion in, 1542
  cosmetic evaluation in, 1537–1538
  facial analysis in, 1538
  functional considerations in, 1541
  hemitransfixion in, 1542
  incisions in, 1541–1543
  intercartilaginous incision in, 1542–1543
  intracartilaginous incision in, 1543
  Killian incision in, 1542
  marginal incision in, 1543
  nasal analysis in, 1538, 1539f
  nasal dorsum assessment in, 1539, 1541
  nasal dorsum augmentation in, 1546–1547
  nasal dorsum reduction in, 1546
  nasal tip definition in, 1539–1540
  nasal tip projection in, 1539–1540, 1548–1550
  nasal tip rotation in, 1540, 1550
  nasal tip shape in, 1550–1551
  nasofrontal angle assessment in, 1538, 1539f
  osteotomies in, 1547
  partial transfixion in, 1542
  postoperative management in, 1551
  psychiatric stability and, 1537
  rim incision in, 1543
  septoplasty in, 1543–1545
  sequencing in, 1541–1543
  skin assessment for, 1538
  symmetry assessment for, 1538–1541
  transcolumellar incision in, 1543
  turbinectomy in, 1545
rhytidectomy
  complications in, 1564–1566
  facial nerve injury in, 1565
  flap development in, 1560–1563
  hematoma in, 1564–1565
  history of, 1555–1556
  neurosensory disturbances after, 1566
  overview of, 1555
  patient evaluation for, 1556–1557
  requirements, 1556t
  skin closure in, 1563
  skin slough in, 1565–1566
  superficial-plane, 1557–1563
  surgical technique, 1557–1563
Counseling, prenatal, for cleft lip and palate, 948–949
Coxsackie virus, 798
CPAP. See Continuous positive airway pressure (CPAP)
Cranial bone graft, 909
Cranial fractures, anterior, in pediatric facial trauma, 583–589
Cranial neural crest, 1191–1192
Cranial sutures. See Dysostosis syndromes
Cranial truncations, 1194
Cranial vault
  aesthetic unit, posterior, in dysostosis syndromes, 999–1000
  dead space, in dysostosis syndrome surgery, 1002–1004
Craniofacial defects, dental implants for, 224
Craniofacial development
  anteroposterior orthopedic treatment in, 1220–1227
  cranial base in, 1202–1203

cranial vault in, 1201–1202
dental development in, 1207–1209
embryonic, 1189–1197
environmental factors in, 1214–1216
facial development in, 1209–1210
facial formation in, 1192–1194
factors influencing, 1211–1216
fetal, 1197–1200
final tissue differentiation in, 1196–1197
fontanelles in, 1201f
genetic analysis of, 1194–1195
genetic factors in, 1211–1212, 1213–1214
germ layer formation in, 1189
in adulthood, 1210–1211
mandible in, 1206–1207
nasomaxilla in, 1203–1206
neural crest in, 1191–1192
neural tube formation in, 1189–1190
neurocranium formation in, 1195–1196
orthopedics for modification of, 1217–1228
ossification in, 1196
postnatal, 1200–1211
postnatal factors in, 1213–1216
prenatal, 1189–1200
prenatal environment and, 1212–1213
prenatal factors in, 1211–1213
skeletal development in, 1200–1207
sutures in, 1201f
transverse orthopedic treatment in, 1218–1220
vertical orthopedic treatment in, 1227–1228
viscerocranium development in, 1195–1196
Craniofacial dysostosis syndromes
  airway in, 997–998
  brain growth and, 996
  cephalometric analysis in, 1000
  dentition in, 998
  extremity anomalies in, 998
  FGFR gene in, 996
  frontoforehead aesthetic unit in, 998–999
  functional considerations in, 996–998
  genetic aspects of, 996
  hearing in, 998
  history of surgical management of, 1000–1002
  hydrocephalus in, 997
  intracranial pressure and, 996
  maxillary-nasal base aesthetic unit in, 1000
  morphologic considerations in, 998–1000
  obstructive sleep apnea in, 997–998
  occlusion in, 998
  orbitonasozygomatic aesthetic unit in, 1000
  overview of, 995
  posterior cranial vault aesthetic unit in, 999–1000
  surgical management of, 1000–1004
    cranial vault dead space management in, 1002–1004
    incision placement for, 1002
    soft tissue management in, 1004
  timing of intervention for, 1002
  vision and, 996
Craniofacial implants
  abutment connections in, 313–314
  autogenous reconstruction and, 303–304
  collaboration with, 305
  computer-guided treatment planning for, 305–306
  extraoral, 307
  for complex maxillofacial defects, 312–313
  for nasal defects, 310–312
  for orbital defects, 308–310

for unusual maxillofacial defects, 313
healing period for, 313–315
history of, 303
hyperbaric oxygen and, 315
impression taking with, 313–314
infections with, 314–315
intranasal, 307–308
intraoral, 307–308
long-term maintenance of, 320
longevity of, 315
management of skin tissue around extraoral abutments, 319–320
nasal, 305
orbital, 304–305
osteotomy in, 308
overlying soft tissues and, 306–307
pretreatment criteria, 305
prosthetic considerations, 315–319
radiation and, 315
residual bony volume and, 305
retention components, 319
soft tissue reactions with, 314–315
surgical considerations, 307–308
surgical technique, 305–313
technical considerations with, 304–305
temporal, 304
transition line in, 307
Craniofacial prostheses, 315–319
auricular considerations, 316–317
color of, 319
construction of, 318–319
nasal, 319
surgical considerations, 316–317
templates for, 317–318
tinting of, 319
with cranial implants, 316
without cranial implants, 316
Craniosynostosis. See also Dysostosis syndromes
bilateral coronal, 981, 985
brain development and, 980
classification of, 980–983
definition of, 979, 995
diagnosis of, 980
functional considerations with, 979–980
intracranial hypertension with, 979
management principles, 983–984
metopic, 981–982, 985–988
multidisciplinary team approach in, 983–984
nonsyndromic, 979–992
psychiatric disorders and, 980
sagittal, 982, 988–991
surgical considerations for, 984–991
unilateral coronal, 980–981, 984–985
unilateral lambdoid, 983, 991
visual impairment in, 979
Crouzon's syndrome, 996, 1004–1014, 1204f. See also Dysostosis syndromes
Crouzon's syndrome with acanthosis nigricans, 996
Crown fracture, 393–394
Crown infraction, 392
Crown-root fracture, 394
Cryosurgery, for skin cancer, 755
CT. See Computed tomography (CT)
Cupid's bow, 1612
Curettage and electrodesiccation, for skin cancer, 755–756
Curve of Spee, 1258–1259, 1266
Curve of Wilson, 1267
Cushing's syndrome, 34
Cuspid-molar position, 1267

Cymba concha, 1600f
Cysts
aneurysmal bone, 663, 832
branchial cleft, 833
dermoid, 832–833
ganglion, in temporomandibular joint, 1045
median mandibular, 667
nasolabial, 666–667
nasopalatine duct, 667
odontogenic
calcifying, 633–635
classification of, 626t
dentigerous, 626–628
glandular, 632–633
overview of, 625–626
salivary gland, 781–782
thyroglossal duct, 833
traumatic bone, 667–668
Cytokines, implant surface treatment with, 238
Cytology, exfoliative, in oral disease diagnosis, 619
Cytomegalovirus, 798

D
D-tubocurarine, 59t
Davis method, for otoplasty, 1601–1603, 1604f
Débridement, of temporomandibular joint, 1107
Debridement, wound, 9–10
Dedo classification of facial profiles, 1557t
Deep sedation, 63t
Deep temporal medial artery, 1600f
Deep venous thrombosis, oral cancer and, 698
Defibrillators, automatic implantable cardioverter, 23
Dehiscence, wound, 9
Delta sleep, 1493
Deltopectoral flap, 888
Dental caries, impacted third molars and, 101
Dental caries, third molar extraction and, 101
Dental implants
abutment fracture with, 225
abutments in, 208–209
aesthetic zone and, 210–211
biomechanical considerations in, 201–209
bone loss and, 239–246
bone volume assessment for, 202
bruxism and, 202
cemented, single-tooth, 211–212
complications with, 224–225
cone beam CT evaluation of, 184–187, 187–191, 191–197, 198f, 203–204
contemporary techniques for, 218–222
crown-to-implant ratio with, 205, 206f
distances in, 202f
early placement of, 219
fixed detachable prostheses, 218
fixed partial dentures, 212–216
cantilevered, 215–216
in aesthetic zone, 212–214
in anterior mandible, 214
in posterior mandible, 215
in posterior maxilla, 214–215
for craniofacial defects, 224
for mandible defects, 222–223
for maxillary defects, 223
fracture of, 225
history of, 206–207
hyperbaric oxygen therapy and, 202
immediate placement of, 218–219
immediate restoration, 220–221

impressions for, 209
in full-arch restorations, 206
in growing child, 170–171
inferior alveolar nerve injury and, 922
maintenance of, 225–226
mandibular hard tissue preparation for, 269–281
mandibular site preparation for
  for full-arch reconstruction, 274–279
  for segmental defects, 272–274
    anterior, 273–274
    posterior, 274
  for single tooth defects, 269–273
    mandibular canine-bicuspid, 271
    mandibular incisor, 269–271
    molar, 272
maxillofacial prostheses, 222–224
Morse taper in, 207, 208f
occlusion and, 205–206
osseointegration of
  abutment positions and, 249–250
  biology of, 229–248
  biomechanics of, 238–248
  bone loss and, 239–246
  bruxism and, 252–253
  cantilevers and, 251–252
  clenching and, 252–253
  early loading failure and, 246–248
  history of, 229
  implant materials and, 229–231
  implant surfaces and, 231–238
    acid etching of, 233–234
    additive, 234–236
    alterations to, 232–238
    bioactive proteins and, 237–238
    bisphosphonates for, 238
    blasting of, 233, 234
    bone morphogenic proteins and, 237–238
    calcium phosphate treatment of, 237
    cytokines and, 238
    fluoride treatment of, 237
    hydrophilic, 236
    hydrophobic, 236
    hydroxyapatite coating of, 234–235
    laser etching of, 236
    nanotechnology in, 237
    oxidation for, 235–236
    pharmacologic coatings for, 238
    subtractive, 233
    surface energy, 236
    titanium plasma spray for, 234
  mandibular edentulism and, 256–260
  masticatory dynamics and, 253
  maxillary edentulism and, 253–256
  mechanical risk factors and, 251
  number of plants and, 248–249
  parafunctional habits and, 252–253
  science of, 248–260
  treatment planning, 248–260
  with titanium, 229
  with zirconia, 229–231
osteoporosis and, 202
overdentures
  implant-retained, 216–217
  implant-supported, 217–218
patient factors in, 201–202
peri-implant biology with, 201
periodontal disease and, 202
preprosthetic surgery for

alveolar distraction osteogenesis in, 153–155
alveolar preservation in, 134–136
alveolar ridge discrepancies in, 150–151
alveolar ridge extension procedures in, 142–147
alveoloplasty in, 136
anesthesia in, 130
bone grafts and, 132–134
bone regeneration and, 131–132
CT evaluation for, 129–130
edentulism and, 123–125
exostoses treatment in, 136
fibrous inflammatory hyperplasia in, 140
genial tubercle reduction in, 137
hard tissue augmentation in, 148–155
hard tissue examination for, 126–128
hard tissue recontouring in, 134–139
history of, 123
hypermobile tissue in, 140
inferior border augmentation, 151–152
inflammatory papillary hyperplasia in, 140
inlay grafts in, 149–150
interpositional grafts in, 149, 150f, 152, 153f
labial frenectomy in, 140–142
lingual frenectomy in, 142
lip-switch, in preprosthetic surgery, 145, 146f
mandibular augmentation in, 151–152, 153f
mandibular vestibuloplasty in, 145, 146f, 147f
maxillary augmentation in, 148–150
maxillary vestibuloplasty in, 143–144
medical considerations in, 125–130
mylohyoid ridge reduction in, 139
onlay grafts in, 149
pedicled grafts in, 152, 153f
radiographic evaluation for, 128–130
ridge-split osteoplasty in, 148–149
sinus lifts in, 149–150
soft tissue examination for, 126–128
soft tissue recontouring in, 139–140
submucous vestibuloplasty in, 142–143
tori removal in, 138–139
treatment planning considerations in, 130–131
tuberosity reduction in, 136–137
radiation exposure and, 202
radiographic bone loss with, 225
radiographic evaluation for, 202–204
radiotherapy and, 224
screw loosening with, 225
screw-retained, single-tooth, 211–212
selection of, 206–209
single-tooth replacement, 210–212
soft tissue complications with, 224–225
soft tissue evaluation for, 201–202
soft tissues management with
  abutment connection, 284, 285f
  acellular dermal matrix with grafting, 299–300
  augmentation of, 287
  epithelialized palatal graft and, 288–290
  flap management considerations, 283–286
  grafting and, 286–287, 287–300
  integration of, 283
  lateral flap advancement and, 286
  nonsubmerged implant placement, 284, 285f
  papilla regeneration and, 285–286
  resective contouring and, 285
  subepithelial connective tissue grafting, 290–295
  submerged implant placement, 283–284
  surgical maneuvers and, 285–286
  vascularized interpositional periosteal connective tissue flap, 295–299

success criteria, 226
surfaces of, 231–238
    acid etching of, 233–234
    additive, 234–236
    alterations to, 232–238
    bioactive proteins and, 237–238
    bisphosphonates for, 238
    blasting of, 233, 234
    bone morphogenic proteins and, 237–238
    calcium phosphate treatment of, 237
    cytokines and, 238
    fluoride treatment of, 237
    hydrophilic, 236
    hydrophobic, 236
    hydroxyapatite coating of, 234–235
    laser etching of, 236
    nanotechnology in, 237
    oxidation for, 235–236
    pharmacologic coatings for, 238
    subtractive, 233
    surface energy, 236
    titanium plasma spray for, 234
surgical installation stability with, 219–220
surgical stents and, 204–205
Dentigerous cysts, 626–628
Dentoalveolar fracture
    classification of, 390–392
    Ellis classification, 392f
    etiology of, 388
    history in, 388–389
    history of, 387
    in pediatric patients, 589
    incidence of, 388
    maxillofacial examination for, 389–390
    physical examination for, 388–389
    radiography for, 390
    treatment of, 400–403
Dentoalveolar surgery, in pediatric patients, 159–175
Dentures
    fixed detachable, 218
    fixed partial, 212–216
        cantilevered, 215–216
        in aesthetic zone, 212–214
        in anterior mandible, 214
        in posterior mandible, 215
        in posterior maxilla, 214–215
        techniques for, 221–222
    overdentures
        implant-retained, 216–217
        implant-supported, 217–218
        techniques for, 221–222
Depressor septi nasi muscle, 1532f
Depressor supercilii, 1575
Dermal substitutes, 13–14
Dermatochalasia, 1516
Dermoid cysts, 832–833
Descending palatine artery, 1534f
Desflurane, 54t, 57, 57f
Development
    brain, craniosynostosis and, 980
    craniofacial
        anteroposterior orthopedic treatment in, 1220–1227
        cranial base in, 1202–1203
        cranial vault in, 1201–1202
        dental development in, 1207–1209
        embryonic, 1189–1197
        environmental factors in, 1214–1216
        facial development in, 1209–1210

facial formation in, 1192–1194
factors influencing, 1211–1216
fetal, 1197–1200
final tissue differentiation in, 1196–1197
fontanelles in, 1201f
genetic analysis of, 1194–1195
genetic factors in, 1211–1212, 1213–1214
germ layer formation in, 1189
in adulthood, 1210–1211
mandible in, 1206–1207
nasomaxilla in, 1203–1206
neural crest in, 1191–1192
neural tube formation in, 1189–1190
neurocranium formation in, 1195–1196
orthopedics for modification of, 1217–1228
ossification in, 1196
postnatal, 1200–1211
postnatal factors in, 1213–1216
prenatal, 1189–1200
prenatal environment and, 1212–1213
prenatal factors in, 1211–1213
skeletal development in, 1200–1207
sutures in, 1201f
transverse orthopedic treatment in, 1218–1220
vertical orthopedic treatment in, 1227–1228
viscerocranium development in, 1195–1196
Diabetes
    as surgical comorbidity, 32–33
    wound healing and, 10
Diabetes insipidus, 34
Diazepam, 46–47, 46f
Digastric branch, of facial nerve, 359f
Digital videography, 1244
Dilator naris anterior muscle, 1532f
Diploic visual fields, 489f
Diplopia, 496–497
    in zygomatic complex fractures, 477–478
Direct healing, of bone, 7
Discharge, postoperative, 86–87
Diskopexy, arthroscopic, in temporomandibular joint,
    1109–1116
Distraction histogenesis, 1467
Distraction osteogenesis (DO)
    activation period in, 1472–1473
    alveolar, 153–155, 1487, 1488f
    biological basis of, 1469–1470
    bone segment separation in, 1476–1477
    complications in, 1469–1470
    consolidation period in, 1473
    definition of, 1467
    device choice in, 1473–1474
    device removal in, 1473
    for end-stage temporomandibular joint disease, 1176–1178
    future of, 1487–1488
    histogenesis in, 1467
    history of, 1467, 1468–1469
    in cleft lip and palate, 1461–1464, 1469
    indications for, 1468t
    latency period in, 1471–1472
    mandibular, 1480–1483, 1484f, 1485f
    maxillary, 1483–1487
    orthodontics for, 1477–1480
    patient evaluation for, 1473–1477
    principles of, 1470–1473
    protocols, 1472t
    surgical technique in, 1470–1471
    vector planning in, 1473–1477, 1478f
    velopharyngeal incompetence and, 1469

Distribution, drug, 44
DO. *See* Distraction osteogenesis (DO)
Dog bites, 581
Dorsal nasal artery, 1533*f*
Down syndrome, 88
Doxacurium, 59*t*
Droperidol, 61*f*
Ductal papilloma, 787
Duke activity status index, 18*t*
Dynamic forces, in fixation, 378–379
Dysostosis syndromes
    airway in, 997–998
    brain growth and, 996
    cephalometric analysis in, 1000
    dentition in, 998
    extremity anomalies in, 998
    FGFR gene in, 996
    frontoforehead aesthetic unit in, 998–999
    functional considerations in, 996–998
    genetic aspects of, 996
    hearing in, 998
    history of surgical management of, 1000–1002
    hydrocephalus in, 997
    intracranial pressure and, 996
    maxillary-nasal base aesthetic unit in, 1000
    morphologic considerations in, 998–1000
    obstructive sleep apnea in, 997–998
    occlusion in, 998
    orbitonasozygomatic aesthetic unit in, 1000
    overview of, 995
    posterior cranial vault aesthetic unit in, 999–1000
    surgical management of, 1000–1004
        cranial vault dead space management in, 1002–1004
        incision placement for, 1002
        soft tissue management in, 1004
    timing of intervention for, 1002
    vision and, 996
Dysrhythmia, cardiac, 18*t*

E
Ear. *See also* Craniofacial prostheses
    anatomy of, 1597–1599
    blood supply to, 570*f,* 1599
    deformities, 1599–1601
    embryology of, 1597
    in pediatric facial trauma, 569–571
    in temporomandibular joint derangement surgery, 1150
    nerves in, 1599
    otoplastic surgery for
        aesthetic complications in, 1607
        anatomy in, 1597–1599
        complications of, 1606–1607
        Davis method for, 1601–1603, 1604*f*
        hematoma in, 1606
        keloid formation in, 1607
        Mustarde method for, 1603–1606
        narrowed meatus after, 1607
        perichondritis in, 1606
        scapha buckling after, 1607
        scarring in, hypertrophic, 1607
        surgical techniques in, 1601–1606
        telephone ear deformity after, 1607
    protruding, 1601
    soft tissue trauma in, 367, 368*f,* 369*f*
Ecchymoses, 816
Ecstasy, 68–69
Ectoderm, 1190*f*
Edentulous arch, single-tooth replacement and, 210

Edentulous patient
    alveolar bone in, 123–124
    functional effects of edentulism in, 124–125
    restorations for, 216–218
Edrophonium, 60*t*
Elderly patients. *See* Geriatric patients
Electrical stimulation, for temporomandibular disorder, 1057
Electrodesiccation, for skin cancer, 755–756
Electrosurgery, for temporomandibular disorder, 1085–1086
Elimination, of drugs, 45
Ellis classification, 392*f*
Embryo, 1190*f*
Embryonic craniofacial development, 1189–1197
Emphysema, 24–25
Enamel fracture, 392
Endocrine disease, 32–34
Endoderm, 1190*f*
Endoscopy
    for forehead and brow lift, 1586–1590
    for frontal fracture, 530
    for orbital fracture, 507
Enflurane, 56*f,* 57*f*
Enophthalmos, with zygomatic complex fractures, 477
Enzyme induction, 45
Ephilis, 811
Epidermolysis bullosa aquisita, 809
Epilepsy, 35
Epiphora, after orthognathic surgery, 1450–1451
Epithelial neoplasms, of head and neck, 833–834
Epithelial odontogenic tumors, 822–824
Epithelialization, in wound healing, 5–6
Epstein-Barr virus, 798
Epulis, congenital, 830
Erythema areata migrans, 802
Erythema migrans, 802
Erythema multiforme, 809–811
Etching, of implant surfaces
    acid, 233–234
    laser, 236
Ewing's sarcoma, 834
Examination
    dental, 1257–1258
    for dentoalveolar fracture, 388–389
    for maxillary fracture, 457–458
    for orbital fracture, 487–491
    for pediatric facial trauma, 565–567
    for zygomatic complex fractures, 467
    in preoperative assessment, 17
    macroaesthetic, 1245–1246, 1252–1254
    miniaesthetic, 1254, 1256–1257
    neurological, in trauma, 343–344
    systematic clinical, 1244–1260
    transverse facial proportions in, 1248–1252
    vertical facial proportions in, 1246–1248
Exarticulations, dental, 397–400
Exercise therapy, for temporomandibular disorder, 1055–1056
Exfoliative cytology, in oral disease diagnosis, 619
Exostoses, treatment of, in preprosthetic surgery, 136
Exposure, of impacted teeth, 103–105
External ballistics, 546
External carotid artery, 1600*f*
Extraction wounds, healing of, 8
Extremities
    assessment of, in trauma, 354
    in dysostosis syndromes, 998
Eye lid(s)
    anatomy of, 1516–1522
    blepharoplasty for

anatomy in, 1516–1522
    complications in, 1527–1529
    dry eyes after, 1529
    nomenclature in, 1515–1516
    overview of, 1515
    patient evaluation for, 1523–1525
    postoperative care for, 1526–1527, 1528f
    surgical procedures in, 1525–1526
  blood supply, 1522
  in pediatric facial trauma, 571–574
  innervation of, 1522
  lacerations, 497–498
  layers, 486t
  soft tissue trauma in, 364–366
Eyes, importance of, 1515

F
Face
  aesthetic subunits of, 877–878
  buttresses of, 594
Face lift
  complications in, 1564–1566
  facial nerve injury in, 1565
  flap development in, 1560–1563
  hematoma in, 1564–1565
  history of, 1555–1556
  neurosensory disturbances after, 1566
  overview of, 1555
  patient evaluation for, 1556–1557
  requirements, 1556t
  skin closure in, 1563
  skin slough in, 1565–1566
  superficial-plane, 1557–1563
  surgical technique, 1557–1563
Facebow transfer, model surgery and, 1296–1297
Facial artery, 1533f, 1579f
Facial asymmetry
  acquired, 1396–1397
  bone scans in evaluation of, 1398–1399
  case examples, 1403–1409
  clinical patient assessment in, 1397–1399
  congenital anomalies in, 1394–1395
  CT assessment of, 1398
  delayed treatment approach to, 1399
  developmental, 1395–1396
  etiology of, 1393–1394
  in condylar trauma, 1396–1397
  in congenital hemifacial hyperplasia, 1395
  in degenerative joint disease, 1397
  in facial hemiatrophy, 1395–1396
  in hemifacial microsomia, 1394, 1395f
  in hemimandibular hyperplasia, 1396
  in juvenile idiopathic arthritis, 1397
  in plagiocephaly, 1395
  orthodontic considerations in, 1399–1401
  overview of, 1393
  radiographic assessment in, 1397–1398
  stereolithographic modeling of, 1398
  surgical treatment of, 1399–1409
Facial clefting, complex, repair of, 959–960
Facial complex, widening of, in panfacial fractures, 602–605
Facial development, 1209–1210
Facial fillers, injectable, 1610–1612
Facial fracture, in pediatric patients, 581–583
Facial hemiatrophy, 1395–1396
Facial implants, 1615–1617
Facial nerve, 1580

anatomy of, 358f, 359f, 1582f
  in gunshot wounds, 559
  in temporomandibular joint derangement surgery, 1129
  injury
    in rhytidectomy, 1565
    in temporomandibular arthroscopy, 1118–1119
Facial profile classification, 1557t
Facial prominences, 1192–1194
Facial proportions
  transverse, 1248–1252
  vertical, 1246–1248
Facial trauma, in pediatric patients
  airway in evaluation of, 566
  airway injury in, 567–568
  anterior cranial fractures in, 583–589
  antibiotic ointments for, 580–581
  breathing in evaluation of, 566
  cheek in, 577–579, 580f
  circulation in evaluation of, 566
  dentoalveolar injuries in, 589
  disability in evaluation of, 566
  ear in, 569–571
  exposure in, 566–567
  eyelid in, 571–574
  facial fracture in, 581–583
  growth disturbance from, 590
  head injuries, 567–568
  history in, 565
  lacrimal apparatus in, 571–574
  lip in, 579–580
  mandible fracture in, 588
  mandibular body fracture in, 589
  mandibular condyle fracture in, 588–589
  mandibular symphysis fracture in, 589
  maxillary fracture in, 587–588
  mouth in, 579–580
  naso-orbitoethmoid fracture in, 585
  neck in, 567–568
  nose in, 574, 575f
  oral cavity in, 579–580
  perioperative management, 568
  physical evaluation in, 565–567
  regional soft tissue wounds in, 569–580
  scalp in, 575–577
  silicone agents for, 581
  soft tissue injuries in, 568–569
  wound care adjuncts for, 580–581
  zygomaticomaxillary complex fracture in, 587
Factor XII, 4
Familial gigantiform cementoma, 656
Fasting, preoperative, 66–67
Feeding, with cleft lip and palate, 949–950
Fentanyl, 46f, 48f, 49
FGFR gene, in dysostosis syndromes, 996
Fibro-osseous neoplasms, 656, 827–829
Fibrosis, temporomandibular joint, 1100
Fibrous dysplasia, 653–655, 827
Fibrous inflammatory hyperplasia, 140
Fillers, facial, 1610–1612
Fine-needle aspiration (FNA), in oral disease diagnosis, 619
Firearm terminology, 548–550
Fistula formation, in orthognathic surgery, 1436
Fixation
  biomechanic studies vs. clinical outcomes, 376–377
  bone plates in, 379
  for mandibular condyle fracture, 445–446
  for mandibular fractures, 374f, 414–416

for maxillary fracture, 459–460
for maxillary osteotomy, 1380
for zygomatic complex fractures, 472–475, 476
lag screw, 381–382
load-bearing, 377–378
load-sharing, 377–378
locking plate-screw systems in, 379–381
nonrigid internal, 373–375
one-point *vs.* two-point, 379
plate fatigue in, 382–383
regional dynamic forces in, 378–379
rigid internal, 373
rigidity in, 376
selection of, 376
single *vs.* multiple mandibular fractures in, 383–385
Fixed detachable prostheses, 218, 221–222
Fixed partial dentures (FPDs), 212–216
    cantilevered, 215–216
    in aesthetic zone, 212–214
    in anterior mandible, 214
    in posterior mandible, 215
    in posterior maxilla, 214–215
    techniques for, 221–222
Flail chest, 334–336
Flap(s)
    advancement, 879–880
    anterolateral thigh, 903–904
    blood supply, 878
    complications, 890–891
    deltopectoral, 888
    design, 879
    hyperbaric oxygen therapy and, 890–891
    iliac crest flee, 914–917
    interpolation, 884–886
    lateral arm free, 905–906
    latissimus dorsi myocutaneous, 889–890, 900–901, 905
    local, 879–886
    microvascular soft tissue, 901–906
    nomenclature, 878–879
    pectoralis major myocutaneous, 886–887, 898–900
    principles, 877–878
    radial artery fasciocutaneous, 901–902
    rectus abdominis myocutaneous, 904–905
    regional, 886–890, 894–901
    rotation, 880–881
    scapula, 914
    sternocleidomastoid, 889
    submental island, 894–895
    temporalis, 888–889, 895–898
    transposition, 881–884
    trapezius myocutaneous, 889
    types of, 879–890
    vascularized, 909–917
Floor-of-mouth lowering, in preprosthetic surgery, 145, 146*f,* 147*f*
Florid cemento-osseous dysplasia, 655–656
Fluids, as anesthetic concept, 75–76
Flumazenil, 46*f,* 47
Fluoride, implant surface treatment with, 237
FNA. *See* Fine-needle aspiration (FNA)
Focal cemento-osseous dysplasia, 655
Fontanelles, 1201*f*
Forces, in fixation, 378–379
Forehead
    bony landmarks in, 1572–1573
    fascial anatomy in, 1573–1577
    in dysostosis syndromes, as aesthetic unit, 998–999
    muscle anatomy in, 1573–1577

nerves in, 1577–1583
soft tissue trauma in, 364
transpalpebral, 1590–1591
vasculature in, 1577–1583
Forehead cosmetic surgery
    adjunctive procedures in, 1591–1592
    aesthetic considerations in, 1571–1583
    anatomic considerations in, 1571–1583
    botulinum toxin-assisted, 1591
    complications of, 1592–1593
    coronal lift, 1585
    direct lift, 1590
    endoscopic, 1586–1590
    micropigmentation in, 1591–1592
    midforehead lift, 1590
    postoperative care for, 1592
    preoperative evaluation for, 1583–1585
    pretrichial lift, 1585–1586
    skin resurfacing in, 1591
    surgical preparation for, 1583–1585
    temporal lift, 1590
    trichophytic lift, 1585–1586
Fractional laser resurfacing, 1617–1620
Fracture
    alveolar
        classification of, 390–392
        Ellis classification, 392*f*
        etiology of, 388
        history in, 388–389
        history of, 387
        in pediatric patients, 589
        incidence of, 388
        maxillofacial examination for, 389–390
        physical examination for, 388–389
        radiography for, 390
        treatment of, 400–403
    anterior table, 528
    cranial, anterior, in pediatric patients, 583–589
    crown, 393–394
    crown-root, 394
    edentulism and risk of, 125
    enamel, 392
    facial, in pediatric patients, 581–583
    frontal sinus
        anatomy in, 519–522
        anterior table fracture in, 528
        classification of, 524–525
        clinical findings in, 522–524
        complications of, 531–532
        deformity correction, 532–534
        endoscopy in, 530
        imaging of, 524
        medical therapy, postoperative, 531
        naso frontal outflow tract evaluation in, 527–528
        naso frontal outflow tract obstruction in, 529
        naso-orbitoethmoid complex reconstruction in, 530–531
        orbital roof reconstruction in, 528
        osseous recovery in, 526–527
        patient evaluation in, 522–525
        physiology in, 519–522
        posterior table, 528
        sinus obliteration in, 529–530
        supraorbital bar reconstruction in, 528
        surgical access in, 526
        treatment of, 525–531
    jaw, third molar impaction and risk of, 102
    mandible

anatomical distribution of, 409*f*
angle, 425–427
bilateral, 427, 428*f*
biomechanical considerations in, 410
body, 421–425, 589
classification of, 409
closed treatment of, 417
comminuted, 428, 429*f*
complications of, 432–433
diagnosis of, 416–417
edentulous atrophic, 428–432
epidemiology of, 408–409
hardware selection for, 418–420
historical perspectives on, 407–408, 410–414
in pediatric patients, 588
infection with, 432–433
load-bearing fixation for, 377*f*
malunion with, 433
nonunion with, 433
operative management of, 417–432
parasymphysis, 421–425
pediatric, 432
preoperative management of, 417
rigid fixation schemes for, 374*f*
single *vs.* multiple, 383–385
splinting for, 410–412
surgical approach for, 418
symphysis, 421–425, 589
teeth in line of, 420–421
treatment of, 410–414
wiring for, 412–414, 417–418
mandibular condyle
anatomic types of, 443–444
bruxism and, 451
chronic pain and, 451
closed treatment of, 445–446
condylar head, 444
condylar neck, 443, 444*f*
deviation on opening with, 442–443
disc injury in, 451
evidence-based approach to, 452
facial asymmetry in, 1396–1397
functional anatomic alterations with, 442–444
functional anatomy in, 441–442
glenoid fossa fracture and, 451
in pediatric patients, 588–589
infection risk and, 450–451
intercuspation and, 442
laterognathia and, 442
masseteric hypertrophy and, 451
mouth opening limitation with, 443
occlusal considerations in, 451
occlusal prematurity with, 442
osteoarthrosis and, 451
outcomes in, 447–452
overview of, 441
patient age and, 450
patient compliance and, 450
patient gender and, 450
ramus shortening and, 451–452
scarring and, 451
subcondylar, 443
systemic disease and, 450
treatment of, 444–452
maxillary
anatomy in, 456–457
avulsive, 461

clinical examination for, 457–458
complications of, 462–463
diagnosis of, 457–458
fixation for, 459–460
high-force, 461
history of, 455
in geriatric patients, 461
in pediatric patients, 587–588
Le Fort classification, 455–456
pediatric patients in, 461–462
surgical splints for, 460–461
treatment of, 458–463
nasal
classification of, 541
complications with, 542–543
CT for, 540–541
diagnostic tools for, 539–541
nasal complex evaluation in, 540
overview of, 539
postoperative care for, 542–543
radiography for, 539–541
reduction of, 542
sense of smell and, 542
surgical anatomy of, 539
surgical management of, 541–542
naso-orbitoethmoid fracture
anatomy in, 519–522
anterior table fracture in, 528
classification of, 524–525
clinical findings in, 522–524
complications of, 531–532
deformity correction, 532–534
endoscopy in, 530
imaging of, 524
in pediatric patients, 585
medical therapy, postoperative, 531
naso frontal outflow tract evaluation in, 527–528
naso frontal outflow tract obstruction in, 529
naso-orbitoethmoid complex reconstruction in, 530–531
orbital roof reconstruction in, 528
osseous recovery in, 526–527
patient evaluation in, 522–525
physiology in, 519–522
posterior table, 528
sinus obliteration in, 529–530
supraorbital bar reconstruction in, 528
surgical access in, 526
treatment of, 525–531
of dental implants, 225
orbital
acute repair of, 507–515
anatomy in, 483–487
clinical examination for, 487–491
configurations, 487
CT of, 492
decision diagram, 503*f*
endoscopic approach, 507
imaging of, 492–493
indications for surgical repair of, 502
inferior orbital approach, 504–505
lateral orbital approach, 504–505
medial orbital approach, 505–507
MRI of, 492–493
nonoperative management of, 499–502
operative management of, 502–514
superior orbital approach, 505–506
surgical approaches for, 502–507

panfacial
  airway management in, 599
  anatomic considerations in, 594–596
  complications with, 602–605
  definition of, 593
  dental fractures in, 594–595
  etiology of, 593
  facial buttresses and, 594
  fracture management in, 599–602
  historic perspective on, 593
  imaging of, 596–597
  intercanthal region in, 596
  key landmarks in, 594
  mandible in, 594–595
  sequence of treatment for, 599–602
  soft tissue resuspension for, 599
  sphenozygomatic suture in, 595–596
  surgical approaches for, 597–599
  widening of facial complex in, 602–605
posterior table, 528
root, 394
tooth, after extraction of third molars, 114
zygomatic arch, 470–471
zygomaticomaxillary complex, in pediatric patients, 587
Freckle, 811
Frenectomy
  for prominent maxillary labial frenulum, 171
  labial, in preprosthetic surgery, 140–142
  lingual
    for high lingual frenum, 172–175
    in preprosthetic surgery, 142
Frontal artery, 1600*f*
Frontal bone, 520–521
Frontal nerve, 1519*f*
Frontal sinus
  embryology, 519
  neurovascular structures in, 521
  osteology, 520–521
  physiology, 520
Frontal sinus fracture
  anatomy in, 519–522
  anterior table fracture in, 528
  classification of, 524–525
  clinical findings in, 522–524
  complications of, 531–532
  deformity correction, 532–534
  endoscopy in, 530
  imaging of, 524
  medical therapy, postoperative, 531
  naso frontal outflow tract evaluation in, 527–528
  naso frontal outflow tract obstruction in, 529
  naso-orbitoethmoid complex reconstruction in, 530–531
  orbital roof reconstruction in, 528
  osseous recovery in, 526–527
  patient evaluation in, 522–525
  physiology in, 519–522
  posterior table, 528
  sinus obliteration in, 529–530
  supraorbital bar reconstruction in, 528
  surgical access in, 526
  treatment of, 525–531
Frontalis muscle, 1517*f,* 1576*f*
Frontoforehead aesthetic unit, in dysostosis syndromes, 998–999
Frontozygomatic branch, 358*f*
Full stomach, emergency treatment on, 67
Full-arch restoration, dental implants and, 206
Fungal infections, 798–801

G
Ganglion cysts, in temporomandibular joint, 1045
Gastric emptying, 66–67
GCS. *See* Glasgow Coma Scale (GCS)
Gender, mandibular condyle fracture, 450
Gene therapy, wound healing and, 13
General anesthesia, definition of, 63*t*
Genetics
  in cleft lip and palate, 947–948
  in craniofacial development, 1194–1195, 1211, 1213–1214
  in dysostosis syndromes, 996
Genial tubercle, reduction of, in preprosthetic surgery, 137
Genioplasty, 1350–1358, 1412, 1414*t*
Genitourinary tract assessment, in trauma, 353–354
Geographic tongue, 802
Geriatric patients
  anesthetic considerations with, 72–74
  cardiovascular considerations with, 73
  general surgical considerations with, 39–40
  hepatic system in, 73–74
  impacted teeth in, 103
  intravenous drug pharmacology in, 84
  maxillary fracture in, 461
  pulmonary considerations with, 73
  urinary system in, 73–74
Germ layer formation, 1189
GFR. *See* Glomerular filtration rate (GFR)
Ghost cell tumor, malignant epithelial odontogenic, 643
Giant cell lesions, 660–663, 826–827
Giant cell tumor, 662
Glands of Krause, 1517*f*
Glandular odontogenic cyst, 632–633
Glasgow Coma Scale (GCS), 34, 35*t,* 327, 327*t*
Glenoid fossa perforation, in temporomandibular
  arthroscopy, 1120
Globulomedullary lesion, 666
Glomerular filtration rate (GFR), 27
Glucocorticoids, 86
Glycopyrrolate, 60*t*
Golden retriever, 1083, 1085*f*
Goldman visual field test, 489*f*
Gonorrhea, 796, 1043–1044
Gorham's disease, 671
Gorham-Stout syndrome, 671
Graft-*versus*-host disease, 805–806
Grafts
  bone
    calvarial bone for, 969–970
    cone beam CT in augmentation assessment, 187–191
    cranial, 909
    for gunshot wounds, 559–561
    for panfacial fractures, 599
    for temporomandibular joint disease, end-stage, 1174–1176
    for zygomatic complex fractures, 477
    iliac crest in, 907–909, 969
    in alveolar cleft repair
      allogenic bone for, 970
      bone morphogenic protein in, 970
      bone sources in, 969–972
      dental *vs.* chronologic age in, 967
      lateral incisors and, 967
      orthodontics and, pre- *vs.* postsurgical, 970–972
      patient size and, 968
      primary, 966
      rationale for, 965
      secondary, 966–969
      social issues with, 968

surgical technique for, 972–974
timing of, 966–969
nonvascularized, 906–909
preprosthetic surgery and, 132–134, 149–150
inlay, 149–150
interpositional, 149, 150f, 152, 153f
onlay, 149
rib for, 969t
tibial, 909, 969t
connective tissue, subepithelial, for dental implants,
290–295
nerve
allografts in, 937
harvesting sites for, 937
skin
full thickness, 8
healing of, 8
in skin cancer, 757–768
split thickness, 8
soft tissue, in implant therapy, 286–287, 287–300
epithelialized palatal, 288–290
subepithelial connective tissue, 290–295
with acellular dermal matrix, 299–300
Great auricular nerve, 1600f
Greater palatine artery, 1534f
Growth assessment, craniofacial, 1216–1217
Growth factors, wound healing and, 12–13
Growth modification, orthopedic treatment for, 1217–1228
Gunshot wounds
airway in management of, 551–552
ammunition type and, 547t
as cause of death, 545
ballistics of, 546
bone grafting for, 559–561
circumstances of, 545–546
classification of, 550
closed vs. open fracture management in, 559–561
contamination of, 558
controversies in management of, 559–561
delayed vs. early management of, 559–561
demographics of, 545–546
energy of, 546–548
facial nerve in, 559
firearm terminology in, 548–550
fragmentation in, 547
from shotguns, 550–551
hemorrhage control in, 552, 553f
history of, 545
infection of, 558
late reconstruction of, 561
management of, 551–558
neck injury in, penetrating, 554–555
nutrition and, 555
operative procedure for, 556–558
overview of, 363–364
penetration in, 547
permanent cavity in, 547
salivary ducts in, 559
temporary cavity in, 547
wounding power of, 546–548

H

HA. See Hydroxyapatite (HA) coating
Hageman factor, 4
Half-time, context sensitive, 45, 46f
Halothane, 54t, 56f, 57, 57f
Handguns, 548, 549
Hasner's valve, 487

HBO. See Hyperbaric oxygen therapy (HBO)
Head
congenital masses and cysts in, 832–833
deep spaces of, 842t
skin cancer in
lasers for, 756
melanoma, 749–751
biopsy strategies, 751t
clinical description, 749–751
histologic description, 749–751
risk factors, 749
survival rates, 751t
nonmelanoma, 743–749
basal cell carcinoma, 746
chemotherapy for, 756
cryosurgery for, 755
curettage and electrodesiccation for, 755–756
environmental factors, 745
epidemiology of, 743
etiology of, 743–746
grafting in, 757–768
immunologic factors, 744
interferons for, 756
management of, 751–768
Mohs' micrographic surgery for, 753–755
photodynamic therapy for, 756
predisposing lesions, 744
prevention of, 745–746
radiation therapy for, 755
retinoids for, 756
squamous cell carcinoma, 746–749
standard excision of, 752
syndromes in, 744
Head assessment, in trauma, 344–348
Healing
advances in, 12–14
age and, 11–12
by first intention, 3
by second intention, 3
by third intention, 3
complications, 8–9
debridement and, 9–10
dehiscence and, 9
dermal substitutes in, 13–14
diabetes and, 10
gene therapy and, 13
growth factors and, 12–13
hemostasis and, 9–10
hyperbaric oxygen therapy and, 11
immunocompromise and, 10–11
in extraction wounds, 8
infections in, 8–9
inflammatory phase of, 4–5, 4f
mucosal substitutes and, 13–14
nutrition and, 12
of bone, 6–7, 7f, 375f, 376f
of nerves, 6
of skin grafts, 8
optimization of, 9–12
perfusion and, 10
process, 3
proliferative phase of, 5–6, 5f
proliferative scarring in, 9
radiation injury and, 11
remodeling phase of, 6
response, 3–6
specialized, 6–8
trauma minimization in, 9

Hearing, in dysostosis syndromes, 998
Heart blocks, 21–22
Heart rate, 18
Heart valve replacement, 20–21
Helical crus, 1600f
Helix, 1600f
Hemangioma, 816, 830–831
Hemarthrosis, in temporomandibular arthroscopy, 1120
Hematoma, 816
Hematopoietic reticuloendothelial tumors, 829–830
Hemifacial microsomia (HFM), 1394, 1395f
Hemimandibular hyperplasia, 1396
Hemophilia A, 30–31
Hemophilia B, 30–31
Hemorrhage
    class I, 340
    class II, 340–341
    class III, 341
    class IV, 341
    in gunshot wounds, 552, 553f
    in trauma, 338–339, 340f, 341f
    retrobulbar, with zygomatic complex fractures, 479
Hemostasis, wound healing and, 9–10
Hemothorax, 333–334
Hepatic system, in geriatric patients, 73–74
Herbst appliance, 1499
Herpes simplex virus, 796–797
HFM. See Hemifacial microsomia (HFM)
Histamine antagonists, 86
HIV. See Human immunodeficiency virus (HIV)
Hodgkin's disease, 829–830
Hofmann elimination, 45
Holmium:yttrium-aluminum-garnet laser, 1086
Horizontal ramus osteotomies, 1343–1347
Horner's muscle, 1520
Howell classification, 127f
HTN. See Hypertension (HTN)
Human bites, 363
Human immunodeficiency virus (HIV)
    as surgical comorbidity, 37, 38
    maxillofacial infections and, 846–847
    salivary glands in, 783
    wound healing and, 10
Hyaluronic acid
    as facial filler, 1610–1611
    for temporomandibular disorder, 1107
Hydrocephalus, in dysostosis syndromes, 997
Hydromorphone, 49
Hydroxyapatite (HA) coating, 234–235
Hyperbaric oxygen therapy (HBO)
    craniofacial implants and, 315
    dental implants and, 202
    flaps and, 890–891
    for osteoradionecrosis, 869–870
    wound healing and, 11
Hypercoagulable diseases, 31–32
Hypermobility, temporomandibular
    classification of, 1166–1167
    etiology of, 1167
    treatment considerations with, 1167–1169
Hyperparathyroidism, 662
Hypertension (HTN)
    as surgical comorbidity, 22–23, 22t
    intracranial
        craniosynostosis and, 979
        in dysostosis syndromes, 996
Hypertensive emergency, 22
Hyperthermia, malignant, 36, 55

Hyperthyroidism, 33
Hyphema, with zygomatic complex fractures, 478
Hypodontia, in pediatric patients, 168–169
Hypomobility, temporomandibular
    ankylosing spondylitis and, 1159
    classification of, 1155
    clinical presentation of, 1155–1156
    complications associated with treatment of, 1162–1166
    etiology of, 1155, 1156t
    imaging assessment of, 1156
    inflammatory causes, 1159–1160
    orthognathic surgery and, 1160
    physical therapy for, postoperative, 1166
    post-traumatic, 1156–1157
    postcraniotomy, 1159
    postinfectious, 1157–1158
    radiation therapy and, 1158–1159
    rheumatologic causes, 1159–1160
    scleroderma and, 1159–1160
    treatment considerations with, 1160–1162
Hypothyroidism, 33
Hypoventilation, 23
Hypovolemic shock, 340–343

I
Iliac crest free flap, 914–917
Iliac crest, for bone grafts, 907–909, 969
Imaging. See also Radiography
    for dentoalveolar fracture, 390
    for gunshot wounds, 555–556
    of frontal sinus fracture, 524
    of gunshot wounds, 555–556
    of orbital fracture, 492–493
    of panfacial fractures, 596–597
    of zygomatic complex fractures, 467–468
    three-dimensional
        for mandibular diagnostics, 191–197, 198if
        of mandibular implants, 184–187
        of maxillary canine impaction, 181–183
        overview of, 179–180
        to assess potential graft augmentation, 187–191
Immunocompromise
    as surgical comorbidity, 37–38
    maxillofacial infections and, 846–847
    wound healing and, 10–11
Impacted teeth
    bonding of, 103–105
    clinical evaluation of, 100
    comorbidities and, 103
    contraindications for treatment of, 102–103
    etiology of, 97–99
    exposure of, 103–105
    first molar, 167–168
    in geriatric patients, 103
    in pediatric patients, 103, 159–168
    incidence of, 97–99
    mandibular premolars, in pediatric patients,
        163–165, 166f
    maxillary canine
        cone beam CT of, 181–183
        in pediatric patients, 160–163
    maxillary incisor, in pediatric patients, 165–167
    maxillary premolars, in pediatric patients, 163–165, 166f
    overview of, 97
    removal of, 106–107
    second molar, 167–168
    surgery for, 103–113
    third molars

adjacent teeth root reabsorption and, 102
alveolar osteitis after extraction of, 114–115
antibiotics in extraction of, 112–113
bleeding after extraction of, 113–114
dental caries and, 101
dental prostheses and, 102
incidence and etiology of, 99–100
indications for removal of, 101–102
jaw fracture risk and, 102
mandibular incisor crowning and, 101–102
nerve disturbances after removal of, 115
odontogenic cysts and tumors and, 102
orthodontic considerations with, 101–102
orthognathic surgery and, 102
pain after extraction of, 114
pain from, 102
pericoronitis and, 101
periodontal healing after extraction of, 116–117
periodontitis and, 101
postoperative complications after extraction of, 114–116
postoperative course for, 113–114
rare complications for, 115–116
steroids in extraction of, 112–113
stiffness after extraction of, 114
surgery for, 107–113
swelling after extraction of, 114
tooth fracture after extraction of, 114
transplantation for, 105–106
treatment of, 100–113
unerupted *vs.*, 97
uprighting of, 105
Implants
craniofacial
abutment connections in, 313–314
autogenous reconstruction and, 303–304
collaboration with, 305
computer-guided treatment planning for, 305–306
extraoral, 307
for complex maxillofacial defects, 312–313
for nasal defects, 310–312
for orbital defects, 308–310
for unusual maxillofacial defects, 313
healing period for, 313–315
history of, 303
hyperbaric oxygen and, 315
impression taking with, 313–314
infections with, 314–315
intranasal, 307–308
intraoral, 307–308
long-term maintenance of, 320
longevity of, 315
management of skin tissue around extraoral abutments, 319–320
nasal, 305
orbital, 304–305
osteotomy in, 308
overlying soft tissues and, 306–307
pretreatment criteria, 305
prosthetic considerations, 315–319
radiation and, 315
residual bony volume and, 305
retention components, 319
soft tissue reactions with, 314–315
surgical considerations, 307–308
surgical technique, 305–313
technical considerations with, 304–305
temporal, 304
transition line in, 307

dental
abutment fracture with, 225
abutments in, 208–209
aesthetic zone and, 210–211
biomechanical considerations in, 201–209
bone loss and, 239–246
bone volume assessment for, 202
bruxism and, 202
cemented, single-tooth, 211–212
complications with, 224–225
cone beam CT evaluation of, 184–187, 187–191, 191–197, 198*f*, 203–204
contemporary techniques for, 218–222
crown-to-implant ratio with, 205, 206*f*
distances in, 202*f*
early placement of, 219
fixed detachable prostheses, 218
fixed partial dentures, 212–216
cantilevered, 215–216
in aesthetic zone, 212–214
in anterior mandible, 214
in posterior mandible, 215
in posterior maxilla, 214–215
for craniofacial defects, 224
for mandible defects, 222–223
for maxillary defects, 223
fracture of, 225
history of, 206–207
hyperbaric oxygen therapy and, 202
immediate placement of, 218–219
immediate restoration, 220–221
impressions for, 209
in full-arch restorations, 206
in growing child, 170–171
inferior alveolar nerve injury and, 922
maintenance of, 225–226
mandible hard tissue preparation for, 269–281
mandibular site preparation for
for full-arch reconstruction, 274–279
for segmental defects, 272–274
for single tooth defects, 269–273
maxillofacial prostheses, 222–224
Morse taper in, 207, 208*f*
occlusion and, 205–206
osseointegration of
abutment positions and, 249–250
biology of, 229–248
biomechanics of, 238–248
bone loss and, 239–246
bruxism and, 252–253
cantilevers and, 251–252
clenching and, 252–253
early loading failure and, 246–248
history of, 229
implant materials and, 229–231
implant surfaces and, 231–238
mandibular edentulism and, 256–260
masticatory dynamics and, 253
maxillary edentulism and, 253–256
mechanical risk factors and, 251
number of plants and, 248–249
parafunctional habits and, 252–253
science of, 248–260
treatment planning, 248–260
with titanium, 229
with zirconia, 229–231
osteoporosis and, 202
overdentures

implant-retained, 216–217
implant-supported, 217–218
patient factors in, 201–202
peri-implant biology with, 201
periodontal disease and, 202
preprosthetic surgery for
    alveolar distraction osteogenesis in, 153–155
    alveolar preservation in, 134–136
    alveolar ridge discrepancies in, 150–151
    alveolar ridge extension procedures in, 142–147
    alveoloplasty in, 136
    anesthesia in, 130
    bone grafts and, 132–134
    bone regeneration and, 131–132
    CT evaluation for, 129–130
    edentulism and, 123–125
    exostoses treatment in, 136
    fibrous inflammatory hyperplasia in, 140
radiation exposure and, 202
radiographic bone loss with, 225
radiographic evaluation for, 202–204
radiotherapy and, 224
screw loosening with, 225
screw-retained, single-tooth, 211–212
selection of, 206–209
single-tooth replacement, 210–212
soft tissue complications with, 224–225
soft tissue evaluation for, 201–202
soft tissues management with
    abutment connection, 284, 285f
    acellular dermal matrix with grafting, 299–300
    augmentation of, 287
    epithelialized palatal graft and, 288–290
    flap management considerations, 283–286
    grafting and, 286–287, 287–300
    integration of, 283
    lateral flap advancement and, 286
    nonsubmerged implant placement, 284, 285f
    papilla regeneration and, 285–286
    resective contouring and, 285
    subepithelial connective tissue grafting, 290–295
    submerged implant placement, 283–284
    surgical maneuvers and, 285–286
    vascularized interpositional periosteal connective tissue flap,
        295–299
success criteria, 226
surfaces of, 231–238
    acid etching of, 233–234
    additive, 234–236
    alterations to, 232–238
    bioactive proteins and, 237–238
    bisphosphonates for, 238
    blasting of, 233, 234
    bone morphogenic proteins and, 237–238
    calcium phosphate treatment of, 237
    cytokines and, 238
    fluoride treatment of, 237
    hydrophilic, 236
    hydrophobic, 236
    hydroxyapatite coating of, 234–235
    laser etching of, 236
    nanotechnology in, 237
    oxidation for, 235–236
    pharmacologic coatings for, 238
    subtractive, 233
    surface energy, 236
    titanium plasma spray for, 234

surgical installation stability with, 219–220
surgical stents and, 204–205
midface, 1615–1617
Implants, dental
    mandibular site preparation for
        for segmental defects
            anterior, 273–274
            posterior, 274
        for single tooth defects
            mandibular canine-bicuspid, 271
            mandibular incisor, 269–271
            molar, 272
    osseointegration of
        implant surfaces and
            acid etching of, 233–234
            additive, 234–236
            alterations to, 232–238
            bioactive proteins and, 237–238
            bisphosphonates for, 238
            blasting of, 233, 234
            bone morphogenic proteins and, 237–238
            calcium phosphate treatment of, 237
            cytokines and, 238
            fluoride treatment of, 237
            hydrophilic, 236
            hydrophobic, 236
            hydroxyapatite coating of, 234–235
            laser etching of, 236
            nanotechnology in, 237
            oxidation for, 235–236
            pharmacologic coatings for, 238
            subtractive, 233
            surface energy, 236
            titanium plasma spray for, 234
Impressions
    for dental implants, 209
    model surgery and, 1296
Incisor(s)
    alveolar cleft grafting and, 967–968
    compensation, 1258
    inclination, 1265
    mandibular
        site preparation for correction of single missing, 269–271
    mandibular, third molar impaction and, 101–102
    maxillary, impaction of, in pediatric patients, 165–167
Induction agents, 50–52. See also Sedation
    barbiturates, 52–54
    in pediatric patients, 82
    ketamine, 52
    methohexital, 53–54
    pentobarbital, 54
    propofol as, 50–51
    thiopental, 53
Infection(s)
    in mandibular condyle fracture, 450–451
    in orthognathic surgery, 1437
    in temporomandibular arthroscopy, 1120
    in temporomandibular joint derangement surgery, 1150
    maxillofacial
        airway compromise in, 845–846
        antibiotic administration for, 853–854
        antibiotics for, 852–853
        culture testing in, 851
        deep spaces in, 843t
        drainage timing in, 851
        frequent patient evaluation in, 854–856
        HIV and, 846–847

hospital admission indications for, 847*t*
host defenses in, 846–847
immune system compromise and, 846–847
incision timing in, 851
location of, 842
medical support for, 851–852
overview of, 841
rate of progression of, 842–844
sensitivity testing in, 851
setting of care for, 847–848
severity of, 841–846
severity scores of, 844*t*
stages of, 844*t*
surgical drainage of, 848–851
surgical treatment of, 848–851
treatment failure in, 854*t*
of temporomandibular joint, 1043–1044
temporomandibular hypomobility from, 1157–1158
with craniofacial implants, 314–315
with gunshot wounds, 558
with mandibular fracture, 432–433
wound healing and, 8–9
Infections, wound healing and, 8–9
Infectious stomatitis, 795–801
Inferior alveolar canal, radiographic predictors of tooth proximity to, 920*t*
Inferior alveolar nerve injury
microneurosurgery for
approximation in, 936
clinical evaluation for, 919
clinical neurosensory testing and, 925–929
coaptation in, 936
demographics in, 920–923
entubulation techniques in, 938
exposure in, 934
external neurolysis in, 934–935
indications for, 931–932
internal neurolysis in, 935
medicolegal issues in, 938–939
nerve grafts in, 937
nerve stump preparation in, 935–936
nerve trauma classification and, 924–925, 926, 926*f,* 926*t*
neurorrhaphy in, 936–937
overview of, 919–920
postsurgical management, 938
referral indications, 930*t*
success rates of, 932
treatment algorithms in, 930–933
trigeminal nerve anatomy in, 923–924
trigeminal nerve physiology in, 923–924
Inferior oblique muscle, 1517*f*
Inferior rectus muscle, 1517*f*
Inferior tarsal muscle, 1517*f*
Inflammatory papillary hyperplasia, in preprosthetic surgery, 140
Inflammatory phase, of wound healing, 4–5, 4*f*
Inflammatory resorption, of root, 395
Infrahyoid muscles, in temporomandibular joint, 1040
Infraorbital artery, 1533*f*
Infratrochlear artery, 1579*f*
Inhalation abuse, 69
Inhalation anesthetics, 54–57
desflurane, 57
disadvantages of, 78
halothane, 57
in pediatric patients, 77–78, 82–84
nitrous oxide, 55–56
potent, 56–57
sevoflurane, 56–57

Injectable facial fillers, 1610–1612
Injury Severity Score, 327–328
Inlay grafts, in preprosthetic surgery, 149–150
Insulin therapy, 32
Intercanthal region, in panfacial fractures, 596
Intercuspation, mandibular condyle fracture and, 442
Internal ballistics, 546
Internal fixation
biomechanic studies *vs.* clinical outcomes, 376–377
bone plates in, 379
for mandibular condyle fracture, 446–447
for mandibular fractures, 374*f,* 414–416
for maxillary fracture, 459–460
for maxillary osteotomy, 1380
for zygomatic complex fractures, 472–475, 476
lag screw, 381–382
load-bearing, 377–378
load-sharing, 377–378
locking plate-screw systems in, 379–381
nonrigid, 373–375
nonrigid internal, 373–375
one-point *vs.* two-point, 379
plate fatigue in, 382–383
regional dynamic forces in, 378–379
rigid, 373
rigid internal, 373
rigidity in, 376
selection of, 376
single *vs.* multiple mandibular fractures in, 383–385
Internal maxillary artery, 1600*f*
Interorbital space, 521
Interpolation flaps, 884–886
Interpositional grafts, in preprosthetic surgery, 149, 150*f,* 152, 153*f*
Intracranial hypertension
in craniosynostosis, 979
in dysostosis syndromes, 996
Intranasal route, for pediatric sedation, 78
Intubation, of pediatric patients, 70–71
Inverted-L ramus osteotomy, 1328–1331
Iontophoresis, for temporomandibular disorder, 1057–1058
Iron-deficiency anemia, 29
Isoflurane, 54*t,* 56, 56*f,* 57*f*

J
Jackson-Weiss syndrome, 996. *See also* Dysostosis syndromes
Jaw fracture, third molar impaction and risk of, 102
JIA. *See* Juvenile idiopathic arthritis (JIA)
Juvenile aggressive ossifying fibroma, 656
Juvenile idiopathic arthritis (JIA), facial asymmetry in, 1397

K
Kaposi's sarcoma, 816
Keratocyst, odontogenic, 628–632
Keratosis, seborrheic, 813–814
Ketamine, 52, 52*f,* 79–81
Ketorolac tromethamine, 57–58
Kidney disease, 27–28
Kiesselbach's plexus, 1534*f*

L
Labial frenectomy
for prominent frenum, 171
in preprosthetic surgery, 140–142
Labial frenum
mandibular, 171–172
Labial frenum, prominent maxillary, 171–175
Lacerations

eyelid, 497–498
soft tissue, 362
Lacrimal apparatus
in frontal sinus anatomy, 521–522
in pediatric facial trauma, 571–574
Lacrimal gland, 1519*f*
Lacrimal gland prolapse, 1516
Lacrimal injuries, 497–498
Lacrimal nerve, 1519*f*
Lacrimal system, 486–487, 1522
Lag screw fixation, 381–382
Lambdoid synostosis, 983, 991. *See also* Craniosynostosis
Lamella
anterior, 1518–1519
middle, 1519
posterior, 1519–1522
Langerhans' cell histiocytosis, 665–666, 829
Laryngospasm, 84–86
Laser etching, of implant surfaces, 236
Laser resurfacing, 1617–1620
Laser-assisted uvulopalatoplasty, 1502
Lasers, for skin cancer, 756
Lateral arm free flap, 905–906
Lateral canthal tendon, 1519*f*
Lateral nasal artery, 1533*f*
Lateral pterygoid muscle, in temporomandibular joint, 1039–1040
Laterognathia, mandibular condyle fracture and, 442
Latham appliance, 952
Latissimus dorsi myocutaneous flap, 889–890, 900–901, 905
Le Fort classification, 455–456
Legal issues, nerve injury and, 938–939
Lentigo, 811–812
Leukemia, 29
Levator aponeurosis, 1517*f,* 1519*f*
Levator labii superioris alaeque nasi muscle, 1532*f*
Levator muscle, 1517*f*
Levator palpebrae superioris, 486, 1519*f*
Lichen planus, 802–804
Lichenoid drug eruption, 804*t*
Lichenoid reactions, 802–804
Linear IgA bulbous dermatosis, 809
Lingual frenectomy
for high lingual frenum, 172–175
in preprosthetic surgery, 142
Lingual nerve injury
microneurosurgery for
approximation in, 936
clinical evaluation for, 919
clinical neurosensory testing and, 925–929
coaptation in, 936
demographics in, 920–923
entubulation techniques in, 938
exposure in, 934
external neurolysis in, 934–935
indications for, 931–932
internal neurolysis in, 935
medicolegal issues in, 938–939
nerve grafts in, 937
nerve stump preparation in, 935–936
nerve trauma classification and, 924–925, 926, 926*f,* 926*t*
neurorrhaphy in, 936–937
overview of, 919–920
postsurgical management, 938
referral indications, 930*t*
success rates of, 932
treatment algorithms in, 930–933
trigeminal nerve anatomy in, 923–924

trigeminal nerve physiology in, 923–924
Lip cancer
anatomic considerations in, 728–729
cervical lymphadenectomy in, 736–737
epidemiology of, 727–728
etiology of, 727–728
evaluation of, 729–730
management of, 729–737
reconstruction in, 732–736
surgical treatment of, 730–732
treatment results in, 737–738
Lip-switch vestibuloplasty, in preprosthetic surgery, 145, 146*f*
Lip-tooth-gingival relationships, 1255
Lip(s)
cleft
classification of, 948
embryology of, 947
etiology of, 947–948
facial asymmetry in, 1395
feeding concerns with, 949–950
genetics in, 947–948
goals of repair, 945
history of, 946–947
management of children with, 945
orthognathic surgery for
distraction osteogenesis in, 1461–1464, 1469
history of, 1456
maxilla development in, 1454–1456
maxillary hyperplasia in, 1456
maxillary osteotomies in, 1458–1459
orthodontics and, 1454–1456
palatal splints and, 1457–1458
postsurgical considerations in, 1464–1465
surgical considerations in, 1460–1461
velopharyngeal considerations in, 1465
prenatal counseling for, 948–949
repair, 951–959
for bilateral cleft lip, 954–955
for cleft palate, 955–959
for complex facial clefting, 959–960
for unilateral cleft lip, 952–953
lip adhesion in, 952
outcome assessment, 960
presurgical orthopedics in, 951–952
presurgical taping in, 951–952
treatment planning and timing in, 950–951
filler injection for, 1611–1612
in pediatric facial trauma, 579–580
oral cancer in, 704–705
soft tissue trauma in, 370
Liver disease, 28
Liver, in geriatric patients, 73–74
Load-bearing fixation, 377
Load-sharing fixation, 377–378
Lobule (ear), 1600*f*
Local anesthetics, for temporomandibular disorder, 1054
Local flaps, 879–886
Locking plate-screw systems, 379–381
Lockwood's ligament, 1520
Lorazepam, 46*f,* 47
LSD. *See* Lysergic acid diethylamide (LSD)
Lupus erythematosus, 804–805
Luxation, periodontal
extrusive, 397
intrusive, 396
lateral, 397
Lyme disease, 1044

Lymphoma, 29–30
  Burkitt's, 829
  non-Hodgkin's, 829
Lysergic acid diethylamide (LSD), 69

M

Macroaesthetic examination, 1245–1246, 1252–1254
Macrophages, in wound healing, 4–5
Magnetic resonance imaging (MRI)
  in oral cancer, 686–687
  in oral disease diagnosis, 618
  of orbital fracture, 492–493
Mahan's sign, 1073, 1076*f*
Malignant hyperthermia, 36, 55
Mallampati classification, 26*t*, 64*f*
Malpractice claims, nerve injury and, 938–939
Mandible
  defects, 222–223
  in craniofacial development, 1206–1207
  in oral cancer, 709–710
  in panfacial fractures, 595
  in temporomandibular joint, 1034
Mandible fracture
  anatomical distribution of, 409*f*
  angle, 425–427
  bilateral, 427, 428*f*
  biomechanical considerations in, 410
  body, 421–425
    in pediatric patients, 589
  classification of, 409
  closed treatment of, 417
  comminuted, 428, 429*f*
  complications of, 432–433
  diagnosis of, 416–417
  edentulous atrophic, 428–432
  epidemiology of, 408–409
  hardware selection for, 418–420
  historical perspectives on, 407–408, 410–414
  in pediatric patients, 588
  infection with, 432–433
  load-bearing fixation for, 377*f*
  malunion with, 433
  nonunion with, 433
  operative management of, 417–432
  parasymphysis, 421–425
  pediatric, 432
  preoperative management of, 417
  rigid fixation schemes for, 374*f*
  single *vs.* multiple, 383–385
  splinting for, 410–412
  surgical approach for, 418
  symphysis, 421–425
    in pediatric patients, 589
  teeth in line of, 420–421
  treatment of, 410–414
  wiring for, 412–414, 417–418
Mandibular asymmetry, 1251
Mandibular atrophy, 124*f*
Mandibular augmentation, in preprosthetic surgery, 151–152, 153*f*
Mandibular blocks, nerve injury from, 921
Mandibular canine, site preparation for correction of single missing, 271
Mandibular condyle fracture
  anatomic types of, 443–444
  bruxism and, 451
  chronic pain and, 451
  closed treatment of, 445–446
  condylar head, 444

condylar neck, 443, 444*f*
  deviation on opening with, 442–443
  disc injury in, 451
  evidence-based approach to, 452
  facial asymmetry in, 1396–1397
  functional anatomic alterations with, 442–444
  functional anatomy in, 441–442
  glenoid fossa fracture and, 451
  in pediatric patients, 588–589
  infection risk and, 450–451
  intercuspation and, 442
  laterognathia and, 442
  masseteric hypertrophy and, 451
  mouth opening limitation with, 443
  occlusal considerations in, 451
  occlusal prematurity with, 442
  osteoarthrosis and, 451
  outcomes in, 447–452
  overview of, 441
  patient age and, 450
  patient compliance and, 450
  patient gender and, 450
  ramus shortening and, 451–452
  scarring and, 451
  subcondylar, 443
  systemic disease and, 450
  treatment of, 444–452
Mandibular distraction osteogenesis, 1480–1483, 1484*f*, 1485*f*
Mandibular fossa, 1034
Mandibular incisors
  site preparation for correction of single missing, 269–271
Mandibular incisors, third molar impaction and crowning of, 101–102
Mandibular labial frenum, 171–172
Mandibular molars, site preparation for correction of single missing, 272
Mandibular nonunion, in orthognathic surgery, 1434
Mandibular orthognathic surgery
  anatomic considerations in, 1321–1323
  anterior subapical osteotomies in, 1347–1348
  bilateral sagittal split osteotomy in, 1331–1343, 1430, 1438, 1445–1446, 1449–1450
  C ramus osteotomy in, 1328–1331
  distal segment lingual plate fracture in, 1444
  for obstructive sleep apnea, 1502–1503, 1506
  history of, 1317–1321
  horizontal osteotomy of symphysis, 1350–1358
  horizontal ramus osteotomies in, 1343–1347
  inverted-L osteotomy in, 1328–1331
  muscles in, 1322–1323
  nerves in, 1321–1322
  osteotomy techniques in, 1323–1358
  physiologic considerations in, 1321–1323
  posterior subapical osteotomy in, 1348–1349
  ramus osteotomies in, 1323–1324
  soft tissue changes in, 1412, 1414*t*, 1416*t*
  subapical osteotomies in, 1347–1349
  total subapical alveolar osteotomy in, 1349–1350
  unanticipated osteotomy fractures in, 1442–1444
  vascular supply in, 1321
  vertical ramus osteotomy in, 1324–1328, 1430–1431, 1438–1439, 1444–1445
Mandibular premolars, impaction of, in pediatric patients, 163–165, 166*f*
Mandibular site preparation
  for full-arch reconstruction, 274–279
  for segmental defects, 272–274
    anterior, 273–274
    posterior, 274
  for single tooth defects, 269–273

mandibular canine-bicuspid, 271
mandibular incisor, 269–271
molar, 272
Mandibular symphysis
as graft harvesting site, 969*t*
fracture of, 421–425, 589
in pediatric patients, 589
horizontal osteotomy of, 1350–1358
Mandibular tori, removal of, in preprosthetic surgery, 138–139
Mandibular vestibuloplasty, in preprosthetic surgery, 145, 146*f*, 147*f*
Marginal arcade, 1579*f*
Marginal mandibular branch, of facial nerve, 358*f*, 359*f*
Marijuana, 67–68
Masseter muscle, in temporomandibular joint, 1039
Mastication, osseointegration and, 253
Maxillary artery
in temporomandibular joint derangement surgery, 1130–1131
injury, in temporomandibular arthroscopy, 1120
Maxillary augmentation, in preprosthetic surgery, 148–150
Maxillary canines, impacted
cone beam CT of, 181–183
in pediatric patient, 160–163
Maxillary defects, 223
Maxillary distraction osteogenesis, 1483–1487
Maxillary fracture
anatomy in, 456–457
avulsive, 461
clinical examination for, 457–458
complications of, 462–463
diagnosis of, 457–458
fixation for, 459–460
high-force, 461
history of, 455
in geriatric patients, 461
in pediatric patients, 587–588
Le Fort classification, 455–456
pediatric patients in, 461–462
surgical splints for, 460–461
treatment of, 458–463
Maxillary incisors, impaction of, in pediatric patients, 165–167
Maxillary labial frenum, prominent, 171–175
Maxillary nonunion, in orthognathic surgery, 1432–1434
Maxillary orthognathic surgery
anterior maxillary osteotomy in, 1380–1382
anterior maxillary repositioning in, 1378–1379
basic principles of, 1366
dissection in, 1370–1371
exposure in, 1370–1371
for obstructive sleep apnea, 1504–1505
historical perspectives on, 1365–1366
in cleft lip and palate, 1458–1459
incisions in, 1370–1371
inferior maxillary repositioning in, 1379–1380
model surgery in, 1366–1367
modified Le Fort osteotomies in, 1387–1389
osseous structures in, 1367–1368
osseous surgery in, 1371–1376
posterior maxillary osteotomy in, 1382–1384
posterior maxillary repositioning in, 1379–1380
rigid internal fixation in, 1380
segmental procedures in, 1376–1378
soft tissue changes associated with, 1412–1413, 1415*t*, 1416*t*
soft tissue envelope in, 1369–1370
superior maxillary repositioning in, 1378
surgical anatomy in, 1367–1370
surgical techniques in, 1370–1380
surgically assisted rapid palatal expansion in, 1384–1387

total maxillary alveolar osteotomy in, 1384
unanticipated maxillary fractures in, 1447–1448
vascular structures in, 1368–1369
zygomatic osteotomy in, 1387–1389
Maxillary premolars, impaction of, in pediatric patients, 163–165, 166*f*
Maxillary tori, removal of, in preprosthetic surgery, 138–139
Maxillary tuberosity, reduction of, in preprosthetic surgery, 136–137
Maxillary vestibuloplasty, in preprosthetic surgery, 143–144
Maxillary-nasal base aesthetic unit, in dysostosis syndromes, 1000
Maxillofacial infection
airway compromise in, 845–846
antibiotic administration for, 853–854
antibiotics for, 852–853
culture testing in, 851
deep spaces in, 843*t*
drainage timing in, 851
frequent patient evaluation in, 854–856
HIV and, 846–847
hospital admission indications for, 847*t*
host defenses in, 846–847
immune system compromise and, 846–847
incision timing in, 851
location of, 842
medical support for, 851–852
overview of, 841
rate of progression of, 842–844
sensitivity testing in, 851
setting of care for, 847–848
severity of, 841–846
severity scores of, 844*t*
stages of, 844*t*
surgical drainage of, 848–851
surgical treatment of, 848–851
treatment failure in, 854*t*
Maxillofacial prostheses, 222–224
Maxillomandibular asymmetry, 1252
McCune-Albright syndrome, 827–828
MCT. *See* Medial canthal tendon (MCT)
MDMA, 68–69
Medial canthal tendon (MCT), 521, 1519*f*
Medial pterygoid muscle, in temporomandibular joint, 1039
Median mandibular cyst, 667
Melanocytic nevi, 813
Melanoma, 749–751, 814–815
biopsy strategies, 751*t*
clinical description, 749–751
histologic description, 749–751
risk factors, 749
survival rates, 751*t*
Melanotic macule, 812
Melanotic neuroectodermal tumor of infancy, 830
MELD. *See* Model for End-Stage Liver Disease (MELD)
Meperidine, 48*f*, 49
Mesenchymal neoplasms, in head and neck, 834
Mesenchymal odontogenic tumors, 824–826
Mesenchymal tumors
benign, 826–829
of childhood, 659–660
Metastasizing pleomorphic adenoma, 786
Methohexital, 51*f*, 53–54
Metopic synostosis, 981–982. *See also* Craniosynostosis
MG. *See* Myasthenia gravis (MG)
Microneurosurgery
approximation in, 936
clinical evaluation for, 919
clinical neurosensory testing and, 925–929
coaptation in, 936

demographics in, 920–923
entubulation techniques in, 938
exposure in, 934
external neurolysis in, 934–935
indications for, 931–932
internal neurolysis in, 935
medicolegal issues in, 938–939
nerve grafts in, 937
nerve stump preparation in, 935–936
nerve trauma classification and, 924–925, 926, 926f, 926t
neurorrhaphy in, 936–937
overview of, 919–920
postsurgical management, 938
referral indications, 930t
success rates of, 932
treatment algorithms in, 930–933
trigeminal nerve anatomy in, 923–924
trigeminal nerve physiology in, 923–924
Micropigmentation, 1591–1592
Microvascular soft tissue flaps, 901–906
Midazolam, 46f, 47, 81–82
Middle lamella, 1519
Midface implants, 1615–1617
Midline defects, 1194
Miniaesthetic examination, 1254, 1256–1257
Mitral stenosis (MS), 20
Model for End-Stage Liver Disease (MELD), 28
Model surgery, for orthognathics
centric relation bite registration in, 1297–1298
dental impressions in, 1296
facebow transfer and, 1296–1297
for mandibular surgery, 1299–1301
for maxillary surgery, 1301–1309, 1366–1367
marking and measuring in, 1299–1309
mounting for, 1298–1299
overview of, 1295
presurgical clinical database in, 1295–1296
presurgical records in, 1296–1298
splint fabrication in, 1309–1310
three-dimensional, 1310–1315
traditional immediate preoperative analytical, 1295–1315
Modulus of elasticity, 240
Mohs' micrographic surgery, 753–755
Molars
first, impacted, 167–168
mandibular, site preparation for correction of single missing, 272
second, impacted, 167–168
third, impacted
adjacent teeth root reabsorption and, 102
alveolar osteitis after extraction of, 114–115
antibiotics in extraction of, 112–113
bleeding after extraction of, 113–114
dental caries and, 101
dental prostheses and, 102
incidence and etiology of, 99–100
indications for removal of, 101–102
jaw fracture risk and, 102
mandibular incisor crowning and, 101–102
nerve disturbances after removal of, 115
odontogenic cysts and tumors and, 102
orthodontic considerations with, 101–102
orthognathic surgery and, 102
pain after extraction of, 114
pain from, 102
pericoronitis and, 101
periodontal healing after extraction of, 116–117
periodontitis and, 101

postoperative complications after extraction of, 114–116
postoperative course for, 113–114
rare complications for, 115–116
steroids in extraction of, 112–113
stiffness after extraction of, 114
surgery for, 107–113
swelling after extraction of, 114
tooth fracture after extraction of, 114
transplantation of, 170
Monitoring
anesthesia, 74–75
respiratory, 74–75
Morphine, 48–49
Morse taper, 207, 208f
MRI. See Magnetic resonance imaging (MRI)
MS. See Mitral stenosis (MS)
Mucoepidermoid carcinoma, 788, 836
Mucosal examination, light-based adjuncts for, 617
Mucosal substitutes, 13–14
Mucous membrane pemphigoid, 808–809
Muenke's syndrome, 996. See also Dysostosis syndromes
Muller's muscle, 1517f
Multiple myeloma, 29–30
Mumps, 783, 834
Muscarinic receptor antagonists, 86
Muscle relaxants, for temporomandibular disorder, 1054, 1055t
Muscular dystrophy, 88–89
Mustarde method, for otoplasty, 1603–1606
Myasthenia gravis (MG), 36
Myeloproliferative disease, 29
Mylohyoid ridge, reduction of, in preprosthetic surgery, 139
Myocardial infarction, 18t

N
Nalbuphine, 50
Naloxone, 50
Nanotechnology, in implant surface modification, 237
Nasal complex
in nasal fracture, 540
in pediatric facial fracture, 585
Nasal dorsum, 1539, 1541
Nasal dorsum reduction, 1546
Nasal fracture
classification of, 541
complications with, 542–543
CT for, 540–541
diagnostic tools for, 539–541
nasal complex evaluation in, 540
overview of, 539
postoperative care for, 542–543
radiography for, 539–541
reduction of, 542
sense of smell and, 542
surgical anatomy of, 539
surgical management of, 541–542
Nasal implants, 305
Nasal pit, 1192f
Nasal secretions, 523t
Nasal surgery, for obstructive sleep apnea, 1500–1501
Nasal tip, 1539–1540, 1547–1551
Nasal valve, 1536–1537
Naso frontal outflow tract (NFOT)
obstruction, 529
patency, 524
Naso-orbitoethmoid fracture
anatomy in, 519–522
anterior table fracture in, 528

classification of, 524–525
clinical findings in, 522–524
complications of, 531–532
deformity correction, 532–534
endoscopy in, 530
imaging of, 524
in pediatric patients, 585
medical therapy, postoperative, 531
naso frontal outflow tract evaluation in, 527–528
naso frontal outflow tract obstruction in, 529
naso-orbitoethmoid complex reconstruction in, 530–531
orbital roof reconstruction in, 528
osseous recovery in, 526–527
patient evaluation in, 522–525
physiology in, 519–522
posterior table, 528
sinus obliteration in, 529–530
supraorbital bar reconstruction in, 528
surgical access in, 526
treatment of, 525–531
Nasociliary nerve, 1519f
Nasofrontal angle, 1538, 1539f
Nasolabial angle, 1540
Nasolabial cysts, 666–667
Nasolabial folds, fillers for, 1611
Nasolacrimal apparatus, soft tissue trauma in, 364–366
Nasopalatine duct cyst, 667
Nausea, postoperative, 60, 65, 85–86
Neck
congenital masses and cysts in, 832–833
deep spaces of, 842t
dissection in oral cancer, 713–716
therapeutic, 717
in pediatric facial trauma, 567–568
penetrating injury to, in gunshot wounds, 554–555
skin cancer in
lasers for, 756
melanoma, 749–751
biopsy strategies, 751t
clinical description, 749–751
histologic description, 749–751
risk factors, 749
survival rates, 751t
nonmelanoma, 743–749
basal cell carcinoma, 746
chemotherapy for, 756
cryosurgery for, 755
curettage and electrodesiccation for, 755–756
environmental factors, 745
epidemiology of, 743
etiology of, 743–746
grafting in, 757–768
immunologic factors, 744
interferons for, 756
management of, 751–768
Mohs' micrographic surgery for, 753–755
photodynamic therapy for, 756
predisposing lesions, 744
prevention of, 745–746
radiation therapy for, 755
retinoids for, 756
squamous cell carcinoma, 746–749
standard excision of, 752
syndromes in, 744
soft tissue trauma in, 370–371
Negative-pressure pulmonary edema (NPPE), 26
Neostigmine, 60t

Nerve blocks
diagnostic, 929
mandibular, nerve injury from, 921
Nerve grafts
allografts in, 937
harvesting sites for, 937
Nervous tissue, healing of, 6
Neural crest defects, 1194–1195
Neural crest, cranial, 1191–1192
Neural plate, 1190f
Neural tube defects, 1194
Neural tube formation, 1189–1190
Neurocranium formation, 1195–1196
Neurofibroma, 669, 830
Neurogenic tumors, 669–670, 830
Neurologic disease, 34–36
Neurologic trauma
as surgical comorbidity, 34–35
classification of, 924–925, 926, 926f, 926t
in orthognathic surgery, 1437–1440
in temporomandibular joint derangement surgery, 1150
legal issues and, 938–939
Neuroma, traumatic, 669–670
Neuromuscular blocking medications, 58–59
Neuropathy, optic, with zygomatic complex fractures, 478–479
Neuropraxia, 6, 924, 926f, 926t, 938, 944
Neurosensory testing, 925–929
Neurosurgery, micro-
approximation in, 936
clinical evaluation for, 919
clinical neurosensory testing and, 925–929
coaptation in, 936
demographics in, 920–923
entubulation techniques in, 938
exposure in, 934
external neurolysis in, 934–935
indications for, 931–932
internal neurolysis in, 935
medicolegal issues in, 938–939
nerve grafts in, 937
nerve stump preparation in, 935–936
nerve trauma classification and, 924–925, 926, 926f, 926t
neurorrhaphy in, 936–937
overview of, 919–920
postsurgical management, 938
referral indications, 930t
success rates of, 932
treatment algorithms in, 930–933
trigeminal nerve anatomy in, 923–924
trigeminal nerve physiology in, 923–924
Neurotmesis, 6, 925, 926f, 926t, 944
Neurotoxins, 1609–1610
Nevi, 813
Nevoid basal cell carcinoma syndrome, 629t, 631–632
New York Heart Association classification, 19
Nitrous oxide, 54t, 55–56, 57f
Non-Hodgkin's lymphoma, 829
Non-REM sleep, 1493–1494
Noncompetitive antagonists, 44
Nondepolarizing agents, 58–59
Nonrigid internal fixation, 373–375
Nonsteroidal anti-inflammatory drugs (NSAIDs), for temporomandibular disorder, 1052
Normocytic anemia, 29
Nose
anatomy of, 1531–1537
blood supply of, 1532–1533

bone in, 1533–1535
cartilage in, 1533–1535
in pediatric facial trauma, 574, 575*f*
musculature of, 1532
musculoaponeurotic system in, 1532
nerves in, 1535–1536
rhinoplasty for
  alar base reduction in, 1551, 1552*f*
  alar width in, 1541
  anatomy in, 1531–1537
  anesthesia for, 1541
  complete transfixion in, 1542
  cosmetic evaluation in, 1537–1538
  facial analysis in, 1538
  functional considerations in, 1541
  hemitransfixion in, 1542
  incisions in, 1541–1543
  intercartilaginous incision in, 1542–1543
  intracartilaginous incision in, 1543
  Killian incision in, 1542
  marginal incision in, 1543
  nasal analysis in, 1538, 1539*f*
  nasal dorsum assessment in, 1539, 1541
  nasal dorsum augmentation in, 1546–1547
  nasal dorsum reduction in, 1546
  nasal tip definition in, 1539–1540
  nasal tip projection in, 1539–1540, 1548–1550
  nasal tip rotation in, 1540, 1550
  nasal tip shape in, 1550–1551
  nasofrontal angle assessment in, 1538, 1539*f*
  osteotomies in, 1547
  partial transfixion in, 1542
  postoperative management in, 1551
  psychiatric stability and, 1537
  rim incision in, 1543
  septoplasty in, 1543–1545
  sequencing in, 1541–1543
  skin assessment for, 1538
  symmetry assessment for, 1538–1541
  transcolumellar incision in, 1543
  turbinectomy in, 1545
skin in, 1531–1532
soft tissue in anatomy of, 1531–1532
soft tissue trauma in, 367
surface anatomy of, 1531
Nosocomial pneumonia, 25
Notochord, 1190*f*
Notochordal process, 1190*f*
NPO, 66–67
Nutrition
  gunshot wounds and, 555
  oral cancer and, 699
  wound healing and, 12

O

Obesity, as surgical comorbidity, 38–39, 66
Obstructive sleep apnea (OSA)
  cephalometric examination in, 1496–1497
  clinical manifestations of, 1495
  complications of surgery for, 1507–1508
  continuous positive airway pressure for, 1500
  CT in, 1497
  diagnosis of, 1496–1498
  differential diagnosis of, 1494–1495
  Herbst appliance for, 1499
  history of, 1495
  in dysostosis syndromes, 997–998

  medical treatment of, 1498–1500
  nasal surgery for, 1500–1501
  oral appliances for, 1498–1500
  orthognathic surgery for, 1502–1506
  oxygen therapy for, 1498
  physical examination in, 1496
  physical findings in, 1495
  polysomnography in, 1497
  progesterone for, 1498
  protriptyline for, 1498
  site of obstruction in, 1497–1498
  surgical treatment of, 1500–1506
  tongue-retaining device for, 1499
  tracheostomy for, 1500
  uvulopalatopharyngoplasty for, 1501–1502
  uvulopalatoplasty for, 1502
Occlusal appliances, for temporomandibular disorder, 1059–1060
Occlusion
  dental implants and, 205–206
  in dysostosis syndromes, 998
  mandibular condyle fracture and, 442, 443
  orthognathic surgery and discrepancies in, 1448–1450
Ocular injury, 493–499
Oculomotor nerve, 1519*f*
Odontogenic cysts
  calcifying, 633–635
  classification of, 626*t*
  dentigerous, 626–628
  glandular, 632–633
  overview of, 625–626
Odontogenic keratocyst, 628–632
Odontogenic myxoma, 645–645, 824–825
Odontogenic tumors
  adenomatoid, 648–649
  ameloblastic carcinoma, 642, 643*f*
  ameloblastic fibroma, 644
  ameloblastoma, 637–641
    malignant, 642
    multicystic, 637–639
    peripheral, 640–641
    solid, 637–639
    unicystic, 639–640
  calcifying epithelial, 647–648
  classification of, 635*t*
  clear cell odontogenic carcinoma, 643
  epithelial, 822–824
  ghost cell, malignant epithelial, 644
  malignant, 641–644
  mesenchymal, 824–826
  mixed, 635–636
  odontoma, 644–645
  overview of, 625–626
  primary interosseous squamous cell carcinoma, 643
Odontoma, 644–645, 825–826
On Point system, 1081–1082
Oncocytomas, 787
Ondansetron, 61*f*
One-point fixation, 379
Onlay grafts, in preprosthetic surgery, 149
Open bite malocclusion, after orthognathic surgery, 1448–1449
Open pneumothorax, 331–333
Open reduction and internal fixation (ORIF)
  of mandibular condyle fracture, 445–446
  of zygomatic complex fractures, 472–475, 476
Ophthalmia, sympathetic, 495–496
Ophthalmic artery, 1519*f*
Opioids

as outpatient anesthesia, 47–50
as perioperative analgesia, 57
Optic nerve, 1519*f*
Optic neuropathy, with zygomatic complex fractures, 478–479
Optic placode, 1192*f*
Optimized problem list, synthesis of, 1261–1262
Oral administration, for pediatric induction, 78
Oral appliances, for obstructive sleep apnea, 1498–1500
Oral cancer
  alcohol and, 698
  biopsy of, 687–688
  cervical lymph node levels in, 685–686
  cervical lymph nodes in, 711–713
  chemoprevention for, 704
  chemotherapy for, 701–704
  deep venous thrombosis and, 698
  diagnosis, 687–688
  distant metastasis assessment in, 687
  ethnicity and, 677*t*
  etiology of, 678–679
  follow-up surveillance, 717–719
  future treatments for, 719
  histology of, 693–694
  in alveolus, 708–709
  in buccal mucosa, 705
  in floor of mouth, 708
  in gingiva, 708–709
  in lip, 704–705
  in palate, 709
  in retromolar trigone, 706
  in tongue, 706–708
  mandible in, 709–710
  MRI in, 686–687
  neck dissection in, 713–716
    therapeutic, 717
  overview of, 677–678
  panendoscopy in, 695–696
  perioperative issues with, 698–699
  PET in, 687
  premalignant disease in, 679–683, 694–695
  primary lesion assessment, 684–685
  radiation for, 699–701
  recurrence of, 717–719
  regional metastasis assessment in, 685–687
  risk factors, 678
  sentinel node biopsy in, 716–717
  staging, 687
  surgery for, 696–699
  treatment choice for, 696
  ultrasound in, 687
Oral cavity, in pediatric facial trauma, 579–580
Oral disease
  border of, 614–615
  character of, 614
  clinical examination in, 613–615
  clinical presentation of, 616
  consistency of, 614
  diagnosis development in, 615–617
  diagnostic process for, 611–615
  differential diagnosis of, 611–622
  distribution of, 615
  final diagnosis of, 617–621
  history in, 613, 616
  imaging of, 617–619
  location of, 616
  microscopic diagnosis of, 621
  molecular evaluation in, 619

  morphology of, 614
  pathogenesis of, 616
  patient follow-up in, 621–622
  site of, 613
  size of, 614
  symptoms of, 615
  tissue analysis in, 619
Oral melacanthoma, 812–813
Oral mucosa, pigmented lesions, 811–817
Orbicularis oculi, 486, 1576*f*
Orbicularis oculi hypertrophy, 1516
Orbicularis oris muscle, 1532*f*
Orbital canals, 485*t*
Orbital defects, 308–310
Orbital fissures, 485*t*
Orbital floor
  in orbital anatomy, 483–484
  in pediatric facial fracture, 585–587
Orbital fracture
  acute repair of, 507–515
  anatomy in, 483–487
  clinical examination for, 487–491
  configurations, 487
  CT of, 492
  decision diagram, 503*f*
  endoscopic approach, 507
  imaging of, 492–493
  indications for surgical repair of, 502
  inferior orbital approach, 504–505
  lateral orbital approach, 504–505
  medial orbital approach, 505–507
  MRI of, 492–493
  nonoperative management of, 499–502
  operative management of, 502–514
  superior orbital approach, 505–506
  surgical approaches for, 502–507
Orbital implants, 304–305
Orbital ligament, 1573
Orbital roof
  in cranial fractures, in pediatric patients, 585
  in orbital anatomy, 483
Orbital septum, 486, 1517*f,* 1519*f*
Orbital walls, 483
Orbitonasozygomatic aesthetic unit, in dysostosis syndromes, 1000
ORIF. *See* Open reduction and internal fixation (ORIF)
ORN. *See* Osteoradionecrosis (ORN)
Orthodontic camouflage, 1228–1229
Orthodontics
  facial asymmetry and, 1399–1401
  for distraction osteogenesis, 1477–1480
  for orthognathic surgery
    arch length in, 1263–1264
    arch width analysis in, 1265–1266
    clinical examination in, 1263–1270
    curve of Spee in, 1266
    curve of Wilson in, 1267
    cuspid-molar position in, 1267
    dental model analysis in, 1263–1270
    dental problems in, 1267
    periodontal status in, 1268–1269
    tongue assessment in, 1269–1270
    tooth ankylosis in, 1267–1268
    tooth arch symmetry in, 1267
    tooth size analysis in, 1264–1265
Orthodontics, alveolar cleft repair and, 970–972
Orthognathic database
  collection, 1240–1244

overview of, 1239
problem list and, 1261–1262
Orthognathic surgery
    alar base in, 1441
    auriculotemporal syndrome after, 1451
    avascular necrosis in, 1431–1432
    cleft
        distraction osteogenesis in, 1461–1464
        history of, 1456
        maxilla development in, 1454–1456
        maxillary hyperplasia in, 1456
        maxillary osteotomies in, 1458–1459
        orthodontics and, 1454–1456
        palatal splints and, 1457–1458
        postsurgical considerations in, 1464–1465
        surgical considerations in, 1460–1461
        velopharyngeal considerations in, 1465
    dental injury in, 1435
    epiphora after, 1450–1451
    facial scars after, 1451
    fistula formation in, 1436
    for obstructive sleep apnea, 1502–1506
    infection in, 1437
    internal nasal valve in, 1440–1441
    lateral cephalometric prediction in, 1411–1421
    mandibular
        anatomic considerations in, 1321–1323
        anterior subapical osteotomies in, 1347–1348
        bilateral sagittal split osteotomy in, 1331–1343, 1430, 1438, 1445–
            1446, 1449–1450
        C ramus osteotomy in, 1328–1331
        distal segment lingual plate fracture in, 1444
        history of, 1317–1321
        horizontal osteotomy of symphysis, 1350–1358
        horizontal ramus osteotomies in, 1343–1347
        inverted-L osteotomy in, 1328–1331
        muscles in, 1322–1323
        nerves in, 1321–1322
        osteotomy techniques in, 1323–1358
        physiologic considerations in, 1321–1323
        posterior subapical osteotomy in, 1348–1349
        proximal segment buccal plate fracture in, 1442–1444
        ramus osteotomies in, 1323–1324
        soft tissue changes in, 1412, 1414*t*, 1416*t*
        subapical osteotomies in, 1347–1349
        total subapical alveolar osteotomy in, 1349–1350
        unanticipated osteotomy fractures in, 1442–1444
        vascular supply in, 1321
        vertical ramus osteotomy in, 1324–1328, 1430–1431, 1438–1439,
            1444–1445
    mandibular hemorrhage in, 1430
    mandibular nonunion, 1434
    mandibular sensory injuries in, 1438–1439
    maxillary
        anterior maxillary osteotomy in, 1380–1382
        anterior maxillary repositioning in, 1378–1379
        basic principles of, 1366
        dissection in, 1370–1371
        exposure in, 1370–1371
        historical perspectives on, 1365–1366
        in cleft lip and palate, 1458–1459
        incisions in, 1370–1371
        inferior maxillary repositioning in, 1379–1380
        model surgery in, 1366–1367
        modified Le Fort osteotomies in, 1387–1389
        osseous structures in, 1367–1368
        osseous surgery in, 1371–1376

        posterior maxillary osteotomy in, 1382–1384
        posterior maxillary repositioning in, 1379–1380
        rigid internal fixation in, 1380
        segmental procedures in, 1376–1378
        soft tissue changes associated with, 1412–1413, 1415*t*, 1416*t*
        soft tissue envelope in, 1369–1370
        superior maxillary repositioning in, 1378
        surgical anatomy in, 1367–1370
        surgical techniques in, 1370–1380
        surgically assisted rapid palatal expansion in, 1384–1387
        total maxillary alveolar osteotomy in, 1384
        unanticipated fractures in, 1447–1448
        vascular structures in, 1368–1369
        zygomatic osteotomy in, 1387–1389
    maxillary hemorrhage in
        acute, 1427–1429
        delayed, 1429–1430
    maxillary nonunion in, 1432–1434
    maxillary sensory injuries in, 1437–1438
    models for
        centric relation bite registration in, 1297–1298
        dental impressions in, 1296
        facebow transfer and, 1296–1297
        for mandibular surgery, 1299–1301
        for maxillary surgery, 1301–1309
        marking and measuring in, 1299–1309
        mounting for, 1298–1299
        overview of, 1295
        presurgical clinical database in, 1295–1296
        presurgical records in, 1296–1298
        splint fabrication in, 1309–1310
        three-dimensional, 1310–1315
        traditional immediate preoperative analytical, 1295–1315
    motor nerve injury in, 1439–1440
    nasal considerations in, 1440–1442
    nasal forms alterations in, 1440–1441
    nerve injury in, 1437–1440
    occlusal discrepancies after, 1448–1450
    orthodontics for
        arch length in, 1263–1264
        arch width analysis in, 1265–1266
        clinical examination in, 1263–1270
        curve of Spee in, 1266
        curve of Wilson in, 1267
        cuspid-molar position in, 1267
        dental model analysis in, 1263–1270
        dental problems in, 1267
        periodontal status in, 1268–1269
        tongue assessment in, 1269–1270
        tooth ankylosis in, 1267–1268
        tooth arch symmetry in, 1267
        tooth size analysis in, 1264–1265
    periodontal injury in, 1435
    salivary gland injury in, 1451
    septal deviation in, 1440
    sinus considerations in, 1440–1442
    sinus disease after, 1441–1442
    soft tissue changes associated with, 1411–1422
    temporomandibular hypomobility and, 1160
    temporomandibular joint dysfunction and, 1447
    vascular complications of, 1427–1432
    vascular compromise in, 1431–1432
        management of, 1436–1437
    wisdom teeth impaction and, 102
Orthognathic treatment planning, 1239–1240
Orthopedics, for growth modification, 1217–1228
OSA. *See* Obstructive sleep apnea (OSA)

Osseointegration
    abutment positions and, 249–250
    biology of, 229–248
    biomechanics of, 238–248
    bone loss and, 239–246
    bruxism and, 252–253
    cantilevers and, 251–252
    clenching and, 252–253
    early loading failure and, 246–248
    history of, 229
    implant materials and, 229–231
    implant surfaces and, 231–238
        acid etching of, 233–234
        additive, 234–236
        alterations to, 232–238
        bioactive proteins and, 237–238
        bisphosphonates for, 238
        blasting of, 233, 234
        bone morphogenic proteins and, 237–238
        calcium phosphate treatment of, 237
        cytokines and, 238
        fluoride treatment of, 237
        hydrophilic, 236
        hydrophobic, 236
        hydroxyapatite coating of, 234–235
        laser etching of, 236
        nanotechnology in, 237
        oxidation for, 235–236
        pharmacologic coatings for, 238
        subtractive, 233
        surface energy, 236
        titanium plasma spray for, 234
    mandibular edentulism and, 256–260
    masticatory dynamics and, 253
    maxillary edentulism and, 253–256
    mechanical risk factors and, 251
    number of plants and, 248–249
    parafunctional habits and, 252–253
    science of, 248–260
    treatment planning, 248–260
    with titanium, 229
    with zirconia, 229–231
Ossifying fibroma, 656
Osteoarthritis, in temporomandibular joint, 1102
Osteoblastoma, 656–657, 828
Osteochondroma, 658–659
Osteoid osteoma, 656–657, 828
Osteoma, 657–658
Osteomyelitis
    clinical presentation of, 862–865
    microbiology of, 862
    overview of, 861
    pain in, 862
    pathogenesis of, 862
    surgical options for, 867–868
    treatment of, 866–867
Osteonecrosis
    bisphosphonate-related, of jaws, 870–873
    osteoradionecrosis, 868–870
Osteoplasty, ridge-split, in preprosthetic surgery, 148–149
Osteoporosis, dental implants and, 202
Osteoradionecrosis (ORN), 868–870
Otic placode, 1192*f*
Otoplastic surgery
    aesthetic complications in, 1607
    anatomy in, 1597–1599
    complications of, 1606–1607

Davis method for, 1601–1603, 1604*f*
    hematoma in, 1606
    keloid formation in, 1607
    Mustarde method for, 1603–1606
    narrowed meatus after, 1607
    perichondritis in, 1606
    scapha buckling after, 1607
    scarring in, hypertrophic, 1607
    surgical techniques in, 1601–1606
    telephone ear deformity after, 1607
Outpatient anesthesia. *See also* Sedation
    alfentanil as, 49
    attention deficit hyperactivity disorder and, 87
    autism and, 87
    benzodiazepines in, 45–47
    cerebral palsy and, 88
    diazepam as, 46–47
    Down syndrome and, 88
    fentanyl as, 49
    fluids in, 75–76
    flumazenil as, 47
    hydromorphone, 49
    in geriatric patients, 72–74
    in pediatric patients, 69–72
    in preprosthetic surgery, 130
    induction agents for, 50–52
    inhalation, 54–57
        in pediatric patients, 77–78
    laryngospasm and, 84–86
    lorazepam as, 47
    meperidine as, 49
    midazolam as, 47
    monitoring in, 74–75
    morphine as, 48–49
    muscular dystrophy and, 88–89
    nalbuphine as, 50
    naloxone as, 50
    opioids in, 47–50
    patient positioning and, 76
    perioperative complications, 84–86
    pharmacodynamics in, 43–44
    pharmacokinetics in, 44–45
    recovery from, 86–87
    remifentanil as, 49
    sufentanil as, 49
    triazolam as, 47
Overdentures
    implant-retained, 216–217
    implant-supported, 217–218
    techniques for, 221–222
Oxidation, of implant surfaces, 235–236
Oxygen therapy, for obstructive sleep apnea, 1498
Oxygenation, in trauma, 336

P
Pacemakers, 23
Paget's disease, 670–671
Pain
    from wisdom tooth extraction, 114
    from wisdom tooth impaction, 102
    in osteomyelitis, 862
    mandibular condyle fracture and, 451
    sympathetically maintained, in temporomandibular disorder, 1064–1065
Palatal graft, epithelialized, for dental implants, 288–290
Palate
    cleft
        classification of, 948

embryology of, 947
etiology of, 947–948
facial asymmetry in, 1395
feeding concerns with, 949–950
genetics in, 947–948
goals of repair, 945
history of, 946–947
management of children with, 945
orthognathic surgery for
   distraction osteogenesis in, 1461–1464, 1469
   history of, 1456
   maxilla development in, 1454–1456
   maxillary hyperplasia in, 1456
   maxillary osteotomies in, 1458–1459
   orthodontics and, 1454–1456
   palatal splints and, 1457–1458
   postsurgical considerations in, 1464–1465
   surgical considerations in, 1460–1461
   velopharyngeal considerations in, 1465
prenatal counseling for, 948–949
repair, 951–959
   for bilateral cleft lip, 954–955
   for cleft palate, 955–959
   for complex facial clefting, 959–960
   for unilateral cleft lip, 952–953
   lip adhesion in, 952
   outcome assessment, 960
   presurgical orthopedics in, 951–952
   presurgical taping in, 951–952
   treatment planning and timing in, 950–951
oral cancer in, 709
surgically assisted rapid expansion of, 1384–1387
Palpebral muscle, 1520
Pancuronium, 59*t*
Panendoscopy, in treatment planning for oral cancer, 695–696
Panfacial fractures
airway management in, 599
anatomic considerations in, 594–596
complications with, 602–605
definition of, 593
dental fractures in, 594–595
etiology of, 593
facial buttresses and, 594
fracture management in, 599–602
historic perspective on, 593
imaging of, 596–597
intercanthal region in, 596
key landmarks in, 594
mandible in, 594–595
sequence of treatment for, 599–602
soft tissue resuspension for, 599
sphenozygomatic suture in, 595–596
surgical approaches for, 597–599
widening of facial complex in, 602–605
Papillary cystadenoma lymphomatosum, 787
Papillary hyperplasia, inflammatory, 140
Parafunction, osseointegration and, 252–253
Paraneoplastic pemphigus, 808
Parietal artery, 1600*f*
Parry-Romberg syndrome, 1395–1396
Patient exposure, in trauma, 344
Patient positioning, 76
PCP. *See* Phencyclidine hydrochloride (PCP)
PE. *See* Pulmonary embolus (PE)
Pectoralis major myocutaneous flap, 886–887, 898–900
Pediatric patients
anatomic considerations in, 70–72
anesthetic considerations in, 69–72

cardiac output in, 71–72
cardiovascular system in, 71–72
dental implants in, 170–171
dentoalveolar surgery in, 159–175
endotracheal intubation of, 70–71
facial trauma in
   airway in evaluation of, 566
   airway injury in, 567–568
   anterior cranial fractures in, 583–589
   antibiotic ointments for, 580–581
   breathing in evaluation of, 566
   cheek in, 577–579, 580*f*
   circulation in evaluation of, 566
   dentoalveolar injuries in, 589
   disability in evaluation of, 566
   ear in, 569–571
   exposure in, 566–567
   eyelid in, 571–574
   facial fracture in, 581–583
   growth disturbance from, 590
   head injuries, 567–568
   history in, 565
   lacrimal apparatus in, 571–574
   lip in, 579–580
   mandible fracture in, 588
   mandibular body fracture in, 589
   mandibular condyle fracture in, 588–589
   mandibular symphysis fracture in, 589
   maxillary fracture in, 587–588
   mouth in, 579–580
   naso-orbitoethmoid fracture in, 585
   neck in, 567–568
   nose in, 574, 575*f*
   oral cavity in, 579–580
   perioperative management, 568
   physical evaluation in, 565–567
   regional soft tissue wounds in, 569–580
   scalp in, 575–577
   silicone agents for, 581
   soft tissue injuries in, 568–569
   wound care adjuncts for, 580–581
   zygomaticomaxillary complex fracture in, 587
femoral vein access in, 77, 77*f*
first molar impaction in, 167–168
general surgical considerations in, 40
hypodontia in, 168–169
impacted teeth in, 103, 159–168
induction agents in, 82
inhalation anesthesia in, 77–78, 82–84
intramuscular route of administration in, 78
ketamine in, 79–81
mandibular fracture in, 432
mandibular premolar impaction in, 163–165, 166*f*
maxillary canine impaction in, 160–163
maxillary fracture in, 461–462
maxillary incisor impaction in, 165–167
maxillary premolar impaction in, 163–165, 166*f*
maxillofacial pathology in
   odontogenic, 821–826
   overview of, 821
midazolam in, 81–82
nasal route of administration in, 78
oral route of administration in, 78
psychological assessment for, 72
rectal route of administration in, 79
respiratory system in, 70
salivary gland disease in, 834–836
second molar impaction in, 167–168

sedation in
routes of administration for, 76–79
sedative techniques in, 76–84
supernumerary teeth in, 168
upper respiratory infections in, 71
Peel, chemical, 1613–1615
Pemphigus vulgaris, 807–808
Pentobarbital, 51*f*, 54
Perfusion, tissue, wound healing and, 10
Periapical cemento-osseous dysplasia, 655
Pericoronitis, impacted third molars and, 101
Periodontal concussion, 395
Periodontal displacement, 395–396
Periodontal extrusive luxation, 397
Periodontal intrusive luxation, 396
Periodontal lateral luxations, 397
Periodontal subluxation, 396
Periodontal tissue injury, 394–397
Periodontitis
impacted third molars and, 101
implants and, 202
Perioperative analgesic medications, 57–58
Peripheral arcade, 1579*f*
PET. *See* Positron emission topography (PET)
Petechia, 816
Pfeiffer's syndrome, 996, 1023–1024. *See also* Dysostosis syndromes
Pharmacodynamics, 43–44
Pharmacokinetics, 44–45
Phencyclidine hydrochloride (PCP), 69
Phenobarbital, 51*f*
Phenothiazines, 85–86
Phonophoresis, for temporomandibular disorder, 1057
Photodynamic therapy, for skin cancer, 756
Physical status classification, 17*t*
Physical therapy, for temporomandibular disorder, 1054–1058
Pigmented lesions, 811–817
Pindborg tumor, 647–648
Pipecuronium, 59*t*
Pituitary disease, 34
Plagiocephaly, 1395
Plain radiography, for zygomatic complex fractures, 468–469
Platelets, in wound healing, 4, 4*f*
Pleomorphic adenoma, 786, 836
Pneumonia, 25
Pneumothorax
open, 331–333
tension, 333, 334*f*
Polymorphous low-grade adenocarcinoma, 788
Polysomnography, in obstructive sleep apnea, 1497
PONV. *See* Postoperative nausea and vomiting (PONV)
Positioning, patient, 76
Positron emission topography (PET)
in oral cancer, 687
in oral disease diagnosis, 619
Posterior auricularis muscle, 1600*f*
Posterior cranial vault aesthetic unit, in dysostosis syndromes, 999–1000
Posterior ethmoidal artery, 1534*f*
Posterior lamella, 1519–1522
Posterior table fracture, 528
Postinflammatory melanosis, 812
Postoperative nausea and vomiting (PONV), 60–61, 65, 85–86
Postoperative recovery and discharge, 86–87
Prealbumin, wound healing and, 12
Prechordal plate, 1189, 1190*f*
Pregnancy
as surgical comorbidity, 40–41, 67
prenatal counseling in, for cleft lip and palate, 948–949
testing, 67

Preload, 18
Premature ventricular contractions (PVCs), 21
Premolars, maxillary, impaction of, in pediatric patients, 163–165, 166*f*
Prenatal counseling, for cleft lip and palate, 948–949
Prenatal craniofacial development, 1189–1200
Preoperative assessment, 64–74
airway in, 26
blood disorders and, 28–32
cardiovascular disease and, 18–26
classifications in, 17–18
endocrine disease in, 32–34
examination in, 17
goal of, 17
in geriatric patients, 39–40
liver disease and, 28
neurologic disease and, 34–36
renal disease, 27–28
respiratory disease and, 23–26
Preoperative fasting, 66–67
Preprosthetic surgery
alveolar distraction osteogenesis in, 153–155
alveolar preservation in, 134–136
alveolar ridge discrepancies in, 150–151
alveolar ridge extension procedures in, 142–147
alveoloplasty in, 136
anesthesia in, 130
bone grafts and, 132–134
bone regeneration in, 131–132
CT evaluation for, 129–130
edentulism and, 123–125
exostoses treatment in, 136
fibrous inflammatory hyperplasia in, 140
floor-of-mouth-lowering procedures in, 145, 146*f*, 147*f*
genial tubercle reduction in, 137
hard tissue augmentation in, 148–155
hard tissue examination for, 126–128
hard tissue recontouring in, 134–139
history of, 123
hypermobile tissue in, 140
inferior border augmentation, 151–152
inflammatory papillary hyperplasia in, 140
inlay grafts in, 149–150
interpositional grafts in, 149, 150*f*, 152, 153*f*
labial frenectomy in, 140–142
lingual frenectomy in, 142
lip-switch, in preprosthetic surgery, 145, 146*f*
mandibular augmentation in, 151–152, 153*f*
mandibular vestibuloplasty in, 145, 146*f*, 147*f*
maxillary augmentation in, 148–150
maxillary vestibuloplasty in, 143–144
medical considerations in, 125–130
mylohyoid ridge reduction in, 139
onlay grafts in, 149
pedicled grafts in, 152, 153*f*
radiographic evaluation for, 128–130
ridge-split osteoplasty in, 148–149
sinus lifts in, 149–150
soft tissue examination for, 126–128
soft tissue recontouring in, 139–140
submucous vestibuloplasty in, 142–143
tori removal in, 138–139
treatment planning considerations in, 130–131
tuberosity reduction in, 136–137
Preseptal orbicularis muscle, 1517*f*
Pretarsal orbicularis muscle, 1517*f*
Pretrichial forehead and brow lift, 1585–1586
Primary interosseous squamous cell carcinoma, 643
Primary survey, trauma, 328–344

Primitive knot, 1190*f*

Primitive streak, 1190*f*

Procerus muscle, 1532*f*, 1575, 1576*f*

Progesterone, for obstructive sleep apnea, 1498

Proliferative phase, of wound healing, 5–6, 5*f*

Promethazine, 61*f*

Propofol, 46*f*, 50–51

Prostheses

craniofacial, 315–319

auricular considerations, 316–317

color of, 319

construction of, 318–319

nasal, 319

surgical considerations, 316–317

templates for, 317–318

tinting of, 319

with cranial implants, 316

without cranial implants, 316

dental

abutment fracture with, 225

abutments in, 208–209

aesthetic zone and, 210–211

biomechanical considerations in, 201–209

bone loss and, 239–246

bone volume assessment for, 202

bruxism and, 202

cemented, single-tooth, 211–212

complications with, 224–225

cone beam CT evaluation of, 184–187, 187–191, 191–197, 198*f*, 203–204

contemporary techniques for, 218–222

crown-to-implant ratio with, 205, 206*f*

distances in, 202*f*

early placement of, 219

fixed detachable prostheses, 218

fixed partial dentures, 212–216

cantilevered, 215–216

in aesthetic zone, 212–214

in anterior mandible, 214

in posterior mandible, 215

in posterior maxilla, 214–215

for craniofacial defects, 224

for mandible defects, 222–223

for maxillary defects, 223

fracture of, 225

history of, 206–207

hyperbaric oxygen therapy and, 202

immediate placement of, 218–219

immediate restoration, 220–221

impressions for, 209

in full-arch restorations, 206

in growing child, 170–171

inferior alveolar nerve injury and, 922

maintenance of, 225–226

mandibular hard tissue preparation for, 269–281

mandibular site preparation for

for full-arch reconstruction, 274–279

for segmental defects, 272–274

for single tooth defects, 269–273

maxillofacial prostheses, 222–224

Morse taper in, 207, 208*f*

occlusion and, 205–206

osseointegration of

abutment positions and, 249–250

biology of, 229–248

biomechanics of, 238–248

bone loss and, 239–246

bruxism and, 252–253

cantilevers and, 251–252

clenching and, 252–253

early loading failure and, 246–248

history of, 229

implant materials and, 229–231

implant surfaces and, 231–238

mandibular edentulism and, 256–260

masticatory dynamics and, 253

maxillary edentulism and, 253–256

mechanical risk factors and, 251

number of plants and, 248–249

parafunctional habits and, 252–253

science of, 248–260

treatment planning, 248–260

with titanium, 229

with zirconia, 229–231

osteoporosis and, 202

overdentures

implant-retained, 216–217

implant-supported, 217–218

patient factors in, 201–202

peri-implant biology with, 201

periodontal disease and, 202

preprosthetic surgery for

alveolar distraction osteogenesis in, 153–155

alveolar preservation in, 134–136

alveolar ridge discrepancies in, 150–151

alveolar ridge extension procedures in, 142–147

alveoloplasty in, 136

anesthesia in, 130

bone grafts and, 132–134

bone regeneration and, 131–132

CT evaluation for, 129–130

edentulism and, 123–125

exostoses treatment in, 136

fibrous inflammatory hyperplasia in, 140

radiation exposure and, 202

radiographic bone loss with, 225

radiographic evaluation for, 202–204

radiotherapy and, 224

screw loosening with, 225

screw-retained, single-tooth, 211–212

selection of, 206–209

single-tooth replacement, 210–212

soft tissue complications with, 224–225

soft tissue evaluation for, 201–202

soft tissues management with

abutment connection, 284, 285*f*

acellular dermal matrix with grafting, 299–300

augmentation of, 287

epithelialized palatal graft and, 288–290

flap management considerations, 283–286

grafting and, 286–287, 287–300

integration of, 283

lateral flap advancement and, 286

nonsubmerged implant placement, 284, 285*f*

papilla regeneration and, 285–286

resective contouring and, 285

subepithelial connective tissue grafting, 290–295

submerged implant placement, 283–284

surgical maneuvers and, 285–286

vascularized interpositional periosteal connective tissue flap, 295–299

success criteria, 226

surfaces of, 231–238

acid etching of, 233–234

additive, 234–236

alterations to, 232–238

bioactive proteins and, 237–238

bisphosphonates for, 238
blasting of, 233, 234
bone morphogenic proteins and, 237–238
calcium phosphate treatment of, 237
cytokines and, 238
fluoride treatment of, 237
hydrophilic, 236
hydrophobic, 236
hydroxyapatite coating of, 234–235
laser etching of, 236
nanotechnology in, 237
oxidation for, 235–236
pharmacologic coatings for, 238
subtractive, 233
surface energy, 236
titanium plasma spray for, 234
surgical installation stability with, 219–220
surgical stents and, 204–205
for obstructive sleep apnea, 1498–1500
Prostheses, dental
mandibular site preparation for
for segmental defects
anterior, 273–274
posterior, 274
for single tooth defects
mandibular canine-bicuspid, 271
mandibular incisor, 269–271
molar, 272
osseointegration of
implant surfaces and
acid etching of, 233–234
additive, 234–236
alterations to, 232–238
bioactive proteins and, 237–238
bisphosphonates for, 238
blasting of, 233, 234
bone morphogenic proteins and, 237–238
calcium phosphate treatment of, 237
cytokines and, 238
fluoride treatment of, 237
hydrophilic, 236
hydrophobic, 236
hydroxyapatite coating of, 234–235
laser etching of, 236
nanotechnology in, 237
oxidation for, 235–236
pharmacologic coatings for, 238
subtractive, 233
surface energy, 236
titanium plasma spray for, 234
Prosthetic heart valve replacement, 20–21
Protriptyline, for obstructive sleep apnea, 1498
Pseudogout, in temporomandibular joint, 1101
Pseudoptosis, 1516
Psychiatric disorders, craniosynostosis and, 980
Psychological assessment, of pediatric patients, 72
Psychotherapy, for temporomandibular disorder, 1058–1059
Pterygoid muscles, in temporomandibular joint, 1039–1040
Pulmonary edema, 26
Pulmonary embolus (PE), 25–26
Purpura, 816

R
Radial artery fasciocutaneous flap, 901–902
Radiation injury
craniofacial implants and, 315
dental implants and, 202
wound healing and, 11

Radiography. *See also* Imaging; *specific modalities*
for dental implant pre-evaluation, 202–204
for nasal fracture, 539–540
for preprosthetic surgery, 128–130
Radionuclide imaging, in oral disease diagnosis, 618–619
Radiotherapy
dental implants and, 224
for oral cancer, 699–701
for skin cancer, 755
osteoradionecrosis and, 868–870
temporomandibular hypomobility after, 1158–1159
Radix, 1598
Ranulas, 835
Rapid ventricular response (RVR), 21
Reconstruction
flaps in
advancement, 879–880
anterolateral thigh, 903–904
blood supply, 878
complications, 890–891
deltopectoral, 888
design, 879
hyperbaric oxygen therapy and, 890–891
iliac crest free, 914–917
interpolation, 884–886
lateral arm free, 905–906
latissimus dorsi myocutaneous, 889–890, 900–901, 905
local, 879–886
microvascular soft tissue, 901–906
nomenclature, 878–879
pectoralis major myocutaneous, 886–887, 898–900
principles, 877–878
radial artery fasciocutaneous, 901–902
rectus abdominis myocutaneous, 904–905
regional, 886–890, 894–901
rotation, 880–881
scapula free, 914
sternocleidomastoid, 889
submental island, 894–895
temporalis, 888–889, 895–898
transposition, 881–884
trapezius myocutaneous, 889
types of, 879–890
overview of, 893–894
techniques for
hard tissue, 906–917
soft tissue, 894–907
Recontouring
hard tissue, in preprosthetic surgery, 134–139
soft tissue, in preprosthetic surgery, 139–140
Rectal administration, for pediatric sedation, 79
Rectus abdominis myocutaneous flap, 904–905
Recurrent aphthous stomatitis, 801–802
Regeneration, bone, 131–132
Regional flaps, 886–890, 894–901
Relaxation, for temporomandibular disorder, 1058
Relaxed skin tension lines (RSTLs), 877
REM sleep, 1493–1494
Remifentanil, 48f, 49
Remodeling phase, of wound healing, 6
Renal disease, 27–28
Renal failure, 27
Replacement resorption, of root, 395
Resective contouring, 285
Resorption
classification of, 127f
root

inflammatory, 395
replacement, 395
surface, 395
root canal
inflammatory, 395
internal replacement, 395
Respiratory disease, 23–26
Respiratory monitoring, 74–75
Respiratory system, in geriatric patients, 73
Resurfacing, 1591, 1617–1620
Retinoids, for skin cancer, 756
Retrobulbar hemorrhage, with zygomatic complex fractures, 479
Retromolar trigone, oral cancer in, 706
Revised Trauma Score, 327
Rheumatoid arthritis, in temporomandibular joint, 1100–1101, 1159
Rhinoplasty
alar base reduction in, 1551, 1552f
alar width in, 1541
anatomy in, 1531–1537
anesthesia for, 1541
complete transfixion in, 1542
cosmetic evaluation in, 1537–1538
facial analysis in, 1538
functional considerations in, 1541
hemitransfixion in, 1542
incisions in, 1541–1543
intercartilaginous incision in, 1542–1543
intracartilaginous incision in, 1543
Killian incision in, 1542
marginal incision in, 1543
nasal analysis in, 1538, 1539f
nasal dorsum assessment in, 1539, 1541
nasal dorsum augmentation in, 1546–1547
nasal dorsum reduction in, 1546
nasal tip definition in, 1539–1540
nasal tip projection in, 1539–1540, 1548–1550
nasal tip rotation in, 1540, 1550
nasal tip shape in, 1550–1551
nasofrontal angle assessment in, 1538, 1539f
osteotomies in, 1547
partial transfixion in, 1542
postoperative management in, 1551
psychiatric stability and, 1537
rim incision in, 1543
septoplasty in, 1543–1545
sequencing in, 1541–1543
skin assessment for, 1538
symmetry assessment for, 1538–1541
transcolumellar incision in, 1543
turbinectomy in, 1545
Rhytidectomy
complications in, 1564–1566
facial nerve injury in, 1565
flap development in, 1560–1563
hematoma in, 1564–1565
history of, 1555–1556
neurosensory disturbances after, 1566
overview of, 1555
patient evaluation for, 1556–1557
requirements, 1556t
skin closure in, 1563
skin slough in, 1565–1566
superficial-plane, 1557–1563
surgical technique, 1557–1563
Rib, as bone grafting source, 969t
Ridge-split osteoplasty, in preprosthetic surgery, 148–149
Rifles, 548, 549

Rigid internal fixation, 373
Rocuronium, 59t
Root canal resorption
inflammatory, 395
internal replacement, 395
Root fracture, 394
Root resorption
inflammatory, 395
replacement, 395
surface, 395
Rostral neuropore, 1191f
Rotation flaps, 880–881
RSTLs. See Relaxed skin tension lines (RSTLs)
RVR. See Rapid ventricular response (RVR)

S
Sagittal synostosis, 982, 988–991. See also Craniosynostosis
Saliva, composition of, 775t, 776t
Salivary ducts, in gunshot wounds, 559
Salivary gland disease
autoimmune, 783–784
complications in surgical treatment of, 789
cystic, 781–782, 835
diagnostic modalities for, 773–778
general considerations in, 773
in HIV infection, 783
in pediatric patients, 834–836
inflammatory, 782–783
neoplastic, 785–789, 835–836
nonneoplastic, 778–784
obstructive, 778–781
Salivary gland infections, 783
Salivary gland injury, after orthognathic surgery, 1451
SARPE. See Surgically assisted rapid palatal expansion (SARPE)
Sathre-Chotzen syndrome, 1025. See also Dysostosis syndromes
Scalp
blood supply to, 570f
in pediatric facial trauma, 575–577
soft tissue trauma in, 364
Scapha buckling, 1607
Scaphoconchal angle, 1598
Scaphoid fossa, 1598, 1600f
Scapula free flap, 914
Scarring, after orthognathic surgery, 1451
Schwannoma, 669
Scleroderma, temporomandibular hypomobility and, 1159–1160
Scopolamine, 60t
Screw loosening, with dental implants, 225
Seborrheic keratosis, 813–814
Secobarbital, 51f
Secondary assessment, in trauma, 344–354
Sedation
conscious, 63t
deep, 63t
femoral vein access for, 77, 77f
goals of, 63–64
in pediatric patients, 76–84
intramuscular route of administration for, 78
ketamine for, 79–81
level of, 63
midazolam for, 81–82
minimal, 63t
nasal route for, 78
oral route of administration for, 78
rectal route for, 79
routes of administration for, in pediatric patient, 76–79
transmucosal route for, 78–79

Seddon nerve injury classification, 926*t*

Seizures, 35

Sentinel node biopsy, 716–717

Sentinel vein, 1578, 1580*f*

Septic arthritis, in temporomandibular joint, 1043–1044

Septoplasty, 1543–1545

Serotonin receptor antagonists, 86

Serum, 523*t*

Sevoflurane, 54*t*, 56–57, 57*f*

Shock, hypovolemic, 340–343

Shotguns, 548, 550–551. *See also* Gunshot wounds

Shunting, 23

Sialoadenitis, acute suppurative, 783

Sialography, in oral disease diagnosis, 618

Sialolithiasis, 778–781

Sickle cell anemia, 29

Silicone agents, in pediatric facial trauma, 581

Single-tooth replacement, 210–212

    cemented, 211

    edentulous arch and, 210

    in aesthetic zone, 210–211

    mandibular, site preparation for, 269–273

    screw-retained, 211–212

Sinus lifts, in preprosthetic surgery, 149–150

Sinusitis, 857–858

Skin biomechanics, 758

Skin cancer

    lasers for, 756

    melanoma, 749–751, 814–815

        biopsy strategies, 751*t*

        clinical description, 749–751

        histologic description, 749–751

        risk factors, 749

        survival rates, 751*t*

    nonmelanoma, 743–749

        basal cell carcinoma, 746

        chemotherapy for, 756

        cryosurgery for, 755

        curettage and electrodesiccation for, 755–756

        environmental factors, 745

        epidemiology of, 743

        etiology of, 743–746

        grafting in, 757–768

        immunologic factors, 744

        interferons for, 756

        management of, 751–768

        Mohs' micrographic surgery for, 753–755

        photodynamic therapy for, 756

        predisposing lesions, 744

        prevention of, 745–746

        radiation therapy for, 755

        retinoids for, 756

        squamous cell carcinoma, 746–749

        standard excision of, 752

        syndromes in, 744

Skin grafts

    full thickness, 8

    healing of, 8

    in skin cancer, 757–768

    split thickness, 8

Skin peel, 1613–1615

Skin resurfacing, 1591

Skin slough, in rhytidectomy, 1565–1566

Skin tension lines, relaxed, 877

Skin, pigmented lesions of, 811–817

Skull assessment, in trauma, 344–348

Sleep apnea

    central, 1494

    classification of, 1494

    differential diagnosis of, 1494–1495

    mixed, 1494

    obstructive

        cephalometric examination in, 1496–1497

        clinical manifestations of, 1495

        complications of surgery for, 1507–1508

        continuous positive airway pressure for, 1500

        CT in, 1497

        diagnosis of, 1496–1498

        differential diagnosis of, 1494–1495

        Herbst appliance for, 1499

        history of, 1495

        in dysostosis syndromes, 997–998

        medical treatment of, 1498–1500

        nasal surgery for, 1500–1501

        oral appliances for, 1498–1500

        orthognathic surgery for, 1502–1506

        oxygen therapy for, 1498

        physical examination in, 1496

        physical findings in, 1495

        polysomnography in, 1497

        progesterone for, 1498

        protriptyline for, 1498

        site of obstruction in, 1497–1498

        surgical treatment of, 1500–1506

        tongue-retaining device for, 1499

        tracheostomy for, 1500

        uvulopalatopharyngoplasty for, 1501–1502

        uvulopalatoplasty for, 1502

    syndrome, 1494–1495

Sleep stages, 1493–1494

Smile, excessive gingival display on, 1255

Smith-Nephew system, 1082, 1083*f*

Smoking, 65

Soft tissues

    in implant therapy

        abutment connection, 284, 285*f*

        acellular dermal matrix with grafting, 299–300

        augmentation of, 287

        epithelialized palatal graft and, 288–290

        flap management considerations, 283–286

        grafting and, 286–287, 287–300

        integration of, 283

        lateral flap advancement and, 286

        nonsubmerged implant placement, 284, 285*f*

        papilla regeneration and, 285–286

        resective contouring and, 285

        subepithelial connective tissue grafting, 290–295

        submerged implant placement, 283–284

        surgical maneuvers and, 285–286

        vascularized interpositional periosteal connective tissue flap, 295–299

    trauma

        abrasions, 362

        anatomic evaluation for, 358

        animal bites, 363

        avulsive injuries, 362–363

        basic repair technique, 358–362

        contusions, 362

        gunshot wounds, 363–364

        human bites, 363

        in ear, 367, 368*f*, 369*f*

        in eyelid, 364–366

        in forehead, 364

        in lip, 370

        in nasolacrimal apparatus, 364–366

in neck, 370–371
in nose, 367
in pediatric facial trauma, 568–569
in scalp, 364
lacerations, 362
management principles, 357
postoperative wound care for, 371
regional considerations, 364–371
repair sequence, 358–362
types of injuries, 362–364
Somites, 1190, 1191*f*
Sphenopalatine artery, 1534*f*
Sphenozygomatic suture, in panfacial fractures, 595–596
Spinal cord assessment, in trauma, 350–352
Splinting
for mandibular fracture, 410–412
for maxillary fracture, 460–461
model surgery and, 1309–1310
Squamous cell carcinoma, in skin cancer, 746–749
Stabilization appliance, for temporomandibular disorder, 1059–1060
Stafne's bone defect, 668–669
Stents, surgical, implants and, 204–205
Stereolithography, in facial asymmetry evaluation, 1398
Sternocleidomastoid flap, 889
Sternomastoid muscle, 1600*f*
Steroids
in third molar extraction, 112–113
wound healing and, 10–11
Stomach, full, 67
Stomatitis
areata migrans, 802
chronic ulcerative, 806
infectious, 795–801
noninfectious, 801–811
Stomodeum, 1192*f*
Stress reduction, for temporomandibular disorder, 1058
Stylohyoid branch, of facial nerve, 359*f*
Subapical osteotomies, 1347–1349
Subluxation, periodontal, 396
Submental island flap, 894–895
Submentovertex view, 469
Submucous vestibuloplasty, in preprosthetic surgery, 142–143
Substance abuse, as surgical comorbidity, 38, 67–69
Succinylcholine, 58, 59*t*, 85
Sufentanil, 46*f*, 48*f*, 49
Sunderland nerve injury classification, 926*t*
Superficial temporal artery, 1579*f*, 1600*f*
Superior auricularis muscle, 1600*f*
Superior crus, 1600*f*
Superior labial artery, 1533*f*, 1534*f*
Superior oblique muscle, 1519*f*
Superior orbital fissure syndrome, with zygomatic complex fractures, 479
Superior rectus muscle, 1517*f*, 1519*f*
Supernumerary teeth, in pediatric patients, 168
Suprahyoid muscles, in temporomandibular joint, 1040
Supraorbital artery, 1533*f*, 1579*f*
Supratrochlear artery, 1533*f*, 1579*f*
Supratrochlear nerves, 1579–1580
Supraventricular tachycardia (SVT), 21
Surface resorption, of root, 395
Surgically assisted rapid palatal expansion (SARPE), 1384–1387
Survey, primary trauma, 328–344
Sutures, cranial, 1201*f*. *See also* Craniosynostosis; Dysostosis syndromes
SVT. *See* Supraventricular tachycardia (SVT)
Sympathetic ophthalmia, 495–496
Sympathetically maintained pain, in temporomandibular disorder, 1064–1065

Synostosis, cranial. *See also* Dysostosis syndromes
bilateral coronal, 981, 985
brain development and, 980
classification of, 980–983
definition of, 979
diagnosis of, 980
functional considerations with, 979–980
intracranial hypertension with, 979
management principles, 983–984
metopic, 981–982, 985–988
multidisciplinary team approach in, 983–984
nonsyndromic, 979–992
psychiatric disorders and, 980
sagittal, 982, 988–991
surgical considerations for, 984–991
unilateral coronal, 980–981, 984–985
unilateral lambdoid, 983, 991
visual impairment in, 979
Synovectomy, for temporomandibular disorder, 1108
Synovial chondromatosis, 658–659, 1045, 1100
Synovitis, temporomandibular joint, 1100
Synovium, in temporomandibular joint, 1034–1036
Syphilis, 795–796

T
Tachycardia
supraventricular, 21
ventricular, 21
Taper, Morse, 207, 208*f*
Tarsus, 1517*f*
Taste, assessment of, 928–929
Tattoos, 816–817
TCA. *See* Trichloroacetic acid (TCA)
Teeth. *See also specific teeth*
ankylosis, 1267–1268
development of, 1207–1209
impacted
bonding of, 103–105
clinical evaluation of, 100
comorbidities and, 103
contraindications for treatment of, 102–103
etiology of, 97–99
exposure of, 103–105
first molar, 167–168
in geriatric patients, 103
in pediatric patients, 103, 159–168
incidence of, 97–99
mandibular premolars, in pediatric patients, 163–165, 166*f*
maxillary canine
cone beam CT of, 181–183
in pediatric patients, 160–163
maxillary incisor, in pediatric patients, 165–167
maxillary premolars, in pediatric patients, 163–165, 166*f*
overview of, 97
removal of, 106–107
second molar, 167–168
surgery for, 103–113
third molars
adjacent teeth root reabsorption and, 102
alveolar osteitis after extraction of, 114–115
antibiotics in extraction of, 112–113
bleeding after extraction of, 113–114
dental caries and, 101
dental prostheses and, 102
incidence and etiology of, 99–100
indications for removal of, 101–102
jaw fracture risk and, 102

mandibular incisor crowning and, 101–102
nerve disturbances after removal of, 115
odontogenic cysts and tumors and, 102
orthodontic considerations with, 101–102
orthognathic surgery and, 102
pain after extraction of, 114
pain from, 102
pericoronitis and, 101
periodontal healing after extraction of, 116–117
periodontitis and, 101
postoperative complications after extraction of, 114–116
postoperative course for, 113–114
rare complications for, 115–116
steroids in extraction of, 112–113
stiffness after extraction of, 114
surgery for, 107–113
swelling after extraction of, 114
tooth fracture after extraction of, 114
transplantation for, 105–106
treatment of, 100–113
unerupted *vs.,* 97
uprighting of, 105
in dysostosis syndromes, 998
mandibular fracture, in line of, 420–421
nonrestorable, 210
size analysis, 1264–1265
supernumerary, 168
transplantation of, 105–106, 169–170
unerupted, impacted *vs.,* 97
Telangiectasia, 815
Telecanthus, 498–499
Telephone ear deformity, 1607
Temporal bone, in temporomandibular joint, 1033–1034
Temporal implants, 304
Temporal lift, 1590
Temporalis fascia, 1576–1577
Temporalis flap, 888–889, 895–898
Temporalis muscle, 1038, 1576–1577
Temporofacial nerve, 1600*f*
Temporomandibular arthroscopy
abraders in, 1085
advantages of, 1070
anatomy in, 1087–1090
anterior recess in, 1099–1100
anti-inflammatory management after, 1116
antibiotics after, 1116
armamentarium for, 1082–1085
articular disk in, 1095–1098
biopsy forceps in, 1082, 1084*f*
cannulas in, 1082
chondromalacia grading in, 1102–1104
complications of, 1118–1121
contraindications, 1070
danger zones in, 1086–1087
diagnostic sweep in, 1092–1100
diet after, 1116
disk reduction for, 1109
electrosurgery in, 1085–1086
facial nerve trauma in, 1118–1119
fibrocartilage scuffing in, 1119
for anterior release, 1108–1109
for botulinum toxin A delivery, 1107
for débridement, 1107
for diskopexy, 1109–1116
for hyaluronic acid delivery, 1107
for lysis and lavage, 1105–1107
for medication delivery, 1107

for posterior scarification/cauterization, 1109
for second puncture, 1104–1105
for steroid delivery, 1107
for synovectomy, 1108
fossa puncture in, 1090–1091
full-radius shaver in, 1085
glenoid fossa perforation in, 1120
goals of, 1069
hemarthrosis in, 1120
history of, 1069
immediate preoperative steps for, 1090
indications for, 1070
infection from, 1120–1121
instrument failure in, 1121
insufflation in, 1090
intermediate zone in, 1098–1099
laser in, 1086
maxillary artery damage in, 1120
medial synovial drape in, 1092–1093
meniscus mender in, 1082–1083, 1084*f*
nerve injury in, 1118–1119
On Point system for, 1081–1082
operative procedures in, 1104–1116
outflow needle puncture in, 1091
pain management after, 1116
palpation of anatomy in, 1090
patient evaluation for, 1070–1072
physical examination for, 1072–1078
physiotherapy after, 1117–1118
portals of entry for, 1086
postoperative patient management in, 1116
postoperative rehabilitation for, 1117–1118
probes in, 1082, 1084*f*
pterygoid shadow in, 1093–1094
retrodiskal synovium in, 1094
shavers in, 1083
Smith-Nephew system for, 1082, 1083*f*
technique for, 1090–1102
trigeminal nerve trauma in, 1119
vestibulocochlear trauma in, 1119
video, 1080–1082
whisker shaver in, 1085
Temporomandibular disorder (TMD). *See also* Temporomandibular joint
derangement
acupressure for, 1058
acupuncture for, 1058
analgesics for, 1051
anterior release for, 1108–1109
anterior repositioning appliance for, 1060
anti-inflammatory medications for, 1051–1053
antidepressants for, 1053–1054
antihistamines for, 1053
anxiolytics for, 1053
assessment form, 1071–1072, 1074*f*–1075*f*
biofeedback for, 1058
corticosteroids for, 1052–1053
débridement for, 1107
definition of, 1049
deformities in, 1073–1076
diet in, 1050
disk reduction for, 1109
diskopexy for, 1109–1116
electrical stimulation for, 1057
end-stage
autogenous bone grafting for, 1174–1176
overview of, 1173–1174
transport distraction osteogenesis for, 1176–1178

etiology of, 1049, 1073–1077
exercise therapy for, 1055–1056
imaging in, 1073
intra-articular botulinum toxin for, 1107
intra-articular hyaluronic acid for, 1107
intra-articular steroids for, 1107
iontophoresis for, 1057–1058
local anesthetics for, 1054
locking in, 1073
lysis and lavage for, 1105–1107
Mahan's sign in, 1073, 1076f
mouth opening in, 1072
muscle relaxants for, 1054, 1055t
noise in, 1072
nonsteroidal anti-inflammatory drugs for, 1052
nonsurgical therapy for, 1050–1064
occlusal adjustment for, 1060
occlusal appliances for, 1059–1060
orthognathic surgery and, 1447
pain assessment in, 1072–1073
panoramic radiograph in, 1073
pharmacotherapy for, 1050–1054
phonophoresis for, 1057
physical therapy for, 1054–1058
posterior scarification/cauterization for, 1109
psychotherapy for, 1058–1059
range of motion in, 1072
relaxation for, 1058
second puncture for, 1104–1105
stabilization appliance for, 1059–1060
stress reduction techniques for, 1058
sympathetically maintained pain in, 1064–1065
synovectomy for, 1108
thermal agents for, 1056–1057
treatment considerations in, 1049–1050
trigger point injections for, 1058
ultrasound therapy for, 1057
Temporomandibular hypermobility
    classification of, 1166–1167
    etiology of, 1167
    treatment considerations with, 1167–1169
Temporomandibular hypomobility
    ankylosing spondylitis and, 1159
    classification of, 1155
    clinical presentation of, 1155–1156
    complications associated with treatment of, 1162–1166
    etiology of, 1155, 1156t
    imaging assessment of, 1156
    inflammatory causes, 1159–1160
    orthognathic surgery and, 1160
    physical therapy for, postoperative, 1166
    post-traumatic, 1156–1157
    postcraniotomy, 1159
    postinfectious, 1157–1158
    radiation therapy and, 1158–1159
    rheumatologic causes, 1159–1160
    scleroderma and, 1159–1160
    treatment considerations with, 1160–1162
Temporomandibular joint (TMJ)
    articular disk in, 1036
    articular disorders of, 1041–1043
    articular dysfunction in, 1102
    as compound joint, 1033
    as diarthrodial joint, 1033
    benign tumors of, 1045
    biomechanics of, 1040
    bony structures in, 1033–1034

cartilage in, 1034–1035
chondrocalcinosis in, 1101
classification of, 1033
fibrosis, 1100
ganglion cysts in, 1045
infections of, 1043–1044
infrahyoid muscles in, 1040
inframandibular muscle group in, 1040
innervation of, 1037–1038
joint stenosis in, 1101–1102
lateral pterygoid muscle in, 1039–1040
ligaments in, 1036–1037
malignant tumors in, 1045
mandible in, 1034
masseter muscle in, 1039
medial pterygoid muscle in, 1039
musculature of, 1038–1040
neoplastic disease in, 1044–1045
nonarticular disorders of, 1040–1041
osteoarthritis in, 1102
pathology, 1040–1045
pseudogout in, 1101
pterygoid muscles in, 1039–1040
replacement
    alloplastic, 1178–11182
    bioengineered tissue for, 1178
    indications for, 1173t
retrodiskal tissue in, 1036
rheumatoid arthritis in, 1100–1101, 1159
septic arthritis in, 1043–1044
suprahyoid muscles in, 1040
supramandibular muscle group in, 1038–1040
synovial chondromatosis in, 1100
synovial tumors in, 1045
synovitis in, 1100
synovium in, 1034–1036
temporal bone in, 1033–1034
temporalis muscle in, 1038
vascular supply of, 1037–1038
villonodular synovitis in, 1100
Temporomandibular joint derangement. *See also* Temporomandibular
    disorder (TMD)
    anchored disc phenomenon in, 1125
    bruxism and, 1124
    clinical course of, 1123–1124
    diagnosis of, 1124–1126
    disc displacement in, 1125
    etiologic factors in, 1124
    goals of surgery for, 1128
    imaging of, 1125–1126
    indications for surgery, 1128
    joint incoordination in, 1125
    joint laxity and, 1124
    joint lubrication and, 1124
    outcomes assessment in, 1128
    pathophysiology of, 1123–1124
    surgery for, open, 1129–1150
        anatomy in, 1129
        auriculotemporal nerve in, 1130
        capsular incisions in, 1134–1135
        complications of, 1148–1150
        disc repair in, 1140–1142
        disc replacement in, 1144–1147
        disc repositioning in, 1135–1140
        discectomy in, 1142–1144
        endaural approach for, 1132
        facial nerve in, 1129

fascial layers in, 1129
maxillary artery in, 1130–1131
modified mandibular condylotomy in, 1147–1148
neurologic injury in, 1150
perioperative complications, 1150
postauricular approach for, 1132–1134
postoperative management for, 1148
preauricular approach for, 1131–1132
procedures in, 1135–1150
superficial temporal vessels in, 1130
vascular injury in, 1150
wound closure in, 1135
trauma and, 1124
Temporoparietal fascia, 1576*f*
Tenon's capsule, 1517*f*
TENS, for temporomandibular disorder, 1057
Tension lines, relaxed skin, 877
Tension pneumothorax, 333, 334*f*
Terminal ballistics, 546
Test(s)
clinical neurosensory, 925–929
Goldman visual field, 489*f*
pregnancy, 67
taste, 928–929
Thiamylal, 51*f*
Thigh flap, anterolateral, 903–904
Thiopental, 46*f*, 51*f*, 53
Three-dimensional imaging
for mandibular diagnostics, 191–197, 198if
of mandibular implants, 184–187
of maxillary canine impaction, 181–183
overview of, 179–180
to assess potential graft augmentation, 187–191
Three-dimensional virtual model surgical simulation, 1310–1315
Thrombocytopenia, 30
Thyroglossal duct cyst, 833
Thyroid disease, 32
TIAs. *See* Transient ischemic attacks (TIAs)
Tibial bone graft, 909, 969*t*
Tip-defining point, 1534
Tissue perfusion, wound healing and, 10
Titanium
osseointegration and, 229
plasma spray, 234
TMAO. *See* Total maxillary alveolar osteotomy (TMAO)
TMD. *See* Temporomandibular disorder (TMD)
TMJ. *See* Temporomandibular joint (TMJ)
Tongue
assessment, in orthodontics for orthognathic surgery, 1269–1270
geographic, 802
oral cancer in, 706–708
Tongue-retaining device (TRD), for obstructive sleep apnea, 1499
Topical chemotherapy, for skin cancer, 756
Tori, 671–673
maxillary and mandibular, removal of, in preprosthetic surgery, 138–139
Torus mandibularis, 672–673
Torus palatinus, 671–672
Total mandibular subapical alveolar osteotomy, 1349–1350
Total maxillary alveolar osteotomy (TMAO), 1384
Total midface deformity, 1006–1012, 1015
Tracheostomy, for obstructive sleep apnea, 1500
Tragus, 1600*f*
Transient ischemic attacks (TIAs), 35
Transmucosal route of administration, for pediatric sedation, 78–79
Transplantation
for impacted teeth, 105–106
of teeth, 169–170

Transport distraction osteogenesis, for end-stage temporomandibular joint disease, 1176–1178
Transposition flaps, 881–884
Transverse artery, 1600*f*
Transverse facial artery, 1579*f*
Transverse facial characteristics, 1255–1256
Transverse facial proportions, 1248–1252
Transverse nasalis muscle, 1532*f*
Trapezius myocutaneous, 889
Trauma
abdomen assessment in, 352–353
airway maintenance in, 328–330
algorithm, 329*f*
bleeding control in, 338–339, 340*f*, 341*f*
breathing in initial survey for, 330–336
cervical spine control in, 328–330
chest assessment in, 348–349
circulation in initial survey for, 336–343
extremities assessment in, 354
facial nerve
in rhytidectomy, 1565
in temporomandibular arthroscopy, 1118–1119
flail chest, 334–336
fracture
alveolar
classification of, 390–392
Ellis classification, 392*f*
etiology of, 388
history in, 388–389
history of, 387
in pediatric patients, 589
incidence of, 388
maxillofacial examination for, 389–390
physical examination for, 388–389
radiography for, 390
treatment of, 400–403
anterior table, 528
cranial, anterior, in pediatric patients, 583–589
crown, 393–394
crown-root, 394
edentulism and risk of, 125
enamel, 392
facial, in pediatric patients, 581–583
frontal sinus
anatomy in, 519–522
anterior table fracture in, 528
classification of, 524–525
clinical findings in, 522–524
complications of, 531–532
deformity correction, 532–534
endoscopy in, 530
imaging of, 524
medical therapy, postoperative, 531
naso frontal outflow tract evaluation in, 527–528
naso frontal outflow tract obstruction in, 529
naso-orbitoethmoid complex reconstruction in, 530–531
orbital roof reconstruction in, 528
osseous recovery in, 526–527
patient evaluation in, 522–525
physiology in, 519–522
posterior table, 528
sinus obliteration in, 529–530
supraorbital bar reconstruction in, 528
surgical access in, 526
treatment of, 525–531
jaw, third molar impaction and risk of, 102
mandible

anatomical distribution of, 409*f*
angle, 425–427
bilateral, 427, 428*f*
biomechanical considerations in, 410
body, 421–425, 589
classification of, 409
closed treatment of, 417
comminuted, 428, 429*f*
complications of, 432–433
diagnosis of, 416–417
edentulous atrophic, 428–432
epidemiology of, 408–409
hardware selection for, 418–420
historical perspectives on, 407–408, 410–414
in pediatric patients, 588
infection with, 432–433
load-bearing fixation for, 377*f*
malunion with, 433
nonunion with, 433
operative management of, 417–432
parasymphysis, 421–425
pediatric, 432
preoperative management of, 417
rigid fixation schemes for, 374*f*
single *vs.* multiple, 383–385
splinting for, 410–412
surgical approach for, 418
symphysis, 421–425, 589
teeth in line of, 420–421
treatment of, 410–414
wiring for, 412–414, 417–418
mandibular
    anatomical distribution of, 409*f*
    angle, 425–427
    bilateral, 427, 428*f*
    biomechanical considerations in, 410
    body, 421–425
    classification of, 409
    closed treatment of, 417
    comminuted, 428, 429*f*
    complications of, 432–433
    diagnosis of, 416–417
    edentulous atrophic, 428–432
    epidemiology of, 408–409
    hardware selection for, 418–420
    historical perspectives on, 407–408, 410–414
    infection with, 432–433
    load-bearing fixation for, 377*f*
    malunion with, 433
    nonunion with, 433
    operative management of, 417–432
    parasymphysis, 421–425
    pediatric, 432
    preoperative management of, 417
    rigid fixation schemes for, 374*f*
    single *vs.* multiple, 383–385
    splinting for, 410–412
    surgical approach for, 418
    symphysis, 421–425
    teeth in line of, 420–421
    treatment of, 410–414
    wiring for, 412–414, 417–418
mandibular condyle
    anatomic types of, 443–444
    bruxism and, 451
    chronic pain and, 451
    closed treatment of, 445–446

condylar head, 444
condylar neck, 443, 444*f*
deviation on opening with, 442–443
disc injury in, 451
evidence-based approach to, 452
facial asymmetry in, 1396–1397
functional anatomic alterations with, 442–444
functional anatomy in, 441–442
glenoid fossa fracture and, 451
in pediatric patients, 588–589
infection risk and, 450–451
intercuspation and, 442
laterognathia and, 442
masseteric hypertrophy and, 451
mouth opening limitation with, 443
occlusal considerations in, 451
occlusal prematurity with, 442
osteoarthrosis and, 451
outcomes in, 447–452
overview of, 441
patient age and, 450
patient compliance and, 450
patient gender and, 450
ramus shortening and, 451–452
scarring and, 451
subcondylar, 443
systemic disease and, 450
treatment of, 444–452
maxillary
    anatomy in, 456–457
    avulsive, 461
    clinical examination for, 457–458
    complications of, 462–463
    diagnosis of, 457–458
    fixation for, 459–460
    high-force, 461
    history of, 455
    in geriatric patients, 461
    in pediatric patients, 587–588
    Le Fort classification, 455–456
    pediatric patients in, 461–462
    surgical splints for, 460–461
    treatment of, 458–463
nasal
    classification of, 541
    complications with, 542–543
    CT for, 540–541
    diagnostic tools for, 539–541
    nasal complex evaluation in, 540
    overview of, 539
    postoperative care for, 542–543
    radiography for, 539–541
    reduction of, 542
    sense of smell and, 542
    surgical anatomy of, 539
    surgical management of, 541–542
naso-orbitoethmoid fracture
    anatomy in, 519–522
    anterior table fracture in, 528
    classification of, 524–525
    clinical findings in, 522–524
    complications of, 531–532
    deformity correction, 532–534
    endoscopy in, 530
    imaging of, 524
    in pediatric patients, 585
    medical therapy, postoperative, 531

naso frontal outflow tract evaluation in, 527–528
naso frontal outflow tract obstruction in, 529
naso-orbitoethmoid complex reconstruction in,
  530–531
orbital roof reconstruction in, 528
osseous recovery in, 526–527
patient evaluation in, 522–525
physiology in, 519–522
posterior table, 528
sinus obliteration in, 529–530
supraorbital bar reconstruction in, 528
surgical access in, 526
treatment of, 525–531
nonoperative management of, 499–502
of dental implants, 225
orbital
  acute repair of, 507–515
  anatomy in, 483–487
  clinical examination for, 487–491
  configurations, 487
  CT of, 492
  decision diagram, 503f
  endoscopic approach, 507
  imaging of, 492–493
  indications for surgical repair of, 502
  inferior orbital approach, 504–505
  lateral orbital approach, 504–505
  medial orbital approach, 505–507
  MRI of, 492–493
  nonoperative management of, 499–502
  operative management of, 502–514
  superior orbital approach, 505–506
  surgical approaches for, 502–507
panfacial
  airway management in, 599
  anatomic considerations in, 594–596
  complications with, 602–605
  definition of, 593
  dental fractures in, 594–595
  etiology of, 593
  facial buttresses and, 594
  fracture management in, 599–602
  historic perspective on, 593
  imaging of, 596–597
  intercanthal region in, 596
  key landmarks in, 594
  mandible in, 594–595
  sequence of treatment for, 599–602
  soft tissue resuspension for, 599
  sphenozygomatic suture in, 595–596
  surgical approaches for, 597–599
  widening of facial complex in, 602–605
posterior table, 528
root, 394
tooth, after extraction of third molars, 114
zygomatic arch, 470–471
zygomaticomaxillary complex, in pediatric patients, 587
genitourinary tract assessment in, 353–354
Glasgow Coma Scale and, 327
gunshot wounds
  airway in management of, 551–552
  ammunition type and, 547t
  as cause of death, 545
  ballistics of, 546
  bone grafting for, 559–561
  circumstances of, 545–546
  classification of, 550

closed vs. open fracture management in, 559–561
contamination of, 558
controversies in management of, 559–561
delayed vs. early management of, 559–561
demographics of, 545–546
energy of, 546–548
facial nerve in, 559
firearm terminology in, 548–550
fragmentation in, 547
from shotguns, 550–551
hemorrhage control in, 552, 553f
history of, 545
infection of, 558
late reconstruction of, 561
management of, 551–558
neck injury in, penetrating, 554–555
nutrition and, 555
operative procedure for, 556–558
overview of, 363–364
penetration in, 547
permanent cavity in, 547
salivary ducts in, 559
temporary cavity in, 547
wounding power of, 546–548
head assessment in, 344–348
hemorrhage in, 338–339, 340f, 341f
hemothorax, 333–334
history of, 387
hypovolemic shock in, 340–343
in pediatric patients
  facial
    airway in evaluation of, 566
    airway injury in, 567–568
    anterior cranial fractures in, 583–589
    antibiotic ointments for, 580–581
    breathing in evaluation of, 566
    cheek in, 577–579, 580f
    circulation in evaluation of, 566
    dentoalveolar injuries in, 589
    disability in evaluation of, 566
    ear in, 569–571
    exposure in, 566–567
    eyelid in, 571–574
    facial fracture in, 581–583
    growth disturbance from, 590
    head injuries, 567–568
    history in, 565
    lacrimal apparatus in, 571–574
    lip in, 579–580
    mandible fracture in, 588
    mandibular body fracture in, 589
    mandibular condyle fracture in, 588–589
    mandibular symphysis fracture in, 589
    maxillary fracture in, 587–588
    mouth in, 579–580
    naso-orbitoethmoid fracture in, 585
    neck in, 567–568
    nose in, 574, 575f
    oral cavity in, 579–580
    perioperative management, 568
    physical evaluation in, 565–567
    regional soft tissue wounds in, 569–580
    scalp in, 575–577
    silicone agents for, 581
    soft tissue injuries in, 568–569
    wound care adjuncts for, 580–581
    zygomaticomaxillary complex fracture in, 587

injury severity assessment, 325–328
Injury Severity Score in, 327–328
lacrimal, 497–498
maxillary artery, in temporomandibular arthroscopy, 1120
maxillofacial area assessment in, 349–350
mortality from, 325
mortality prediction in, 327t
mortality rates, 328t
neck assessment in, 349–350
neurologic
    as surgical comorbidity, 34–35
    classification of, 924–925, 926f, 926t
    in orthognathic surgery, 1437–1440
    in temporomandibular joint derangement surgery, 1150
    legal issues and, 938–939
    microneurosurgery for
        approximation in, 936
        clinical evaluation for, 919
        clinical neurosensory testing and, 925–929
        coaptation in, 936
        demographics in, 920–923
        entubulation techniques in, 938
        exposure in, 934
        external neurolysis in, 934–935
        indications for, 931–932
        internal neurolysis in, 935
        medicolegal issues in, 938–939
        nerve grafts in, 937
        nerve stump preparation in, 935–936
        nerve trauma classification and, 924–925, 926, 926f, 926t
        neurorrhaphy in, 936–937
        overview of, 919–920
        postsurgical management, 938
        referral indications, 930t
        success rates of, 932
        treatment algorithms in, 930–933
        trigeminal nerve anatomy in, 923–924
        trigeminal nerve physiology in, 923–924
neurologic examination for, 343–344
ocular, 493–499
open pneumothorax, 331–333
oxygenation in, 336
patient exposure in, 344
primary survey for, 328–344
score, 327
secondary assessment for, 344–354
skull assessment in, 344–348
soft tissue
    abrasions, 362
    anatomic evaluation for, 358
    animal bites, 363
    avulsive injuries, 362–363
    basic repair technique, 358–362
    contusions, 362
    gunshot wounds, 363–364
    human bites, 363
    in ear, 367, 368f, 369f
    in eyelid, 364–366
    in forehead, 364
    in lip, 370
    in nasolacrimal apparatus, 364–366
    in neck, 370–371
    in nose, 367
    in pediatric facial trauma, 568–569
    in scalp, 364
    lacerations, 362
    management principles, 357

postoperative wound care for, 371
    regional considerations, 364–371
    repair sequence, 358–362
    types of injuries, 362–364
spinal cord assessment in, 350–352
temporomandibular hypomobility from, 1156–1157
tension pneumothorax, 333, 334f
triage decision scheme for, 326f
vestibulocochlear nerve, in temporomandibular arthroscopy,
    1119
Traumatic bone cyst, 667–668
Traumatic neuroma, 669
TRD. See Tongue-retaining device (TRD)
Triazolam, 47
Trichloroacetic acid (TCA), 1613–1615
Trichophytic forehead and brow lift, 1585–1586
Trigeminal nerve
    anatomy of, 923–924
    fibers, 924t
    injury
        in temporomandibular arthroscopy, 1119
        microneurosurgery for
            approximation in, 936
            clinical evaluation for, 919
            clinical neurosensory testing and, 925–929
            coaptation in, 936
            demographics in, 920–923
            entubulation techniques in, 938
            exposure in, 934
            external neurolysis in, 934–935
            indications for, 931–932
            internal neurolysis in, 935
            medicolegal issues in, 938–939
            nerve grafts in, 937
            nerve stump preparation in, 935–936
            nerve trauma classification and, 924–925, 926, 926f, 926t
            neurorrhaphy in, 936–937
            overview of, 919–920
            postsurgical management, 938
            referral indications, 930t
            success rates of, 932
            treatment algorithms in, 930–933
            trigeminal nerve anatomy in, 923–924
            trigeminal nerve physiology in, 923–924
        nonsurgical treatment of, 929–930
    physiology of, 923–924
Trigeminal neuralgia, 930
Trigger point injections, for temporomandibular disorder, 1058
Trismus, with zygomatic complex fractures, 479
Tuberculosis, 795
Tumors
    congenital gingival granular cell, 830
    hematopoietic reticuloendothelial, 829–830
    in temporomandibular joint, 1044–1045
    mesenchymal, benign, 826–829
    neurogenic, 669–670, 830
    odontogenic
        adenomatoid, 648–649
        ameloblastic carcinoma, 642, 643f
        ameloblastic fibroma, 644
        ameloblastoma, 637–641
            malignant, 642
            multicystic, 637–639
            peripheral, 640–641
            solid, 637–639
            unicystic, 639–640
        calcifying epithelial, 647–648

classification of, 635*t*
clear cell odontogenic carcinoma, 643
epithelial, 822–824
ghost cell, malignant epithelial, 644
malignant, 641–644
mesenchymal, 824–826
mixed, 635–636
odontoma, 644–645
overview of, 625–626
primary interosseous squamous cell carcinoma, 643
salivary gland, 785–789
Turbinectomy, 1545
Two-point fixation, 379

U
Ultrasonography
in oral cancer, 687
in oral disease diagnosis, 618
in temporomandibular disorder therapy, 1057
Unerupted teeth, impacted *vs.,* 97
Upper respiratory infections, in pediatric patients, 71
Uprighting, of impacted teeth, 105
Urinary system, in geriatric patients, 73–74
Urine output, 27
Uvulopalatopharyngoplasty, for obstructive sleep apnea, 1501–1502
Uvulopalatoplasty, laser-assisted, for obstructive sleep apnea, 1502

V
Valvular heart disease, 20
Varicella-zoster virus, 798
Varix, 815
Vascular malformations, 663–669, 831–832
Vecuronium, 59*t*
Velopharyngeal incompetence (VPI), 1469
Ventilation-perfusion mismatching, 23
Ventilator-associated pneumonia, 25
Ventricular arrhythmias, 21
Ventricular tachycardia, 21
Vertical facial characteristics, 1255
Vertical facial proportions, 1246–1248
Vertical ramus osteotomy, 1324–1328, 1430–1431, 1438–1439, 1444–1445
Vestibulocochlear nerve, injury to, in temporomandibular arthroscopy, 1119
Vestibuloplasty
lip-switch, in preprosthetic surgery, 145, 146*f*
mandibular, in preprosthetic surgery, 145, 146*f,* 147*f*
maxillary, in preprosthetic surgery, 143–144
submucous, in preprosthetic surgery, 142–143
Video arthroscopy, 1080–1082
Villonodular synovitis, 1100
Viscerocranium formation, 1195–1196
Vision
craniosynostosis and, 979
in dysostosis syndromes, 996
Visual impairment, 493–495
Vomiting, postoperative, 60, 65, 85–86
VPI. *See* Velopharyngeal incompetence (VPI)

W
Wallerian degeneration, 6
Wandering rash of tongue, 802
Warfarin therapy, 31
Warthin's tumor, 787
Waters' view, 468

Whitnall's ligament, 1520
Whitnall's tubercle, 484–485
Wiring, for mandibular fracture, 412–414
Wisdom teeth, impacted
adjacent teeth root reabsorption and, 102
alveolar osteitis after extraction of, 114–115
antibiotics in extraction of, 112–113
bleeding after extraction of, 113–114
dental caries and, 101
dental prostheses and, 102
incidence and etiology of, 99–100
indications for removal of, 101–102
jaw fracture risk and, 102
mandibular incisor crowning and, 101–102
nerve disturbances after removal of, 115
odontogenic cysts and tumors and, 102
orthodontic considerations with, 101–102
orthognathic surgery and, 102
pain after extraction of, 114
pain from, 102
pericoronitis and, 101
periodontal healing after extraction of, 116–117
periodontitis and, 101
postoperative complications after extraction of, 114–116
postoperative course for, 113–114
rare complications for, 115–116
steroids in extraction of, 112–113
stiffness after extraction of, 114
surgery for, 107–113
swelling after extraction of, 114
tooth fracture after extraction of, 114
Wound care, for soft tissue trauma, 371
Wound healing
advances in, 12–14
age and, 11–12
by first intention, 3

by second intention, 3
by third intention, 3
complications, 8–9
debridement and, 9–10
dehiscence and, 9
dermal substitutes in, 13–14
diabetes and, 10
gene therapy and, 13
growth factors and, 12–13
hemostasis and, 9–10
hyperbaric oxygen therapy and, 11
immunocompromise and, 10–11
in extraction wounds, 8
infections in, 8–9
inflammatory phase of, 4–5, 4*f*
mucosal substitutes and, 13–14
nutrition and, 12
of bone, 6–7, 7*f,* 375*f,* 376*f*
of nerves, 6
of skin grafts, 8
optimization of, 9–12
perfusion and, 10
process, 3
proliferative phase of, 5–6, 5*f*
proliferative scarring in, 9
radiation injury and, 11
remodeling phase of, 6
response, 3–6
specialized, 6–8
trauma minimization in, 9

X

X-ray
    for zygomatic complex fractures, 468–469
    in oral disease diagnosis, 617–618

Y

Yolk sac, 1190*f*

Z

Zirconia, osseointegration with, 229–231
Zone of adherence, 1573
Zygomatic arch fractures, 470–471
Zygomatic complex fractures
    asymmetry with, 477
    bone grafting in, 477
    classification of, 469
    complications of, 477–479
    diagnosis of, 466–469
    diplopia with, 477–478
    enophthalmos in, 477
    high-energy, 472
    history in, 467
    hyphema with, 478
    infraorbital paresthesia in, 477
    internal fixation of, 472–475
    low-energy, 471
    malunion with, 477
    middle-energy, 471
    open reduction and internal fixation of, 474–475
    optic neuropathy with, 478–479
    orbital floor management in, 475–477
    physical examination in, 467
    radiographic evaluation for, 467–468
    retrobulbar hemorrhage with, 479
    superior orbital fissure syndrome with, 479
    surgical anatomy in, 465–466
    surgical treatment of, 469–477
    trismus with, 479
    Waters' view for, 468
Zygomaticofacial artery, 1579*f*
Zygomaticomaxillary complex (ZMC), fracture, in pediatric
    patients, 587